Reproductive Medicine
Challenges, Solutions and Breakthroughs

Reproductive Medicine
Challenges, Solutions and Breakthroughs

Editors

Sulbha Arora MD DNB
Consultant Fertility Specialist
Rotunda Fertility Clinic and Keyhole Surgery Center
Mumbai, Maharashtra
India

Rubina Merchant PhD
Embryologist
Rotunda–The Center for Human Reproduction
Mumbai, Maharashtra
India

Gautam N Allahbadia
MD DNB FNAMS FCPS DGO DFP FICMU FICOG
Medical Director
Rotunda–The Center for Human Reproduction
Rotunda IVF and Keyhole Surgery Center
Rotunda Blue Fertility Clinic and Keyhole Surgery Center
Rotunda Fertility Clinic and Keyhole Surgery Center
Mumbai, Maharashtra
India

Foreword
Hananel EG Holzer

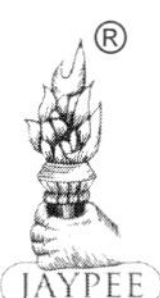

JAYPEE BROTHERS MEDICAL PUBLISHERS (P) LTD
New Delhi • London • Philadelphia • Panama

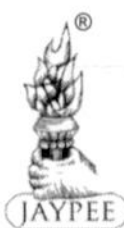 **Jaypee Brothers Medical Publishers (P) Ltd.**

Headquarters

Jaypee Brothers Medical Publishers (P) Ltd.
4838/24, Ansari Road, Daryaganj
New Delhi 110 002, India
Phone: +91-11-43574357
Fax: +91-11-43574314
Email: jaypee@jaypeebrothers.com

Overseas Offices

J.P. Medical Ltd.
83, Victoria Street, London
SW1H 0HW (UK)
Phone: +44-2031708910
Fax: +02-03-0086180
Email: info@jpmedpub.com

Jaypee-Highlights Medical Publishers Inc.
City of Knowledge, Bld. 237, Clayton
Panama City, Panama
Phone: +507-301-0496
Fax: +507-301-0499
Email: cservice@jphmedical.com

Jaypee Medical Inc.
The Bourse
111, South Independence Mall East
Suite 835, Philadelphia
PA 19106, USA
Phone: + 267-519-9789
Email: joe.rusko@jaypeebrothers.com

Jaypee Brothers Medical Publishers (P) Ltd.
17/1-B, Babar Road, Block-B
Shaymali, Mohammadpur
Dhaka-1207, Bangladesh
Mobile: +08801912003485
Email: jaypeedhaka@gmail.com

Jaypee Brothers Medical Publishers (P) Ltd.
Bhotahity, Kathmandu, Nepal
Phone: +977-9741283608
Email: kathmandu@jaypeebrothers.com

Website: www.jaypeebrothers.com
Website: www.jaypeedigital.com

Inquiries for bulk sales may be solicited at: jaypee@jaypeebrothers.com

Reproductive Medicine: Challenges, Solutions and Breakthroughs

First Edition: **2014**

ISBN : 978-93-5025-778-4

Printed at Sanat Printers, Kundli

Dedicated to

*The Indo-French Friendship
and
Academic Collaboration*

Contributors

Abraham Golan MD FRCOG
Professor
Director and Chairman
Department of Obstetrics and Gynecology
Edith Wolfson Medical Center, Holon
Head of Obstetrics and Gynecology
Sackler Faculty of Medicine
Tel Aviv University
Tel Aviv, Israel

Adusumilli Rajyalakshmi MSc
Senior Embryologist
Dr Rama's Institute for Fertility
Hyderabad, Andhra Pradesh, India

Akanksha Allahbadia MBBS
Observer Fellow
Rotunda—The Center for Human Reproduction
Mumbai, Maharashtra, India

Alain Audebert MD
Institut Greenblatt France
Bordeaux, France

Alon Shrim MD
Consultant
The Fetal Medicine Unit
Department of Obstetrics and Gynecology
The Sheba Medical Center
Tel-Hashomer, Israel

Amelie Gervaise MD
Departments of Obstetrics and Gynecology
Histology-Embryology and Cytogenetics and
Biology and Genetics of Reproduction
Antoine Béclère Hospital
Assistance Publique-Hôpitaux de Paris
Clamart Cedex
Univ Paris-Sud, Hôpital Kremlin Bicêtre
Le Kremlin Bicêtre Bicêtre, France

Amit Shah MD MRCOG
Consultant
Homerton Fertility Centre
Homerton University Hospital
London, UK

Amiya Mukherjee PhD
(Clinical Embryology)
Senior Embryologist
Harley Street Fertility Centre
London, UK

Andrea Borini MD
Director
Tecnobios Procreazione—Center for
Reproductive Health
Bologna, Italy

Anil Chittake DGO DNB
Fellowship in Endoscopy and ART
Associate ART Consultant and Endoscopist
Ruby Hall Clinic
Pune, Maharashtra, India

Anil Gudi MD MRCOG
Consultant and Director
Homerton Fertility Centre
Homerton University Hospital
London, UK

Aniruddha Malpani MD
Medical Director
Malpani Infertility Clinic
Mumbai, Maharashtra, India

Anjali Gupta MBBS MS
Infertility Specialist/Obstetrician and
Gynecologist
Clinical Research Fellow—Gynecological
Endoscopy
Vardhman Trauma and Laparoscopy Centre
Pvt Ltd, Muzaffarnagar
Uttar Pradesh, India

Anne-Claire Donnadieu MD
Departments of Obstetrics and Gynecology
Histology-Embryology and Cytogenetics
Biology and Genetics of Reproduction
Antoine Béclère Hospital
Assistance Publique-Hôpitaux de Paris
Clamart Cedex, France

Anoop Kumar Gupta MD DGO FCPS
DNBE
Infertility Specialist
Honorary and Head
Department of Gynecology
MT Agarwal Municipal General Hospital
Mumbai
Maharashtra, India

Antoine Torre MD
Department of Obstetrics and Gynecology
Reproductive Medicine and Biology and
Genetics of Reproduction
Antoine Béclère Hospital
Assistance Publique-Hôpitaux de Paris
(AP-HP), Clamart Cedex
Univ Paris-Sud, Hôpital Kremlin Bicêtre
Le Kremlin Bicêtre, Bicêtre
Endocrinologie et Génétique de la
Reproduction et du Développement, France

Arie Lissak MD
Head, Minimally Invasive Unit
Department of Obstetrics and Gynecology
Carmel Medical Center
Haifa, Israel

Arpita Ray MD MRCOG
Senior Clinical Fellow
Homerton Fertility Centre
Homerton University Hospital
London, UK

Avi Tsafrir MD
Gynecologist and Infertility Specialist
In vitro Fertilization Unit
Department of Obstetrics and Gynecology
Shaare-Zedek Medical Center
Jerusalem, Israel

Aygul Demirol MD
Associate Professor
Medical Director
Gurgan Clinic Women Health, Infertility
and IVF Center
Ankara, Turkey

Benjamin Fisch MD PhD
Director
Infertility and IVF Unit
Rabin Medical Center—Beilinson Hospital
Professor of Obstetrics and Gynecology
Sackler Faculty of Medicine
Tel-Aviv University
Tel-Aviv, Israel

Bhavana Agarwal Mittal DNB DGO FNB
(Reproductive Medicine) MNAMS
Infertility and IVF Specialist
Pushpanjali Crosslay Hospital
Ghaziabad, Uttar Pradesh, India

Boussion F MD
Sonographist
Department of Gynecologic Surgery and
Department of Prenatal Diagnosis
Department of Obstetrics and Gynecology
University Hospital
Angers, France

Cagri Beyazyurek Msc
(Molecular Biology and Genetics)
Preimplantation Genetic Diagnosis
Assisted Reproduction Techniques and
Reproductive Genetics Centre
Genetics Department
Istanbul Memorial Hospital
Istanbul, Turkey

Carmen Martinez Jover MD PhD
Infertility Writer and Painter
International PR
Mexican Institute of Infertility
Nuevo León México, Mexico

Catala Laurent MD
Hospital Surgeon
Department of Gynecologic Surgery
Department of Obstetrics and Gynecology
University Hospital
Angers, France

Catherine Rongières MD
Praticien Hospitalier
Hôpitaux Universitaires de Srrasbourg
Schiltigheim, France

Céline Lefebvre Lacoeuille MD
Hospital Surgeon
Department of Gynecologic Surgery
Department of Obstetrics and Gynecology
University Hospital
Angers, France

C Ferretti
Departments of Obstetrics and Gynecology
and Reproductive Medicine
Antoine Béclère Hospital
Assistance Publique-Hôpitaux de Paris
Clamart Cedex, France

Charles H Koh MD FRCOG FACOG
Microsurgeon, Obstetrician and Gynecologist
Reproductive Specialty Center
Columbia St Mary's Hospital
Milwaukee, Wisconsin, USA

Charulata Chatterjee MSc
Lead Embryologist
Dr Rama's Institute for Fertility
Hyderabad, Andhra Pradesh, India

Claire Basille MD
Departments of Obstetrics and Gynecology
Histology, Embryology and Cytogenetics
Biology and Genetics of Reproduction
Antoine Béclère Hospital
Assistance Publique-Hôpitaux de Paris
Clamart Cedex, France

Cristina Lagalla BSc
Tecnobios Procreazione—Center for
Reproductive Health
Bologna, Italy

Daniel B Williams MD
Reproductive Endocrinolgy and Infertility
Houston Fertility Institute
Volunteer Clinical Professor of Obstetrics and
Gynecology
University of Texas Medical School at
Houston, Texas, USA

Daniel Humberto Méndez Lozano MD
Departments of Obstetrics and Gynecology
Reproductive Medicine and Biology and
Genetics of Reproduction
Clamart, and Université Paris XI
Le Kremlin-Bicêtre, France

Daniel S Seidman MD
Associate Professor
Department of Obstetrics and Gynecology
Sheba Medical Center, Tel-Hashomer
Sackler School of Medicine
Tel-Aviv University
Tel-Aviv, Israel

David Stockheim MD
Consultant Obstetrician and Gynecologist
Department of Obstetrics and Gynecology
Sheba Medical Center
Tel-Hashomer, Israel

Deepu Rajkamal Selvaraj MS
Fertility Research Centre, GG Hospital
Chennai, Tamil Nadu, India

Devendra Patil MS
Resident in Urology
Lilavati Hospital
Mumbai, Maharashtra, India

Dharmesh Kapadia
Nadkarni Hospital and Test-tube
Baby Centre, Killa Pardi
Valsad, Gujarat, India

Durga G Rao MRCOG
Fellowship in Reproductive Endocrinology
and Infertility (McGill University, Canada)
Medical Director
Oasis—Centre for Reproductive Medicine
Hyderabad, Andhra Pradesh, India

Edi Vaisbuch MD
Obstetrician and Gynecologist
Department of Obstetrics and Gynecology
Kaplan Medical Center
Affiliated to the Hebrew University and
Hadassah School of Medicine
Jerusalem, Israel

Elizabeth Ball MD PhD MRCOG
Consultant Obstetrician and Gynaecologist
Royal London Hospital
London, UK

Ernesto Bosch Aparicio MD PhD
Medical Director
Human Reproduction Unit
Instituto Valenciano de Infertilidad
Valencia, Spain

Estelle Feyereisen MD
Departments of Obstetrics and Gynecology
Histology Embryology and Cytogenetics
Biology and Genetics of Reproduction
Antoine Béclère Hospital Assistance
Publique-Hôpitaux de Paris
Clamart Cedex, France

Fabrice G Petit PhD
Chargé de recherches INSERM
Department of Endocrinology and Genetics
of Reproduction and Development
Antoine Béclère Hospital, Assistance
Publique-Hôpitaux de Paris
Clamart Cedex, France

Gautam N Allahbadia
MD DNB FNAMS FCPS DGO DFP FICMU
FICOG
Medical Director
Rotunda—The Center for
Human Reproduction
Rotunda IVF and
Keyhole Surgery Center
Rotunda Blue Fertility Clinic and
Keyhole Surgery Center
Rotunda Fertility Clinic and
Keyhole Surgery Center
Mumbai, Maharashtra, India

Geetha Haripriya MD DGO FRCOG
Medical Director
Prasanth Fertility Research Centre
Chennai, Tamil Nadu, India

Gérard Chaouat MD PhD
Director of Research Emeritus CNRS
Department of Endocrinology and Genetics
of Reproduction and Development
Antoine Béclère Hospital
Clamart Cedex, France

Guy Israel Seidman LLM SJD
Associate Professor of Law
Radzyner School of Law
The Interdisciplinary Center
Herzliya, Israel

Hemant Bhanudas Nemade MS DNB
(Surgery), FCPS (Surgery), DNB (Urology)
FRCS (Urology)
Surgical Fellow (Onco-urology)
The Royal Marsden NHS Foundation Trust
London, UK

Henry Mateo Sanez MD
Medical Director
Instituto Mexicano de Infertilidad (IMI)
Ensenada, Baja California
México City, México

Hervé Fernandez MD PhD
Professor
Departments of Obstetrics and Gynecology
Histology Embryology and Cytogenetics
Biology and Genetics of Reproduction
Antoine Béclère Hospital Assistance
Publique-Hôpitaux de Paris
Univ Paris-Sud
Hôpital Kremlin Bicêtre
Le Kremlin Bicêtre
Department of Endocrinology
Genetics and Reproduction and
Development
Clamart Cedex, France

Humberto Aguirre Famania MD
Medical Director
Instituto Mexicano de Infertilidad (IMI)
Puerto Vallarta, Jalisco
México City, México

Jacob Farhi MD
Senior Physician
Infertility and IVF Unit
Rabin Medical Center-Beilinson Hospital
Senior Lecturer, Obstetrics and Gynecology
Sackler Faculty of Medicine
Tel-Aviv University
Tel-Aviv, Israel

Jagarlamudi Vijayalakshmi DGO
Obstetrician and Gynecologist
Dr Rama's Institute for Fertility
Hyderabad, Andhra Pradesh, India

Jayant G Mehta MD
Scientific Director
Reproductive Care
Morden Surrey, UK

Jeanine Ohl MD
Praticien hospitalier
Hôpitaux Universitaires de Srrasbourg
Schiltigheim, France

Jorge Eduardo Montoya Sarmiento
MD
Medical Director
Instituto Mexicano de Infertilidad (IMI)
Mazatlán, Sinaloa
México City, México

Jude Jose MD MRCOG
Senior Clinical Fellow
Homerton Fertility Centre
Homerton University Hospital
London, UK

Jyothi Pillai
Consultant Obstetrician and Gynecologist
Bangalore Assisted Conception Centre
Bangalore, Karnataka, India

Kaberi Banerjee MD MRCOG
Consultant-Centre of Reproductive Medicine
and IVF
Moolchand Medcity
New Delhi, India

Kalyani Patel DNB
Fellow in Reproductive Medicine (ICOG)
Consultant-Reproductive Medicine and
Infertility
Rotunda—The Centre for Human Reproduction
Mumbai, Maharashtra, India

Kamal Ojha MD MRCOG
Consultant Obstetrician and Gynaecologist
St George's Hospital
London, UK

Kamala Selvaraj MD DGO PhD
Associate Director
Fertility Research Centre
GG Hospital
Chennai, Tamil Nadu, India

Kamini A Rao MD
Medical Director
Bangalore Assisted Conception Centre
Bangalore, Karnataka, India

Kemal Ozgur MD
Consultant Gynecologist and Obstetrician
Antalya IVF
Antalya, Turkey

Kishore Nadkarni MS FCPS MNAMS
Medical Director
Surgeon and Male Infertility Specialist
Nadkarni Hospital and Test-tube Baby Centre
Killa Pardi Valsad
Gujarat, India

KK Gopinathan MD DGO
Infertility Specialist
Department of Infertility
PVS Hospital (P) Ltd
Calicut, Kerala, India

Kulvinder Kochar Kaur MD
(Obstetrics and Gynecology)
Professor
Reproductive Endocrinologist and Infertility
Specialist, Medical Director
Rotunda Virk—Center for Human Reproduction
Jalandhar, Punjab, India

Lakhbir Dhaliwal MD DGO
Professor and Head
Department of Obstetrics and Gynecology
Postgraduate Institute of Medical Education
and Research (PGIMER)
Chandigarh, India

L Gindes
Department of Obstetrics and Gynecology
Sheba Medical Center, Tel-Hashomer
Sackler School of Medicine
Tel-Aviv University
Tel-Aviv, Israel

Lakshmi Ravikanti MD
Senior Registrar
Waikato Hospital and Fertility Associates
Hamilton, New Zealand

Lata Kamble MD MRCOG
Locum Consultant
Homerton Fertility Centre
Homerton University Hospital
London, UK

Luis Arturo Ruvalcaba Castellón MD
Director General and CEO
Instituto Mexicano de Infertilidad (IMI)
Guadalajara, Jalisco
Endoscopia Ginecológica, Cirugía Robótica
Técnicas de Reproducción Asistida
Centro Médico Puerta de Hierro
México City, México

Madhusree Ghosh MBBS DNB (Obstetrics
and Gynaecology)
Specialist Registrar
Department of Obstetrics and Gynaecology
St George's Hospital
London, UK

Late Mandakini Parihar MD DGO
Director, Mandakini IVF Center
Hon Associate Professor (Obstetrics and
Gynecology)
KJ Somaiya Medical College and Hospital
Chairperson, Family Welfare Committee FOGSI
President, Navi Mumbai Obstetrics and
Gynecology Society
Consultant, Wockhardt Hospital
Mumbai, Maharashtra, India

Mandeep Singh MD (Med) DM (STD)
Neuroconsultant Neurologist and Physician
Swami Satyanand Hospital
Baradari, Jalandhar, India

Manisha Joshi MSc
(Reproductive Endocrinology and
Physiology) Diploma (Clinical Research)
Clinical Research Associate
ReGenesis Center of Assisted Reproduction
Endoscopy and Fetal Medicine
Reliance Life Sciences Pvt Ltd
Mumbai, Maharashtra, India

Manisha Palep Singh MD MRCOG
Consultant Gynecologist
Subspecialist in Reproductive Medicine
and Surgery
St Mary's University Teaching Hospital
CMMC NHS Trust
Manchester, UK

Manisha Takhtani MD FNB
Consultant Fertility Specialist
Rotunda Fertility Clinic and Keyhole Surgery
Center, Andheri, Mumbai, Maharashtra, India

Marco Antonio Flores Miranda MD
Fellowship in Reproductive Medicine
Concibe Reproducción Asistida
México City, México

Marialuisa Partisani MD
Praticien Hospitalier
Hôpitaux Universitaires de Srrasbourg
Schiltigheim, France

Marie Petitbarat PhD
Ingénieur de recherches
Department of Endocrinology and Genetics
of Reproduction and Development
Antoine Béclère Hospital
Assistance Publique-Hôpitaux de Paris
Clamart Cedex, France

Martha Isolina García Amador MD
Teaching Chief
Instituto Mexicano de Infertilidad (IMI)
Guadalajara, Jalisco, México City, México

Maruthini D MRCOG
Clinical Research Fellow
Assisted Conception Unit, Leeds General Infirmary
Leeds, UK

M Eftekhar MD
Assistant Professor
(Obstetrics and Gynecology)
Fellowship in Infertility
Sabzevar University of Medical Science
Sabzevar, Iran

Meena Chimote MD
Obstetrician and Gynecologist
Vaunshdhara Assisted Conception Center
Nagpur, Maharashtra, India

Meenakshi Bharath MD, DGO
Consultant Infertility Specialist
CART Fertility Clinic
Bangalore, Karnataka, India

Mete Isikoglu MD
IVF Practitioner
Obstetrician and Gynecologist
Gelecek–The Center for Human Reproduction
Lara Antalya, Turkey

Micha Baum MD
Consultant Obstetrician and Gynecologist
Department of Obstetrics and Gynecology
Sheba Medical Center
Tel-Hashomer, Israel

Michael Grynberg MD
Chef de Clinique Assistant
Departments of Obstetrics and Gynecology
and Reproductive Medicine
Antoine Béclère Hospital Assistance
Publique-Hôpitaux de Paris, Clamart, France

Mirudhubashini Govindarajan FRCSC
Director
Assisted Reproductive Technology Center
Women's Center
Coimbatore, Tamil Nadu, India

Mohinder Kochhar MD
Senior Consultant
Centre of IVF and Human Reproduction
Sir Ganga Ram Hospital
New Delhi, India

Mona Rahmati MD
Doctoral Fellow
Department of Endocrinology and Genetics
of Reproduction and Development
Antoine Béclère Hospital, Assistance
Publique-Hôpitaux de Paris
Clamart Cedex, France

Murat Berkkanoglu MD
Consultant Gynecologist and Obstetrician
Antalya IVF
Antalya, Turkey

Murat Seleker MSc
Embryologist
Antalya IVF
Dokuma Antalya, Turkey

Mybodi Karimzadeh MD
Professor of Obstetrics and Gynecology
Fellowship of Infertility
Pioneer of Infertility Treatment in Iran
Member of Iranian Board of Obstetrics and
Gynecology, Shahid Sadoughi Medical
University, Yazd, Iran

Natachandra Chimote MD
Obstetrician and Gynecologist
Vaunshdhara Assisted Conception Center
Nagpur, Maharashtra, India

Nathalie Ledée MD PhD
Chef d'équipe INSERM
Department of Endocrinology and Genetics
of Reproduction and Development
Antoine Béclère Hospital
Assistance Publique-Hôpitaux de Paris
Clamart Cedex, France

Neri Laufer MD
Gynecologist and Infertility Specialist
IVF Unit
Department of Obstetrics and Gynecology
Hadassah Hebrew University Medical Center
Jerusalem, Israel

Nikhil D Datar MD DNB FCPS FICOG LLB
DGO DHA
Health Right Activist Medicolegal Consultant
Chairman Medicolegal Cell Association of
Medical Consultants
Consultant Gynecologist
Dr Balabhai Nanavati Hospital
Hinduja Health Care Surgical Hospital
Datar Nursing Home
Yashada Maternity and Surgical Home
Honorary Gynaecologist
Dr RN Cooper Hospital
Mumbai, Maharashtra, India

Nirmalendu Nath PhD
Former Head
Department of Biochemistry
Nagpur University
Nagpur, Maharashtra, India

Nutan Jain MS
Director
Vardhman Trauma and Laparoscopy Centre
Pvt Ltd, Muzaffarnagar
Uttar Pradesh, India

Padma Rekha Jirge MRCOG FICOG
Scientific Director, Shreyas Hospital
Kolhapur, Maharashtra, India

Paul PG MBBS DGO
Endoscopic Surgeon
Paul's Hospital, Kaloor
Kochi, Kerala, India

Philippe Descamps MD PhD
Professor
Hospital Surgeon (Department of
Gynecologic Surgery)
Chief, Department of Obstetrics and Gynecology
University Hospital, Angers
Senior Lecturer
University of Angers
Department of Obstetrics and Gynecology
University Hospital, Angers, France

Priya Selvaraj MD MNAMS MCE
Assistant Director
Fertility Research Centre, GG Hospital
Chennai, Tamil Nadu, India

Purnima Nadkarni MD DGO FCPA
Medical Director
Obstetrician, Gynecologist and Infertility
Specialist, Nadkarni Hospital and Test-tube
Baby Centre
Gujarat, India

Rajeev Kumar MCh
Assistant Professor of Urology
All India Institute of Medical Sciences
New Delhi, India

Rajesh V Darade MBBS DNB FICS [USA]
FCPS FICMCH FICOG [Mumbai] DGO DFP
DGOCPS MNAMS [Delhi], Endoscopic Surgeon
Vaishnavi Hospital and Endoscopy Centre
Postgraduate Institute
Associate Professor and Head of Unit
Department of Obstetrics and Gynecology
Government Medical College
Latur, Maharashtra, India

Ramadevi Papolu MD
Infertility Specialist
Dr Rama's Institute for Fertility
Hyderabad, Andhra Pradesh, India

Renato Fanchin MD PhD
Professor
Chief of the Division of Reproductive Medicine
Department of Obstetrics and Gynecology
Hôpital A Béclère, University Paris, Clamart
France

René Frydman MD
Professor
Hôpital FOCH de Suresnes
Department of Obstetrics and Gynecology
Suresnes, France

Rivka Peltz MD
Consultant
The Fetal Medicine Unit
Department of Obstetrics and Gynecology
The Sheba Medical Center
Tel-Hashomer, Israel

Robab Taheripanah MD
Associated Professor (Obstetrics and
Gynecology)
Fellowship in Infertility
Infertility and Reproductive Health Research
Center (IRHRC), Shahid Beheshti Medical
University, Tehran, Iran

Ronit Machtinger MD
Infertility Specialist
Department of Obstetrics and Gynecology
Sheba Medical Center
Tel-Hashomer, Israel

Roy Mashiach MD
Reproductive Surgeon
Sheba Medical Center, Ramat-Gan, Israel

RS Sharma PhD
Scientist F and Deputy Director General
Division of Reproductive Health and Nutrition
Indian Council of Medical Research
New Delhi, India

Rupin Shah MS (Surgery) MCh (Urology)
Consultant Andrologist and Microsurgeon
Lilavati Hospital and Research Centre
Mumbai, Maharashtra, India

Sandeep Talwar MBBS DNB
(Obstetrics and Gynecology)
Senior Consultant and Head
IVF and Reproductive Medicine
BLK Superspeciality Hospital
New Delhi, India

Sandra Cubillos Gracía
Embryologist
IVF Lab Director
Concibe Reproducción Asistida
México City, México

Sandra De la Garza MD PhD
President
Mexican Infertility Association
Nuevo León México, Mexico

Sanjeev Khot MD DGO DNB
IVF Consultant
ReGenesis Center of Assisted Reproduction
Endoscopy and Fetal Medicine
Reliance Life Sciences Pvt Ltd
Mumbai, Maharashtra, India

Satyen Kasabwala MD DGO
Endoscopic Surgeon, Anand Hospital
Navsari, Gujarat, India

Sedighe Ghandi MD
Assistant Professor (Obstetrics and Gynecology)
Fellowship in Infertility
Sabzevar University of Medical Science
Sabzevar, Iran

Semra Kahraman MD PhD
Professor
Director of ART and Genetics Center
Istanbul Memorial Hospital
Istanbul, Turkey

Shalini Gainder MD DGO
Assistant Professor
Department of Obstetrics and Gynecology
Postgraduate Institute of Medical Education
and Research (PGIMER)
Chandigarh, India

Shelly Tse DCR DMU
Senior Radiographer
Concept Fertility Clinic
London, UK

Shevach Friedler MD
Associate Professor
Department of Obstetrics and Gynecology
Sackler School of Medicine, Tel-Aviv University
Infertility and IVF Unit
Assaf Harofeh Medical Center, Israel
Sackler School of Medicine
Tel-Aviv University, Tel-Aviv, Israel

Shimon Ginath MD
Instructor
Division of Urogynecology and Pelvic Floor
Surgery
Department of Obstetrics and Gynecology
Edith Wolfson Medical Center, Holon
Sackler Faculty of Medicine
Tel Aviv University, Tel-Aviv, Israel

Shlomo Lipitz MD
Professor and Director
The Fetal Medicine Unit
Department of Obstetrics and Gynecology
The Sheba Medical Center
Tel-Hashomer, Israel

Shweta Goel MBBS MS
Infertility Specialist/Obstetrician and Gynecologist
Clinical Research Fellow-Gynecological
Endoscopy
Vardhman Trauma and
Laparoscopy Centre Pvt Ltd
Muzaffarnagar, Uttar Pradesh, India

Silvio Cuneo Pareto MD
Director
Concibe Reproducción Asistida
México City, México

Stefan Kostadinov MD FCAP
Staff Perinatal Pathologist
Departments of Pathology and Pediatrics
Women and Infants Hospital
Assistant Professor of Pathology (Clinical)
The Warren Alpert Medical School of Brown
University
Providence, Rhode Island, USA

Sujata Kar MD DNB
(Obstetrics and Gynecology)
Director
Kar Clinic and Hospital Pvt Ltd
Bhubaneshwar, Orissa, India

Suleyman Guven MD
Assistant Professor
Karadeniz Technical University , School of
Medicine, Department of Obstetrics and
Gynecology, Trabzon, Turkey

Late Sulochana Gunasheela FRCS
(Edinburgh) FRCOG (London)
Gunasheela IVF Centre
Bangalore, Karnataka, India

Sunita Tandulwadkar MD FICOG FICS
Diploma in Endoscopy (USA, Germany)
Head, Department of Obstetrics and Gynecology
Chief
IVF and Endoscopy Centre
Ruby Hall IVF and Endoscopy Centre
Gynecological Endoscopist
Poona Hospital and Research Centre
Aditya Birla Memorial Hospital
Pune, Maharashtra, India

Surendra Sharma PhD MD
Departments of Pathology and Pediatrics
Women and Infants Hospital
Brown Medical School
Providence, Rhode Island, USA

Surveen Ghumman MD
(Obstetrics and Gynecology)
Senior Specialist
Safdarjang Hospital
New Delhi, India

Sylvie Dubanchet
Assistant Ingénieur de Recherches INSERM
Endocrinologie et Génétique de la
Reproduction et du Développement
Hôpital Antoine Béclère
Clamart Cedex, France

Timur Gurgan MD
Professor and Section Head
Reproductive Endocrinology and Infertility
Andrology Unit
Department of Obstetrics and Gynecology
School of Medicine, Hacettepe University
Ankara, Turkey

Tony Thomas MD MRCOG
Consultant Obstetrician and Gynecologist
Walsall Manor Hospital
Walsall Healthcare NHS Trust
Walsall, West Midlands
England, UK

Verinica Bianchis PhD
ESHRE Senior Embryologist
Tecnobios Procreazione—Center for
Reproductive Health
Bologna, Italy

Ved Prakash Singh MD
Consultant
Waikato Hospital, Hamilton
Associates Medical Director Fertility
Associates Hamilton
Hamilton, New Zealand

Vineeta Kharb MD FNB
Student
Reproductive Medicine
Ruby Hall Clinic
Pune, Maharashtra, India

Vivek Salunke MD
(Obstetrics and Gynecology)
Gynecological Endoscopic Surgeon
Nalini Endoscopy Unit
Mumbai, Maharashtra, India

Xavier Deffieux MD PhD
Departments of Obstetrics and Gynecology
Histology Embryology and Cytogenetics
Biology and Genetics of Reproduction
Antoine Béclère Hospital Assistance
Publique-Hôpitaux de Paris
Clamart Cedex, France

Yadava Bapurao Jeve MS DNB MSc
(Reproductive Medicine) MRCOG
Specialist (Obstetrics and Gynecology)
University Hospitals of Leicester, UK

Yaron Zalel MD
Associate Professor
Specialist in Obstetrics and Gynecology
and Ultrasound
Department of Obstetrics and Gynecology
and Ultrasound Unit
Sheba Medical Center, Tel-Hashomer
Sackler School of Medicine
Tel-Aviv University
Tel-Aviv, Israel

Yuval Kaufman BSc MD
Clinical Consultant
Head of the Multidisciplinary Center for the
Treatment of Endometriosis
Department of Obstetrics and Gynecology
Carmel Medical Center
Haifa, Israel

Zion Hagay MD
Professor and Chairman
Obstetrician and Gynecologist
Department of Obstetrics and Gynecology
Kaplan Medical Center
Affiliated to the Hebrew University and
Hadassah School of Medicine
Jerusalem, Israel

Thirty-five years after the birth of Louise Brown, numerous textbooks discussing reproduction and Assisted Reproductive Techniques (ART) have been published. Is a new textbook actually needed? Merely by reading the Title and the Table of Contents of *"Reproductive Medicine: Challenges, Solutions and Breakthroughs",* a comprehensive, practical guide, that question would evidently be answered.

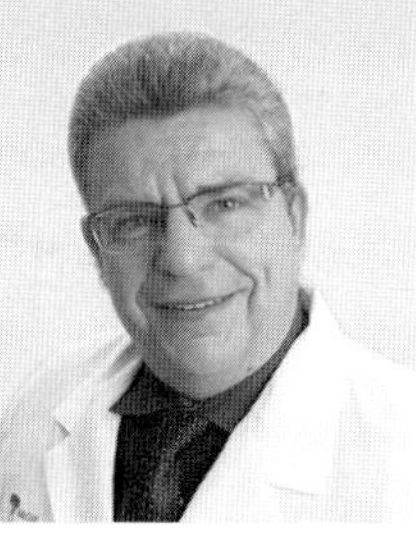

From basic discussions of evaluation and treatment of the female partner before ART, gonadotropin preparation in infertility treatment, and the choice of the starting dose in *in vitro* fertilization (IVF) through more specific issues in Reproductive Surgery and practical questions in ART to highly advanced techniques, the textbook will be a useful resource to many.

Medical students, residents and fellows will find the basic approach to infertility and infertility care. Specialists in Obstetrics and Gynecology will find useful information on the basic approach and treatments; when, why and for what should patients be referred to more highly specialized facilities. Reproductive surgeons will find excellent reviews on gynecological endoscopy. Reproductive endocrinologists and Infertility specialists, who often encounter practical questions, such as management of a persistently thin endometrium, addition of luteinizing hormone in controlled ovarian stimulation protocols using recombinant follicle-stimulating hormone (FSH), rationale for the use of insulin-sensitizing drugs in polycystic ovary syndrome (PCOS) or the use of Aspirin in ART protocols, would, with no doubt, benefit from those chapters in the textbook. All of the above would probably be intrigued by questions such as: Do we need Hysterosalpingography in the times of 3D/4D USG?

Our partners, the Embryologists, Andrologists and Urologists, will find sections discussing their contributions to our patients care, but would also benefit from all other sections for a more comprehensive interdisciplinary care.

Administrative managers are an integral part of reproductive centers. They share responsibilities for the everyday running of the clinics and for planning the future. They will find special interests in the sections concerning: Marketing and Advertising in IVF and ART regulation, but could also benefit from the textbook's other sections.

Third party reproduction, an area of assisted reproduction that involves more than one party in the process of realizing the birth of a child, essentially gamete (oocyte, sperm) donation, embryo donation, and surrogacy, is bound to raise many ethical and philosophical questions and dilemmas with regard to the future child. Indeed, many of these are intertwined in the different sections of the textbook.

Two-thirds of the world's population currently lives in countries where reproductive care is available. Over four million children have been born as a result of ART. Societies are called to establish rules and regulations for those highly advanced techniques. The policy-makers are usually not medical experts. However, they must acquire some basic knowledge in that field. This textbook will help them to better understand the field of Reproductive Medicine and will allow them to constitute well-informed, scientifically-based policies.

Excellent authors from many parts of the globe have contributed to this comprehensive, 'State of the Art' textbook. This could certainly be expected, considering the vast experience and extensive, useful and exciting publications by the enthusiastic editors of the textbook, Gautam N Allahbadia, Sulbha Arora and Rubina Merchant in the field of Infertility and ART, and the impressive intiative by Dr Gautam Allahbadia in organizing numerous clinical, academic and research-oriented national and international conferences. One could hardly wait to add the textbook to one's library.

Hananel EG Holzer MD
Director
Reproductive Endocrinology and Infertility Division
Department of Obstetrics and Gynecology
McGill University, Montreal, Quebec
Canada

> *"To follow knowledge like a sinking star,*
> *Beyond the utmost, bound of human thought."*
>
> **—*Ulysses*, Alfred Lord Tennyson**

A whole new world has opened up in the field of making miracles. And, it takes many man-hours of many medical men to try to do what the Lord did at leisure after he made the world. This textbook encapsulates the achievements of our peers, who have not let a seemingly little thing like nature get in the way of dreams. The field of Assisted Reproductive Techniques (ART) encapsulates a whole wing of Modern Medicine, including General Gynecologists, Sonologists, Laparoscopic Surgeons, Embryologists, Andrologists, Counselors and ART Practitioners, covering various different specialities that form a jigsaw puzzle, with each adding a missing piece. In spite of being a part of this path-breaking field, even we, as scientists, must pause and absorb the magnitude of it all.

In vitro fertilization (IVF) is not a perfect science and we are constantly faced with the question 'what next?' What else can be done to help the most complex cases? How can we improve success rates? How can we build on the existing knowledge and improve our techniques? These are some of the questions the textbook aims to answer. By inviting stalwarts in the field of ART to share their experiences and insights, we hope to create the opportunity for inspiration that encourages others to perpetuate the legacy.

Gynecologists, ART Practitioners and especially, students of Infertility rely heavily on the experience and publishing of others to improve their own techniques. Reproductive Medicine is a young science and as such, all innovations are happening in our lifetime by our seniors, peers and even by young stars in the field. In this comprehensive compilation, *Reproductive Medicine: Challenges, Solutions and Breakthroughs*, we aim to offer an easy approach to current concepts and advances on far-ranging topics by experts from several countries, pioneering in Fertility studies.

The fourteen distinct sections of the textbook deal with every aspect of Reproductive Medicine. The textbook begins with an in-depth analysis of diagnostic techniques and fertility-enhancing endoscopic procedures. Ovarian Stimulation Protocols are covered next, followed by a section on Contemporary Clinical Management. Various assisted reproductive techniques, as well as their complications, are addressed in the next sections. There are also sections on the ART Laboratory, Preimplantation Genetic Diagnosis, Current Concepts in the field of Male Infertility, Ultrasound, Regulation of ART and Marketing and Advertising of ART Centers.

The textbook does not just skim through these topics; instead, it takes a deeper look at issues and concerns and examines them as a reader would. These topics will bring you in touch with current advances as we continue to take great strides in the field of Reproductive Medicine. The Editors would like to thank the exemplary panel of doctors, who have contributed to this volume, and particularly, acknowledge the efforts of Dr Mandakini Parihar and Dr Sulochana Gunasheela who, unfortunately, are not with us today to enjoy this enriching edition that they contributed to.

The wealth of knowledge and humanity that my very good friend and colleague, Mandakini, and the doyen of ART, Dr Sulochana Gunasheela, who has always helped me at all the stages of my career, have left behind, will always live on!

—Gautam N Allahbadia

Sulbha Arora   Rubina Merchant   Gautam N Allahbadia

Acknowledgments

We would like to acknowledge the encouragement and support of Professor René Frydman, without whose presence, the Indo-French Congress and this textbook would have remained a dream.

You see things, and you say,
"Why?"
But I dream things that never were, and I say,
"Why not?"

–George Bernard Shaw

Contents

Section 7 PREIMPLANTATION GENETIC DIAGNOSIS

Section 9 CURRENT CONCEPTS IN THE TREATMENT OF MALE INFERTILITY

Section 14 THE FUTURE OF ART

Gynecological Endoscopy

Philosophy of Endoscopy in Infertility

Vivek Salunke, Rajesh V Darade

OVERVIEW

The tale of evolution of endoscopy is by no means less than an epic by itself. It is in fact, the story of a revolution, the seed of whose philosophy was sowed as far back as 4,600 years ago. This long journey, with many turns and turbulences, has probably reached the grand finale in the present era of state of art minimally invasive surgeries and robotics. This is the fruit of centuries of tedious battles by scientists and doctors and the pioneers of endoscopy, who had the foresight to apply and develop scientific knowledge with the courage to judiciously experiment and evolve, and to challenge the deeply rooted ideology of open surgery.

Infertility affects more than 80 million people worldwide. One in 10 couples experience primary or secondary infertility. Although infertility is not a public health problem, it is indeed, a central issue in the lives of those suffering from it. Though irrational, many societies evaluate the potential of a woman through her reproductive capacity and this attaches the stigmata of barrenhood to those who cannot achieve it. Unstable marriages, peer and social pressures, domestic violence and ostracism mar the suffering of an infertile woman. Developments in the field of infertility through endoscopy and assisted reproductive technique (ART) have infused hopes in such people to resolve their infertility through the most minimally invasive means and coupled with with the maximum chances of success.

The present chapter attempts to trace the journey of development in endoscopy, particularly with reference to infertility that has led to its present position as a method par excellence.

INTRODUCTION

How do we categorize 'Endoscopy'? What is Endoscopy anyways? A revolution or an evolution? A more accurate definition, however, places endoscopy firmly in the category of a new philosophy, one-rooted in what is now referred to as minimally invasive surgery. Interestingly, it is not a modern phenomenon. It dates back to almost 4,600 years.

Hippocrates had specifically instructed physicians to avoid invasive methods as much as possible, allowing instead, the body's own healing process to take effect, as the former approach was certainly influenced by a high mortality rate due to infection and hemorrhage. Nevertheless, in reviewing the history of medicine, we can see that the philosophy of minimally invasive medicine has been an integral part of medicine for thousands of years. The late 19th and the early 20th century, favored a form of surgical intervention dominated by "big incisions". Open surgical approaches were soon codified as gold standards of "classical surgery", a point that later served to interfere substantially with the progress of endoscopy. While facing such institutionalized beliefs about classical surgery, the story of endoscopy was related to individuals responsible for its progress, whose courage and tenacity envisioned a path of progress beyond technical limitations.

For these reasons alone, taking a moment to review the endoscopy development process will help us to recognize how dominant ideologies or cultural influences act as such profound forces in shaping the practice of medicine.

Ancient Indian Perspective

A strong pro-minimally invasive approach is exemplified in the ancient text *Sushruta Samhita* in the chapter 25, which states that the surgeon should take care of the patient as his own son and the use of surgical equipment in excess can cause harm and grave injury to the body. Chapter 5 clearly states that surgical incisions should be made swiftly and the smaller the incision the better.

History of Endoscopy in Infertility

1970: Steptoe and Edwards[1] primed the ovaries with gonadotropins and used the laparoscope to recover preovulatory oocytes.

1972: Maathius et al.[2] reported that laparoscopic investigation was preferable to hysterosalpingography.

1975: Moghissi and Sim[3] found that 19 percent of patients with normal hysterosalpingography had pathology at laparoscopy.

1984: Asch et al.[4] reported a pregnancy following translaparoscopic gamete intrafallopian transfer (GIFT).

Endometriosis

1983: Keye et al.[5] used argon lasers in the treatment of endometriosis.

1986: Carbon dioxide lasers were used to treat endometriosis by Davis. Nezat et al.[6] reported encouraging conception rates when treatment was for infertility as well as pain.

1987: Lamaro used the Nd: YAG laser.

CLINICAL DISCUSSION

Endoscopy in Infertility

Currently, laparoscopy is perceived as a minimally invasive surgical technique that both provides a panoramic and magnified view of the pelvic organs and allows surgery at the time of diagnosis. Endoscopic reproductive surgery, intended to improve fertility, may include surgery on the uterus, ovaries, pelvic peritoneum and on the Fallopian tubes.

Endoscopic Tubal Surgery

Procedures included under endoscopic tubal surgeries are salpingo-ovariolysis, salpingostomy and tubal reanastomosis. Adhesions involving the Fallopian tubes have been implicated as the cause of infertility. In a control study, examining the role of salpingo-ovariolysis, 69 infertile women were subjected to this procedure and 78 women with a similar degree of adhesions were not treated.[7] The cumulative pregnancy rate at 24 months follow-up was significantly higher in the treated women compared to the untreated group, (45% versus 16%, respectively). In one study, 167 patients with pelvic adhesions, suffering from an inability to conceive, underwent operative laparoscopy and adhesiolysis. According to the severity of adhesions, patients were categorized by diagnostic laparoscopy as mild (group 1), moderate (group 2), and severe (group 3). After laparoscopic adhesiolysis, all the

patients were followed up for one year. Pregnancies occurred in 51 (70.8%), 28 (48.3%) and 8 (21.6%) patients in groups 1, 2 and 3, respectively.

Salpingo-ovariolysis, as a fertility-enhancing procedure is done by separating adnexal adhesions with laparoscopic scissors, electrocautery, or lasers. Endoscopic surgery is more precise for excision of such adhesions as it avoids damage to the surrounding vital structures. An increased rate of adhesion formations has been reported in patients undergoing reproductive surgery via laparotomy.[8,9] In their study, Nezhet et al.[10] demonstrated that endoscopic reproductive surgery was very effective in reducing peritoneal adhesions and was associated with a low frequency of postoperative adhesions recurrence and mostly avoided the formation of *de novo* adhesions at most surgical sites.[10]

Hydrosalpinx is a chronic pathological condition of the Fallopian tube and a major cause of infertility, the main caused being pelvic inflammatory disease, previous abdominal operations, history of peritonitis and tuberculosis and endometrioses.[11,12] Laparoscopy provided both the certain diagnoses and treatment of hydrosalpinx at the same sessions. One meta-analysis demonstrated deleterious effects of hydrosalpinx on achieving pregnancy in women undergoing *in vitro* fertilization (IVF). It was shown that the clinical pregnancy rate was 50 percent lower and the miscarriage rate was more than two-fold higher in patients with hydrosalpinx.[13] The proposed mechanism by which embryotoxicity occurs begins with the leakage of fluid from the hydrosalpinx into the uterine cavity. This fluid may not only be harmful to the embryos but may have an adverse effect on the uterine receptivity and implantation mechanisms. A Cochrane review confirmed that the odds of pregnancy were increased with laparoscopic salpingectomy prior to IVF.[14] All these data demonstrate that laparoscopic surgery for hydrosalpinges is a preferred procedure for improving pregnancy rates. Proximal tubal obstruction is found in 10 to 25 percent cases of tubal infertility. It is most commonly due to salpingitis isthmica nodosa (SIN). Cornual implantation, done endoscopically, is rarely preformed nowadays except in very specialized centers. Diseases of the distal tube could be secondary to any pelvic inflammatory condition including infection, endometriosis, or may occur postsurgically. Tubal preservation surgery for distal tubal lesions includes salpingostomy and fimbrioplasty. Patency of the distal tube does not necessarily equate with normality of the tubal mucosa. Fimbrioscopy and salpingoscopy are procedures to ascertain the quality of fimbriae and endosalpinx, respectively and determine the prognosis of future fertility.[12] Laparoscopic tubo-tubal anastomosis is done for reversal of tubal ligation. The success of the surgery depends on the type of tubal ligation procedure performed, total tubal length before reversal, patient's age and ovarian function.

Laparoscopic Myomectomy

Uterine fibroids can affect 30 to 40 percent of reproductive aged women. It has been observed that pregnancy rates are lower in patients presenting with myomas. Approximately 50 percent of women with myomas conceive after myomectomy.[15] Depending on the locations of myomas, a hysteroscopic or laparoscopic approach is used to remove them. As fertility preservation is the primary goal of myomectomy, laparoscopy gives a distinct advantage over laparotomy. The incidence of adhesions following open myomectomy is 100 percent as compared to 36 to 67 percent following laparoscopic myomectomy.[16-20] Dubuisson et al.[20] studied the risk of adhesions after laparoscopic myomectomy. Second-look procedures were performed in 45 of 271 laparoscopic myomectomy patients. Additional laparoscopy procedures were performed at the time of laparoscopic myomectomy in 19 patients (42.2%). Overall, the postoperative adhesion rate was 35.6 percent, with 16.7 percent of the myomectomy sites affected. Most importantly, the adnexal adhesions rate was 24.4 percent, with 11 percent being bilateral. In patients without associated laparoscopic procedures, the adhesion rates were even lower with an overall adhesions rate of 26.9 percent and an adnexal adhesions rate of 11.5 percent, none of which was bilateral. One of the concerns regarding laparoscopic myomectomy has been adequate reconstruction and healing of the uterine defect, with subsequent ability of the uterus to withstand pregnancy and labor. The excessive use of electrocautery contributes to myometrial necrosis and impaired wound healing. Few studies have evaluated the effect of myomas on pregnancy rates after assisted reproductive technique (ART). Elder Geva et al.[21] compared 106 ART cycles in patients with uterine fibroids and 318 ART cycles in patients without uterine fibroids and concluded that implantation and pregnancy rates were significantly lower in patients with intramural and submucosal fibroids, even those with no deformation in the uterine cavity.[21] Stovall et al.[22] showed that even after patients with submucosal fibroids are excluded, the presence of fibroids reduces the efficacy of ART.[22] Therefore, infertile women with intramural fibroids should be subjected for myomectomies earlier.

Endoscopy in Endometriosis

About 30 to 70 percent of infertile women have been reported to have endometriosis.[23] Severe endometriosis, associated with pelvic adhesions and distortion of the pelvic anatomy, would result in infertility. However, the impact of mild to moderate endometriosis on fertility could be explained by ovulatory dysfunction, endocrine abnormality, inflammatory and immunological abnormalities. Laparoscopy is the best surgical approach for treating endometriosis. Superficial peritoneal endometriosis is fulgurated or excised. For larger lesions more than 5 mm, excision is a better option. For endometriomas, drainage and removal of the cyst wall should be tried. The IVF success rates in infertile patients with endometriosis are lower compared to women undergoing IVF for other indications. Barnhart, et al.[24] investigated the IVF outcome in patients with endometriosis.[24] It was demonstrated that patients with endometriosis have more than a 50 percent reduction in pregnancy rate after IVF compared with women with tubal factor infertility. Data suggest that the presence of endometriosis affects multiple aspects of the reproductive cycle, including oocyte quality, embryogensis and endometrial receptivity, which may result in lower implantation rates.[25-27] The Practice Committee of ASRM developed a report in May 2004. According to their recommendations, when laparoscopy is performed, the surgeon should consider safely ablating or excising visible lesions of endometriosis. In women with stage I and II endometriosis-associated infertility, expectant management or superovulation with intrauterine insemination (IUI) can be considered for younger patients. Older patients, more than 35 years, should be treated with superovulation /IUI or *in vitro* fertilization-embryo transfer (IVF-ET). In women, with stage III and IV endometriosis-associated infertility, conservative surgical therapy with laparoscopy and possible laparotomy are indicated.

Advances in endoscopic surgery have revolutionized our approaches to gynecological surgery. Endoscopic surgery for infertile patients has a major role to play, and if performed by an endoscopic surgeon experienced in fertility-enhancing surgeries, better results can be obtained.[28]

CONCLUSION

Advances in endoscopy have revolutionized our approach to gynecological surgery. Surgery, pertaining to the reproductive organs, can and should be approached laparoscopically, especially in the context of infertility. It is evident that endoscopic surgery, when performed by an expert endoscopist, is efficacious and produces as good and probably, better results when compared to open surgery.

Laparoscopy is not merely a technological advancement but a paradigm shift in the way of looking at 'treatment'. The shift towards minimal invasion reflects a deeper, philosophical commitment to minimal pain in all aspects— physical, mental and social. An exemplary case in point is the laparoscopic approach to infertility treatment. In most societies, where womanhood is synonymous to motherhood, infertility is accompanied by enormous psychological and social pressures, which are exacerbated by the physical trauma of open surgery. In such a context, laparoscopy comes as a much awaited change by virtue of being a more holistic and humane approach to treatment.

REFERENCES

1. Steptoe PC, Edwards RG. Laparoscopic recovery of preovulatory human oocytes after priming of ovaries with gonadotrophins. Lancet 1970;l:683-9.
2. Maathuis JB, Horbach JG, van Hall EV. A comparison of the results of hysterosalpingography and laparoscopy in the diagnosis of fallopian tube dysfunction. Fertil Steril 1972;23:428-31.
3. Moghissi KS, Sim GS. Correlation between hysterosalpingography and pelvic endoscopy for the evaluation of tubal factor. Fertil Steril 1975;26:1178-81.
4. Asch RH, Ellsworth LR, Balmaceda JP, Wong PC. Pregnancy after translaparoscopic gamete intrafallopian transfer. Lancet 1984;2:1034-5.
5. Keye WR Jr, Matson GA, Dixon J. The use of the argon laser in the treatment of experimental endometriosis. Fertil Steril 1983;39:26-9.
6. Nezhat C, Crowgey SR, Garrison CP. Surgical treatment of endometriosis via laser laparoscopy. Fertil Steril 1986;45:778-83.
7. Tulandi T, Collins JA, Burrows E, et al. Treatment dependent and treatment independent pregnancy among women with periadnexal adhesions. Am J Obstet Gynecol 1990;162:354.
8. Risberg B. Adhesions: preventive strategies. Eur J Surg 1997;577(suppl):32-9.
9. Brill AI, Nezhat F, Nezhat CH, Nezhat C. The incidence of adhesions after prior laparotomy: a laparoscopic appraisal. Obstet Gynecol 1995;85:269-72.
10. Nezhat CR, Nezhat FR, Metzget DA, Luciano AA. Adhesion reformation after reproductive surgery by videolaseroscopy. Fertill Steril 1990;53:1008-11.
11. Bontis JN, Dinas KD. Management of Hydrosalpinx; reconstructive surgery of IVF. Ann NY Acad Sci 2000;900:260-71.
12. Nezhat F, Winer WK, Nezhat C. Fimbrioscopy and salpingoscopy in patients with minimal to moderate pelvic endometriosis. Obstet Gynecol 1990;75:15-7.
13. Zeyneloglu HB, Arici A, Olive DL. Adverse effects of hydrosalpinx on pregnancy rates after *in vitro* fertilization – embryo transfer. Fertil Steril 1998;70:492.
14. Johnson NP, Mak W, Sowter MC. Laparoscopic salpingectomy for women with hydrosalpinges enhances the success of IVF: a Cochrane review. Hum Reprod 2002;17:543.
15. Verkauf BS. Myomectomy for fertility enhancement and preservation. Fertil Steril 1992;58:1-15.
16. Tulandi T, Murray C, Guralnick M. Adhesion formation and reproductive outcome after myomectomy and second-look laparoscopy. Obstet Gynecol 1993;82:213-5.
17. Nezhat C, Nezhat F, Silfen SL. Laproscopic myomectomy. Int J Fertil 1991;36:275-80.
18. Hasson HM, Rotman C, Rana N. Laproscopic myomectomy. Obstet Gynecol 1992;80:884-8.
19. Mais V, Agossa S, Guerriero S, Mascia M, Solla E, Melis GB. Laproscopic versus abdominal myomectomy: a prospective, randomized trial to evaluate benefits in early outcome. Am J Obstet Gynecol 1996;174:654-8.
20. Dubuisson JB, Fauconnier A, Chapron C, Krieker G, Norgaard C. Second look after laparoscopic myomectomy. Hum Reprod 1998;13:2102-6.
21. Elder-Geva T, Meagher S, Healy DL, MacLachlan V, Breheny S, Wood C. Effect of intramural, subserosal and submucosal uterine fibroids on the outcome of assisted reproductive technology treatment. Fertil Steril 1998;70:687-91.
22. Stovall DW, Parrish SB, Van Voorish BJ, Hahn SJ, Sparks AET, Syrop CH. Uterine leiomyomata reduce the efficacy of assisted reproduction cycles:results of matched follow-up study. Hum Reprod 1998;13:192-7.
23. Donnez J, Wyns C, Nisolle M. Does ovarian surgery for endometriomas impair the ovarian response to gonadotropin. Fertil Steril 2001;76:662-5.
24. Bernhart K, Dunsmoor-Su R, Coutifaris C. Effect of endometriosis on *in vitro* fertilization. Fertil Steril 2002;77:1148-55.
25. Elsheikh A, Milingos S, Loutradis D, Kallipolitis G, Michalas S. Endometrosis and reproductive disorders. Ann N Y Acad Sci 2003;997:247-54.
26. Buyalos RP, Agarwal SK. Endometriosis - associated infertility. Curr Opin Obstet Gynecol 2000;12:377-81.
27. Winkle CA. Evaluation and management of women with endometriosis, Obstet Gynecol 2003;102:397-408.
28. Bulent B, Mahdavi A, Shahmohamady B, Nezhat C. Role of laparoscopic surgery in infertility. MEFSJ 2005;10:94-104.

Hysteroscopic Markers of Genital Tuberculosis

Sunita Tandulwadkar, Bhavana Agarwal Mittal

OVERVIEW

In women presenting with infertility, the prevalence of genital tuberculosis was found to be about 10 percent in India. The incidence of infertility in genital tuberculosis varies between 40 and 60 percent. While primary tuberculosis of the genital tract is rare, secondary tuberculosis can occur secondary to tuberculous lesions in the lungs (the most common) or extrapulmonary tuberculosis. Most patients are either asymptomatic or may have only constitutional symptoms. Infertility may be the only reason for which the patient may present to a gynecologist. The diagnostic dilemma arises from a varied clinical presentation, diverse results on imaging and endoscopy, and the availability of a battery of bacteriological, serological and histopathological tests, which are often required for the collective evidence for the diagnosis of genital tuberculosis. Not all tests are required in all the patients and the choice depends on the clinical presentation.

Hysterosalpingography (HSG) is contraindicated in genital tuberculosis as it may flare up subclinical infection. Usually, diagnosis is made retrospectively when HSG is incidentally performed in infertile patients. Hysteroscopy has a role in diagnosis, therapy (adhesiolysis, metroplasty) and monitoring the response to treatment. The hysteroscopic findings may be normal, reveal a pale-looking endometrium, presence of granulomas, poor distensibility, or the cavity may be partially or completed obliterated with adhesions or a small shrunken cavity.

Microscopic examination of acid fast bacillus (AFB) requires the presence of at least 10,000 organisms in the sample. Culture is more sensitive, requiring as little as 100 organisms/mL, while polymerase chain reaction (PCR) may be positive with only 1 to 10 organisms/mL.

The commonly used screening tests are adenosine deaminase (ADA), Mycobacterium IgG, IgM ad IgA antibodies, AFB smear by fluorescent microscopy and AFB smear by Ziehl-Neelsen (ZN) staining. The confirmatory tests are RNA detection by transcription-mediated amplification (TMA) method (improved PCR) and radiometric culture by BACTEC.

INTRODUCTION

The Problem of Tuberculosis

There are 8 million annual cases of tuberculosis worldwide, of which, 95 percent occur in the developing countries. In India, 40 percent of the adults are infected with tuberculosis. The greatest burden of tuberculosis is in adults aged 15 to 54 years. Globally, the HIV epidemic is increasing the number of tuberculosis cases and accelerating the spread of the disease.[1] Multidrug resistant (MDR) and extreme drug resistant (XDR) tuberculosis are also a cause of serious concern.[2]

World Health Organization's Global Tuberculosis Program (WHO, GTB) declared tuberculosis as a global emergency in 1993 and promoted the Directly Observed Treatment Short (DOTS) course strategy. The Revised National Tuberculosis Control Program (RNTCP) of India incorporated the DOTS strategy, covering 87 percent of the population in 2004.

Genital Tuberculosis

Female genital tract tuberculosis was first described by Morgagni in 1744 on an autopsy of a young lady who died of tuberculous peritonitis, while a detailed study of its course and treatment was reported by Hager in 1886.[3] The exact incidence of genital tuberculosis is not accurately known as it is under reported due to asymptomatic cases and lack of reliable confirmatory investigations.[4,5] The reported incidence in India varies from 1 to 19 percent. A prevalence of 2.3 percent tuberculous endometritis has been observed in the asymptomatic population.[6] In women presenting with infertility, the prevalence of genital tuberculosis was found to be about 10 percent in India.[7-10] The incidence of infertility in genital tuberculosis varies between 40 and 60 percent.[11]

CLINICAL DISCUSSION

Pathogenesis

Causative Organism

Tuberculosis is caused by the *Mycobacterium tuberculosis* complex (*M. tuberculosis, M. bovis, M. africanum* or atypical *Mycobacteria sp.*).

Mode of Spread

Primary tuberculosis of the genital tract is rare. It involves the vulva and cervix and may occur by direct contact with infective material or be sexually transmitted.

Secondary tuberculosis can occur secondary to tuberculous lesions in the lungs (the most common) or extrapulmonary tuberculosis. It can spread via the bloodstream, lymphatics and directly from neighboring organs. The closer to menarche the primary infection occurs, the more likely it is that pelvic tuberculosis will follow.

Sites of Genital Tuberculosis

- Fallopian tubes (90–100%)
- Endometrium (50–80%)
- Ovaries (20–30%)
- Cervix (5–15%)
- Vulva or vagina (1% of cases).[4,5,7]

Endometrial Tuberculosis

Macroscopically

- The endometrial appearance may be unremarkable due to repeated menstruation, minimizing the disease
- Caseation and ulceration
- Slight distortion to complete obliteration of the cavity due to adhesions
- Asherman's syndrome genital tuberculosis appears to be an important and common cause of Asherman's syndrome in India, causing oligomenorrhea or amenorrhea with infertility.[12]

Microscopically

- Tuberculous granulomas with or without caseation, epithelioid cells and Langhans cells containing birefringent crystals

- Focal collection of lymphocytes
- Dilated glands
- Destruction of epithelium

CASE STUDIES

Clinical Presentation

Most patients are asymptomatic or may have only constitutional symptoms. Upto 11 percent cases of genital tuberculosis are silent with no constant clinical signs of illness.[13,14] Infertility may be the only reason for which the patient may present to a gynecologist. It may be primary in 75 percent of cases and secondary in 14 percent cases following an abortion, ectopic or normal delivery. The reason for infertility is involvement of the Fallopian tubes (blocked and damaged tubes), endometrium (non-receptive and damaged endometrium) and ovarian damage.[7,9,15] Timely diagnosis will facilitate treatment and help in successful future pregnancies.

Majority of the patients (50–85%) may have normal menstruation. However, women may present with menstrual disorders, such as dysmenorrhea, menorrhagia or menometrorrhagia, due to tuberculous endometritis and also with amenorrhea (7%) due to destruction of the endometrium. Amenorrhea may be primary, following peritoneal tuberculosis in childhood or secondary, following scanty periods. The patient may also complain of pain in the abdomen or of vague abdominal discomfort.

Diagnosis

Being a paucibacillary disease, the demonstration of *M. tuberculosis* is not possible in all cases and a high index of suspicion is required. The diagnostic dilemma arises from a varied clinical presentation, diverse results on imaging and endoscopy, and the availability of a battery of bacteriological, serological and histopathological tests, which are often required to obtain collective evidence for the diagnosis of genital tuberculosis.[10,16] Not all tests are required in all the patients and the choice depends on the clinical presentation.

- Complete blood count along with raised erythrocyte sedimentation rate (ESR) is a non-specific marker of tuberculosis but can support the clinical suspicion of the disease.
- Chest X-ray may detect coexisting pulmonary disease.
- Tuberculin testing indicates *Mycobacterium* infection but not tuberculous disease. It has a sensitivity of 55 percent and specificity of 80 percent.
- Enzyme-linked immunosorbent assay (ELISA), to detect 38-kDa antigen of *M. tuberculosis,* or monoclonal antibody-based sandwich ELISA, is rapid, inexpensive and simple to perform but has a low sensitivity (50–66%) and specificity.
- Other tests include detection of *Mycobacterium* IgG, IgM and IgA antibodies (98% specificity, 40% sensitivity) and adenine deaminase activity (ADA) in body fluids.

Hysterosalpingography

Hysterosalpingography (HSG) is contraindicated in genital tuberculosis as it may flare up a subclinical infection. Usually, diagnosis is made retrospectively when HSG is incidentally performed in infertile patients.

The synechie and intrauterine adhesions in tuberculosis are characteristically irregular, angulated and stellate-shaped with well-demarcated borders. Unilateral scarring may cause a pseudounicornuate uterus appearance. Scarring may lead to a T-shaped uterus. An asymmetric, small-sized uterine cavity is usually due to tuberculosis.[3,17] Venous and lymphatic extravasation is a good indicator of endometrial tuberculosis but it is not very specific.

The findings may be classified as follows:

Group I–   No abnormality on HSG
          Tubal occlusion present
          Superficial endometrium involved

Group II–   Uterine cavity smaller than normal
           Tubes usually occluded in the cornual region
           Fine irregularity of the endometrial cavity

Group III– Progressive destruction of the endometrium and myometrium

Group IV– Extensive obliteration of the uterine cavity, utero-lymphatic and uterovenous extravasation.

Role of Hysteroscopy

- For diagnosis
- Adhesiolysis and metroplasty
- Monitoring the response to treatment.

Findings (Figs 2.1 to 2.8)

- Normal hysteroscopy findings (if no endometrial tuberculosis or early stage tuberculosis) with bilateral open ostia.
- Pale looking endometrium
- Presence of granulomas
- Poor distensibility
- Cavity may be partially or completed obliterated with adhesions
- Small shrunken cavity.

One has to be careful in performing hysteroscopy in genital tuberculosis as the cervix is often constricted and dilatation is difficult with chances of perforation and false passage.

In an observational study, the hysteroscopy showed normal findings in 30 percent of the patients, flimsy adhesions in 20 percent, thick adhesions in 15 percent, and an obliterated cavity with inability to see the ostia or blocked ostia in 25 percent.[18] In another study, diagnostic hysteroscopy in genital tuberculosis showed that 11 (18.9%) patients had uterine

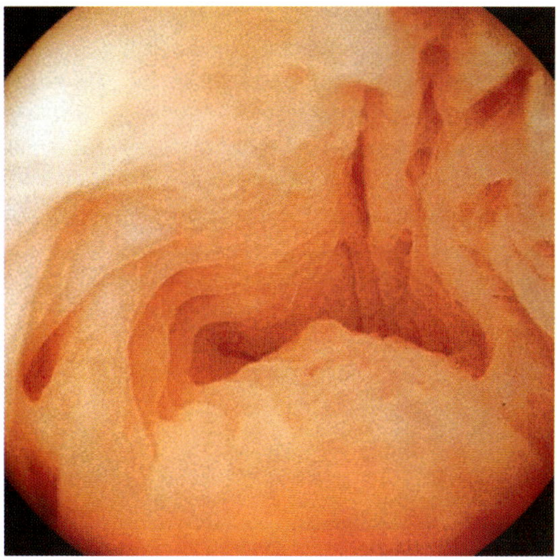

Fig. 2.1: Normal cervical canal

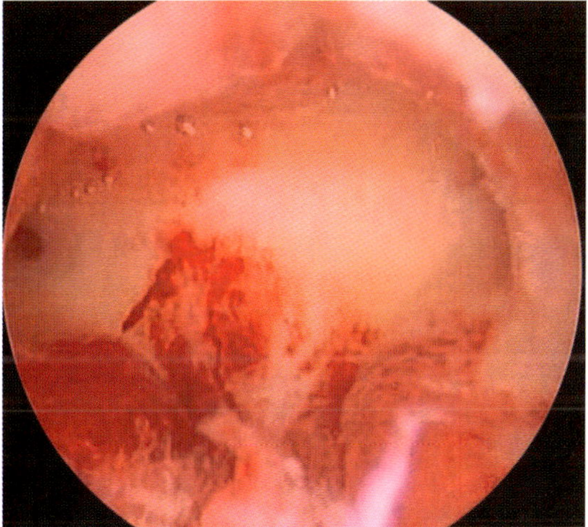

Fig. 2.2: Panoramic view from internal os

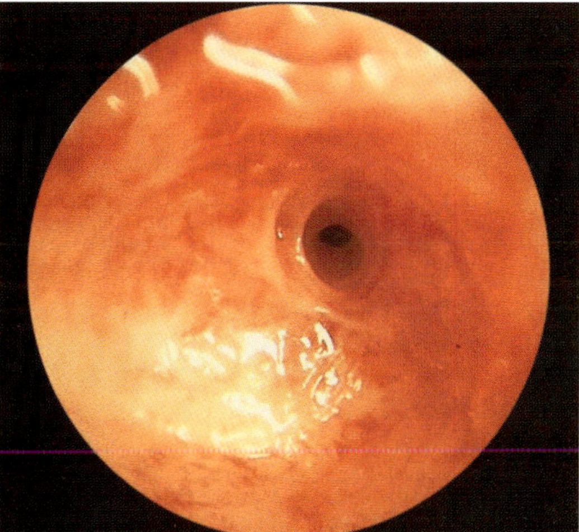

Fig. 2.3: Extensive stenosis of cervical canal

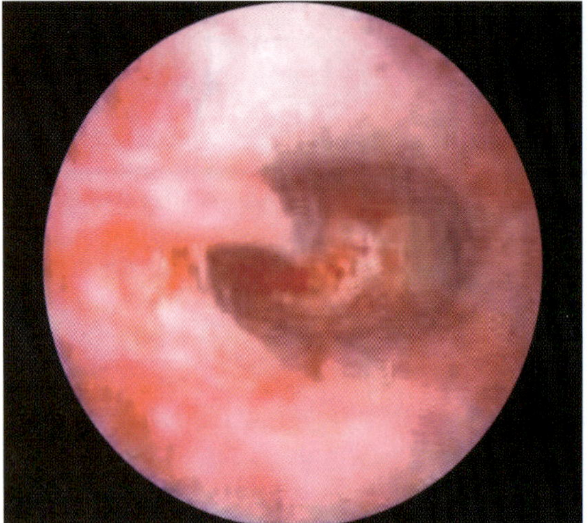

Fig. 2.4: Small uterine cavity with long cervical canal

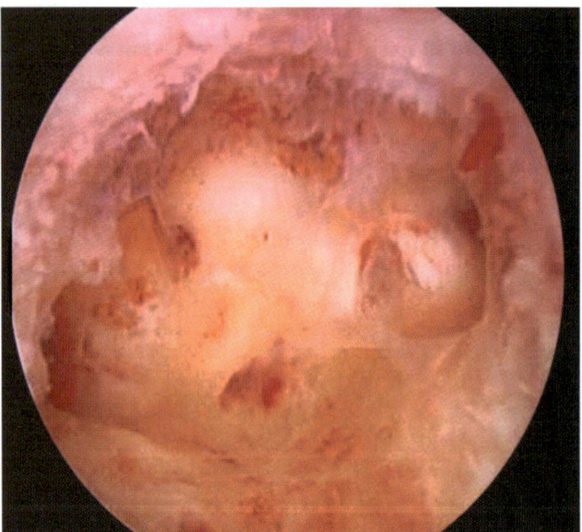

Fig. 2.5: Flimsy uterine adhesions

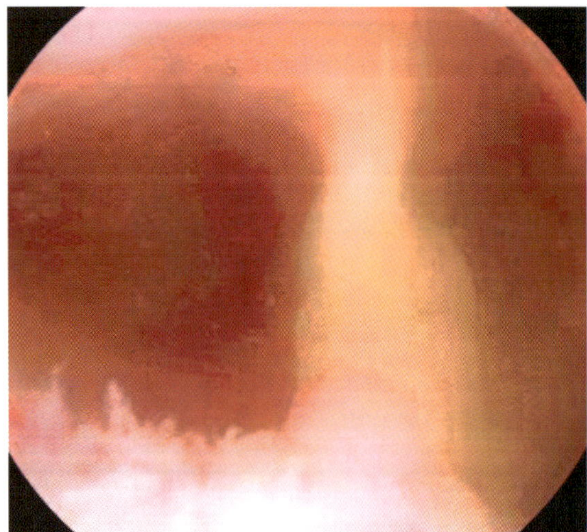

Fig. 2.6: Uterine adhesion band

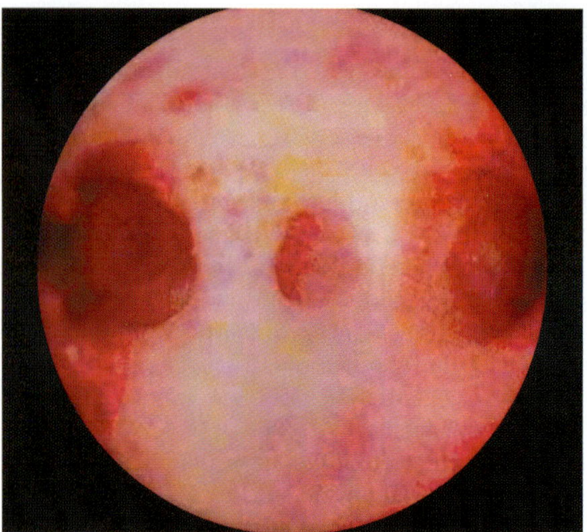

Fig. 2.7: Multiple uterine adhesion bands

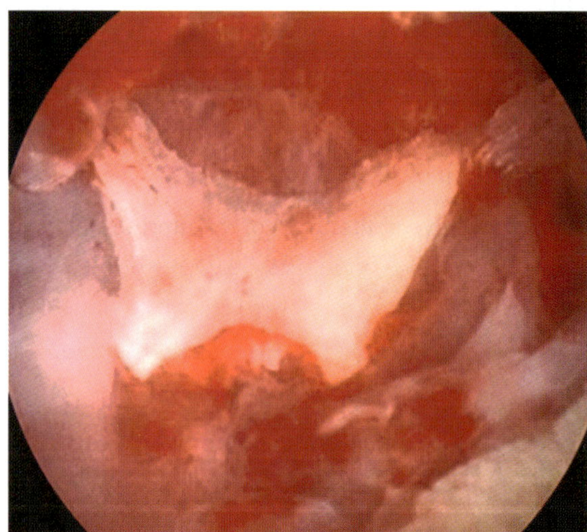

Fig. 2.8: Dense uterine adhesions

adhesions and 1 patient had a pale endometrium.[19] In a study on hysteroscopic findings in women with primary infertility due to genital tuberculosis, the hysteroscopic findings were normal in 20.5 percent cases, adhesions were grade-2 in 15.1 percent cases, grade-2a in 1.4 percent cases, grade-3 in 15.1 percent cases, grade-3b in 8.2 percent cases, and grade-4 in 38.4 percent cases.[20]

Endometrial biopsy: Curettage from the cornual regions or aspirate should ideally be done in the premenstrual phase. Pseudopregnancy, with progesterone to prevent cyclical shedding and subsequent biopsy, may show tuberculous follicles (Kistner method). The sample is subjected to smear examination (ZN staining, Pap flouorescein staining or Rhodamine rapid staining) for acid fast bacillus (AFB), culture on Lowenstein–Jensen (LJ) media and guineapig inoculation, which takes 6 to 8 weeks to provide results.

Histopathological examination of the specimen yields higher results (28–69.5%) than traditional culture methods (12–29.4%).[10,12] Early unsuspected cases show few tuberculous follicles, which are best evident in the premenstrual phase of the cycle. They usually start from the cornual region as a result of spread from the Fallopian tubes and may also be a diffuse process involving a major part of the endometrium. There may be replacement of the endometrium by granulation tissue and hyalinized connective tissue. The areas of caseation may involve the myometrium.

The radiometric culture (BACTEC 460), based on generation of radioactive carbon dioxide from palmitic acid, has a higher sensitivity (80–90%) with quicker results (2–3 weeks). It is particularly suitable for drug sensitivity testing in MDR tuberculosis. Deoxyribonucleic acid (DNA) finger-printing is done from BACTEC for diagnosis of false positive cultures.

Absence of signs of tuberculous endometritis in any biopsy is not proof of absence of genital tuberculosis because:
- Tuberculous endometritis is seen in only 50 to 60 percent of cases of genital tuberculosis
- Nonrepresentative tissue samples
- Improper processing of the sample
- Stage of the disease
- Effect of HIV coinfection.

TB-PCR-DNA

This is a rapid, sensitive and specific molecular biological method for detecting mycobacterial DNA. PCR assays target various gene segments, including a 65 kDa protein encoding gene, the IS 6110 element and the mpt64 gene. It detects live as well as dead bacteria and has a testing time of 8 to 12 hours. PCR is more sensitive (43.1–56%) than histopathology and culture for detecting genital tuberculosis.[10,21,22]

Microscopic examination of AFB requires the presence of at least 10,000 organisms in the sample. Culture is more sensitive, requiring as little as 100 organisms/mL while PCR may be positive with only 1 to 10 organisms/mL.[22] However, PCR has some disadvantages:
- It can give false negative results due to high salt or heparin concentrations in the specimen.
- As it cannot distinguish between live and dead bacilli, there is a small risk of false positive results.
- It may not be able to differentiate between infection and disease.
- Antituberculosis treatment (ATT) should not be started on the basis of positive PCR unless there is some other clinical, histopathological or laparoscopic evidence of the disease.
- The positive predictive value is less than 75 percent due to problems of contamination.
- It should not be used as a therapy monitoring tool, as it detects both live and dead bacilli.

RNA Detection by Transcription-mediated Amplification-improved PCR

It detects live bacteria (nucleic acid detected is RNA). It has no false positive results and no issues of contamination. Testing time is 3 hours. It can be used as a therapy-monitoring tool, because it detects live bacteria. It has a positive predictive value of 100 percent.

In our own prospective study to evaluate the role of pilot office hysteroscopy in patients undergoing *in vitro* fertilization (IVF)/intracytoplasmic sperm injection (ICSI), 237 patients with no suspicion of uterine and cervical pathology underwent pilot hysteroscopy. Endometrial biopsy for TB-PCR-RNA by the transcription-mediated amplification (TMA) method was also undertaken, as the incidence of pelvic tuberculosis in infertile women in India is 40 percent. Office hysteroscopy helped to detect intrauterine adhesions secondary to tuberculosis or endometritis. Endometrial samples, taken in the same sitting and sent for TB-PCR-RNA by the TMA method, allowed us to detect live tuberculous bacilli, which could result in implantation failure. TB-PCR-RNA by the TMA method was positive in 2.5 percent of the cases (unpublished data).

The commonly used screening tests are ADA, *Mycobacterium* IgG, IgM and IgA antibodies, AFB smear by fluorescent microscopy and AFB smear by ZN staining. The confirmatory tests are RNA detection by the TMA method (improved PCR) and radiometric culture by BACTEC.

Recent Advances

Newer tests, like Gen-Probe Amplified *Mycobacterium tuberculosis* Direct Test (MTD) and Amplicor, have also been developed but are not widely available. MTD for *Mycobacterium tuberculosis*, and Amplicor *Mycobacterium* for Mycobacteria (AMP-M. TB for *M. tuberculosis*, AMP-M. av for *M. avium* and AMP-M. in for *M. intracellulare*) are used for the detection of the relevant *Mycobacterium* species. MTD and AMP-M. TB are more sensitive than the conventional culture method, and MTD is more sensitive than AMP-M. TB but needs more careful treatment to avoid contamination.[23]

CONCLUSION

The high incidence of genital tuberculosis in India, and of infertility in women afflicted with genital tuberculosis, warrants prompt diagnosis of the disorder. Varied clinical presentation, diverse imaging results and the availability of a battery of bacteriological, serological and histopathological tests, often required for collective evidence for the diagnosis of genital tuberculosis, usually creates a diagnostic dilemma. Hence, the choice of test used must be guided by the clinical presentation. ADA, *Mycobacterium* IgG, IgM and IgA antibodies, AFB smear by fluorescent microscopy and AFB smear by ZN staining are commonly used screening tests, however, advanced molecular diagnostic techniques, such as RNA detection by the TMA method (improved PCR), and radiometric culture by BACTEC may be required for confirmation. Hysteroscopy has an important role in diagnosis, management and monitoring the response to treatment but HSG should be avoided in genital tuberculosis as it may flare up subclinical infection.

REFERENCES

1. Central TB. Division-General of Health Services (DGHS). Ministry of Health and Family Welfare. Government of India, New Delhi (June 2000).
2. DeAngelis CD, Flanagin A. Tuberculosis-a global problem requiring a global solution. JAMA 2005;293:2793-4.
3. Kumar S. Tuberculosis in pregnancy. In: Sharma SK, Mohan A, (Eds) Tuberculosis, Ist edn. New Delhi: Jaypee; 2001. pp. 304-10.
4. Kumar S. Female genital tuberculosis. In: Sharma SK, Mohan A, (Eds). Tuberculosis, Ist edn. New Delhi: Jaypee; 2001.pp.311-24.
5. Sharma JB. Female genital tuberculosis revisited. Obstet Gynecol Today 2007;XII:61-3.
6. Bazaz-Malik G, Maheshwari B, Lal N. Tuberculous endometritis: a clinicopathological study of 1000 cases. Br J Obstet Gynecol 1983;90:84-6.
7. Schaefer G. Female genital tuberculosis. Clin Obstet Gynecol 1976;19:223-39.
8. Deshmukh KK, Lopez JA, Naidu TAK, Gaurkhede MD. MV Place of laparoscopy in pelvic tuberculosis in infertile women. Arch Gynecol 1985;237:197-200.
9. Chhabra S, Saharan K, Pohane D. Pelvic tuberculosis continues to be a disease of dilemma-case series. Indian J Tuberc 2010;57: 90-4.
10. Jindal UN. An algorithmic approach to female genital tuberculosis causing infertility. Int J Tuberc Lung Dis 2006;10:1045-50.
11. Tripathy SN. Laparoscopic observations of pelvic organs in pulmonary tuberculosis. Int J Gynaecol Obstet 1990;32:129-31.
12. Sharma JB, Roy KK, Pushparaj M, Gupta N, Jain SK, Malhotra N, Mittal S. Genital tuberculosis: an important cause of Asherman's syndrome in India. Arch Gynecol Obstet 2008; 277:37-41.
13. Falk V, Ludviksson K, Agren G. Genital tuberculosis in women. Analysis of 187 newly diagnosed cases from 47 Swedish hospitals during the ten-year period 1968 to 1977. Am J Obstet Gynecol 1980;138 (7 Pt 2):974-7.
14. Arora R, Asmita. Female genital tract tuberculosis. In: Arora VK, Arora Raksha (Eds). Practical approach to tuberculosis management. 1st edn. Jaypee Brothers Medical Publishers (P) Ltd., New Delhi; 2006.pp.113-9.
15. Sharma JB, Roy KK, Pushparaj M, Kumar S, Malhotra N, Mittal S. Laparoscopic findings in female genital tuberculosis. Arch Gynecol Obstet 2008;278:359-64.
16. Jassawala MJ. Genital tuberculosis—a diagnostic dilemma. J Obstet Gynecol India 2006;56:203-4.
17. Chavhan GB, Hira P, Rathod K, Zacharia TT, Chawla A, Badhe P, Parmar H. Female genital tuberculosis: hysterosalpingographic appearances. Br J Radiol 2004;77:164-9.
18. Sharma JB, Roy KK, Kumar S, Malhotra N, Chawla P, (unpublished data).
19. Singh N, Sumana G, Mittal S. Genital tuberculosis: a leading cause for infertility in women seeking assisted conception in North India. Arch Gynecol Obstet 2008;278:325-7.
20. Sharma JB, Roy KK, Pushparaj M, Kumar S. Hysteroscopic findings in women with primary and secondary infertility due to genital tuberculosis. Int J Gynecol Obstet 2009;104:49-52.
21. Abebe M, Lakew M, Kidane D, Lakew Z, Kiros K, Harboe M. Female genital tuberculosis in Ethiopia. Int J Gynecol Obstet 2004;84:241-6.
22. Bhanu NV, Singh UB, Chakraborty M, Suresh N, Arora J, Rana T, Takkar D, Seth P. Improved diagnostic value of PCR in the diagnosis of female genital tuberculosis leading to infertility. J Med Microbiol 2005;54(Pt 10):927-31.
23. Sato A, Sonobe T, Okazaki M, Umeda B. Evaluations of MTD and Amplicor *Mycobacterium* for direct detection of mycobacteria from clinical specimens. [Article in Japanese] Kekkaku 1999;74:433-9.

Hysteroscopic Intratubal Sterilization

Hervé Fernandez, Anne-Claire Donnadieu, Claire Basille, Xavier Deffieux, Estelle Feyereisen, Amelie Gervaise

OVERVIEW

Minimally-invasive surgery has made substantial advances in recent years. Among these procedures, tubal sterilization by laparoscopy remains the most common and is most often performed as a day surgery. Conceptus recently developed a tubal micro-insert, Essure®, that avoids the risks of laparoscopy.

The Essure® device is an expanding spring micro-insert, 2 mm in diameter and 4 cm in length; it consists of a flexible stainless steel inner coil, a dynamic outer coil made of nickel titanium alloy (Nitinol), and a layer of polyethylene terephthalate fibers that induce localized tissue in-growth, with fibrosis and occlusion of the tubal lumen in one to three months.

The device is placed through a 5 Fr operative channel 30° hysteroscope, with saline distension medium, into the proximal section of the Fallopian tube; optimal positioning of the insert occurs when 3 to 8 loops of the spring remain visible. The procedure can be performed in the operating theater or the physician's office and does not require general anesthesia.

Patients are instructed to continue or begin temporary alternative contraception for three months to ensure that the device is retained and that the fibrotic reaction and tubal occlusion occur. Pelvic radiography (X-Ray abdomen and/or hysterosalpingography) is performed to verify that the micro-inserts have been retained within the pelvic cavity in an appropriate position.

On the other hand, ultrasound detects the Essure® device, which is highly echogenic and thus, stands out from the surrounding structures, and three-dimensional (3D) ultrasound may be recommended for assessing device position after placement.

Furthermore, combining Essure® hysteroscopic sterilization and operative hysteroscopy is a new approach to optimize the efficacy of endometrial ablation and permanent contraception.

INTRODUCTION

Minimally-invasive surgery has made substantial advances in recent years. Among these procedures, tubal sterilization by laparoscopy remains the most common and is most often performed as a day surgery. Conceptus recently developed a tubal micro-insert that avoids the risks of laparoscopy: Essure® (Essure Permanent Birth Control System, Conceptus, Inc., San Carlos, CA). The Essure® device was approved in November 2001 by the European Health Office and a year later by the United States Food and Drug Administration. Its development in France, was authorized by L. 2001 to 588 of 4 July 2001 (Journal Officiel n°156, dated 7 July 2001), which regulated sterilization for contraceptive purposes.

The Essure® device is an expanding spring micro-insert, 2 mm in diameter and 4 cm in length; it consists of a flexible stainless steel inner coil, a dynamic outer coil made of nickel titanium alloy (Nitinol), and a layer of polyethylene terephthalate (PET) fibers that induce localized tissue in-growth, with fibrosis and occlusion of the tubal lumen in one to three months.

Since the first attempts, a lot of scientific publications confirmed the development of the surgical technique. The successful bilateral placement of the device has shown a steady increase from 1999 to 2005 (Fig. 3.1). Moreover, with experience and the new catheter, the procedure time has decreased from 18 minutes to less than 10 minutes (Fig. 3.2).[1-3]

CLINICAL DISCUSSION

Instrumentation and Technique

A hysteroscope with a 5 Fr working channel is used to perform the procedure without dilating the cervical canal. The so-called "Bettocchi" hysteroscope (Karl Storz, Germany),

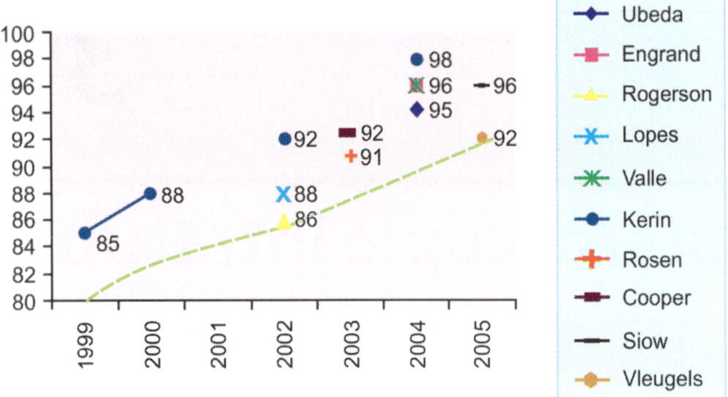

Fig. 3.1: Successful bilateral placement (%)

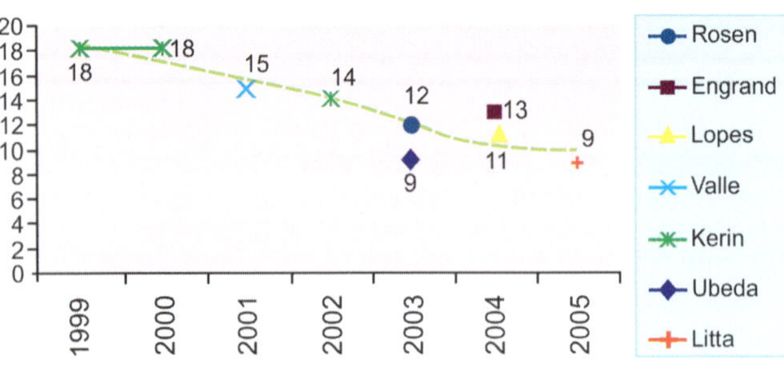

Fig. 3.2: Procedure time (%)

available in sizes of 4.2 or 4.9 mm, is the most optimal scope to be used when choosing the vaginal hysteroscopic approach. These scopes have an oval design that matches the oval-shaped internal ostium of multiparous women. These small hysteroscopes have a 5 Fr-working channel in which the Essure® device fits.

The patient is positioned in the lithotomy position. The operating table is elevated such that the surgeon can sit relaxed with flexed elbows and shoulders. The hips of the patient are flexed to an angle of more than 90 degrees with the table in order to facilitate the surgeon to move the hysteroscope to the lateral sides even in obese women.

Procedure time is the most important factor to be discussed with the patient. The hysteroscopy should be scheduled right after the period, by withdrawal bleeding or regular menstruation, before the onset of the proliferative stage. With increasing thickness of the endometrium, the small tubal orifices cannot be localized properly. Moreover, the later sterilization is planned, the more probable it is that edema of the endometrium will impair vision of the tubal ostia.

Patients should be informed about the procedure details, specifically regarding the introduction of the scope without a speculum and without local anesthesia. Patients may be accompanied by their husbands or friends. The more information a patient receives, the more she can accept limited feelings of discomfort or slight cramps.

Premedication

Non-steroidal anti-inflammatory drugs (NSAIDs) (i.e. Diclofenac 100 mg) are given as suppositories 1 or 2 hours prior to the procedure. The premedication 1 hour ahead of hysteroscopy may be combined with any analgesic agent (i.e. Paracetamol 1000 mg). The transvaginal approach involves the introduction of the hysteroscope without prior administration of local anesthesia. The Essure procedure is recommended without anesthesia. For example, the experience in Cordoba, Spain on 973 patients, shows that more and more surgeons use the Bettocchi technique and avoid IV sedation and local anesthesia (Table 3.1). Very rarely, dilation and, as a consequence, local anesthesia is required. In this case, a speculum has to be brought into position and the cervix has to be grasped by the tenaculum. Local anesthesia is injected and around the cervix clockwise at 2, 5, 7 and 11 o'clock positions. The needle may be slightly bent to facilitate introduction of anesthesia in the upper cervical canal at the level of the internal ostium, Lidocaïne (1%) or Ropivacaïne may be used as anesthetic agents.

To prevent any discomfort to the patient and to reduce the risk of iatrogenic trauma to genital tissues that may stimulate prostaglandin release, the speculum and tenaculum may be avoided.

The scope is introduced in the vagina and the posterior vaginal fornix filled with normal saline. One has to be aware that the vaginal axis of a woman in lithotomy position is almost vertical, at an angle of 45° to 60°. By using a speculum, this axis is artificially reduced to 180°, which is not natural.

Once the posterior vaginal section is filled with normal saline, the scope is retracted slowly until, at 12 o'clock, the

Table 3.1: Anesthesia				
	No/few difficulties during the procedure	*Successful placement rate*	*No/little pain during the procedure*	*Patients very satisfied with the procedure*
Group with local anesthesia (434 patients)	81.80%	98.40%	95.7%	92.5%
Group without any anesthesia (539 patients)	90%	99.10%	97.5%	95%

external ostium becomes visible. The scope is introduced under direct vision into the cervical canal. Due to the inflow pressure of the normal saline, the cervix will be distended. The oval-shaped internal ostium can be easily passed by 90 degrees on-axis rotation.

Patients may feel some cramps or pain, but they accept the discomfort for a short while after having been explained what the problem is and what you intend to do. Moreover, the patient is given the option to observe the procedure on the monitor screen, which facilitates the explanation.

Before the hysteroscope is brought into the vagina, a plastic sheet has to be placed in the rubber stopcock of the working channel. This sheet facilitates introduction of the very thin and vulnerable device. Two sheets are sterile-packed separately, together with the two devices.

As soon as the device is introduced into the cavity, both the tubal ostia should be localized. The procedure can be initiated only if both the ostia are visible. The tube in which the anticipated approach may be associated with a higher incidence of difficulty needs to be blocked first because in case this tube cannot be blocked, the other easier approach can be omitted. In this way, opening both sterilized and separately packed devices can be avoided if the first ostium appears blocked.

After the first device has been placed and the windings inside the cavity have been counted, the assistant introduces the second device as quickly as possible, while the surgeon turns the scope to the other tube. The more dexterous and proficient the operating surgeon is, the lesser the stimulus that induces prostaglandin release. In this way, the risk for tubal spasm of the contralateral tube can be reduced.

The devices are advanced in the tubes as far as the black mark on the outer sheeth of the device reaches the tubal orifice. Once the black spot is in place, the hysteroscope has to be fixed very precisely with both hands; the device-handpiece, together with the scope, must be grasped to prevent movement of the device in relation to the position of the hysteroscope. While turning the wheel on the hand-piece the outer sheet with the black spot is retracted and brought outside the view of the surgeon. At the moment this wheel blocks, an orange connecting piece can be seen by the surgeon. This is another landmark for a good position. Once this orange piece is in the view of the surgeon, the Nitinol spring, which is curled around the central guiding catheter, becomes visible. With the later in view, a thickness of the spring can be seen at the tubal ostium. This small thickness is another landmark and indicates where the PET fibers are fixed to the spring. In case one sees this thickness, the most optimal position is reached. A small correction of the position can be achieved by carefully pushing and pulling the device forward or backward. After pushing on the button of the hand-piece, one can turn the wheel further backwards,

retracting the outer sheet and releasing the spring. This spring will be uncurled now and will partly act as a screw, turning a little bit further into the tubal ostium. After the wheel on the hand-piece blocks again, one has to wait a few seconds just to allow the spring to settle itself firmly in the tube. After a few seconds the guiding catheter can be detached from the spring by turning the hand-piece 5 times or more counter-clockwise and carefully pulling it out.

Problem Solving and Troubleshooting

Spasm of the Tube

A pinpoint tubal ostium indicates a spasm of the tubes and the device will not slip into the ostium. The woman often explains that she feels uterine cramps. Do not apply force and reduce the pressure to relax the uterus. Wait several minutes and as soon as the patient indicates that she does not feel anymore cramps, dilate the cavity and try to place the device. Intravenous medication, like NSAID, does not always relax the tubes. In case the device cannot be placed for this reason, the patients may be asked to return later on the same day or the next cycle.

Prevention: Avoid any stressful situation and prostaglandin release. Plan the procedure straight after the periods within 10 days. Advice breakfast or any meal before hand. Premedication is necessary.

Abnormal Position of the Tube

The angle of entry of tube with the uterus can be greater than 90 degrees, causing difficulties in the introduction of the device. Moreover, an irregularity in the tube can cause resistance during introduction. Do not use force, but try to introduce the device by turning the screwing movements of the scope, using the slightly bent tip of the device. By turning the scope, the angle of direction of the device and the inlet of the tube can be manipulated. Reducing the pressure in the cavity might be helpful in changing the position of the tube. Most important is to take your time.

Intrauterine pathology, like a fibroid in the tubal corner, may hide the tubal ostium. In these cases, it must be known that introduction might be difficult and the depth of placement cannot be controlled visually.

Retraction after Release of the Device

After releasing the device, a few seconds wait is required to enable the spring to fully expand and fix in the tube before unlocking the introducer by at least 5 turning movements to the left.

Shallow Insertion Depth

After releasing the device, it may be extruded out of the tubal ostium, either during removal of the introducer or later on at home, which may result in a shallow, inadequate insertion depth. This may occur inadvertently during the afore-mentioned procedure and may go unnoticed until incorrect placement is diagnosed either by ultrasound or by means of an X-ray or hysterosalpingography (HSG).

Excessive Insertion Depth

In case the placement is too deep, the Essure® device will be localized in the distal tubal part, outside the uterine wall. Due to less intense contact with the PET, fibers, lesser and later tubal fibrosis will occur. Moreover, the device might be expelled by tubal contractions into the abdominal cavity. This problem can occur when less than 3 windings are visible after placement of the device and often happens at the beginning of the learning curve. The situation can be prevented by fixing the hysteroscope precisely during the retraction of the outer sheath once the device is introduced correctly. During the retraction of the outer sheath the hysteroscopic view of the tubal area should be kept the same and the black tip of the retracting outer sheath should be brought outside this view.

At the end of the placement, the orange colored connection piece should be outside the tubal ostium, with at least 5 curled windings between this orange part and the tube. The place where the PET fibers are fixed proximally can be recognized as a thickened part; this part, just located in the tubal ostium, indicates the most optimal positioning.

Bleeding after the Procedure

On the day of the procedure, some minimal blood loss may be expected. Some women have spotting after the procedure during the first cycle. After the next period, no abnormal bleeding has been reported.

Postoperative Complaints

All women have slight abdominal discomfort for a few hours after sterilization. These complaints do not exceed their menstrual discomfort, requiring no more than one dose of home medication. In case the patient needs more medication, and the pain hampers normal social life, she must consult the surgeon who did the procedure.

Total or Partial Perforation

Although the Essure® device will always be introduced in the ostium of the tube, due to abnormal position or sharp angle of the tube with the outline of the uterus, or contraction of the tube, the proximal tip of the device can perforate the tube. Patients feel more pain as usual at the moment of placement or have prolonged complaints the day after. At laparoscopy, the tip of the tube can be found outside the tubo-cornual junction. Sometimes, a partial perforation is found; the tip is still subserosal, i.e. it lies under the covering peritoneum of the tube.

In case of a difficult procedure, which takes more than 15 minutes or, during which more force is used, a control X-ray should be done. On this X-ray, sometimes an abnormal position, like a curling device can be seen. On the hysterosalpingogram, performed three months later, the tubes seem to be blocked, i.e. no passage is seen but at the tubo-cornual junction, leakage might be recorded at the place of the perforation. On the ultrasound, this problem can not be suspected as the reflection of the device is still within the outline of the uterus. Prevention is done by avoidance of any force in case the device does not slip smoothly into the tubal ostium.

Regret after the Sterilization

Due to the characteristics of this method reanastomosis of the tubes is impossible. Only *in vitro* fertilization (IVF) can offer a chance for a pregnancy. Results of IVF treatment after Essure® sterilization are not available yet, although case reports of Essure® placements in women with hydrosalpinges, who underwent IVF treatment, show that the IVF outcome may not be hampered by the Essure® devices. Good patient counseling is essential to avoid later regrets.

Efficacy of Sterilization

The efficacy of sterilization must be assessed three months after the procedure. Histological studies have proven that 100 percent of all tubes after a normal procedure will be blocked at that time. Thus, in case of an uncomplicated procedure, only proof of a correct position is sufficient; transvaginal ultrasound is the ultimate diagnostic method to do so, but in other cases, the X-ray and HSG are needed.

X-ray Abdomen

An X-ray of the pelvis can prove the presence of the Essure® device. The position of both devices in relation to each other indicates whether they have been placed properly. The X-ray may address the following:
- The visible trailing length of the micro-insert at the conclusion of the device placement is < 3 coils or > 8 coils.
- Identification of the tubal ostium was compromised due to poor distension, poor illumination, or visualization secondary to endometrial debris.
- Concern of possible perforation due to excessive force required on delivery catheter, sudden loss of resistance or no visible trailing length of the micro-insert.

- Since placement, the patient has been complaining of persistent uterine cramping and/or bleeding spotting.
- The four white spots on the X-ray have to be on one line, straight or slightly bent; if one spot cannot be placed on the line of the other 3 spots, a HSG should be performed and/ or laparoscopy done to exclude any partial perforation.

Hysterosalpingography

Three months following the Essure® micro-insert placement procedure, the patient can be scheduled for a HSG. The HSG is performed to evaluate: 1) micro-insert location, and 2) Fallopian tube occlusion. The position on HSG is correct when the distal end of the inner coil is within the tube, with less than 50 percent of the length of the inner coil trailing into the uterine cavity, or the proximal end of the inner coil appears to be up to 30 mm into the tube from where contrast fills the uterine cornua.

The true indication of HSG stays in discussion; systematically in US and in case of misinterpretation of X-ray or ultrasound in Europe.

Transvaginal Ultrasound

On transvaginal ultrasound, the Essure® device can be seen by the ultrasonic reflection of the Nitinol windings. The location of the device can be checked in relation to the cavity and the outline of the uterus.

Three studies have evaluated ultrasonography (USG) to verify device position and propose this examination instead of pelvic radiography at the 3-month check-up. The first study, a case series of 15 women in Australia[4] found that ultrasound was an appropriate imaging modality. In the second, Kerin et al.[3] who conducted both the phase II and pivotal trials of Essure®, evaluated this practice on 37 patients and then confirmed their findings in 145 cases.[3] Another Australian study on 99 patients reached the same

conclusion.[5] The ultrasound examination can be performed by the gynecologist, and results are available immediately (Fig. 3.3).

We recommend the routine use of volume contrast (3D) mode for ultrasound assessment. This procedure is no longer time-consuming: acquisition takes only a few seconds. It is then possible to reconstruct any desired plane. In contrast to 2D ultrasound, using 3D techniques and a vaginal probe allows quick and easy visualization of the coronal plane. The 3D reconstructed coronal view is ideally suited for the detection of Essure® devices and confirmation of their correct placement on both sides (Fig. 3.4). The resolution of the 5 mm thick image is excellent. This procedure improves the patient's comfort and saves time for both her and the physician. We propose a didactic classification of device location that makes it possible to evaluate surgical practices (Figs 3.5A to D). For women

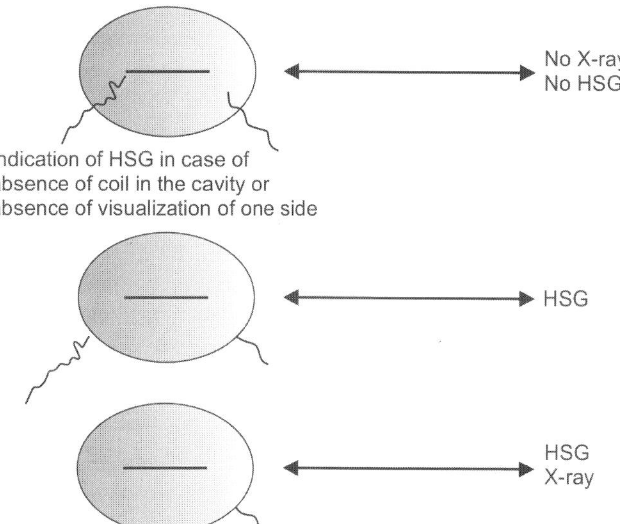

Fig. 3.3: Predictive value of USG

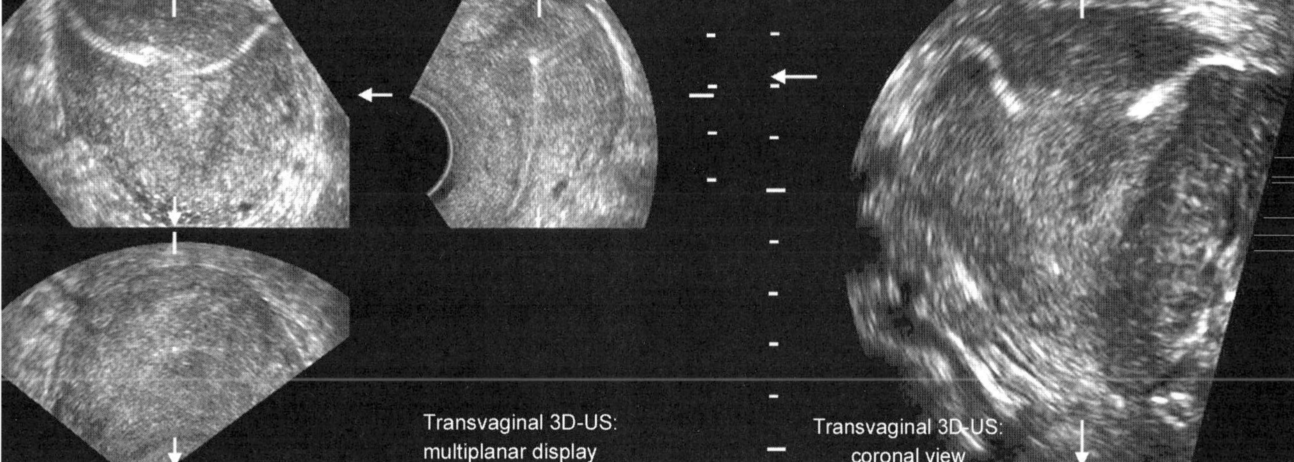

Fig. 3.4: 3D ultrasound central

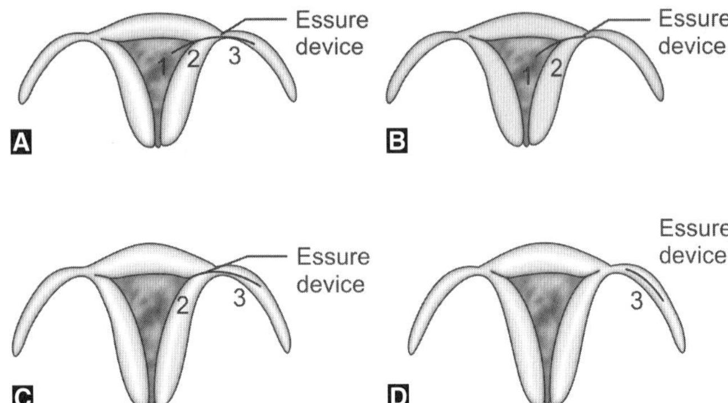

Figs 3.5A to D: Examples of Essure® device placement: 1. uterine cavity portion, 2. intramural portion, 3. tubal portion; (A) Optimal placement is 1-2-3; (B) Proximal placement with intramural portion 1-2; (C) Distal placement with intramural portion 2-3. Efficiency depends on the fibrosis, especially in the intramural part, so portion 2 seems to be essential; (D) Distal incorrect placement 3

with an enlarged uterus, we recommend image acquisition in a frontal plane, rather than two separate images, each of half the uterus. Given the ease of ultrasound visualization of the intrauterine loops, saline hysterosonography offers many disadvantages and no advantages; our experience shows that it is not a sensitive approach for assessing tubal permeability.

We looked to see whether ultrasound could establish fibrosis around the device and thus, confirm its contraceptive efficacy. We did not, however, find any specific sign of fibrosis; this absence was consistent with the macroscopic absence of any specific tissue differentiation. Parietal edema of the tubes was present in some but not all cases and thus, cannot serve as a protocol criterion.

Very recently, a Canadian study used 3D ultrasound together with conventional ultrasound imaging to assess device location for the last 34 patients of a 50-patient cohort.[6] They concluded, as we do, that it improves sensitivity. To our knowledge, there are no studies comparing 2D and 3D ultrasound scans. We hope that this report stimulates such a study. The use of volume contrast, of course, depends on the availability of this machine and the experience of its operator.

Combined Hysteroscopic Sterilization and Operative Hysteroscopy

Operative hysteroscopy, such as endometrial ablation or myomectomy, could be proposed in the same operative time as hysteroscopic sterilization.

The micro-insert will conduct energy if directly or closely contacted by an active electrosurgical device, and then, there is a risk of patient injury. It is known that second generation global auto-ablasive systems that employ radiofrequency energy (like Novasure) should not be used in women with Essure® micro-inserts in place. Using such energy will cause significant damage to the surrounding tissue if an active radiofrequency instrument comes into direct contact with the Essure® micro-inserts.

Bench and clinical studies have demonstrated that thermal endometrial ablation of the uterus can safely and effectively be performed with the Gynecare Thermachoice Uterine Balloon System immediately following Essure® micro-insert placement. However, no specific studies have been conducted to evaluate Essure® expulsion or contraception rates following combined Essure® Thermachoice procedures.

There are also no data regarding the use of endometrial resection (by monopolar or bipolar energy) or endometrial destruction with the Essure® micro-inserts in place.

Endometrial destruction is indicated for the treatment of abnormal uterine bleeding (functional or intrauterine lesions like polyps or fibroma) for women with no desire of pregnancy. Nevertheless, it should not be considered as a permanent contraceptive procedure and patients should be advised to continue to use protective measures. Could Essure® micro-insert be a good choice for these patients?

We conducted a retrospective continuous study, between December 2004 and February 2006. The analysis was by intention to treat. All patients were treated consecutively by the same medical shift. All study participants were seeking permanent contraception for personal or medical reasons and had proven menorrhagia. A complete medical history was obtained. A physical and pelvic examination was conducted. Premalignant uterine lesions were excluded by a previous biopsy of the endometrium.

An Essure® device placement procedure was attempted on each Fallopian tube. The choice of procedure for endometrial destruction among the four available options depended on the choice of the medical staff in accordance with menorrhagia etiology.

As this study was not based on a randomized clinical trial, effectiveness was estimated from patients' answers during the follow-up examination and radiologic results. Treatment success was defined by the confirmation of satisfactory location of the micro-inserts, absence of menorrhagia and non-requirement for a second procedure. Patients who reported having undergone a second procedure, or who were menorrhagic were considered as treatment failures.

Satisfaction with the procedure was scored as 1 (fully satisfied), 2 (partially satisfied) and 3 (not at all satisfied). No patients were lost to follow-up.

Overview of Technologies and Technical Characteristics

Current flow in monopolar surgery is from an active electrode, through tissue and returned to the generator via a large surface area plate. Glycocolle is used as the distension fluid and to conduct energy. Current flow in bipolar surgery is passed through the tissue placed in between the two electrodes. The patient's body is not part of the electrical circuit. This is safer and presents no risk of injuries to the patient. The distension fluid is physiologic serum. We also proceeded with endometrectomy using monopolar energy before Essure® micro-insert placement and bipolar energy after Essure® placement.

The Therma Choice Uterine Balloon System is a software-controlled device that accomplishes endometrial ablation using thermal energy from heated sterile fluid (5% dextrose in water) within a silicon balloon. It consists of a controller and single-use sterile catheter and umbilical cable. No cervical distension is required. The Essure® micro-insert can be inserted with the usual rigid 3 mm outside-diameter hysteroscope. The Essure® micro-insert could be in place before or after that procedure.

The HTA makes use of USP 0.9 percent saline for uterine distension and a single-use, polycarbonate sheath with inflow and outflow channels through which a standard, 3 mm outside-diameter, rigid hysteroscope is inserted.

The Novasure System consists of a disposable device, radiofrequency (RF)-control and foot switch. RF energy delivery averages 90 seconds, but treatment is limited to 2 minutes in all cases. Cervical distension up to a diameter of 8 mm is required for the two previous procedures.

The Essure® micro-insert should be placed after the endometrial resection by monopolar energy and endometrial ablation by Novasure. These procedures require a previous cervical distension (up to 8 or 10 mm). To introduce the Essure® micro-insert as a secondary procedure a specific bridge was necessary to decrease the lost of fluid from the opened cervix.

Results

A total of 23 patients were included in the study, of which, 14 patients underwent thermal ablation by Thermachoice, 4 underwent a radiofrequency ablation by Novasure, 2 underwent thermal ablation by HTA and 2 underwent endometrial resection (one by monopolar and one by bipolar energy) (Fig. 3.6).

The mean age of the patients undergoing tubal sterilization was 43 years old (range 30–49 years). Definitive tubal sterilization was medically indicated in 30 percent (7/23) of cases and in 70 percent (16/23) of cases as a patient request.

The mean postoperative follow-up was 14 months.[4-6] Hysteroscopy was indicated in 14 cases (60%) for functional menorrhagia and in 9 cases (40%) for organic menorrhagia (polyps or fibroids).

The procedure was carried out under general anesthesia in 92 percent (21/23) of cases under rachianesthesia and local anesthesia in 4 percent (1/23) of the cases, respectively. The mean operating time was 43 minutes.[4-6]

Effectiveness of Micro-inserts Placement

The Fallopian tubes could be successfully cannulated in 87 percent (20/23) of cases. The three cases of failure were due to non-visualization of the tubal ostia since the beginning of the hysteroscopic procedure and were not secondary to the endometrial ablation or resection. The first two failures occurred during the initial stages of our experience with the technique.

Endometrial destruction could not explain placement failures, all the same, visualization of tubal ostia post-endometrial ablation was difficult and Essure® micro-insert placement required an experienced physician. No patient injury was described during the study.

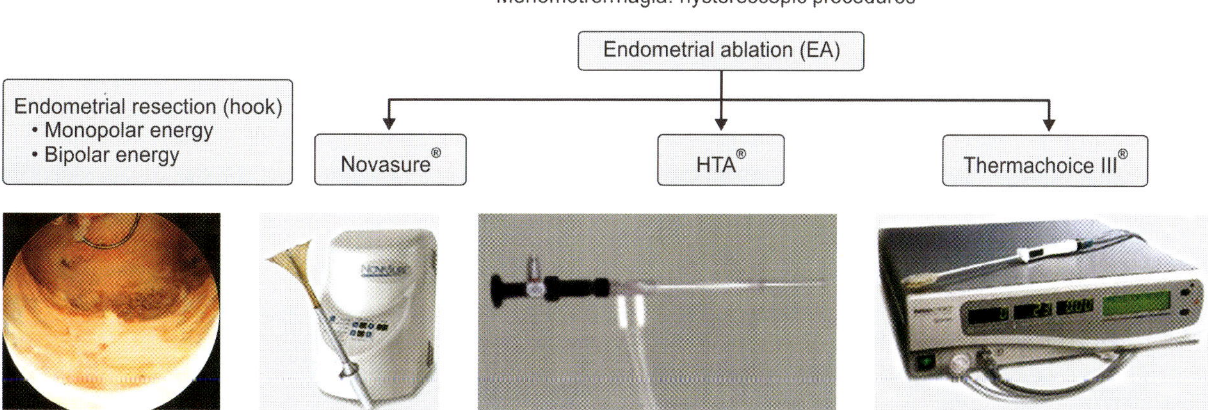

Fig. 3.6: Endometrial destruction: surgical techniques

Adequate bilateral occlusion was confirmed by ultrasound and X-ray at follow-up in 20 patients 3 months later. No pregnancy has been described in patients with effective insertion of Essure® micro-implants.

About Menorrhagia

Only 3 patients failed or were unsatisfied with the endometrial procedure due to persistent of abnormal uterine bleeding and dysmenorrhea. Two of them had successful complementary treatment by progesterone and one underwent a hysterectomy three months later. All the patients who were satisfied with the results of the procedure (78.5%) experienced hypomenorrhea without the need for contraception.

The better practice calls for placing Essure® micro-insert at the beginning of the hysteroscopy owing to the risk of masking the tubal ostia by thermal ablation. This is possible with the thermal ablation by Thermachoice and HTA and resection by bipolar energy but not with ablation by radiofrequency energy (Novasure) or monopolar energy. In these cases, the Essure® micro-insert should be inserted after the thermal ablation. Though the tubal ostia were more difficult to visualize, however, it was still possible to insert the micro-implants with satisfactory results 3 months later in our study. In our study, like the previous studies, uterine balloon ablation appeared to be easier to perform, making the technique readily reproducible, especially by those with limited expertise in hysteroscopic surgery, and thus, more widely applicable and safer when combined with Essure® micro-insert placement.

The 13 percent failure rate observed in our study was close to the 12 percent failure rate reported by previous studies.[1,7]

In our study, the principle cause of failure was non-visualization of the tubal ostia since the beginning of the intervention, confirming the importance of programming the surgical procedure during the early proliferative phase of menstrual cycle. Failure to conform to this rule will result in decreased visualization of the Fallopian tube ostia and could be the main reason for failure of the procedure.

Performing endometrial ablation immediately following placement of Essure® micro-inserts may increase the risk of post-ablation tubal sterilization syndrome, a rare condition that has been reported in women with a history of tubal sterilization who underwent endometrial ablation.[7] We have not observed this syndrome in our clinical experience with a maximal follow-up of 27 months.

The incidence of pregnancy after endometrial destruction is low and is reported to be 0.7 percent. Seventy-four-pregnancies have been reported after various methods of endometrial destruction. We previously reviewed the records of the patients considered "fertile" in a consecutive series of 206 patients, treated by intrauterine balloon ablation for dysfunctional uterine bleeding; three pregnancies were observed among 58 patients (5.2%), with two spontaneous abortions and a placenta accreta at 26 weeks. The risk of pregnancy is estimated at 0.7 percent after hysteroscopic endometrial resection.[8] It is evident from the results of this study that Essure® sterilization is a good contraceptive choice that can be performed during the same operative time as endometrial ablation. These implants can be placed during the same procedure as endometrial ablation, with general, regional, or even local (for thermal ablation) anesthesia.

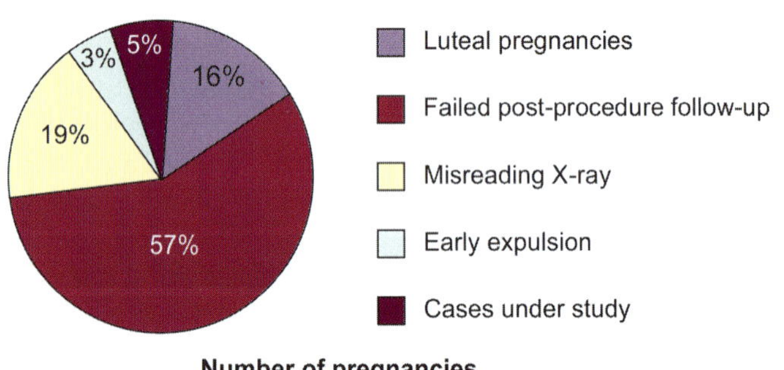

No pregnancy due to failure of properly placed Essure® implants
There were 64 pregnancies following 50000 procedures—Rate: 1.28/1000

Fig. 3.7: Pregnancies: AAGL, Nov 2006

Table 3.2: Recommendations to avoid pregnancies (AAGL November 2006)
1. Give an efficient contraceptive until the 3 months follow-up.
2. Perfom the procedure during days 7 to 14 of the proliferative phase of the menstrual cycle for women who have regular cycles and who use an efficient contraceptive.
Do not perfom the procedure at the end of the cycle.
3. Perform X-ray of the abdomen after 3 months without preparation (or a 2D/3D echography: except protocol) and if you have any doubts, add a hysterography.
4. See the patient after 3 months with her X-ray to confirm the placement and the efficiency of the Essure® device.

CONCLUSION

Essure® sterilization is an effective technique (Fig. 3.7).

It is essential to follow the recommendations to avoid pregnancies (Table 3.2).

In the 21st century, hysteroscopic sterilization is becoming the gold standard.

ACKNOWLEDGMENT

MPH Vleugels, Rivierenland Hospital, Tiel Netherlands.

REFERENCES

1. Kerin JF, Cooper JM, Price T, Herendael BJ, Cayuela-Font E, Cher D, et al. Hysteroscopic sterilization using a micro-insert device: results of a multicenter Phase II study. Hum Reprod 2003;18:1223-30.
2. Cooper JM, Carignan CS, Cher D, Kerin JF. Microinsert nonincisional hysteroscopic sterilization. Obstet Gynecol 2003;102:59-67.
3. Kerin JF, Munday DN, Ritossa MG, Pesce A, Rosen D, Cooper JM, et al. Essure hysteroscopic sterilization: results based on utilizing a new coil catheter delivery system Microinsert nonincisional hysteroscopic sterilization. Hysteroscopic sterilization using a micro-insert device: results of a multicenter Phase II study. The safety and effectiveness of a new hysteroscopic method for permanent birth control: results of the first Essure pbc clinical study. J Am Assoc Gynecol Laparosc 2004;11:388-93.
4. Tteoh M, Meagher S, Kovacs G. Ultrasound detection of the Essure permanent birth control device: a case series. Aust N Z J Obstet Gynaecol 2003;43:378-80.
5. Weston G, Bowditch J. Office ultrasound should be the first-line investigation for confirmation of correct ESSURE placement. Aust N Z J Obstet Gynaecol 2005;45:312-5.
6. Thiel JA, Suchet IB, Lortie K. Confirmation of Essure micro-insert tubal coil placement with conventional and volume-contrast imaging three-dimensional ultrasound. Fertil Steril 2005;84:504-8.
7. Lo JS, Pickersgill A. Pregnancy after endometrial ablation: English literature review and case report. J Minim Invasive Gynecol 2006;13:88-91.
8. Gervaise A, de Tayrac R, Fernandez H. Contraceptive information after endometrial ablation. Fertil Steril 2005; 84:1746-7.

Ovarian Drilling by Transvaginal Fertiloscopy for the Treatment of Polycystic Ovary Syndrome

Hervé Fernandez, Amélie Gervaise, René Frydman

OVERVIEW

Ovarian drilling by transvaginal fertiloscopy with bipolar electrosurgery appears to be an effective minimally invasive procedure in patients with polycystic ovary syndrome (PCOS) resistant to Clomiphene citrate without complications. We attempted to evaluate the efficacy of ovarian drilling by transvaginal fertiloscopy, using bipolar energy for the treatment of PCOS in 80 women with Clomiphene-resistant PCOS in a prospective study (Canadian Task Force II) at a University teaching hospital and private clinic. Regular and ovulatory cycles were recovered in 89 percent (73/80) of the patients during a mean follow-up of 18.1 months (± 6.4). The cumulative pregnancy rate was 59 percent (44/75) for spontaneous and stimulated cycles (n=30) and 38.7 percent (29/75) imputed to drilling alone. The mean time to conceive was 3.9 months (range 1–11.8). There were 8 miscarriages (18%) and no ectopic or multiple pregnancies.

INTRODUCTION

Polycystic ovary syndrome (PCOS) is reported to affect around 7 percent of women.[1] Presence of ovarian dysfunction (oligoanovulation), hyperandrogenism and polycystic ovary morphology (Fig. 4.1) are the most common characteristics (Rotterdam consensus).[2]

Ultrasonographic criteria to define a polycystic ovary include more than 12 follicles, 2 to 9 mm per ovary, whatever the distribution (Rotterdam consensus 2004, Jonard 2003, Balen 2003). Infertility, due to chronic anovulation, is the most common reason for women to seek medical assistance.

Antiestrogen therapy remains the first-line approach for women with PCOS, and clomiphene citrate (CC) successfully induces ovulation in more than 80 percent of the anovulatory women treated with it. The cumulative pregnancy rates after 6 months are disappointing (30–60%) and the miscarriage rate is high (30–40%).[3,4] Despite treatment with incremental doses of CC, 15 to 20 percent of women remain anovulatory. Approximately, 50 percent of patients with ovulatory cycles will fail to conceive.[2,5]

Clomiphene-resistant women may be treated with gonadotropin therapy or surgically. Gonadotropin treatment in these patients offers a cumulative pregnancy rate above 50 percent after 4 to 6 cycles (Fig. 4.1) with insufficient data

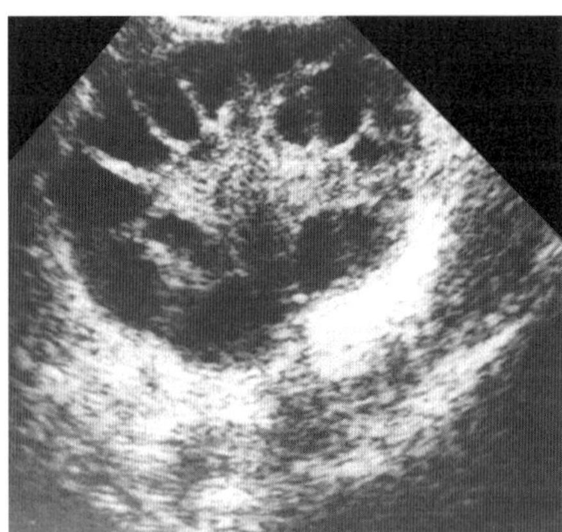

Fig. 4.1: PCOS—sonography

to show a difference with laparoscopic ovarian drilling,[6] but that is associated with an increased risk of severe ovarian hyperstimulation syndrome (OHSS), miscarriage and multiple pregnancies.[7] Several dose regimens have been used, with the low dose step-up regimen considered as the most efficient and safest for use.[8]

Other treatment options, such as metformin therapy or ovarian drilling, have been recommended. Metformin therapy is reported to improve ovarian function in women

Table 4.1: Surgery—historical evidence. It is working !...

Laparotomy

- 1935 : Bilateral ovarian wedge resection (Stein and Leventhal)
- 1982 : Unilateral ovariectomy (Hamerlynck)
- 2003 : Drilling (Yildirim)

Laparoscopy

- 1975 : Biopsies (Yuzpe et Rioux)
- 1984 : Ovarian electrocautery (Gjonnaess)
- 1989 : Vaporization laser (Daniell and Miller)
- 1992 : Bilateral ovarian wedge resection by laser (Ostrzenski)
- 1993 : Bilateral ovarian wedge resection by monopolar energy (Campo)
- 1996 : Drilling by bipolar energy (Merchant)

Fertiloscopy

- 1972 : Bilateral ovarian wedge resection by culdoscopy (Paldi)
- 1999 : Drilling by bipolar energy (Fernandez)

with PCOS, with a restored ovulation rate of approximately 60 to 80 percent.[9] Metformin appears safe, may decrease the incidence of type-2 diabetes and coronary heart disease and is inexpensive. Nowadays, Metformin is given initially in the treatment of PCOS, alone or in addition with CC.[10] Hence, the surgical approach is used only after failure of the medical approach with CC and/or metformin.[11]

Since the first surgical treatment by bilateral ovarian wedge resection with laparotomy (Table 4.1), a variety of surgical options has been applied during laparoscopy for the treatment of PCOS; these include biopsy alone, cauterization, multielectrocoagulation and laser surgery.[12] The main risk of these procedures is the high frequency of adhesions and their association with postoperative mechanical sterility.[13] Nonetheless, the cumulative pregnancy rate after ovarian surgery for PCOS exceeds 50 percent, and the risk of multiple pregnancies and OHSS is lower than with gonadotropin therapy.[14,15] Farquhar et al.[16] found that the pregnancy rates after laparoscopic ovarian diathermy are comparable to those after three cycles of ovulation induction with gonadotropins. Moreover, women pretreated with ovarian drilling appear to achieve a significantly better ongoing pregnancy rate after *in vitro* fertilization-embryo trasfer (IVF-ET),[17] with less risk of OHSS. The decrease in luteinizing hormone (LH) levels after ovarian drilling has been suggested as a mechanism of the improved outcome. However, a systematic review of published studies failed to demonstrate a decrease in miscarriage rate after ovarian drilling.[18]

Technological developments have made new procedures for ovarian drilling possible. These include sonographic transvaginal ovarian drilling,[19] minilaparoscopic ovarian drilling under local anesthesia,[20] and transvaginal hydrolaparoscopy.[21,22] We previously published a short series of cases treated with ovarian drilling using bipolar electrosurgery. We now present a full evaluation of the effectiveness and risks of this procedure after a substantially longer follow-up. Moreover, the reproducibility of the procedure has been evaluated in two different departments.[23]

MATERIALS AND METHODS

Patients

This report includes 80 infertile patients diagnosed with PCOS based on the criteria laid down at the 1990 National Institutes of Health Development Conference.[24] The patients were treated in two centers, a University teaching hospital in Paris and a private endoscopic center in Lyon (France) between November 1998 and December 2001. The diagnosis of PCOS was based on oligoanovulatory cycles, a ratio of luteinizing hormone (LH) to follicle-stimulating hormone (FSH) >2.0 and/or the characteristic appearance of the ovaries on ultrasonography (increased volume of stroma and ovary and > 10 cysts < 8 mm along the periphery).[25]

The mean (± SD) body mass index was 24.7 ± 6.3. Eighteen of the patients were hirsute. None had biological signs of hyperthyroidism or adrenal hyperplasia. Before surgery, 25 patients were amenorrheic (cycle duration > 120 days), 40 were oligomenorrheic (cycle duration 46–120 days), and 15 had cycles of up to 45 days. All patients had polycystic ovaries on ultrasonography and/or a typical hormonal profile (mean LH: FSH ratio 1.9 ± 0.6). No male factor infertility was added.

Ovarian drilling by transvaginal hydrolaparoscopy was proposed after a failure of 6 cycles of CC therapy despite incremental doses (200 mg/day for 5 days). In this study, the failure of CC therapy was defined as failure to conceive despite ovulation with CC (n = 50 cases), or in the absence of ovulation (n = 30 cases). All the patients had bilateral tubal patency on hysterosalpingography.

If no pregnancy was observed 6 months after the procedure, we proposed stimulation with CC and recombinant follicle stimulating hormone (r-FSH) in association with intrauterine insemination. The cumulative pregnancy rate was computed with the life table method, with the first pregnancy achieved (spontaneous or after induction of ovulation) as the end point. Pregnancies achieved after IVF-ET were excluded from the cumulative pregnancy rate. All patients were seen at 3, 6, 9, and 12 months after surgery, as well as at some later visits. No systematic post-treatment hormonal data were recorded for this study.

We did not seek a new Institutional Review Board (IRB) approval for this study because we routinely performed this surgical procedure in both the institutions for our initial study,[21] and we only asked for an extension of the IRB.

The Procedure

The Balloon Introducer (Figs 4.2 and 4.3)

The Watrelot balloon introducer has a 5-Fr operative channel,[26] includes a central channel for the scope (2.9 mm with its sheath or 4 mm without it) and an auxilliary channel for a 5-Fr instrument. A 5-mL distal balloon prevents unintended withdrawal and maintains the introducer in the pouch of Douglas.

The Bipolar Electrode

We used two electrosurgical devices (Versapoint,Versapoint-Gynecare Inc., Menlo Park, CA, and Ovadrill, Erbe-Soprano, Lyon, France), both of which use bipolar current in a saline environment. A bipolar probe (5 Fr in diameter and 360 mm in

length) is connected to a generator with power settings from 1 to 200 W. The conductivity of the saline solution is used to advance the two electrodes along the axis of the instrument. The high level of energy delivered produces steam around the distal active electrode and vaporizes the tissue. The two electrosurgical devices delivered the same energy and we used power settings up to 130 W.

Surgical Procedure (Figs 4.4A and B)

Under general anesthesia, the patients were placed in the gynecologic position, in dorsal lithotomy with the legs in standard stirrups. A veress needle was used to instill 300 mL of normal saline solution into the peritoneal cavity through the posterior vaginal fornix. A 2 to 9 mm scope, with a 30° lens (Karl Storz, SA, Germany), was inserted through the sheath

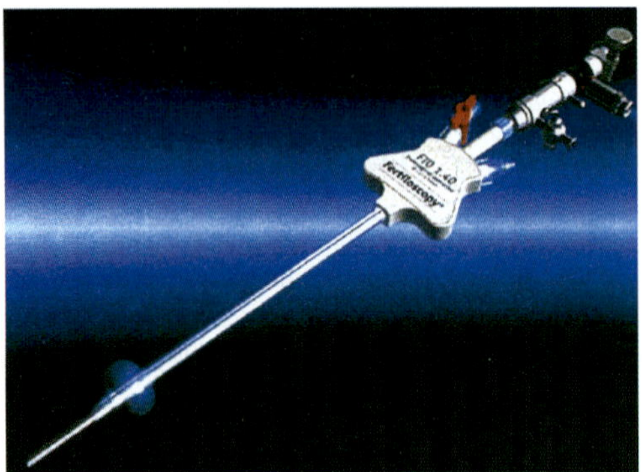

Fig. 4.2: Instruments

- Veress needle
- Balloon introducer with a 5-FR operative channel *(FTO 1–40 Soprano, SA, France)*
- 2.9 mm scope with 30° lens *(K Storz, SA, Germany)*
- Bipolar electrosurgical probe *(Versapoint-Gynecare Inc, Menlo-Park, CA, USA)*

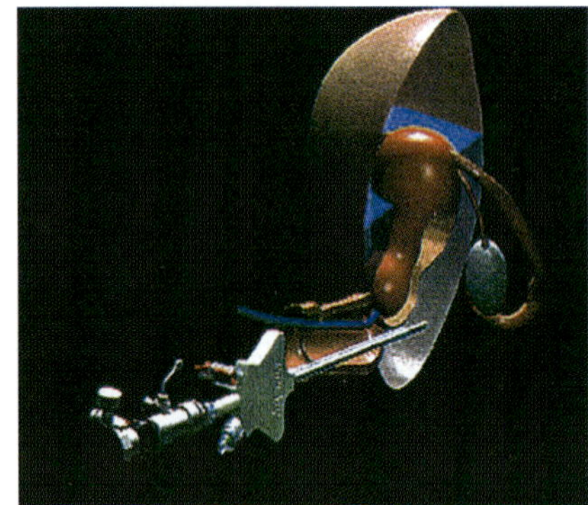

Fig. 4.3: Surgical procedure

- General anesthesia
- Patient in gynecologic position
- Instillation of 300 mL normal saline solution in the peritoneal cavity through the posterior vaginal fornix
- Insertion of balloon introducer in the pouch of Douglas
- Insertion of scope and inspection

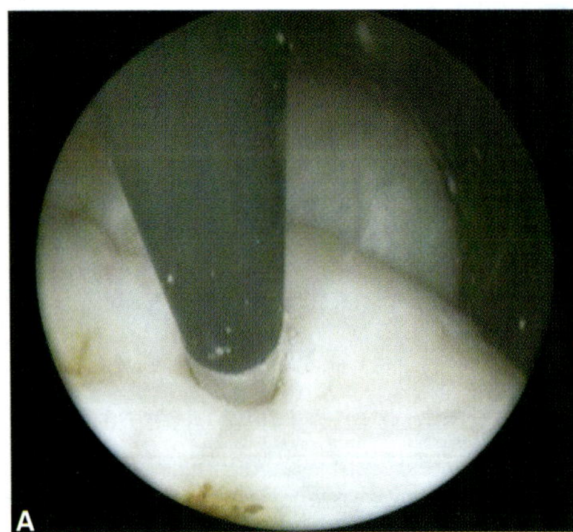

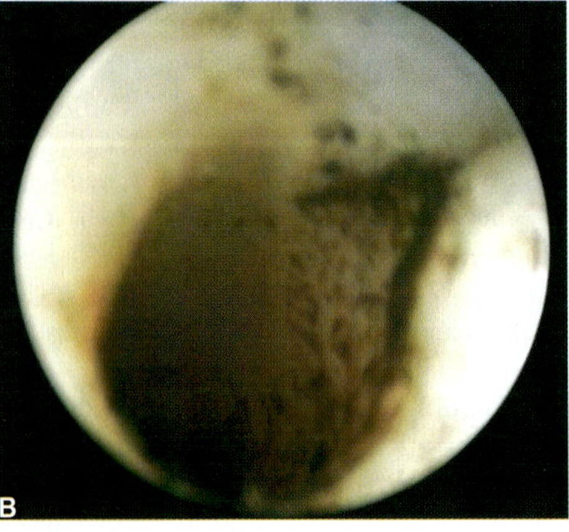

Figs 4.4A and B: Surgical procedures: (A) Bipolar electrosurgical probe is introduced through the auxilliary channel; (B) Using this probe, portions of the ovarian cortex were ablated (drilled) at 4 to 8 points

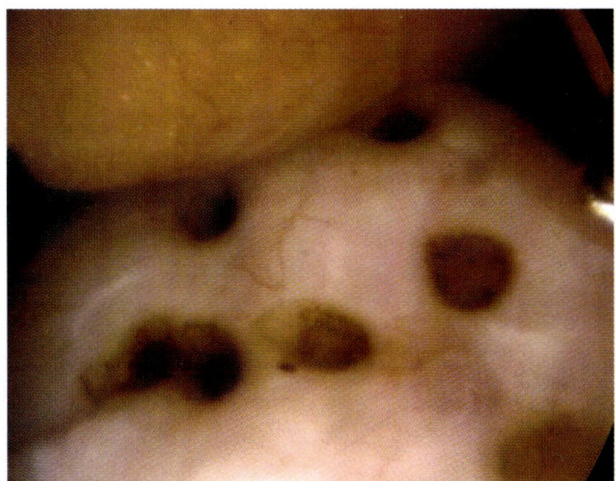

Fig. 4.5: Final aspect of ovarian drilling

Table 4.2: Pretreatment clinical and demographic data in 80 patients undergoing ovarian drilling by transvaginal hydrolaparoscopy

• Age (y) ± 8D	30.5 ± 3.7
• BMI	24.7 ± 6.3
• FSH (mIU/mL)	5.6 ± 2.3
• LH (mIU/mL)	9.3 ± 3.7
• Testosterone (ng/mL)	0.8 ± 0.4
• Duration of infertility (months)	34.7 ± 22.4
• Mean operative time (minutes)	18 ± 3
• Dye test positive	80
• Hysteroscopy (n)	75
• Mean follow-up (months)	18.1 ± 6.4

of 4 mm and was introduced into the pouch of Douglas. The posterior aspect of the uterus was examined first followed by the ovary and Fallopian tube on each side.

We introduced the bipolar electrosurgical probe through the auxilliary channel of the sheath. We used this probe to ablate (drill) 10 to 15 points in the ovarian cortex, with a power setting of 130 W. The number of diathermy points was determined by the ovarian accessibility. The depth of insertion was 10 mm up to the return electrode located on the shaft of the bipolar electrode. Figure 4.5 depicts the final aspect of ovarian drilling. Bipolar energy reduces the area of damage. If necessary, a dye test, salpingoscopy, and hysteroscopy may be performed with the same scope.

Patients received antibiotic prophylaxis with amoxicillin and clavulanic acid, as usually proposed in our department in case of surgery by the vaginal route. Patients were informed that it might be necessary to perform a laparoscopy.

RESULTS

Ovarian drilling was performed by transvaginal hydrolaparoscopy in all patients and no laparoscopic conversion was required. Table 4.2 presents the clinical and demographic data.

No immediate or late complications occurred. All the procedures were performed on an outpatient basis. One dose each of Ketoprofen (100 mg) and of Paracetamol (1 g) were systematically given postoperatively. In all, 73 patients (89%) recovered regular and ovulatory cycles, determined by basal body temperature monitoring. Three patients were lost to follow-up and 2 patients divorced few months after the procedure.

To date, 44 pregnancies have occurred: 29 were spontaneous and directly imputed to drilling alone (38.7%) and 15 were achieved after stimulation and intrauterine insemination performed in 30 patients. The cumulative pregnancy rate for spontaneous and stimulated cycles was

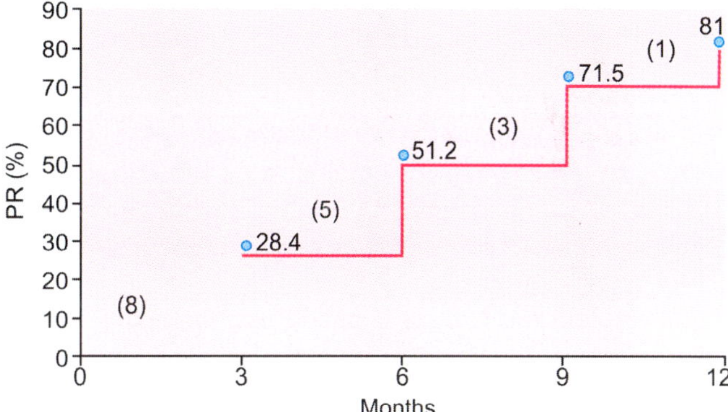

Fig. 4.6: Cumulative pregnancy rate () N pregnancy

59 percent (44/75), being 28.4, 51.2, 71.5 and 81 percent after 3, 6, 9, 12 months, respectively (Fig. 4.6) and mean time to conceive was 3.9 months (range 1–11.8 months). All the patients had a follow-up ≥ 18 months.

There were 8 miscarriages (18%), and 36 patients delivered live-born infants. No ectopic pregnancies occurred and no multiple pregnancies were observed despite the need for stimulation 6 months after the surgical procedure.

The pregnancy rate was similar irrespective of the cause of failure to conceive, i.e. absence of ovulation after CC therapy or despite ovulation with CC with absence of pregnancy.

CLINICAL DISCUSSION

Polycystic ovary syndrome involves a spectrum of etiologies with various clinical manifestations. While CC appears as the first-line approach, combined with weight loss, it results in pregnancies in fewer than half of all the patients. At the time of this study, we did not propose treatment for associated hyperinsulinemia. However, in lieu of the current efficacy and

Table 4.3: Surgical treatment for PCOS (Campo 1998)			
	Patients (N)	*Ovulatory cycle*	*Spontaneous pregnancy rate*	*Cumulative pregnancy rate*
Laparotomy Ovarian resection	679	81.6 (53–94)	50.0 (0–5)	55.3 (12–85)
Laparoscopy Electrosurgery	720	79.7 (30–100)	51.5 (20–88)	63.6 (20–88)
Laparoscopy Laser	322	71.5 (61–100)	43.7 (0–75)	53.1 (0–75)
Laparoscopy Biopsy or resection	82	82.6 (73–94)	48.7 (42–57)	55.0 (50–58)
Total patients	1803	1007	891	1055
Results		78.1	49.4	58.5

safety of Metformin, this treatment must be proposed before the surgical procedure.[11]

Our results confirm, in a large series with a long follow-up, the feasibility of ovarian drilling by transvaginal fertiloscopy. The pregnancy rate was similar to that obtained with ovarian drilling by laparoscopy[15,27] (Table 4.3). We suggest this minimally invasive surgery after initial CC therapy and/or Metformin in two situations: (i) as an alternative to long-term low-dose stimulation with FSH; and (ii) for patients who hyper-respond to CC or to gonadotropin therapy. It is also an appropriate initial treatment for patients, who must have endoscopy to investigate a tubo-adnexal infertility factor.

Factors in favor of surgery include a durable effect, mono-follicular cycle restoration, no increased risk of multiple pregnancies, no OHSS. The combination of ovarian drilling and gonadotropin therapy for intrauterine insemination or IVF-ET reduces the number of cycle cancellations, the quantity of medication required, dominant follicles and OHSS.[28] The exact mechanism underlying the drilling procedure has not been clearly elucidated, although it has been suggested that decreases in local and circulating levels of androgens, induced by destruction of the ovarian capsule and subcapsular cysts, plays a role. It is thought that the decreased androgen levels reduce the secretion rate and activity of LH, normalize the LH: FSH ratio, and allow follicular development with ovulation. Zullo, et al.[20] showed that ovarian drilling was followed by significant decreases in LH, testosterone and androstenedione.[20]

The bipolar technique provides maximum safety and optimizes the localization of tissue destruction. Ten to fifteen drillings seem to be adequate.

Arguments against a surgical approach are the intrinsic morbidity associated with laparoscopy and the potential for formation of postoperative adhesions. Few complications of transvaginal hydrolaparoscopy (THL) have occurred, none severe. Transvaginal hydrolaparoscopy can be performed under local analgesia, as Gordts et al.[29] and Watrelot et al.[26] have proposed, but not in operative procedures that use electric current.[22] Zullo et al.[20] proposed minilaparoscopic ovarian drilling under local anesthesia but the benefit of this procedure compared with a short general anesthesia is not clear.

The excellent results observed for ovarian drilling by THL encourage the routine use of this procedure in patients with PCOS resistant to CC therapy. Moreover, the procedure is less expensive than laparoscopy. However, despite the excellent results with ovarian drilling, the results observed in our series after IVF-ET were disappointing in terms of the clinical pregnancies (2/15) as the cases included in this series were poor responders, despite the ovarian drilling. Ferraretti, et al.[19] obtained good results with this procedure in patients with PCOS who underwent IVF treatment.[19] Repeated ovarian drilling seems to be effective in women, who previously responded to the first procedure.[30]

A randomized trial comparing THL and laparoscopy could determine whether both methods are equivalent in terms of pregnancy rates and surgical complications.

Bipolar energy combines the advantage of the use of energy without its principal drawback. It vaporizes tissues as a laser does but with ease of a monopolar electrode and with greater intrinsic safety. The number of pregnancies observed in this series confirmed the obvious benefits of avoiding multiple pregnancies and hyperstimulation, reported after medical treatment. The minimal risks of the procedure are clearly outweighed by the inconvenience of and need for monitoring with gonadotropins. However, a sufficiently powered rando-mized trial comparing ovarian stimulation with IUI and ovarian drilling with more data appear appropriate.

A long-term follow-up is necessary to evaluate the duration of effect of the fertiloscopy procedure, but the morphological effects of drilling by laparoscopy appear to be sustained for up to 9 years.[31] The decreased morbidities of fertiloscopy and bipolar energy, used for the drilling, suggest that this procedure could become the surgical gold standard for the treatment of PCOS.

CONCLUSION

Hence, ovarian drilling is an option for the management of female infertility associated with PCOS, especially as a second line treatment after the failure of Clomiphene citrate treatment.

REFERENCES

1. Balen A, Michelmore K. What is polycystic ovary syndrome? Are national views important? Hum Reprod 2002;17:2219-27.
2. The Rotterdam ESHRE/ASRM-sponsored workshop group. Revised 2003 consensus on diagnostic criteria and long-term health risks related to polycystic ovary syndrome (PCOS). Hum Reprod 2004;19:41-7.
3. European Society of Human Reproduction and Embryology (ESHRE). Female infertility: treatment options for complicated cases. Hum Reprod 1997;12:1191-6.
4. Kousta E, White SM, Franks S. Modern use of clomiphene citrate in induction of ovulation. Hum Reprod Update 1997;3: 359-65.
5. Nugent D, Vanderkerckhove P, Hughes E, et al. Gonadotrophin therapy for ovulation induction in subfertility associated with polycystic ovary syndrome. Cochrane Database Syst Rev 2000; CD000410.
6. Tadokoro N, Vollenhoven B, Clark S, Baker G, Kovacs G, Burger H, Healy D. Cumulative pregnancy rates in couples with anovulatory infertility compared with unexplained infertility in an ovulation induction program. Fertil Steril 1997;9:1939-44.
7. Fahri J, Homburg R, Lerner A, Ben Rafael Z. The choice of treatment for anovulation associated with polycystic ovary syndrome following failure to conceive with clomiphene. Hum Reprod 1993;8:1367-71.
8. Christin-Maitre S, Hugues JN. A comparative randomized multicentric study comparing the step-up versus step-down protocol in polycystic ovary syndrome. Hum Reprod 2003;18: 1626-31.
9. Fleming R, Hopkinson ZE, Wallace AM, Greer IA, Sattar N. Ovarian function and metabolic factors in women with oligomenorrhea treated with metformin in a randomized double-blind placebo- controlled trial. J Clin Endocrinol Metab 2002; 87:569-74.
10. Barbieri RL. Metformin for the treatment of polycystic ovary syndrome. Obstet Gynecol 2003;101:785-93.
11. Pirwany I, Tulandi T. Laparoscopic treatment of polycystic ovaries: is it time to relinquish the procedure? Fertil Steril 2003; 80:241-51.
12. Cohen J. Laparoscopic procedures for treatment of infertility related to polycystic ovarian syndrome. Hum Reprod Update 1996;2:337-44.
13. Adashi EY, Rock JA, Guzick D, Wentz AC, Jones GS, Jones HW Jr. Fertility following bilateral ovarian wedge resection: a critical analysis of 90 consecutive cases of the polycystic ovary syndrome. Fertil Steril 1981;36:320-25.
14. Gadir AA, Mowafi RS, Alnaser HM. Ovarian electrocautery versus human menopausal gonadotrophins and pure follicle stimulating hormone therapy in the treatment of patients with polycystic ovarian disease. Clinical Endocrinol 1990; 33:585.
15. Campo S. Ovulatory cycles, pregnancy outcome and complications after surgical treatment of polycystic ovary syndrome. Obstet Gynecol Surv 1998;53:297-308.
16. Farquhar CM, Williamson K, Gudex G, Jonhson NP, Garland J, Sadler L. A randomized controlled trial of laparoscopic ovarian diathermy versus gonadotropin therapy for women with clomiphene citrate-resistant polycystic ovary syndrome. Fertil Steril 2002;78:404-11.
17. Cohen J. Laparoscopic surgical treatment of infertility related to polycystic ovary syndrome. In: Kovacs GT. (Eds) Polycystic ovary syndrome. Cambridge: Cambridge University Press; 2000. pp. 144-58.
18. Farquhar C, Vandekerckhove P, Arnot M, Lilford R. Laparoscopic drilling by diathermy or laser for ovulation induction in anovulatory polycystic ovary syndrome. Cochrane Database Syst Rev 2000; CD001122.
19. Ferraretti AP, Gianaroli L, Magli M, Iammarrone E, Feliciani E, Fortini D. Transvaginal ovarian drilling: a new surgical treatment for improving the clinical outcome of assisted reproductive technologies in patients with polycystic ovary syndrome. Fertil Steril 2001;76:812-6.
20. Zullo F, Pellicano M, Zupi E, Guida M, Mastrantonio P, Nappi C. Minilaparoscopic ovarian drilling under local anesthesia in patients with polycystic ovary syndrome. Fertil Steril 2000;74: 376-9.
21. Fernandez H, Alby JD, Gervaise A, De Tayrac R, Frydman R. Operative transvaginal hydrolaparoscopy for treatment of polycystic ovary syndrome: a new minimally invasive surgery. Fertil Steril 2001;75:607-11.
22. Shibara H, Hirano Y, Kikuchi K, et al. Postoperative endocrine alterations and clinical outcome of infertile women with polycystic ovary syndrome after transvaginal hydrolaparoscopic ovarian drilling. Fertil Steril 2006;85:244-6.
23. Fernandez H, Watrelot A, Alby JD, Kadoch J, Gervaise A, de Tayrac R, Frydman R. Fertility after ovarian drilling by transvaginal fertiloscopy for treatment of polycystic ovary syndrome. J Am Assoc Gynecol Laparosc 2004;11:374-8.
24. Zawedzki JK, Dunaif A. Diagnostic criteria for polycystic ovary syndrome: towards a rational approach. In: Dunaif A, Givens JR, Haseltine FP, et al. (Eds) Polycystic ovary syndrome. Boston, Blackwell Scientific, 1992. pp. 377-84.
25. Dewailly D, Ardaens Y, Robert Y. Ultrasound in the polycystic ovary syndrome (PCOS). In: Azziz JENaDD R, (Eds) Androgen excess disorders in women. Philadelphia: Lipincott-Raven; 1997. pp. 269-78.
26. Watrelot A, Dreyfus JM, Andine JP. Evaluation of the performance of fertiloscopy in 160 consecutive infertile patients with no obvious pathology. Hum Reprod 1999;14:707-11.
27. Kriplani A, Manchanda R, Agarwal N, Nayar B. Laparoscopic ovarian drilling in clomiphene citrate-resistant women with polycystic ovary syndrome. J Am Ass Gynecol Laparosc 2001; 8:511-8.

28. Farhi J, Soule S, Jacobs HS. Effect of laparoscopic ovarian electrocautery on ovarian response and outcome of treatment with gonadotropins in clomiphene citrate-resistant patients with polycystic ovary syndrome. Fertil Steril 1995;64:930-5.

29. Gordts S, Campo R, Rombauts L, Brosens IA. Transvaginal hydrolaparoscopy as an outpatient procedure for infertility investigation. Hum Reprod 1998;13:99-103.

30. Amer SAKS, Li TC, Cooke ID. Repeated laparoscopic ovarian diathermy is effective in women with anovulatory infertility due to polycystic ovary syndrome. Fertil Steril 2003;79:1211-5.

31. Amer SAKS, Banu K, Li TC, Cooke ID. Long-term follow-up of patients with polycystic ovary syndrome after laparoscopic ovarian drilling: endocrine and ultrasonographic outcomes. Hum Reprod 2002;11:2851-7.

Laparoscopic Ovarian Cauterization: How Many Punctures are Optimal?

Sandeep Talwar

OVERVIEW

Several techniques of laparoscopic ovarian surgery, such as operative laparoscopy, cautery or LASER to drill multiple holes through the ovarian capsule, have been used to induce ovulation in patients with polycystic ovary syndrome (PCOS). This is known as laparoscopic electrocauterization of ovarian stroma (LEOS) or ovarian drilling.

Laparoscopic ovarian surgery has replaced ovarian wedge resection as a surgical treatment for Clomiphene citrate-resistant PCOS patients. Wedge resection of ovaries was described by Stein Leventhal in 1935 when polycystic ovaries were diagnosed during laparotomy.[1] Figures 5.1 to 5.3 illustrate the anatomic appearance of polycystic ovaries while Figure 5.4 illustrates the ultrasound appearance of polycystic ovaries. However, wedge resection went out of favor in 1970 owing to the recognition of significant postoperative adhesion formation and unsustainable favorable pregnancy rates.

Laparoscopic electrocautery is most widely used due to its simplicity, effectiveness, relative safety and low cost.

INTRODUCTION

The commonly used methods for laparoscopic surgery include: (i) monopolar electrocautery[2] and (ii) LASER.[3] In the first reported series of 63 patients, ovarian cautery resulted in ovulation in 90 percent of the patients and conception in 70 percent of a total 62 women treated.[2] The pregnancy outcome was the same as that observed in the normal population.[4]

CLINICAL DISCUSSION

Endocrine Changes following LEOS

Laparoscopic ovarian drilling is associated with following endocrine changes:

- Decrease in serum testosterone levels.
- Decreases in luteinizing hormone (LH) pulse amplitude without a change in the LH pulse frequency.[5]
- Decrease in serum androgen levels due to the destruction of androgen-producing ovarian stroma and drainage of follicles, which have high androgen levels.
- Rise in follicle-stimulating hormone (FSH) levels.

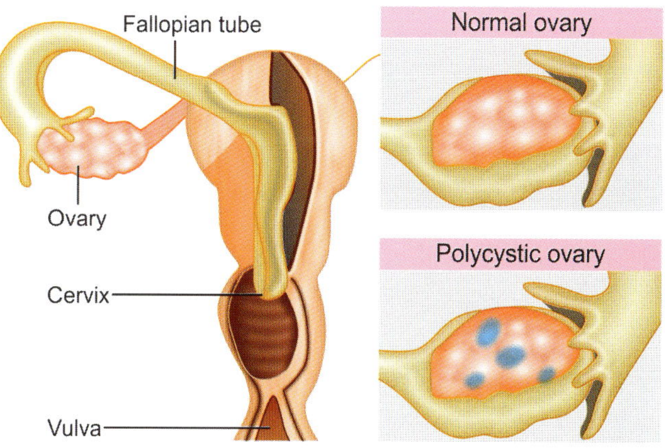

Fig. 5.1: Comparison between polycystic and normal ovaries

- Normalization of LH: FSH ratio.
- Decrease in extra-ovarian production of estrone.
- Attenuation of gonadotropin-releasing hormone (GnRH)-stimulated LH.[6]
- Correction in the disturbance in ovary-pituitary feedback.[7]

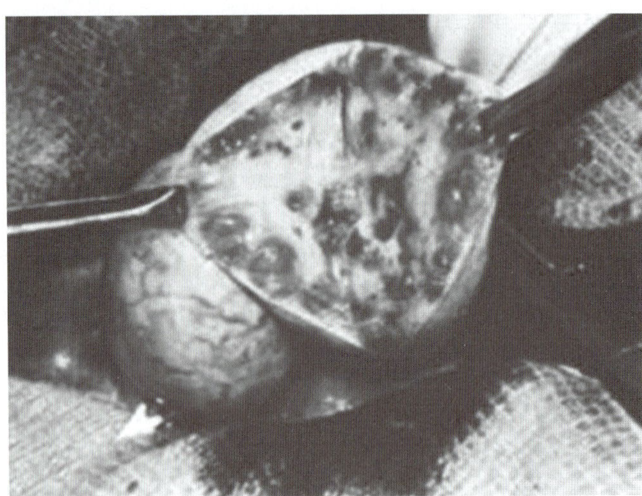

Fig. 5.2: Cross-section of the ovary demonstrating polycystic ovaries

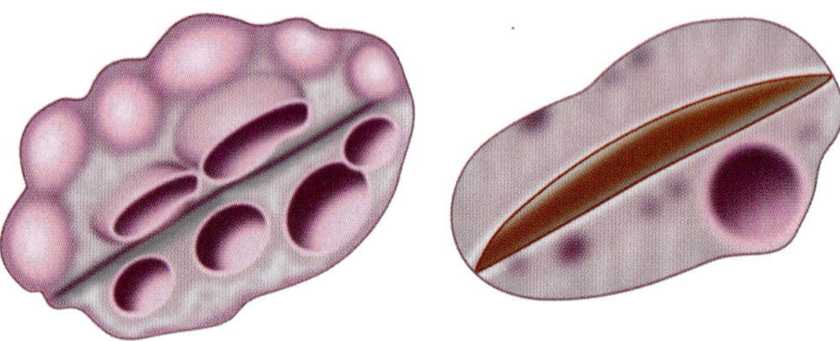

Fig. 5.3: Polycystic ovary

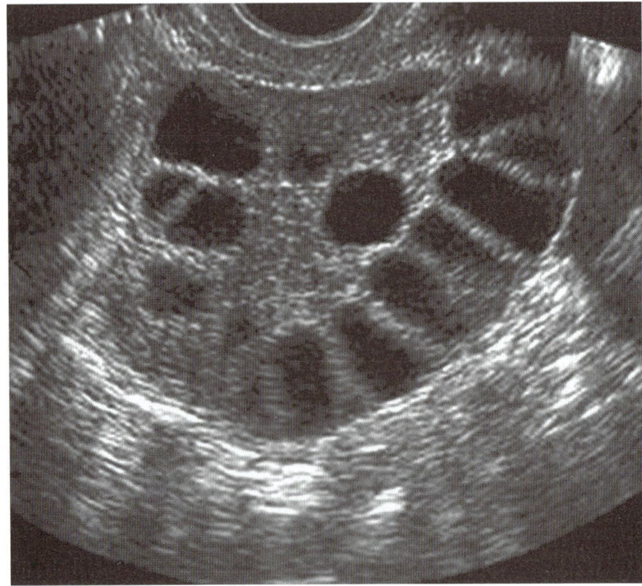

Fig. 5.4: Ultrasound appearance of polycystic ovaries

Ovarian Stromal Blood Flow Changes after LEOS in Women with PCOS

In a study by Parsanezhad et al.[8] color Doppler changes in ovarian stroma were recorded and serum concentration of FSH, LH and testosterone were measured in 52 women with polycystic ovaries before and after ovarian diathermy. Six to ten weeks after laparoscopic ovarian drilling (LOD), there was a significant decrease in the serum LH and testosterone concentrations, and mean peak systolic velocity ($p = 0.001$), and a significant increase in the pulsatility index (PI) ($p = 0.001$) and resistance index(RI) ($p = 0.001$). There was a significant negative correlation between PI and LH ($r = -0.43$, $p = 0.001$), PI and testosterone ($r = -0.40$, $p = 0.001$) and PI and LH/ FSH ratio ($r = -0.53$, $p = 0.001$). The PI increased significantly after LOD and 73 percent women ovulated. The ovarian stromal blood flow velocity declined after LOD in women with PCOS and there was a dramatic fall in the ovarian blood flow parallel with LH and testosterone levels and LH/ FSH ratio 6 to 10 weeks after surgery. Results show that Doppler indices of ovarian stromal blood flow significantly changed after LOD and these changes significantly correlated with hormonal changes and subsequent ovulation. The data suggests that measurement of ovarian stromal blood flow by color Doppler may be of value in predicting the prognosis of PCOS after LOD.[8]

Laparoscopic Ovarian Drilling

An insulated unipolar electrode is used. The needle is inserted perpendicularly to the ovarian surface and 40 W of current is employed for 4 seconds. During the procedure, it is important to hold the ovary away from bowel and other vital structures to avoid thermal injury (Fig. 5.5).

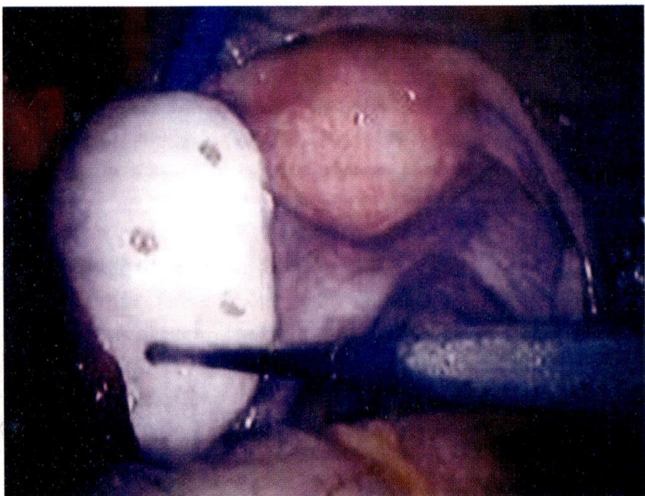

Fig. 5.5: Laparoscopic ovarian drilling

How Many Punctures to be Made?

There are no differences in results with either the monopolar electrocautery or the LASER method. Gjonnaess et al.[2] cauterized the ovary at 5 to 8 points for 5 to 6 sec at each point with 300 to 400 W. There was mild-to-moderate adhesion formation in 10 percent patients.[2] Neather and co-workers[9] treated patients with 5 to 20 points per ovary with 400 W for approximately 1 second. The rate of adhesions was 16.6 percent.[9] The rate of periovarian adhesions increased with the number of punctures. An additional concern is possibility of ovarian destruction leading to ovarian failure.[10]

In a study to compare the biochemical, clinical and reproductive results after LEOS in 63 Clomiphene-resistant patients, 5 punctures per ovary versus 10 punctures per ovary were analyzed. All the parameters were same in both the groups. 5 instead of ≥10 punctures were sufficient for improving the clinical and reproductive outcomes.[11] The current recommendation is the the cauterization of the ovary at 4 points using 40 W for 4 seconds.[12] Fewer than 4 punctures on each ovary results in poor pregnancy rates. Tubal evaluation with laparoscopy is recommended.

Complications of LEOS

Complications following LEOS include periadenexal adhesion formation and premature ovarian failure. Precautions must be taken not to cauterize near the ovarian hilum.

Results after Surgery

In a retrospective study on 112 Clomiphene-resistant anovulatory women with PCOS, who underwent LEOS, the reproductive outcome and adhesion formation was studied. Ovulation occurred spontaneously in 73 percent of the patients. The cumulative probability of conception at 12, 18 and 24 months after surgery was 54, 68 and 72 percent, respectively. Out of the 15 women who had a second look laparoscopy, 11 were found free of adhesions and 4 had periadnexal adhesions that were filmy, minimal and observed on the ovarian surface only.[13] Results of controlled studies showed that 82 percent patients ovulated with operation and 63 percent conceived, either spontaneously or after treatment.

Hence with LEOS, there is a high rate of spontaneous ovulation and subsequent medical induction becomes easier. According to a Cochrane Database review, conducted in 2001, ongoing pregnancy rates compared favorably with gonadotropins. Multiple pregnancy rates were reduced with LEOS in 4 arms of trial as compared to gonadotropins (OR 0.16, 95% CI 0.03, 0.98). There was no difference in abortion rates.[14]

LEOS versus Gonadotropins

According to Cochrane Database Review, 2005, LEOS compared favorably with ovulation induction with gonadotropins in clomiphene-resistant PCOS.[14] There was no difference in live births or ongoing pregnancies in both groups, OR was 1.04 and 1.16 respectively. Multiple pregnancy rates were lower with ovarian drilling than with gonadotropins (1% vs 16%, OR 0.13, 95% CI: 0.03 to 0.59). No difference in miscarriage rates was observed between the two groups (OR 0.81, 955% 0.36, 1.86). Thus, there was no difference in pregnancy rates between the two groups but a reduction in the multiple pregnancy rates in women undergoing LEOS makes it a more attractive procedure.

Cost of LEOS versus Gonadotropins

The cost of LEOS is one-third of gonadotropins with similar pregnancy rates. Hence it is more cost effective.[15]

Recent Advances

LASER ovarian surgery: Four different modalities of LASER, including Nd:YAG, CO_2, Argon and KTP have been used to perform ovarian drilling in women with PCOS. Nd:YAG LASER is delivered via a fine quartz fiber and can be used in a contact and noncontact mode. It is used to make punctures or to coagulate a wedge-like area. The CO_2 LASER has been used to drill 10 to 40 craters in the ovarian tissue and to vaporize the subcapsular follicles. With Argon and KTP LASERs, contact mode is used, all subcapsular cysts can be vaporized and 20 to 40 punctures can be made.[16-19]

LASER versus Ovarian Surgery

Electrocautery is superior to LASER for following reasons: (i) it is more effective than LASER in achieving ovulation and pregnancy, (ii) it is associated with lesser adhesion formation compared to LASER, (iii) it is less expensive and easy to handle, and (iv) the effect of diathermy lasts longer than LASER.[9,16,19]

CONCLUSION

Key Points for Clinical Practice

- Laparoscopic ovarian surgery achieves ovulation rates of 70 to 80 percent in women with Clomiphene-resistant PCOS.
- Clomiphene citrate remains first-line therapy for ovulation induction in PCOS.
- Gonadotropin therapy and laparoscopic ovarian diathermy are equally effective in Clomiphene-resistant patients.
- Laparoscopic surgery should be performed by appropriately trained surgeons.

- Minimum amount of ovarian damage should be caused.
- Diathermy is recommended at 4 points on each ovary.
- An appropriate amount of ovarian damage will sensitize the ovary to FSH, whether endogenous or exogenous.
- Laparoscopic ovarian surgery requires less monitoring than gonadotropin therapy and does not carry the risks of multiple pregnancy or ovarian hyperstimulation syndrome.
- Tubal patency may be assessed at the same time as laparoscopic ovarian surgery.
- The risks of laparoscopic ovarian surgery include the risk of an anesthetic, periovarian adhesions and ovarian destruction or failure.

REFERENCES

1. Stein IF, Leventhal ML. Amenorrhoea associated with bilateral polycystic ovaries. Am J Obstet Gynecol 1935;29:181-91.
2. Gjonnaess H. Polycystic ovarian syndrome treated by ovarian electrocautery through the laparoscope. Fertil Steril 1984;41: 20-25.
3. Daniell JF, Miller N. Polycystic ovaries treated by laparoscopic LASER vaporization. Fertil Steril 1989;51:232-6.
4. Gjoannaess H. The course and outcome of pregnancy after ovarian electrocautery with PCOS: the influence of body weight. Br J Obstet Gynaecol 1989;96:714-9.
5. Abdel Gadir A, Khatim MS, Mowagi RS, Alnaser HMI, Alzaid HGN, Shaw RW. Hormonal changes in patients with polycystic ovarian disease after ovarian electrocautery or pituitary desensitization. Clin Endocrinol 1990;32:749-54.
6. Rossmanith WG, Keckstein J, Spatzier K, Lauritzen C. The impact of ovarian LASER surgery on the gonadotrophin secretion in women with polycystic ovarian disease. Clin Endocrinol 1991;34:223-30.
7. Balen AH, Jacobs HS. A prospective study comparing unilateral and bilateral laparoscopic ovarian diathermy in women with the polycystic ovary syndrome. Fertil Steril 1994;62:921-5.
8. Parsanezhad ME, Bagheri MH, Alborzi S, Schmidt EH. Ovarian stromal blood flow changes after laparoscopic ovarian cauterization in women with polycystic ovary syndrome. Hum Reprod 2003;18:1432-7.
9. Naether OG, Baukloh V, Fischer R, Kowalczyk T. Long-term follow-up in 206 infertility patients with polycystic ovarian syndrome after laparoscopic electrocautery of the ovarian surface. Hum Reprod 1994;9:2342-9.
10. Cohen BM. LASER laparoscopy for polycystic ovaries. Fertil Steril 1989;52:167-8.
11. Malkawi HY, Qublan HS. Laparoscopic ovarian drilling in the treatment of polycystic ovary syndrome: how many punctures per ovary are needed to improve the reproductive outcome? J Obstet Gynaecol Res 2005;31:115-9.
12. Armar NA, McGarrigle HH, Honour J, Holownia P, Jacobs HS, Lachelin GC. Laparoscopic ovarian diathermy in the management of anovulatory infertility in women with polycystic ovaries: endocrine changes and clinical outcome. Fertil Steril 1990;53:45-9.
13. Felemban A, Tan SL, Tulandi T. Laparoscopic treatment of polycystic ovaries with insulated needle cautery: a reappraisal. Fertil Steril 2000;73:266-9.
14. Farquhar C, Lilford RJ, Marjoribanks J, Vandekerckhove P. Laparoscopic ovarian drilling by diathermy or LASER for ovulation induction in anovulatory polycystic ovary syndrome. Cochrane database Syst Rev 2005;20:CD001122.
15. Farquhar CM. An economic evaluation of laparoscopic ovarian diathermy versus gonadotrophin therapy for women with clomiphene citrate resistant polycystic ovary syndrome. Hum Reprod 2004;19:1110-15.
16. Gürgan T, Kişnişçi H, Yarali H, Develioğlu O, Zeyneloğlu H, Aksu T. Evaluation of adhesion formation after laparoscopic treatment of polycystic ovarian disease. Fertil Steril 1991; 56:1176-8.
17. Keckstein G, Rossmanith W, Spatzier K, Schneider V, Börchers K, Steiner R. The effect of laparoscopic treatment of polycystic ovarian disease by CO_2-LASER or Nd:YAG LASER. Surg Endosc. 1990;4:103-7.
18. Keckstein J. Laparoscopic treatment of polycystic ovarian syndrome. Baillieres Clin Obstet Gynaecol 1989;3:563-81.
19. Kojima E, Yanagibori A, Otaka K, Hirakawa S. Ovarian wedge resection with contact Nd:YAG LASER irradiation used laparoscopically. J Reprod Med 1989;34:444-6.

Laparoscopic Recanalization after Tubal Sterilization

Alain Audebert

OVERVIEW

Sterilization is the first method of family planning used worldwide. Contrary to contraceptive methods, the limitation of procreation is permanent and definitive, suggesting that patients undergoing this procedure be carefully selected because the rate of demand for reversal varies from 1 to 3 percent. Various methods of tubal sterilization have been proposed. The laparoscopic approach, until recently, has been the most popular, with different techniques of tubal occlusion being used. Hysteroscopic methods, which are safer and simpler to perform, thus with expanding applications, do not however, enable surgical reversal.

Selection of patients, following a complete infertility work-up of both partners, and especially ovarian reserve and psychological assessments, is mandatory prior to offering surgical reversal.

Microsurgery by laparotomy emerged during the seventies and the technology has since been standardized and rapidly become the gold standard. With trained operators, an 80 percent delivery rate for reversal of clip sterilization in younger patients may be obtained without any associated factor of hypofertility. In the late eighties, *in vitro* fertilization (IVF) not only became widely available but also simpler to perform with improved results. Laparoscopic reversal of sterilization, requiring specific micro-instrumentation, became available in the nineties. In properly selected patients, with trained operators, the results of published series with this technology are similar to those obtained previously by laparoscopy. However, no comparative truly controlled studies are available to compare both the surgical approaches. Considering the well-known advantages of the laparoscopic route, this approach should be recommended and discussed with patients as an alternative to IVF, when available.

INTRODUCTION

Sterilization is the first method of family planning used worldwide.[1] Contrary to contraception, sterilization is the permanent and definitive limitation of procreation. This is the reason why some patients will seek to have their fertility restored, usually after facing a dramatic event. The rates of demand for sterilization reversal usually vary from 1 to 3 percent.[2] The objective of this short review is to evaluate the role of laparoscopic tubal recanalization as an alternative to the laparotomic microsurgical approach, still considered as the gold standard, and IVF.

PREREQUISITES

Reasons for Reversal Demand

As previously quoted, it is estimated that 1 to 3 percent of sterilized women do regret the procedure for various reasons, and a large proportion of them will demand a recanalization.[1]

The reasons for regret are well-known and have not changed during the last two decades. The reasons for recanalization are presented in Table 6.1 and two successive personal unpublished series, are compared. The first survey was realized in 1986 for patients operated by microsurgical laparotomy, and the second one, established in 2002, was done in a series of patients operated by laparoscopy.

Table 6.1: Main reasons for the demand for sterilization reversal		
Reasons	*Series 1986* *(123 cases)*	*Series 2002* *(70 cases)*
Divorce	72%	74.3%
Husband's death	1.6%	4.4%
Child's death	5.7%	2.8%
Desire for a new child	9.0%	7.1%
Unaware	2.4%	2.8%
Regrets	10.0%	8.6%

Divorce is the reason most frequently claimed, as has been previously reported.[2,3]

If dramatic unexpected familial events are also frequent reasons, it appears surprising that more than 10 percent of women were not aware of the definitive limitation of procreation or had regrets without real immediate plans to have a new child. These facts should lead to routinely consider two practical issues:

Prevention

Ideally, the first measure to undertake should be preventive. A strict selection of patients requesting sterilization should be performed, taking into account the well-known risk factors for reversal demand: young age, childless, emergency situations and couple instability (50%). Sterilization would not be recommended for some couples presenting with these factors, and additionally, in emergency situations, such as voluntary abortion, and during the period at risk of child death, such as immediate postpartum. These issues are presently even more crucial with the rapid development of newer methods of hysteroscopic sterilization, such as Essure® microimplants,[4] because this procedure is a contraindication for surgical tubal recanalization.

Psychological Background

Women who ask for tubal recanalization have a frequently strong feeling of culpability, especially in case of divorce. This feeling leads them to prefer in first line, surgical restoration of their fallopian tubes instead of IVF, in order not to involve their new partner, frequently younger. In some cases, the new partner is not even informed about the previous sterilization. Indeed, the motivations have also to be clearly evaluated before performing surgery and are major issues in the counseling.

CLINICAL DISCUSSION

Method of Tubal Sterilization

The method of tubal sterilization that has been used since the eighties has not markedly changed.[5] The routine sterilization methods used vary in their success rates after surgical restoration. Non-standardized techniques, such as tubal electrocoagulation or the Pomeroy technique, bear a risk of excessive tubal destruction in order to be more efficient, and consequence a reduced chance of pregnancy after surgery, or a longer delay to pregnancy if the restored tube is significantly shorter.[5] It has also been shown that the site of tubal occlusion affects the expected results, the best results being obtained after istmo-isthmic anastomosis (Table 6.2). The so-called 'mechanical' methods, such as the Yoon band or Filshie clip, offer the best reversal potential and thus, should be presently recommended.[6]

It is thus, important to know which method of sterilization has been previously performed. Surprisingly, some patients are unaware of the method and do not have the surgical report. A simple abdominal X-ray can easily identify the mechanical methods, but for other methods with a poorer prognosis, there is no means of identifying them before surgery.

Presurgical Infertility Investigations

As for any other cause of infertility, a minimal work-up of the couple is required in order to identify the associated factors, which, in some cases, will limit the choice of treatment for restoring fecundity. The gynecological history of patients is carefully analyzed and a clinical examination is performed on both partners. Any risk factor or contraindication for pregnancy should be identified initially. Three investigations are routinely performed:

i.   *Ovarian reserve:* In our experience, most of the women are aged more than 37 to 40 years and thus, an assessement of the ovarian reserve is performed in the first line and will, in some cases, arrest further investigations, except if oocyte donation is accepted after proper counseling.

Ovarian reserve assessment is usually performed with follicle-stimulating hormone (FSH), estradiol and inhibin B assays on the third day of the cycle with or without an ovarian follicular count, done by vaginal ultrasonographic examination.

ii. *Semen analysis:* A proper semen analysis, according to accepted recommendations,[7] is performed, even if the new partner had previously procreated with another woman. In case of a severe male factor, IVF

Table 6.2: Meta-analysis of published reports after microsurgical recanalization according to the method of tubal sterilization			
Method	*No. of cases (n)*	*Deliveries (%)*	*Abortions (%)*	*Ectopic pregnancies (%)*
---	---	---	---	---
Pomeroy	467	50.0	–	2.6
Electrocoagulation	347	45.5	–	4.6
Yoon band	176	176	6.0	5.0
Filshie clips	100	82.0	4.5	3.0

with intracytoplasmic sperm injection (ICSI) is then the recommended procedure.

iii. *Hysterosalpingography (HSG):* Hysterosalpingography is routinely performed in order to exclude any uterine abnormality (leiomyoma, etc.), mainly to identify the site of tubal occlusion and to evaluate the proximal portion of the occluded tube. It is not rare to find polyps or endometrioid lesions that significantly reduce the success of surgery. In addition, clips or bands will easily be identified. If an abnormality of the uterine cavity is suspected, a hysteroscopic assessement is then required.

Other Occasional Investigations

Some other investigations may be required, depending on the past history or the results of the clinical examination. Hormonal assays may be performed if an ovulatory disturbance is suspected. According to the sexual lifestyle and the local endemy, it may be wise to assess the serology for *Chlamydia trachomatis*. This serology is a good marker for additional tubal alterations,[8] and the present recommended threshold value for positivity is 1/16.[9]

Classical Therapeutic Tools

Tubal Microsurgery

Ever since its emergence during the seventies, microsurgery as a technology was standardized and became the gold standard.[10,11] Technical aspects have been accurately and extensively described by Gomel,[12] and have not changed so far. The results of microsurgery, according to the method of sterilization, are reported in Table 6.2. Most of the pregnancies were obtained during the first year following surgery. It appears that there is a trend to achieve better results with surgery for women aged more than 40 years of age in comparison to what is observed for IVF. For women aged more than 40 years of age, the results are still acceptable, with pregancy rates around 45 to 52 percent.[13,14] In contrast, for IVF, the results decrease significantly with a delivery rate of 8.2 percent per cycle.[15] In addition, spontaneous abortion rates and multiple pregnancy rates appear lower after surgery.[16] However, there is still no randomized study comparing surgery to IVF to validate this assumption.[17]

Factors affecting the results have been identified; unilateral recanalization and associated hypofertility conditions decrease the pregnancy rates. Recently, a large series of 1118 cases in which 56.6 percent of the cases were sterilized by laparoscopic electrocoagulation, with pregnancy and delivery rates of 54.8 and 32.7 percent, has been published.[18]

In Vitro Fertilization

In vitro fertilization (IVF) is the main therapeutic alternative to microsurgery by laparotomy. Initially, IVF was developed for definitive tubal occlusions. The results vary greatly between centers, depending especially upon the type of selection applied to patients undergoing the procedure: it is thus, difficult to find a proper control group, since, as noted earlier, there is no real controlled study comparing the results of surgery versus the results of IVF. This is also true for patients previously sterilized, hence, comparisons are difficult to be done.

In France, an IVF register is operative for many years and provides data on large numbers (several hundred of thousands) of attempts, giving the average results observed yearly in this country. From this data, it is possible to calculate a theoretical cumulative success rate of delivery after 4 attempts; this theoretical rate is 52 percent.[19]

However, in routine practice, not all patients will undergo the 4 assumed trials. In one French center performing IVF, the average delivery rate was 21.2 percent per attempt.[20] In a series of 503 IVF cycles, performed for tubal disease, the observed delivery rate for 4 trials was 44.4 percent.[21] In the same center, an evaluation of the cost per baby born indicates that operative laparoscopy for distal tubal lesions is cheaper than IVF,[21] despite the fact that the results of surgery are lower for distal lesions in comparison with recanalization. A more recent Canadian study has arrived at the same conclusions.[22]

It must also be remembered that IVF carries a risk of multiple pregnancy, and probably, a higher rate of spontaneous abortions. Finally, we have assumed that for older women, more than 40 years of age, the results of surgery are not affected, contrary to IVF. All these facts must be taken into account when counseling the patients.

Laparoscopic Tubal Recanalization

The first tubal recanalization by laparoscopy was reported in 1989.[23] During the following years, this approach was increasingly used worldwide, technical aspects have been properly standardized and specific instrumentation developed.[24]

Technical Aspects

The first step is to carry out a proper pelvic assessement in order to exclude associated lesions and to identify the method of sterilization and the site of tubal occlusion.

The proximal stump is then sectioned with scissors or a specific transector. Appropriate minute hemostasis is achieved with a fine bipolar forceps or micro-electrode. The quality of the mucosa and the muscularis is assessed and a transuterine retrograde patency test is performed with methylene blue. The same procedure is applied to the distal stump, with an anterograde patency test. The mesosalpinx is sutured in order to reduce the tension between the two stumps.

Anastomosis can then be performed with fine sutures (7 or 8 zero), involving the mucosa and the muscularis layers. Usually, the number of stitches is limited to 4, starting at the 6 'o' clock position. Various alternative techniques have been described. Several stitches are also placed on the serosa to complete the anastomosis. The same procedure is applied for each Fallopian tube.[24] Finally, the transuterine patency test is performed and the pelvis is carefully washed as for any laparoscopic procedure.

The use of a preventive methods to reduce the formation of postoperative adhesions is debated for this procedure, but usually carries a low risk.

As previously noted, alternative techniques have been proposed, but they have usually been used for a limited number of cases and need to be further evaluated. Among them is the 'one stitch technique',[25] the use of tubal stents or biological glue, the use of titanium clips in order to avoid stitches,[26,27] or robotic assistance.[25,29]

Results

Several observational series have been published, but in many cases, the number of procedures are limited and the reported rates of success show marked variations.[24,28,30-39] A meta-analysis of the published results of laparoscopic tubal recanalization, involving 506 cases, provides some indication of the results listed in Table 6.3.

A large reported series included 186 cases with a one year follow-up. The mean age of the patients was 35 years and the delay between sterilization and recanalization was 8.5 years. However, 15 patients, who were lost to follow-up, were excluded from the analysis. The pregnancy and delivery rates were 84.9 and 69.5 percent, respectively. The abortion and ectopic pregnancy rates were 15.5 and 3.2 percent, respectively.[35]

No controlled study comparing the results of the microsurgical laparotomy approach and the laparoscopic approach has been published. One study retrospectively compared these two approaches,[39] with 44 cases being performed by laparotomy and 37 by laparoscopy (5 cases were excluded for analysis). The pregnancy rates were very similar: 80 percent for laparotomy and 80.5 percent for laparoscopy.[39]

It thus appears that the laparoscopic approach provides very similar results in comparison with microsurgery by laparotomy, when performed on selected patients by a trained operator with adequate instrumentation.

Practical Management

In routine practice, the choice of the therapeutic management, when all methods are available, depends firstly, on the wishes of the couple after complete and clear counseling and secondly, on the eventual associated subfertility factor.

As previously mentioned, the choice of the patient is not always rational and, in our experience, many women want their tubal function restored.

IVF with ICSI is indeed, the recommended procedure when marked deterioration in semen quantity and quality is identified. Moreover, surgery cannot be performed in cases where it is contraindicated, or in rare cases, when severe pelvic lesions (adhesions or endometriosis) are suspected. Moderate associated lesions, identified at laparoscopy, can be treated during surgery, but may reduce the results. IVF may also be preferable if the couple desires only one child.

For the majority of cases, laparoscopic recanalization is a favored procedure when considering the advantages and the risk of laparoscopy (including the cost) and the satisfactory results to be expected. This is true irrespective of the age of the patients and may be more beneficial for patients aged more than 40 years. IVF may be offered after failure of surgery (after a delay of 12 months) in patients younger than 40 years. In contrast, the surgical approach may be considered after failure of IVF.[40]

The demands for sterilization reversal are the result, in the majority of cases, of a dramatic familial event. In some cases, risk factors are present at the time of sterilization and prevention of failures in such cases, requires a careful selection of patients to be sterilized.

The two main therapeutic alternatives to be discussed with the couple are surgical recanalization and IVF. The laparoscopic approach appears to provide similar results in comparison with microsurgery by laparotomy, if performed by adequately trained operators.

A careful assessment of the motivations and wishes of the couple, and a minimal investigation of other fertility parameters, is mandatory before proceeding with the treatment.

In the majority of cases, the laparoscopic approach can be recommended because of the advantages of laparoscopy, the limited risks, the lower cost and satisfactory results with a pregnancy rate of 80 percent, which is close to the natural fertility.

Table 6.3: Meta-analysis of published results of laparoscopic tubal recanalization (506 cases)		
	Mean %	*% Variations*
Pregnancies	77.5	31.0–83.0
Abortions	13.6	7.1–21.7
Ectopic pregnancies	4.3	3.2–16.7
Deliveries	59.4	25.0–63.3

REFERENCES

1. Wilcox LS, Chu SY, Eaker ED, Zeger SL, Peterson HB. Risk factors for regret after tubal sterilization: 5 years of follow-up in a prospective study. Fertil Steril 1991;55:927-33.
2. Wilson RM. Why 103 women asked for reversal of sterilization? Br Med J 1977;2:305-7.
3. Leader A, Galan N, George R, Taylor PJ. A comparison of definable traits in women requesting reversal of sterilization and women satisfied with sterilization. Am J Obstet Gynecol 1983; 145:198-202.
4. Kerin JF, Carignan CS, Cher D. The safety and effectiveness of a new hysteroscopic method for permanent birth control: results of the first Essure PBC clinical study. Aust N Z J Obstet Gynaecol 2001;41:364-70.
5. Audebert A. Techniques des anastomoses pour reperméabilisation tubaire après stérilisation in "Techniques microchirurgicales de la stérilité", Masson; Paris, 1982;1:126-32.
6. Audebert A. La stérilisation féminine et masculine: une alternative à la contraception. in "La contraception", D. Serfaty éditeur, Douin, Paris 1992;1:623-43.
7. WHO. WHO Laboratory Manual for the Examination of Human Semen and Sperm-cervical Mucus Interaction. 3rd edn. Cambridge University Press, Cambridge (UK) 1992;1:107.
8. Mol BW J, Dijkman B, Wertheim P. The accuracy of serum chlamydial antibodies in the diagnosis of tubal pathology: a meta-analysis. Fertil Steril 1997;67:1031-7.
9. Land JA, Evers JLH, Goossens VJ. How to use Chlamydia antibody testing in subfertility patients? Hum Reprod 1998;13: 1094-8.
10. Gomel V. Microsurgical reversal of female sterilization: a reappraisal. Fertil Steril 1980;33:587-97.
11. Winston RML. Microsurgical tubocornual anstomosis for reversal of sterilization. Lancet 1997;1:284.
12. Gomel V. Microsurgery in female infertility. Little, Brown and Company, Boston 1983;1:111-24.
13. Glock JL, Kim AH, Hulka JF, Hunt RB, Trad FS, Brumsted JR. Reproductive outcome after tubal reversal in women 40 years of age or older. Fertil Steril 1996;65:863-5.
14. Trimbos-Kemper TC. Reversal of sterilization in women over 40 years of age a multicenter survey in the Netherlands. Fertil Steril 1990;53:575-7.
15. Templeton A, Morris JK, Parslow W. Factors that affect outcome of *in vitro* fertilisation treatment. Lancet 1996;48:1402-6.
16. Royal College of Obstetricians and Gynaecologists. The management of infertility in secondary care. Evidence-based clinical guidelines No.3. RCGO Press, London 1998.
17. Yossry M, Aboulghar M, D'Angelo A, Gillett W. *In vitro* fertilisation versus tubal reanastomosis (sterilisation reversal) for subfertility after tubal sterilisation. Cochrane Database Syst Rev. 2006;3:CD004144.
18. Kim SH, Shin CJ, Kim JG, Moon SY, Lee JY, Chang YS. Microsurgical reversal of tubal sterilization: a report on 1,118 cases. Fertil Steril 1997;68:865-70.
19. FIVNAT, bilan de l'année 2000. Vol. 1; 2002, Publication FIVNAT, Laboratoire Organon, Paris.
20. Pouly JL, Mage, Pouly-Vye P, Janny L, Canis M, Bruhat MA. Stérilité tubaire: FIV ou chirurgie? Job Gyn 1997;6:1-4.
21. Pouly JL, Janny L, Pouly-Vye P, et al. Cumulative delivery rate after *in vitro* fertilization for tubal infertility. Ref Gynecol Obstet 1995;3(Suppl.):224-30.
22. Hawkins J, Dube D, Kaplow M, Tulandi T. Cost analysis of tubal anastomosis by laparoscopy and by laparotomy. J Am Assoc Gynecol Laparosc 2002;9:120-4.
23. Sedbon E, De La Jolinieres JB, Boudouris O, Madelenat P. Tubal desterilization through exclusive laparoscopy. Hum Reprod 1989;4:158-9.
24. Koh CH. Laparoscopic microsurgical tubal anastomosis. Endoscopic surgery for gynaecologists. In: Sutton C, Diamond M (Eds). WB Saunders Company Ltd, London. 1998;1:176-85.
25. Dubuisson JB, Swolin K. Laparoscopic tubal anastomosis (the one stitch technique): preliminary results. Hum Reprod 1995; 10:2044-6.
26. Stadtmauer L, Sauer M. Outpatient reversal of sterilization with laparoscopically placed titanium staples. Am Assoc Gynecol Laparosc 1996;3(Suppl):S47.
27. Wiegerinck MA, Roukema M, van Kessel PH, Mol BW. Sutureless reanastomosis by laparoscopy versus microsurgical reanastomosis by laparotomy for sterilization reversal: a matched cohort study. Hum Reprod 2005;20:2355-8.
28. Falcone T, Goldberg JM, Margossian H, Stevens L. Robotic-assisted laparoscopic microsurgical tubal anastomosis: a human pilot study. Fertil Steril 2000;73:1040-2.
29. Degueldre M, Vandromme J, Huong PT, Cadiere GB. Robotically assisted laparoscopic microsurgical tubal reanastomosis: a feasibility study. Fertil Steril 2000;74:1020-3.
30. Lee CL, Lai YM, Huang HY, Soong YK. Laparoscopic rescue after tubal anastomosis failure. Hum Reprod 1995;10:1806-9.
31. Stadtmauer L, Sauer MV. Reversal of tubal sterilization using laparoscopically placed titanium staples: preliminary experience. Hum Reprod 1997;12:647-9.
32. St George LI, Kapila HB, Lahoud RH. Laparoscopic tubotubal reanastomosis. Med J Aust 1997;167:367-8.
33. Yovich J, Chau E. Intrauterine pregnancies following laparoscopic tubal reanastomosis. Med J Aust 1998;168:524-5.
34. Koh CH, Janik GM. Laparoscopic microsurgery: current and future status. Curr Opin Obstet Gynecol 1999;11:401-17.
35. Yoon TK, Sung HR, Kang HG, et al. Laparoscopic tubal anastomosis: fertility outcome in 202 cases. Fertil Steril 1999;72:1121-6.
36. Bissonnette F, Lapensee L, Bouzayen R. Outpatient laparoscopic tubal anastomosis and subsequent fertility. Fertil Steril 1999;72: 549-52.
37. Barjot PJ, Marie G, Von Theobald P. Laparoscopic tubal anastomosis and reversal of sterilization. Hum Reprod 1999;14: 1222-5.
38. Katz E, Donesky BW. Laparoscopic tubal anastomosis: a pilot study. J Reprod Med 1994;39:497-8.
39. Cha SH, Lee MH, Kim JH, Lee CN, Yoon TK, Cha KY. Fertility outcome after tubal anastomosis by laparoscopy and laparotomy. J Am Assoc Gynecol Laparosc 2001;8:348-52.
40. Sitko D, Commenges-Ducos M, Roland P, Papaxanthos-Roche A, Horovitz J, Dallay D. IVF following impossible or failed surgical reversal of tubal sterilization. Hum Reprod 2001;16: 683-5.

Does Surgery for Endometriosis Improve the ART Outcomes?

Lakshmi Ravikanti, Ved Prakash Singh

INTRODUCTION

Endometriosis is a chronic, complex, yet relatively common gynecological disorder, reportedly affecting >70 million adult and adolescent females worldwide. Endometriosis affects an estimated 10 to 15 percent of all women of reproductive age, 20 to 50 percent of all women with infertility, and 25 to 70 percent of women and adolescents with chronic pelvic pain (CPP) or pelvic pain and dysmenorrhea. Common among adolescents as well as adults, endometriosis has been observed in females as young as 10 years of age. Although the published incidence rates also vary among adolescents with CPP, one study estimated an incidence of 12 percent among girls between 11 to 13 years of age.[1]

How Much do We Know About Endometriosis?

Endometriosis remains one of the final frontiers in gynecology. As far as the issue of endometriosis-related infertility is concerned, there are more questions than answers. For example:

- If endometriosis causes infertility, does removal of endometriosis increase fertility? Do results differ in patients with the stage of endometriosis?
- Do assisted reproductive technique (ART) increase fertility in endometriosis?
- Is the *in vitro* fertilization (IVF) outcome affected in endometriosis? If it is affected, is it due to poor endometrial receptivity or poor oocyte quality?
- Which ART is optimal?
- Which is better, surgery or ART?
- Does surgery before ART improve the outcome?

CLINICAL DISCUSSION

Is the IVF Outcome Affected in Endometriosis?

The answer appears to be yes. In a large meta-analysis of 22 studies, Barnhart et al.[2] clearly showed that women with endometriosis are less likely to conceive with IVF when compared to women with tubal disease with an odds ratio of 0.56. This study concluded that patients with endometriosis-associated infertility, undergoing IVF, respond with significantly decreased levels of all markers of the reproductive process, suggesting that the effect of endometriosis is not exclusively on the receptivity of the endometrium but perhaps, also on the development of the oocyte and embryo. The IVF outcomes were worse in women with severe endometrioisis when compared to those with mild endometriosis, with an odds ratio of 0.60 (Fig. 7.1).[2]

How does Endometriosis Affect the Outcome of IVF?

There has been much debate in the literature whether the IVF outcomes in endometriosis-related infertility are poorer due to reduced implantation of embryos, i.e. poor endometrial receptivity or a reduction in oocyte quality. Two elegant studies have addressed this issue.

Diaz et al.[3] used healthy donor oocytes and introduced sibling oocytes into healthy recipients and recipients with endometriosis. They found no statistically significant difference in the implantation rate or livebirth in the two groups, indicating that uterine receptivity is not impaired in patients with endometriosis.[3]

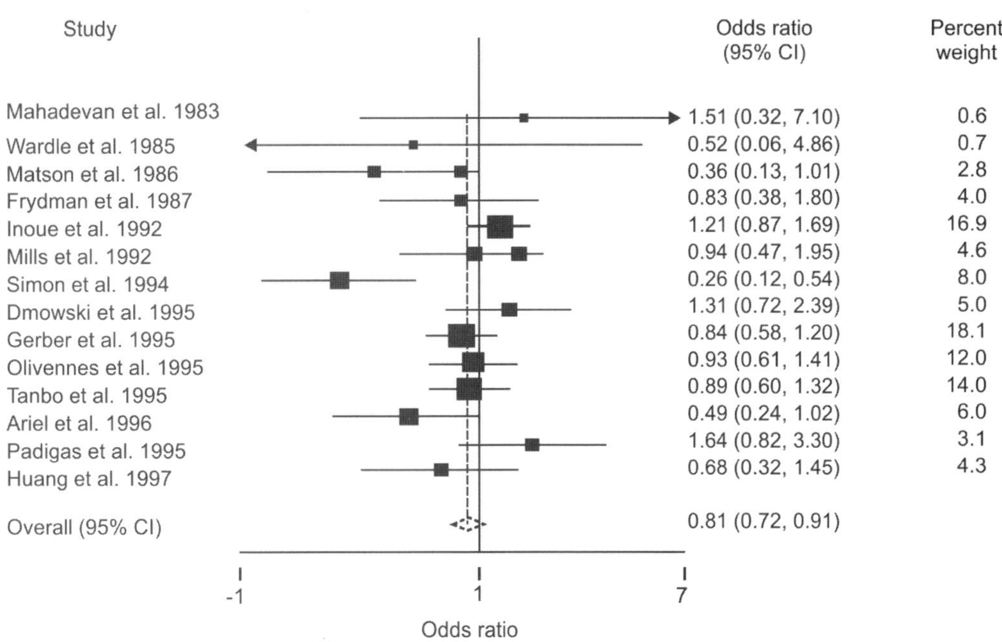

Fig. 7.1: IVF outcomes in women with endometriosis *(Adopted from Barnhart K, Dunsmoor-Su R, Coutifaris C. Effect of endometriosis on in vitro fertilization. Fertil Steril 2002;77:1148-55)*

In another well-designed study by Simon et al.[4], the IVF outcomes in patients following oocyte donation from donors with endometriosis was compared to that following oocyte donation from donors without endometriosis. The recipients who received oocytes from donors with endometriosis had significantly lower pregnancy rates. This study demonstrates the likelihood of poor oocyte quality as the key reason why IVF pregnancy rates are lower in patients with endometriosis.[4]

Management Options in Endometriosis-related Infertility

- *Expectant management:* A study by Soliman et al.[5] showed that none of the six women with endometriosis, who were followed up expectantly, got pregnant compared to 33 percent of the women in the IVF group who conceived.[5] It is therefore, unwise to manage these patients expectantly.[5]
- *Endometriosis and controlled ovarian hyperstimulation (COH)/intrauterine insemination (IUI):* Tummon et al.[6] demonstrated the well-known fact to us that superovulation and IUI improves the chances of conception up to 30 percent in 4 cycles compared to 10 percent in the non-treatment group. They also concluded that the pregnancy rate plateaus after 4 cycles (Fig. 7.2).[6]
- *Surgical therapy-issues:* Surgical therapy has become a standard approach in symptomatic patients with endometriosis. However, there are very few randomized controlled studies comparing the various techniques as well the outcomes from surgery versus no surgery,

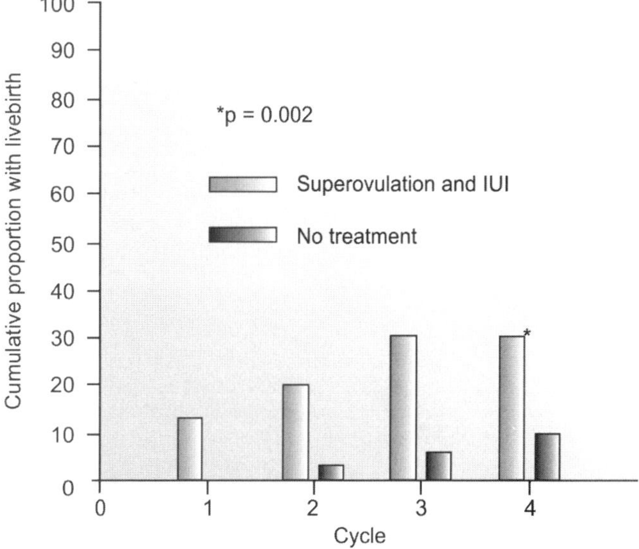

Fig. 7.2: Comparison in cumulative livebirth rates following COH/IUI and no treatment in patients with endometriosis-associated infertility. *(Adopted from: Tummon IS, Asher LJ, Martin JS, Tulandi T. Randomized controlled trial of superovulation and insemination for infertility associated with minimal or mild endometriosis. Fertil Steril 1997;68:8-12)*

particularly in the area of endometriosis-related infertility. In the studies available, there is often a lack of description of follow-up and fecundity rates. There is a difference in surgical techniques in different studies. Excision of endometriosis can be complete or partial depending on the surgeon's experience and surgical skills. There is an increasing recognition of "atypical" lesions.

There are very few randomized controlled trials but many observational studies indicating that surgery for endometriosis improves the likelihood of spontaneous conception when compared to medical or expectant management. In a meta-analysis, Adamson et al.[7] showed that the crude pregnancy rate was 38 percent higher following surgery compared to medical therapy or expectant management.[7] Though this study was not controlled for the endometriosis stage, another meta-analysis by Hughes et al.[8] that was controlled for stage, showed higher pregnancy rates (OR 2.67) in favor of surgery compared to medical treatment or expectant management.[8]

The Endo Can study by Marcoux et al.[9] (Fig. 7.3) is one of the few randomized controlled trials that showed benefit in surgically treating stage 1 and stage 2 endometriosis. In this study, the authors randomized 341 infertile women, 20 to 39 years of age, with minimal and mild endometriosis. In their 34-week follow-up, 30.7 percent of women conceived in the laparoscopic resection or ablation group compared to 17.7 percent in the laparoscopy only group. The corresponding rates of fecundity were 4.7 and 2.4 per 100 person-months. These results were statistically significant (p = 0.006).[9]

Hence, surgery for endometriosis-related infertility is useful for stages 1 and 2 endometriosis, but what remains to be determined is whether the improvement in fertility is worth the risk of surgery in endometriosis stages 3 and 4. As mentioned earlier, there are no randomized controlled trials (RCTs) to guide us in American Fertility Staging (AFS) Stage 3 and 4 endometriosis-related infertility in the absence of significant symptoms. Let us consider two cases from our series with different presentations to illustrate the dilemmas we face in our day-to-day practice.

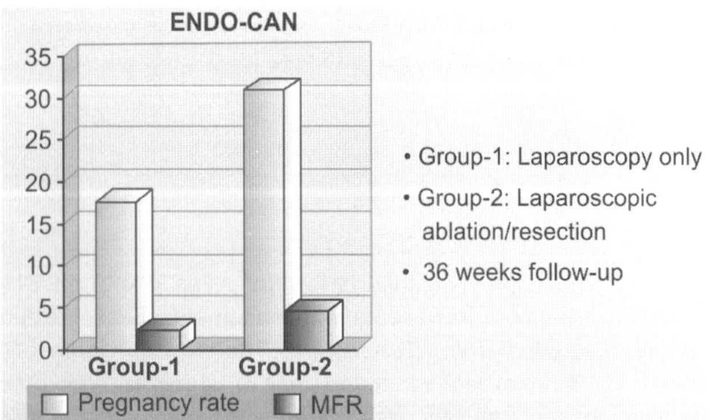

Fig. 7.3: Comparison of pregnancy outcomes in patients with minimal and mild endometriosis following laparoscopic surgery *(Adopted from Marcoux S, Maheux R, Berube S. The Canadian Collaborative Group on Endometriosis. Laparoscopic Surgery in Infertile Women with Minimal or Mild Endometriosis. N Eng J Med 1997;337:217-222)*

Case 1

A 34-year-old woman presented with primary infertility of 4 years. She had regular periods and minimal dysmenorrhea on the first day of her period. She had no dyspareunia or bowel-related symptoms. Her partner's semen analysis was normal. Diagnostic laparoscopy diagnosed AFS Stage 3 endometriosis and patent tubes with no adhesions. Transvaginal scan revealed a 3 cm endometrioma on the left ovary. We faced the dilemma of whether to proceed to IUI, do an IVF or perform surgical treatment of endometriosis. The considerations and thought process are presented in Figure 7.4.

We discussed with her that if she opts to have surgery, she will have, roughly, a 30 percent chance of conceiving naturally. Developing symptoms are matter of time and there would be a lower risk of infections, if she needs ovum pick-up (OPU) in future. Surgery may improve the quality of oocytes but there may be associated risks with surgery.

With IVF, she has 45 percent chance of conceiving with one cycle and 70 percent with two cycles. However, there is an associated cost factor and emotional impact that she would have to deal with. The IVF has fewer complications compared to surgery. She opted to have IVF and had a successful outcome.

Case 2

A 38-year-old presented with primary infertility of 2 years. She had irregular periods and complaints of severe dysmenorrhea, mild dyspareunia, but no dyschezia.

She underwent diagnostic laparoscopy at a different center with suboptimal views and unconfirmed endometriosis. On per vaginal examination, we found nodularity in the pouch of Douglas (POD) and tenderness. On transvaginal examination, we found a 4 cm endometrioma on the right ovary and a 2 cm endometrioma on the left ovary. The dilemma we faced here was whether to perform an IUI, IVF or offer another laparoscopy. We proceeded to perform a laparoscopic

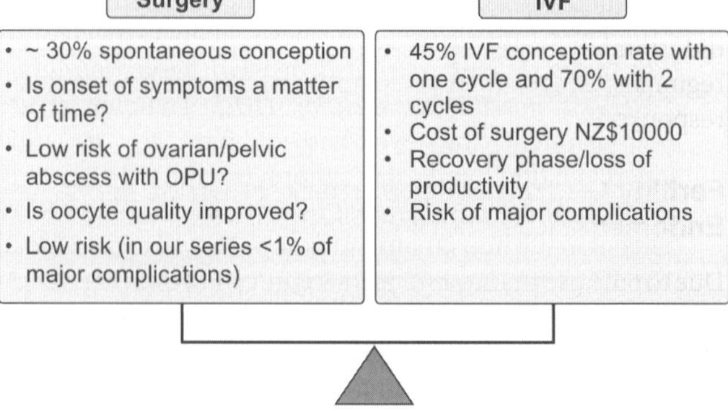

Fig. 7.4: Comparison between surgery and IVF for endometriosis-related infertility

excisional surgery for endometriosis. The patient was asymptomatic at 3-months follow-up in the clinic. She conceived spontaneously at 6 months and delivered a baby boy. She remained asymptomatic at 6 months postpartum.

Does Endometrioma Affect IVF?

Surgery for endometrioma prior to IVF is the "gold standard". There are many observational studies supporting an improvement in IVF outcome following the removal of endometriomas but no randomized trials to prove it. In a retrospective case control study by Garcia-Velasco et al.[10] in 2004, 189 women with endometriomas underwent IVF treatment. Of these, 56 women proceeded directly to IVF and 133 first underwent surgery followed by IVF. The authors observed no significant difference in pregnancy rates, indicating that treating endometriomas prior to IVF does not improve success rates following IVF.[10]

Endometrioma: Excision or Ablation

In a systemic review by Hart et al.[11] in 2005, it was noted that there were no randomized studies on the management of endometriomata by laparotomy, but 2 randomized studies on the laparoscopic management of endometrioma >3 cm. They concluded from that study that laparoscopic excision of the cyst wall of the endometrioma provides a more favorable outcome than drainage and ablation with regard to the recurrence of the endometrioma, recurrence of symptoms and subsequent spontaneous pregnancy in women who were previously subfertile. However, they found no data to indicate the best surgical approach in women planning to undergo assisted reproductive techniques.[11]

Prolonged GnRH Agonist Therapy Prior to an IVF Cycle in Endometriosis Patients

In a recent prospective, randomized controlled trial by Surrey et al.[12] in 2002, prolonged use of gonadotropin-releasing hormone (GnRH) agonist before *in vitro* fertilization-embryo transfer (IVF-ET) in patients with endometriosis resulted in significantly higher ongoing pregnancy rates than did standard controlled ovarian hyperstimulation (COH) regimens. They also observed no deleterious effect on ovarian response.[12]

Fertility Outcome after Surgery for Grade III / IV Endometriosis in our Practice

Due to the lack of reliable data for stage 3 and 4 endometriosis-related infertility, we are compelled to rely on our experience and observational studies. This prompted us to undertake a retrospective audit of our own experience in this area. We looked at all the cases of endometriosis excision over 5 years, performed by a single surgeon or under his direct supervision.

There were 261 cases that were operated between 2001 to 2006 out of which 208 were AFS stage 3 and 4.

We included a total number of 208 patients in the study. Of these, 168 women presented with pain only, 34 women with pain and infertility and 6 of them with infertility alone. All the 6 women who presented with infertility alone had endometriomas on ultrasound scan. In the pain only group, 148 women were followed-up, while the remaining 20 failed to attend the follow-up appointments. In the pain and infertility group, 31 patients were followed-up. In the infertility group, all the women attended the follow-up appointment (Fig. 7.5).

In all, we could follow-up 185 women. In the pain only group 11.5 percent conceived despite infertility not being an issue that they presented with initially. In the pain and infertility group 38.7 percent conceived spontaneously. One woman in this group had an ectopic pregnancy 12 months after her surgery. In the infertility only group, 16.6 percent conceived (Fig. 7.6). In this group, we found that all the women had endometriomas at the surgery.

Additional Procedures Required and Complications

We needed to perform elective bowel resection in 13 women for the pain only group. One woman had partial bladder resection for a bladder lesion of endometriosis causing urinary symptoms. Our complication rate was comparable to other studies. We had one intraoperative rectal injury that was managed laparoscopically with no consequence, one abdominal wall hematoma, requiring return to the theater, one small bowel obstruction and one case of primary hemorrhage, requiring blood transfusion. Overall, the complication rate was 2 percent.

Keys to a Successful Endometriosis Unit

In our view, a successful endometriosis unit needs a multidisciplinary team with two gynecologists, one colorectal surgeon, anesthesiologist, counselor, trained theater staff,

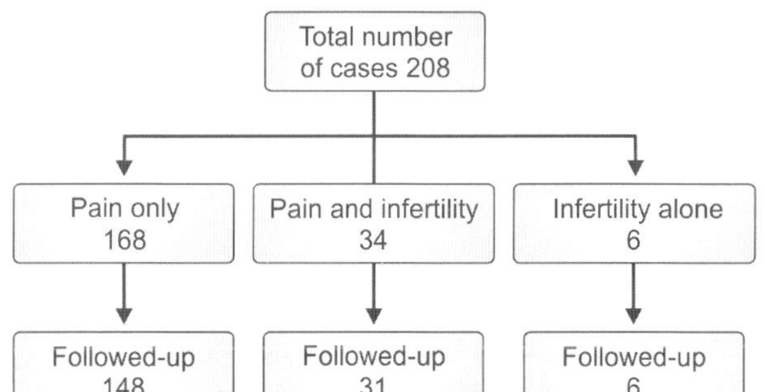

Fig. 7.5: Patient statistics in stage 3 and 4 endometriosis-related infertility patients undergoing endometriosis excision

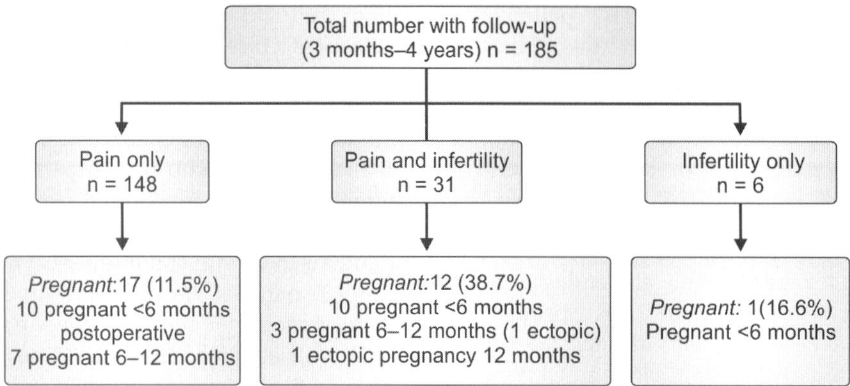

Fig. 7.6: Pregnancy outcome following endometriosis excision in patients with stage 3 and 4 endometriosis-related infertility

adequate equipment like monopolar hook diathermy, bipolar forceps, harmonic scalpel, rectal probe, RUMI manipulator, and endo GIA staplers.

In our unit, the stoma nurse and the surgeons see the patient preoperatively and explain the surgery and its risks to her. We perform bowel preparation for all the grade 3 and 4 endometriosis patients prior to laparoscopic excision. Consistency in technique is ensured. The surgical procedure is recorded and the findings of the surgery adequately documented. Our results are regularly audited on a 6-monthly basis.

CONCLUSION

- The management of endometriosis-related infertility is complex.
- Surgical treatment of stage I and II endometriosis should be undertaken at the time of initial assessment.
- Surgical management of large endometriomas >3 cm should be managed prior to IVF.
- Surgical excision of infertility related to stage III and IV endometriosis in the absence of pain symptoms remains controversial in the absence of reliable prospective studies. If surgery in this situation is undertaken, the patient should be given detailed counseling regarding the risks and benefits of the surgery. Such a surgery should be performed in a multidisciplinary specialist center.
- Pretreatment with GnRHa 3 to 6 months prior to IVF in patients with stage III/IV endometriosis may have potential benefits.

REFERENCES

1. Gao X. Economic burden of endometriosis, Presented at the American College of Obstetricians and Gynecologists at 54th Annual Clinical Meeting, Washington DC.
2. Barnhart K, Dunsmoor-Su R, Coutifaris C. Effect of endometriosis on *in vitro* fertilization. Fertil Steril 2002;77:1148-55.
3. Diaz I, Navarro J, Blasco L, Simon C, Pellicer A, Remohi J. Impact of stage III-IV endometriosis on recipients of sibling oocytes: matched case control study. Fertil Steril 2000;74:31-4.
4. Simon C, Gutiérrez A, Vidal A, de los Santos MJ, Tarín JJ, Remohí J, Pellicer A. Outcome of patients with endometriosis in assisted reproduction: results from *in vitro* fertilization and oocyte donation. Hum Reprod 1994;9:725-9.
5. Soliman S, Daya S, Collins J, Jarrell J. A randomized trial of *in vitro* fertilization versus conventional treatment for infertility. Fertil Steril 1993;59:1239-44.
6. Tummon IS, Asher LJ, Martin JS, Tulandi T. Randomized controlled trial of superovulation and insemination for infertility associated with minimal or mild endometriosis. Fertil Steril 1997;68:8-12.
7. Adamson GD, Pasta DJ. Surgical treatment of endometriosis-associated infertility: meta-analysis compared with survival analysis. Am J Obstet Gynecol 1994;171:1488-1504.
8. Hughes EG, Fedorokow DM, Collins JA. A quantitative overview of controlled trials in endometriosis-associated infertility. Fertil Steril 1993;59:963-70.
9. Marcoux S, Maheux R, Berube S. The Canadian Collaborative Group on Endometriosis. Laparoscopic Surgery in Infertile Women with Minimal or Mild Endometriosis. N Eng J Med 1997;337:217-22
10. Garcia-Velasco JA, Mahutte NG, Corona J, Zuniga V, Giles J, Arici A, Pellicer A. Removal of endometriomas before *in vitro* fertilization does not improve fertility outcomes: a matched, case-control study. Fertil Steril 2004;81:1194-7.
11. Hart R, Hickey M, Maouris P, Buckett W, Garry R. Excisional surgery versus ablative surgery for ovarian endometriomata: a Cochrane Review. Hum Reprod 2005;20:3000-7.
12. Surrey ES, Silverberg KM, Surrey MW, Schoolcraft WB. Effect of prolonged gonadotropin-releasing hormone agonist therapy on the outcome of *in vitro* fertilization-embryo transfer in patients with endometriosis. Fertil Steril 2002;78:699-704.

Radical Excision of Endometriosis Improves the Fertility Outcome

Nutan Jain, Shweta Goel, Anjali Gupta

OVERVIEW

Endometriosis has been directly related to pelvic pain, dysmenorrhea, dyspareunia and infertility. Laparoscopy has emerged as a major player in the diagnosis, especially surgical management of deep infiltrating endometriosis. The goal of laparoscopic treatment is radical excision of all visible and palpable disease that is, excising large, superficial and deep lesions and excising in toto, smaller lesions. The implants, seen on the pelvic side wall peritoneum, are just the tip of iceberg. Opening the peritoneum exposes all the implants, which can then be excised from the base. This leaves a very clear pelvis with normalization of the tuboperitoneal relationship.

Complete adhesiolysis, cul-de-sac dissection, rectal mobilization, lateral clearing between the uterosacral ligaments and rectum, excision of the involved vagina with an adenomyotic nodule with a 0.5 cm disease-free margin helps in not only clearing of the diseases but alot in postoperative pain relief, return of fertility and lastly, in the quality of life. For a localized adenomyoma, adenomyomectomy is performed similar to myomectomy by laparoscopic ultrasonic energy. Though the plane of cleavage is not well-defined, coring is done by harmonic shears and reconstruction by interrupted vertical mattress sutures. To prevent postoperative adhesion formation, meticulous hemostasis, working in the correct anatomical plane, gentle handling of tissues, copious irrigation and lavage should be done.

All the patients are routinely followed up by active fertility management with controlled ovarian hyperstimulation (COH) and intrauterine insemination (IUI). Very severe grades of endometriosis are referred for *in vitro* fertilization (IVF).

Thus, all visible and palpable lesions of the disease must be excised for the patient to reap any real benefits, to avoid persistence of lesions and to minimize the rate of recurrence following surgery.

INTRODUCTION

Endometriosis is an enigmatic disease. It remains unresolved whom it affects, how it affects remaining the foremost cause of infertility and pelvic pain. In the recent times, alot of attention has been given to elucidating the exact nature, etiopathology and disease symptomatology in relation to chronic pelvic pain and infertility. Endometriosis has been directly related to pelvic pain, dysmenorrhea, dyspareunia, and infertility, and laparoscopy has emerged as a major player in the diagnosis and especially, the surgical management[1] of deep infiltrating endometriosis. Medical therapy is found be ineffective[2] and temporary with a recurrence rate as high as 76 percent,[3] whereas surgical treatment is highly effective in relieving pelvic pain, dyspareunia and infertility.[4,5]

In the pelvis, three different types of endometriosis are recognized:[6-9]

1. Peritoneal[10]
2. Ovarian[11,12]
3. Rectovaginal septum[13-16]

Peritoneal endometriosis is recognized as red lesions and brown-black lesions, red lesions being the more active form of the disease. This is often causative of pelvic pain, infertility or both.

In this chapter, we shall discuss the etiology, pathophysiology, diagnosis and laparoscopic management of infiltrating endometriosis.[17,18]

CLINICAL DISCUSSION

Radical Excision of Grade I Endometriosis

It has been unequivocally accepted that rather than vaporization or fulguration, radical excision gives better

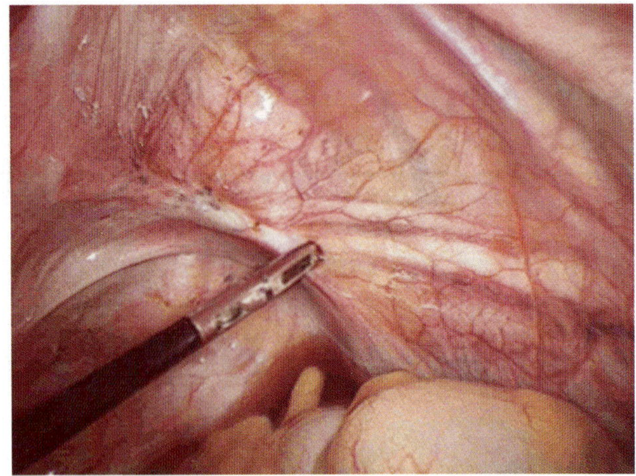

Fig. 8.1A: Blue-black endometriotic implants on right uterosacral ligaments

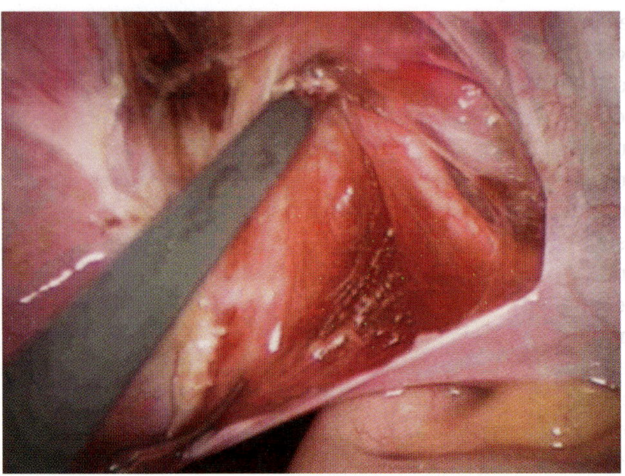

Fig. 8.1B: Dissection of endometriotic implants with ureter comes in view

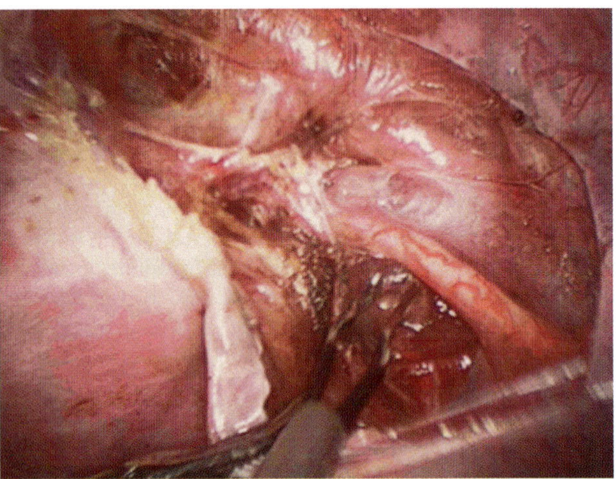

Fig. 8.1C: All endometriotic implants fulgurated on posterior surface of ureter

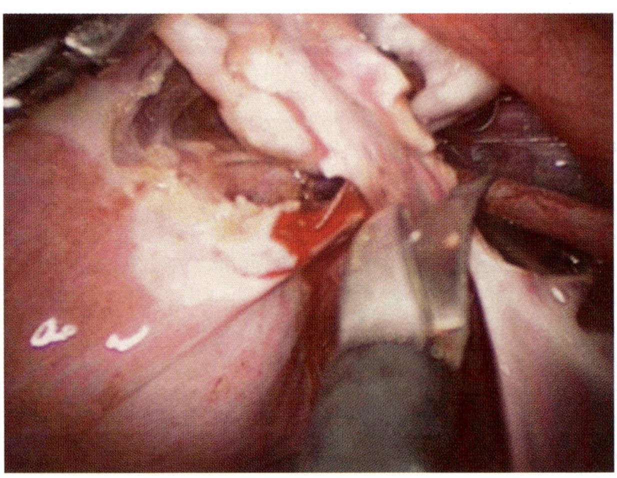

Fig. 8.1D: Excision of endometriotic implants

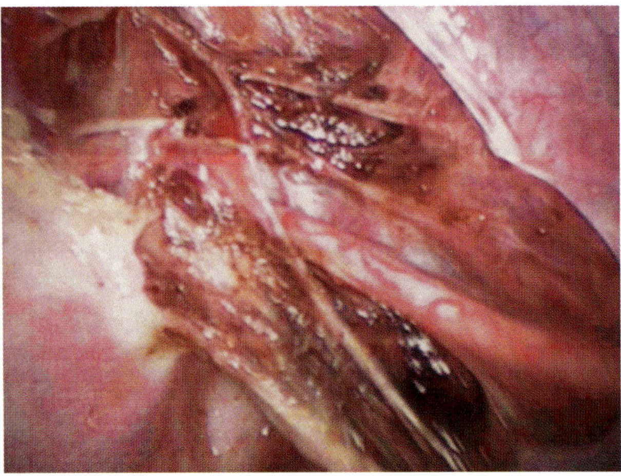

Fig. 8.1E: Complete excision of endometriotic implants, ureter seen free

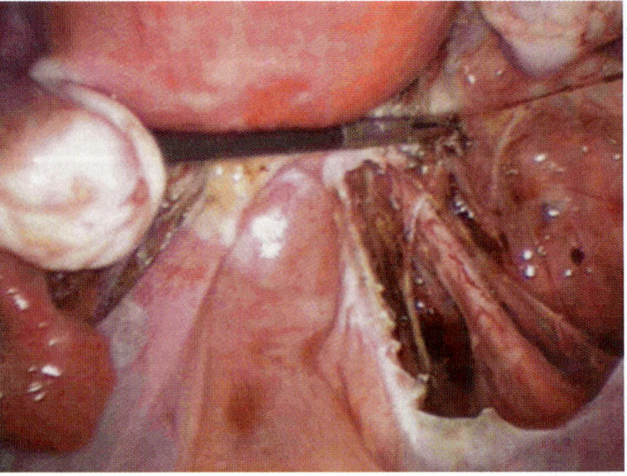

Fig. 8.1F: Excision of endometriotic implants on both pelvic side walls

results; the standard technique is to carry out a four-port laparoscopy. The lesions are identified and initial adhesiolysis is carried out as deemed necessary. Once the pelvis is clear, then the implants are picked up with a tooth grasper and the implants excised using monopolar cautery and sharp dissecting scissors. This gives a neat, clean base and minimizes bleeding. Before attempting any excision using monopolar cautery, the ureter should be identified and preferably, the peritoneum medial to the ureter should be opened. This itself exposes many more endometriotic implants in the deeper retroperitoneal plane. The implants seen on the pelvic side wall peritoneum are just the tip of the iceberg. Opening the peritoneum exposes all the implants, which can then be excised from the base. All the covering peritoneum is also excised by using copious suction irrigation lavage and a micro-bipolar diathermy forceps. Hemostasis is readily achieved. At the end of the procedure, the ureter is clearly exposed and all the endometriotic implants and the pelvic side wall peritoneum is excised. This leaves a very clean pelvis with normalization of the tuboperitoneal relationship. All the implants on the uterosacral ligaments are also excised (Figs 8.1A to F). This goes a long way in relieving pain also in patients with early endometriosis. To prevent postoperative adhesion formation, a meticulous hemostasis is mandatory. Working in the correct anatomical plane, gentle handling of tissues and copious irrigation and lavage are supportive in reducing adhesion formation and facilitating a good fertility outcome. We additionally instill 4 percent Icodextrin 1000 mL solution after clearing the pelvis of all blood, clots, char and debris. These patients fare well postoperatively. Fertility concerns are addressed by postoperative active management of infertility by controlled ovarian hyperstimulation (COH) and intrauterine insemination (IUI).

Ovarian endometriomas present a different spectrum of the same disease. They are formed by the invagination of the ovarian cortex at the point of superficial endometriotic implants. This is the theory postulated by Hughesdon.[11] This causes a severe type of disease, often associated with pelvic mass and infertility.

The third and most severe form of the disease has been defined by Donnez et al.[13-16] as adenomyosis of the rectovaginal septum. It is characterized by complete or partial obliteration of the cul-de-sac (Figs 8.2A and B) with symptomatology being severe dysmenorrhea, dyspareunia, dyschezia and non-cyclic pelvic pain and infertility.

The concept of adenomyotic nodule was advanced by Cullen in 1920,[19] while infiltrating endometriosis of the rectovaginal area was described by Sampson in 1927.[20] In 1974, Novak and Woodruff[21] verified that the lesion was a combination of fibromuscular tissue within which resided the glands and stroma of endometriosis. Sampson described cul-de-sac obliteration as "extensive adhesion in cul-de-

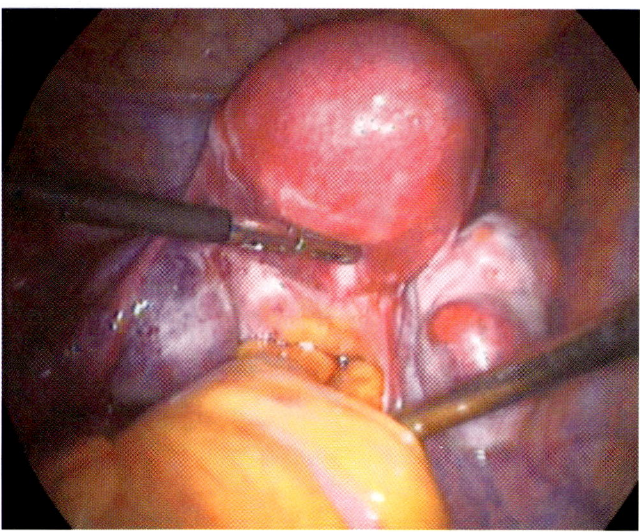

Fig. 8.2A: Partial obliteration of the cul-de-sac

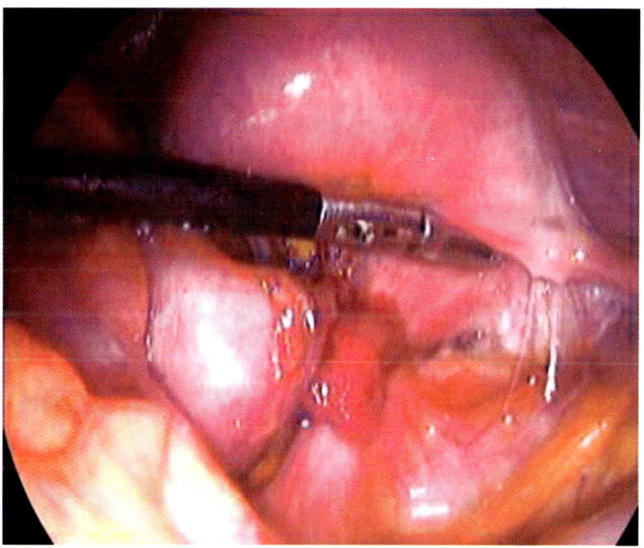

Fig. 8.2B: Complete obliteration of the cul-de-sac

sac", obliterating its lower portion and uniting the cervix, or the lower portion of the uterus to the rectum. Adenoma of the endometrial type invades the cervical and the uterine tissue and probably also, to a lesser degree, the anterior wall of the rectum. In this situation, deep retrocervical adenomyosis is present beneath the peritoneum.

Deep Rectovaginal Endometriosis

Diagnosis: The diagnosis of deep rectovaginal endometriosis can be made by patient history and examination. In the history, information regarding infertility, deep dyspareunia, severe congestive dysmenorrhea, dyschezia, i.e. rectal

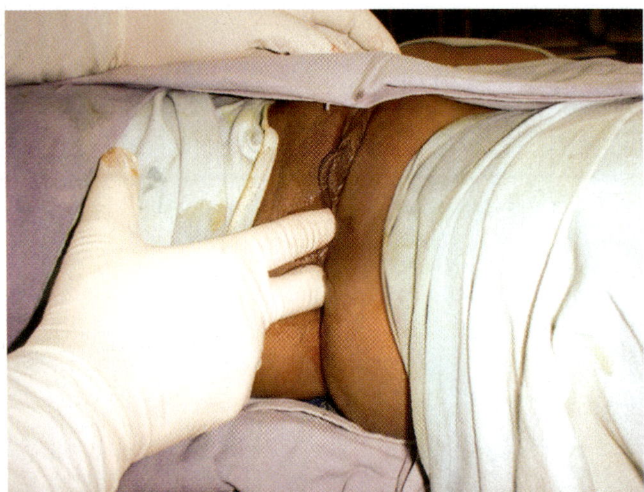

Fig. 8.3: Bimanual pelvic examination

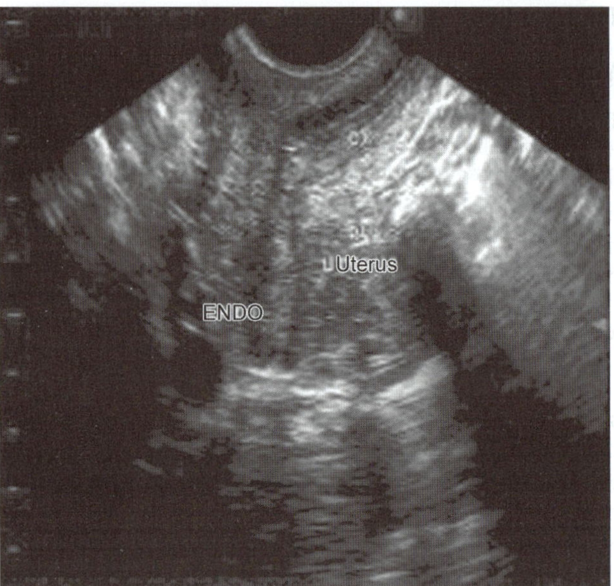

Fig. 8.4A: Adenomyosis and fixed retroversion

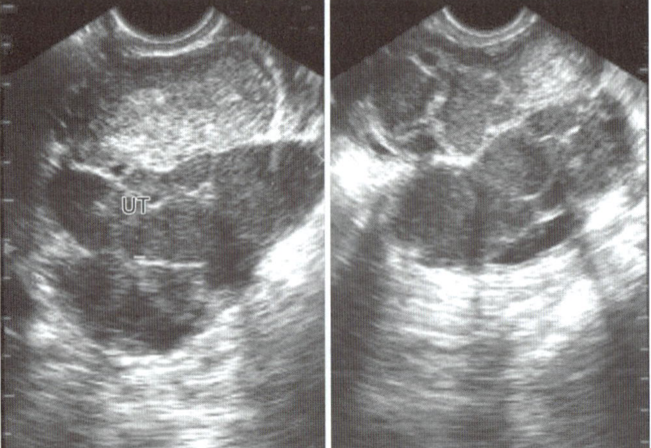

Fig. 8.4B: Fixed retroversion with endometrioma

symptoms comprising of the urgency to defecate and feeling of incomplete evacuation and rectal pain during defecation, is obtained from the patient. This symptom is quite pathognomonic of deep infiltrating endometriosis. The patient could present with rectal bleeding cyclically with menstruation if the rectal mucosa is fully infiltrated and involved in endometriosis. Some patients may present continuous pelvic pain, worsening during periods, while they remain infertile.

Evaluation: Tenderness in the posterior fornix at a routine pelvic examination gives a clue. Lateral fornices could be tender if co-existent endometrioma is also present. Per speculum examination shows the typical blue, black lesions puckering the posterior vaginal wall. These are quite suggestive of full-length penetration of vaginal wall with deep endometriosis.

Bimanual pelvic examination: This is a very important way to diagnose deep infiltrating endometriosis. The patient is typically examined during the menstrual cycle and the index finger is in the vagina, while the lubricated middle finger is in the rectum (Fig. 8.3). Between these two fingers the rectovaginal nodule is easily palpated, more so, during menstruation when it becomes tender and more prominent.

Ultrasonography: Sonography, especially transvaginal, is very useful. It shows definite signs such as:
- The presence of adenomyosis and fixed retroversion (Fig. 8.4A).
- Adherent ovaries on the back surface of the uterus without the presence of big endometriomas (Fig. 8.4B).

- Tenderness on maneuvering a vaginal probe. In my hands, these are the most important diagnostic tools, which have a high correlation with preoperative transvaginal sonography and intra-operative findings.
- *Transrectal Sonography:* More recently, transrectal sonography, using a small part, high frequency transducer has been more favored. Transrectal sonography has a sensitivity and specificity of 97 percent and 96 percent, respectively for the identification of vaginal and rectal wall infiltration. The patient is given soap water enema one hour prior to the transrectal sonography to empty out the fecal contents. This sonography gives the best delineation of the extent of rectal involvement and size of the adenomyotic nodule.

Treatment Options

Medical Management

Though ovarian suppression, either by Danazol or gonado-tropin-releasing hormone (GnRH) agonist, is done, owing to the lack of histopathology of this lesion in the glandular epithelium and of the high proportion of fibromuscular tissue, it is less effective and recurrences are high with a higher incidence of side effects of the drugs used.

Surgical Management

It can be offered by laparotomy, laparoscopy or micro-surgery depending upon the surgeon's skill and existing infrastructural facilities such as the presence of a colorectal surgeon, urologist, etc. Surgical management by laparoscopy offers distinctive advantages:

- Visualization of peritoneal endometriosis and retro-peritoneal access at laparotomy is poor, which becomes much improved by video laparoscopy.
- Resection and repair of bowel, bladder and ureter is a major part of resection of deep endometriosis and has been possible only by superior magnification offered by a laparoscope.

Technique of laparoscopic radical excision: The goal of laparoscopic treatment is the radical excision of all visible and palpable disease. It includes excising large, superficial and deep lesions and excising in toto, smaller lesions.

Aim of surgery: Separation of the anterior rectum from the posterior vagina and the excision or ablation of the endometriosis in that area.

Surgical technique: All cases are done under general anesthesia with endotracheal intubation. The patient is laid in steep Trendelenburg position with a modified lithotomy position. A thorough bowel preparation, including a mechanical bowel preparation, like peglac, is mandatory. The anesthetist should not use nitrous oxide in the anesthesia protocol as nitrous oxide bloats up the bowel and makes dissection in rectovaginal space hazardous. Four-ports are utilized, two for the surgeon standing on the left of the patient according to the concept of working in the ipsilateral style, i.e. lower left lateral port and upper left para-umbilical port. The right lower port is usually for the assistant and is utilized for suction, irrigation and a grasper (Fig. 8.5).

Preparation at the vaginal-end (Fig. 8.6):
- Strong uterine elevator like RUMI.
- Rectal probe placed *in situ*.
- Sponge in posterior vagina, mounted over a ring forceps.

This arrangement allows for a very stout anteversion required to create a cleavage plane between the uterus and rectum. The rectal probe safeguards the integrity of the rectum

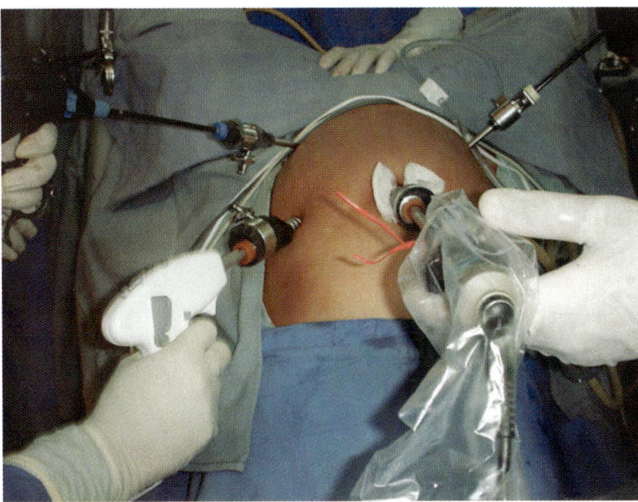

Fig. 8.5: Four-ports placement

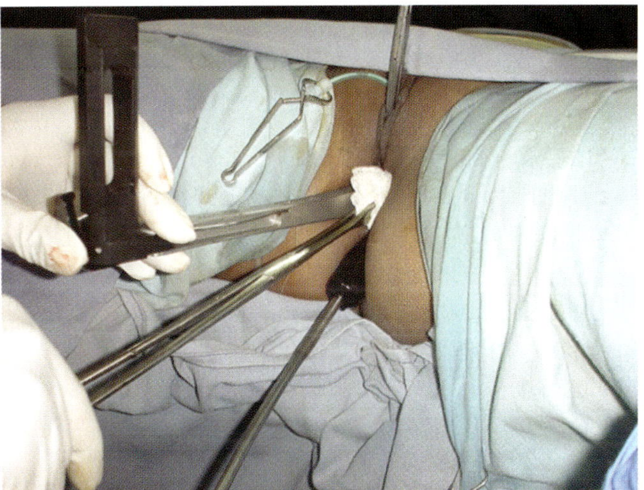

Fig. 8.6: Placing the rectal probe, vaginal probe and uterine elevator

during sharp and blunt dissection. The posterior fornix sponge delineates the vagina from the rectum and facilitates the mobilization of the rectum from the posterior vagina. This arrangement is readied before starting any dissection in the rectovaginal space.

Mode of electrosurgery used for dissection: Various modalities could be used to separate the rectum from the posterior uterus and cervix:
- Aqua dissection.
- Blunt hook scissors (Figs 8.7A and B).
- Electrosurgery-unipolar current.
- Laser CO_2 or KTP.

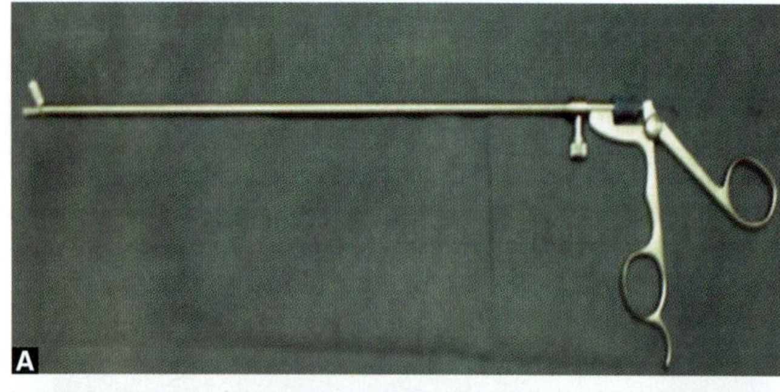

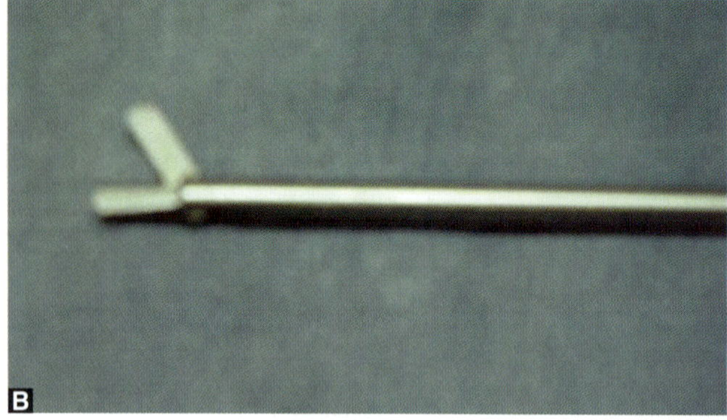

Figs 8.7A and B: Blunt hook scissor

This is subject to availability and surgeon preference. Lasers and blunt hook scissors are mostly used. Dr Redwine prefers to use monopolar cautery.

Exact surgical technique: Deep fibrotic nodular adenomyosis, involving the cul-de-sac, requires an excision of the nodular tissue from the posterior vagina, rectum, and posterior cervix and uterosacral ligaments. Donnez et al.[13-16] described that attention is first directed towards complete dissection of the anterior rectum throughout its area of involvement till the loose fibro-fatty tissue of the rectovaginal space is reached. To begin with, the peritoneum covering the cul-de-sac is opened between the adenomyotic lesion and the rectum (Figs 8.8A to C) so the rectum is first freed from the loose areolar tissue of the rectovaginal septum prior to excising and or vaporizing visible and palpable deep endometriosis. This is possible even when the anterior rectal wall is involved. The dissection is carried out by blunt hook scissors till the rectum is mobilized and identified below the lesion.

The next step is the lateral clearing between the uterosacral ligament and rectum (Fig. 8.9) as this usually carries abundant afferent nervous fibers responsible for severe pain symptoms. This procedure not only clears the disease, but also plays an important role in postoperative pain relief and future fertility concerns.

Ablation of endometriotic implants: Vaporization or fulguration of all endometriotic implants on the back surface of the uterus, cervix, and uterosacral ligaments is carried out after

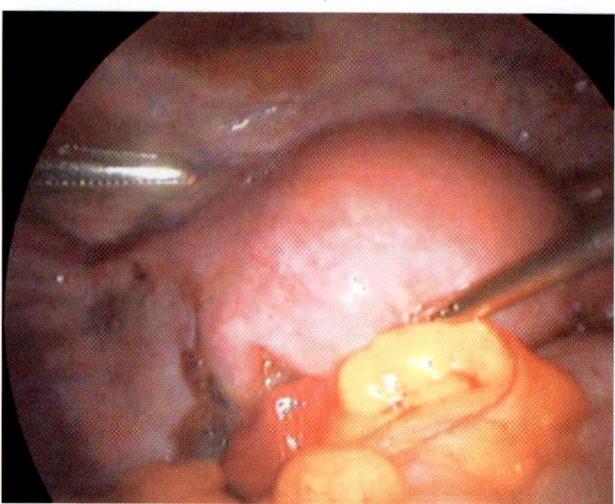

Fig. 8.8A: Fixed retroversion

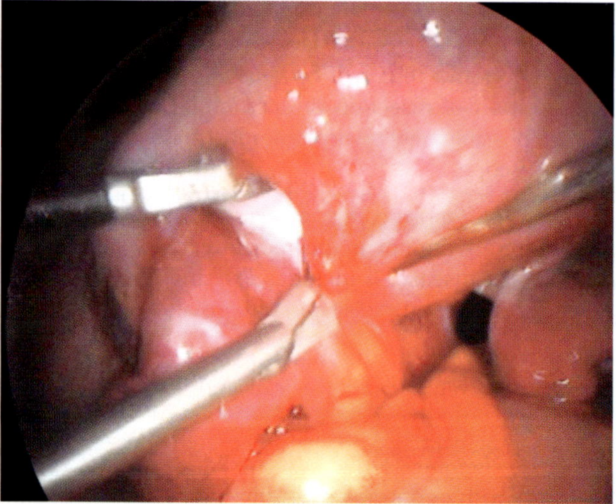

Fig. 8.8B: Rectal mobilization using blunt scissor

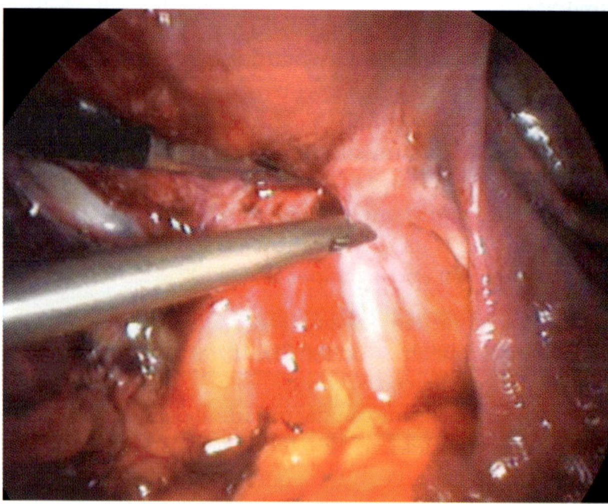

Fig. 8.8C: Rectal mobilization in progress

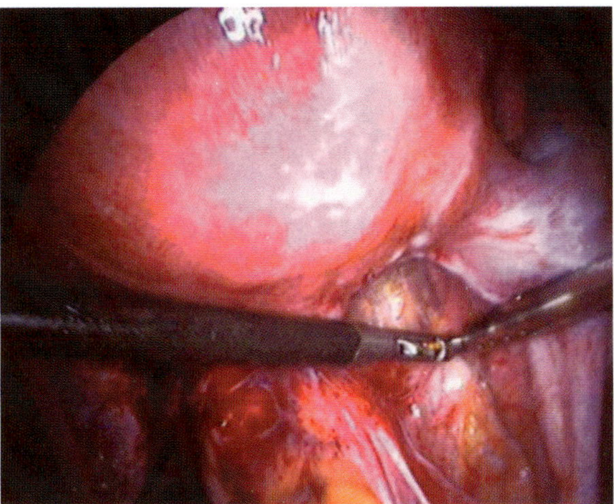

Fig. 8.9: Lateral clearing between the uterosacral ligament and rectum

rectal mobilization and lateral clearing using microbipolar forceps. Thorough suction irrigation and lavage is performed and complete hemostasis achieved (Figs 8.10A and B).

After this, attention is paid to the posterior vagina. If it is involved, excision of the involved vagina with the adenomyotic nodule is essential with a 0.5 cm disease-free vaginal margin around the nodule. En-bloc laparoscopic excision is done by using monopolar cautery on the sponge already inserted deep in the posterior vagina. Now, after complete rectal mobilization and the adenomyotic nodule being fully exposed, we put a sponge in vagina and prepare to excise the nodule in toto. Laser or monopolar hook can be used. All visible adenomyotic implants and nodules are excised along with a 5 mm disease-free margin. En-bloc laparoscopic excision right up to the vaginal wall is carried out and the pneumoperitoneum is maintained using a sponge in the vagina. The excised nodule is removed with a 10 mm claw forceps passed through a CCL extractor placed in the vagina (Figs 8.11A to F). The colpotomy wound is closed laparoscopically, employing 1 to 0 vicryl on curved needle (Figs 8.12A to F). After thorough suction irrigation and lavage, a suture is passed through the lower vaginal margin, then through the upper vaginal margin and the knot is secured by taking two throws of the suture. This is further reinforced by another knot by taking a single throw. Ipsilateral port placement works very well. A continuous closure from one end to the other is done and the hiatus closed completely. At the end, the suture is tied by utilizing the curve of the needle and taking two throws of the suture. The left needle holder then takes another single wrap and by pulling the sutures in opposite direction, a secure surgeon's knot is completed. Two liters of fluid are left in the peritoneal cavity. A cystoscopy is performed at the end of the procedure to check the integrity of the ureter after such an extensive procedure. Postoperative recovery and pain relief

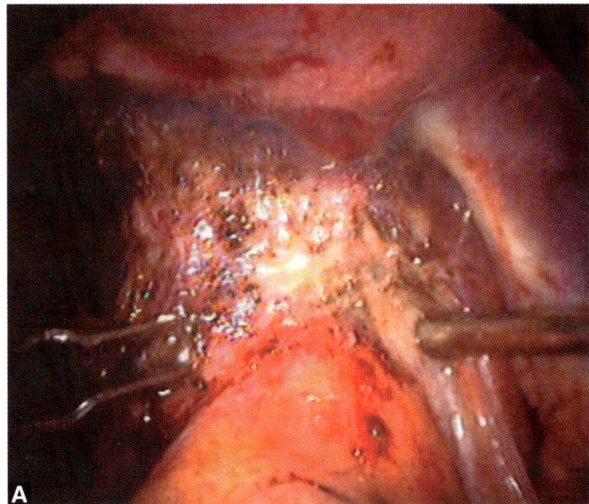

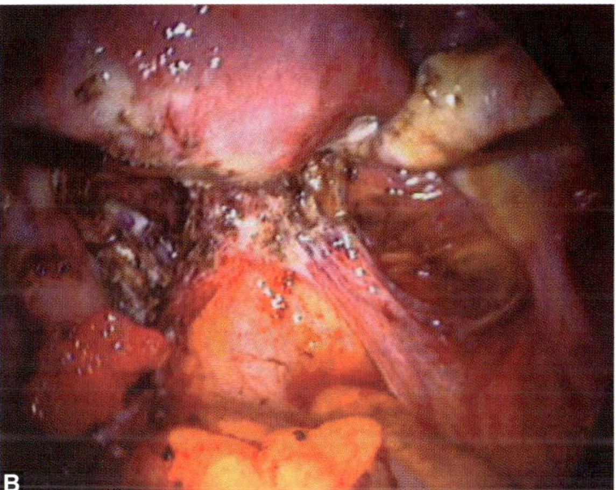

Figs 8.10A and B: Ablation of all endometriotic implants

are very good. Several literature reports of rectovaginal nodule excision by various authors have appeared. Full thickness rectal lesion resections were carried out and repaired with sutures in the series of Reich and associates.[22]

The point of rectal excision, partial or full thickness, remains debatable and essentially dependent on operator skill. Donnez,[23] his series of 1125 cases, feels that bowel resection is usually unnecessary except in cases of bowel occlusion and rectal bleeding. In such a case, resection of the rectosigmoid should be carried out,[23] while full thickness rectal lesions can be successfully repaired with sutures as in the series of Reich and associates.[22] Redwine and Wright[4] and Koh and Janik[24] are also proponents of more drastic radical excision involving the anterior rectum. While coming to the Indian scenario, this radical treatment is not so easily possible due to the lack of patient understanding of the disease, difficulty in obtaining consent and explanation for the need of colostomy in the eventuality of a mishap in radical rectal excision. Hence, most of us in India prefer to remain "radical reproductive

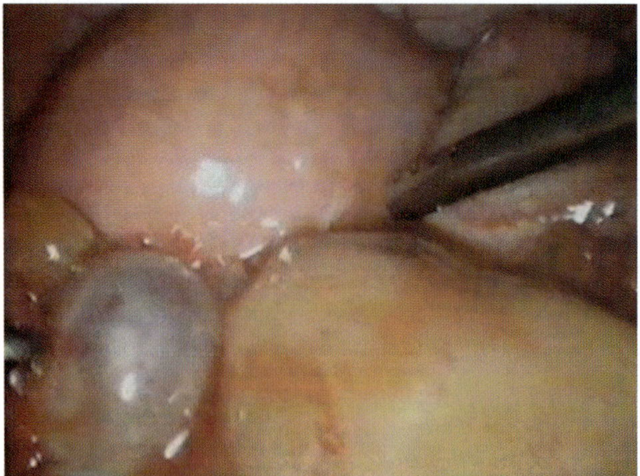

Fig. 8.11A: Total obliteration of pouch of Douglas

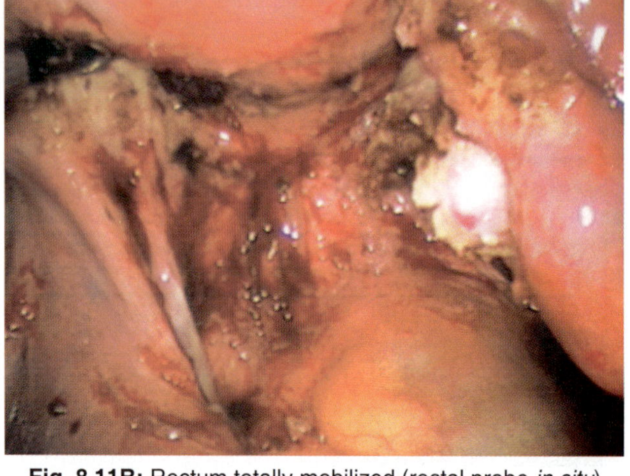

Fig. 8.11B: Rectum totally mobilized (rectal probe *in situ*) from the rectovaginal nodule

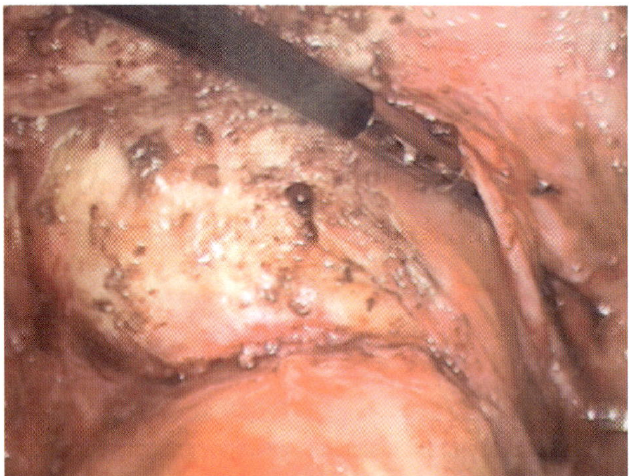

Fig. 8.11C: Appearance of rectovaginal nodule

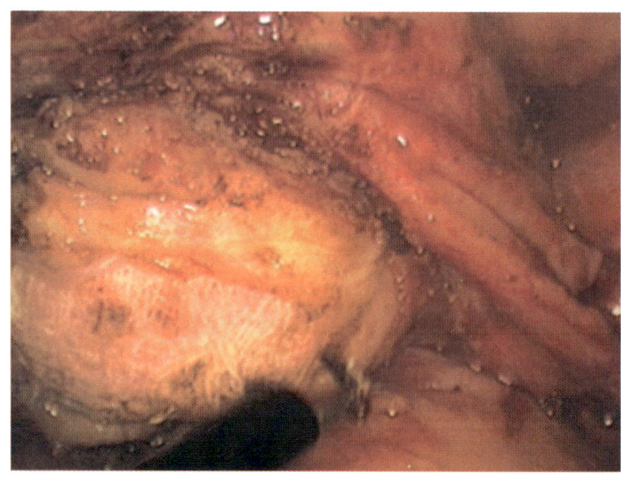

Fig. 8.11D: Incision by monopolar cautery for excision of adenomyotic nodule over a sponge in vagina

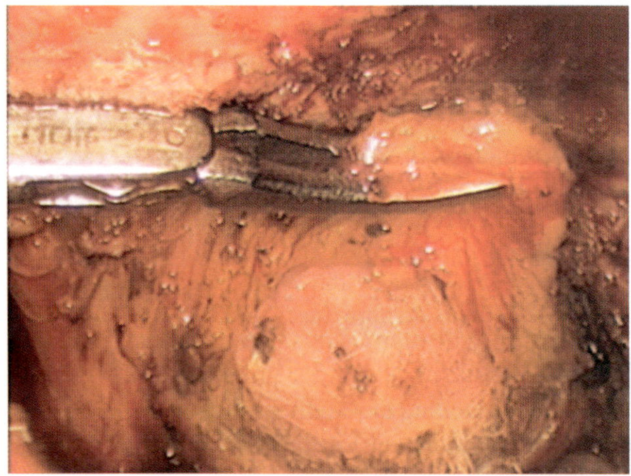

Fig. 8.11E: Continuing excision of adenomyotic nodule

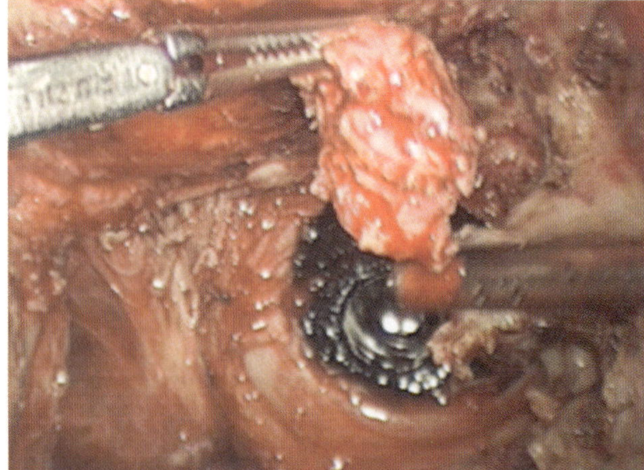

Fig. 8.11F: Complete excision and removal of adenomyotic nodule through CCL extractor and 10 mm claw forceps placed in vagina

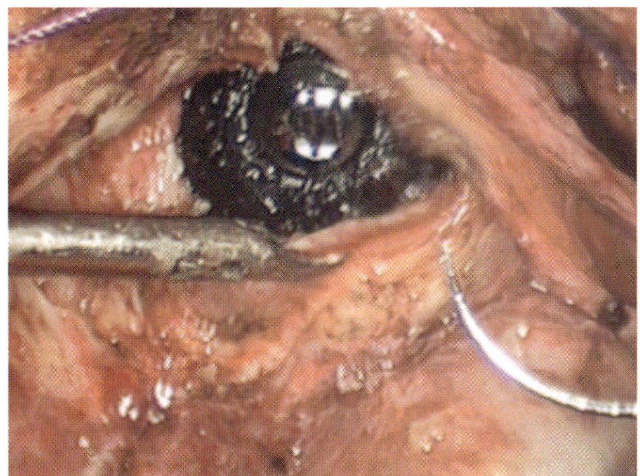

Fig. 8.12A: After rectovaginal nodule excision beginning curve needle suturing

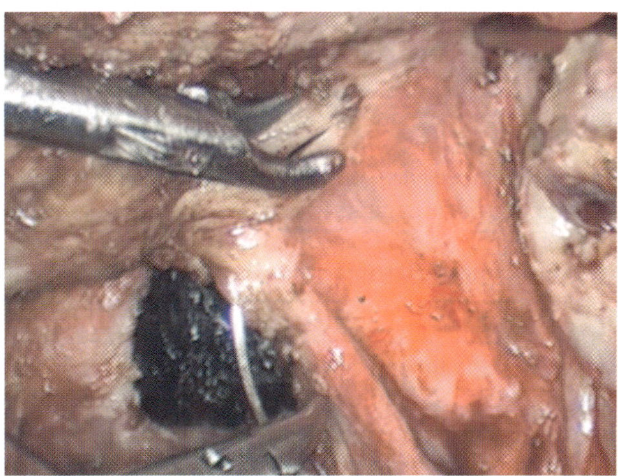

Fig. 8.12B: Passing the first suture through the lower and upper vagina flap

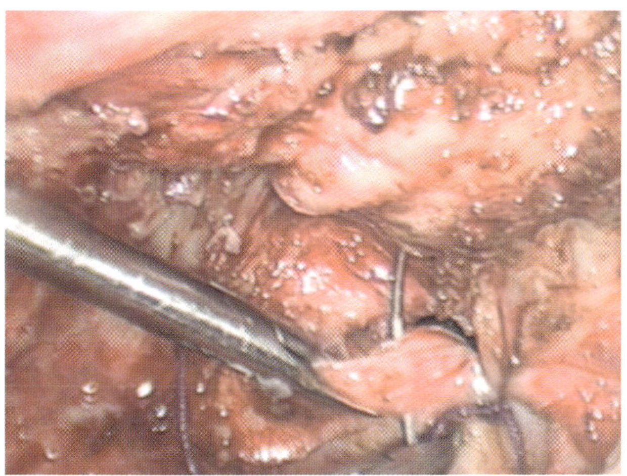

Fig. 8.12C: Progressive bite in the lower vagina flap

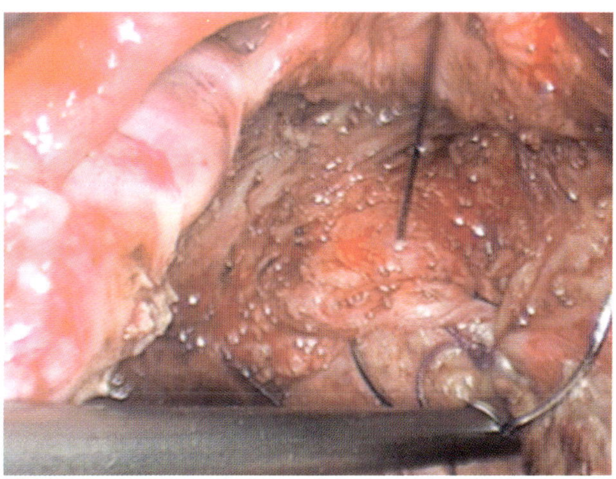

Fig. 8.12D: Continuous closure of colpotomy incision

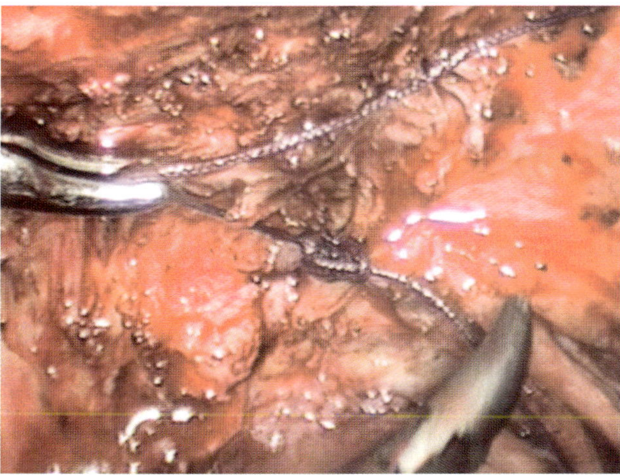

Fig. 8.12E: Tying the secure surgeons knot

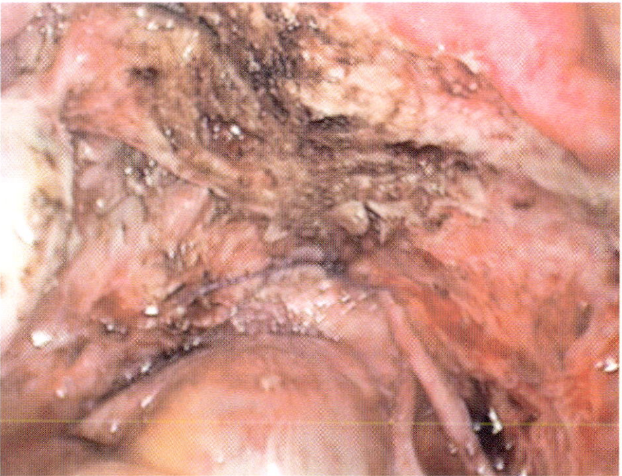

Fig. 8.12F: Final appearance of vaginal closure after rectovaginal nodule excision

surgeons" and mobilize the rectum from the posterior uterus, do the lateral clearing and ablate all endometriotic implants, refraining from radical rectal resection and anastomosis till absolutely necessary for rectal symptoms like cyclic rectal bleeding and/or severe dyschezia. Rectal excision, as a part of treatment for pelvic pain, is not commonly practised. We see more and more patients with infertility rather than pelvic pain, hence, the rationale against rectal nodule excision.

Risk for the rectal injury is real. Several case reports appear in literature. Donnez,[23] in his series cites seven rectal perforations out of 1125 cases. All the perforations were diagnosed at the time of laparoscopy. In 3 cases, the rectum was repaired by laparotomy and in the others, by colpotomy. In our series, we had one rectal perforation due to undue misdirected force on the rectal probe by the assistant during the final stage of the surgery during suction irrigation while the operating table was in reverse Trendelenburg position. This was repaired by laparoscopic double layer closure. This was accomplished by using 2 to 0 vicryl utilizing continuous curved needle suturing. The patient underwent smooth postoperative recovery with four days of IV supplementation and a nasogastric tube. There was no other postoperative complication.

Adenomyomectomy

Adenomyomectomy or debulking of a large adenomatous uterus can also be easily performed by laparoscopically using harmonic energy (Figs 8.13A to F). The preferred instrument is an ultrasonic long hook. A vertical incision is preferred as it

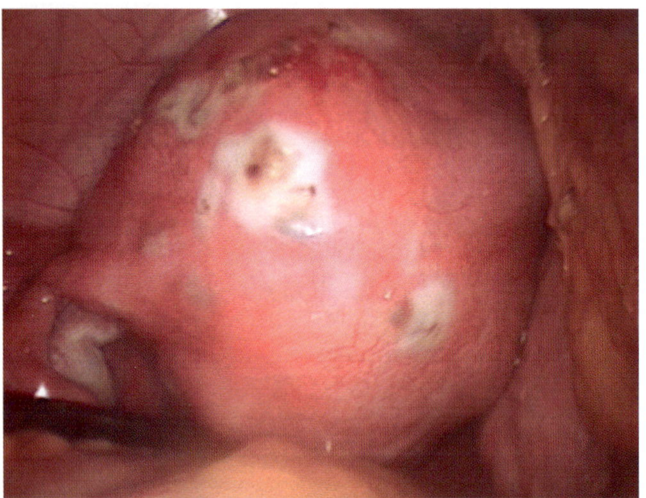

Fig. 8.13A: Initial appearance of adenomyosis

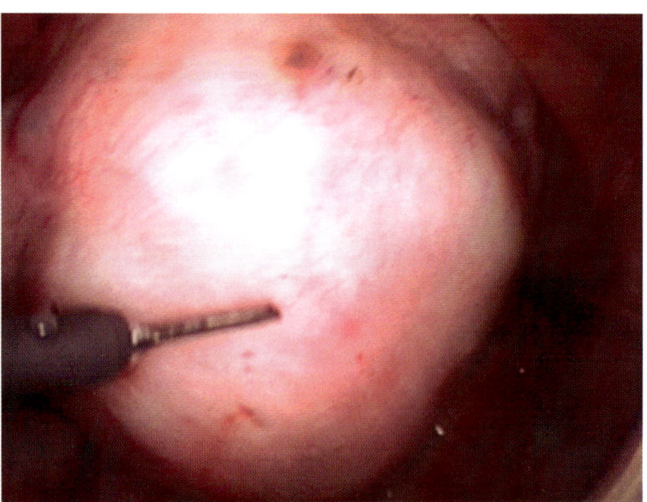

Fig. 8.13B: Injecting vasopressin

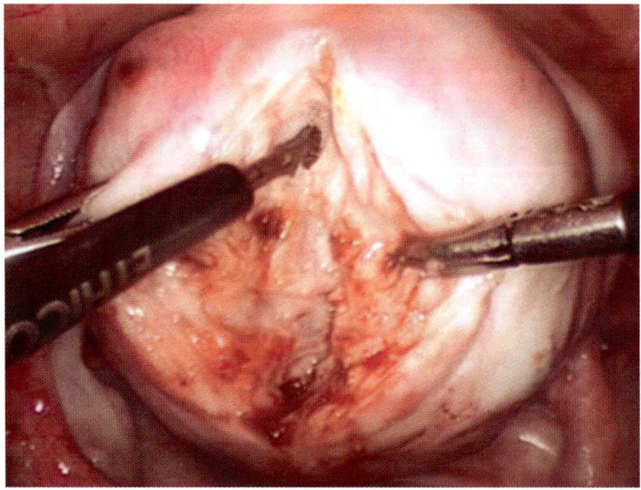

Fig. 8.13C: Vertical incision with the harmonic scalpel

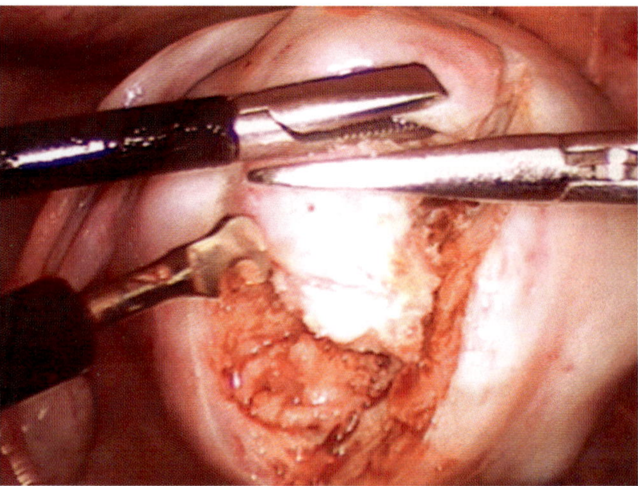

Fig. 8.13D: Beginning cutting of adenomyoma

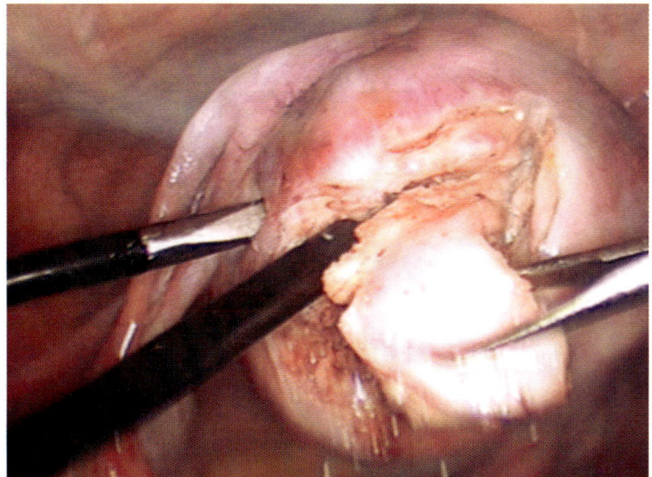

Fig. 8.13E: Adenomyomectomy in progress

Fig. 8.13F: Adenomyoma cutting on the other side by the harmonic scalpel

helps in coring out large chunks of adenomyotic tissue. Thick, fibrotic tissue of adenomyosis cuts well with the ultrasonic hook without causing smoke or char.

Gross debulking of the uterus is carried out. If a localized adenomyoma is present, then an adenomyomectomy similar to myomectomy is carried out. Though the plane of cleavage is not handy, coring out is carried out by harmonic shears or the hook blade. Hemostasis is easily obtained. Uterine reconstruction is best obtained by interrupted vertical mattress sutures, using 1 to 0 polyglactin suture material (Figs 8.14A to F). Attempts at meticulous closure, like for a myoma, in continuous fashion, is not possible due to very firm tissue dealt with for approximation. Postoperatively, patients benefit greatly in terms of symptoms of dysmenorrhea, dyspareunia and infertility. Several case reports from all over

are coming in favor of this type of laparoscopic surgery and benefit in infertility management.

Results

As with most surgical treatments, randomized controlled trials of radical excision of deep infiltrating endometriosis are not available, however, observational, comparative data and prospective clinical studies are encouraging.[25] In a retrospective study of 21 patients with resection of deep uterosacral ligament lesions, 84.2 percent had improvement in symptoms of dysmenorrhea, 94.1 percent had improvement in deep dyspareunia, and 77 percent had improvement in chronic pelvic pain.[26] The postoperative fertility rate achieved by Redwine and Wright[4] was 43

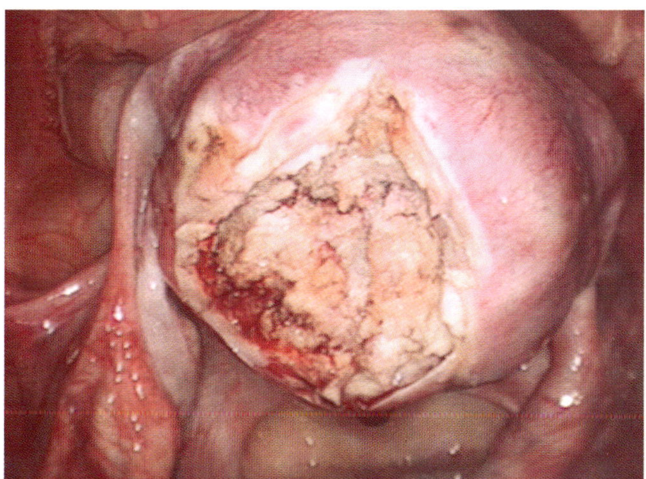

Fig. 8.14A: Uterus after debulking of adenomyosis

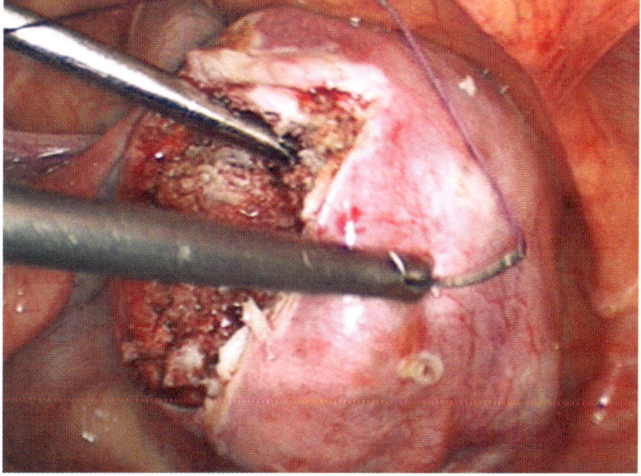

Fig. 8.14B: Passing deep suture with 1.0 vicryl taper cut needle

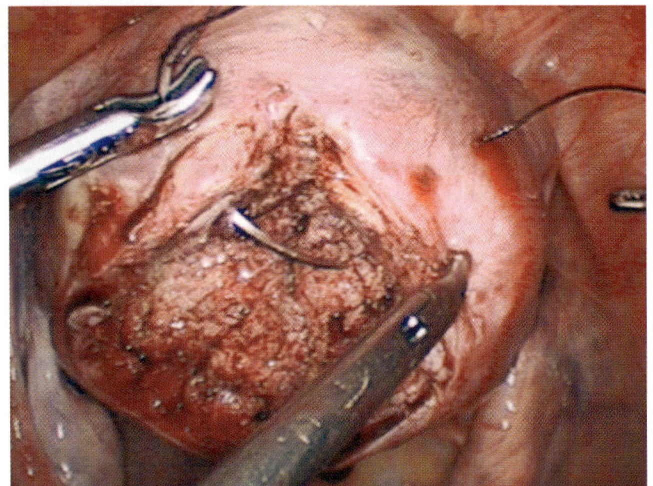

Fig. 8.14C: Passing mattress suture

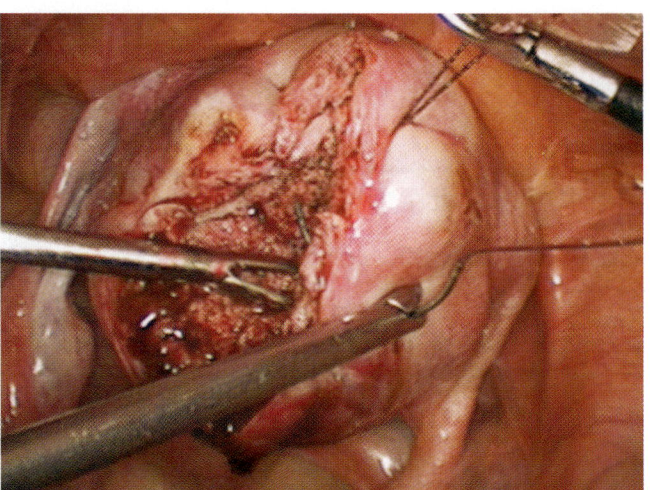

Fig. 8.14D: First knot tied and starting the second suture

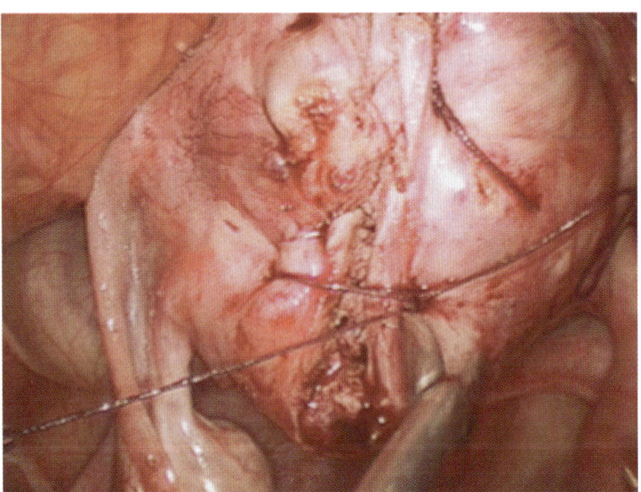

Fig. 8.14E: Tying the knot

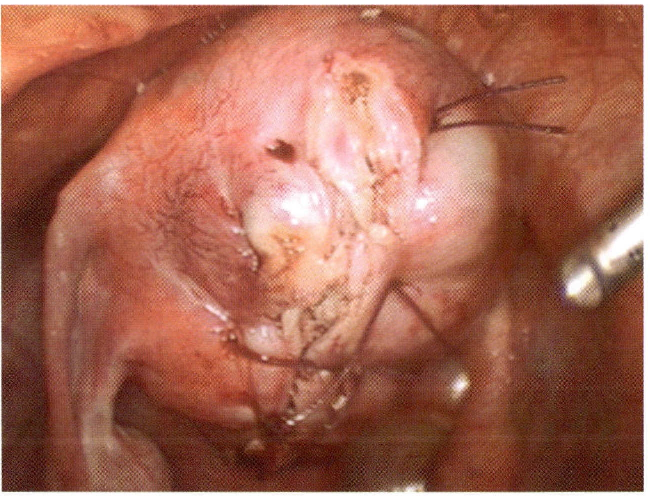

Fig. 8.14F: Final appearance of adenomyomectomy

percent. Similar good results for infertility outcome and pain relief have been reported by Koh and Janik,[24] Reich et al.[22] and Cannis and Martin.[27] We have done about 210 cases of superficial and deep endometriosis, treated exclusively by excision, in the last 30 months. There were no intraoperative or postoperative complications. In all the cases, cold scissors dissection and excision was carried out. A microbipolar forceps at low setting was employed for hemostasis. All the microsurgical principles for infertility surgery were strictly followed. A pregnancy rate of around 53 percent was achieved in all grades of excisional management. The pregnancy rates depend not only on the surgical technique but are also affected by variables like the duration of infertility, age of the patient and husband, and semen analysis parameters. All the patients are routinely followed-up by active infertility management with controlled ovarian hyperstimulation (COH) and intrauterine insemination (IUI). Very severe grades of endometriosis with alot of tubal damage are referred for *in vitro* fertilization (IVF). These results of excision of endometriosis are better than our previous results of fulguration and diathermy dessication.

CONCLUSION

In conclusion, deep infiltrating disease should be considered an adenomyoma different from mild and cystic ovarian endometriomas and deserves special treatment by a special surgical team and expertise. Radical resection of deep infiltrating endometriosis, according to Redwine, is "a feast for a surgeon who loves challenges", undoubtedly, not for the less experienced or chicken-hearted laparoscopist. Rectovaginal endometriosis remains the domain of skillful, select laparoscopic surgeons. This treatment is best offered by laparoscopy and with an established multispeciality team consisting of an expert gynecological endoscopist and a good operation theater team. Clinical results, in terms of pain relief and fertility outcome, are encouraging in all stages of the disease, hence, highly recommended as a surgical option, though one that requires greater skill.

REFERENCES

1. Kwok A, Lam A, Ford R. Deeply infiltrating endometriosis: implications, diagnosis, and management. Obstet Gynecol Survey 2001;56:168-77.
2. Fedele L, Bianchi S, Zanconato G, Tozzi L, Raffaelli R. Gonadotropin-releasing hormone agonist treatment for endometriosis of the rectovaginal septum. Am J Obstet Gynecol 2000;183:1462-7.
3. Shaw RW. Treatment of endometriosis. The Lancet 1992;340:1267-71.
4. Redwine DE, Wright JT. Laparoscopic treatment of complete obliteration of the cul-de-sac associated with endometriosis: long-term follow-up of en bloc resection. Fertil Steril 2001;76:358-65.
5. Redwine DD. Conservative laparoscopic excision of enodmetriosis by sharp dissection: life-table of reoperation and persistent or recurrent disease. Fertile Steril 1991;56:628-34.
6. Donnez J, Nisolle M, Casanas-Roux F. Three-dimensional architectures of peritoneal endometriosis. Fertil Steril 1992;57:980-3.
7. Nisolle M, Donnez J. Peritoneal endometriosis, ovarian endometriosis, and adenomyotic nodules of the rectovaginal septum are three different entities. Fertil Steril 1997;68:585-96.
8. Donnez J, Nisolle M. Appearances of peritoneal endometriosis. In Proceedings of The 3rd International Laser Surgery Symposium, Brussels, 1988.
9. Nisolle M, Paindaveine B, Bourdon A, Berlière M, Casanas-Roux F, Donnez J. Histologic study of peritoneal endometriosis in infertile women. Fertil Steril 1990;53:984–8.
10. Nisolle M, Casanas-Roux, Anaf V, Mine JM, Donnez J. Morphometric study of the stromal vascularization in peritoneal endometriosis. Fertil Steril 1993;59:681-4.
11. Hughesdon PE. The structure of endometrial cysts of the ovary. J Obstet Gynecol Br Empire 1957;64:481-7.
12. Donnez J, Nisolle M, Gillet N, Smets M, Bassil S, Casanas-Roux F. Large ovarian endometriomas. Hum Reprod 1996;11:641-64.
13. Donnez J, Nisolle M, Casanas-Roux F, et al. Laparoscopic treatment of rectovaginal septum endometriosis. In Donnez J, Nisolle M (Eds). An Atlas of Laser Operative Laparoscopy and Hysteroscopy. Carnforth, UK: Parthenon Publishing 1994: 75-85.
14. Donnez J, Nisolle M. Advanced laparoscopic surgery for the removal of rectovaginal septum endometriotic and adenomyotic nodules. Baillieres Clin Obstet Gynecol 1995;9:769-74.
15. Donnez J, Nisolle M, Casanas-Roux F, Bassil S, Anaf V. Rectovaginal septum endometriosis or adenomyosis: laparoscopic management in a series of 231 patients. Hum Reprod 1995;10:630-5.
16. Donnez J, Nisolle M, Gillenot S, Smets M, Bassil S, Casanas-Roux F. Rectovaginal septum adenomyotic nodules: a series of 500 cases. Br J Obstet Gynecol 1991;104:1009-13.
17. Soysal Me, Soysal S, Vicdan K. Laparoscopically assisted definitive treatment of severe endometriosis. Int J Gynecol Obstet 2001;72:191-2.
18. Redwine DB. Endometriosis persisting after castration: clinical characteristics and result of surgical management. Obstet Gynecol 1994;83:405-13.
19. Cullen TS. Distribution of adenomyoma containing uterine mucosa. Arch Surg 1920;1:215-82.
20. Sampson JA. Peritoneal endometriosis due to menstural dissemination of endometrial tissue into peritoneal cavity. Am J Obstet Gynecol 1927;14:422.
21. Novak ER, Woodruff JD. Pelvic endometriosis. Novak's Gynecologic and Obstetrics Pathology; 1974. p. 506.
22. Reich H, McGlynn F, Salvat J. Laparoscopic treatment of cul-de-sac obliteration secondary to retrocervical deep fibrotic endometriosis. J Reprod Med 1991;36:516-22.
23. Donnez J. Laparoscopic treatment of rectovaginal septum adenomyosis; State of the Art Atlas of Endoscopic Surgery in Infertility and Gynecology 2004;16:181.
24. Koh CH, Janik GM. The surgical management of deep rectovaginal endometriosis. Curr Opin Obstet Gynecol 2002;14: 357-64.
25. Jacobson TZ, Barlow DH, Garry R, Koninckx P. Laparoscopic surgery for pelvic pain associated with endometriosis. Cochrane Database Syst Rev 2001;4:CD001300.
26. Donnez J, Nisolle M, Gillerot, Smets M, Bassil S, Casanas-Roux F.. Rectovaginal septum adenomyotic nodules: a series of 500 cases. Br J Obstet Gynaecol 1997;104:1014-8.
27. Martin DC. Laparoscopic and vaginal colpotomy for the excision of infiltrating cul-de-sac endometriosis. J Reprod Med 1988; 33:806-8.

Laparoscopic Myomectomy: Is it Worth it?

Yuval Kaufman, Arie Lissak

OVERVIEW

Uterine fibroids are the most common gynecological tumors in women with a prevalence of 20 to 40 percent during their reproductive years. The most common symptoms include menorrhagias, hypermenorrhea and pelvic mass symptoms. Their occurrence depends on the number, size and location of the leiomyomas. Treatment options vary from medical treatment to minimally invasive procedures and open abdominal surgery. Myomectomy is the procedure of choice for women with symptomatic fibroids who wish to retain childbearing potential or those who wish to preserve their uterus for psychological purposes. Laparoscopic myomectomy is considered an advanced laparoscopic procedure. A great deal of laparoscopic suturing and hemostasis control is necessary to complete the procedure. Hence, both surgical skill and experience are required. Success depends not only on the surgeon but also on proper patient selection. After determining patient expectations, a thorough assessment of the number, size and location of the myomas is mandatory. Laparoscopic myomectomy has been shown to be associated with less postoperative pain, shorter hospital stay and a shorter recovery from surgery when compared to laparotomic myomectomy, however, the duration of surgery and blood loss are no different. With laparoscopic myomectomy, the conversion rate to laparotomy is low and postoperative adhesions are less common. There is no proven risk for uterine rupture during a subsequent pregnancy and the risk for a clinically significant myoma recurrence is similar to the risk following an open myomectomy. Therefore, laparoscopic myomectomy should be the procedure of choice for properly selected patients.

INTRODUCTION

Uterine leiomyomas are benign smooth muscle tumors that form within the myometrium of the uterus. Also known as uterine fibroids, they are the most common of gynecological tumors with a prevalence that varies with age, race and method of diagnosis. During the reproductive years, leiomyomas can be found in 20 to 40 percent of the women.[1] As their prevalence increases with age, ultrasound screening shows a cumulative rate of up to 70 percent of white women and 80 percent of African-Americans by the age of 50.[2] Symptomatic leiomyomas peak during the perimenopausal years due to the effect of unopposed estrogen caused by anovulatory cycles followed by a decline during menopause when hormonal effects are minimal.[3] In the United States alone, there were 198,000 hysterectomies performed due to fibroid uteri out of 598,000 (33%) during 1999. At the same time, only 30,000 myomectomies were performed.[4]

The majority of women with leiomyomata is asymptomatic, with only 20 to 50 percent of those who have one or more leiomyomas experiencing any symptoms directly related to the tumor.[5] Symptoms are varied (Table 9.1) and depend on the number, size and location of the leiomyomas. The most common symptoms are menorrhagias or hypermenorrhea, which can lead to anemia. Pelvic mass symptoms are caused by pelvic pressure and increased abdominal girth. They depend on the size and location of the myomas in relation to the adjacent organs causing, mostly, urinary and gastrointestinal symptoms as well as abdominal discomfort. Pain is less commonly encountered and can be related to a pedunculated myoma in torsion or cervical dilatation due to a cervical myoma. During pregnancy, pain can be related to a red degeneration of the myoma.

Leiomyomas are an uncommon cause of infertility. Although they can be found in 27 percent of infertile women, they appear to be associated with infertility in only 5 to 10 percent of the cases and are a sole cause for infertility in only 2 to 3 percent of these women.[5,6] The exact pathogenesis is unknown but may be related to mechanical, vascular or immunological factors.[5] Possible mechanical factors

Table 9.1: Possible symptoms resulting from uterine leiomyomas	
Abnormal uterine bleeding	*Pregnancy-related*
Menorrhagias	Spontaneous miscarriage
Hypermenorrhea	Recurrent pregnancy loss
Anemia	Red degeneration
Urinary symptoms	Intrauterine growth restriction
Frequency	Preterm delivery
Incontinence	Premature rupture of membranes
Outflow obstruction	Placental abruption
Hydronephrosis	Pre-eclampsia
Gastrointestinal symptoms	Malpresentation
Constipation	Increased rate of cesarean delivery
Tenesmus	Postpartum hemorrhage
Rectal pressure	Decreased Apgar score
Pelvic pain	Fetal anomalies (limb reduction, head deformities, torticolis)
Infertility	

include obstruction of the tubal ostia, sperm blockage by a cervical myoma, alteration of the endometrial contour and the persistence of endometrial blood clots interfering with sperm transport and embryo implantation. Vascular disturbances can be at the endometrial or subendometrial level, reducing endometrial receptivity. These changes can eventually cause endometrial thinning, ulceration and inflammation, releasing cytokines and growth factors, which can inhibit embryo implantation. Infertility is mostly associated with submucosal myomas and a debate exists whether intramural and sub-serosal myomas can be a cause of infertility. Some studies have concluded that there is no reduction in implantation and pregnancy rates with intramural and subserous myomas, whereas other studies claim there is a connection.[5] A causal relationship has not been found, but a recent prospective study of *in vitro* fertilization (IVF) patients with a mechanical factor and uterine myomas showed an increase in pregnancy rate from 15 to 33 percent for women undergoing laparoscopic myomectomy. All patients had 1 to 5 myomas that were not submucosal, with at least one myoma over 5 centimeters in diameter.[7]

Obstetric complications related to leiomyomas are mostly caused by aberrant placentation causing placental insufficiency, placental abruption, preterm labor and premature rupture of membranes.[5] Their mass effect can also cause malpresentation and dystocia when located near the cervix. Myomas that increase in size are more prone to undergo red degeneration. Due to the heterogeneity of myomas, they behave differently to the hormonal influences of pregnancy, with some myomas increasing in size, whereas others decreasing or remaining static. If there is an increase in size, it is usually found during the first trimester.[8]

CLINICAL DISCUSSION

The variety of treatment methods for symptomatic leiomyomas has increased with the years, with some forms of treatment gaining more popularity than others. Treatment methods (Table 9.2) include expectant management, medical treatment and surgical intervention, including minimally invasive procedures. Factors to consider when deciding on the type of treatment include aspects that are related to the patient's status and desires, as well as elements related to the leiomyomas. Demographic aspects include age, medical status, obstetric history as well as future family planning, extent and severity of symptoms, signs of pending menopause, willingness to undergo invasive procedures and the patient's desire for uterine preservation or removal. Elements related to the leiomyomas include size, location, position (submucosal, intramural and subserosal), the number of myomas and the growth rate of the myomas. Treatment should be tailored after the patient is made aware of all the relevant therapeutic possibilities and gives an informed consent.

Medical treatment is usually of limited value because of an insufficient decrease in myoma size, an increase to pretherapy size after discontinuation of treatment and because of potential side effects. The most studied formulas are gonadotropin-releasing hormone (GnRH) agonists, which are considered the most successful of medical treatments. GnRH agonists can be administered for several cycles before performing myomectomy (especially hysteroscopic) in order to decrease the size of the myomas by up to 60 to 70 percent. This may allow surgery to be less extensive[9,10] although it is believed by some investigators that GnRH agonists can

Table 9.2: The different forms of treatment for uterine leiomyomas	
Medical management	*Minimally invasive techniques*
• Estrogen/progestin	• Thermomyolysis
• Progestin only	• Cryomyolysis
• GnRH agonist	• MRI-guided high-frequency ultrasound (HIFUS)
• GnRH antagonist	
• Aromatase inhibitors	***Surgery***
• Raloxifene	• Uterine artery embolization
• Mifepristone	• Myomectomy
• Asoprisnil	– Laparoscopic
• Androgens	– Hysteroscopic
• Levonorgestrel-releasing intrauterine device	– Open
	• Hysterectomy
	– Laparoscopic
	– Vaginal
	– Abdominal

distort the myoma-uterus interface and make the dissection more difficult.[1] Long-term treatment may cause symptoms of hypoestrogenism, including hot flushes, headaches vaginal dryness, depression and osteoporosis. Discontinuation of treatment causes myomas to increase to their original size within 3 months.

Other medical treatments, such as aromatase inhibitors, have been investigated less extensively but may have promising results in the future. One interesting option is the Levonogestrel-releasing intrauterine device (IUD) called Mirena (Scherring, Germany). This type of IUD has been shown to significantly reduce menstrual bleeding without causing any major side effects.[11,12] Although a fibroid uterus with an enlarged or distorted uterine cavity is considered a contraindication for the use of Mirena (due to possible ineffective contraception), some studies have investigated its effect on myomas and have shown a reduction in size, as well as a significant reduction in menstrual bleeding,[11] but these are only small clinical trials.

Minimally invasive procedures are gaining increasing popularity due to their lower complication rates and shorter hospital stay. Minimally invasive techniques for treating fibroid uteri include myolysis and laparoscopic myomectomy or hysterectomy. Myolysis is done by creating focal tissue damage followed by necrosis within the myoma, causing it to shrink or completely degenerate. Thermomyolysis can be done by using either a laser or a bipolar electrical probe. To access the myoma, laparoscopy is required. Cryomyolysis is performed by using probes cooled up to −90°C by liquid nitrogen or differential gas exchange. Both myolysis techniques have been shown to reduce myoma volume by about 50 to 60 percent and are reserved for women with no desire for future fertility.[13] There have been reports of uterine rupture with thermomyolysis. Magnetic resonance imaging (MRI) guided, high-frequency ultrasound (HIFUS) is another non-invasive modality to shrink myomas. It is done by using multiple ultrasound beams that concentrate within the target area, causing destruction of the lesion. This treatment is still considered quasi-experimental and is not used for women who desire future fertility. Another important technique for women who wish to avoid surgery is selective uterine artery embolization (UAE). This technique has been used by invasive radiologists to control extensive uterine bleeding, usually in relation to cesarean sections. UAE has shown good results with fibroid uteri, including up to 90 percent symptom resolution.[14] There have been reports of significant post-procedural pain and infection. Amenorrhea and premature ovarian failure have also been reported and in women who have conceived following embolization and there were more cases of spontaneous abortions, preterm delivery, abnormal placentation and postpartum hemorrhage when compared to myomectomy.[15] The American College of Obstetrics and Gynecologists recommended in 2004 that UAE should be considered investigational or relatively contraindicated in women wishing to retain fertility.[16] The Randomized Trial of Embolization versus Surgical Treatment for Fibroids (REST) has recently reported the results of a comparison between UAE and open hysterectomy or myomectomy. The study showed similar rates of minor complications and major adverse events for both types of procedures. UAE was associated with faster recovery and resumption of usual activities, but also a higher rate of secondary intervention after 1 year to treat persistent or recurrent symptoms.[17] This study has been criticized for its methodology, but mainly for the fact that most of the surgical procedures were hysterectomies done by laparotomy (43 out of 51 patients) with 8 open myomectomies and no laparoscopic procedures. This can definitely contribute to a slower recovery rate when compared to UAE.[17]

Successful ligation has also been reported by laparoscopic surgical ligation of the uterine arteries either by vascular clips[18] or bipolar coagulation.[19] Another interesting option is the non-incision temporary uterine clamp, which is placed on both vaginal fornices under Doppler guidance without entering the peritoneum.[20] Unfortunately, this device has never been commercialized due to troubling complications, such as clamping of the ureters, during the procedure.

Abdominal hysterectomy has been shown to improve the quality of life for women with uterine myomas, relieving them from symptoms, such as bleeding, pelvic pressure, pain and urinary incontinence,[21-23] without impairing sexuality. Although hysterectomy still remains the surgical treatment of choice for women who have completed their childbearing, there is an increase in demand for more conservative approaches for women opting to avoid surgical intervention or those who want to retain their uteri. However, hysterectomy is still considered the procedure of choice when there is an increased possibility of malignancy, as suggested by MRI or computerized tomography (CT) imaging, or when myomectomy is likely to fail due to a uterus with an extensive number of myomas.

Myomectomy is the procedure of choice for women with symptomatic fibroids, who wish to retain childbearing potential, or those who wish to keep their uterus for psychological purposes. Submucosal myomas can be treated by hysteroscopy (or vaginal surgery in cases of a pedunculated myoma. Intramural and subserosal fibroids require an abdominal laparoscopic or open approach.

CASE STUDIES

Laparoscopic minimal invasive surgery has proven its benefits in many fields, including gynecological surgery. Today, it is considered the goldstandard choice for many procedures such as salpingostomy or salpingectomy for ectopic pregnancy, salpingo-oophorectomy and most cases of hysterectomy. Its major limitation is the need for extensive experience and expertise to perform advanced laparoscopic surgery. Surgical centers that have these abilities can perform complex procedures such as radical hysterectomy or pelvic exanterations by laparoscopy. Laparoscopic myomectomy is considered a level IV procedure according to the guidelines formed by the European Society for Human Reproduction and Embryology (ESHRE) Committee of Special Interest Group on Reproductive Surgery.[24] This is the highest skill level and it includes other procedures, including treatment of severe and retroperitoneal endometriosis, oncologic procedures and more. Since its first description by Semm and Mettler in 1980,[25] laparoscopic myomectomy has become more common and more feasible with the improvement of technical skills. Today, a successful laparoscopic myomectomy depends chiefly on the number, size and location of the myomas as well as the surgeon's laparoscopic surgical skills. Laparoscopic myomectomy has been shown to be associated with less postoperative pain, shorter hospital stay and a shorter recovery from surgery when compared to myomectomy done by laparotomy.[26] The cut-off criteria for a successful laparoscopic myomectomy in terms of number and size of myomas have been escalating. Based on their experience as well as previous studies, Dubuisson and his colleagues[27] set the feasibility cut-off point at 2 to 3 subserous or intramural myomas with an average size smaller than 9 cm. Since then, successful myomectomies have been performed on myomas that reach up to 20 centimeters in diameter[28] and uteri that are equivalent to 16 weeks of pregnancy or larger.[29] Fine imaging studies are required in order to assess per case feasibility of laparoscopic myomectomy. This is usually done by transvaginal sonography although MRI is an excellent tool for describing the number, size and location of the myomas and for discriminating between a myoma and adenomyosis.

When evaluating the safety and efficacy of laparoscopic myomectomy vs myomectomy performed by laparotomy, there are several factors that must be considered:

- Surgery duration
- Amount of blood loss
- Conversion to laparotomy
- Postoperative adhesions
- The risk of uterine rupture
- Myoma recurrence.

- *Surgery duration:* The first trials published on laparoscopic myomectomy showed a considerably longer duration of surgery when compared to laparotomy. More recent publications show that the laparoscopic surgery time for myomectomy has decreased substantially and has now become comparable to laparotomy in selected patients.[4,26,30-33] A study done by Mais and colleagues,[26] comparing myomectomy done by laparoscopy vs laparotomy, showed no significant difference in surgery duration (100 minutes, vs 93 minutes, respectively). This study included patients with no more than 4 myomas with a maximal diameter of the largest myoma being 3 to 6 centimeters. The inclusion criteria were selected following a pilot study that showed a significantly increased operative time when there were more than 4 myomas and the largest myoma had a mean diameter larger than 6 centimeters. Another comparative study, done by Seracchioli et al.[32] included patients with uteri that had at least one myoma greater than 5 centimeters in diameter but no more than a total of three myomas. This study also showed no difference in operative time between the two groups. In a prospective study of 368 patients with 768 myomas, the mean operative duration was 100 minutes.[33] In a another study, proving the feasibility of laparoscopic myomectomy for large myomas, Malzoni and his colleagues[34] performed myomectomy in women with uteri containing myomas ranging from 5 to 18 centimeters with a mean size of 8 centimeters.[34] Their average operative time was 95 minutes (with a range of 58 to 180 minutes) with only a 1.4 percent conversion rate to laparotomy. Mettler and colleagues[35] performed laparoscopic myomectomy on patients with uteri containing a mean myoma diameter of 4 centimeters. Their mean surgical duration was 90 minutes (with a range of 25 to 215 minutes). Therefore, most recent studies have an average operating time of 90 to 100 minutes for laparoscopic myomectomy, which is no longer than an average open myomectomy.

- *Amount of blood loss:* Laparoscopic myomectomy is associated with less blood loss than open myomectomy. A study comparing both types of myomectomies showed a greater drop in hemoglobin level following open myomectomy (2.17 g/dL vs 1.33 g/dL).[32] The study also showed more postoperative fever and longer hospital stays when myomectomy was done by laparotomy. Landi and colleagues[33] showed a decrease in hemoglobin level of 1.4 g/dL when using vasopressin.[33]

- *Conversion to laparotomy:* The rate of conversion from laparoscopy to laparotomy during myomectomy has been reported between 0 percent and 11 percent. Dubuisson and his colleagues[36] reported a conversion rate of 11.3 percent. Conversion was performed when there was a lack of a clear myoma-uterus cleavage plane, when there was concern for insufficient sutures over the uterine defect and when there was excessive bleeding that was difficult to control and would lead to blood transfusion.[36] A fibroid size larger than 5 centimeters, an intramural location of the myoma, anterior location of the largest fibroid and preoperative GnRH administration have been reported as independent risk factors for conversion. A retrospective chart analysis of 351 patients showed an average conversion rate to laparotomy of 0.6 percent during myomectomy.[37] The conversion rate was influenced by the experience of the performing surgeon. Landi and colleagues[33] had no conversions to laparotomy during laparoscopic myomectomy.[33] They did not use GnRH agonists since they claim it makes myomectomy more difficult, mainly due to loss of a clear cleavage plane of the myoma-uterus interface. Others[35] claim that performing laparoscopic myomectomy six weeks after cessation of a GnRH agonist causes shrinkage of the myomas without the loss of a cleavage plane. They claim that the estrogen that is secreted during this period causes an increase in myoma vascularization, making it easier to enucleate it.[35] For cases of difficulty during suturing or increased hemorrhage, a laparoscopically assisted myomectomy can be performed. This approach includes enucleation of the myomas by laparoscopy and suturing of the uterine defects by minilaparotomy.[38]

- *Postoperative adhesions:* Postoperative intraperitoneal adhesions are considered very common after open myomectomy, even with the use of adhesion preventive barriers. Laparoscopic myomectomy has been found to substantially reduce adhesions. Dubuisson and his colleagues[27] analyzed studies that have performed a second-look laparoscopy after myomectomy. They found that the frequency of adhesions was 51.1 percent after laparoscopic myomectomy and 89.6 percent after open myomectomy. The percentage of patients with adnexal adhesions was 30.5 percent vs 68.9 percent, respectively.[27] Fewer postoperative adhesions following laparoscopy have also been found after surgery due to a tubal ectopic pregnancy.[39] Risk factors for adhesions include addition of a second surgical procedure during laparoscopic myomectomy, evidence of adhesions that existed before the current surgery and a posterior location of the myoma.[40]

- *The risk of uterine rupture:* It is estimated that the risk of uterine rupture during pregnancy or delivery following open myomectomy is between 0.002 percent and 5 percent.[41] Since laparoscopic myomectomy is a relatively new procedure, the risk of rupture following this procedure remains unknown. Uterine dehiscence or rupture has been reported in 11 cases following laparoscopic myomectomy.[4] In a series of 100 cases Dubuisson and his colleagues[27] reported one case of uterine rupture.[27] Nine other studies, including a total of 156 patients, had no cases of uterine rupture. Possible causes for rupture include inadequate approximation of the myomectomy margins or hematomas within the myometrium, causing impaired scar healing. Another possible cause is necrosis due to excessive electrocautery, causing impaired vascularization within the uterus. A study that compared laparoscopic vs open myomectomy showed no case of uterine rupture in both groups following myomectomy.[30]

An elective cesarean section has classically been recommended when the uterine cavity has been entered during myomectomy. Others recommend performing a cesarean section if over 50 percent of the myometrium has been penetrated since the myometrium gives the uterus its tensile strength.[15]

- *Myoma recurrence:* An ultrasonographic study has found myomas recurring in up to 50 percent of patients within 5 years following myomectomy done by laparotomy.[42] Another study has estimated symptomatic recurrence in 15 to 30 percent of patients within 10 years of open myomectomy.[43] It has been speculated that the loss of ability to palpate the uterus during laparoscopy may lead to an incomplete removal of small myomas and eventually, to a higher rate of myoma recurrence. Rosetti and colleagues[44] performed a prospective randomized study of 81 patients undergoing either laparoscopic or open myomectomy.[44] They followed the patients sonographically every 6 months for at least 40 months and found a recurrence of myomas larger than 1 cm in 27 percent of women after laparoscopic myomectomy, and in 23 percent of women following open myomectomy. None of the women required reoperation or any other procedure as a result of the recurrence. Seracchioli and colleagues[32] also found no difference with regard to recurrence with a 21 percent rate for both the groups.[32]

CONCLUSION

Women who are being counseled regarding treatment options for leiomyomata should be made aware of all the different options. Hysterectomy remains the procedure of choice for women who have completed their childbearing and do not desire to retain their uterus. If myomectomy is required, a minimal invasive approach would be a good choice if the patient is an appropriate candidate. A successful laparoscopic myomectomy depends mostly on two factors. First, the surgeon should be able to decide truly and accurately whether the patient is suitable for this kind of procedure or are the chances for conversion to laparotomy high. A feasibility investigation should include a good ultrasound or MRI scan that describes the exact size and location of all myomas within the uterus. Second, the surgeon has to be highly skilled and experienced with advanced laparoscopic surgery. Surgical expertise is a crucial factor for success. For a suitable patient, in the right hands, laparoscopic myomectomy has proven to be a safer procedure than open myomectomy, with less postoperative pain, shorter hospital stay and a shorter recovery from surgery. Surgery duration and blood loss are no different. The conversion rate to laparotomy is low and postoperative adhesions are less common. There is no proven risk for uterine rupture during a subsequent pregnancy and the risk for a clinically significant myoma recurrence is similar to the risk following open myomectomy. Laparoscopic myomectomy has evolved from being a bold and risky procedure to becoming a logical and widely accepted procedure that can be done in most gynecological endoscopic surgery rooms performing advanced laparoscopic surgery.

REFERENCES

1. Wallach EE, Vlahos NF. Uterine myomas: an overview of development, clinical features, and management. Obstet Gynecol 2004;104:393-406.
2. Day Baird D, Dunson DB, Hill MC, et al. High cumulative incidence of uterine leiomyoma in black and white women: ultrasound evidence. Am J Obstet Gynecol 2003; 188:100-7.
3. Flake GP, Andersen J, Dixon D. Etiology and pathogenesis of uterine leiomyomas: a review. Environ Health Perspect 2003; 111:1037-54.
4. Parker WH. Laparoscopic myomectomy and abdominal myomectomy. Clin Obstet Gynecol 2006;49:787-97.
5. Bukulmez O, Doody KJ. Clinical features of myomas. Obstet Gynecol Clin North Am 2006;33:69-84.
6. Practice committee of the American Society of Reproductive Medicine. Myomas and reproductive function. Fertil Steril 2004;82(suppl 1):S111-6.
7. Bulleti C, DE Ziegler D, Levi Setti P, et al. Myomas, pregnancy outcome, and *in vitro* fertilization. Ann N Y Acad Sci 2004;1034:84-92.
8. Lev-Toaff AS, Coleman BG, Arger PH, et al. Leiomyomas in pregnancy: sonographic study. Radiology 1987;164:375-80.
9. Andreyko JL, Blumenfeld Z, Marshal LA, et al. Use of an agonistic analog of gonoadotropin-releasing hormone (nafarelin) to treat leiomyomas: assessment by magnetic resonance imaging. Am J Obstet Gynecol 1988; 158:903-10.
10. Maheux R, Lemay A, Merat P. Use of intranasal luteinizing hormone-releasing hormone agonist in uterine leiomyomas. Fertil Steril 1987;47:229-33.
11. Hurskainen R, Paavonen J. Levonogestrel-releasing intrauterine system in the treatment of heavy menstrual bleeding. Curr Opin Obstet Gynecol 2004;16:487-90.
12. Stewart A, Cummins C, Gold L, Jordan R, Phillips W. The effectiveness of the levonogestrel-releasing intrauterine system in menorrhagia: a systematic review. BJOG 2001;108:74-86.
13. Zupi E, Sbracia M, Marconi D, Munro M. Myolysis of uterine fibroids: is there a role?. Clin Obstet Gynecol 2006;49:821-33.
14. Spies JB, Ascher SA, Roth AR, et al. Uterine artery embolization for leiomyomata. Obstet Gynecol 2001;98:29-34.
15. Goldberg J, Pereira L. Pregnancy outcomes following treatment for fibroids: uterine fibroid embolization versus laparoscopic myomectomy. Curr Opin Obstet Gynecol 2006;18:402-6.
16. ACOG. Uterine artery embolization. Committee opinion No. 293. Obstet Gynecol 2004;103:403-4.
17. Edwards RD, Moss JG, Lumsden MA, et al. Committee of the Randomized Trial of Embolization versus Surgical Treatment for Fibroids. Uterine-artery embolization versus surgery for symptomatic uterine fibroids. N Engl J Med 2007;356:360-70.
18. Lee PI, Chang YK, Yoon JB. Preliminary experience with uterine artery ligation for symptomatic uterine leiomyomas. J Am Assoc Gynecol Laparosc 1999;6:S27-S28.
19. Lui WM, Ng HT, Wu YC, Yen YK, Yuan CC. Laparoscopic bipolar coagulation of uterine vessels: a new method for treating symptomatic fibroids. Fertil Steril 2001;75:417-22.
20. Istre O. Uterine artery occlusion for the treatment of symptomatic fibroids: Endoscopic, radiological and vaginal approach. Minim Invasive Ther Allied Technol 2005;14: 167-74.
21. Weber AM, Walters MD, Scover LR. MR. Functional outcomes and satisfaction after abdominal hysterectomy. Am J Obstet Gynecol 1999;181:530-35.
22. Kjerulff KH, Langenberg PW, Rhodes JC, et al. Effectiveness of hysterectomy. Obstet Gynecol 2000;95:319-26.
23. Rowe MK, Kanouse DE, Mittman BS, Bernstein SJ. Quality of life among women undergoing hysterectomies. Obstet Gynecol 1999;93:915-21.
24. Chapron C, Devroey P, Dubuisson JB, et al. (Committee of special interest group on reproductive surgery). ESHRE guidelines for training, accreation and monitoring in gynaecological endoscopy. Fertil Steril 1997;12:867-8.
25. Semm K, Mettler L. Technical progress in pelvic surgery via operative laparoscopy. Am J Obstet Gynecol 1980;138:121-7.
26. Mais V, Ajossa S, Guerriero S, et al. Laparoscopic versus abdominal myomectomy: a prospective randomized trial to evaluate benefits in early outcome. Am J Obstet Gynecol 1996;174:654-8.
27. Dubuisson JB, Fauconnier A, Babaki-Fard K, Chapron C. Laparoscopic myomectomy: a current view. Hum Reprod Update 2000;6:588-94.
28. Damiani A, Melgrati L, Marziali M, Sesti F, Piccione E. Laparoscopic myomectomy for very large myomas using an isobaric (gasless) technique. JSLS 2005;9:434-8.
29. West S, Ruiz R, Parker WH. Abdominal myomectomy in women with very large uterine size. Fertil Steril 2006;85:36-9.
30. Olive DL, Lindheim SR, Pritts EA. Conservative surgical management of uterine myomas. Obstet Gynecol Clin North Am 2006;33:115-24.
31. Malzoni M, Sizzi O, Rossetti A, Imperato F. Laparoscopic myomectomy: a report of 982 procedures. Surg Technol Int 2006;15:123-9.
32. Seracchioli R, Rossi S, Govoni F, et al. Flamigni C. Fertility and obstetric outcome after laparoscopic myomectomy of large myomata: a randomized comparison with abdominal myomectomy. Hum Reprod 2000;15:2663-8.
33. Landi S, Zaccoletti R, Ferrari L, Minneli L. Laparoscopic myomectomy: technique, complications and ultrasound scan evaluations. J Am Assoc Gynecol Laparosc 2001;8:231-40.
34. Malzoni M, Rotond M, Perone C, et al. Fertility after laparoscopic myomectomy of large uterine myomas: operative technique and preliminary results. Eur J Gynaecol Oncol 2003;24:79-82.
35. Mettler L, Schollmeyer T, Shelat NR, Jonat W. Update on laparoscopic myomectomy. Online publication - Gynecol Surg 2005;2:173-7.

36. Dubuisson JB, Fauconnier A, Babaki-Fard K, et al. Laparoscopic myomectomy: predicting the risk of conversion to an open procedure. Hum Reprod 2001;16:1726-31.

37. Altgassen C, Kuss S, Berger M, et al. Complications in laparoscopic myomectomy. Surg Endosc 2006;20:614-8.

38. Nezhat C, Nezhat F, Bess O, Nezhat CH, Mashiach R. Laparoscopically assisted myomectomy: a report of a new technique in 57 cases. Int J Fertil Menopausal Stud 1994;39:39-44.

39. Lundorff P, Hahlin M, Kallfelt B, Thorburn J, Lindblom B. Adhesion formation after laparoscopic surgery in tubal pregnancy: a randomized trial versus laparotomy. Fertil Steril 1991;55:911-5.

40. Dubuisson JB, Fauconnier A, Chapron C, et al. Second-look after laparoscopic myomectomy. Hum Reprod 1998;13:2102-6.

41. Falcone T, Bedaiwy MA. Minimally invasive management of uterine fibroids. Curr Opin Obstet Gynecol 2002;14:401-7.

42. Fedele L, Parazzini F, Luchini L, et al. Recurrence of fibroids after myomectomy: a transvaginal ultrasonographic study. Hum Reprod 1995;10:1795-6.

43. Candiani GB, Fedele L, Parazzini F, Villa L. Risk of recurrence after myomectomy. Br J Obstet Gynaecol 1991;98:385-9.

44. Rossetti A, Sizzi O, Soranna L, Mancuso S, Lanzone A. Fertility outcome: long-term results after laparoscopic myomectomy. Gynecol Endocrinol 2001;15:129-34.

Laparoscopic Hysterectomy in the Frozen Pelvis

Paul PG, Tony Thomas, Satyen Kasabwala

OVERVIEW

Frozen pelvis refers to the surgical condition where reproductive organs and adjacent structures are distorted by extensive adhesive disease and fibrosis, which obscure the normal anatomic landmarks and surgical planes, making dissection extremely difficult and increasing the risk of damage to vital organs.[1] Hysterectomy in a frozen pelvis, whether by laparotomy or laparoscopy, is a challenging surgical condition. The overall keys to success in such cases depend on the knowledge in the pelvic anatomy and operative experience involving varying degrees of pelvic distortion. The surgeon should have the flexibility to change the course of surgery when a particular pathway proves too risky. He should have a realistic expectation that the operation will be difficult and fraught with hazards, and patience to take things as slowly as necessary. Laparoscopic hysterectomy is now performed for severe pelvic adhesions or severe endometriosis as surgical techniques have improved and surgeons have gained more experience. We describe our experience in performing laparoscopic hysterectomy in the frozen pelvis due to severe endometriosis or pelvic adhesions. It includes some cases, where a previous laparotomy has failed.

INTRODUCTION

Causes for Frozen Pelvis

The common causes of extensive pelvic disease leading to a frozen pelvis are:

Infection: Adhesions and fibrosis, secondary to infectious processes, such as salpingitis, tubo-ovarian abscess, infected pelvic hematoma, and ruptured appendix, can create severe pelvic adhesions. Abdominal Koch's can cause extensive pelvic adhesions.

Surgery: The type of surgery a patient has undergone may provide important clues to potential problems. Laparotomic myomectomies and surgery for endometriosis can also cause gross adhesions. Residual ovaries and remnant ovaries after abdominal hysterectomy may require extensive dissection of the ureter and bowel.

Benign and malignant growths: Severe endometriosis can lead to a frozen pelvis. Malignant growths of the adnexa, such as ovarian carcinoma, can necessitate en bloc resection of portions of the gastrointestinal tract along with the tumor.

Radiation therapy: When a woman has undergone radiation, pelvic structures are commonly adherent to the uterus and each other, making hysterectomy a challenge. The intestines and urinary tracts also must be handled with great care. Even a small degree of intraoperative trauma to these structures can lead to postoperative complications including fistula formation.

Patient Evaluation

The potential for a frozen pelvis, as well as its causes, can usually be identified by taking a careful history and documenting previous surgeries or pelvic problems. When evaluating a patient, it is important to determine which of the above etiological conditions exist and a physical examination also helps to reveal the possible cause. The type of laparotomy scars and drain sites will give a clue to the difficulty of the previous surgery. Be alert for any anatomic changes apparent at the pelvic examination, which should include a rectovaginal assessment. If a lesion is palpated, an attempt must be made to define its size and determine whether it is fixed or mobile. Additionally, it must be ascertained whether the cul-de-sac is free, the uterus can be lifted out of the pelvis, and the disease process is predominantly uterine, adnexal, or involves the adjacent organs.

Preoperative transvaginal sonography will be of immense value.[2] Magnetic resonance imaging may be worthwhile in some cases. It is particularly important to learn preoperatively whether there is hydronephrosis and involvement of the ureters.

Other diagnostic steps, such as cystoscopy and sigmoidoscopy, can be performed at the time of diagnostic laparoscopy or postponed until the actual surgery.

CLINICAL DISCUSSION

Preparation for Surgery

The patient must be given as much information as possible about potential problems with pelvic structures such as the ureters, bowel, and bladder. She must be advised that other surgeons may be called into assist or to help repair damage to surrounding structures.

In anticipation of possible enterolysis or intestinal tract surgery, all patients should undergo preoperative bowel preparation.

An intraoperative ureteral catheterization should be planned if gross pelvic side wall pathologies like severe endometriosis are diagnosed. The use of catheters helps the surgeon to identify the ureters intraoperatively and may therefore, prevent their injury.

Postoperative wound infections and deep venous thrombosis, with the potential for life-threatening pulmonary embolization, are both significantly increased in patients, who undergo pelvic surgery. The prophylactic use of antibiotics and low-molecular-weight heparin is recommended.[3-5]

Surgical Technique

Abdominal Entry

The most important step of the surgery is the abdominal entry. We create a pneumoperitoneum with a veress needle at the Palmer's point. The primary trocar entry is with a Ternamian endotip (Figs 10.1 and 10.2) at the umbilicus, Palmer's point or 5 cm above the pelvic mass.

Omental and Bowel Adhesiolysis

After entering the abdomen, the pelvic structures and their location in relation to one another are identified. Omental adhesions to parietal peritoneum are very common. Omental adhesions to parietal peritoneum are released with scissors, a unipolar hook electrode or a harmonic scalpel. A combination of blunt and sharp dissection is necessary in dense adhesions to visualize the presence of the intestine behind the omental adhesions.

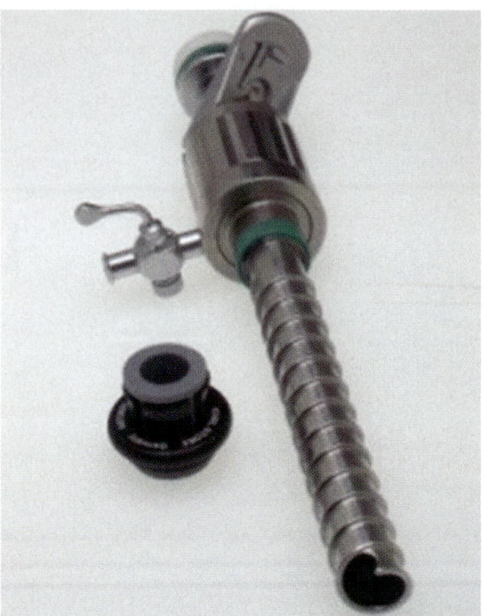

Fig. 10.1: Ternamian endotip for primary trocar entry into the peritoneal cavity

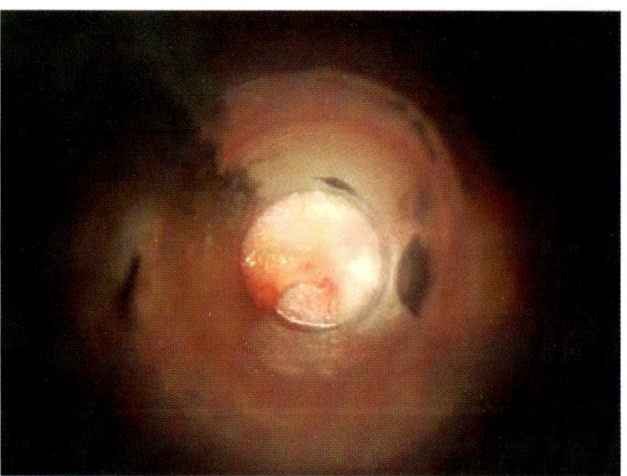

Fig. 10.2: Sheath visualized through the endotip during primary trocar entry

Bowel adhesiolysis is difficult if there is no space between the peritoneum and bowel (Fig. 10.3). Dissection is done with a hook electrode, scissors or harmonic scalpel in this situation. A combination of sharp and blunt dissection can make a space between the bowel and abdominal wall. Cutting close to the peritoneum is safer (Fig. 10.4).

Identify Landmarks

After omental or intestinal adhesions have been separated, the small and large intestines are moved from the pelvis. Uterine manipulation with a suitable manipulator will allow the surgeon to identify the pelvic structures more clearly. We use a Clermont Ferrand uterine manipulator (Karl Storz) for hysterectomies. The following pelvic structures: uterine

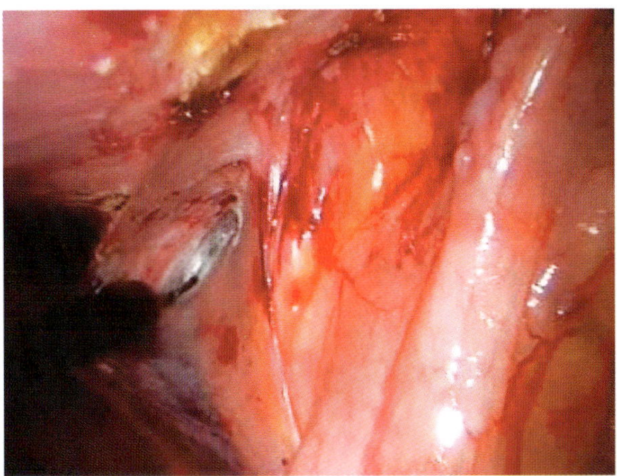

Fig. 10.3: Small bowel loops adherent to parietal peritoneum

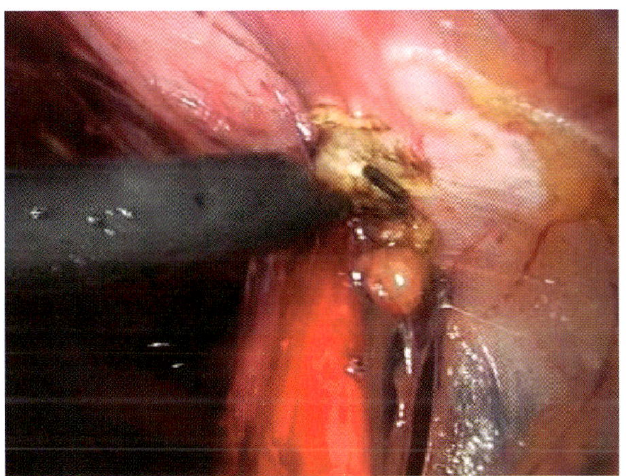

Fig. 10.4: Bowel adhesiolysis from parietal peritoneum. Hook electrode cuts more towards parietal peritoneum

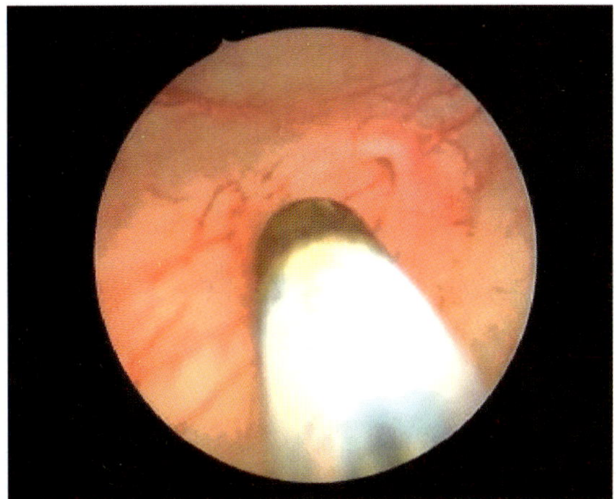

Fig. 10.5: Ureteric catheterization with illuminated catheter

patient with a frozen pelvis. The retroperitoneal approach makes it possible to reach around structures that are fixed in the pelvis, to identify the blood supply and other vital structures, and to proceed safely. Several entry sites are possible. In the frozen pelvis, the round ligament is the ideal location. This ligament must be identified and divided as it enters the internal ring, and the peritoneum cephalad incised along the course of the IP ligaments.

Adnexal Mobilization and Division of Infundibulopelvic Ligament

In severe endometriosis, the adnexa are released from the pelvic side wall with blunt and sharp dissection. Dissection starts from a normal area in the pelvis and the adnexal is released from the pelvic side wall by sharp and blunt dissection. The ureter is identified on both sides before coagulating the IP ligament. This technique is possible in a good number of cases.

Ureter Identification

The position of the ureter must never be assumed without confirming it; a major deviation of its course can occur secondary to pathologic processes in the pelvis. The ureter can be identified by direct visualization, peristalsis, and palpation with a probe. Near the level of the pelvic brim, on the left side of the body, the ureter will be closer to the IP ligament than it is on the right side, due to the location of the sigmoid colon and its mesentery on the left side, which elevates the ureter in the ventral direction.

Rarely, an illuminated ureteric catheter is placed if ureters cannot be clearly identified. Ureteric catheterization can be done with an operating hysteroscope with little training (Fig. 10.5). The illuminated ureteric catheter can be visualized laparoscopically by reducing the laparoscopic light (Fig. 10.6).

fundus, round ligaments, infundibulopelvic (IP) ligaments, posterior cul-de-sac, anterior cul-de-sac, prevesical peritoneum, and pelvic brim, are then identified. These structures may be difficult to recognize and to mobilize because of fibrosis and adhesions in the frozen pelvis.

Entry into the Retroperitoneum

Once the pelvic structures have been identified, the approach to the retroperitoneum must be determined. This decision is important because the blood supply to the uterus and adnexa lies in the retroperitoneum, as do the ureters, which must be identified and kept under direct vision during coagulation and division of the infundibulopelvic (IP) ligaments and dissection of the peritoneum around the uterus.

Retroperitoneal entry and elaboration of the retroperitoneal spaces are keys to the safe performance of a difficult hysterectomy or removal of retained adnexa in a

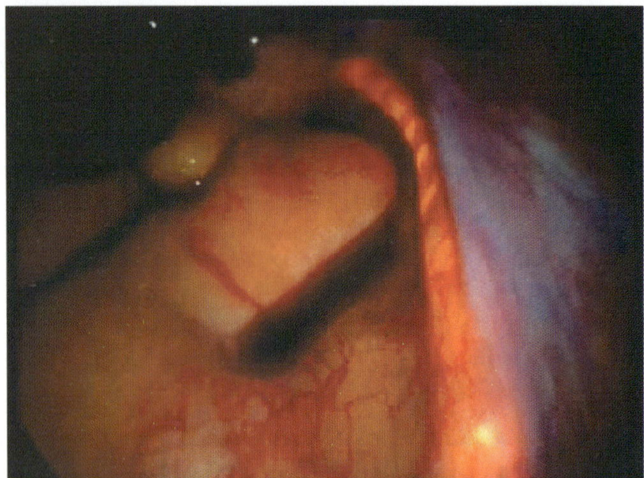

Fig. 10.6: Illuminated catheter visible at the pelvic brim

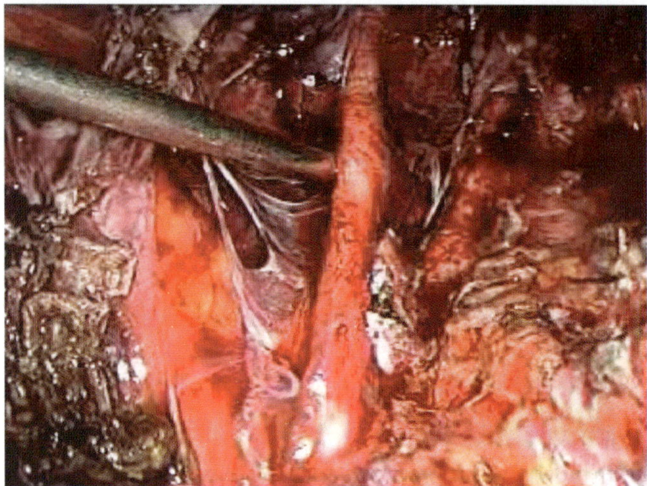

Fig. 10.7: Left ureter after separation of the adherent adnexa

It also makes the ureters rigid for palpation and dissection (Fig. 10.7).

Bladder Separation

A history of surgery in the area of the bladder, such as cesarean section or bladder advancement with uterine suspension, may leave the bladder adherent to or hard to separate from the cervix and vagina. Normally, the vesicouterine peritoneum is flexible, mobile, and easy to free from the cervix and vagina. A history of disease processes, such as endometriosis, infection, or tumors, makes this dissection difficult, with a real risk of inadvertent cystotomy.

One technique to make this dissection easier and safer is to enter the retroperitoneum laterally near the round ligament. In this location, the bladder may not have been involved in the prior dissection, and the tissue may be more areolar and less dense than it is in the midline. The bladder is then separated from the cervix by a hook electrode or harmonic scalpel, remaining close to the cervix. The fornix bulger of uterine manipulator can help in deciding the limit of bladder dissection. Very rarely, filling the bladder with 200 cc of saline can help in identifying the bladder limit (Figs 10.8 and 10.9).

Coagulation and Division of Uterine Vessels

Once the bladder separation is done, uterine vessels are identified at the isthmus and skeletonized. The vessels are coagulated with bipolar forceps and divided. Since the ureters are already identified, this step of laparoscopic hysterectomy is similar to any other hysterectomy.

Cul-de-sac Obliteration

In the pelvis, the posterior cul-de-sac is bounded laterally by the uterosacral ligaments, posteriorly by the rectum and

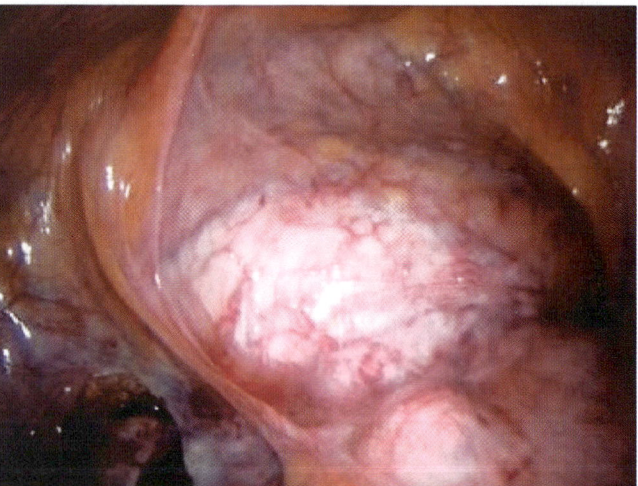

Fig. 10.8: Bladder is filled with 200 cc of saline to visualize the bladder limits

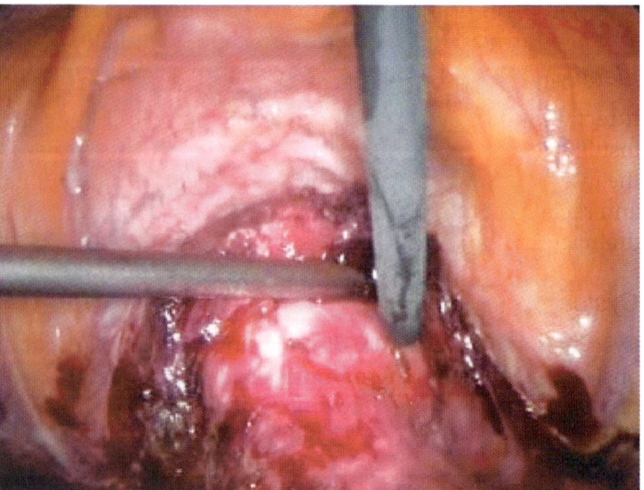

Fig. 10.9: After bladder separation

sacrum, and caudally by the vagina but these relationships are usually lost in the frozen pelvis. Extensive inflammatory disease, tumors of the tubes and ovaries, extensive pelvic endometriosis, and prior infection due to a ruptured appendix can obscure the normal confines of the cul-de-sac. Freeing the peritoneal attachments both, anteriorly and posteriorly, as well as at the sides of the pelvis, allow elevation of the uterus with the manipulator. Then the ureter, uterine vasculature, and supporting ligaments can be identified. Dissection becomes simpler after this point.

However, when the rectum is densely adherent, as it is often in the frozen pelvis, dissection can become difficult with a real danger of rectal perforation. A basic principle in any hysterectomy is to remain close to the uterus, staying near the posterior surface of the uterus and cervix and using both blunt and sharp dissection. This eventually makes it possible to find a reasonable plane to enter the rectovaginal space at the superior portion of the cul-de-sac between the uterosacral ligaments. The tissue below this level is not usually involved in the frozen pelvis and will give way readily once the uterosacral ligaments are divided. It is unnecessary to operate beyond this level to any great extent because the surgery already extends distal to the cervicovaginal junction.

In some circumstances, it may be necessary to open the vagina anteriorly to define the relationship between the posterior cervix and adherent bowel (Fig. 10.10). The hysterectomy is completed in a retrograde fashion. The adherent rectum is then separated from the uterus by sharp dissection in small steps (Fig. 10.11).

Vaginal Closure and Hemostasis

The vagina is now closed laparoscopically after removing the specimen vaginally. The vaginal angle sutures incorporate the uterosacral and cardinal ligaments for vault support (Fig. 10.12). The peritoneal cavity is lavaged with saline and complete hemostasis is ensured. A drain is kept in the pelvis overnight.

Identifying Bowel Injury

If rectal injury is suspected, the submersed rectosigmoid is insufflated with air (Fig. 10.13). Bubbles signal a breach in the integrity of the bowel wall. If the bowel has been prepped, and rectal enterotomy occurs during dissection, closure and drainage are the only necessary steps.

Cystoscopy

Cystoscopy is performed to look for any bladder injury and observe the urine reflux from both ureteric orifices.

Results

We describe our experience in performing laparoscopic hysterectomy in the frozen pelvis due to severe endometriosis

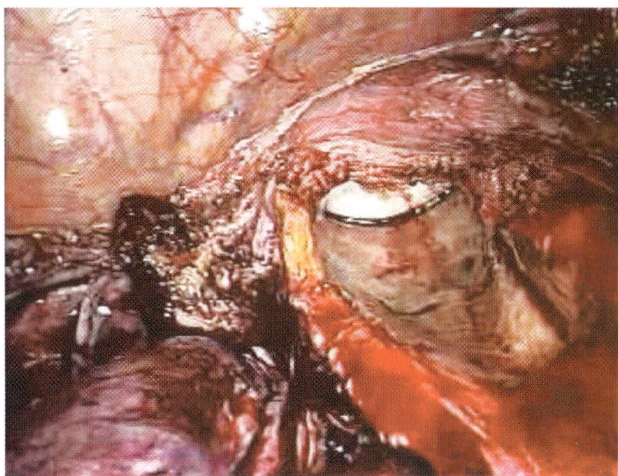

Fig. 10.10: Anterior vagina is incised and posterior vagina still attached to uterus

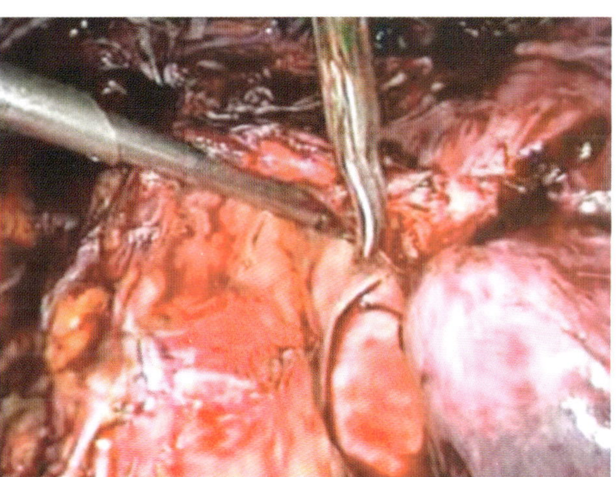

Fig. 10.11: Dividing the rectal adhesions to the uterus after separating the cervix from the vagina

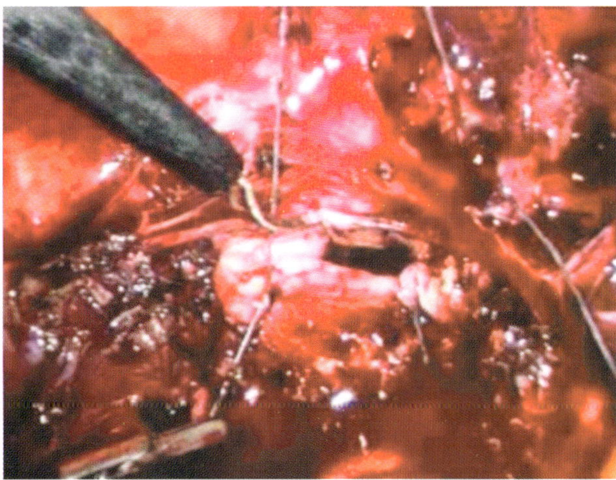

Fig. 10.12: Suturing the vaginal vault after hysterectomy

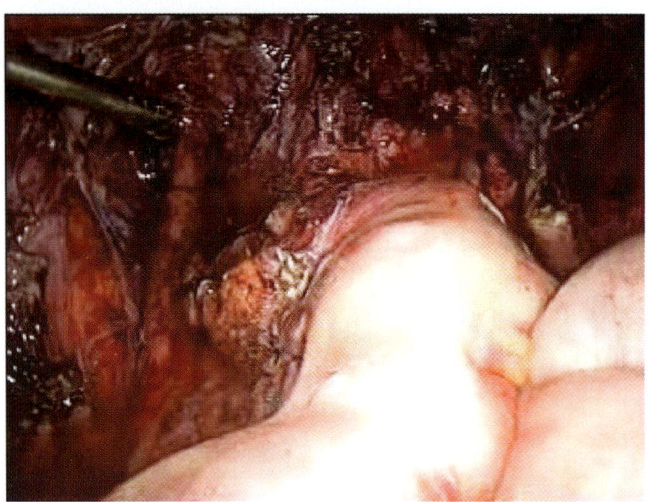

Fig. 10.13: Rectum inflated with air to look for injury

or pelvic adhesions. There were 16 cases, all of which had a history of previous surgery for endometriosis: Four patients had two laparotomies, 8 had one laparotomy, 1 had three laparoscopic surgeries, 4 had two laparoscopic surgeries, and 5 had one laparoscopic surgery. There were 4 cases, where a previous laparotomy had failed to complete hysterectomy. All the patients had a frozen pelvis and endometriosis with or without adenomyosis. Laparoscopic adhesiolysis with total laparoscopic hysterectomy with bilateral/unilateral salpingo-oophorectomy was done for all. In one patient, the biopsy report revealed a well-differentiated adenocarcinoma of the tubal stump. The average duration of surgery was 2 hours 30 minutes. Blood loss was less than 500 mL. No blood transfusion was given for any patient. There was no bowel or bladder injury in this series. Postoperative hospital stay was 2 to 3 days. Three patients had postoperative fever, which was treated with antibiotics.

CONCLUSION

Hysterectomy in the frozen pelvis, whether performed by the open or laparoscopic route, is a difficult surgical procedure. A good preoperative evaluation and planning helps the surgeon to prepare for a difficult hysterectomy and organize intraoperative urological or gastrointestinal surgical consultation. The surgical technique has to be modified for a particular case and the surgeon should be prepared to change the course of surgery. It is possible and safe to perform total laparoscopic hysterectomy in cases of frozen pelvis by experienced surgeons.

REFERENCES

1. Donald P Goldstein, Michael J Callahan. Surgical strategies to untangle a frozen pelvis. OBG Management 2007;19:03.
2. Brosens I, Puttemans P, Campo R, Gordts S, Brosens J. Non-invasive methods of diagnosis of endometriosis. Curr Opin Obstet Gynecol 2003;15:519-22.
3. Polk HC Jr. Continuing refinements in surgical antibiotic prophylaxis. Arch Surg 2005;140:1066-7.
4. Fejgin MD, Lourwood DL. Low-molecular-weight heparins and their use in obstetrics and gynecology. Obstet Gynecol Surv 1994;49:424-6.
5. Löfgren M. Postoperative infections and antibiotic prophylaxis for hysterectomy in Sweden: a study by the Swedish National Register for Gynecologic Surgery. Acta Obstet Gynecol Scand 2004;83:1202-7.

Complications of Laparoscopic Hysterectomy

Edi Vaisbuch, Zion Hagay

OVERVIEW

Ever since the laparoscopic approach to hysterectomy was first performed by Harry Reich in 1988, this technique has become a standard of care for treating benign uterine pathologies in many centers worldwide. Laparoscopic hysterectomy offers the patient many potential advantages over the classic abdominal hysterectomy, however, because it requires higher surgical expertise, it also carries some hazards. Overall, the reported incidence of gynecologic laparoscopy-related complications varies between 0.1 and 10 percent. The associated risk factors for such complications include the extremes of age and body mass index, previous abdominal surgeries, presence of intra-abdominal adhesions, level of surgical complexity, and probably the most significant, the surgeon experience. The potential complications can be classified as intra- and postoperative, anesthesia or laparoscopy-related. This chapter discusses the potential complications of LH and strategies to minimize them, especially during the surgeon learning curve.

INTRODUCTION

Hysterectomy is the most common of all gynecologic operations. Until the late 1980s, there were two available approaches for hysterectomy: abdominal or vaginal. The laparoscopic approach to hysterectomy is relatively new and was first performed by Harry Reich in 1988.[1] Since then, laparoscopic hysterectomy (LH) has gained widespread interest and has become a standard of care for treating benign uterine pathology in many centers worldwide. Laparoscopic hysterectomy has become an alternative to abdominal hysterectomy with many potential advantages to the patient, but because the laparoscopic approach to hysterectomy requires higher surgical expertise, it also carries some hazards. Possibly, this is the reason that after nearly two decades from the first LH, there are many countries where the majority of hysterectomies are still done by the abdominal route. Nowadays, for the expert laparoscopic surgeon, there are only a few indications left to perform abdominal hysterectomy. Laparoscopic hysterectomy is not supposed to be an alternative to the vaginal route, which is probably the preferred route for hysterectomy, whenever it is easily feasible.[2]

Options of Laparoscopic Hysterectomy

Laparoscopic hysterectomy may be performed in different ways depending on the degree of laparoscopic use during hysterectomy and the degree of complexity. The main terminologies used under the umbrella of laparoscopic hysterectomy are:

Laparoscopic-assisted vaginal hysterectomy (LAVH): With this technique, the upper uterine ligaments are disconnected using laparoscopy and the hysterectomy completed vaginally. LAVH is the simple type of laparoscopic hysterectomy preferred when vaginal hysterectomy can be done but the surgeon expects it would be hard to have the adnexas removed as in cases of expected adhesions, endometriosis or ovarian masses.

Laparoscopic supracervical hysterectomy (LSH): As with subtotal abdominal hysterectomy, the uterus is cut with the cervix left attached to the vagina. The uterus is removed from the abdominal cavity by morcellation. The main potential advantage with LSH is a lower risk for ureter damage. A possible disadvantage is when morcellating a non-identified cancerous uterus.

Total laparoscopic hysterectomy (TLH): The uterus is completely disconnected laparoscopically and removed through the vagina. The vagina can be closed laparoscopically.

Potential Advantages and Disadvantages of Laparoscopic Hysterectomy

Laparoscopic hysterectomy has many potential advantages. From the patient's point of view, there is shorter hospital stay, faster return to normal activities, reduced postoperative pain, fewer infections, febrile and ileus complications.[2-7] From the surgeon's point of view, the magnification of the surgical field leads to better assessment of the anatomy with better control for complete hemostatsis, leading to lower intraoperative blood loss. The price, at least during the learning curve, is longer operation time[3,7-12] with a higher rate of major complications, especially those involving the urinary tract, when compared to abdominal or vaginal hysterectomy.[2,10,12,13]

Indications for Laparoscopic Hysterectomy

Except for advanced gynecologic cancers, where there is still lack of evidence for the safety of laparoscopic surgery, the indications for LH are nowadays more likely to those of abdominal hysterectomy, depending mainly on the surgeon experience.

CLINICAL DISCUSSION

Complications of Laparoscopic Hysterectomy

Although there are important advantages of LH over the classic abdominal hysterectomy, it is important to remember that there are some potential complications. The reported incidence of complications related to gynecologic laparoscopies is 0.1 to 10 percent.[14] A multi-center survey from France reported a complication rate of 0.46 percent and a mortality rate of 3.3/100,000 in 29,996 laparoscopic procedures.[15] Over 50 percent of these complications occurred during the laparoscopic entry rather during the procedure itself.[16] A recently published large multicenter study from 28 centers throughout the UK and two in South Africa (EVALUATE trial) compared abdominal, vaginal and laparoscopic hysterectomy and found that LH was associated with a higher rate of major complications (11.1%) when compared to abdominal hysterectomy (6.2%).[12] In a meta-analysis of 27 trials with a total of 3643 participants, it was found that only urinary tract injuries were more frequent with LH when compared to abdominal hysterectomy (odds ratio 2.61; 95% CI 1.22-5.60).[2]

The risk factors of laparoscopic surgery include the extremes of age and body mass index (BMI), previous abdominal surgeries, presence of adhesions as after pelvic inflammatory disease or endometriosis, level of surgical complexity, such as surgery for large uterus or malignancy, but probably, the most vital is the surgeon experience. It is imperative to remember that there is a learning curve even for the skilled surgeons. A learning curve of 30 laparoscopic hysterectomies was found to correlate with a lower complication rate.[8,17]

Generally, the potential complications are classified as intraoperative and postoperative. Complications can be anesthesia-related or laparoscopy-related. The laparoscopy-related complications can be further subdivided into those that are related to entry and the laparoscopic approach and those related to the surgical procedure itself.

Intraoperative Complications

- *Conversion to laparotomy:* This can itself be classified as a major complication of laparoscopic surgery but without the laparoscopic option, the patient would have a primary laparotomy anyway. Conversion to laparotomy can be due to several reasons as equipment failure, technical surgical difficulties, unexpected intra-abdominal disease or adhesions or major intraoperative complications, such as massive bleeding, requiring immediate intervention. Therefore, every patient scheduled for laparoscopic hysterectomy must sign an informed consent for laparotomy too.

- *Complications of anesthesia specifically related to laparoscopy:* Laparoscopic procedures are associated with physiological cardiopulmonary changes, mainly related to the increased intra-abdominal pressure, patient position due to the need for prolonged Trendelenburg position during pelvic surgery (both leading to displacement of the diaphragm upward), excessive systemic carbon dioxide (CO_2) absorption that should be overwhelmed by increased minute ventilation and the length of the surgery.[18] Anesthetic management during laparoscopic surgery must accommodate to the special surgical requirements and allow for the mentioned physiological changes that are generally well-tolerated by healthy and young people but can lead to complications especially in the obese, elderly or patients with limited cardiopulmonary reserve.[19] Whenever, an anesthesia-related problem, such as acute cardiopulmonary collapse, fall in blood pressure or respiratory failure, arises, besides the routine evaluation by the anesthesiologist, the insufflations should be stopped immediately, intra-abdominal pressure reduced and a complete laparoscopic survey of the abdomen made to rule out injury to a major blood vessel, allowing the anesthesiologist to fortify the patient.

- *Complications related to laparoscopy:*
  - *Complications related to entry:* More than 50 percent of the complications related to laparoscopy occur during the laparoscopic entry rather than during

the procedure itself.[16] The potential complications related to entry and insufflation for developing a pneumoperitoneum are subcutaneous or preperitoneal emphysema, that are relatively common but benign complications, injury to the abdominal wall vessels or intra-abdominal large vessels, injuries to the viscera, mainly the bowel, but also the bladder or stomach and postoperative incisional hernias. Risk factors for entry complications are prior surgeries and intra-abdominal diseases, increasing the chance of adhesions, and non-obese patients. An overdistended non-catheterized bladder or improper overdistention of the stomach during anesthesia can further increase the risk. There are two main approaches to entry, one with the Veress needle, that is a blind procedure to enter the peritoneum, and the 'open' technique of Hasson.[20] Other techniques are available and under trial as the direct vision trocars. The open technique is more time consuming and is probably safer for reducing the risk of subcutaneous emphysema and major vessels injury but not bowel injury. Insertion of the primary trocar is also a blind procedure, but the secondary trocars are introduced under vision. Low intra-abdominal pressure, uncontrolled entry or improper direction of insertion of the primary trocar can result in injuries to large blood vessels or viscera. Although secondary trocars are inserted under vision, complications can occur with injuries to the inferior epigastric arteries that run beneath the rectal muscles being the most common.

i.   *Vessel injury:* The reported rate of vessel injury related to entry is about 0.2/1000,[21] but the reported incidence of intraoperative hemorrhage requiring conversion to laparotomy is up to 2 to 3 percent and it is probably related to the surgeon experience. Fortunately, catastrophic vascular injuries to aorta, vena cava or iliac arteries are rare and immediate laparotomy is crucial. As mentioned, the 'open' technique for entry as an alternative to the 'closed' technique might be safer in terms of large vessel injury although because of the rarity of the event and the non-randomized trials, this is hard to prove.

ii. *Gas emboli:* Despite the large number of gynecological laparoscopies performed, gas emboli are only rarely reported.[22] Accidental insufflation into a penetrating unrecognized injury to a blood vessel may lead to gas emboli and without proper immediate recognition, resuscitation to death.

iii. *Bowel injury:* Bowel injury is an uncommon event with a cited general incidence of 0.4/1000,[21] but probably increases with advanced laparoscopic surgery and is obviously higher when previous abdominal surgeries exists since the main association is with extensive intraperitoneal adhesions. It may occur as a result of insertion of the Veress needle, placement of a trocar, trauma during dissection or electrosurgical injury. The main problem with bowel injury is that it can be missed intraoperatively. Delayed diagnosis is life-threatening and one of the main reasons for laparoscopy-related death, thus a high index of suspicion is crucial. Generally, traumatic injury becomes symptomatic 24 to 72 hours postoperatively but electrosurgical injury may present itself after 4 to 10 days.

iv. *Urinary tract injuries:* Injury to the bladder and ureter can occur in every laparoscopy but with a higher incidence in advanced pelvic surgery as for endometriosis or LH[2] and hence, are discussed as complications related to hysterectomy.

– *Complications related to laparoscopic hysterectomy:* The main concern when arguing against the laparoscopic approach to hysterectomy besides the longer procedure duration, is the higher reported incidence of major complications, mainly involving the bladder and ureter when compared to the abdominal or vaginal route.[12]

i.   *Bladder injury:* Bladder injury is relatively common. The prevalence of bladder injury in the evaluate study was 2 percent (18 cases out of 920 laparoscopic hysterectomies), whereas the prevalence in the abdominal and vaginal route was 1 percent and 1.2 percent, respectively.[12] The bladder can be injured during trocar placement or during dissection of the bladder from the uterus and cervix. The injury can be either blunt or thermal. The most important thing is intraoperative detection and repair of the injury. Cystoscopy and bladder filling with blue dye can assist in suspected injury. In our LH series, we had two cases (1.2%) of bladder injury in the laparoscopic hysterectomy group and one (0.85%, P-not significant) in the abdominal hysterectomy group.[23]

ii. *Ureter injury:* Injuries to the ureter are relatively uncommon with an incidence of less than 1 percent. In the EVALUATE study, it was 0.6 percent after laparoscopic hysterectomy (6 cases out of 920), whereas no such case was reported after abdominal or vaginal hysterectomy.[12] Injury to the ureter can occur at the pelvic brim, near the infundibulopelvic ligament and at the pelvic side wall, where the ureter passes beneath the uterine artery but mainly during the ligation of the uterine arteries or during the vaginal part of LAVH. The risk is greater in the presence of endometriosis, pelvic adhesions or large pelvic masses, where the normal anatomy is distorted. Potential injury can be from wrong suturing, kinking, transection or thermal injury. To reduce the risk of such complications, routine exposure of the ureter, by retroperitoneal dissection to visualize its entire course is advisable. The sooner the injury is identified, the better it may be for limiting the extent postoperative morbidity, but unfortunately, ureteral injuries, especially thermal injuries, cannot easily be identified intraoperatively. For this reason, although not considered by all as a must, we support and advocate routine cystoscopy with intravenous indigo-carmine injection after every LH, even in the most uneventful operation. Thermal injury to the ureter can easily be missed and should be suspected postoperatively when deviation from normal recovery exists.

Postoperative Complications

Hematoma formation: Intraperitoneal hematomas, especially vaginal cuff hematomas is not an uncommon complication, responsible for anemia, postoperative pain and febrile morbidity. Antibiotics and time are generally enough for spontaneous resolution of the hematomas but rarely, drainage is required due to persistent pain or fever. We had one case of persistent symptomatic (pain) pelvic hematoma requiring drainage, two weeks post-TLH, in a woman under dialysis due to chronic renal failure.

Ileus: Postoperative ileus is relatively uncommon with a cited incidence of less than 1 percent.

Infection: Infection morbidity after laparoscopic surgery mainly includes urinary tract infections, wound infection and pelvic abscess formation. Absolute hemostasis, evacuation of large clots and copious irrigation may help to further decrease postoperative infection. We give one dose of second generation Cephalosporin as prophylactic antibiotics to every patient after induction of anesthesia. At the beginning of our experience, we had one woman who underwent explorative laparotomy with bilateral salpingectomy due to post LAVH pelvic infection.

Thromboembolism: This is relatively common in gynecological surgery. Compression of the pelvic veins due to the intra-abdominal pressure can result in a higher incidence of thromboembolic event following laparoscopy, but on the other hand, there is a shorter convalescence time with early mobilization. For minimizing the incidence, we use the intermittent compressive device in every case with the addition of prophylactic low molecular weight heparin according a protocol built according to risk factors such as age, obesity, general health status and expected complexity of the procedure. There has been no such complication in our series.

Fistula formation: There are several possible fistula complications: vesicovaginal, vesicoperitoneal, urethrovaginal. Rectal fistulas are rather infrequent. We had one case of vesicovaginal fistula that was diagnosed and treated three weeks post TLH.

Incisional hernia: The reported incidence of incisional hernias is relatively low with an incidence of 21/100,000 as reported by the American Association of Gynecologic Laparoscopists.[24] The incidence might be higher in more complicated procedures, when multiple or larger diameter ports are needed for complex instruments. Closure of the fascia with large trocar incisions (>10 mm) can reduce the risk but not eliminate it.

Port site metastases: Tumor seeding with port site metastases after laparoscopic surgery has been reported in almost all gynecologic malignancies. The reported incidence of port site metastases is 1 to 2 percent,[25,26] with an even higher incidence after laparoscopic surgery for ovarian cancer.[27] For reducing the incidence, it is essential to try and avoid tumor morcellation, and if needed, morcellation or removal of the specimen should be performed in a retrieval bag to prevent spillage into the peritoneal cavity or along the port site tract even when malignancy is not suspected.

Neuropathy: Peripheral neuropathy can occur, especially from nerve compression as consequences of wrong positioning of the patient. The hands should be placed fastened along the body. Because working in the pelvis is easier and probably safer to the bowel many surgeons ask for deep Trendelenburg, and wrong placement of the shoulder restraints can compress the brachial plexus.

The Evolution of Laparoscopic Hysterectomy at Kaplan Medical Center

We started performing the first laparoscopic assisted vaginal hysterectomy in 1998. In the beginning, the women were selected carefully, so that the operation could be performed without significant complications. We used the open technique of Hasson for achieving a pneumoperitoneum, using a 10 mm trocar at the umbilicus and two 5 mm trocars at the right and left lower quadrants. Initially, LAVH was performed, disconnecting the infundibulopelvic and broad ligaments laparoscopically with vaginal completion of uterus disconnection by cutting the uterine arteries and the sacro-uterine ligaments. After gaining experience and reviewing our results of the first 50 LAVH operations, we moved one step further, dealing with the uterine arteries laparoscopically and completing a SLH with morcellation of the uterus.

Following a case of post-SLH diagnosis of uterine sarcoma, we decided to further proceed to TLH, avoiding the need for intra-abdominal uterine morcellation, although there was no evidence yet for a worse prognosis in such cases. LAVH was reserved for selected cases of genital prolapse with uterus myomatosus and/or adnexal pathology, where vaginal hysterectomy was considered to be technically difficult.

For evaluating our results, we compared the intraoperative and short-term postoperative results of 169 laparoscopic hysterectomies (LAVH, LSH and TLH) during and after completing the learning curve to that of the classic total abdominal hysterectomy (TAH).[23] More than 90 percent of the laparoscopic hysterectomies were performed by the same team of surgeons. The conversion rate was 1.8 percent, with three of the intended LAVH converted to TAH, two just after insertion of the laparoscope due to severe adhesions, and another after a bladder tear. There were no statistically significant differences between the two groups for age, BMI, previous abdominal surgery, first postoperative day hemoglobin drop and complication rate. Operation time was significantly longer for LH when compared to TAH (156±40 and 91.2±33 minutes, respectively) but with a shorter hospital stay (3.9 and 6.55 days, respectively). We had no cases of death, sepsis, massive pulmonary emboli or permanent neurological deficit in either of the groups. Seven (4.2%) women in the LH group (4 after LAVH, one after STLH and two after TVH) compared to 6 (5%) women in the TAH group had excessive blood loss that required blood transfusion. One woman in the LH group had an explorative laparotomy with bilateral salpingectomy due to post LAVH pelvic infection. We had two cases of bladder injury (one repaired laparoscopically during TLH and the second during LAVH, requiring conversion to laparotomy) and one woman had a vesicovaginal fistula, diagnosed and repaired 3 weeks post-TLH.

We concluded that LH is as safe as abdominal hysterectomy, takes longer to perform and can be carried out with a reasonable complication rate even during the learning curve. Some investigators reported that LAVH involves a high rate of major complications during the initial learning period of the surgeon.[10,13] Others concluded that LAVH is a safe procedure even when performed by a variety of surgeons with different skill levels.[28] According to our experience, the rate of major complications during the initial learning period of LH was low and similar to TAH (2.4% vs 2.5%, respectively). When comparing the first 30 LH with the later operations, we found in the late group, a trend to lower the total complication rate (30% vs 16.7%, p=0.08) with a significantly shorter hospital stay (4.75±1.4 vs. 3.7±1.4 days; p<0.05). After a plateau in the learning curve is reached, the operating time decreased and became similar for laparoscopic and abdominal hysterectomy.[29,30]

RECENT ADVANCES

Robot-assisted Laparoscopic Hysterectomy

Recently, robotic technology has been introduced in gynecologic surgery and several studies have demonstrated that robot-assisted hysterectomy is feasible and probably has, at least, comparable outcomes to TLH.[31-35] The potential advantages of robotic surgery include improved visualization of the operative field with increased dexterity, allowing more precise movements, thus, potentially allowing more complex operations to be performed with greater precision.[31,34] However, the operating costs of robotic surgery are relatively high and randomized clinical trials are needed to further evaluate the benefits and the cost-effectiveness of this new technology over the conventional LH. Detailed description and discussion on robotic surgery is beyond the scope of this chapter.

CONCLUSION

When introducing a new surgical technique, the learning curve is a critical period, especially with regard to complications, and especially where other options that are well-established and known exist. The goal must be minimum complications during the learning curve and for that, the operation time should be the last concern, with efforts made to perform surgeries by the same team until enough experience is gathered to introducing the technique to more surgeons. Doing so, laparoscopic hysterectomy can be safely performed even during the learning curve with a relatively low and reasonable complication rate. As experience is gained, the operation time as well as the complication rate and hospital stay will further decrease.

Laparoscopy is only another surgical technique and the target should be that every surgeon able to perform an abdominal or vaginal hysterectomy should be familiar with or be able to do a LH when appropriate. Otherwise, many women who could benefit from the advantages of LH will have an abdominal hysterectomy.

REFERENCES

1. Reich H, De Caprio J, McGynn F. Laparoscopic hysterectomy. J Gynecol Surg 1989;5:213-6.
2. Johnson N, Barlow D, Lethaby A, Tavender E, Curr E, Garry R. Methods of hysterectomy: systematic review and meta-analysis of randomised controlled trials. BMJ 2005;330:1478.
3. Olsson JH, Ellstrom M, Hahlin M. A randomized prospective trial comparing laparoscopic and abdominal hysterectomy. Br J Obstet Gynaecol 1996;103:345-50.
4. Meikle SF, Nugent EW, Orleans M. Complications and recovery from laparoscopic-assisted vaginal hysterectomy compared with abdominal and vaginal hysterectomy. Obset Gynecol 1997;89: 304-11.
5. Nezhat C, Childers J, Nezhat F Nezhat CH, Seidman DS. Major retroperitoneal vascular injury during laparoscopic surgery. Hum Reprod 1997;12:480-3.

6. Phipps JH, Jhon M, Nayak S. Comparison of laparoscopically assisted vaginal hysterectomy and bilateral salpingo-oophorectomy with conventional abdominal hysterectomy and bilateral salpingo-oophorectomy. Br J Obstet Gynaecol 1993;100: 698-700.

7. Raju KS, Barry JA. A randomized prospective study of laparoscopic vaginal hysterectomy versus abdominal hysterectomy each with bilateral salpingo-oophorectomy. Br J Obstet Gynecol 1994;101:1068-71.

8. Mäkinen J, Johansson J, Tomás C, Tomás E, Heinonen PK, Laatikainen T, et al. Morbidity of 10110 hysterectomies by type of approach. Hum Reprod 2001;16:1473-8.

9. Summitt RL, Stovall TG, Steege JF, Lipscomb GH. A multicenter randomized comparison of laparoscopically assisted vaginal hysterectomy and abdominal hysterectomy in abdominal hysterectomy candidates. Obstet Gynecol 1998;92:321-6.

10. Boike GM, Elfstrand EP, DelPriore G, Schumock D, Holley HS, Lurain JR. Laparoscopically assisted vaginal hysterectomy in a university hospital: Report of 82 cases in comparison with abdominal and vaginal hysterectomy. Am J Obstet Gynecol 1993;168:1690-701.

11. Richardson RE, Bournas N, Magos AL. Is laparoscopic hysterectomy a waste of time? Lancet 1995;345:36-41.

12. Garry R, Fountain J, Brown J, Manca A, Mason S, Sculpher M, et al. EVALUATE hysterectomy trial: a multicentre randomised trial comparing abdominal, vaginal and laparoscopic methods of hysterectomy. Health Technology Assessment 2004;8:1-154.

13. Visco AG, Barber MD, Myers ER. Early physician experience with laparoscopically assisted vaginal hysterectomy and rates of surgical complications and conversion to laparotomy. Am J Obstet Gynecol 2002;187:1008-12.

14. Magrina, JF. Complications of laparoscopic surgery. Clin Obstet Gynecol 2002;45:469-80.

15. Chapron C, Querleu D, Bruhat MA, Madelnat P, Fernandez H, Pierre F, et al. Surgical complications of diagnostic and operative gynaecological laparoscopy: a series of 29,966 cases. Human Reprod 1998;13:867-72.

16. Jansen FW, Kapiteyn K, Trimbos-Kemper T, Hermens J, Trimbos JB. Complications of laparoscopy: a prospective multicentre observational study. Br J Obstet Gynaecol 1997;104:595-600.

17. Altgassen C, Michels W, Schneider A. Learning laparoscopic-assisted hysterectomy. Obstet Gynecol 2004;104:308-13.

18. O'Malley C, Cunningham AJ. Physiologic changes during laparoscopy. Anesthesiol Clin North America 2001;19:1-19.

19. Joshi GP. Complications of laparoscopic surgery. Anesthesiol Clin North America 2001;19:89-105.

20. Hasson HM. Modified instruments and methods for laparoscopy. Am J Obstet Gynecol 1971;110:886-90.

21. Garry R. Laparoscopic surgery. Best Pract Res Clin Obstet Gynaecol 2006;20:89-104.

22. Hynes SR, Marshall L. Venous gas embolism during gynaecological laparoscopy. Can J Anaesth 1992;39:748-9.

23. Vaisbuch E, Goldchmit C, Ofer D, Agmon A, Hagay Z. Laparoscopic hysterectomy versus total abdominal hysterectomy: A comparative study. Eur J Obstet Gynecol Reprod Biol 2006;126:234-8.

24. Montz FJ, Holschneider CH, Munro MG. Incisional hernia following laparoscopy: a survey of the American Association of Gynecologic Laparoscopists. Obstet Gynecol 1994;84:881-4.

25. Childers JM, Aqua KA, Surwit EA, Hallum AV, Hatch KD. Abdominal-wall tumor implantation after laparoscopy for malignant conditions. Obstet Gynecol 1994;84:765-9.

26. Nagarsheth NP, Rahaman J, Cohen CJ, Gretz H, Nezhat. The incidence of port-site metastases in gynecologic cancers. JSLS 2004;8:133-9.

27. Huang KG, Wang CJ, Chang TC, Liou JD, Hsueh S, Lai CH, et al. Management of port site metastasis after laparoscopic surgery for ovarian cancer. Am J Obstet Gynecol 2003;189:16-21.

28. Johns DA, Carrera B, Jones J, DeLeon F, Vincent R, Safely C. The medical and economic impact of laparoscopically assisted vaginal hysterectomy in a large, metropolitan, not-for-profit hospital. Am J Obstet Gynecol 1995;172:1709-19.

29. Perino A, Cucinella G, Venezia R, Castelli A, Cittadini E. Total laparoscopic hysterectomy versus total abdominal hysterectomy: an assessment of the learning curve in a prospective randomized study. Hum Reprod 1999;14:2996-9.

30. Marana R, Busacca M, Zupi E, Garcea N, Paparella P, Catalano GF. Laparoscopically assisted vaginal hysterectomy versus total abdominal hysterectomy: a prospective, randomized, multicenter study. Am J Obstet Gynecol 1999;180(2 Pt 1): 270–5.

31. Nezhat FR, Datta MS, Liu C, Chuang L, Zakashansky K. Robotic radical hysterectomy versus total laparoscopic radical hysterectomy with pelvic lymphadenectomy for treatment of early cervical cancer. JSLS 2008;12:227-37.

32. Chen CC, Falcone T. Robotic gynecologic surgery: past, present, and future. Clin Obstet Gynecol 2009;52:335-43.

33. Shashoua AR, Gill D, Locher SR. Robotic-assisted total laparoscopic hysterectomy versus conventional total laparoscopic hysterectomy. JSLS 2009;13:364-9.

34. Matthews CA, Reid N, Ramakrishnan V, Hull K, Cohen S. Evaluation of the introduction of robotic technology on route of hysterectomy and complications in the first year of use. Am J Obstet Gynecol 2010;203:499.e1-5.

35. Sert MB, Eraker R. Robot-assisted laparoscopic surgery in gynaecological oncology; initial experience at Oslo Radium Hospital and 16 months follow-up. Int J Med Robot 2009;5: 410-4.

Making Hysteroscopic Surgery Safer

Abraham Golan, Shimon Ginath

OVERVIEW

Intrauterine pathology, such as intrauterine polyps, submucus leiomyomas or endometrial carcinomas, may present with irregular or increased vaginal bleeding, or as intrauterine adhesions or septae, presenting as infertility. The diagnosis and treatment of these pathological conditions has undergone significant changes in the last decade. Previously, the diagnosis was based on ultrasonography (USG) and hysterosalpingography (HSG), and treatment consisted of curettage and hysterectomy. Today, this is based on hysteroscopy for diagnosis and management. The use of monopolar electrical energy with glycine or mannitol as the distention medium was the practice in surgical hysteroscopy. Recently, with the development of the bipolar electric system, the use of a physiological solution as distention medium has become feasible. This has significantly reduced the potential complications reflected to the distention medium, probably becoming the preferred method for surgical hysteroscopy.

INTRODUCTION

History

Bozzini was the first to use an endoscope in 1806 in Frankfurt.[1] He used an aluminum tube, illuminated by a wax candle, which directed light into the internal cavities of the body. The Vienna Medical Society, however, did not share his enthusiasm and highly disapproved his activity.[2] The first successful diagnostic and operative hysteroscopy was reported by Pantaleoni in 1869. He used a modified cystoscope and a kerosene lamp for a light source in a 60-year-old woman with postmenopausal bleeding and diagnosed an intrauterine polyp, eventually managed by cauterization with silver nitrate.[3] The difficulty in distending the uterus due to its thick wall and its small cavity was the reason for the slow development of diagnostic hysteroscopy.[4] Nitze, a German urologist, used a new functional cystoscope in 1877, using an overheated glowing platinum wire as an illumination source, thus improving vision.[5] In 1907, David evaluated the uterine cavity with a cystoscope.[6] In 1914, Heineberg introduced a water-irrigating system with inflow and outflow channels to improve intrauterine visualization[7] and in 1925, Rubin was the first to use CO_2 as a distension medium, which became more popular only later with the introduction of the CO_2

insufflators.[8] Seymour, in 1926, developed a continuous-flow irrigation system, and also introduced an additional operating channel through which surgical instruments could be passed.[9] The invention of the cold light source by Fourestiere et al.[10] in 1943, that transmitted light via optical cables and prevented the dissipation of heat inside the uterine cavity, and the invention of the rod-lens system by Hopkins in 1959, were the next two major steps in the development of hysteroscopy.[11] During the 1980s, the visual examination of the uterine cavity was performed with a diagnostic hysteroscope with a total diameter of at least 5 mm, consisting of a 4 mm rod-lens system scope inserted in a simple sheath. Miniaturization of the scopes occurred during the 1990s. New scopes were introduced with much smaller diameters ranging between 1.2 and 3 mm and operative sheaths with external diameters of less than 5 mm.[12] During these years, the CO_2 medium for diagnostic hysteroscopy was replaced by normal physiological solution.

Hysteroscopic Technique

Hysteroscopy can be either diagnostic or operative. Diagnostic hysteroscopy is performed for the evaluation of the uterine cavity and exclusion (Fig. 12.1) or confirmation of

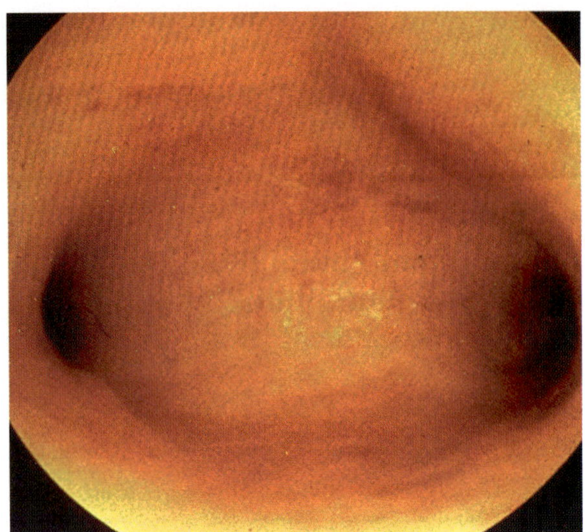

Fig. 12.1: Normal endometrial cavity at diagnostic hysteroscopy

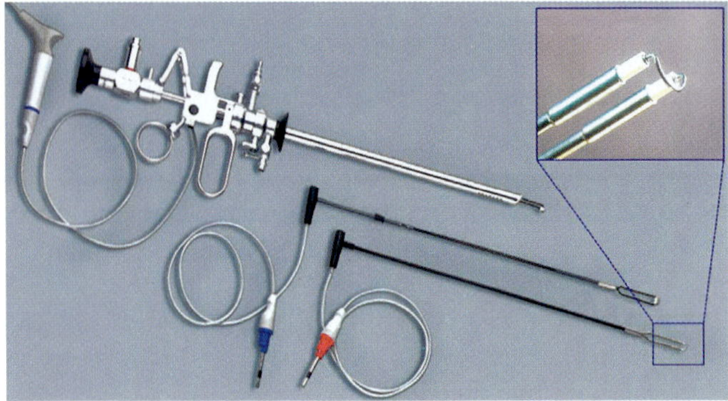

Fig. 12.2: The bipolar system—VersaPoint. In the magnified square-loop resecting electrode

intrauterine pathology. Operative hysteroscopy is the surgical removal of such pathology.

A diagnostic hysteroscope consists of an optical telescope with a diameter of about 3.5 mm, surrounded by a sheath, which increases the diameter to 4 to 5 mm and allows the circulation of the distension fluid, usually normal saline. Various view angles, ranging from 0° to 12° or 30°, exist, depending on the preference of the operator. Dilatation of the cervix is sometimes necessary. To avoid dilatation a 'no touch' hysteroscopic procedure was pioneered by Bettocchi and Salvaggi[13] in 1997 and further practised and investigated by our group.[14] It is performed without medication, cervical dilatation and use of a vaginal speculum or cervical tenaculum. The 5 mm hysteroscope is introduced into the vagina and advanced through the cervical canal into the uterine cavity. In a randomized controlled study, we found that compared to the traditional diagnostic hysteroscopy, the "no touch" approach appears to be less painful and better accepted by the patients.[14] Operative hysteroscopy can be performed with various instruments, including scissors, fiber lasers (Nd: YAG, Ho: YAG) and electrical. Operating a special electrosurgical resectoscope, one can use electrodes that can cut, vaporize, resect, or coagulate tissue. Loop electrodes are widely used for resection of myomas and polyps and for endomyometrial resection and ablation. Ball-shaped and barrel-shaped electrodes are available for coagulation of the endometrium.[15]

In conventional operative hysteroscopy, monopolar electrodes are used, in which the electrical current enters the tissue through a relatively small active electrode and returns through a much larger electrode or grounding pad placed at a remote site.[15]

Glycine, an amino acid widely used by the urologists for cystoscopy, was chosen as a non-conductive distention medium to be used in operative hysteroscopy using monopolar electrical current. However, it was soon noticed that its hypo-osmotic nature carries inherent grave danger. When absorbed excessively it may induce water intoxication, which may lead to cerebral edema due to a gradient between the circulation and the brain, with possible fatal outcome.[16]

A major development in this issue was the introduction of bipolar electrosurgery (VersaPoint, Gynecare, Somerville, NJ, USA and ERA sleeve, Conceptus, San Carlos, CA, USA) in normal saline solution during the late nineties (Fig. 12.2).[16-18] The electrosurgical system consists of a high-frequency dedicated electrosurgical generator and co-axial bipolar electrodes designed to cut, desiccate (coagulate) and vaporize tissue. The return electrode is in close proximity to the active electrode, providing an efficient path of electron flow while minimizing the undesired spread of electrons throughout the conductive distention medium. Activation of the bipolar system creates a high resistance vapor pocket around the active tip of the electrode to maintain a high-power density (Fig. 12.3). On contact of the vapor pocket with the uterine tissue, electrosurgical current passes through the low-impedance path and vaporization is begun.[16] Using the VersaPoint hysteroscope system, we have accumulated a large experience in resection of uterine septa, lysis of adhesions, and resection of leiomyomas or polyps. Since the report of the first 116 such operations in 2001, we have treated hundreds of cases with such intrauterine pathologies using bipolar electrical energy in normal physiological solution without any complication.[16]

Distention Media

Although we have already described the hysteroscopic technique, we feel this subject deserves a special attention. In order to visualize the uterine cavity and the endometrium,

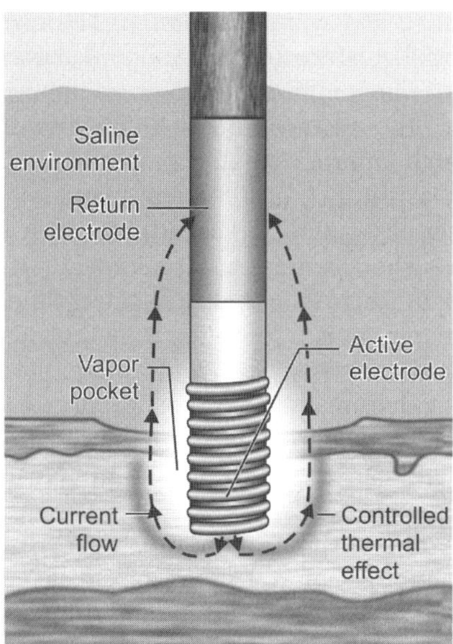

Fig. 12.3: Mechanism of vaporization of VersaPoint bipolar system. Energy is delivered from the generator through the active electrode. Vapor pocket is created, which upon contact with tissue, causes instantaneous cellular rupture. Energy then seeks the path of least resistance to the return electrode. *(Source: Golan A, Sagiv R, Berar M, Ginath S, Glezerman M. Bipolar electrical energy in physiologic solution—a revolution in operative hysteroscopy. J Am Assoc Gynecol Laparosc. 2001;8:252-8)[16]*

the surgeon must dilate it with a suitable distention medium. Currently available distention media include carbondioxide (CO_2) gas, high-viscosity and low-viscosity fluids, but to date, none of these completely meets the characteristics of the ideal medium.

Gaseous distention is suitable only for diagnostic procedures because the risk of gas embolus is too great when blood vessels are breached during therapeutic hysteroscopy. The formation of bubbles of CO_2 mixed with blood is another obstacle to intrauterine surgery. Of the gaseous agents that have been used, CO_2 is closest to the ideal because it is highly soluble and rapidly dissolves in the bloodstream. To reduce the risk of gas embolism, which is proportional to the flow of infused gas, the gaseous insufflation equipment used for hysteroscopy must therefore, limit the flow rate to less than 100 mL/min, with a maximal distending pressure limited to 100 mm Hg.[19] Sutton[19] states that as long as the intrauterine pressure does not exceed 40 to 50 mm Hg, and the flow rate does not exceed 60 mL/minute, the CO_2 distention is extremely safe.

For distention of the uterine cavity by a fluid medium, the distention system has to be capable of generating inflow pressures of 80 to 110 mm Hg.[20] As blood vessels are opened during surgery, there is a significant risk of inadvertent absorption of the irrigant. The results of such an observation vary depending on the amount and the type of fluid.

The most popular fluid distention media used in operative hysteroscopy in the presence of monopolar diathermy are 1.5 percent glycine, sorbitol, and dextran 70. These media, however, still carry risks of causing a dilutional hypo-osmolarity if absorption is excessive[15,21] (Table 12.1). A special advance was the development of electrocautery hysteroscopic bipolar system operating in physiologic irrigation media.[16-18]

Dextran 70 is a clear high-viscosity solution of 32 percent dextran in 10 percent dextrose in water. (Hyskon, Kabia Pharmacia, Piscataway, NJ) with a molecular weight of 70,000. Advantages of Dextran 70 for uterine distention result from its high viscosity, which renders the medium immiscible

Table 12.1: Distention media for hysteroscopy[22]			
Class	*Example*	*Advantages*	*Disadvantages*
Gas	CO_2	Excellent visibility	Requires hysteroscopic insufflator
		Low cost	Unsatisfactory with active bleeding or operative procedures
		Neatness	
High-viscosity fluid	Dextran 70	Immiscible with blood	Pulmonary edema
			Anaphylaxis: 1/10,000
			Foul instruments
Low-viscosity fluid			
Hypotonic	Glycine	Low cost	Hyponatremic hypervolemia
	Sorbitol	Continuous-flow system	Pulmonary edema
	Mannitol		Cerebral edema
Isotonic	Normal saline	Low cost	Pulmonary edema
		Continuous-flow system	Cannot be used with standard monopolar electrodes
		No hyponatremic hypervolemia	

with blood, allowing clear intrauterine visualization even in the presence of moderate bleeding. It is electrolyte-free and therefore, non-conductive and suitable for electrocautery. Diagnostic examinations rarely require the use of more than 100 mL, whereas operative procedures may require 200 to 500 mL. To minimize the potential for intravascular absorption and resultant pulmonary edema, infusion pressures should not exceed 150 mm Hg, and operative time should be limited to 45 minutes.[22] Technical disadvantages of Dextran 70 result from its tendency to crystallize when dried and to caramelize when heated, thus clogging hysteroscopic sheaths and channels. Instruments must be rinsed thoroughly in hot water immediately after use to avoid permanent damage. Its use is less common now because of its hydrophilic nature; if it accidentally enters the circulation, its high molecular weight pulls with it at least six times its volume of fluid and cases of fluid overload with pulmonary edema and left heart failure have been reported.[23] Cases of disseminated intravascular coagulopathy (DIC), adult respiratory distress syndrome (ARDS) and fatal anaphylactic reactions have also been described.[19] We believe that there is no place today for the use of Dextran as a distention medium, neither for diagnostic nor for operative hysteroscopy.

Glycine is a low-viscosity 1.5 percent solution of the amino acid glycine. It is non-conductive and non-hemolytic, and has good optical properties. It is important to note that it is hypotonic relative to extracellular fluid, however, with an osmolarity of 200 mmol/L. Because glycine is electrolyte-free, excessive systemic absorption can result in hyponatremia, hypokalemia, hypocalcemia, and hypo-osmolarity.[24] Glycine has an intravascular half-life of 85 minutes. It is absorbed intracellularly and metabolized, leaving excessive free water extracellularly. If this water is not eliminated, hypo-osmolar hyponatremia may result. Due to the wandering of water along its osmotic and hydrostatic gradients extravascularly and across the blood-brain barrier, non-cardiogenic pulmonary edema and hypotension may result. The resulting cerebral edema can cause increased intracranial pressure. As a result, systemic arterial blood pressure increases, accompanied by reflex bradycardia to maintain cerebral perfusion pressure. As intracranial pressure increases further, cerebral perfusion pressure decreases, resulting in reduced cerebral blood flow and cerebral ischemia, creating a vicious cycle of further brain swelling and reduced blood flow. Seizures can occur, and as swelling continues, an increased brain volume of only 5 percent within the cranium can lead to herniation and death.[21]

The picture is further complicated because glycine itself is an inhibitory neurotransmitter within the central nervous system (CNS) and also potentiates the excitatory neuro-transmitter N-methyl-D-aspartate (NMDA) by potentiation of its receptor activity, which can contribute to seizure activity.[25] In addition, a major metabolite of glycine by oxidative deamination is ammonia, and this could also contribute to the CNS symptomatology.[26]

Sorbitol (2.7%) with mannitol (0.54%) is available as a commercial mixture (Cytal, Abbott Laboratories, North Chicago, IL) with a minimal effect on serum electrolytes and osmolality.[27] It is a low-viscous solution without electrolytes and although appropriate for monopolar electrocautery, it also carries the risk of dilutional hyponatremia because of excessive absorption.[28] The advantage of sorbitol over glycine is its short half-life of 35 minutes. It is metabolized in the liver to fructose and glucose. Over 90 percent of the absorbed mannitol is freely filtered by the kidneys and can cause osmotic diuresis. This could offset the potential for fluid overload from systemic absorption of the irrigating fluid. Higher concentrations of mannitol can cause visual distortion and can crystallize on the hysteroscope, causing surgical difficulties.

Glycine and sorbitol/manitol solutions are still in use by many hysteroscopists. Due to their disadvantage of low osmolarity, special care and monitoring are mandatory during such operations.

Physiologic solutions, which are non-toxic, non-hemolytic, and electrolytically in balance with the extracellular fluid, carry less risk if systemically absorbed. Until recently, the conductive nature of solutions, such as saline or lactated Ringer's, has limited their use during electrocautery because the dissipation of current through the irrigation fluid prevents generation of sufficient current density to allow effective dissection or ablation. This has limited their use for diagnostic or surgical laser surgery. Recently, special systems have been developed, which allow bipolar electrosurgery in physiologic distention media.[16] Although fluid overload can still occur, and careful monitoring of fluid balance is still required, especially in patients with cardiac or renal insufficiency, complications of hyponatremia and hypo-osmolarity are not a problem. We are convinced that using such bipolar systems in physiological solution is the optimal method today for operative hysteroscopy.

Fluid Management Systems

Fluid is delivered to the hysteroscope by means of gravity or by a pump. It is imperative to monitor the exact inflow and outflow of the fluid to prevent complications from excessive fluid absorption. Excessive absorption of hypotonic solutions can result in severe complications from hyponatremia or fluid overload. Istre et al.[29] showed that it is the fluid deficit, which expresses the amount of fluid retained by the patient that correlates directly with the fall in serum electrolytes during operative hysteroscopy using hypotonic solutions and not the total volume of fluid used or the operating time.

It is imperative to maintain a proper balance between a pressure that allows an adequate flow, distention, and visualization and a pressure that does not permit over absorption of the distention medium into the patient's body. Fluid absorption increases significantly when intrauterine pressure exceeds the mean arterial pressure (70 mm Hg).

Table 12.2: Osmolality of serum and commonly used distention media[22,92]	
Distention media	*Osmolality (mOsm/L)*
Normal serum osmolality	290
Glycine 1.5%	200
Sorbitol 3% Mannitol 0.5%	178
Normal saline	304

Distention of the uterine cavity usually requires an average pressure of 40 to 60 mm Hg, therefore, it is crucial to carefully monitor fluid inflow and outflow.[30]

The simplest irrigation system delivers fluid using gravity. The height of the fluid container above the uterus determines the maximum intrauterine pressure.

Hysteroscopic pumps that maintain a constant intrauterine pressure and control flow rates by varying fluid outflow rates create less fluid absorption than older systems that maintain a continuous flow regardless of the intrauterine pressure.[31] These hysteroscopic pump systems have separate controls for both flow rate and intrauterine pressure, calculating the difference between input and output.

The accurate measurement of this fluid deficit determines the volume that has been absorbed by the patient. Continuous monitoring of this fluid deficit is simultaneously presented by weighing the inflow container and outflow canister. It is however, important to remember that this does not account for fluid that is lost in the drapes or on the floor. The osmolality of serum and commonly used distention media is presented in Table 12.2.

CLINICAL DISCUSSION

Clinical Use and Recent Advances

Intrauterine Adhesions

Intrauterine adhesions (IUA), although not necessarily common, are being increasingly recognized, with a wider use of hysteroscopy for the assessment of subfertile women. They are characterized by variable degrees of fibrosis and scarring of the upper part of the cervical canal or the uterine cavity, forming, at times, connections between the opposite walls of the uterus. Joseph Asherman, an Israeli gynecologist, was the first to describe in detail these adhesions, its etiology, its frequency and its related presentation and typical roentgenologic picture. Asherman related the etiology of the condition, presenting by amenorrhea to curettage after delivery, miscarriage, molar pregnancy, or intrauterine, which probably inflicted injury to the basal endometrium.[32,33] It is not easy to determine the incidence of IUA. The degree of awareness of the physician, the widely diverging numbers of abortions in different parts of the world, the high incidence of genital tuberculosis (TB) in some countries and the criteria set

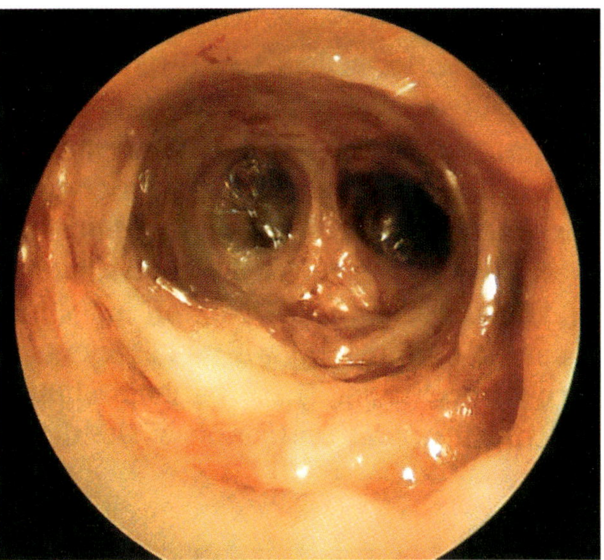

Fig. 12.4: Intrauterine adhesions

in defining IUA are all contributing factors to this difficulty.[34] The estimated overall prevalence might be in the range of 1.5 percent of all patients subjected to hysterosalpingogram, and as high as 25 percent in selected groups.[35]

Adhesions may originate in the endometrium, myometrium or connective tissue. Therefore, it can resemble endometrial tissue or be myofibrous or merely fibrous adhesions.[34]

The majority of patients with Asherman's syndrome have alterations in the duration and amount of the menstrual flow and a varying degree of dysmenorrhea and subfertility. The most frequent complaint is amenorrhea or hypomenorrhea of variable duration. A history of postpartum or postabortal curettage causing menstrual abnormalities, especially if repeated, should alert the clinician to the possibility of intrauterine adhesions.[36]

The progesterone challenge test, resulting in failure of withdrawal bleeding, may be helpful in amenorrheic patients with a biphasic basal body temperature curve.[37]

Although hysterosalpingography (HSG) may be helpful in the diagnosis, it has a significant false positive and false negative rates.[38] Hysteroscopy confirms the presence, the extent and the degree of adhesions,[37] and in fact, is the diagnostic gold standard for the detection and assessment of IUA.

Central adhesions appear at hysteroscopy as columns connecting the opposite uterine walls. Marginal adhesions may present like curtains, which may hide a cornu and create an asymmetry of the uterine cavity (Fig. 12.4).

Various classifications of intrauterine adhesions have been suggested. The European Society classification,[39] and the American Fertility Society classification (Table 12.3)[40] are the most accepted ones.

Table 12.3: American Fertility Society, 1988 classification of intrauterine adhesions[40]

Extent of cavity involved	< 1/3	1/3 – 2/3	> 2/3
	1	2	4
Type of adhesions	Filmy	Filmy and dense	Dense
	1	2	4
Menstrual pattern	Normal	Hypomenorrhea	Amenorrhea
	0	2	4

Prognostic classification:

Stage I (mild)	1–4
Stage II (moderate)	5–8
Stage III (severe)	9–12

Treatment of IUA

Operative hysteroscopy is the method of choice for the treatment of IUA. It is the least aggressive intervention for the healthy endometrium. Lysis of adhesions under direct vision is safer and more complete than blind curettage or hysterotomy. Hysteroscopy permits the scar tissue to be cut and spares the normal endometrium. The mere touch of the endoscope is sometimes sufficient. If not, the adhesions can be divided mechanically, utilizing scissors, electrosurgery or laser. Synechiae in columns are easily removed, while fibrous marginal synechiae, are more difficult to break down and their removal might carry the risk of uterine perforation. Adhesiolysis should start caudally and proceed upwards, until the normal anatomy of the endometrial cavity is restored. Lysis should begin with central and filmy adhesions, whereas marginal and dense ones should be cut afterwards. Visualization of both the tubal ostia and the achievement of a normalized uterine fundus represent the desired outcome of the procedure.[41]

Postoperative adhesion reformation is of concern. Insertion of an intrauterine device (IUD) or a balloon catheter to maintain the separation between the traumatized uterine walls and immediate treatment with estrogens to stimulate rapid growth of the atrophic and damaged endometrium has been suggested by some authors. There is wide consensus regarding the use of postoperative hormonal therapy, however no real evidence for its efficacy exists.[41]

The success rate in establishing normal menstruation in patients treated for IUA ranges from 73 to 92 percent. Successful fertility outcome after hysteroscopic treatment has been correlated with the type of adhesions and the extent of uterine cavity occlusion, ranging from a term pregnancy rate of 81.3 percent in patients with mild disease to 31.9 percent in patients with severe disease.[42] Patients treated for moderate or severe adhesions should be considered at risk during pregnancy and closely followed up, particularly in the early stages of pregnancy and following delivery. Placental insertion abnormalities, such as placenta acreta, increta or percreta, may occur.

Endometrial Polyps

Endometrial polyps are pedunculated masses composed of endometrium that result from focal proliferation of stromal and glandular tissue that lines the uterus and may be present with bleeding. The etiology of endometrial polyps is believed to be related to estrogen stimulation. Late menopause, the use of estrogen-containing hormone replacement therapy and Tamoxifen are considered risk factors for its development.

The prevalence of endometrial polyps depends upon the population being studied. The incidence of endometrial polyps in asymptomatic premenopausal women older than 30 has been reported to be 10 percent.[43] However, the incidence in perimenopausal women with abnormal uterine bleeding was 13 to 35 percent.[44,45] Polyps occur in all age groups but are most commonly found in women between age 40 and 49 years[46] (Figs 12.5A and B).

Late luteal phase endometrium is thick and has a polypoidal appearance, which can often be thought to be abnormal, hence, it is important to be aware and to record the exact timing in menstrual cycle when the diagnostic hysteroscopy is performed.[19]

The likelihood of an endometrial polyp harboring malignancy is small, even with symptomatic irregular bleeding. The average risk of developing atypical hyperplasia or adenocarcinoma of the endometrium is reported as 2.9 percent (Table 12.4).[47-52] Consensus as to which polyp should be removed is lacking. Ben-Arie et al.[47] suggested removal of a polyp during menopause irrespective of the existence of symptomatology, and in premenopausal years, for women with symptomatic polyps or polyps larger than 1.5 cm. Demonstrating similar rates of malignancy among symptomatic and asymptomatic patients, they concluded that the presence of symptoms irrespective of menopause was not a predictor of cancer.[47]

Shushan et al.[51] reported 5 cases of malignancy/premalignancy among 300 cases of endometrial polyps. All were symptomatic. Menopausal status, however, was of no significance, and they stated that no specific hysteroscopic image could characterize a malignant polyp. Machtinger et al.[48] in a series of 438 patients who underwent hysteroscopic polypectomy, found a positive correlation between malignancy and premalignancy and menopause and abnormal uterine bleeding (AUB). Ten of the 11 patients with malignancy/premalignancy in their series had AUB (4.3%) compared to one asymptomatic patient (0.5%). Ten of them were postmenopausal compared to only one premenopausal patient (5% vs 0.4%, respectively). They thought that because of the low incidence of malignancy/premalignancy in asymptomatic women (especially premenopausal), surgical intervention is not warranted in the asymptomatic premenopausal group.

We removed endometrial polyps by operative hysteroscopy in 1124 women and found 23 (2.0%) cases of

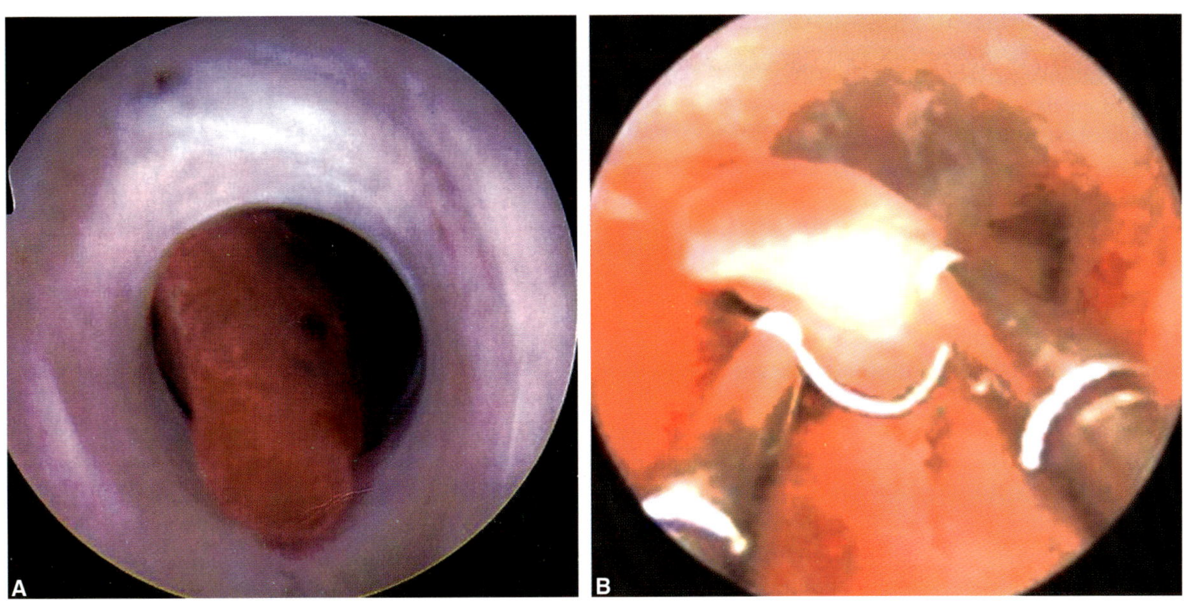

Figs 12.5A and B: (A) Endometrial polyp protrudes through the internal cervical os.
(B) Resection of endometrial polyp using a loop resecting electrode

Table 12.4: Prevalence of atypical hyperplasia and carcinoma in endometrial polyps			
	Atypical hyperplasia	*Carcinoma*	*Total*
Savelli et al. 2003[50]	16/509 (3.1%)	4/509 (0.8%)	20/509 (3.9%)
Ben-Arie et al. 2004[47]	14/402 (3.5%)	13/402 (3.2%)	27/402 (6.7%)
Shushan et al. 2004[51]	1/300 (0.3%)	4/300 (1.3%)	5/300 (1.6%)
Preutthipan et al. 2005[49]	1/240 (0.4%)	0/240 (0%)	1/240 (0.4%)
Machtinger et al. 2005[48]	5/430 (1.1%)	6/438 (1.4%)	11/438 (2.5%)
Lieng et al. 2007[92]	3/411 (0.7%)	11/411 (2.7%)	14/411 (3.4%)
Ferrazzi et al. 2009[93]	31/1922 (1.6%)	33/1922 (1.7%)	64/1922 (3.3%)
Golan et al. 2010[52]	9/1124 (0.8%)	14/1124 (1.2%)	23/1124 (2.0%)
Total	**80/5346 (1.5%)**	**85/5346 (1.6%)**	**165/5346 (3.1%)**

premalignant and malignant lesions.[52] To the best of our knowledge, this is the largest reported series of endometrial polyps removed surgically by operative hysteroscopy from one medical center. We found that such premalignant and malignant lesions can be found in either symptomatic or asymptomatic women and irrespective of their menopausal status. In view of these results, we strongly advocate hysteroscopic polypectomy in all cases of endometrial polyps, regardless of the age, symptomatology, or menopausal status.[52]

Any size polyp can be removed during hysteroscopy by grasping the stalk at its base and cutting or avulsing it from the uterine wall. Broad-based sessile polyps may be removed using the resectoscope or the operating hysteroscope with laser.

Uterine Leiomyomas

Leiomyomata of the uterus are one of the most common tumors in women, with an increasing incidence through reproductive age, and clonal in origin.[53] These are firm, round or oval-shaped well-differentiated smooth muscle cell tumors. They often appear singular but are generally multiple, varying in dimensions and locations. Uterine leiomyoma can occur within the myometrial layer (intramural) of the uterus, in the inner aspect of the myometrium (submucosal) and outside the myometrium (subserosal). They are estrogen-dependant tumors and can grow under the influence of this hormone to quite a remarkable size. This is supported by the fact that fibroids usually increase in size during pregnancy

Table 12.5: Classification of submucous leiomyoma (Fig. 12.6)[55]	
Type 0	Pedunculated submucous leiomyoma without intramural extension.
Type 1	Sessile submucous leiomyoma with less than 50% intramural extension.
Type 2	Sessile submucous leiomyoma with greater than 50% intramural extension.

and shrink either postpartum, after menopause or also after downregulation with gonadotropin-releasing hormone agonists (GnRHa).

Myomas, and especially those of the submucous variety, are an important cause for abnormal uterine bleeding, leading to surgical intervention.

Transvaginal ultrasound examination can reveal an intrauterine lesion but, occasionally, differentiation between a submucous leiomyoma and an endometrial polyp is difficult. Hysteroscopy remains the most definitive method of diagnosis. It provides information about the number of the leiomyomas, their size, and their location.[54] They usually have a whitish appearance and are relatively avascular although occasionally, they do have large blood vessels coursing over the surface.

Hysteroscopic classification of the location of submucous leiomyomas was suggested by Wamsteker and de-Blok[55] and later adopted by the European Society of Hysteroscopy. (Table 12.5, Fig. 12.6). The deeper the fibroid penetrates the myometrium, the more advanced is the type in the classification.

Hysteroscopic removal of submucous myomas is indicated in women with abnormal uterine bleeding, with recurrent pregnancy wastage and with reproductive failure attributed to the presence of a myoma.

Preoperative treatment with a GnRHa is recommended in women with large submucous myomas (≥4 cm) and in those with severe anemia to facilitate surgery by reductions in the size and vascularity of both the uterus and the myoma. GnRHa therapy is best started in the midluteal phase of the cycle to minimize its initial stimulatory effects. This can be given up to 3 months.

The hysteroscope is inserted into the uterine cavity under direct vision via a video camera, using the resectoscope. The myoma is shaved gradually into small tissue chips by drawing the loop electrode steadily toward the objective lens, using a unipolar or bipolar current (depending on the distention media).[56] A pedunculated myoma can be removed by cutting the basis of the pedicle. (Fig. 12.7). However, the removal of a sessile leiomyoma can be more difficult. The protruding dome of the leiomyoma is resected by the resectoscope. This is carried out until the level of normal surrounding endometrium is reached. The remnant intramyometrial

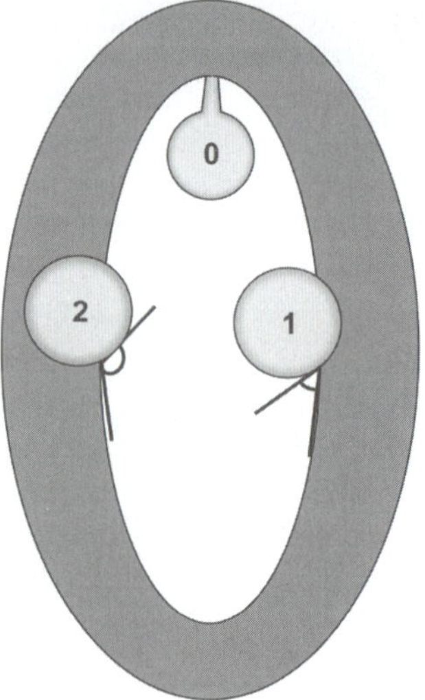

Fig. 12.6: Classification of submucous leiomyoma. The degree of intramural extension is assessed by observing the angle of the fibroid with the endometrium at the attachment to the uterine wall. The wider the angle the deeper is the intramural extension

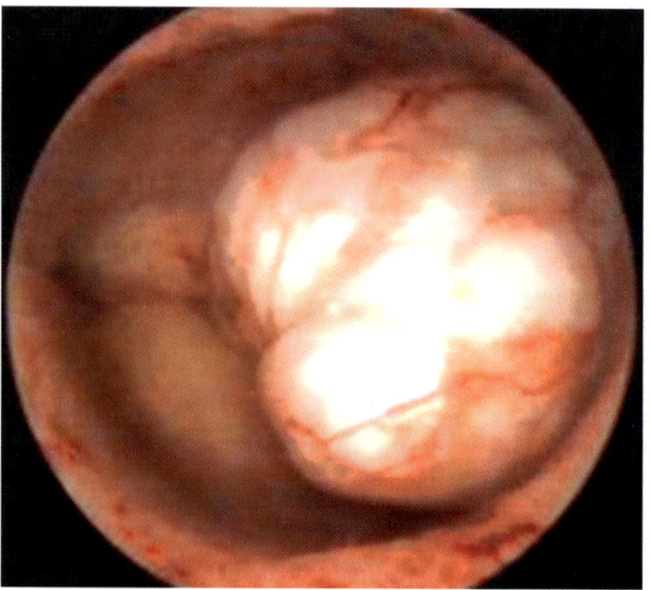

Fig. 12.7: Intracavitary myoma (submucous myoma type 0)

leiomyoma node can be handled by several different methods. Donnez et al.[57] proposed a two-step procedure combined with GnRHa therapy. The protruding portion was removed and the intramural portion remained untouched until further surgery. After additional GnRHa therapy for 8 weeks, the intramural portion becomes submucous and again protruded inside the uterine cavity; possibly because the GnRHa-induced uterine shrinkage provoked the protrusion of the remaining portion. This technique is the safest option because it does not involve cutting into the myometrium; however, the extended GnRHa treatment and repeated hysteroscopies can cause greater distress in patients.[57] Loffer[58] even reported that the remainder of the myoma was squeezed out of the depth of the wall by contractions of the uterus during the removal of tissue chips.[58] This observation suggests the possibility that an intramural leiomyoma can be squeezed into the uterine cavity if the power of the uterine contraction exceeds the intrauterine pressure. Implication of this concept by injection of prostglandins, such as PGF-2α, to induce uterine contractions, enabled extrusion of the intramural myoma into the uterine cavity and easy shaving of the remnant leiomyoma in one-step without cutting deeply into the myometrium.[59,60] The shrunken uterine cavity consequent to PGF-2α injection may interfere temporarily with visualization and therefore, it is necessary to wait to restart the resection until the contractions weaken. When all of these procedures can be carried out in the uterine cavity, the risk of uterine perforation is decreased.

Hysteroscopic resection of submucous leiomyoma is a relatively safe procedure. Uterine perforation during the operation was reported as 1.6 percent in a recent large case series.[61] Fecundity improves following resection with 59 percent of infertile patients conceiving postoperatively.[62] In women undergoing in vitro fertilization (IVF) treatment, pregnancy rates per embryo transfer significantly improved following hysteroscopic resection.[63]

Uterine Septum

It can be estimated that about 1 percent of the female fertile population has a uterine septum.[64] Uterine septum results from an incomplete resorption of the adjacent walls of the two fused Müllerian ducts. It can be partial or complete. According the American Fertility Society classification of Müllerian anomalies, a septate uterus is defined as complete when the septum reaches the internal os.[40] The outer surface of the uterine fundus seems normal. It was always believed that the septum effects fertility by defective implantation on an avascular septum. Dabirashrafi et al.[65] found that biopsies from the septum compared with biopsy specimens obtained away from the septum were composed of more muscle fibers and less connective tissue. Sparac et al.[66] reported similar findings following histological examination of intrauterine septa resected hysteroscopically and by ultrasonic Doppler flow studies.[66]

The incidence of septate uterus is higher in women with selected reproductive difficulties, particularly recurrent abortion and preterm labor. The prevalence of uterine anomalies in patients with repeated pregnancy loss is 12.6 percent, and septate uterus can be identified in about one-third of these patients,[41] a proportion that is certainly higher than that of the general population.[67] Septate uterus is mainly associated with the highest

incidence of first and second trimester recurrent miscarriage and preterm deliveries. Homer et al.[68] in a large meta-analysis of 19 studies of pregnancies in women with untreated septate uterus, reported a miscarriage rate of 79 percent and a preterm delivery rate of 9 percent.[68] However, the prevalence of Müllerian defects in infertile patients is 3.4 percent,[64] which is very similar to that found in the fertile population, suggesting that such defects, and with septate uterus in particular, have little influence on fecundity.[69]

The parallel performance of hysteroscopy and laparoscopy represents the gold standard for the definitive diagnosis of a septate uterus. However, visualization of the uterine fundus can also be achieved with non-invasive methods, such as ultrasound or magnetic resonance imaging (MRI) when HSG or hysteroscopy raises the suspicion of a septum.[41]

There is consensus regarding the need to correct a septate uterus when the reproductive history of the patient includes repeated abortions and/or preterm delivery. On the other hand, there are controversies regarding the appropriateness of performing metroplasty in infertile patients, or in patients with an incidental finding of this anomaly.

Operating on a uterine septum means making an incision, not resection, because once divided, the fibromuscular tissue that constitutes the septum immediately retracts to about the level of the endometrium. This can be done with either mechanical scissors, electrosurgery or laser energy. Surgery is started with access to the endometrial cavity and visualization of each tubal ostium, followed by an equidistant incision between the anterior and posterior uterine wall, extending the incision of the septum from the apex to the uterine fundus. The determination of the end point is achieved when the hysteroscope can be moved freely from one tubal ostium to the other and when both ostia are simultaneously visible from the level of the internal cervical os (Figs 12.8A and B).

No occurrence of postoperative intrauterine adhesionsis is the rule in these cases. In a large multi-center Italian study, not even one case of intrauterine adhesions was detected in 973 cases of hysteroscopic resection of uterine septum.[70]

The effectiveness of hysteroscopic metroplasty is based only on case control studies and there are no of randomized trials comparing outcomes of treated and non-treated patients. Reviewing 16 studies, Homer et al.[68] found that hysteroscopic metroplasty in women with a septate uterus improved subsequent reproductive outcome. The miscarriage rate dropped from 88 to 14 percent (p < 0.001), the preterm delivery rate dropped from 9 to 6 percent (p = 0.051), while the term delivery rate increased from 3 to 80 percent (p < 0.001).[68]

Endometrial Ablation for Abnormal Uterine Bleeding

Abnormal uterine bleeding (AUB) affects approximately 20 to 25 percent of otherwise healthy premenopausal women. The

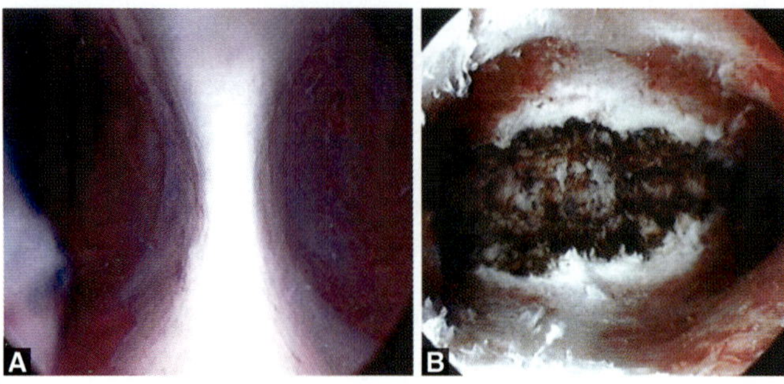

Figs 12.8A and B: (A) Uterine septum; (B) Endometrial cavity immediately after cutting of the septum with bipolar VersaPoint spring

prevalence of AUB increases with age and peaks during the fifth decade just before menopause. AUB may result in iron deficiency anemia, affect quality of life, and account for up to 30 to 35 percent of all hysterectomies.[71]

Traditionally, treatment of AUB included medical therapies, dilatation and curettage (D&C), and hysterectomy. Endometrial ablation is a procedure that destroys the endometrium by thermal energy or resection.

Hysteroscopic endometrial ablation was introduced by Lindemann[72] in 1971 as an alternative to hysterectomy for those patients with AUB and benign pathology who are unable or unwilling to tolerate traditional therapies. Prior to ablation, it is imperative to exclude premalignant and malignant endometrial conditions, polyps, or leiomyomas in the uterine cavity. Endometrial ablation should not be offered to women who wish to preserve their fertility or be used for contraception.

There are two methods for performing endometrial ablation: the first-generation of endometrial ablation technology includes laser or electrocoagulation with the use of operative hysteroscopy, whereas the second-generation of endometrial ablation technologies, which are also referred to as "global endometrial ablation technologies" involve the automated destruction of the endometrium with an energy source without the use of operative hysteroscopy.[73]

The endometrium is systematically resected electrosurgically using the loop resectoscope or destroyed by the rollerball or rollerbar electrode.

Garry et al.[74] reported on 600 laser ablations in 524 women. After a mean follow-up of 15 months, successful outcome was reported in 83.4 percent of the women with a hysterectomy rate of 6.8 percent. In a follow-up study that reported on 1000 consecutive endometrial laser ablations, the life table analysis showed that the hysterectomy rate was 21 percent at 6.5 years.[74] Rollerball ablation has evolved to be the most commonly used hysteroscopic ablation technique because it is easy to use and is associated with less risks and complications than the loop electrode.[75]

In a Cochrane review, hysteroscopic endometrial ablation has been proved to be as effective as hysterectomy as an alternative treatment for heavy menstrual bleeding.[76] In another Cochrane comparison of the second-generation techniques with the hysteroscopic ablative techniques (first-generation), surgery was found to be shorter and had less complications of fluid overload, uterine perforation, and cervical lacerations. However, equipment failure, and side effects of nausea, vomiting and uterine cramping were more common in second-generation ablation.[77]

Retained Products of Conception (RPOC)

This is a very common problem in gynecological practice and can be found after incomplete miscarriage, vaginal delivery and even following cesarean section (Fig. 12.9). Curettage of the endometrial cavity was always the classical management. Operative hysteroscopy can be used very efficiently for the removal of the adherent trophoblastic residual tissue. The resectoscope loop is used for mechanical selective removal of the adherent residual tissue without the use of electricity, while interference with the rest of the endometrial surface is avoided. Comparing this method to the traditional curettage for the treatment of RPOC demonstrated similar reproductive outcomes in both groups without any complications.[78]

The hysteroscopic mechanical removal of RPOC using the loop in physiological solution is the common practice in our department in the management of this problem and we have recently reported on 159 such cases with minimal complications.[79] Hysteroscopic removal of retained products of conception is a simple and safe, and most probably, the preferred procedure. It should be considered an alternative to

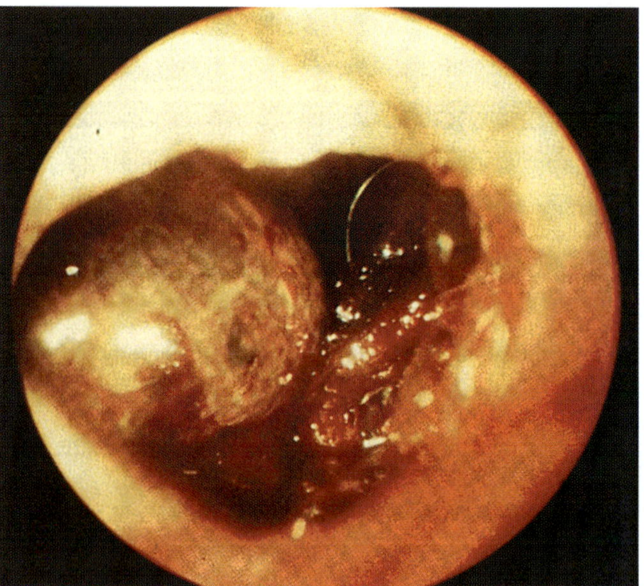

Fig. 12.9: Retained products of gestation

conventional blinded evacuation by curettage. It seems that this procedure preserves the integrity of the uterine cavity while averting additional trauma, and retains reproductive capacity.[79]

Sterilization

Bilateral blockage of the Fallopian tubes by the hysteroscopic route is a practical option for sterilization that avoids the disadvantage and the risks involved in the laparoscopic approach. This approach involves the use of the Essure system. The system includes a coil made from nickel-titanium dacron thread. It is inserted into the uterine ostium on each side through the hysteroscope and induces fibrosis and blockage of the tubes. This can be performed ambulatory without using anesthesia. The reported success rate following the completion of this procedure is over 90 percent. Three months after the procedure, hysterosalpingography is performed for ensuring the blockage of the Fallopian tubes. Sinha et al.[80] reported a complete two-sided block in 99 percent of the cases after 3 months of the procedure and in 100 percent of the cases after 6 months.[80]

Complications of Hysteroscopy

Complications of hysteroscopy can be divided into intra-operative procedure-related or media-related events and postoperative events.

The complication rate of hysteroscopy has been estimated to be in the range of 0.3 percent to 2.7 percent.[81,82] The rate of complications is directly proportional to the type of hysteroscopic procedure performed. The safest procedure is obviously diagnostic hysteroscopy. Myomectomy and resection of uterine septa were reported as procedures with the highest complication rates, whereas polypectomies and endometrial ablations had lower rates of complications.[82] In another study, adhesiolysis had the greatest risk of complications, followed by endometrial resection, myomectomy, and polypectomy. Almost half of the complications were related to cervical entry.[81] Preoperative treatment with GnRH agonist therapy was associated with a 4 to 7 times higher odds of operative complications.

Uterine perforation, occurring in 14.2 per 1000 cases, remains the most common complication reported in most hysteroscopic reviews. The risk of perforation is increased in relation to nulliparity, menopause, GnRH agonist use, previous cone biopsy, markedly retroverted uterus and the use of undue force.[83] When uterine perforation occurs, the procedure must be abandoned. Uterine perforation can be suspected if fluid deficit rises quickly as a result of the fast intraperitoneal accumulation.

In an attempt to avoid complications related to forceful problematic cervical dilatation, intravaginal administration of misoprostol before surgery has been used.[84,85]

Diagnostic hysteroscopic procedures can be performed with carbon dioxide or fluid, whereas operative procedures should never be performed using carbon dioxide because of the high risk of carbon dioxide embolism due to open venous channels associated with a vascular endometrium. The incidence of severe non-fatal embolism in carbondioxide diagnostic hysteroscopic procedures is 0.03 percent, and the risk of subclinical embolic events is 0.51 percent.[86] Pulmonary hypertension, hypercarbia, hypoxia, arrhythmias, tachypnea, and systemic hypotension are the most common symptoms of venous or gas embolism.[87] A sudden decrease in end-tidal carbon dioxide appears when cardiovascular collapse from gas embolism is imminent. If suspected, the hysteroscopic procedure should be immediately stopped and 100 percent oxygen given. The patient should be turned to the left lateral decubitus position, and aspiration of gas by a central venous catheter urgently attempted.[83]

Special efforts to reduce the occurrence of air embolism should include avoidance of steep Trendelenburg, purging of the hysteroscope tubing, utilization of a low-pressure hysteroscopic carbon dioxide insufflator and continuous monitoring of the end-tidal carbon dioxide volume.

Due to all the above, normal saline has become the most popular distention medium for diagnostic hysteroscopy worldwide. We have performed thousands of such diagnostic procedures without any complication.

All the fluids used as distention media in hysteroscopic procedures can be associated with complications (Table 12.1). The type of distention medium used in operative and diagnostic hysteroscopy is usually determined by the surgeon and the system in use. Current options include high-viscosity Dextran 70 and low-viscosity fluid hypotonic, electrolyte-free solution (glycine, mannitol–sorbitol), or isotonic, electrolyte-containing solutions (normal saline).

Anaphylactic reactions including acute hypotension, hypoxia, pulmonary edema, fluid overload, fulminant coagulapathies, and anemia are well-described with Dextran 70. Operative hysteroscopy, performed in a monopolar environment, requires a hypotonic electrolyte-free, non-conductive solution including glycine 1.5 percent, or sorbitol 2.7 percent plus mannitol 0.5 percent. When glycine and sorbitol are metabolized, excess of water accumulates, and is associated with hyponatremic hypervolemia. Normally, compensatory mechanisms adapt to move the excess of water and osmotically active cations into extracellular and intracellular spaces. Failure of this compensatory mechanism causes an increase in free water in the brain, hyponatremia and dilutional hypo-osmolality, resulting in cerebral edema, increased intracranial pressure, and cellular necrosis. Mental agitation, apprehension, confusion, nausea and vomiting, visual disturbances, and headache and convulsions follow. If left untreated and unrecognized, bradycardia and hypertension develop, rapidly followed by pulmonary edema, cardiovascular collapse and death. Free ammonia, resulting from metabolized glycine, also contributes to central nervous system disturbance.

The introduction of isotonic, electrolyte-containing and physiological solutions eliminated the possibility of hyponatremic hypervolemia. However, fluid overload, pulmonary edema, and congestive heart failure can still occur.

The amount of fluid absorbed is associated with the surface area of the surgical field, duration of surgery, opened venous channels, type of irrigation fluid used, and intrauterine pressure. Under regional anesthesia, central nervous system complications are more readily apparent than when general anesthesia is used.[83]

Infectious complications of operative hysteroscopy occur in 0.3 to 1.6 percent of cases.[83] Most cases involve urinary tract infections, endometritis, pyometritis and rarely, tubo-ovarian abscess. Women with a history of pelvic inflammatory disease, necrotic residual tissue, long procedures, and extensive endomyometrial destruction are at increased risk.

Delayed complications of hysteroscopy have been recognized months to years after the procedure. Endometrial ablation is not a method of contraception. Pregnancy rates of 0.2 to 1.6 percent have been described, but may be under-reported. The endometrial tissue is quite resilient and may regenerate after endometrial ablation. Sterilization should be recommended when endometrial ablation is performed.[83]

Endometrial ablation is not usually offered for the treatment of abnormal uterine bleeding in women who have endometrial hyperplasia, although this is not in consensus.[88,89]

The risk of dissemination of endometrial cancer cells during hysteroscopy has been debated. Retrospective data shows a correlation between fluid-based hysteroscopy and the presence of cancer cells in the peritoneal cavity.[90] However, in a prospective multicenter study, Kudela and Pilka[91] studied the risk of positive finding of malignant cells in women with endometrial cancer, who underwent a dilatation and curettage or hysteroscopy, performed with a fluid medium. Cul-de-sac aspiration after instrumentation and at the beginning of the subsequent operation demonstrated no increased risk of positive cytology.[91]

Patients experiencing intraoperative complications during hysteroscopic metroplasty or deep resection of intramural fibroids should be informed of the risk of uterine rupture in a subsequent pregnancy and may consider elective cesarean section or at least increased surveillance. Uterine dehiscence, uterine sacculation, and extremely thin myometrium have all been reported after uterine adhesiolysis, uterine perforation during operative hysteroscopy, and leiomyoma resection.[83]

CONCLUSION

This review provides an updated survey of the advances in operative hysteroscopy for the treatment of a variety of intrauterine conditions and demonstrates that it can be very effective and safe, especially with the use of bipolar electrosurgery in a physiologic distention media.

REFERENCES

1. Bozzini P. Lichtleiter, eine Erfindung zur Anschauung innerer Teile und Krankheiten. J Prak Heilk 1806;24:107.
2. Shah J. Endoscopy through the ages. BJU Int 2002;89:645-52.
3. Pantaleoni DC. On endoscopic examination of the cavity of the womb Medical Press Circular 1869;8:26-7.
4. Valle RF. Office hysteroscopy. Clin Obstet Gynecol 1999;42:276-89.
5. Nitze M. Beobachtung-und Untersuchungsmethode fur Harnohre, Harnblase und Rectum. Wien Med Wochenschr 1879;29:649.
6. David JM. De l'endoscopie de l'uterus ares avortement et dans es suites de couches a l'etat pathologique. Bulletin of Society of Obstetrics 1907.
7. Heineberg A. Uterine endoscopy: An aid to precision in the diagnosis of intrauterine disease. Surg Gynecol Obstet 1914;18:513.
8. Rubin IC. Uterine endoscopy, endometroscopy with the aid of uterine insufflation. Am J Obset Gynecol 1925;10:313-27.
9. Seymour H. Endoscopy of the uterus: with description of a hysteroscope. Obstet Gynaecol Br Commonw 1926;6:52-5.
10. Fourestiere M, Gladu A, Vulmiere J. Laperitinioscopy. Presse Medicale 1943;5:46-7.
11. Gow JG. Harold Hopkins and optical systems for urology: an appreciation. Urology 1998;52:152-7.
12. Bettocchi S, Nappi L, Ceci O, Selvaggi L. Office hysteroscopy. Obstet Gynecol Clin North Am 2004;31:641-54, xi.
13. Bettocchi S, Selvaggi L. A vaginoscopic approach to reduce the pain of office hysteroscopy. J Am Assoc Gynecol Laparosc 1997;4:255-8.
14. Sagiv R, Sadan O, Boaz M, Dishi M, Schechter E, Golan A. A new approach to office hysteroscopy compared with traditional hysteroscopy: a randomized controlled trial. Obstet Gynecol 2006;108:387-92.
15. Indman PD. Instrumentation and distention media for the hysteroscopic treatment of abnormal uterine bleeding. Obstet Gynecol Clin North Am 2000;27:305-15, vi.
16. Golan A, Sagiv R, Berar M, Ginath S, Glezerman M. Bipolar electrical energy in physiologic solution: a revolution in operative hysteroscopy. J Am Assoc Gynecol Laparosc 2001;8:252-8.
17. Vilos GA. Intrauterine surgery using a new coaxial bipolar electrode in normal saline solution (Versapoint): a pilot study. Fertil Steril 1999;72:740-3.
18. Isaacson KB, Olive DL. Operative hysteroscopy in physiologic distention media. J Am Assoc Gynecol Laparosc 1999;6:113-8.

19. Sutton C. Hysteroscopic surgery. Best Pract Res Clin Obstet Gynaecol 2006;20:105-37.
20. Magos AL, Lockwood GM, Baumann R, Turnbull AC, Kay JD. Absorption of irrigating solution during transcervical resection of endometrium. Bmj 1990;300:1079.
21. Murdoch JA, Gan TJ. Anesthesia for hysteroscopy. Anesthesiol Clin North America 2001;19:125-40.
22. Cooper JM, Brady RM. Hysteroscopy in the management of abnormal uterine bleeding. Obstet Gynecol Clin North Am 1999;26:217-36.
23. Golan A, Siedner M, Bahar M, Ron-El R, Herman A, Caspi E. High-output left ventricular failure after dextran use in an operative hysteroscopy. Fertil Steril 1990;54:939-41.
24. Agraharkar M, Agraharkar A. Posthysteroscopic hyponatremia: evidence for a multifactorial cause. Am J Kidney Dis 1997; 30:717-9.
25. Pourcho RG, Goebel DJ, Jojich L, Hazlett JC. Immuno-cytochemical evidence for the involvement of glycine in sensory centers of the rat brain. Neuroscience 1992;46:643-56.
26. Hahn RG. Blood ammonia concentrations resulting from absorption of irrigating fluid containing glycine and ethanol during transurethral resection of the prostate. Scand J Urol Nephrol 1991;25:115-9.
27. Moir CL, Mandin H, Brant R. Sorbitol 2.5 percent mannitol 0.54 percent irrigation solution for hysteroscopic endometrial ablation surgery. Can J Anaesth 1997;44:473-8.
28. Kim AH, Keltz MD, Arici A, Rosenberg M, Olive DL. Dilutional hyponatremia during hysteroscopic myomectomy with sorbitol-mannitol distention medium. J Am Assoc Gynecol Laparosc 1995;2:237-42.
29. Istre O, Skajaa K, Schjoensby AP, Forman A. Changes in serum electrolytes after transcervical resection of endometrium and submucous fibroids with use of glycine 1.5 percent for uterine irrigation. Obstet Gynecol 1992;80:218-22.
30. Isaacson K. New developments in operative hysteroscopy. Obstet Gynecol Clin North Am 2000;27:375-83.
31. Garry R. Safety of hysteroscopic surgery. Lancet 1990;336: 103-14.
32. Asherman J. Traumatic intrauterine adhesions. Br J Obstet Gynaecol 1950;57:892-6.
33. Asherman J. Amenorrhoea traumatica. J Obstet Gynaecol Br Emp 1948;55:23-30.
34. Schenker JG, Margalioth EJ. Intrauterine adhesions: an updated appraisal. Fertil Steril 1982;37:593-610.
35. Dmowski WP, Greenblatt RB. Asherman's syndrome and risk of placenta accreta. Obstet Gynecol 1969;34:288-99.
36. Magos A. Hysteroscopic treatment of Asherman's syndrome. Reprod Biomed Online 2002;4 Suppl 3:46-51.
37. Al-Inany H. Intrauterine adhesions. An update. Acta Obstet Gynecol Scand 2001;80:986-93.
38. Golan A, Eilat E, Ron-El R, Herman A, Soffer Y, Bukovsky I. Hysteroscopy is superior to hysterosalpingography in infertility investigation. Acta Obstet Gynecol Scand 1996;75:654-6.
39. Wamsteker K, DeBlok S. Diagnostic hysteroscopy: technique and documentation. New York: Lippincott Williams and Wilkins Publishers; 1995.
40. The American Fertility Society classifications of adnexal adhesions, distal tubal occlusion, tubal occlusion secondary to tubal ligation, tubal pregnancies, mullerian anomalies and intrauterine adhesions. Fertil Steril 1988;49:944-55.
41. Fedele L, Bianchi S, Frontino G. Septums and synechiae: approaches to surgical correction. Clin Obstet Gynecol 2006; 49:767-88.
42. Valle RF, Sciarra JJ. Intrauterine adhesions: hysteroscopic diagnosis, classification, treatment, and reproductive outcome. Am J Obstet Gynecol 1988;158:1459-70.
43. Clevenger-Hoeft M, Syrop CH, Stovall DW, Van Voorhis BJ. Sonohysterography in premenopausal women with and without abnormal bleeding. Obstet Gynecol 1999;94:516-20.
44. Goldstein SR, Zeltser I, Horan CK, Snyder JR, Schwartz LB. Ultrasonography-based triage for perimenopausal patients with abnormal uterine bleeding. Am J Obstet Gynecol 1997;177: 102-8.
45. Mihm LM, Quick VA, Brumfield JA, Connors AF, Jr., Finnerty JJ. The accuracy of endometrial biopsy and saline sonohysterography in the determination of the cause of abnormal uterine bleeding. Am J Obstet Gynecol 2002;186: 858-60.
46. Silberstein T, Saphier O, van Voorhis BJ, Plosker SM. Endometrial polyps in reproductive-age fertile and infertile women. Isr Med Assoc J 2006;8:192-5.
47. Ben-Arie A, Goldchmit C, Laviv Y, Levy R, Caspi B, Huszar M, Dgani R, Hagay Z. The malignant potential of endometrial polyps. Eur J Obstet Gynecol Reprod Biol 2004;115:206-10.
48. Machtinger R, Korach J, Padoa A, Fridman E, Zolti M, Segal J, et al. Transvaginal ultrasound and diagnostic hysteroscopy as a predictor of endometrial polyps: risk factors for premalignancy and malignancy. Int J Gynecol Cancer 2005;15:325-8.
49. Preutthipan S, Herabutya Y. Hysteroscopic polypectomy in 240 premenopausal and postmenopausal women. Fertil Steril 2005;83:705-9.
50. Savelli L, De Iaco P, Santini D, et al. Histopathologic features and risk factors for benignity, hyperplasia, and cancer in endometrial polyps. Am J Obstet Gynecol 2003;188:927-31.
51. Shushan A, Revel A, Rojansky N. How often are endometrial polyps malignant? Gynecol Obstet Invest 2004;58:212-5.
52. Golan A, Cohen-Sahar B, Keidar R, Condrea A, Ginath S, Sagiv R. Endometrial polyps: symptomatology, menopausal status and malignancy. Gynecol Obstet Invest 2010;70:107-12.
53. Nowak RA. Fibroids: pathophysiology and current medical treatment. Baillieres Best Pract Res Clin Obstet Gynaecol 1999;13:223-38.
54. Tulandi T, al-Took S. Endoscopic myomectomy. Laparoscopy and hysteroscopy. Obstet Gynecol Clin North Am 1999;26:135-48, viii.
55. Wamsteker K, de-Blok S. Diagnostic hysteroscopy: technique and documentation. London: WB Saunders; 1993.
56. Murakami T, Tamura M, Ozawa Y, Suzuki H, Terada Y, Okamura K. Safe techniques in surgery for hysteroscopic myomectomy. J Obstet Gynaecol Res 2005;31:216-23.
57. Donnez J, Gillerot S, Bourgonjon D, Clerckx F, Nisolle M. Neodymium: YAG laser hysteroscopy in large submucous fibroids. Fertil Steril 1990;54:999-1003.
58. Loffer FD. Removal of large symptomatic intrauterine growths by the hysteroscopic resectoscope. Obstet Gynecol 1990;76: 836-40.

59. Murakami T, Shimizu T, Katahira A, Terada Y, Yokomizo R, Sawada R. Intraoperative injection of prostaglandin F2alpha in a patient undergoing hysteroscopic myomectomy. Fertil Steril 2003;79:1439-41.

60. Indman PD. Use of carboprost to facilitate hysteroscopic resection of submucous myomas. J Am Assoc Gynecol Laparosc 2004;11:68-72.

61. Agostini A, Cravello L, Bretelle F, Shojai R, Roger V, Blanc B. Risk of uterine perforation during hysteroscopic surgery. J Am Assoc Gynecol Laparosc 2002;9:264-67.

62. Ubaldi F, Tournaye H, Camus M, Van der Pas H, Gepts E, Devroey P. Fertility after hysteroscopic myomectomy. Hum Reprod Update 1995;1:81-90.

63. Narayan R, Rajat, Goswamy K. Treatment of submucous fibroids, and outcome of assisted conception. J Am Assoc Gynecol Laparosc 1994;1:307-11.

64. Grimbizis GF, Camus M, Tarlatzis BC, Bontis JN, Devroey P. Clinical implications of uterine malformations and hysteroscopic treatment results. Hum Reprod Update 2001;7:161-74.

65. Dabirashrafi H, Bahadori M, Mohammad K, et al. Septate uterus: new idea on the histologic features of the septum in this abnormal uterus. Am J Obstet Gynecol 1995;172:105-07.

66. Sparac V, Kupesic S, Ilijas M, Zodan T, Kurjak A. Histologic architecture and vascularization of hysteroscopically excised intrauterine septa. J Am Assoc Gynecol Laparosc 2001;8:111-6.

67. Golan A, Schneider D, Avrech O, Raziel A, Bukovsky I, Caspi E. Hysteroscopic findings after missed abortion. Fertil Steril 1992;58:508-10.

68. Homer HA, Li TC, Cooke ID. The septate uterus: a review of management and reproductive outcome. Fertil Steril 2000;73: 1- 14.

69. Acien P. Reproductive performance of women with uterine malformations. Hum Reprod 1993;8:122-6.

70. Colacurci N, De Placido G, Perino A, Mencaglia L, Gubbini G. Hysteroscopic metroplasty. J Am Assoc Gynecol Laparosc 1998;5:171-4.

71. Lefebvre G, Allaire C, Jeffrey J, et al. SOGC clinical guidelines. Hysterectomy. J Obstet Gynaecol Can 2002;24:37-61.

72. Lindemann HJ. Eine neue unteruchungsmethode fur die hysteroscopie. Endoscopy 1971;3:194-201.

73. Vilos GA. Hysteroscopic and nonhysteroscopic endometrial ablation. Obstet Gynecol Clin North Am 2004;31:687-704, xi.

74. Garry R, Fuller TA, Segal S. Laser photovaporization of endometrium for the treatment of menorrhagia. Obstet Gynecol 1981;85:14-9.

75. Overton C, Hargreaves J, Maresh M. A national survey of the complications of endometrial destruction for menstrual disorders: the MISTLETOE study. Minimally Invasive Surgical Techniques-Laser, EndoThermal or Endorescetion. Br J Obstet Gynaecol 1997;104:1351-9.

76. Lethaby A, Shepperd S, Cooke I, Farquhar C. Endometrial resection and ablation versus hysterectomy for heavy menstrual bleeding. Cochrane Database Syst Rev 2000:CD000329.

77. Lethaby A, Hickey M, Garry R. Endometrial destruction techniques for heavy menstrual bleeding. Cochrane Database Syst Rev 2005:CD001501.

78. Cohen SB, Kalter-Ferber A, Weisz BS, Zalel Y, Seidman DS, Mashiach S, et al. Hysteroscopy may be the method of choice for management of residual trophoblastic tissue. J Am Assoc Gynecol Laparosc 2001;8:199-202.

79. Golan A, Dishi M, Shalev A, Keidar R, Ginath S, Sagiv R. Operative hysteroscopy to remove retained products of conception: novel treatment of an old problem. J Minim Invasive Gynecol 2011;18:100-103.

80. Sinha D, Kalathy V, Gupta JK, Clark TJ. The feasibility, success and patient satisfaction associated with outpatient hysteroscopic sterilisation. BJOG 2007;114:676-83.

81. Jansen FW, Vredevoogd CB, van Ulzen K, Hermans J, Trimbos JB, Trimbos-Kemper TC. Complications of hysteroscopy: a prospective, multicenter study. Obstet Gynecol 2000;96:266-70.

82. Propst AM, Liberman RF, Harlow BL, Ginsburg ES. Complications of hysteroscopic surgery: predicting patients at risk. Obstet Gynecol 2000;96:517-20.

83. Bradley LD. Complications in hysteroscopy: prevention, treatment and legal risk. Curr Opin Obstet Gynecol 2002;14:409-15.

84. Fung TM, Lam MH, Wong SF, Ho LC. A randomised placebo-controlled trial of vaginal misoprostol for cervical priming before hysteroscopy in postmenopausal women. Bjog 2002;109:561-5.

85. Preutthipan S, Herabutya Y. Vaginal misoprostol for cervical priming before operative hysteroscopy: a randomized controlled trial. Obstet Gynecol 2000;96:890-4.

86. Brandner P, Neis KJ, Ehmer C. The etiology, frequency, and prevention of gas embolism during CO(2) hysteroscopy. J Am Assoc Gynecol Laparosc 1999;6:421-8.

87. Munro MG, Weisberg M, Rubinstein E. Gas and air embolization during hysteroscopic electrosurgical vaporization: comparison of gas generation using bipolar and monopolar electrodes in an experimental model. J Am Assoc Gynecol Laparosc 2001;8:488-94.

88. Vilos GA, Harding PG, Ettler HC. Resectoscopic surgery in 10 women with abnormal uterine bleeding and atypical endometrial hyperplasia. J Am Assoc Gynecol Laparosc 2002;9:138-44.

89. Vilos GA, Harding PG, Ettler HC. Resectoscopic surgery in women with abnormal uterine bleeding and nonatypical endometrial hyperplasia. J Am Assoc Gynecol Laparosc 2002;9: 131-7.

90. Revel A, Tsafrir A, Anteby SO, Shushan A. Does hysteroscopy produce intraperitoneal spread of endometrial cancer cells? Obstet Gynecol Surv 2004;59:280-4.

91. Kudela M, Pilka R. Is there a real risk in patients with endometrial carcinoma undergoing diagnostic hysteroscopy (HSC)? Eur J Gynaecol Oncol 2001;22:342-4.

92. Lieng M, Qvigstad E, Sandvik L, Jorgensen H, Langebrekke A, Istre O. Hysteroscopic resection of symptomatic and asymptomatic endometrial polyps. J Minim Invasive Gynecol 2007;14:189-94.

93. Ferrazzi E, Zupi E, Leone FP, Savelli L, Omodei U, Moscarini M, et al. How often are endometrial polyps malignant in asymptomatic postmenopausal women? A multicenter study. Am J Obstet Gynecol 2009;200:235 e1-6.

Resection of the Uterine Septum or *In Vitro* Fertilization: What Comes First?

Murat Berkkanoglu, Kemal Ozgur

OVERVIEW

Lack of resorption of the mid-line septum between the two Müllerian ducts results in defects that range from a slight mid-line septum to a complete division of the endometrial cavity. The septate uterus is associated with a high incidence of reproductive failure and obstetric complications, including first and second trimester recurrent miscarriage, premature delivery, abnormal fetal presentation, intrauterine growth retardation (IUGR), and infertility.

There are various diagnostic tools with differing accuracies to identify the uterine septum. Among these diagnostic tools, hysteroscopy not only provides a diagnostic approach but also a treatment option. Hysteroscopic metroplasty is a simple technique with minimal intraoperative and postoperative morbidity.

Although there are currently no well-randomized, controlled studies regarding the management of the septate uterus, recent studies have demonstrated improvement in subsequent reproductive outcomes after metroplasty including miscarriage and preterm delivery. The role of hysteroscopic metroplasty in patients with primary infertility is controversial. However, removal of the septum before assisted reproductive treatment is usually recommended to reduce the possibility of poor reproductive outcome.

RATIONALE

Among the congenital abnormalities of the Müllerian ducts, the septate uterus is the most common type. Although it is associated with a poor reproductive outcome, it is the type which is most amenable to simple hysteroscopic treatment. Therefore, the known adverse reproductive outcomes and various treatment indications of the septate uterus are reviewed in this chapter.

INTRODUCTION

Congenital abnormalities of the Müllerian ducts are relatively common and are encountered with an incidence of 2 to 4 percent in fertile women and 3 percent in infertile women.[1-3] Lack of resorption of the mid-line septum between the two Müllerian ducts results in defects that range from a slight mid-line septum to a complete division of the endometrial cavity. In addition, since both the urinary and genital systems develop from a common mesodermal ridge, it is not surprising that Müllerian anomalies are associated with urologic malformations.

Apoptosis has been proposed as a mechanism by which the uterine septum regresses.[4] Absence of some apoptotic molecules, such as Bcl-2, may result in failure of regression of the septum.

The uterine septum was believed to consist of fibromuscular tissue with more connective tissue and fewer muscle fibers in the septum.[5] However, a recent study, based on the biopsy specimens obtained from the different points in the septum, has shown that there is less connective tissue and more muscle fibers in the septum.[6] An electron microscopic study has also shown that septal endometrium has defective development.[7] This may result in a decrease in the sensitivity to steroid hormones.

Clinical Discussion

Diagnosis

There are various diagnostic tools to identify the uterine septum with different accuracies. These include hysterosalpingography (HSG), ultrasonography (USG), sonohysterography, three-dimensional ultrasonography

(3D USG), hysteroscopy, magnetic resonance imaging (MRI) and combined hysteroscopy and laparoscopy.

Hysterosalpingography can detect a two-chambered uterus with a typical "Y"-shape image, and allow the assessment of the size and the extent of a septum.[8] However, it is not always easy to differentiate a septate uterus from a bicornuate or didelphic uterus. Hysterosalpingography has a diagnostic accuracy of only 55 percent in differentiating between a septate and a bicornuate uterus.[9] Furthermore, HSG may not detect minor septal defects.

Ultrasonography is another diagnostic tool that is especially useful in pregnant women. On transabdominal ultrasonography, a septate uterus is seen as two cavities without sagittal notching and with a fundal myometrium. Transvaginal ultrasonography provides a better assessment in the diagnosis of the septate uterus. The fundal myometrial thickness and cornual myometrial thickness can be measured at the mid-sagittal plane during transvaginal ultrasonography. If the difference between the fundal myometrial thickness and the cornual myometrial thickness is more than 5 mm, it could denote a partial or complete septate uterus.[10]

Sonohysterography involves the instillation of fluid into the uterine cavity under transabdominal or preferably transvaginal ultrasonographic examination. It provides a good contour of the endometrial cavity. As in transvaginal ultrasonography, the fundal and cornual myometrial thicknesses can be measured in the mid-sagittal plane. If the difference between these two parameters is more than 4.4 mm, it could denote a partial or complete septate uterus.[10]

Three-dimensional ultrasonography is also a very useful tool in diagnosis of Müllerian anomalies and has an accuracy of 92 percent for the diagnosis of septate uterus.[11]

Magnetic resonance imaging (MRI) provides a very accurate diagnosis of Müllerian anomalies. It has a sensitivity and specificity of 100 percent in the diagnosis of the septate uterus.[12] When compared with USG, MRI may yield slightly better diagnostic information on uterine morphology. However, disadvantages of MRI include a higher cost and lower accessibility. Therefore, its use is usually confined to referral centers.

Hysteroscopy is very useful in assessing the endometrial cavity. It is regarded as the gold standard in the diagnosis of congenital Müllerian anomalies, especially when combined with laparoscopy.[13,14] In addition, it provides a treatment option for the septate uterus.

Adverse Reproductive Outcome

Among the different types of structural uterine anomalies, the septate uterus is the most common[15,16] and associated with the poorest reproductive outcome, with fetal survival rates of 6 to 28 percent and a high rate of spontaneous miscarriages (>60%).[17-19] The septate uterus is also associated with

recurrent miscarriages, premature delivery, abnormal fetal presentation and intrauterine growth retardation (IUGR).

Septa have also been claimed to be an etiologic factor for infertility. Decrease in sensitivity of the endometrium covering the septa to preovulatory changes may be the cause of infertility.[7]

Treatment

Surgical correction of the septate uterus was traditionally performed by transabdominal metroplasty. This treatment required a long postoperative interval (3 to 6 months) before conception. During this procedure, the full thickness of the uterine fundus was damaged. Therefore, it was associated with a significant risk of scar rupture. This mode of therapy dictates that the mode of delivery in a subsequent pregnancy be by cesarean section.

Since the first introduction of the hysteroscopic approach for the treatment of septate uterus in 1974,[20] hysteroscopic metroplasty has become an outstanding technique for the treatment of the septate uterus. This method has universally replaced transabdominal metroplasty. Although hysteroscopic exicision of a uterine septum leaves an injured area within the endometrial cavity, it is rapidly covered by nearby healthy endometrium. Mencaglia and Tantini[13] demonstrated healing of the injured area within one month of postoperative hysteroscopy.[13] Furthermore, we have shown that initiating an intracytoplasmic sperm injection-embryo transfer (ICSI-ET) cycle just after the hysteroscopic procedure does not result in any impairment in implantation or pregnancy rate compared to that initiated two or more months after the operation.[21] Therefore, if a conception is planned after hysteroscopic resection of uterine septum, there is no reason to delay attempts.

The hysteroscopic approach for the septate uterus can be performed using microscissors, electrosurgery, or laser. The most important factor in the hysteroscopic surgery is deciding when to stop the incision. In one study, it was shown that leaving a small residue of less than 1 cm does not impair the reproductive outcome,[22] failing which, there could be a risk of damage to the myometrial tissue over the fundal area, possible perforation and subsequent uterine rupture during pregnancy.

Indications

There is a high prevalence of septate uterus in women with recurrent (≥ 3) miscarriages.[23,24] Hysteroscopic metroplasty has been shown to improve subsequent reproductive outcome. There are several studies showing a dramatic fall in the overall miscarriage rate from 90 to 80 percent to 13 to 4.5 percent.[5,25,26] However, all these studies are non-randomized and therefore, open to bias. At present, hysteroscopic metroplasty is offered to women with recurrent miscarriages. Though hysteroscopic metroplasty may be controversial if there is a history of only one miscarriage, many clinicians still advocate the treatment in this group.[5]

Septate uterus could be associated with preterm delivery, as well. Hysteroscopic metroplasty has been shown to reduce the incidence of preterm delivery from 10 percent to 5 percent.[5,25,26] Therefore, metroplasty should be offered to reduce the likelihood of a recurrence. However, if there is a history of term delivery, this condition lessens the reproductive importance of the septate uterus.

Whether the septate uterus is a cause of infertility is controversial. Furthermore, the role of hysteroscopic metroplasty in patients with primary infertility is controversial. A crude pregnancy rate of approximately 48 percent may be achieved after hysteroscopic metroplasty.[27]

CONCLUSION

Among congenital uterine abnormalities, the septate uterus is associated with the highest incidence of reproductive failure and obstetric complications, including first and second trimester recurrent miscarriages, premature delivery, abnormal fetal presentation, IUGR and infertility.

Besides being a diagnostic tool, hysteroscopy provides a treatment option for the septate uterus. It is a simple technique with minimal intraoperative and postoperative morbidity. In the absence of any prospective, randomized, controlled studies, most retrospective series compared the reproductive outcome before and after surgery. Such an approach is less than ideal. However, observational studies do provide some information. At present, hysteroscopic metroplasty is offered to women with recurrent miscarriages or a history of preterm delivery. Advancing age, especially over 35 years, is associated with inherent adverse reproductive effects and therefore, may necessitate early intervention. In women with long-standing unexplained infertility, hysteroscopic removal of the septum may be considered.

Sometimes, hysteroscopy and laparoscopy are performed in women for other reasons. During the procedure, if a septate uterus is discovered, septal incision is advised and may be performed at the same time.[13,28,29]

The hysteroscopic procedure is now used more liberally in women with only one miscarriage or unexplained infertility. Therefore, many IVF centers recommend removal of the septum before assisted reproductive treatment to reduce the possibility of miscarriage.[15]

REFERENCES

1. Acien P. Incidence of Müllerian defects in fertile and infertile women. Hum Reprod 1997;12:1372.
2. Ashton D, Amin HK, Richart RM, Neuwirth RS. The incidence of asymptomatic uterine anomalies in women undergoing transcervical tubal sterilization. Obstet Gynecol 1988;72:28-30.
3. Sorensen S. Estimated prevalence of Müllerian anomalies. Acta Obstet Gynecol Scand 1988;67:441-5.
4. Lee DM, Osathanondh R, Yeh J. Localization of Bcl-2 in the human fetal Müllerian tract. Fertil Steril 1998;70:135-40.
5. Fayez JA. Comparison between abdominal and hysteroscopic metroplasty. Obstet Gynecol 1986;68:399-403.
6. Dabirashrafi H, Bahadori M, Mohammad K, Alavi M, Moghadami-Tabrizi N, Zandinejad K, Ghafari V. Septate uterus: new idea on the histologic features of the septum in this abnormal uterus. Am J Obstet Gynecol 1995;171:105-7.
7. Fedele L, Bianchi S, Marchini M, Franchi D, Tozzi L, Dorta M. Ultrastructural aspects of endometrium in infertile women with septate uterus. Fertil Steril 1996;65:750-2.
8. Barbot J. Hysteroscopy and hysterography. Obstet Gynecol Clin North Am 1995;22:591-603.
9. Reuter KL, Daly DC, Cohen SM. Septate versus bicornuate uteri: errors in imaging diagnosis. Radiology 1989;172:749-52.
10. Berkkanoglu M, Ozgur K, Isikoglu M. Uterine subseptus: a quentification is lacking. Conjoint meeting of the ASRM 61st annual meeting and the CFAS 51st annual meeting, Montreal, Quebec, Canada, October 15 to 19, 2005.
11. Wu MH, Hsu CC, Huang KE. Detection of congenital Müllerian duct anomalies using three-dimensional ultrasound. J Clin Ultrasound 1997;25:487-92.
12. Fischetti SG, Politi G, Lomeo F, Garozzo G. Magnetic resonance in the evaluation of Müllerian duct anomalies. Radiol Med (Torino) 1995;89:105-11.
13. Mencaglia L, Tantini C. Hysteroscopic treatment of septate and arcuate uterus. Gynaecol Endosc 1996;5:151-4.
14. Letterie GS, Haggerty M, Lindee G. A comparison of pelvic ultrasound and magnetic resonance imaging as diagnostic studies for müllerian tract abnormalities. Int J Fertil Menopausal Stud 1995;40:34-8.
15. Raga F, Bauset C, Remohi J, Bonilla-Musoles F, Simon C, Pellicer A. Reproductive impact of congenital Müllerian anomalies. Hum Reprod 1997;12:2277-81.
16. Nasri MN, Setchell ME, Chard T. Transvaginal ultrasound for diagnosis of uterine malformations. Br J Obstet Gynaecol 1990;97:1043-5.
17. Heinonen PK, Saarikoski S, Pystynen P. Reproductive performance of women with uterine anomalies. Acta Obstet Gynecol Scand 1982;61:157-60.
18. Golan A, Langer R, Bukovsky I, Caspi E. Congenital anomalies of the Müllerian system. Fertil Steril 1989;51:747-55.
19. Green LK, Harris RE. Uterine anomalies. Frequency of diagnosis and associated obstetric complications. Obstet Gynecol 1976; 47:427-9.
20. Edstrom K. Intrauterine surgical prodecures during hysteroscopy. Endoscopy 1974;6:175-81.
21. Berkkanoglu M, Isikoglu M, Ozgur K. When to perform ICSI/ET cycle after hysteroscopic surgery for uterine septum. Conjoint meeting of the ASRM 61st annual meeting and the CFAS 51st annual meeting, Montreal, Quebec, Canada, October 15 to 19, 2005.
22. Fedele L, Bianchi S, Marchini M, Mezzopane R, DiNola G, Tozzi L. Residual uterine septum of less than 1 cm after hysteroscopic metroplasty does not impair reproductive outcome. Hum Reprod 1996;11:727-9.

23. Raziel A, Arieli S, Bukovsky I, Caspi E, Golan A. Investigation of the uterine cavity in recurrent aborters. Fertil Steril 1994; 62:1080-2.

24. Clifford K, Rai R, Watson H, Regan L. An informative protocol for the investigation of recurrent miscarriage: preliminary experience of 500 consecutive cases. Hum Reprod 1994;9: 1328-32.

25. Cararach M, Penella J, Ubeda A, Labastida R. Hysteroscopic incision of the septate uterus: scissors versus resectoscope. Hum Reprod 1994;9:87-97.

26. Pabuccu R, Atay V, Urman B, Ergun A, Orhon E. Hysteroscopic treatment of septate uterus. Gynaecol Endosc 1995;4:213-5.

27. Homer HA, Li TC, Cooke ID. The septate uterus: a review of management and reproductive outcome. Fertil Steril 2000;73: 1-14.

28. Fedele L, Bianchi S. Hysteroscopic metroplasty for the septate uterus. Obstet Gynecol Clin North Am 1995;22:473-89.

29. Daly DC, Maier D, Soto-Albors CE. Hyesteroscopic metroplasty: six years' experience. Obstet Gynecol 1989;73:201-5.

Ovarian Stimulation Protocols

Gonadotropin Preparations in Infertility Treatment

Mybodi Karimzadeh, Robab Taheripanah, Sedighe Ghandi, M Eftekhar

OVERVIEW

Gonadotropin therapy in various forms has been used to restore ovulation in anovulatory women. Only after the introduction of IVF, have gonadotropins been applied to stimulate multiple follicle development. The latter treatment overrides the physiologic selection of a single dominant follicle by extending the time during which serum follicle-stimulating hormone (FSH) concentrations remain above the threshold level required for follicular recruitment and ongoing maturation. The availability of a number of mature oocytes suitable for IVF procedures improves the likelihood of achieving fertilization, of generating good quality embryos, and of a successful pregnancy. Human menopausal gonadotropins (hMG) was successfully used to induce ovulation. The lack of purity and the limited batch-to-batch consistency may have negatively affected clinical results. Increasing efforts were made to separate and purify the individual components of urinary gonadotropin preparations by various physiological, chemical and immunologic means. Monoclonal antibodies were used to produce highly purified urinary FSH from bulk hMG. This increased purity, reduced the total amount of injected protein and allowed for subcutaneous administration. Product consistency also enabled pharmacokinetic and pharmacodynamic analysis, and facilitated more patient-specific treatment plans adjusted to individual responses. The problem of the short supply of high-quality gonadotropins was solved by the advent of recombinant DNA technology, which permitted the large-scale production of pure recombinant human gonadotropin preparations. These recombinant molecules are structurally very similar to native pituitary FSH and the final product is highly purified, with a high specific *in vivo* bioactivity. The relatively short elimination half-life and rapid metabolic clearance of current FSH preparations requires that daily injections are administered to maintain steady state FSH levels above the threshold level during ovarian stimulation. The development of FSH analogs, with a longer half-life and a slower absorption to peak serum levels may be more helpful to render an extended injection-free period than to increase the initial dose of current FSH preparations. The main advantages of less frequent dosing are an increase in patient convenience, fewer chances for mistakes during drug administration and improved compliance, which is particularly relevant during long-term treatment. An additional benefit is that long-acting agents induce more stable serum levels of a drug compared with repeated dosing using a short-acting agent.

INTRODUCTION

Infertility treatments have become available due to developments in the characterization and purification of hormones. For more than 30 years, human menopausal gonadotropins (hMGs) have been applied in the treatment of human infertility. Clinical indications include ovulation induction and ovarian stimulation in assisted reproduction techniques. During the last decade, there has been a substantial increase in the use of infertility drugs. The current strategies are aimed at increasing the safety and convenience of infertility therapy, while keeping the costs at reasonable levels. The last decade of the 20th century witnessed a potential milestone in the treatment of infertility as the previously urine-derived gonadotropins were increasingly replaced by gonadotropins produced through recombinant technologies. This progression in ovulation induction and/or assisted reproduction techniques is the subject of this chapter.

HISTORICAL OVERVIEW

It is nearly 100 years since ablation experiments in dogs provided the first empiric evidence of a role for the pituitary gland in the regulation of gonadal function.[1] Animal pituitary extracts with both FSH and LH-like activities such as pregnant mares' serum gonadotropin (PMSG) were used until the late 1960s for ovulation induction in women with gonadotropin insufficiency. These products were eventually withdrawn from clinical use due to their antigenic potential, although PMSG is still used experimentally in laboratory animals and for ovulation induction in cattle.[2]

In 1927, Ashheim and Zondek discovered a substance in the urine of pregnant women with the same action as the gonadotropic factor in the anterior pituitary.[3] They coined this substance 'gonadotropin' or 'prolan'. Furthermore, they believed that there were two distinct hormones prolan A and prolan B. In 1930, Zondek reported that gonadotropins were also present in the urine of postmenopausal women and Cole and Hart found gonadotropins in the serum of pregnant mares in the same year.[4,5] However, Cartland and Nelson were able to produce a purified extract of this hormone in 1937.[6]

After years of experiment, it has gradually become apparent that the pituitary factor was needed for the production of mature follicles and that the use of gonadotropin extracts from nonprimate sources was of limited clinical value owing to development of autoantibodies that neutralized their therapeutic effect. In 1947, Piero Donini, a chemist at the Pharmaceutical Institute, Sereno, in Rome, tried to purify hMG from postmenopausal urine. The first urine extract of gonadotropin contained luteinizing hormone (LH) and FSH and was named Pergonal.[7]

The first successful induction of ovulation with FSH derived from human pituitary glands was described by Gemzell et al. in 1958. The first pregnancy was achieved with Pergonal treatment in a patient with secondary amenorrhea in 1961. Urinary FSH (Metrodin) and highly purified FSH have become available with the development of new technologies using specific monoclonal antibodies to bind the FSH and LH molecules in the hMG material in such a way that unknown urinary proteins could be removed.[8]

A final step in the purification of FSH was achieved when in the mid-1990s that recombinant FSH (r-FSH) was introduced to the market. Recombinant FSH is in its amino acid sequence identical to human FSH, though carbohydrate side chain attachments responsible for the pharmacodynamics do differ to some extent from human pituitary FSH.[9]

History of drug development and technology for infertility treatment:

1927: The discovery of pituitary hormone controlling ovarian functions.

1937-1948: Non-primate gonadotropins and human chorionic gonadotropin (hCG) used to treat infertile women.

1950: First hMG extracted from the urine of postmenopausal women.

1959: Purification and clinical use of pituitary and urine gonadotropins.

1960: Clinical use of Clomiphene citrate.

1966: Use of Clomiphene citrate and gonadotropin becomes common practice.

1970: Development of radioimmunoassay for measuring hormone levels.

1978: Ultrasound imaging of ovarian follicles.

1984: Use of gonadotropin releasing hormone (GnRH) agonist in infertility treatment.

1985: Further purification of urinary gonadotropins.

1990: Use of recombinant gonadotropins.[7]

CLINICAL DISCUSSION

Pituitary Gonadotropins

Follicle stimulating hormone (FSH) and luteinizing hormone (LH) are two anterior pituitary gonadotropin hormones that control gonadal function. Both hormones are synthesized and secreted by the same pituitary cells and it has been shown that both are influenced by gonadotropin-releasing hormone (GnRH), a single hypothalamic hormone.[10]

FSH and LH together play a central role in regulation the menstrual cycle and ovulation. Therefore, a basic knowledge of gonadotropin control of ovulation induction is an essential requirement for a proper understanding of ovulation-induction techniques using exogenously administered gonadotropins.

Gonadotropins are glycoproteins with molecular weights of approximately 30, 000 Da and contain fructose, mannose, galactose acetylglucosamine and N-acetylneuraminic acid as carbohydrate moieties.[11] The sialic acid content varies widely among the glycoprotein hormones, from 20 residues in human chorionic gonadotropin (hCG) and five in FSH to only one or two in human LH. These differences are largely responsible for the variation in the isoelectric points of gonadotropins, leading to the differences in molecular weight and biologic activities of the hormones isolated from various sources. The higher the sialic acid content, the longer the biologic half-life, and thus, an increased amount in urinary gonadotropins is responsible for its significantly longer half-life compared with that of the pituitary LH or FSH.[12]

The gonadotropin hormones comprise of two hydrophobic, non-covalently associated α and β-subunits.[11] All the gonadotropins share a common α-subunit of 92 amino acid residues in the same sequence, with five disulfide bonds, as well as two carbohydrate moieties.[11] However, the β-chains are unique and after linkage to the α-chain, determine specific hormone function.[12] The three-dimensional structure of each subunit is maintained by internally cross-linked disulfide bonds. Gonadotropin hormones may be dissociated into several component subunits by denaturing agents. The subunits are practically without biological activity, but the hormonal activity is regenerated by recombination of the subunits. Gonadotropic LH and FSH, together with thyroid-stimulating hormone (TSH) and hCG, belong to the family of glycoprotein hormones. They all are composed of two non-covalently linked subunits, α and β. The α-subunit is common to all glycoprotein hormones, whereas the β-subunits confer the hormonal specificity.[13] The β-subunits of FSH, LH, and hCG are unique to each hormone and determine their biological specificity. They have amino acid chains of variable lengths and contain six disulfide bonds.[11]

Follicle Stimulating Hormone

Follicle stimulating hormone (FSH) is a globular glycosylated protein with a molecular weight of 28,000 to 30,000 Dalton, consisting of one α and one β-subunit. It shares a common α-subunit with LH, hCG and thyroid stimulating hormone (TSH). Individually, neither subunit has only biological activity. The four α-subunits have significant amino acid homology with one another and have probably evolved from a common precursor. The amino acid sequence determination of the α-subunit was reviewed by Sairam. It consists of 92 amino acid with a molecular weight of 14,600 Dalton, and is stabilized by five disulfide bonds.[14]

The FSH β-subunit contains six disulfide bonds. Similar to the α-subunit, oligosaccharides are N-linked at two asparagine residues. Neuraminic acid is always the terminal oligosaccharide and there are no N-acetylgalactosamine residues. Both LH and FSH β-subunits are found in the same cells within the anterior pituitary.[15] Removal of sialic acid residues from the proteins reduces their plasma-half-lives because the liver binds sialoglycoproteins and removes them from the circulation.[16] The implication of the slow clearance rate of serum concentrations of FSH *in vivo* is that they can neither increase nor decrease as rapidly as concentrations of LH.[12]

In the ovary, FSH binds to receptors located on granulosa cells and acts via the 3, 5 cyclic adenosine monophosphate (CAMP)-dependent protein kinase pathway. Follicle stimulating hormone binding to antral and preovulatory follicles increases aromatase activity.[17]

Luteinizing Hormone (LH)

The carbohydrate moieties play an important role in determining the bio-potencies and circulating clearance rates of glycoprotein hormones. Moreover, there is considerable microheterogeneity in glycosylation according to the physiologic state. Although LH and FSH are synthesized by the same gonadotroph cells of the anterior pituitary, very clear differences occur in their glycosylation patterns, with sulfated structures dominating in LH and sialylated ones in FSH. The function of LH is initiated by its binding to the LH

receptor (LHR), a member of the G-protein coupled seven-transmembrane domain receptor family that is primarily expressed in testicular Leydig cells and ovarian theca, granulosa and luteal cells.[18-20] LH-receptor interaction activates a multitude of signaling mechanisms, including adenylate-cyclase, phospholipase C, modulation of Ca^{+2} fluxes and mitogen-activated protein kinase (MAPK).[20-23] The carbohydrate moieties of the α, but not the β-subunit, are involved in LH activation and subsequent signal transduction. The processing of N-linked oligosaccharides of glycoprotein hormones is tissue and dimer specific. Whereas LH and TSH, synthesized in gonadotrophs and thyrotrops, respectively, possess sulfated (SO_4) oligosaccharides and N-acetylgalactosamines at their carbohydrate termini, pituitary FSH and placental hCG bear oligosaccharides terminating with sialic acid and galactose.[20-25] The differences determine the longer circulatory half-lives of FSH and hCG, whereas LH and TSH are cleared faster from the circulation by a hepatic receptor specific for sulfated glycoproteins.[13,25-28] For this reason, the physiological relevance of recombinant gonadotropin preparations depends to a great extent on the nature of their glycosylation.

Midcycle LH Surge

The midcycle LH surge is a key event in the menstrual cycle. Appropriate timing and adequate duration and amplitude of this surge are prerequisites for human female fertility. An adequate surge will lead to several changes at the follicle level that are pivotal for obtaining a pregnancy. First, the surge induces the cumulus oophorus mucinification, allowing the oocyte to be released subsequently from the follicular wall. Second, it provokes the resumption of the oocyte meiosis, that is, from germinal vesicle stage to metaphase II. Reaching the metaphase II meiotic stage is a mandatory step for allowing proper fertilization of the oocyte and embryonic development. Third, the LH surge triggers follicular rupture, expelling the oocyte from the follicle and leading to its capture by the Fallopian tube. Finally, it induces a shift in the granulosa cell steroidogenic process, changing it from a dominating estradiol secretory process towards a progesterone secretory process, forming an active corpus luteum. Three major regulatory factors have been identified to play a role in the induction of the midcycle LH surge, hypothalamic GnRH, the ovarian steroids (estradiol and progesterone), and some less well-characterized peptide hormones such as gonadotropin surge-attenuating factor, (GnSAF).[29]

The Need for a Surrogate LH Surge

In several clinical situations, a surrogate LH surge must be produced because the endogenous feedback mechanisms that produce an endogenous LH surge are absent or impaired. In anovulation resulting from severe gonadotropin deficiency (WHO group 1 anovulation, hypogonadotropic hypogonadism), follicular growth induced by a combined administration of FSH and LH is usually not followed by a spontaneous LH surge. In anovulation resulting from hypothalamic-pituitary dysfunction, which is characterized by residual gonadotropin and estradiol secretion [WHO group 2 anovulation, polycystic ovary syndrome (PCOS)], the restoration of follicular growth by FSH administration does not usually lead to a correct timing and adequate amplitude of the LH surge.[30] Treatment of anovulation with gonadotropins thus requires the production of a surrogate LH surge.

It has been shown that feedback mechanisms are often disrupted in ovulatory patients undergoing multiple follicular stimulation by the administration of pharmacological doses of FSH before assisted reproductive technique (ART).[31-32] This leads to improperly timed LH surges that are often also blunted. The administration of a surrogate LH surge has therefore, become a standard procedure in ART. Moreover, since ART treatment failure has often been attributed to an improper LH surge, most patients are now pretreated with a GnRH agonist or use cotreatment with GnRH antagonist. This treatment abolishes pituitary responsiveness to endogenous GnRH and prevents the occurrence of a spontaneous endogenous LH surge.[32] This has resulted in a significant improvement in the ART treatment outcome.[33]

The Natural LH Surge

The main characteristics of a natural LH surge, as reported in the literature, are summarized in Table 14.1. The natural surge lasts for about 2 days and is made up of an ascending phase, a plateau and a descending phase. LH serum levels, when measured by radioimmunoassay (RIA), are about 10 to 20 times the basal LH levels. Studies analyzing the LH surges show relatively large variations between individuals in terms of duration and amplitude of the LH surge. This might result partially from an insufficiently high sampling frequency. From a clinical point of view, this variation also suggests that patients may have different threshold levels for the LH surge, as is the case for FSH in terms of follicular development. This should be taken into account when designing a therapeutic regimen for inducing a surrogate LH surge that must be effective in most patients. Indeed, in contrast to FSH therapy, no dose adjustment is possible.

A regimen for inducing a surrogate surge needs to be designed based on the therapeutic objective. The regimen for provoking oocyte maturation and luteinization in patients for whom no follicular rupture is required (that is, before ovum pick-up for ART), could be different from one aiming to provoke the full process of ovulation for *in vivo* conception.[34]

Pituitary LH

Human LH preparations, derived from cadaver pituitary glands, were used in the 1960s to trigger final follicular maturation and ovulation in WHO class 1 anovulation treated with hMG. Repeated administrations of pituitary LH were used (i.e. 800 to 1200 IU every 8h for 24h). Continuation of LH administration throughout the luteal phase was shown to be necessary to obtain a pregnancy.[34] This is not surprising considering that these patients are profoundly deficient in both LH and FSH. The pituitary derived preparations are obviously no longer acceptable as therapeutic preparations because of the risk of infectious agent transmission.[35]

Human Menopausal Gonadotropin (hMG)

Human menopausal gonadotropin is a relatively crude hormonal extract from the urine of postmenopausal women which contains both FSH and LH activity and contains 75 IU of FSH and 75 IU of LH *in vivo* bioactivity.

The first hMG was approved in the United States in 1970, for follicular development in anovulatory and oligovulatory women. It remained the mainstay of fertility treatment for almost 20 years.[36]

It was shown by Cook et al.[37] that hMG preparations also consist of up to five different FSH isohormones and up to nine LH species.[37] Part of the LH activity is due to the presence of a third hormone, hCG. Menotropin describes the source of the hormonal activity, but does not indicate the purity of the concentrate. FSH, which is the major active agent, accounts for <5 percent of the local protein content in the extracted urinary gonadotropin products.[38] The specific activity can

Table 14.1: Summary of LH surge characteristics			
LH surge characteristics	*Natural midcycle LH surge*	*hCG (5000 IU IM)*	*GnRH agonist induced surge*
Surge duration (h)	49 ± 9	>96	24–48
Ascending phase (h)	~14	~20	~4
Plateau (h)	~14	0	0
Descending phase (h)	~20	>72	20–36
LH peak value (IU/L)	100–200	–	50–250
Peak: Baseline ratio	10–20	–	10–20

actually be as low as 40 IU FSH/mg protein. There may also be batch-to-batch variations in the FSH:LH ratio. Proprietary preparations of hMG usually have the FSH:LH ratio adjusted to a standardized value, usually 2:1 or 1:1. The specific activity of these products does not usually exceed 150 IU/mg protein. The different proteins found in various hMG preparations include tumor necrosis factor, binding protein I, transferrin, urokinase, epidermal growth factor and immunoglobulin related proteins. These differences may cause variations in patients' responses as sometimes observed when using different batches of the same preparation.[37]

Although hMG preparations have been effective and relatively safe for the last 30 years, local side effects have been reported such as pain and allergic reactions, possibly attributed to immune reactions related to impurities (intact and degraded proteins).[38,39]

Purified Urinary FSH

In the early 1970s, clinicians began to voice the opinion that different patient groups and individuals may need different treatment regimens, with variations in protocols and dosages of FSH and LH. Such individually adjusted treatment regimens would require therapeutic gonadotropin preparations that contained pure gonadotropins or almost pure FSH or LH. Attempts to separate FSH from LH in gonadotropin extracts were pursued via a multitude of modifications in various methods. Butt and his co-workers[40] supplemented the digestion process with the removal of inert proteins by starch gel electrophoresis.[40]

In 1966, Donini and associates combined electrophoresis and chromatography with lyophilization of the elute and its subsequent filtration on a sephadex column.

However, none of the above efforts brought in a real solution, being either too cumbersome, complicated and expensive, or not sufficiently accurate and efficient.[41] New developments in immunological techniques opened a virtually limitless horizon for measuring and producing several hormones including purified FSH. A urinary hMG preparation containing both FSH and LH was filtered through the column; all of the proteins contained in hMG including FSH passed through the column and LH was retained in the column bound by the specific antibodies.[42]

Urofollitropin(u-FSH), a hormone extracted from the urine of postmenopausal women, which contains mostly FSH activity with little LH activity (<1 IU), introduced by Serono in 1983, was found to increase the success of medically assisted reproduction programs in the eighties. In fact, this preparation is derived from hMG using a further stage of extraction and purification in which LH is bound to an antibody, which is chemically bound to a column of sepharose. At the end of this process, the u-FSH contains 85 to 100 percent of the initial FSH activity, but very little of the LH activity. The specific activity is approximately 150 IU FSH/mg protein, but still more than 95 percent of the proteins present are contaminants.[43,44] With only minimal LH activity, the final product, metrodin, contained 150 IU of FSH and 1 IU of LH per mg of proteins. Preparation of purified gonadotropins, coupled with the availability of macromolecules permitting the developments of whole array of efficient immunoabsorbents, enabled the pharmaceutical industry to introduce purified FSH preparation almost free from LH contamination.[42]

Highly Purified Urinary FSH

Further technological advances made it possible to replace polyvalent antibodies with highly specific monoclonal antibodies. The production of purified urinary FSH was essentially a passive process in which LH was separated from bulk material and FSH together with some other urinary proteins was collected and lyophilized for use.[45]

Third-generation gonadotropins, such as highly purified urinary FSH, are produced by a more direct process. The affinity column uses highly specific monoclonal antibodies to selectively bind FSH molecules in the hMG bulk material.[46] The unbound urinary protein and LH pass through the column and are removed leaving pure FSH retained by the column. This is then extracted as a highly purified product devoid of both LH and contaminating urinary proteins. As a result of the improved processing, this highly purified urinary FSH contains less than 0.1 IU of LH activity and less than 5 percent of unidentified urinary proteins with a specific activity of 9000 IU/mg protein, compared to the specific FSH activity of hMG and urinary FSH (urofollitropin) of 150 IU/mg protein.[42]

Because of its high purity, u-hFSH HP could be administered to patients who previously had severe systemic reactions to other crude urinary preparations, resulting in side effect-free ovulatory cycles.[44] The very high purity of the preparation led to reduced batch-to-batch variability.[45]

Recombinant Human FSH (rhFSH) Preparation

Although highly purified urinary FSH is associated with good tolerance and efficacy, the major problem is the growing need to resort to infertility treatments and limitations in the postmenopausal urine as the source. With advances in technology, researchers trended to genetic engineering and hormone production by this method. The application of recombinant DNA technology finally made the production of a pharmaceutical FSH preparation possible, resulting in the approval of rhFSH (Follitropin-α, Gonal-F, Ares-Serono, Geneva, Switzerland) in 1995. Follitropin-α is produced by transfecting Chinese hamster ovary cells with the genes for the α and β-subunits of human FSH.[47]

Table 14.2: Comparison of urinary and recombinant gonadotropin preparations

	hMG	*u-HFSH*	*r-FSH*
Potency	*In vivo* bioassay	*In vivo* bioassay	*In vivo* bioassay
Specific activity (FSH/mg protein)	≈ 150 IU	≈10,000 IU	≈10,000 IU
Protein content (mcg/75 IU)	370–750	6–11	6–11
Active protein content (%FSH) in bulk	<5	>95	99

The secretory products of these cells undergo a six-step purification process to give a final preparation, which is highly pure biochemically (> 99% FSH), structurally identical to native human pituitary FSH and with highly specific activity (approximately 10,000 IU/mg protein) (Table 14.2). Unlike uhFSH, however, Follitropin alpha shows a low level of oxidation or degradation, typically less than 10 percent compared with 30 to 40 percent for uhFSH.[48]

A second r-FSH preparation, follitropin-β (Puregon/Follistim/Nv Organon, Oss, the Netherlands) is also available. The Follitropin-α and Follitropin-β molecules are almost indistinguishable structurally and biochemically except for some minor differences in the percentage of oxidized and degraded isoforms. In addition, it has recently been demonstrated that when administered on an equivalent IU basis, they produce identical ovarian stimulation characteristics.[49]

Is There a Difference in Safety?

Whether recombinant gonadotropins offer an improvement in safety margins over the older urinary products is one of the most crucial questions. Many scientists strongly argued that: (1) a pure (i.e. recombinant) products were in principle preferable to an impure (i.e. urinary) product; (2) human (i.e. urinary) products carried a risk of infection by slow viruses, raising concerns; (3) human products, since impure, carried a risk of immunogenicity and (4) human products had repeatedly been demonstrated to be uneven in biological potency.

These four arguments, all basically favoring medical modernity over older-line products, and all representing basic common sense, carried considerable impact and greatly contributed to the dramatic marketing success of recombinant gonadotropins. These arguments discuss here. It is difficult to argue with the basic premise that purity is preferable to impurity. Yet, impurity affects safety only if it can be demonstrated that any of the potential contaminations adversely affect either the patient's health or the treatments outcome. The outcome comparisons will be discussed below, following the discussion on the safety aspect.

In over 30 years of clinical use of urinary gonadotropins, not a single case of infections contamination has been reported. Even cases of slow viruses should, in such a time span, have clinically become apparent.[50] In contrast, the risk of immunogenicity appears more realistic: Biffoni et al.[51] representatives of one of the major pharmaceutical companies in the field, report that during a conventional IVF cycle, only approximately 0.2 mg of 15 mg or more, of protein, which is administered in the form of a urinary gonadotropin, is either FSH or LH. The rest is a contamination by-product with, at least theoretically, immunogenic potential.[51]

Moreover every practitioner in the field has encountered patients with significant local, allergic reactions, especially with IM administration. A safety study supported by one of the manufacturers of an hMG product with Food and Drug Administration (FDA) approval for both, IM and SC administration, demonstrated actually significantly increased injection site edema and/or reaction with SC administration over IM administration of the same, or a competitor's product.[52] Allergic reactions are of concern, since they can activate immune processes that may be hostile to implantation and increase miscarriage risks.[53]

Biffoni et al.[51] demonstrated that preparations from different manufacturers have different *in vitro* immunological effects, which may reflect a different profile of contaminants.[51] It appears doubtful whether products from the same manufacturer will maintain their immunological profile. Nobody has been able to link the occurrence of antiphospholipid antibodies (APAs) with gonadotropin therapy.[54] However, the allergic reactions can be associated with significant shifts in Th1/Yh2 activities, which can include APA-responses, and which have been closely linked to an increased risk of infertility and pregnancy wastage.[53] Hence, recombinant medications are less immunogenetic than older urinary-derived medication and, at least from this point of view, are preferable.

Uneven biological potency also carries significant risk, since controlled ovarian stimulation can become less predictable. Practitioners in the field have long complained about the varying biopotency of different batches of urinary gonadotropin products. Such reports have, however, remained largely anecdotal. Moreover, while recombinant products may be easier to standardize, variations in biopotency can also occur if this production technique is applied. There is currently no convincing evidence in the literature to favor recombinant over urinary products.

Finally, one also has to consider the biological risk exclusive to recombinant products: such FSH is produced by transfixing a genomic clone into Chinese hamster ovary cells, which then synthesize the FSH protein.[9] As an animal cell product, this creates the theoretical risk of introducing animal viruses into humans. Like the previously noted concern about the introduction of slow viruses through urinary products, pharmaceutical filtering and purification techniques make this, however, only an issue of theoretical concern. In summary, with regards to safety, there was a slight advantage in recombinant products.

Is There a Difference in Outcome?

The literature offers a number of studies on the impact of different gonadotropin preparations on induction of ovulation and ART cycles.

Ovarian Induction Without IVF

In one review, the efficacy, safety, costs and acceptability of recombinant FSH with urinary-derived FSH for ovulation induction was compared. Follitropin-alfa, beta and urinary FSH products appeared to be equally effective in terms of pregnancy rates. Patient safety was also found to be comparable, as the incidence of side effects, including multiple pregnancy, was similar for all FSH products.[55]

As ovarian stimulation protocols have received less attention in IUI, in a new systematic review and meta-analysis, recombinant FSH was compared with highly purified FSH for intrauterine insemination. Recombinant FSH was associated with higher per cycle pregnancy rate than highly purified FSH, when used at the same dose, whereas the pregnancy rates were similar when the dose of recombinant FSH was 50 percent lower.[56]

Ovarian Stimulation for IVF

Many different gonadotropins preparation with more acidic property and urinary are available in market. Many studies were done to evaluate the clinical efficacy and safety of highly purified urinary FSH with acidic properties in IVF cycles. The different gonadotropin preparations and combinations have received a lot of attention in IVF cycles, and a number of articles have been published, in many cases, with conflicting reports,[57,58] possibly resulting from the different inclusion criteria.[59] It seems that high purified hMG performed better than r-FSH in older women and women with poor ovarian response, probably because of exogenous LH activity and/ or relatively higher acidic isoforms of the FSH protein, which may be of relevance for the clinical outcome.[60] On the contrary, the evidence-based Cochrane review showed that the comparison of r-FSH to any of the other gonadotropins, irrespective of the downregulation protocol used, did not result in any evidence of a statistically significant difference in live birth rate. There was also no evidence of a difference in the OHSS rate.[61] In a systematic review, the effectiveness of hMG with recombinant FSH in ovarian stimulation protocols for IVF or ICSI treatment cycles was compared. For all three GnRH-a protocols analyses, there is insufficient evidence of a difference between hMG and r-FSH on ongoing pregnancy or live birth.[62] Hence, the clinical choice of gonadotropin should depend on the availability, convenience and costs, and further research on these comparisons is unlikely to identify substantial differences in effectiveness or safety.

Corifollitropin-alfa

Corifollitropin-alfa is a sustained follicle stimulant composed of the α-subunit of human follicle-stimulating hormone (FSH) and a hybrid β-subunit formed by fusion of the human chorionic gonadotropin β-subunit carboxy terminal peptide with the β-subunit of human FSH.[63] Like the wild-type FSH, corifollitropin-alfa interacts only with the FSH receptor and lacks LH activity. Corifollitropin-alfa is a successful example of the available long-acting, follicle stimulating hormone. Corifollitropin-alfa has a prolonged half-life and a slower absorption rate, but has the same receptor-binding and biological activity as recombinant FSH.[64]

Efficacy

The pharmacokinetic profile of Corifollitropin-alfa after a single injection implies the highest FSH activity during the first two days of stimulation, followed by decreasing FSH activity until treatment with daily FSH is started. As such, the profile mimics the rather high FSH starting dose and, if required, the FSH step-down protocol, as practised in North America, instead of the low starting dose and if needed, the FSH step-up as practised in Europe,[65] may be used. Injection of Corifollitropin-alfa in the early follicular phase of the menstrual cycle results in the ongoing stimulation of the recruited cohort of antral follicles. Therefore, Corifollitropin-alfa is effective in the stimulation of multifollicular growth for IVF, but seems far less suitable for the induction of monofollicular growth, as documented in a first feasibility study in anovulatory women.[66] In this small trial, in several cases, Corifollitropin-alfa induced multifollicular growth even though much lower dosages were tested. To date, there is insufficient data to support the application of this compound for ovulation induction in anovulatory patients or in intrauterine insemination patients.

Different studies have proven the efficiency of a single Corifollitropin-alfa dose to initiate and sustain multiple follicular development in a gonadotropin-releasing hormone antagonist protocol. In a large randomized trial, the ongoing pregnancy rates were assessed after one injection of 150 microgram Corifollitropin-alfa during the first week of stimulation and compared with daily injections of 200IU r-FSH using a standard GnRH antagonist protocol. The results showed that Corifollitropin-alfa is an effective treatment for normal responder patients, resulting in a high ongoing pregnancy rate, equal to that achieved with daily r-FSH.[67]

Recombinant Human LH (rhLH)

Human LH produced by DNA recombinant technology is now available as are human FSH and hCG. Recombinant LH (r-LH) appears to have essentially similar pharmacokinetic characteristics to the pituitary derived hLH. In humans, recombinant hLH was found to have a distribution of about 1 hour and a terminal-t after intravenous administration of around 10 hours. This is similar to the urine-derived LH (hMG) terminal-t, and contrasts with the urine-derived hCG or recombinant hCG, which have a distribution-t of about 5 hours and a terminal-t of about 30 hours. Hence, hCG will remain in the organism about three times longer than LH. In humans, recombinant hLH (r-hLH) has been tested for triggering final follicular maturation before *in vitro* fertilization-embryo transfer (IVF-ET).[68]

Two studies have shown that r-hLH is as effective as hCG (in terms of oocyte recovery), but safer [(in terms of propagating ovarian hyperstimulation syndrome (OHSS)] than hCG when used in assisted reproductive techniques (ART) to induce final follicular maturation and luteinization.[69,70] A single dose of r-hLH ranging between 15000 and 30000 IU gives the highest efficacy/safety ratio in IVF patients.[28] In one systematic review, r-LH was compared with urinary human chorionic gonadotropin (uhCG) for inducing final oocyte maturation and triggering ovulation in assisted conception.[71] There was no statistically significant difference between r-hLH vs uhCG regarding the ongoing pregnancy, live birth rate, pregnancy rate, miscarriage or incidence of OHSS. Recombinant hLH was comparable with 5000 IU urinary hCG in terms of efficacy.

On the other hand, the efficacy of r-hLH together with r-FSH is controversial. Some authors believe that r-hLH combined with r-FSH can promote optimal follicular development, estrogen secretion and endometrial thickness.[72] But Balasch et al.[73] showed it has a negative impact on oocyte maturation and fertilization.[73] In a systematic review, the effectiveness and safety of a combination of recombinant LH and recombinant FSH was compared with recombinant FSH alone in COH protocols for IVF or ICSI cycles. There was no evidence of a statistical difference in pregnancy outcome when LH was used.[74]

Human Chorionic Gonadotropin (hCG)

Human chorionic gonadotropin is an oligosaccharide glycoprotein composed of 244 amino acids with a molecular mass of 36.7 kDa. Its total dimensions are 75 × 35 × 30 angstroms. The alfa subunit is 92 amino acid long chains and has dimensions

60 × 25 × 15 angstroms. It is heterodimeric, with an α-subunit identical to that of LH, FSH, and TSH and β-subunit that is unique to hCG.[75-76]

Human chorionic gonadotropin shares with LH the common biological property of recognizing and activating the same receptor. It is, however, somewhat different from LH in terms of receptor affinity. The binding affinities of urinary and recombinant hCG are about two to four times higher than those of pituitary-derived human LH (hLH) and recombinant hLH. In addition, there are significant differences in terms of pharmacokinetic characteristics; hCG has a terminal half-life about three times longer than urinary hLH and recombinant hLH. Together, these differences indicate that the administration of an equal dose of LH and hCG, assuming all other pharmacokinetic properties to be similar, will lead to a higher and more prolonged biological signal with hCG than with LH.[77,78]

The use of urinary hCG instead of LH to mimic the preovulatory LH surge has been historically justified by the fact that urinary hCG was easier to obtain than LH. Research into the extraction and concentration of the minute amounts of hCG that occur in the urine of pregnant women began in the late 1940s. By the early 1960s, a purified extract of hCG (Profasi®) was made available. For more than 30 years, hCG extracted from urine of pregnant women has provided a therapeutic analog for LH in the induction of midcycle follicular maturation and ovulation in women,[6] and for the treatment of cryptorchidism in boys and hypogonadotropism in men.[7,8] Initially, having a preparation with a prolonged activity was an advantage, because ultrasonography was not available for timing the surge administration and patients generally belonged to the category of WHO group 1 anovulation who require some luteal phase support.

Based on extended experience with urinary hCG, its efficacy and safety, it is anticipated that recombinant hCG will become the reference preparation for inducing a surrogate LH surge in most patients.

The widely accepted dose range for urinary hCG is 5000 to 10,000 IU as a single injection. The surge profile obtained after a single injection of hCG is more prolonged than the natural LH surge practically; after an injection of 10000 IU hCG, serum levels of the hormone were found to be above baseline in all patients up to day 10 after the injection.[79] The efficacy and safety of the surrogate hCG surge are well-established and to date, there are no arguments for questioning its use, at least in most patients.

However, the occurrence of the OHSS, multiple pregnancy and a somewhat low implantation rate after therapy with human menopausal gonadotropin (hMG)-FSH/hCG has drawn clinicians' attention to the prolonged activity of hCG to these adverse outcomes. It is well-established that the amplitude of the response to FSH (that is, the number of growing follicles) will determine the risk of the OHSS and multiple pregnancy.[80] In addition, in patients receiving hCG after controlled ovarian hyperstimulation (COH), preliminary data suggest that progesterone rises more abruptly than in the natural cycle, which may accelerate the secretory changes in the endometrum to the point of phasing out endometrial receptivity, and thus, in some cases, impair the implantation process.[81]

Finally, vasvular endothelial growth factor (VEGF) has been proposed as a key factor of OHSS pathogenesis, and hCG/LH directly stimulates VEGF synthesis by granulosa cells.[82]

Recombinant hCG

Urinary preparations, however, are associated with a number of disadvantages, including an uncontrolled source, lack of purity, and batch-to-batch variation inactivity leading to variable clinical results.[83] Furthermore, the low purity of urinary preparations restricts them to intramuscular injection. The use of biotechnology processes led to continuing improvement in purity and now permits the introduction of the first 99 percent pure recombinant hCG. Recently, hCG, produced *in vitro* by recombinant DNA technology (Ovidrel), has entered the clinical phase of evaluation.

The pharmacokinetic characteristics of the recombinant hCG are very similar to those of the urinary derived hCG. Their terminal half-lives are about 30 hours. Although r-hFSH has been the major advance with respect to recombinant gonadotropins for the induction of ovulation in anovulatory infertility associated with PCOS, rhCG has also been successfully used in such a condition to trigger ovulation when used instead of urinary hCG.[84] In a double-blind, double-dummy, randomized multicenter study, subcutaneous administration of r-hCG and urinary hCG showed equivalent efficacy in ovulation induction, but r-hCG was better tolerated and was associated with significantly higher midluteal serum progesterone levels.[85] In one randomized study, rhCG was compared with u-hCG during ovulation induction in intrauterine insemination cycles.[86] Recombinant hCG was found to be as effective as urinary hCG in achieving pregnancy during COH-IUI cycles. The outcome of pregnancy was similar in both the groups. Randomized clinical trials have shown that rhCG (250 μg SC) is equivalent to 10,000 IU of urinary hCG (SC or IM) in the induction of final follicular maturation and luteinization in women undergoing ART, in terms of the number of oocytes retrieved per patient. In addition, there are potential advantages of r-hCG-compared with urinary hCG in terms of number of mature oocytes retrieved, luteal progesterone serum concentration, and local tolerance when urinary hCG is administered subcutaneously.[87,88]

In one systematic review, r-hCG was compared with u-hCG for inducing final oocyte maturation and triggering ovulation in assisted conception.[71] There was no evidence of difference between urinary and recombinant hCG regarding the ongoing pregnancy, live birth rate, pregnancy rate, miscarriage or incidence of OHSS.

The empty follicle syndrome is a frustrating condition causing expense and inconvenience. The syndrome has been cured in the same cycle. When oocytes were not obtained from follicles in one ovary a second injection of hCG from a totally different batch yielded retrieved oocytes from the other ovary 36 hours later. This would imply that empty follicle syndrome is in many cases, a drug-related problem rather than a clinical dysfunction. This may be related to marked differences in the manufacturing process of urinary hCG. Therefore, it is plausible to postulate that r-hCG proves to be a more reliable ovulation induction agent than urinary hCG.[66,89,90]

Future Directions

Novel drug development in the infertility field is likely to concentrate on less invasive delivery methods, such as the use of long-acting compounds or different routes of administration that may include transdermal, inhaled or oral agents. On the horizon is the development of orally active, low-molecular weight gonadotropins, for which a first proof-of-concept study has been reported in female volunteers.[91]

CONCLUSION

Recombinant gonadotropins represent a very obvious technical progress in comparison with the older urinary gonadotropins. This appears most clearly in their relative ease of administration and in their lack of contaminations. There is, however, no convincing evidence that recombinant FSH improves clinical outcome in either standard ovulation induction or with IVF. Since outcome affects cost, the lower acquisition costs of urinary products represent a very significant factor in choosing a preferred medication. The benefits of the Corifollitropin-alfa regimen should be weighed against the potential risks. The ovarian response induced by Corifollitropin-alfa may decrease with the patient's age and ovarian reserve, the dose of Corifollitropin-alfa cannot be reduced to obtain milder stimulation. Dose reductions during the first week of stimulation cannot be made in case of hyper-response. Therefore, Corifollitropin-alfa may be less suitable for patients with known risk factors for a hyper-response, such as patients with a history of hyper-response to medication, OHSS or patients with PCOS. Finally, it remains to be confirmed that the pregnancy/live birth rate of this new treatment regimen is comparable to that of daily FSH protocols.

REFERENCES

1. Crowe SJ, Cushing H, Homans J. Experimental hypophysectomy. Bull Johns Hopkins Hosp 1910;21:127-67.
2. Lunenfeld B. Historical perspectives in gonadotropin therapy. Hum Reprod Update 2004;10:453-67.
3. Ascheim S, Zondec B. Hypophysenvorderlappen–hormone und ovarial hormone im Harn von schwangeren. Klin wochenscher 1927;6:13-21.
4. Zonde KB. ueber die function des ovariums. Zeitschr Geburtsh gynakol. Klinwochenschr 1930;9:393-6.
5. Cole HH, Hart GH. The potency of blood serum of mares in progressive stages of pregnancy in affecting the sexual maturity of the immature rat. Am J Physiol 1930;93:57-68.
6. Stewart HL, Sano ME. Gonadotropins in IVF. Montgomery TL. J clin Endocrinol 1948;8:175-88.
7. Donini P, Mortenzemolo R. Rassegnadi clinica, Terapiae Scienze Affini. A publication of the Biologic laboratories of the Institute serono) 1949;48:3-48.
8. Lunenfeld B, sulimouicis, Rabau E, E shkol A. L'Induction de lovalution dunsles amenorrheas hypophysaires par undergarment de gonadotrophines. Chroniques. cR Soc francai se de Gynecol 1973;5:1-6.
9. Prevost RR. Recombinant follicle stimulating hormone: New biotechnology for infertility. Pharmacotherapy 1998;18:1001-1010.
10. van Santbrink EJ, Fauser BC. Urinary follicle-stimulating hormone for normogonadotropic clomiphene-resistant anovulatory infertility: prospective, randomized comparison between low dose step-up and step-down dose regimens. J Clin Endocrinol Metab 1997;82:3597-602.
11. Butt WR, K ennedy JF. Structure-activity relationship of protein and polypeptide Hormones. In: Margoulis M, Greenwood PC (Eds). Excerptn Medica, Amsterdam 1971.p.115.
12. Gardner DK, Weissman A, Howles C, Shoham Z. Textbook of Assisted reproductive Techinques. Drug used for controlled ovarian Stimulation. 1st edn, Taylor and Francis 2004.pp.530-36.
13. Pierce JG, parsons TF. Glycoprotein hormones: structure and function. Annu. Rev. Biochem 1981;50:465-95.
14. Sairam MR. Gonadotropin hormones: relationship between structure and function with emphasis on antagonists. In: In Hormonal proteins and peptides. New York: Academic press 1983;11:1-79.
15. Denef C. Paracrine interactions in the anterior pituitary. J Clin Endocrinol Metab 1986;15:1-32.
16. Morell AG, Gregoriadis G, Scheinberg IH, Hickman J, Ashwell G. The role of sialic acid in determining the survival of glycoproteins in the circulation. J Biol Chem 1971;246:1461-7.
17. Dorringtor JH. Moon Ys Armstrong DT. Estradiol-17 B biosynthesis in cultured granulosa cells from hypophysectomized immature rats: stimulation by follicle stimulating hormone. Endocrinology 1975;97:1328-31.
18. McFarland KC, Sprengel R, Phillips HS, Kohler M, Rosemblit N, Nikolics K, Segaloff DL, Seeburg PH. Lutropin-choriogonadotropin receptor: an unusual member of the G protein-coupled receptor family. Science 1989;4;245:494-9.
19. Camp TA, Raha IJO, Mayo KE. cellular localization and hormonal regulation of follicle-stimulating hormone and luteinizing hormone receptor messenger RNAs in the rat ovary Mol. Endocrinol 1991;5:1405-17.
20. Segaloff DL, Ascoli M. The lutropin/choriogonadotropin receptor. 4 years later. Endocr Rev 1993;14:324-47.
21. Zhang FP, Rannikko AS, Manna PR, Fraser HM, Huhtaniemi IT. Cloning and functional expression of the luteinizing hormone receptor complementary deoxyribonucleic acid from the marmoset monkey testis: absence of sequences encoding exon 10 in other species. Endocrinology 1997;138:2481-90.
22. Gudermann T, Birnbaumer M, Birnbaumer L. Evidence for dual coupling of the murine luteinizing hormone receptor to adenylyl cyclase and phosphoinositide breakdown and Ca^{2+} mobilization. Studies with the cloned murine luteinizing hormone receptor expressed in L cells. J Biol Chem 1992;5;267:4479-88.
23. Cameron MR, Foster JS, Bukovsky A, Wimalasena J. Activation of mitogen-activated protein kinases by gonadotropins and cyclic adenosine 5'-monophosphates in porcine granulosa cells. Biol Reprod 1996;55:111-9.
24. Sairam MR. Role of carbohydrates in glycoprotein hormone signal transduction. FASEB J 1989;3:1915-26.
25. Furuhashi M, Suzuki S, Tomoda Y, Suganuma N. Role of the Pro-Leu-Arg motif in glycosylation of human gonadotropin alpha-subunit. Endocrinology 1995;136:2270-75.
26. Jia XC, Oikawa M, Bo M, Tanaka T, Ny T, Boime I, Hsueh AJ. Expression of human luteinizing hormone (LH) receptor: interaction with LH and chorionic gonadotropin from human but not equine, rat, and ovine species. Mol Endocrinol 1991;5:759-68.
27. Baenziger JU, Kumar S, Brodbeck RM, Smith PL, Beranek MC. Circulatory half-life but not interaction with the lutropin/chorionic gonadotropin receptor is modulated by sulfation of bovine lutropin oligosaccharides. Proc Natl Acad Sci USA 1992;1;89:334-8.
28. Green ED, Baenziger JU. Asparagine-linked oligosaccharides on lutropin, follitropin, and thyrotropin. I. Structural elucidation of the sulfated and sialylated oligosaccharides on bovine, ovine, and human pituitary glycoprotein hormones. J Biol Chem 1988;5;263:25-35.
29. Fowler PA, Templeton A. The nature and function of putative gonadotropin surge-attenuating/inhibiting factor (GnSAF/IF). Endocr Rev 1996;17:103-20.
30. Seibel MM, Kamrava MM, McArdle C, Taymor ML. Treatment of polycystic ovary disease with chronic low-dose follicle stimulating hormone: biochemical changes and ultrasound correlation. Int J Fertil 1984;29:39-43.
31. Glasier A, Thatcher SS, Wickings EJ, Hillier SG, Baird DT. Superovulation with exogenous gonadotropins does not inhibit the luteinizing hormone surge. Fertil Steril 1988;49:81-5.
32. Loumaye E. The control of endogenous secretion of LH by gonadotropin-releasing hormone agonists during ovarian hyperstimulation for *in vitro* fertilization and embryo transfer. Hum Reprod 1990;5:357-76.

33. Hughes EG, Fedorkow DM, Daya S, Sagle MA, Van de Koppel P, Collins JA. The routine use of gonadotropin-releasing hormone agonists prior to *in vitro* fertilization and gamete intrafallopian transfer: a meta-analysis of randomized controlled trials. Fertil Steril 1992;58:888-96.

34. Vande Wiele RL, Bogumil J, Dyrenfurth I, Ferin M, Jewelewicz R, Warren M, Rizkallah T, Mikhail G. Mechanisms regulating the menstrual cycle in women. Recent Prog Horm Res 1970;26:63-103.

35. Cochius JI, Burns RJ, Blumbergs PC, Mack K, Alderman CP. Creutzfeldt-Jakob disease in a recipient of human pituitary-derived gonadotropin. Aust N Z J Med 1990;20:592-3.

36. Nichols J, Wochenhauer E, Fein SH, Nardi RV, Marshall DC, Repronex SC. Ovulation Induction Study Group. Subcutaneously administered Repronex in digo-ovulatory female patients undergoing ovulation induction is as effective and well-tolerated as intramuscular human menopausal gonadotropins treatment. Fert. Stert 2001;76:58-66.

37. Cook AS, Webster BW, Terranova PF, Keel BA. Variation in the biologic and biochemical characteristics of human menopausal gonadotropins. Fertil Steril 1988;49:704-12.

38. Howles CM, Loumaye E, Giroud D, Luyet G. Multiple follicular development and ovarian steroidogenesis following subcutaneous administration of a highly purified urinary FSH preparation in pituitary desensitized women undergoing IVF: a multicentre European phase III study. Hum Reprod 1994;9:424-30.

39. Harika G, Gabriel R, Querex C, Wahl P. Hypersensitization to human menopausal gonadotropins with anaphylactic shock syndrome during a fifth *in vitro* fertilization cycle. J Assist Reprod Gen 1994;11:51-3.

40. Butt Wr, Cunningham FJ, Hartree AS. Gonadotropins. Preparation and assayof human pituitary FSH and LH. Proc R Soc Med 1964;57:107-8.

41. Shoham Z. Yuvalor, urinary gonadotropins and recombinant FSH. Ovulation induction 2002. pp.187-94.

42. Peter R. Brindsden, cambridge UK. Historical prospectives in the management of Fertility. Textbook of *in vitro* fertilization and assisted production. First edn 2005. pp.129-48.

43. Giudice E, Crisci C, Eshkol A, Papoian R. Composition of commercial gonadotropin preparations extracted from human postmenopausal urine: characterization of nongonadotropin proteins. Hum Reprod 1994;9:456-7.

44. Li TC, Hindle JE. Adverse local reaction to intramuscular injections of urinary-derived gonadotropins. Hum Reprod 1993; 8(11):1835-6.

45. Rodgers M, McLoughlin JD, Lambert A, Robertson WR, Mitchell R. Variability in the immune reactive and bioactive follicle-stimulating hormone content of human urinary menopausal gonadotropin preparations. Hum Reprod 1995;10:1982-6.

46. Lunenfeld B, Eshkol A. Immunology of follicle-stimulating hormone and luteinizing hormone. Vitam Horm 1969;27:131-97.

47. Howles CM. Genetic engineering of human FSH (Gonal-F). Hum Reprod Update 1996;2:172-91.

48. Howles CM, Wikland M. The use of recombinant human FSH *in vitro* fertilization In: Shohan Z, Howles CM, Jacobs HS (Eds).

female infertility therapy: current practice London: Martin Dunitz 1999. pp. 52-4.

49. Lunenfeld E, Siberstein T. The Art Science of Assisted Reproductive Techniques. 1st edn, Taylor and Francis 2002;50-4.

50. Balen A. Bye–bye urinary gonadotrophins? Is there a risk of prion disease after administration of urinary–derived gonadotropins? Hum Reprod 2002;17:1676-80.

51. Biffoni M, Marcucci I, Ythier A, Eshkol A. Effect of urinary gonadotropin preparations on human *in vitro* immune function. Hum. Reprod 1998;13:2430-34.

52. Tarrytown NY. Ferring Pharmaceuticals Inc 2002; Data on file.

53. Gleicher N. Some thoughts on the autoimmune Reproductive Failure Syndrome (RAFS) and Th–1 versus Th–2 immune responses. Am J Reprod Immunol 2002;48:252-5.

54. Franklin RD, Bronson RA, Kutteh WH. Gonadotropins do not induce antiphospholipid antibodies. Am J Reprod Immunol 1998;40:359-63.

55. Nahuis M, Van der Veen F, Oosterhuis J, Mol BW, Hompes P, Van Wely M. Review of the safety, efficacy, costs and patient acceptability of recombinant follicle-stimulating hormone for injection in assisting ovulation induction in infertile women. Int J Womens Health 2010;9;1:205-11.

56. Matorras R, Osuna C, Exposito A, Crisol L, Pijoan JI. Recombinant FSH versus highly purified FSH in intrauterine insemination: systematic review and meta-analysis. Fert. Stert 2011;95:1937-42.

57. Daya S, Gunby J. Recombinant versus urinary follicle stimulating hormone for ovarian stimulation in assisted reproduction. Hum Reprod 1999;14:2207-15.

58. Al-Inany H, Aboulghar M, Mansour R, Serour G. Meta-analysis of recombinant versus urinary-derived FSH: an update. Hum Reprod 2003;18:305-13.

59. Matorras R, Prieto B, Exposito A, et al. Supplementation with mid-follicular LHin women aged over 35 years undergoing COS in cycles of ICSI: a randomized controlled study. Reprod Biomed Online 2009;19:879-87.

60. Andreeva P. HP-FSH (Fostimon): a matter of choice in women with low ovarian response. Akush Ginekol (Sofiia) 2008;47:56-61.

61. Van Wely M, Kwan I, Burt AL, Thomas J, Vail A, Van der Veen F, Al-Inany HG. Recombinant versus urinary gonadotropin for ovarian stimulation in assisted reproductive technology cycles. Cochrane Database Syst Rev 2011;2. CD005354.

62. Westergaard LW, Bossuyt PM, Van der Veen F, Van Wely M. WITHDRAWN: Human menopausal gonadotropin versus recombinant follicle stimulating hormone for ovarian stimulation in assisted reproductive cycles. Cochrane Database Syst Rev 2011;2. CD003973.

63. Lapolt PS, Nishimori K, Fares FA, Perls E, Boime I, Hsueh AJ. Enhanced stimulation of follicle maturation and ovulatory potential by long-acting follicle-stimulating hormone agonists with extended carboxyl-terminal peptides. Endocrinology 1992; 131:514-20.

64. Loutardis D, Vlismas A, Drakakis P. Corlfollitropin alfa: a novel long-acting recombinant follicle-stimulating hormone agonist for controlled ovarian stimulation. Women's Health 2010; 6:655-64.

65. Macklon NS, Stouffer RL, Giudice LC, Fauser BCJM. The science behind 25 years of ovarian stimulation for *in vitro* fertilization. Endocr Rev 2006;27:170-207.

66. Balen AH, Mulders AG, Fauser BCJM, Schoot BC, Renier MA, Devroey P, Struijs MJ, et al. Pharmacodynamics of a single low dose of long-acting recombinant follicle-stimulating hormone (FSH – carboxy terminal peptide, corifollitropin-alfa) in women with World Health Organization group II anovulatory infertility. J Clin Endocrinol Metab 2004;89:6297-304.

67. Devroey P, Boostanfar R, Koper NP, Mannaerts BM, Lizerman–Boon PC, Fauser BC. A double blind, noninferiority RCT comparing corifollitropin-alfa and recombinant FSH during the first seven days of ovarian stimulation using a GnRH antagonist protocol. Hum Reprod 2009;24:3063-72.

68. Imthurn B, Piazzi A, Loumaye E. Recombinant human luteinizing hormone to mimic midcycle LH surge. Lancet 1996; 3;348: 332-3.

69. The European Recombinant LH Study Group. Human Recombinant Luteinizing Hormone is as effective as, but safer than, urinary human chorionic gonadotropin in inducing final follicular maturation and ovulation in *in vitro* fertilization procedures: Results of a multicenter double-blind study. J Clin Endocrinol Metab 2001;86:2607-18.

70. Manau D, Fabregues F, Arroyo V, Jimenez W, Vanrell JA, Balasch J. Hemodynamic changes induced by urinary human chorionic gonadotropin and recombinant luteinizing hormone used for inducing final follicular maturation and luteinization. Fertil Steril 2002;78:1261-7.

71. Al–Inany HG, Aboulghar M, Mansour R, Proctor M. Recombinant versus urinary human chorionic gonadotropin for ovulation induction in assisted conception. Cochrane Database Syst Rev 2005;18:CD003719.

72. Baer G, Loumaye E. Comparison of recombinant human luteinising hormone (r-hLH) and human menopausal gonadotropin (hMG) in assisted reproductive technology. Curr Med Res Opin 2003;19:83-8.

73. Balasch J, Creus M, Fabregues F, Civico S, Carmona F, Puerto B, Casamitjana R, Vanrell JA. The effect of exogenous luteinizing hormone (LH) on oocyte viability: evidence from a comparative study using recombinant human follicle-stimulating hormone (FSH) alone or in combination with recombinant LH for ovarian stimulation in pituitary-suppressed women undergoing assisted reproduction. J Assist Reprod Genet 2001;18:250-6.

74. Moshtar MH, Van der Veen, Ziech M, Van Wely M. Recombinant Luteinizing Hormone (r-LH) for controlled ovarian hyperstimulation in assisted reproductive cuc;es. Cochrane Database Syst Rev 2007;18:CD005070.

75. Acevedo HF. Human chorionic gonadotropin (hCG), the hormone of life and death: a review. J Exp Ther Oncol 2002; 2:133-45.

76. Wu H, Lustbader JW, Liu Y, Canfield RE, Hendrickson WA. Structure of human chorionic gonadotropin at 2. 6. A resolution from MAD analysis of the selenomethionyl protein. Structure 1994;15;2:545-58.

77. le Cotonnec JY, Porchet HC, Beltrami V, Munafo A. Clinical pharmacology of recombinant human luteinizing hormone: Part I. Pharmacokinetics after intravenous administration to healthy female volunteers and comparison with urinary human luteinizing hormone. Fertil Steril 1998;69:189-94.

78. le Cotonnec JY, Porchet HC, Beltrami V, Munafo A. Clinical pharmacology of recombinant human luteinizing hormone: Part II. Bioavailability of recombinant human luteinizing hormone assessed with an immunoassay and an *in vitro* bioassay. Fertil Steril 1998;69:195-200.

79. Damewood MD, Shen W, Zacur HA, Schlaff WD, Rock JA, Wallach EE. Disappearance of exogenously administered human chorionic gonadotropin. Fertil Steril 1989;52:398-400.

80. Pride SM, James CSY, Yusen BLT. The ovarian hyper stimulation syndrome, semin Reprod Endocrinol 1990;8:247-60.

81. Fanchin R, castracane D, Taieb J. the post hCG hormonal profile in IVF-ET: plasma P increases 3 times more rapidly than in the menstrual cycle but androgens are unaffected. Am Fertil Soc suppl 1993 (abstract).

82. Rizk B, Aboulghar M, Smitz J, Ron-El R. The role of vascular endothelial growth factor and interleukins in the pathogenesis of severe ovarian hyperstimulation syndrome. Hum Reprod Update 1997;3:255-66.

83. Zegers-Hochschild F, Fernandez E, Mackenna A, Fabres C, Altieri E, Lopez T. The empty follicle syndrome: a pharmaceutical industry syndrome. Hum Reprod 1996;10:2262-5.

84. Loumaye E, Martineau I, Piazzi A, O'Dea L, Ince S, Howles C, Decosterd G, Van Loon K, Galazka A. Clinical assessment of human gonadotropins produced by recombinant DNA technology. Hum Reprod. 1996;11 Suppl 1:95-107; discussion 117-9.

85. International Recombinant Human Chorionic Gonadotropin Study Group Induction of ovulation in World Health Organization group II anovulatory women undergoing follicular stimulation with recombinant human follicle-stimulating hormone: a comparison of recombinant human chorionic gonadotropin (rhCG) and urinary hCG. Fertil Steril 2001;75:1111-8.

86. Sakhel K, Khedr M, Schwark S, Ashraf M, Fakih MH, Abuzeid M. Comparizon of urinary and recombinant human chorionic gonadotropin during ovulation induction in intrauterine insemination cycles: a prospective randomized clinical trial. Fert. Stert 2007;87:1357-62.

87. Chang. P, Kenley S, Burns T, Denton G, Currie K, DeVane G, O'Dea L. Recombinant human chorionic gonadotropin (rhCG) in assisted reproductive technology: results of a clinical trial comparing two doses of rhCG (OvidrelR) to urinary hCG (ProfasiR) for induction of final follicular maturation in *in vitro* fertilization-embryo transfer. Fertil Steril 2001;75:67-74.

88. Ludwig M, Doody KJ, Doody KM. Use of recombinant human chorionic gonadotropin in ovulation induction. Fertil Steril 2003;79:1051-9.

89. Ndukwe G, Thornton S, Fishel S, Dowell K, Aloum M, Green S. 'Curing' empty follicle syndrome. Hum Reprod 1997;12:21-3.

90. Penarrubia J, Balasch J, Fabregues F, Crues M, Civico S, Vanrell JS. Recurrent empty follicle syndrome successfully treated with recombinant human chorionic gonadotropin. Hum Reprod 1999;14:1703-6.

91. Mannaerts BMJL. Novel FSH and LH agonists. In: Filicori M. Proceedings of the fourth world congress on ovulation induction (Bologna, 27-29 May 2004). Rome: Aracne Proceedings 2005; 159-72.

The Choice of Starting Dose in *In Vitro* Fertilization

Aygul Demirol, Suleyman Guven

OVERVIEW

Infertility affects approximately 10 to 15 percent of couples. To enhance the chances of conception, techniques in assisted reproductive technique (ART) have been improved and, in the last 5 years, thousands of babies have been delivered after *in vitro* fertilization (IVF) or intracytoplasmic (ICSI) procedures. Currently, follicle-stimulating hormone (FSH) is the most common drug used for ovulation induction. Selecting the optimal starting dose of FSH to retrieve an acceptable number of oocytes is, however, complicated, and numerous predictive biomarkers have been proposed. These biomarkers fall into three main categories: physical characteristics [age, body-mass-index, presence of polycystic ovary syndrome (PCOS), previous ovarian response], ultrasound assessment of ovarian activity (total number of antral follicles, ovarian stromal blood flow, PCO morphology) and hormonal criteria (concentrations of estradiol, basal FSH, inhibin B, anti-Müllerian hormone). A 'standard patient', who is usually defined as a patient aged less than 36 years, with a regular menstrual cycle, a normal basal FSH and normal total antral follicle count (>10 in both the ovaries) is commonly treated with rFSH, 150 IU/day as a starting dosage. Patients with a poor ovarian response require 450 IU/day rFSH. The dosage should be fixed based on clinical and laboratory parameters: patients age, data obtained from previous controlled ovarian hyperstimulation (COH) cycles, body mass index (BMI) and presence of endometriosis.

RATIONALE

The main rationale of this chapter is to answer the common question of how to assess the individual FSH starting dose in assisted reproduction cycles and also to give practical guidelines for calculating the starting FSH dose.

INTRODUCTION

Infertility affects approximately 10 to 15 percent of couples. To enhance the chances of conception, techniques in assisted reproductive technique (ART) have been improved and, in the last 5 years, thousands of babies have been delivered after *in vitro* fertilization (IVF) or intracytoplasmic sperm injection (ICSI) procedures. To obtain an appropriate and controlled ovarian hyperstimulation (COH), clinicians have introduced many drug protocols based on gonadotropin-releasing hormone (GnRH) agonists or antagonists for pituitary downregulation and follicle stimulating hormone (FSH) or human menopausal gonadotropin (hMG) for ovarian stimulation. Currently, FSH is the most common drug used for ovulation induction.[1] FSH is a glycoprotein hormone composed of two peptide subunits:[2] the alpha-subunit, which is common to the gonadotropins, and the beta-subunit, specific for FSH.[3] The alpha-subunit is encoded on chromosome 6, in the 6q12–q21 location;[3,4] the beta-subunit is encoded on chromosome 11, in the 12p13 location.[5] The molecular weight of FSH is around 30 000 Da, of which one-third is from sugar residues. The secreted FSH has a plasma half life about 149 min, which is five times longer than the approximately 30 min for LH.[6] Gonadotropins are water-soluble and highly degradable by enzymes present in the gastrointestinal tract. They must therefore be administered parenterally (intramuscularly or subcutaneously).[7]

Follicle Stimulating Hormone and Folliculogenesis

Follicle stimulating hormone has a key role in reproductive function: in males it is essential for Sertoli cell function and spermatogenesis, and in females, it stimulates the growth of a large preovulatory follicle that, because of its FSH-dependent maturation, is able to ovulate and to form a corpus luteum in response to the midcycle LH surge.[8] Follicle development from the primordial to the pre-ovulatory stage takes several months.[9] The initiation of growth of the primordial follicles takes place continuously and it appears to be independent of pituitary gonadotropins.[8]

Early antral follicles become FSH-responsive and constitute a pool of available follicles that can be stimulated to grow. The final destiny of the majority of these follicles will be atresia, except for a single follicle that will grow until final maturation to the preovulatory stage. At the end of the luteal phase, early antral follicles (2–5 mm in diameter) are present. The granulosa cells of these early antral follicles seem more sensitive to FSH stimulation. During the luteo-follicular transition, due to the demise of the corpus luteum and the subsequent decrease in estrogen production, the FSH serum concentration rises (perimenstrual rise), maintaining a plateau in the first days of the follicular phase. FSH must reach a threshold; a critical concentration of FSH must be achieved to initiate the process of follicular development.[8]

According to the two cell-two gonadotropin theory, both FSH and LH are necessary for ovarian follicular maturation and the production of ovarian steroids. In addition to promoting follicular growth, FSH stimulates the granulosa cells to increase the expression of the cyctochrome P450 enzyme, aromatase,[7,10] while LH promotes the production of androgens from cholesterol and pregnenolone by stimulating 17 alpha hydroxylase activity in the thecal cells. These androgens then diffuse to the granulosa cells where they are converted to estrogens by the activity of the aromatase enzyme.[11] Adequate estrogen production is essential for the provision of an appropriate milieu for successful fertilization and implantation within the female reproductive tract.[7]

CLINICAL DISCUSSION

Choice of Gonadotropins for Superovulation

The first urinary gonadotropin preparation, hMG, that was used in the early days of ART, contained both LH and FSH. Human menopausal gonadotropin was p obtained from the urine of menopausal women by centrifugation and filtration. It was calculated that approximately 4 to 5 liters of urine were needed for each 75 unit ampule, which represents at least 50 liters for each treatment cycle. Modern FSH preparations, such as recombinant human FSH (r-hFSH), contain no LH and the amount of LH in highly purified urinary FSH (u-hFSH HP) or urinaryFSH (u-FSH) preparations is negligible.[1]

Two kinds of r-FSH are available commercially for therapeutic use: Follitropin alpha (Gonal-F, Serono, Switzerland) and Follitropin beta (Puregon, Organon, The Netherlands). Both the drugs are very similar as they have been synthesized with the same recombinant technology, but they differ from one another in the glycosylation and purification procedure.[1]

The characteristics of exogenous FSH preparations are summarized in Table 15.1. There are no confirmed differences in safety, purity, or clinical efficacy among the various available urinary or recombinant gonadotropin products. New, longer acting gonadotropin preparations are under development and hold promise for improving patient satisfaction while maintaining efficacy.[12]

Starting Dose of FSH for COH

Given the physiological role of FSH, the rational basis of COH is to increase the duration that serum FSH concentrations are maintained above the threshold by direct administration of FSH. Selecting the optimal starting dose of FSH to retrieve

Table 15.1: The characteristics of exogenous FSH preparations (modified from reference)[12]

Gonadotropin preparation	FSH activity (IU/ampule)	LH activity (IU/ampule)	% Protein contamination	Source	Route of admission
Human menopausal gonadotropin	75 or 150	75 or 150	>95%, <5%[a]	Urine	IM or SC
Urinary FSH	75 or 150	Negligible	>95%	Urine	IM
Highly purified urinary FSH	75 or 150	Negligible	< 5%	Urine	IM
Recombinant FSH; follitropin alpha	75-150, 300-900[b]	0	Unknown	Transfected Chinese hamster ovary cells	SC
Recombinant FSH; follitropin beta	75-150, 300-900[b]	0	Unknown	Transfected Chinese hamster ovary cells	IM or SC

Abbreviations: IM: intramuscular; SC: subcutaneous.

[a]For Menopur®, [b]For pen formulations.

an acceptable number of oocytes is, however, complicated, and numerous predictive biomarkers have been proposed. Several baseline characteristics have been assessed for their predictive value regarding a woman's ovarian response in her first cycle of stimulation for assisted reproduction. These characteristics fall into three main categories: physical characteristics [age, body-mass-index, presence of polycystic ovary syndrome (PCOS), previous ovarian response], ultrasound assessment of ovarian activity [total number of antral follicles, ovarian stromal blood flow, polycystic ovarian (PCO) morphology] and hormonal criteria (concentrations of estradiol, basal FSH, inhibin B, anti-Müllerian hormone).[13] Recently, Popovic-Todorovic and colleagues[14] developed a scoring system for calculating the FSH starting dose based on four predictors: the total number of antral follicles, total Doppler score, serum testosterone concentrations and smoking habit.[14]

FSH Dosage for the 'Standard Patient'

A 'standard patient' is usually defined as a patient aged <36 years, with a regular menstrual cycle, normal basal FSH and normal total antral follicle count (>10 in both the ovaries). In Scandinavia, such patients are commonly treated with 150 IU/day rFSH. This dose is used in order to achieve a compromise between giving a dose that is high enough to ensure development of a reasonable number of mature follicles, whilst minimizing the risk of ovarian hyperstimulation syndrome (OHSS).[15] The anticipated yield of oocytes varies according to the patient's chronological as well as ovarian age; in women <40 years of age, reports in the literature have considered 8 to 10 oocytes (range 5–14) per stimulation cycle as adequate. Such a yield should result in the availability of sufficient high-quality embryos to allow a choice when transferring one to three embryos.[15,16] The starting dose of FSH needed to obtain multiple follicular selection and growth is usually between 100 IU and 300 IU per day, but there is no real consensus on the optimal starting FSH dose.[17,18]

Although no specific studies have been conducted as such, the clinical practice of administering a higher rFSH dose according to age has been reported. The cut-off value for age is usually 35 years; that is, patients aged <35 years are given 150 IU/day, whilst those aged >35 years are started on a higher rFSH dose (usually 225–300 IU/day). In one study, investigating predictive factors, 18 patients were given 150 to 300 IU/day depending on their age, although the age cut-off values were not stated.

A mild IVF cycle is defined as an ART cycle in which FSH or hMG is administered at lower doses, and/or for a shorter duration in a gonadotropin-releasing hormone (GnRH) antagonist co-treated cycle, or when oral compounds (antiestrogens or aromatase inhibitors) are used either alone or in combination with gonadotropins. The aim is to collect between 2 and 7 oocytes.[19] The novel mild ovarian stimulation approach in young women (under 36 years), with normal ovarian function and a good prognosis, may improve the results of IVF while reducing the high cost associated with the treatment. The comparison of cycle outcome characteristics of 142 first IVF cycles of women aged 30 to 35, who had undergone stimulation with 100 IU or 150 IU of rFSH, revealed similar findings. This study demonstrates that it is possible to develop mild IVF using the long GnRH agonist protocol. Young women with good prognosis respond to a low dose of rFSH (100 IU) in a similar manner to higher doses of rFSH (150 IU). Results in the number of oocytes, embryos and pregnancy rates are similar, and using a significantly lower amount of rFSH allows IVF to be performed at a lower cost. Additionally, it is concluded that a reduction in the number of embryos transferred in young women decreases the twin rate without compromising the pregnancy rate.[20] In one study, it was shown that an increase in the daily recombinant FSH dose from 150 to 250 IU in women between 30 and 39 years of age has only limited benefit. Although there was a tendency for more oocytes retrieved in the 250 IU group (10.2 vs 8.9), the difference was not statistically significant. The difference of 1.3 oocytes in favor of the high-dose group was achieved using an extra 903 IU of recombinant FSH. The slight advantage in number of eggs did not reflect in the number of transferable embryos. The vital pregnancy rates per started cycle in the low-dose and high-dose groups were similar (17.1% and 16.7%, respectively).[21]

Briefly, a significant number of randomized controlled trials (RCTs) were identified that addressed the question of the FSH starting dose in expected normal responders. Using GnRH agonists for pituitary down regulation, five studies[22-26] compared a starting dose of 100 IU with 200 IU and three studies[21,27,28] compared a starting dose of 150 IU with 250 IU. Two studies were identified that used GnRH antagonists for pituitary suppression. One compared a starting dose of 150 IU with 200 IU,[29] whereas the other compared 150 IU with 225 IU.[30] These RCTs suggest that higher starting doses do not lead to improved pregnancy rates, despite a lower cancellation rates.[31] Young et al.[28] reported that approximately five more eggs were retrieved in women aged <33 years in the 225-IU compared with the 150 IU group, but in older women (≥33 years), the number of eggs retrieved in both groups was similar. In view of the above findings, the higher rate of hormone-related side-effects and extra cost associated with the higher dose protocol, it would be reasonable to conclude that most patients should be started on a dose of 150 IU.[31]

FSH Dosage for 'Poor Responders'

Mostly, in a stimulated IVF cycle, when three or fewer follicles are recruited and serum estradiol concentrations are lower than 300 pg/mL (if one follicle) or 500 pg/mL (if two or three follicles) at the time of human chorionic gonadotropin (hCG) administration, the patient is considered as a poor responder.[32] The single most important predictor of ovarian response was antral follicle count (AFC), performed after pituitary downregulation (dAFC); dAFC thresholds of ≤10 predicted poor ovarian response.[33] There is only one RCT that looked at the efficacy of doubling the starting dose in women who were anticipated to respond poorly.[19] Those patients with <5 antral follicles just prior to starting gonadotropins were recruited for the study. Fifty-two patients were randomized to the normal starting dose of 150 IU/day or the higher dose of 300 IU/day. The median number of oocytes and embryos was the same for both groups (three and two, respectively). Sixty-five percent of the patients in group I and 62 percent in group-II experienced a poor response. The ongoing pregnancy rate was 8 percent in group I and 4 percent in group II (P = 0.55).[34] The most extensively employed strategy to improve follicular response in these so-called 'poor responders' involves the use of high doses of gonadotropins. A small number of randomized controlled trials and retrospective studies have evaluated the effectiveness of the high-dose FSH regimes over a 300 IU threshold. The results of these studies have shown these approaches to be of little or no clinical benefit, although both, the costs of treatment and side effects were higher.[35] In a recent retrospective study, the authors evaluated whether increasing the starting dose of FSH stimulation above the standard dose of 150 IU/day in patients with low predicted ovarian reserve can improve IVF outcomes. A total of 122 women aged <36 years in their first cycle of IVF were identified as having a likely low ovarian reserve (serum AMH measurement <14 pmol/L). Thirty-five women were administered the standard dose of 150 IU/day FSH, while the remaining 87 received a higher starting dose (200–300 IU/day FSH). No significant improvement in oocyte and embryo yield or pregnancy rates was observed following an upward adjustment of the FSH starting dose.[36] There are other studies that have examined 450 IU FSH regimens or even more. Three non-randomized studies showed that increasing the dose of hMG up to 450 IU/day in a second cycle did not increase the number of available embryos, nor did it improve the outcome of the treatment cycle compared to the previous cycle in which the patients had been started on a lower hMG dose.[37-39] Land et al.[38] compared the effects of a 450 IU daily regime of hMG in 126 poor responders with their previous response to a 225 IU dose, resulting in a significantly higher number of follicles and oocytes, but a low pregnancy rate (3.2%). The authors concluded that poor responders do not benefit from the higher dose of hMG.[38] In another prospective study, 80 poor responders were treated using a classic flare-up GnRH agonist regimen with 450 to 600 IU/day of hMG from cycle day 3 and resulted in a satisfactory number of retrieved oocytes (10 + 6.6 per cycle), but a low pregnancy rate per transfer of 13.4 percent.[40] Increasing the

dose of FSH during a cycle is not effective in averting a poor response. There is insufficient evidence for an increased FSH dose after a previous poor response. Although not supported by good evidence, most authors seem to be comfortable with a starting dose of 300 IU/day. Similarly, a maximum dose of 450 IU/day seems to be universally accepted.[31]

Obesity and FSH dosage: It has been reported that obese women require increased doses of gonadotropins in ART cycles.[41] The dose of gonadotropins was higher in women with a body mass index (BMI) of ≥25 kg/m^2 (required nearly 210 units more of gonadotropins) in comparison with those with BMI of <25 kg/m^2. The requirement for gonadotropins was higher (nearly 360 more units of gonadotropins required) in obese women (BMI ≥30 kg/m^2 versus BMI <30 kg/m^2).[42] In contrast to the above study findings, it was reported that in younger patients undergoing IVF, BMI has a significant negative impact on fertility that diminishes as patients reach their mid-thirties. After age 36, BMI has a minimal impact on fertility. It appears that it may be appropriate to recommend weight loss prior to IVF in patients under age 36, whereas in older patients, a more immediate and aggressive approach to ART may be warranted.[43]

Individualizing the FSH Dose for Assisted Reproduction: rFSH Normogram

Popovic-Todorovic et al.[14] in 2003, reported a rFSH dosage normogram consisting of the total number of antral follicles on days 2 to 5, total Doppler score on days 2 to 5, total ovarian volume on days 2 to 5, age, and smoking status. Upon the onset of menstrual bleeding in a spontaneous cycle preceding GnRH analog treatment between days 2 and 5 of the cycle, ovarian transvaginal ultrasonography should be performed and each ovary should be examined. The number of antral follicles (<5 mm and <10 mm) is counted. The maximum longitudinal (D1), anteroposterior (D2) and transverse (D3) diameters of each ovary are measured, and the ovarian volume is calculated (D1 × D2 × D3 × 0.523). Ovarian stromal blood flow is also evaluated using power Doppler, and a semi-quantitative score is allocated to each ovary according to the number and area of the power Doppler signals. Score 1 (poor flow) is given in the presence of only a few and scanty signals, suggesting poor vascularization. Score 3 (good flow) is given in the presence of several pronounced power Doppler signals. A score of 2 (moderate flow) is allocated to those ovaries with intermediary findings. The total Doppler score (the sum of scores for each ovary) is analyzed as a predictive factor, the values being 2, 3, 4, 5 and 6. The calculation of total dose based on five parameters is summarized on Table 15.2.[14]

The rFSH dosage normogram is easy to use in a clinical setting. To illustrate the use of the normogram, a 36-year-old

Table 15.2: FSH dosage normogram based on five predictive parameters (modified from reference[14])

Parameters	FSH starting dose (IU/day)
Total number of antral follicles in ovaries (no.)	
<15	90
15–25	60
>25	50
Total ovarian volume (mL)	
<9	90
9–13	60
>13	50
Total Doppler score (no.)	
2–3	30
4	20
5	10
6	0
Age (years)	
>35	20
30–35	10
<30	0
Smoking habits (cigarettes/day)	
>10	20
≤10	10
Non-smoker	0

woman, non-smoker, with 10 antral follicles, ovarian volume of 8 mL, and a Doppler score 4 should be given 220 IU/day of rFSH (20 + 0 + 90 + 90 + 20).

In one prospective, randomized study, the use of individual rFSH doses between 100 and 250 IU/day (calculated using the rFSH dose normogram) was compared with a standard dose of rFSH of 150 IU/day. The authors concluded that an individual dose regimen in a well-defined 'standard' patient population increased the proportion of appropriate ovarian responses and decreased the need for dose adjustments during controlled ovarian stimulation. A higher ongoing pregnancy rate (36% vs 24.4%, p < 0.01) was observed in the individual dose group.[15]

Individualizing the FSH Dose for Assisted Reproduction: A Novel Algorithm

Howles et al.[7] analyzed the predictive factors of ovarian response. According to their study results, basal FSH, BMI, age and number of follicles < 11 mm at screening were the most important variables in ART patients < 35 years of age who were treated with r-hFSH monotherapy. Using these four predictive factors, a follitropin alfa starting dose calculator was developed to select the FSH starting dose required for an optimal response.[7] In a recent study, a centralized interactive voice response system (IVRS) was used to assign the r-hFSH dose, as calculated by the dosing algorithm. The age, height and weight of the patient, serum FSH concentrations in the early follicular phase of an unstimulated cycle, and baseline AFC in the early follicular phase were entered into the IVRS. The variables were entered into the algorithm described by Howles et al.[44] The FSH dose was then assigned in multiples of 37.5 IU. It is notable that the rate of oocyte recovery, implantation and pregnancy was comparable between the low (75 IU and 112.5 IU) and higher (150 IU and above) dose groups. Thus, by using the evidence-based intervention of the algorithm, a good outcome was achieved in a standard long GnRH agonist protocol at doses that would not usually be selected by clinical judgement alone.[13]

Practical Approach for FSH Starting Dosage

The recommended FSH starting dose may be as follows:[45]

First cycle in patients <37 years	:	150 IU/day
First cycle with a baseline scan suggestive of PCOS	:	112 IU/day
First cycle in a 37 to 39 year old patient	:	225 IU/day
First cycle in a patient ≥40 years old	:	300 IU/day
Previous history of normal response (>5 oocytes)	:	150 IU/day
Previous history of OHSS	:	75 IU/day
Previous history of poor ovarian response	:	450 IU/day

BMI >30 kg/m^2 (PCOS excluded) or history of severe endometriosis: the starting dose should be increased by 75 IU/day.

CONCLUSION

A 'standard patient', who is usually defined as a patient aged less than 36 years, with a regular menstrual cycle, a normal basal FSH and normal total antral follicle count (>10 in both ovaries) is commonly treated with rFSH, 150 IU/day as a starting dosage. Patients with a poor ovarian response require a higher dose of 450 IU/day rFSH. The dosage should be fixed based on clinical and laboratory parameters: patient's age, data obtained from previous COH cycles, BMI and the presence of endometriosis.

REFERENCES

1. Palagiano A, Nesti E, Pace L. FSH: urinary and recombinant. Eur J Obstet Gynecol Reprod Biol 2004;115 (Suppl 1):S30-3.
2. Pierce JG, Parsons TF. Glycoprotein hormones: structure and function. Annu Rev Biochem 1981;50:465-95.

3. Boothby M, Ruddon RW, Anderson C, McWilliams D, Boime I. A single gonadotropin alpha-subunit gene in normal tissue and tumor-derived cell lines. J Biol Chem 1981;256:5121-7.

4. Fiddes JC, Goodman HM. Isolation, cloning and sequence analysis of the cDNA for the alpha-subunit of human chorionic gonadotropin. Nature 1979;281:351-6.

5. Watkins PC, Eddy R, Beck AK, Vellucci V, Leverone B, Tanzi RE et al. DNA sequence and regional assignment of the human follicle-stimulating hormone beta-subunit gene to the short arm of human chromosome 11. DNA 1987;6:205-12.

6. Chappel SC. Heterogeneity of follicle stimulating hormone: control and physiological function. Hum Reprod Update 1995; 1:479-87.

7. Howles CM. Role of LH and FSH in ovarian function. Mol Cell Endocrinol 2000;161:25-30.

8. Vegetti W, Alagna F. FSH and folliculogenesis: from physiology to ovarian stimulation. Reprod Biomed Online 2006;12:684-94.

9. Gougeon A. Regulation of ovarian follicular development in primates: facts and hypotheses. Endocr Rev 1996;17:121-55.

10. Richards JS. Hormonal control of gene expression in the ovary. Endocr Rev 1994;15:725-51.

11. Erickson GF, Magoffin DA, Dyer CA, Hofeditz C. The ovarian androgen producing cells: a review of structure/function relationships. Endocr Rev 1985;6:371-99.

12. Practice Committee of American Society for Reproductive Medicine, Birmingham, Alabama. Gonadotropin preparations: past, present, and future perspectives. Fertil Steril 2008;90: S13-20.

13. Olivennes F, Howles CM, Borini A, Germond M, Trew G, Wikland M, et al. Individualizing FSH dose for assisted reproduction using a novel algorithm: the CONSORT study. Reprod Biomed Online 2009;18:195-204.

14. Popovic-Todorovic B, Loft A, Lindhard A, Bangsboll S, Andersson AM, Andersen AN. A prospective study of predictive factors of ovarian response in 'standard' IVF/ICSI patients treated with recombinant FSH. A suggestion for a recombinant FSH dosage normogram. Hum Reprod 2003;18:781-7.

15. Popovic-Todorovic B, Loft A, Bredkjaeer HE, Bangsboll S, Nielsen IK, Andersen AN. A prospective randomized clinical trial comparing an individual dose of recombinant FSH based on predictive factors versus a 'standard' dose of 150 IU/day in 'standard' patients undergoing IVF/ICSI treatment. Hum Reprod 2003;18:2275-82.

16. van der Gaast MH, Eijkemans MJ, van der Net JB, de Boer EJ, Burger CW, van Leeuwen FE, et al. Optimum number of oocytes for a successful first IVF treatment cycle. Reprod Biomed Online 2006;13:476-80.

17. Devroey P, Tournaye H, Van Steirteghem A, Hendrix P, Out HJ. The use of a 100 IU starting dose of recombinant follicle stimulating hormone (Puregon) in in vitro fertilization. Hum Reprod 1998;13:565-6.

18. Kupesic S, Kurjak A. Predictors of IVF outcome by three-dimensional ultrasound. Hum Reprod 2002;17:950-55.

19. Nargund G, Fauser BC, Macklon NS, Ombelet W, Nygren K, Frydman R. The ISMAAR proposal on terminology for ovarian stimulation for IVF. Hum Reprod 2007;22:2801-4.

20. Fernandez-Shaw S, Perez Esturo N, Cercas Duque R, Pons Mallol I. Mild IVF using GnRH agonist long protocol is possible: comparing stimulations with 100 IU vs 150 IU recombinant FSH as starting dose. J Assist Reprod Genet 2009;26:75-82.

21. Latin-American Puregon IVF Study Group. A double-blind clinical trial comparing a fixed daily dose of 150 and 250 IU of recombinant follicle-stimulating hormone in women undergoing in vitro fertilization. Fertil Steril 2001;76:950-6.

22. Hoomans EH, Mulder BB. A group-comparative, randomized, double-blind comparison of the efficacy and efficiency of two fixed daily dose regimens (100- and 200-IU) of recombinant follicle stimulating hormone (rFSH, Puregon) in Asian women undergoing ovarian stimulation for IVF/ICSI. J Assist Reprod Genet 2002;19:470-6.

23. Out HJ, David I, Ron-El R, Friedler S, Shalev E, Geslevich J, et al. A randomized, double-blind clinical trial using fixed daily doses of 100 or 200 IU of recombinant FSH in ICSI cycles. Hum Reprod 2001;16:1104-9.

24. Out HJ, Lindenberg S, Mikkelsen AL, Eldar-Geva T, Healy DL, Leader A, et al. A prospective, randomized, double-blind clinical trial to study the efficacy and efficiency of a fixed dose of recombinant follicle stimulating hormone (Puregon) in women undergoing ovarian stimulation. Hum Reprod 1999;14:622-7.

25. Pruksananonda K, Suwajanakorn S, Sereepapong W, Virutamasen P. Comparison of two different fixed doses of follitropin-beta in controlled ovarian hyperstimulation: A prospective randomized, double blind clinical trial. J Med Assoc Thai 2004;87:1151-5.

26. Tan SL, Child TJ, Cheung AP, Fluker MR, Yuzpe A, Casper R, et al. A randomized, double-blind, multicenter study comparing a starting dose of 100 IU or 200 IU of recombinant follicle stimulating hormone (Puregon) in women undergoing controlled ovarian hyperstimulation for IVF treatment. J Assist Reprod Genet 2005;22:81-8.

27. Out HJ, Braat DD, Lintsen BM, Gurgan T, Bukulmez O, Gokmen O, et al. Increasing the daily dose of recombinant follicle stimulating hormone (Puregon) does not compensate for the age-related decline in retrievable oocytes after ovarian stimulation. Hum Reprod 2000;15:29-35.

28. Yong PY, Brett S, Baird DT, Thong KJ. A prospective randomized clinical trial comparing 150 IU and 225 IU of recombinant follicle-stimulating hormone (Gonal-F*) in a fixed-dose regimen for controlled ovarian stimulation in in vitro fertilization treatment. Fertil Steril 2003;79:308-15.

29. Out HJ, Rutherford A, Fleming R, Tay CC, Trew G, Ledger W, et al. A randomized, double-blind, multicentre clinical trial comparing starting doses of 150 and 200 IU of recombinant FSH in women treated with the GnRH antagonist ganirelix for assisted reproduction. Hum Reprod 2004;19:90-5.

30. Wikland M, Bergh C, Borg K, Hillensjo T, Howles CM, Knutsson A, et al. A prospective, randomized comparison of two starting doses of recombinant FSH in combination with cetrorelix in women undergoing ovarian stimulation for IVF/ICSI. Hum Reprod 2001;16:1676-81.

31. Rombauts L. Is there a recommended maximum starting dose of FSH in IVF? J Assist Reprod Genet 2007;24:343-9.

32. Loutradis D, Vomvolaki E, Drakakis P. Poor responder protocols for in vitro fertilization: options and results. Curr Opin Obstet Gynecol 2008;20:374-8.

33. Khairy M, Clough A, El-Toukhy T, Coomarasamy A, Khalaf Y. Antral follicle count at down-regulation and prediction of poor ovarian response. Reprod Biomed Online 2008;17:508-14.

34. Klinkert ER, Broekmans FJ, Looman CW, Habbema JD, te Velde ER. Expected poor responders on the basis of an antral follicle count do not benefit from a higher starting dose of gonadotrophins in IVF treatment: a randomized controlled trial. Hum Reprod 2005;20:611-5.

35. Siristatidis CS, Hamilton MP. What should be the maximum FSH dose in IVF/ICSI in poor responders? J Obstet Gynaecol 2007;27:401-5.

36. Lekamge DN, Lane M, Gilchrist RB, Tremellen KP. Increased gonadotrophin stimulation does not improve IVF outcomes in patients with predicted poor ovarian reserve. J Assist Reprod Genet 2008;25:515-21.

37. Karande VC, Jones GS, Veeck LL, Muasher SJ. High-dose follicle-stimulating hormone stimulation at the onset of the menstrual cycle does not improve the *in vitro* fertilization outcome in low-responder patients. Fertil Steril 1990;53:486-9.

38. Land JA, Yarmolinskaya MI, Dumoulin JC, Evers JL. High-dose human menopausal gonadotropin stimulation in poor responders does not improve *in vitro* fertilization outcome. Fertil Steril 1996;65:961-5.

39. Pantos C, Thornton SJ, Speirs AL, Johnston I. Increasing the human menopausal gonadotropin dose—does the response really improve? Fertil Steril 1990;53:436-9.

40. Karande V, Morris R, Rinehart J, Miller C, Rao R, Gleicher N. Limited success using the "flare" protocol in poor responders in cycles with low basal follicle-stimulating hormone levels during *in vitro* fertilization. Fertil Steril 1997;67:900-3.

41. Tamer Erel C, Senturk LM. The impact of body mass index on assisted reproduction. Curr Opin Obstet Gynecol 2009;21: 228-35.

42. Maheshwari A, Stofberg L, Bhattacharya S. Effect of overweight and obesity on assisted reproductive technology—a systematic review. Hum Reprod Update 2007;13:433-44.

43. Sneed ML, Uhler ML, Grotjan HE, Rapisarda JJ, Lederer KJ, Beltsos AN. Body mass index: impact on IVF success appears age-related. Hum Reprod 2008;23:1835-9.

44. Howles CM, Saunders H, Alam V, Engrand P. Predictive factors and a corresponding treatment algorithm for controlled ovarian stimulation in patients treated with recombinant human follicle stimulating hormone (follitropin alfa) during assisted reproduction technology (ART) procedures. An analysis of 1378 patients. Curr Med Res Opin 2006;22:907-18.

45. Healy DL, Breheny S, MacLachlan V, Baker G. Basics of ovarian stimulation. In: Gardner DK (Ed). *In vitro* Fertilization: A Practical Approach. New York, USA: Informa Healthcare; 2007. p.50.

Evaluation and Treatment of the Female Partner before ART

Manisha Takhtani, Akanksha Allahbadia, Gautam N Allahbadia

OVERVIEW

Any woman who fails to achieve a successful pregnancy after 12 months or more of regular unprotected intercourse needs diagnostic evaluation for infertility. A thorough evaluation is the most important step in managing any infertile couple as only after completion of this step can the various treatment options be discussed realistically. Diagnostic evaluation should be carried out in a systematic, expeditious and cost-effective manner. A careful history and physical examination can help identify the possible of infertility in a particular couple. Further diagnostic evaluation can then be focussed towards the most likely cause. The basic tests should include tests for ovulation, ovarian reserve and tubal patency. The choice of treatment then depends on the duration of infertility, the underlying pathological cause and the age of the female partner, and is also often related to issues of efficacy, cost, ease of use and side effects. Failure of treatment, which sadly exceeds the success rates, must be discussed before planning further therapy in a particular couple.

INTRODUCTION

Infertility is a common problem with one in every six couples experiencing difficulty in achieving conception at some stage in their reproductive lifespan. In some, the phase may be temporary and they conceive spontaneously after trying for variable periods. However, many others will conceive only after some kind of medical intervention. This is because one or both members of the couple could be subfertile or sterile. Any woman who fails to achieve a successful pregnancy after 12 months or more of regular unprotected intercourse needs diagnostic evaluation for infertility.[1]

Early evaluation after 6 months of futile efforts may be warranted in women who are more than 35 years of age. Also, women with history of oligomenorrhea, amenorrhea, or known or suspected uterine/tubal/peritoneal pathology need an early evaluation.[2-4]

CLINICAL DISCUSSION

Evaluation of the Female Partner

A thorough evaluation is the most important step in managing any infertile couple. Only once this is completed can the various treatment options be discussed realistically. The complete evaluation includes a clinical history and physical examination, routine investigations and hormonal tests.

History and Physical Examination

A detailed history and a thorough physical examination should be carried out for all couples. Several questions with the aim of finding out any obvious cause of infertility, probing into all aspects of each partner's medical, sexual, personal and social life; and occupation should be asked. The World Health Organization has formulated a set of standard questions, which should be asked to all infertile couples.[5,6] The relevant history in a female partner should include the following:

- Duration of infertility and past-treatment and evaluation.
- Menstrual history, including age at menarche, cycle characteristics, premenstrual molimina, dysmenorrhea.
- Coital frequency and sexual dysfunction.
- Past obstetric history.
- Any contraceptive history.
- Past surgery, hospitalization, serious illness.
- Thyroid disease, galactorrhea, hirsutism, pelvic or abdominal pain and dyspareunia.

- Previous abnormal Pap smears.
- Current medications and any drug allergies.
- *Significant family history*: Birth defects, mental retardation, early menopause, infertility.
- Occupation and exposure to any known environmental hazards.
- *History of drug abuse*: Tobacco, alcohol, recreational or illicit drugs.

Like the history, the physical examination is directed to find out any features pointing towards the cause of infertility and should document the following:

- Anthropometric measurements, such as body mass index (BMI) and waist-hip ratio (WHR), help identify subjects with central adiposity. These patients may require further evaluation of hyperandrogenism and hyperinsulinemia that may cause aberrations in ovulation and cause luteal phase deficiency despite medication.
- Thyroid enlargement and tenderness.
- Breast secretions.
- Signs of androgen excess.
- Abdominal mass, tenderness or organomegaly.
- Pelvic examination, including vaginal and cervical abnormalities and discharge, uterine size, shape, position, mobility, adnexal mass or tenderness and cul-de-sac mass, tenderness or nodularity.

Diagnostic Evaluation

This should be carried out in a systematic and cost-effective manner. The couple's preferences, patient's age, duration of infertility and any significant finding on medical history and physical examination should decide the pace and extent of such evaluation. A number of tests can be carried out to assess the functionality of various reproductive organs. These include tests for ovulation, ovarian reserve, testing; tests for, tubal patency, cervical abnormality, uterine malformations or abnormalities and peritoneal factors.

Tests for Ovulation

Ovulatory dysfunction is responsible for 40 percent of infertility in women.[7] The most common cause of anovulation is polycystic ovaries. The other common causes are thyroid dysfunction, hyperprolactinemia, obesity and strenous exercise, or the cause can be obscure in many cases. Tests commonly performed to evaluate ovulatory function include the following:

- *Serial basal body temperature (BBT):* This test is based on the fact that rise in progesterone after ovulation increases the body temperature slightly (approx ±0.5°C). This increase in temperature is usually maintained for 10 days before it falls to normal levels in those who do not conceive. Ovulatory cycles are usually associated with biphasic BBT recordings, whereas anovulatory cycles result in monopahasic patterns. The period of highest fertility spans from seven days prior to the BBT rise. Though it is a simple and inexpensive method for evaluating ovulation, the test is unreliable as some ovulatory women cannot document clearly biphasic BBT patterns[8] and also, the test cannot define the exact time of ovulation and hence, is no longer recommended.
- *Serum progesterone:* These levels should ideally be obtained a week before the expected onset of next menses (e.g. day 21 in a 28-day cycle). A progesterone concentration of >3 ng/mL provides reliable evidence of recent ovulation.[9] Though levels of >10 ng/mL have been used as a measure of adequate luteal phase, this is unreliable as progesterone secretion by the corpus luteum is pulsatile and can vary seven-fold within a few hours span.[10]
- *Urinary LH detection:* This provides indirect evidence of ovulation as the midcycle LH surge precedes ovulation by 1 to 2 days. The period of highest fertility starts from the day of LH surge and the following two days.[11] However, the accuracy and reliability of the test varies with different products and testing may yield false positive and false negative results.[12]
- *Endometrial dating:* Using endometrial biopsy is no longer considered a valid diagnostic method as it lacks accuracy and precision and cannot distinguish fertile from infertile women.[13,14]
- *Transvaginal ultrasound:* It can reveal the size and number of developing follicles. The progressive follicular growth followed by sudden collapse of the follicle, loss of clearly defined follicular margins, presence of internal echoes and fluid in the cul-de-sac are the various signs of recent ovulation.[15]

Tests for Ovarian Reserve

These tests can yield prognostic information, especially in women:

- More than 35 years of age.
- With a family history of early menopause.
- With a single ovary or history of previous ovarian surgery, chemotherapy or pelvic irradiation.
- With unexplained infertility.
- With poor response to ovarian stimulation.

These tests help to predict the response to ovarian stimulation with exogeneous gonadotropins. However, none of these tests when abnormal imply inability to conceive. The routinely performed tests include:

- *Baseline serum FSH and estradiol measurements:* High baseline follicle stimulating hormone (FSH) (>10 to 20 IU/L) is usually associated with poor ovarian response and has been shown to have high specificity (83 to 100%) but a limited sensitivity (10 to 80%) for predicting poor response.[16] Similarly, cycle day 3 estradiol (E2) levels less than 80 pg/mL are indicative of good ovarian reserve.

In women with amenorrhea, serum FSH and estradiol measurements can help distinguish women with ovarian failure (high FSH and low E2), who will need oocyte donation, from those with hypothalamic amenorrhea (low or normal FSH and low E2) who will require exogenous gonadotropin stimulation for ovulation induction.

- *Antral follicle count (AFC):* Basal AFC is one of the best predictors for predicting ovarian response and a low AFC (range 3 to 10) has been associated with poor response to ovarian stimulation and failure to achieve a successful outcome.[17]
- *Serum AMH (anti-Müllerian hormone):* AMH is a substance produced by granulosa cells in ovarian follicles, mainly by the preantral and small antral stages (less than 4 mm diameter) of follicle development. Production decreases and then stops as the follicles grow larger. There is almost no AMH made in human follicles over 8 mm in size. Because of this, the levels are quite constant and the AMH test can be done on any day of a woman's cycle.[18-21] AMH is a useful marker for predicting ovarian aging and the potential for successful *in vitro* fertilization (IVF). The normal values range from 0.7 to 3.5 ng/mL. Reduced serum AMH (<1 ng/mL) is associated with poor response to ovarian stimulation, poor embryo quality and poor pregnancy outcome.[22-25]
- *Dynamic tests:* These include Clomiphene citrate challenge test (CCCT) and GnRH agonist test. There is a need for consensus on the performance of these tests and the definition of normality, if their use is to be continued. However, given the present level of evidence, these tests should be completely abandoned.

Other Hormonal Tests

- *Serum prolactin and thyroid profile:* Approximately 5 percent of women attending the infertility clinic are diagnosed to have thyroid dysfunction.[26] Derangements in the thyroid profile can lead to anovulatory cycles, hence the thyroid profile is an essential part of the infertility work-up. Hyperprolactinemia also causes chronic anovulation and other defects in ovarian function.
- In case of patients with PCOS, diagnosed by ultra-sonography (USG), symptomatology or having features of androgenization, the following tests should also be performed:
  - Fasting serum insulin level
  - Fasting and post-prandial blood sugars
  - DHEAS, androstenedione and testosterone.

Tests for Tubal Patency

Tubal disease is an important cause of female infertility and should be specifically excluded. Tests commonly used to check tubal patency include: hysterosalpingography (HSG), hysterosalpingo-contrast sonography (HyCoSy) and laparoscopy with chromotubation.

- *Hysterosalpingography:* This is a time-honored test for tubal patency. It helps in the evaluation of the uterine cavity and to check tubal patency. It helps to diagnose proximal or distal tubal occlusion, salpingitis isthmic nodosa, fimbrial phimosis and peritubal adhesions. Additionally, uterine malformations, adhesions (Asherman's syndrome), or any alteration in the shape of the uterine cavity by fibroids, polyps, etc. can also be diagnosed. The positive and negative predictive value of HSG in the detection of tubal disease is 38 percent and 94 percent, respectively.[27] It is an inexpensive and reliable screening test. However, it does not reveal any abnormalities in the pelvis, like adhesions or endometriosis, which may be contributing to infertility. A HSG revealing proximal tubal occlusion requires further evaluation to exclude any artefacts resulting from myometrial or tubal contraction or related to catheter position.
- *Hysterosalpingo-contrast sonography:* It is an inexpensive, fast and well-tolerated method of detecting tubal patency. The method has an added advantage that additional information on the uterine cavity, pelvic adhesions and fimbrial movement can be gathered.
- *Diagnostic laparoscopy and hysteroscopy:* It is the gold standard for evaluating the uterus, patency of Fallopian tubes and other pelvic structures, and may be required in certain cases to establish the exact diagnosis.
- *Fluoroscopic/hysteroscopic tubal cannulation:* It confirms any proximal tubal occlusion suggested by HSG/ laparoscopy and also provides a means for possible correction by recanalization.[28]

Cervical Factors

Abnormalities of cervical mucus are rarely the principal or sole cause of infertility. Traditionally, the postcoital test (PCT) was used to diagnose cervical factor infertility. However, as the test is subjective, has poor reproducibility, is inconvenient, and does not predict the inability to conceive, it is no longer recommended.[29,30]

Peritoneal Factors

Endometriosis and pelvic or adnexal masses and adhesions can cause or contribute to infertility. A history and physical examination can raise the suspicion of these diseases. This can be further confirmed by transvaginal sonography (TVS), which can help to diagnose pathologies, like endometriomas, and laparoscopy, which allows direct visualization of pelvic structures. These factors should also be considered in women with otherwise unexplained infertility.

Flow chart 16.1: Schematic evaluation of the female partner

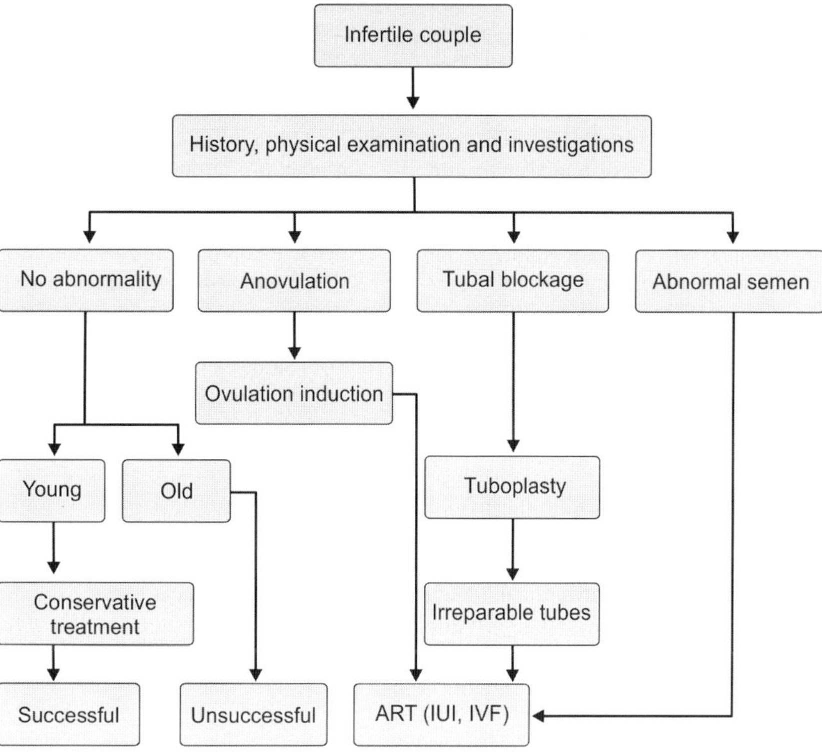

TREATMENT

With the fast advancement in Reproductive Medicine, a wide range of treatment options are available for infertile couples. The choice of treatment depends on the duration of the couple's infertility, which partner is affected, the underlying pathological cause, the age of the female partner and any previous children. The choice of treatment is also often related to issues of efficacy, cost, ease of use and side effects. There are three main types of fertility treatment, including medical treatment (ovulation induction therapy), surgical treatment (laparoscopy and hysteroscopy); and the different assisted reproduction techniques [intrauterine insemination (IUI), *in vitro* fertilization (IVF), intracytoplasmic sperm injection (ICSI)]. Any underlying hormonal disorders, such as thyroid and prolactin disorders, should be addressed first. Flow chart 16.1 shows a simple algorithm for treating infertile couples depending upon the cause of infertility.

CONCLUSION

Diagnostic evaluation before assisted reproductive technique (ART) should be conducted in a systematic, expeditious and a cost-effective manner. A careful history and physical examination can help identify the possible cause of infertility in a particular couple. Further diagnostic evaluation can then be focussed towards the most likely cause. The least invasive methods to diagnose the common causes of infertility should initially be emphasized upon. Failure of treatment, which sadly often exceeds the success rates, must be discussed before planning further therapy in a particular couple.

REFERENCES

1. Practice Committee of American Society for Reproductive Medicines. Definition of infertility and recurrent pregnancy loss. Fertil Steril 2008;90:560.
2. Guttmacher AF. Factors affecting normal expectancy of conception. J Am Med Assoc 1956;161:855-60.
3. Wilcox AJ, Weinberg CR, Baird DD. Timing of sexual intercourse in relation to ovulation. Effects on the probability of conception, survival of the pregnancy, and sex of the baby. N Engl J Med 1995;333:1517-21.
4. Zinaman MJ, Clegg ED, Brown CC, O' Connor J, Selevan SG. Estimates of human fertility and pregnancy loss. Fertil Steril 1993;65:303-9.
5. Rowe PJ, Comhaire FH, Hargreave TB, et al. WHO Manual for the Standardized Investigations, Diagnosis and Management of the Infertile Male. Cambridge; Cambridge University Press, 1993.
6. Rowe PJ, Comhaire FH, Hargreave TB, et al. WHO Manual for the Standardized Investigations, Diagnosis and Management of the Infertile Female. Cambridge; Cambridge University Press, 2000.

7. Mosher WD, Pratt WF. Fecundity and infertility in the United States: incidence and trends. Fertil Steril 1991;56:192-3.

8. Luciano AA, Peluso J, Koch El, Maier D, Kuslis S, Davison E. Temporal relationship and reliability of the clinical, hormonal, and ultrasonographic indices of ovulation in infertile women. Obset Gynecol 1990;75:412-6.

9. Wathen NC, Perry L, Lilford RJ, Chard T. Interpretation of single progesterone measurement in diagnosis of anovulation and defective luteal phase: observations on analysis of the normal range. Br Med J 1984;288:7-9.

10. Filicori M, Butler JP, Crowley WF Jr. Neuroendocrine in regulation of the corpus luteum in the human. Evidence for pulsatile progesterone secretion. J Clin Invest 1984;73:1638-47.

11. Practice Committee of American Society for Reproductive Medicine in collaboration with Society for Reproductive Endocrinology and I. Optimizing natural fertility. Fertil Steril 2008; 90:S1-6.

12. McGovern PG, Myers ER, Silva S, Coutifaris C, Carson SA, Legro RS, et al. Absence of secretory endometrium after false-positive home urine luteinizing hormone testing. Fertil Steril 2004;82:1273-7.

13. Murray MJ, Meyer WR, Zaino RJ, Lessey BA, Novotny DB, Ireland K, et al. A critical analysis of the accuracy, reproducibility, and clinical utility of histologic endrometrial dating in fertile women. Fertil Steril 2004;81:1333-43.

14. Coutifaris C, Myers ER, Guzick DS, Diamond MP, Carson SA, Legro RS, et al. Histological dating of timed endometrial biopsy tissue is not related to fertility status. Fertil Steril 2004;82: 1264-72.

15. de Crespigny LC, O'Herlihy C, Robinson HP. Ultrasonic observation of the mechanism of human ovulation. Am J Obstet Gynecol 1981;139:636-9.

16. Broekmans FJ, Kwee J, Hendriks DJ, Mol BW, Lambalk CB. A systematic review of tests predicting ovarian reserve and IVF outcome. Hum Reprod Update 2006;12:685-718.

17. Hendricks DJ, Mol BW, Bancsi LF, Te Velde ER, Broekmans FJ. Antral follicle count in the prediction of poor ovarian response and pregnancy after *in vitro* fertilization: a meta-analysis and comparison with basal follicle stimulating hormone level. Fertil Steril 2005;83:291-301.

18. Fanchin R, Taieb J, Lozano DH, Ducot B, Frydman R, Bouyer J. High reproducibility of serum anti-Mullerian hormone measurements suggests a multistaged follicular secretion and strengthens its role in the assessment of ovarian follicular status. Hum Reprod 2005;20:923-7.

19. Tsepelidis S, Devreker F, Demeestere I, Flahaut A, Gervy C, Englert Y. Stable serum levels of anti-Mullerian hormone during the menstrual cycle: a prospective study in normo-ovulatory women. Hum Reprod 2007;22:1837-40.

20. La Marca A, Stabile G, Artenisio AC, Volpe A. Serum anti-Mullerian hormone throughout the human menstrual cycle. Hum Reprod 2006;21:3103-7.

21. Hehenkamp WJ, Looman CW, Themmen AP, de Jong FH, Te Velde ER, Broekmans FJ. Anti-Mullerian Hormone levels in the spontaneous menstrual cycle do not show substantial fluctuation. J Chin Endocrinol Metab 2006;91:4057-63.

22. Muttukrishna S, McGarrigle H, Wakim R, Khadum I, Ranieri DM, Serhal P. Antral follicle count, anti-mullerian hormone and inhibin B: predictors of ovarian response in assisted reproductive technology? BJOG 2005;112:1384-90.

23. Muttukrishna S, Suharjono H, McGarrigle H, Sathanandan M. Inhibin B and anti-Mullerian hormone: markers of ovarian response in IVF/ICSI patients? BJOG 2004;111:1248-53.

24. van Rooij IA, Broekmans FJ, te Velde ER, Fauser BC, Bancsi LF, de Jong FH, et al. Serum anti-Mullerian hormone levels: a novel measure of ovarian reserve. Hum Reprod 2002;17:3065-71.

25. Silberstein T, Maclaughlin DT, Shai I, Trimarchi JR, Lambert-Messerlian G, Seifer DB, et al. Mullerian inhibiting substance levels at the time of HCG administration in IVF cycles predict both ovarian reserve and embryo morphology. Hum Reprod 2006;21:159-63.

26. Stratford GA, Barth JH, Rutherford AJ, et al. The value of thyroid function tests in women in the routine investigations of uncomplicated infertility. Hum Fertil 2000;3:203-6.

27. Coppus SF, Opmeer BC, Logan S, van der Veen F, Bhattacharya S, Mol BW. The predictive value of medical history taking and chamydia IgG ELISA antibody testing (CAT) in the selection of subfertile women for diagnostic laproscopy: a clinical prediction model approach. Hum Reprod 2007;22:1353-8.

28. Valle RF. Tubal cannulation. Obstet Gynecol Clin North Am 1995;22:519-40.

29. Griffith CS, Grimes DA. The validity of the post coital test. Am J Obstet Gynecol 1990;162:615-20.

30. Oei SG, Helmerhorst FM, Bloemenkamp KW, Hollens FA, Meerpoel DE, Keirse MJ. Effectiveness of the postcoital test: a randomised controlled trial. BMJ 1998;317:502-5.

Aromatase Inhibitors for Ovulation Induction

Mandakini Parihar, Meenakshi Bharath

INTRODUCTION

One of the most important causes of female factor infertility is anovulation. Management of ovulatory dysfunction and the ability to induce ovulation with the resultant pregnancy was a big milestone in infertility treatments. The commonest cause of anovulation is polycystic ovary syndrome (PCOS). Polycystic ovary syndrome is a common and heterogeneous disorder in women of reproductive age, characterized by chronic anovulation and hyperandrogenism. One problem in understanding the etiology has been the wide variability in clinical manifestations in patients with PCOS. Clomiphene citrate (CC) is the first drug of choice used in the management of anovulatory infertility. Unfortunately, despite the high rates of ovulation, pregnancy rates per cycle remain relatively low with the use of CC. An antiestrogenic effect of clomiphene on the endometrium has been postulated. When CC fails, the only recourse available till now was the use of gonadotropins for the treatment of anovulation. Gonadotropin injections in patients with normogonadotrophic anovulation can be experienced as a time-consuming and ineffective treatment modality with high complication rates.[1]

Mitwally and Casper[1] have shown that the use of CC may be complicated owing to the antiestrogenic effects on endometrial development. To deal with this, patients are increasingly offered 'controlled ovarian stimulation' (COH) combined with intrauterine insemination (IUI) or *in vitro* fertilization (IVF) as the first line of treatment, regardless of the type of infertility.[1] This alteration in treatment strategy is not based on sound scientific evidence and is likely to result in substantially higher multiple pregnancy rates and a major increase in overall treatment costs.[1]

For these reasons, a simple, inexpensive and safe alternative to CC for use in anovulatory women is required. Mitwally and Casper[1] proposed that aromatase inhibitors could replace CC in the future as the new primary treatment for ovulation induction in PCOS patients. Aromatase inhibitors can be used for ovulation induction or ovarian stimulation with higher pregnancy rates compared with CC.

The aim of this chapter is to address the issue of management of anovulatory infertility with aromatase inhibitors, present a review of literature by the Medline and journal search for the different options available for the same, and highlight the current recommendations for treatment.

CLINICAL DISCUSSION

Rationale for the Use of Aromatase Inhibitors in Anovulatory Women

Pharmacological agents used for ovulation induction either block estrogen receptors or block estrogen synthesis and hence, release the hypothalamo-pituitary-ovarian (HPO) axis from the negative feedback effect of plasma estrogen, thereby facilitating follicular growth and ovulation. Aromatase is the enzyme responsible for the conversion of androgens to estrogens. Aromatase inhibitors block the conversion of androgens to estrogen resulting in a relative deficiency of estrogen. This results in increased follicle stimulating hormone (FSH) secretion from the pituitary in the presence of an intact hypothalamo-pituitary-ovarian (HPO) axis.

Clomiphene citrate (CC), an antiestrogen, is a first choice treatment for ovulation induction in women with anovulatory infertility. However, about 25 percent of such women do not respond to CC. Among the 75 percent who ovulate in response to CC, only 20 to 40 percent of them have a successful pregnancy,[1-3] necessitating a simple, inexpensive and safe alternative. Another antiestrogen Tamoxifen, though primarily indicated in breast cancer, is also an established therapy for anovulatory infertility.[4] The poor fertility rates with CC despite successful ovulation induction, possibly attributed to endometrial thinning, necessitated a need to look for alternatives or better ovulation inducing agents.[6,7] With advances in monitoring for ovulation[5] and prompted by the efficacy of Tamoxifen and CC for ovulation, aromatase inhibitors, like Letrozole, have been considered as the next candidates for induction of ovulation. Major clinical studies have reported successful induction of ovulation with Letrozole.[1-3] The use of Letrozole has been known to induce ovulation in 75 to 80 percent women.[1,6,7] In addition to this, the use of Letrozole has not been associated with the undesirable effects of CC.

Mechanism of Action of Letrozole

Letrozole is an aromatase inhibitor that acts by blocking the synthesis of estrogen. It releases the HPO axis from estrogenic inhibition, facilitating follicular growth and culminating in ovulation. Though Letrozole is labeled as an anticancer drug, its use is not associated with the classical adverse effects of an anticancer drug such as bone marrow depression, alopecia, mucosal ulcers and infections. The side effects of Letrozole are generally mild, tolerable and transitory in nature and can be explained on the basis of reduced estrogen levels caused by the drug. Moreover, since this drug is meant to be used for only 5 days in a month for induction of ovulation, the incidence and severity of side effects are anticipated to be lesser compared to its use in breast cancer. The other aromatase inhibitor used in clinical practice for anovulatory infertility is Anastrozole. However, there is very little data available on it and the majority of research reports the use of Letrozole. Hence, for the purpose of this chapter, unless specified, the use of aromatase inhibitor would refer to studies using Letrozole.

Comparison of the Success Rates of Letrozole and Clomiphene Citrate

Several authors found combined controlled ovarian hyperstimulation (COH) and intrauterine insemination (IUI) treatment to be very effective in unexplained and mild male infertility.[8-11] Studies have shown significantly lower estradiol concentrations and more stimulated follicles in cycles stimulated with Letrozole compared to 100 mg CC from day 3 to 7 of the cycle.[12] The estrogen levels in women on aromatase inhibitors were found to be 2 to 3 times lower than those reported in CC cycles.[3,13,14] despite similar LH and FSH profiles.[13,14] However, the endometrial thickness was greater in the aromatase inhibitor cycles[13,14] or unaffected.[3] In a selected population of women with a mean endometrial thickness of 5 mm after CC treatment, Letrozole treatment in the early follicular phase resulted in a significant increase in midcycle endometrial thickness (mean of 9 mm).[2]

Al-Fozan, et al.[13] compared the effect of CC and Letrozole in women undergoing superovulation. There was no difference in pregnancy rates or endometrial thickness between the Letrozole and CC groups in his study. However, interestingly, the miscarriage rate was higher in the CC group. The reason is not clear but is probably due to the difference in mechanisms of action of Letrozole and CC. Fatemi et al.[14] suggest a lower multiple gestation rate with Letrozole, but larger controlled studies examining the effects of Letrozole on the incidence of multiple gestation are needed to confirm these findings.

In all the studies conducted so far, the aromatase inhibitor, Letrozole, was administered as a 5-day regimen, usually from day 3 to 7 of the menstrual cycle, at a dose of 2.5 to 5 mg/day. Mitwally and Casper[15,16] proposed that aromatase inhibitors would replace CC in the future as the new primary treatment for ovulation induction in PCO patients.[15,16]

Combining Gonadotropins and Aromatase Inhibitors

The use of gonadotropins in anovulation has given good results with pregnancy rates varying between 20 to 60 percent. A major disadvantage of gonadotropin treatment is the high cost of treatment. In addition, there is a higher risk of multiple pregnancies and ovarian hyperstimulation syndrome (OHSS) when using gonadotropins, both of which increase the risk to the patient. To reduce the gonadotropin requirement and risk, combination protocols using CC have been in practice.[17] While these protocols were initially popular,[18,19] the use of gonadotropins plus CC has been largely abandoned after reports that CC negatively affects endometrial thickness, subendometrial blood flow, oocyte quality, embryo development, and hence, ultimately the pregnancy rates.[19-21] In a prospective randomized trial, Ransom et al.[22] showed that the endometrium is significantly thinner in the group where CC was used along with gonadotropins. This was even more marked when the number of preovulatory follicles was similar in the only gonadotropins group and the CC + gonadotropins group. Also noteworthy was the fact that fewer pregnancies were achieved in patients treated with CC and gonadotropins. The postulated theory for this negative effect is estrogen receptor suppression by CC that has adverse effects on endometrial maturation as well as cervical mucus.[22]

With reports about the use of aromatase inhibitors, it was suggested that a specific reversible, non-steroidal aromatase inhibitor, like Letrozole or Anastrazole, that suppresses estrogen biosynthesis,[23] can successfully replace CC in superovulation.[2,24] Aromatase inhibitors like CC, increase the endogenous gonadotropin secretion, but unlike CC, they do not result in estrogen receptor depletion. They may also possibly have a local effect by increasing the androgen concentration, the sensitivity of the ovaries to FSH and hence, decreasing the requirement for gonadotropins without negative effects on peripheral estrogen sensitive tissues. Studies have reported that Letrozole co-treatment with gonadotropins is superior to CC plus gonadotropins.[25,26]

Additionally, concomitant treatment of Letrozole with gonadotropins in poor responders results in increased number of preovulatory follicles compared with previous cycles with gonadotropins alone.[26]

Despite the low estrodiol levels owing to the local affects of the potent anti-aromatase effect of Letrozole, there is no negative effect on endometrial thickness. It is postulated that this is due to the relatively short half-life of Letrozole, which allows complete endometrial recovery before implantation. There is a definite decrease in gonadotropin requirements in patients treated with Letrozole plus gonadotropins compared to gonadotropins alone.[25]

Sammour, et al.[27] compared Letrozole with CC along with gonadotropins for superovulation before IUI and found that although fewer follicles developed, a superior uterine environment was achieved and this resulted in better pregnancy rates in the Letrozole group than in the CC group.[27]

Outcome of Pregnancies Achieved with Aromatase Inhibitors

One of the concerns regarding the use of any new agent for fertility treatment is the potential effects it could have on the offspring born. There was a concern raised by an abstract submitted for the ASRM meeting though it was never published. The initial fear about the safety of Letrozole has been set aside by the excellent review by Tulandi et al.[28] who reported no difference in the overall rates of major and minor congenital malformations among the offspring of women who conceived following Letrozole or CC treatments. However, congenital cardiac anomalies were less frequent in the Letrozole group. The concern that Letrozole use for ovulation induction could be teratogenic is unfounded based on their data.[28]

A concern about the safety of Letrozole to the fetus was recently raised in an abstract presentation at the 2005 ASRM meeting.[29] The authors reported the outcome of 170 infants of which, 20 were lost to follow-up. As a result, 150 babies from 130 pregnancies were compared to a control group of over 36,000 infants born from low-risk spontaneously pregnant women in a community hospital. The control population was younger than the Letrozole group. The results of this study, which had several methodological issues, suggested that Letrozole might increase the risk of cardiac and bone anomalies; however, the overall rate of major malformations did not differ between the 2 groups.[29] A further concern regarding potential law suits was raised by the notice issued to all practicing infertility specialist on the website of Novartis, the makers of Femara®.[30]

In their multicenter study, Tulandi et al.[20] reported on the incidence of congenital malformations among 911 babies born after infertility treatment with Letrozole (n = 252), Letrozole + FSH (n = 262), CC (n = 293) or CC + FSH (n = 104). Congenital malformations were encountered in 2.4 percent of newborns in the Letrozole group and 4.8 percent of newborns in the CC group. Major malformations were detected in 1.2 percent of the babies in the Letrozole group and in 3.0 percent of the babies in the CC group. These rates of major anomalies were not statistically different between the two groups and were similar to the quoted rates of anomalies found in the general population (2–3%).[31,32]

It has been suggested by Tulandi, et al.[28] and others[33] that as the half-life of Letrozole is approximately 45 hours (range 30–60 hours), it is completely cleared from the body by the time of embryo implantation as compared to Clomiphene citrate, which remains in the system due to its longer half-life of 5 to 7 days.[33] Letrozole is eliminated as an inactive carbinol metabolite mainly via the kidneys. Thus, exposure to the drug predates the critical fetal development period, casting doubt on the biological plausibility of teratogenicity in the use of the drug for ovulation induction.[28]

CONCLUSION

In summary, the different studies seem to confirm the efficacy of aromatase inhibitors in ovulation induction. The results suggest that the aromatase inhibitor, Letrozole, may be used as an alternative new first-line treatment for ovulation induction in anovulatory infertile patients. However, all the studies conducted so far are in small numbers and only larger randomized control studies will be able to shed light on whether it is time to say goodbye to Clomiphene citrate.

REFERENCES

1. Mitwally MF, Casper RF. Use of an aromatase inhibitor for induction of ovulation in patients with an inadequate response to clomiphene citrate. Fertil Steril 2001;75:305-9.
2. Bart CJ, M Fauser, et al. Revised 2003 consensus on diagnostic criteria and long-term health risks related to polycystic ovary syndrome (PCOS) The Rotterdam ESHRE/ASRM-sponsored PCOS consensus workshop group.
3. Fisher SA, Reid RL, Dean A, Van Vugt, Casper RF. A randomized double-blind comparison of the effects of clomiphene citrate and the aromatase inhibitor letrozole on ovulatory function in normal women. Fertil Steril 2002;78:280-5.
4. Boostanfar R, Jain JK, Mishell DR Jr, Paulson RJ. A prospective randomized study comparing clomiphene citrate with tamoxifen citrate for ovulation induction. Fertil Steril 2001;75: 1024-6.
5. Smith YR, Randolph JF Jr, Christman GM, Ansbacher R, Howe DM, Hurd WW. Comparison of low-technology and high-technology monitoring of clomiphene citrate ovulation induction. Fertil Steril 1998;70:165-8.
6. Mittal S, Chakravarty BN, Ghosh S. Use of Aromatase Inhibitor for ovulation in anovulatory infertile women. Book of Abstracts, AICOG 2003.

7. Parihar M. Will Aromatase Inhibitors replace clomiphene citrate for ovulation induction? Book of Abstracts, AICOG 2002.

8. Davar R, Ashgharnia M, Tayebi M. Comparison of the success rate of letrozole and clomiphene citrate in COH with IUI. Journal of Research in Medical Sciences 2006;11:382.

9. Aboulghar MA, Mansour RT, Serour GI, Amin Y, Abbas AM, Salah IM. Ovarian superstimulation and intrauterine insemination for the treatment of unexplained infertility. Fertil Steril 1993;60:303-6.

10. Van Voorhis BJ, Barnett M, Sparks AE, Syrop CH, Rosenthal G, Dawson J. Effect of the total motile sperm count on the efficacy and cost-effectiveness of intrauterine insemination and *in vitro* fertilization. Fertil Steril 2001;75:661-8.

11. Zayed F, Lenton EA, Cooke ID. Comparison between stimulated *in vitro* fertilization and stimulated intrauterine insemination for the treatment of unexplained and mild male factor infertility. Hum Reprod 1997;12:2408-13.

12. Fisher SA, Reid RL, Van Vugt DA, Casper RF. A randomized double-blind comparison of the effects of clomiphene citrate and the aromatase inhibitor letrozole on ovulatory function in normal women. Fertil Steril 2002;78:280-5.

13. Al Fozan H, Al Khadouri M, Tan SL, Tulandi T. A randomized trial of Letrozole versus Clomiphene citrate in women undergoing superovulation. Fertil Steril 2004;82:1561-3.

14. Fatemi HM, Kolibianakis E, Tournaye H, Camus M, Van Steirteghem AC, Devroey P. Clomiphene citrate versus Letrozole for ovarian stimulation: a pilot study. Reprod Biomed Online 2003;7:543-6.

15. Mitwally MF, Casper RF. Aromatase inhibition: a novel method of ovulation induction in women with polycystic ovarian syndrome. Reprod Technol 2000;10:244-7.

16. Mitwally MF, Biljan MM, Casper RF. Pregnancy outcome after the use of an aromatase inhibitor for ovarian stimulation. Am J Obstet Gynecol 2005;192:381-6.

17. Kemmann E, Jones JR. Sequential clomiphene citrate-menotropin therapy for induction or enhancement of ovulation. Fertil Steril 1983;39:772-9.

18. Jarrell J, McInnes R, Cooke R, Arronet G. Observations on the combination of Clomiphene citrate-human menopausal gonadotropin-human chorionic gonadotropin in the management of anovulation. Fertil Steril 1981;35:634-7.

19. Lu PY, Chen AL, Atkinson EJ, Lee SH, Erickson LD, Ory SJ. Minimal stimulation achieves pregnancy rates comparable to human menopausal gonadotropins in the treatment of infertility. Fertil Steril 1996;65:583-7.

20. Hsu CC, Kuo HC, Wang ST, Huang KE. Interference with uterine blood flow by Clomiphene citrate in women with unexplained infertility. Obstet Gynecol 1995;86:917-21.

21. Laufer N, Pratt BM, DeCherney AH, Naftolin F, Merino M, Markert CL. The *in vivo* and *in vitro* effects of clomiphene citrate on ovulation, fertilization, and development of cultured mouse oocytes. Am J Obstet Gynecol 1983;47:633-9.

22. Ransom MX, Doughman NC, Garcia AJ. Menotropins alone are superior to a Clomiphene citrate and menotropin combination for superovulation induction among Clomiphene citrate failures. Fertil Steril 1996;65:1169-74.

23. Geisler J, Haynes B, Anker G, Dowsett M, Lonning PE. Influence of Letrozole and Anastrozole on total body aromatization and plasma estrogen levels in postmenopausal breast cancer patients evaluated in a randomized, crossover study. J Clin Oncol 2002; 20:751-7.

24. Mitwally MF, Casper RF. Aromatase inhibition reduces gonadotrophin dose required for controlled ovarian stimulation in women with unexplained infertility. Hum Reprod 2003; 18:1588-97.

25. Healey S, Tan SL, Tulandi T, Biljan MM. Effects of Letrozole on superovulation with gonadotropins in women undergoing intrauterine insemination. Fertil Steril 2003;80:1325-9.

26. Mitwally MF, Casper RF. Aromatase inhibition improves ovarian response to follicle-stimulating hormone in poor responders. Fertil Steril 2002;77:776-80.

27. Sammour A, Biljan MM, Tan SL, Tulandi T. Prospective randomized trial comparing the effects of Letrozole (LE) and clomiphene citrate (clomiphene citrate) on follicular development, endometrial thickness and pregnancy rate in patients undergoing super-ovulation prior to intrauterine insemination (IUI) Fertil Steril 2001; 76(Suppl 1):S110.

28. Tulandi T, Martin J, Raedah Al-Fadhli, Kabli N, et al. Congenital malformations among 911 newborns conceived after infertility treatment with letrozole or clomiphene citrate. Fertil Steril 2006;85:1761-5.

29. Biljan MM, Hemmings R, Brassard N. The outcome of 150 babies following the treatment with Letrozole or Letrozole and gonadotropins. Fertil Steril 2005; 84 (supp.1); O-231, Abstract 1033.

30. Fontana PG, Leclerc JM. Contraindication of Femara® (Letrozole) in premenopausal women. http://www.ca.novartis.com/downloads/en/letters/femara_hcp_e_17_11_05.pdf.

31. William's Obstetrics, 22nd edition, Chapter 13. Prenatal Diagnosis and Fetal Therapy. Ed. FG Cunningham, et al. New York, McGraw-Hill Professional, 2005.

32. Health Canada. Congenital Anomalies in Canada - Perinatal Health Report, 2002. http://www.phac-aspc.gc.ca/cac-acc02.

33. Holzer H, Casper R, Tulandi T. A new era of ovulation induction. Fertil Steril 2006;85:277-84.

Intrafollicular Consequences of the Use of Aromatase Inhibitors in ART

Maruthini D, Manisha Palep-Singh

OVERVIEW

Aromatase is a cytochrome P450 containing enzyme complex, which catalyzes the rate-limiting steps in the production of estrogen through hydroxylation of androgens. The inhibitors of this enzyme complex have been used effectively in the management of breast cancer and are now being used in the management of subfertility. Evidence suggests that estrogens directly augment the stimulation of granulosa cell aromatase activity through follicle-stimulating hormone (FSH), which may be one of the mechanisms activating intraovarian positive feedback resulting in selective follicle maturation. This chapter discusses the potential role of aromatase inhibitors in managing various forms of subfertility including their safety profile and success rates.

INTRODUCTION

The use of aromatase inhibitors in the treatment of infertility is currently under extensive research. Aromatase is an indispensable enzyme complex in women, particularly in the premenopausal ovaries. It is responsible for the production of estrogen from androgens such as androstenedione and testosterone. In simple terms, inhibition of aromatase is considered to relatively increase the ovarian androgen concentration, which in turn is believed to have a positive effect on the reproductive function of the ovaries.

Human Aromatase Activity

Circulating estrogen is produced by the ovaries in premenopausal women and by the adipose tissues in postmenopausal women. Aromatase is a cytochrome P450 hemoprotein containing an enzyme complex, which catalyzes the rate-limiting steps in the production of estrone and estradiol through hydroxylation of androstenedione and testosterone respectively.[1] Though, aromatase is found primarily in the human ovaries, it is also present in other tissues such as testis, adipose tissue, placenta, brain, muscle and skin fibroblasts.[2-4]

Aromatase inhibitors (AIs) were first developed when aminoglutethimide was identified to inhibit cytochrome P450 and found to be effective in the treatment of women with advanced breast cancer.[5]

Testolactone was developed as a first-generation AI. Subsequently, the second-generation AIs, such as formestane and fadrazole, became available for clinical use. This was followed by the third-generation inhibitors, namely anastrazole, Letrozole, exemestane and vorozole. These are 1000 to 10,000-fold more potent than aminoglutethimide in the treatment of breast cancer.[6]

There are two groups of AIs according to their structure: steroidal (type 1) and non-steroidal (type 2). The type 1 inhibitors such as testolactone, examestane and formestane are all derivatives of androstenedione and bind irreversibly to the androgen binding site with continuing treatment. The type 2 inhibitors namely, aminoglutethimide, anastrazole, Letrozole, vorozole and fadrozole are non-steroidal. They bind to the heme moiety of the cytochrome P450 enzyme and exert their function.[7]

CLINICAL DISCUSSION

Aromatase Activity in the Ovaries

The aromatase mRNA expression in granulosa cells commences when the follicle reaches a size of 7 mm or above in diameter.[8] Aromatase activity in the ovarian granulosa cells is modulated by the endocrine and paracrine hormones. In a natural menstrual cycle, under the influence of luteinizing hormone (LH), theca cells produce androstenedione and

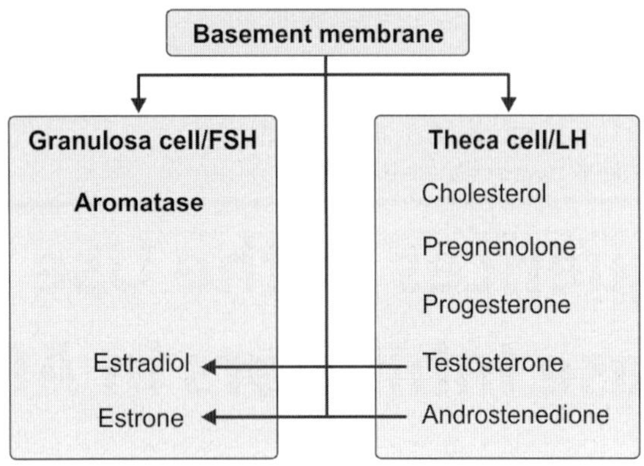

Fig. 18.1: Ovarian hormone synthesis

testosterone from cholesterol through a series of enzymatic reactions. Finally, the aromatase enzyme in the granulosa cells converts the C19 steroids to estradiol. Thus, the granulosa cells are not capable of estradiol synthesis *de novo* but dependent on the androgen substrate supply from theca cells as shown in Figure 18.1.

The aromatase system is dependent on follicle stimulating hormone (FSH) and in the late proliferative phase, also on LH. Follicle stimulating hormone stimulates the granulosa cell production of estrogens. In cultured mouse preantral follicles, androgen treatment stimulates follicle growth.[9] Androgen treatment increases the number of preantral and small antral follicles in monkeys as apoptosis seems to be inhibited and theca/granulosa cell proliferation enhanced.[10,11] In primates, the granulosa cell androgen receptor levels are 4.2 fold higher in immature follicles than in preovulatory follicles.[12] Androgens have been shown to promote follicular FSH sensitivity[13] and also insulin-like growth factor (IGF)-I and IGF-I receptor gene expression,[14] which in turn increase intrafollicular steroidogenesis.[15]

Animal studies have shown that the aromatase activity is important in the process of selection and development of a dominant follicle. It is greater in granulosa cells from the largest follicle than those from smaller follicles.[16] Recent evidence suggests that estrogens directly augment the stimulation of granulosa cell aromatase activity through FSH which may be one of the mechanisms activating intraovarian positive feedback resulting in selective follicle maturation.[17] In humans, the aromatase activity begins to diminish with the oocyte-corona-cumulus complex (OCC complex) maturation. In a study on human menopausal gonadotropin (hMG)/human chorionic gonadotropin (hCG) stimulated cycles, a diminution in aromatase activity was identified in the preovulatory follicles.[18] However, Costa et al.[19] have disproved this recently by showing a significant increase in the intrafollicular ratios of progesterone/estradiol (E2), progesterone/testosterone and E2/testosterone in follicular fluid containing mature oocytes, suggesting a reduction in

C21 to C19 conversion, but not in the aromatase activity.[19] Human follicular fluid showed higher estradiol/testosterone (E2/T) ratio in pregnancy-associated follicles than in follicles in which the oocytes failed to implant or did not cleave.[20]

Modulators of Ovarian Aromatase Activity

The modulation of granulosa cell aromatase system is closely inter-related to follicular development. The transition of primordial follicles to a pool of growing follicles is FSH-independent as these follicles do not express FSH and LH receptors.[21] Once the initial follicular recruitment is achieved, the small antral follicles develop FSH-induced aromatase activity while theca cells commence production of androgens. In early antral follicles, androgens seem to be folliculotropic while, at a later stage, they may exert atretogenic effects by interfering with the aromatase system. It also appears that too high concentrations of androgens could be detrimental to follicular growth.

Polycystic Ovary Syndrome (PCOS) and Aromatase Inhibitors

In polycystic ovaries, the follicular fluid estradiol concentration is low compared to that in dominant follicles in spite of high levels of androstenedione.[22,23] Literature suggests that there is sufficient substrate but reduced aromatization in women with polycystic ovaries. However, recent research indicates a reduced aromatase-stimulating bioactivity to increase P450 aromatase mRNA expression in PCOS. The aromatase-stimulating bioactivity is the combined activity of various intrafollicular endogenous factors such as a high molecular weight FSH receptor binding inhibitor,[24] inhibin-α subunit precursor,[25] insulin-like growth factor binding proteins (IGFBPs),[26] epidermal growth factor (EGF)[27] and tumor necrosis factor (TNF)-α.[28] This means that there is relative aromatase deficiency in the ovary, leading to increased androgens in the hormonal milieu. Due to an increased number of FSH receptors resulting from hyperandrogenism, these polycystic ovaries are sensitive to both exogenous and endogenous rise in gonadotropins, risking the development of ovarian hyperstimulation syndrome (OHSS) and multiple pregnancies. Theoretically, AIs suppress estrogen synthesis in the ovaries and brain resulting in increased FSH to stimulate the ovaries. The AIs do not antagonize the inhibin feedback mechanism on the pituitary. Therefore, the secondary feedback loop continues to work, moderating the FSH rise in response to the aromatase inhibitors, thereby reducing the risk of OHSS. At the same time, the absence of antiestrogenic side effects may be advantageous to the endometrium. Whether a further increase in testosterone and LH concentrations resulting from AIs would be detrimental to these women needs to be addressed by large studies.

Clinical Applications of Aromatase Inhibitors

Ovulation Induction

Aromatase inhibitors have been recently used for the purpose of ovulation induction in the dose of 2.5 to 5 mg for 5 days in the early follicular phase of the cycle. Mitwally et al.[29] explored the impact of aromatase inhibitor activity in the early menstrual phase as compared to that of Clomiphene citrate (CC). They hypothesised that inhibition of estrogen production from all the sources using an aromatase inhibitor would release the hypothalamo-pituitary-ovarian (HPO) axis from the negative feedback, thereby increasing the FSH selection towards stimulation of ovarian follicles.

The selective non-steroidal AIs have a relatively short half-life (45 hours) compared to CC (2 weeks) and thus, seem to be ideal for this purpose.[29] Mitwally et al.[29] conducted a series of clinical trials to assess the efficacy of aromatase inhibitors in ovulation induction. In this study, there were 12 anovulatory PCOS women and 10 ovulatory infertile women. These women had either failed to ovulate or had evidence of an endometrial thickness <5 mm with CC. The mean number of follicles was 2.5 with CC as compared to 2.3 with Letrozole. Overall, four pregnancies were achieved in response to Letrozole. In both the groups, the mean serum E2 concentration was lower on the day of hCG administration in women treated with Letrozole. In the PCOS group, the serum E2 level was 962 pmol/L in the Letrozole treatment cycles as compared with 1638 pmol/L in the CC treatment cycles. In ovulatory patients, the serum E2 level was 719 pmol/L in Letrozole treatment cycles versus 3003 pmol/L in the CC treatment cycles. In spite of the relatively low estrogen levels, Letrozole produced a thicker endometrium than CC. This is explained by the antiestrogenic property of CC, which is absent in Letrozole.

Al-Omari et al.[30] compared 2.5 mg of Letrozole with 1 mg of anastrazole in 18 CC-resistant PCOS women. The endometrial thickness (L: 8.2 mm; A: 6.5 mm), ovulation rate (L: 84.4%; A: 60%) and pregnancy rate (L: 18.8%; A: 9.7%) was higher in the Letrozole group as compared with the Anastrazole group.[30]

In women with PCOS, the efficacy of Letrozole in combination with Metformin has been studied recently in a prospective randomized trial (RCT). A small group of 29 women were recruited into two groups. One group received metformin and CC while the other group received Metformin and Letrozole. There was a significant increase in the full term pregnancy rates in the Letrozole group although there was no difference in the ovulation rates, mean serum E2 levels and clinical pregnancy rates between the two groups.[31]

In 106 women with PCOS, 2.5 mg of Letrozole for 5 days was compared as a first line treatment with a 100 mg of CC for 5 days. The results showed a thicker endometrium and a higher pregnancy rate in the Letrozole group than in the CC group.[32]

Aromatase Inhibitors in Ovulatory Infertility/Superovulation

Intrauterine Insemination (IUI)

A prospective quasi-randomized study showed a comparable efficacy of Letrozole to CC when used for IUI in patients with unexplained infertility, mild endometriosis or borderline male factor infertility.[33] The mean serum E2 concentration was lower in the Letrozole group, however, the mean endometrial thickness (8 mm) and the ovulation rates (81% vs 85%, respectively) were comparable in both the groups. The pregnancy rate (PR) per cycle was 9 percent (5/52) in the Letrozole group and 12 percent (8/67) in the CC group.

A similar study was carried out in 93 ovulatory women. Following initial priming with either Letrozole or CC, the women received gonadotropins until the day of hCG. There was no significant difference in the endometrial thickness, mean number of follicles, pregnancy rates and serum E2 levels between the two groups. The authors concluded that Letrozole results in comparable pregnancies as CC.[34]

A randomized controlled trial comparing 2.5 mg of Letrozole with 5 mg of the same drug in 34 patients reported a higher follicle number and pregnancy rate with the higher dose of Letrozole. There was no increase in the incidence of multiple pregnancies. There was no difference in the endometrial thickness between the two groups.[35]

In vitro Fertilization (IVF)

Aromatase inhibitors have been used in controlled ovarian hyperstimulation (COH) during *in vitro* fertilization (IVF). A small prospective, randomized pilot study by Verprost et al.[36] demonstrated increased median serum LH, FSH, testosterone and androstenedione concentrations in women undergoing antagonist cycles with recombinant FSH and Letrozole compared with FSH alone for IVF/ICSI. The endometrium was significantly thicker in the former group.[36]

Garcia-Velasca et al.[37] carried out a pilot study on 147 poor responders with previously cancelled IVF cycles. Patients were stimulated with either Letrozole followed by a high dose of FSH (Group 1), or high doses of FSH without Letrozole (Group 2) in antagonist cycles. The Letrozole-treated group showed a significantly higher number of follicles and higher implantation rates despite similar doses of FSH for stimulation. The follicular fluid testosterone and androstenedione levels were higher in the Letrozole-treated group compared to the non-Letrozole group (80.3 vs 43.8 pg/mL and 57.9 vs 37.4 mg/mL, respectively).[37] It appears that intraovarian androgens have a profound influence on early follicular growth.

The AIs are used in controlled ovarian stimulation of patients with breast cancer undergoing IVF prior to chemotherapy. The main benefits of AIs in this category of patients are their ability to decrease the dose of FSH required for stimulation and also to relatively decrease the concentration of estrogen during COH. Any other standard protocol and dose of FSH may result in dangerously high levels of estrogen in these women, worsening their prognosis, particularly in those with estrogen-sensitive breast cancers.[38,39]

Do Aromatase Inhibitors Improve Implantation?

Many of the comparative studies have consistently shown a relatively thicker endometrium following the use of AIs, which may be a result of enhanced stromal blood flow thereby, improving the implantation rate. A direct effect of AIs on the endometrium is yet to be proven.

Safety of Aromatase Inhibitors

Aromatase inhibitors are not yet licensed for the treatment of infertility in the UK. The safety profile has been investigated by researchers. Tulandi et al.[40] reviewed 911 patients treated with either CC or Letrozole and compared the congenital malformation rate in both the groups. This study showed no difference in the incidence of major or minor congenital defects in the babies born after Letrozole or CC. Interestingly, it also appears that congenital heart lesions occur much less frequently in the Letrozole group.[40] However, it is generally felt that more methodical research is required to support the safety of AIs before they are widely used.

CONCLUSION

Aromatase inhibitors are a new addition to the medical treatment of infertility. Letrozole and Anastrazole are third-generation AIs that have been used for ovulation induction, superovulation and controlled ovarian hyperstimulation. The AIs are more advantageous than CC for ovulation induction, in terms of reduced estrogen antagonizing side effects. This has been shown as improved endometrial thickness with the use of AIs. Mono-ovulation cannot be guaranteed even with AIs and the risk of multiple pregnancies exists with AIs too. There is a trend for higher pregnancy rates following superovulation with AIs than with Clomiphene. There has been no direct comparison between gonadotropins and AIs for superovulation/IUI. When added to IVF protocols, less gonadotropins are required for ovarian stimulation.

Polycystic ovary syndrome forms a special group by itself, known to have complex endocrine and paracrine abnormalities. The exact mechanism of action of AIs on polycystic ovaries needs to be established beyond doubts by randomized controlled trials before routinely recommending them to this group.

Finally, tissue-specific AIs will be an exciting development and ideal for infertility treatment. This demands advanced research on aromatase inhibitors.

REFERENCES

1. Steinkampf MP, Mendelson CR, Simpson ER. Regulation by follicle-stimulating hormone of the synthesis of aromatase cytochrome P-450 in human granulosa cells. Mol Endocrinol 1987;1:465-71.
2. Bulun SE, Rosenthal IM, Brodie AM, Inkster SE, Zeller WP, DiGeorge AM, et al. Use of tissue-specific promoters in the regulation of aromatase cytochrome P450 gene expression in human testicular and ovarian sex cord tumors, as well as in normal fetal and adult gonads. J Clin Endocrinol Metab 1994;78:1616-21.
3. Berkovitz GD, Brown TR, Fujimoto M. Aromatase activity in human skin fibroblasts grown in cell culture. Steroids 1987;50:281-95.
4. Matsumine H, Hirato K, Yanaihara T, Tamada T, Yoshida M. Aromatization by skeletal muscle. J Clin Endocrinol Metab 1986;63:717-20.
5. Santen RJ, Santner S, Davis B, Veldhuis J, Samojlik E, Ruby E. Aminoglutethimide inhibits extraglandular estrogen production in postmenopausal women with breast carcinoma. J Clin Endocrinol Metab 1978;47:1257-65.
6. Mokbel K. The evolving role of aromatase inhibitors in breast cancer. Int J Clin Oncol 2002;7:279-83.
7. Bhatnagar AS, Hausler A, Schieweck K, Lang M, Bowman R. Highly selective inhibition of estrogen biosynthesis by CGS 20267, a new nonsteroidal aromatase inhibitor. J Steroid Biochem Mol Biol 1990;20;37:1021-7.
8. Jakimiuk AJ, Weitsman SR, Brzechffa PR, Magoffin DA. Aromatase mRNA expression in individual follicles from polycystic ovaries. Mol Hum Reprod 1998;4:1-8.
9. Murray AA, Gosden RG, Allison V, Spears N. Effect of androgens on the development of mouse follicles growing *in vitro*. J Reprod Fertil 1998;113:27-33.
10. Vendola KA, Zhou J, Adesanya OO, Weil SJ, Bondy CA. Androgens stimulate early stages of follicular growth in the primate ovary. J Clin Invest 1998;101:2622-9.
11. Weil SJ, Vendola K, Zhou J, Adesanya OO, Wang J, Okafor J, et al. Androgen receptor gene expression in the primate ovary: cellular localization, regulation, and functional correlations. J Clin Endocrinol Metab 1998;83:2479-85.
12. Hillier SG, Tetsuka M, Fraser HM. Location and developmental regulation of androgen receptor in primate ovary. Hum Reprod 1997;12:107-11.
13. Hillier SG, Tetsuka M. Role of androgens in follicle maturation and atresia. Baillieres Clin Obstet Gynaecol 1997;11:249-60.
14. Vendola K, Zhou J, Wang J, Bondy CA. Androgens promote insulin-like growth factor-I and insulin-like growth factor-I receptor gene expression in the primate ovary. Hum Reprod 1999;14:2328-32.

15. Demeestere I, Gervy C, Centner J, Devreker F, Englert Y, Delbaere A. Effect of insulin-like growth factor-I during preantral follicular culture on steroidogenesis, *in vitro* oocyte maturation, and embryo development in mice. Biol Reprod 2004;70:1664-9.

16. Rhodes FM, Peterson AJ, Jolly PD. Gonadotrophin responsiveness, aromatase activity and insulin-like growth factor binding protein content of bovine ovarian follicles during the first follicular wave. Reproduction 2001;122:561-9.

17. Adashi EY, Hsueh AJ. Estrogens augment the stimulation of ovarian aromatase activity by follicle-stimulating hormone in cultured rat granulosa cells. J Biol Chem 1982;257:6077-83.

18. Polan ML, Laufer N, Ohkawa R, Botero-Ruiz W, Haseltine FP, DeCherney AH, et al. The association between granulosa cell aromatase activity and oocyte-corona-cumulus complex maturity from individual human follicles. J Clin Endocrinol Metab 1984;59:170-4.

19. Costa LO, Mendes MC, Ferriani RA, Moura MD, Reis RM, Silva de Sa MF. Estradiol and testosterone concentrations in follicular fluid as criteria to discriminate between mature and immature oocytes. Braz J Med Biol Res 2004;37:1747-55.

20. Andersen CY. Characteristics of human follicular fluid associated with successful conception after *in vitro* fertilization. J Clin Endocrinol Metab 1993;77:1227-34.

21. Oktay K, Briggs D, Gosden RG. Ontogeny of follicle-stimulating hormone receptor gene expression in isolated human ovarian follicles. J Clin Endocrinol Metab 1997;82:3748-51.

22. San Roman GA, Magoffin DA. Insulin-like growth factor binding proteins in ovarian follicles from women with polycystic ovarian disease: cellular source and levels in follicular fluid. J Clin Endocrinol Metab 1992;75:1010-6.

23. Erickson GF, Magoffin DA, Garzo VG, Cheung AP, Chang RJ. Granulosa cells of polycystic ovaries: are they normal or abnormal? Hum Reprod 1992;7:293-9.

24. Lee DW, Grasso P, Dattatreyamurty B, Deziel MR, Reichert LE, Jr. Purification of a high molecular weight follicle-stimulating hormone receptor-binding inhibitor from human follicular fluid. J Clin Endocrinol Metab 1993;77:163-8.

25. Schneyer AL, Sluss PM, Whitcomb RW, Martin KA, Sprengel R, Crowley WF, Jr. Precursors of alpha-inhibin modulate follicle-stimulating hormone receptor binding and biological activity. Endocrinology 1991;129:1987-99.

26. Duijkers IJ, Willemsen WN, Hollanders HM, Hamilton CJ, Thomas CM, Vemer HM. Follicular fluid hormone concentrations during controlled ovarian hyperstimulation using gonadotropin preparations with different FSH/LH ratios. I. Comparison of an FSH-dominant and a purified FSH preparation. Int J Fertil Womens Med 1997;42:426-30.

27. Mason HD, Margara R, Winston RM, Beard RW, Reed MJ, Franks S. Inhibition of oestradiol production by epidermal growth factor in human granulosa cells of normal and polycystic ovaries. Clin Endocrinol (Oxf) 1990;33:511-7.

28. Rice VM, Williams VR, Limback SD, Terranova PF. Tumour necrosis factor-alpha inhibits follicle-stimulating hormone-induced granulosa cell oestradiol secretion in the human: dependence on size of follicle. Hum Reprod 1996;11:1256-61.

29. Mitwally MF, Casper RF. Use of an aromatase inhibitor for induction of ovulation in patients with an inadequate response to clomiphene citrate. Fertil Steril 2001;75:305-9.

30. Al-Omari WR, Sulaiman WR, Al-Hadithi N. Comparison of two aromatase inhibitors in women with clomiphene-resistant polycystic ovary syndrome. Int J Gynaecol Obstet 2004;85:289-91.

31. Sohrabvand F, Ansari S, Bagheri M. Efficacy of combined metformin-letrozole in comparison with metformin-clomiphene citrate in clomiphene-resistant infertile women with polycystic ovarian disease. Hum Reprod 2006;21:1432-5.

32. Atay V, Cam C, Muhcu M, Cam M, Karateke A. Comparison of Letrozole and clomiphene citrate in women with polycystic ovaries undergoing ovarian stimulation. J Int Med Res 2006;34:73-6.

33. Bayar U, Tanriverdi HA, Barut A, Ayoglu F, Ozcan O, Kaya E. Letrozole vs. clomiphene citrate in patients with ovulatory infertility. Fertil Steril 2006;85:1045-8.

34. Jee BC, Ku SY, Suh CS, Kim KC, Lee WD, Kim SH. Use of Letrozole versus clomiphene citrate combined with gonadotropins in intrauterine insemination cycles: a pilot study. Fertil Steril 2006;85:1774-7.

35. Al-Fadhli R, Sylvestre C, Buckett W, Tan SL, Tulandi T. A rando- mized trial of superovulation with two different doses of Letrozole. Fertil Steril 2006;85:161-4.

36. Verpoest WM, Kolibianakis E, Papanikolaou E, Smitz J, Van Steirteghem A, Devroey P. Aromatase inhibitors in ovarian stimulation for IVF/ICSI: a pilot study. Reprod Biomed Online 2006;13:166-72.

37. Garcia-Velasco JA, Moreno L, Pacheco A, Guillen A, Duque L, Requena A, et al. The aromatase inhibitor Letrozole increases the concentration of intraovarian androgens and improves *in vitro* fertilization outcome in low responder patients: a pilot study. Fertil Steril 2005;84:82-7.

38. Oktay K, Hourvitz A, Sahin G, Oktem O, Safro B, Cil A, et al. Letrozole reduces estrogen and gonadotropin exposure in women with breast cancer undergoing ovarian stimulation before chemotherapy. J Clin Endocrinol Metab 2006;91:3885-90.

39. Oktay K, Buyuk E, Libertella N, Akar M, Rosenwaks Z. Fertility preservation in breast cancer patients: a prospective controlled comparison of ovarian stimulation with tamoxifen and Letrozole for embryo cryopreservation. J Clin Oncol 2005;23:4347-53.

40. Tulandi T, Martin J, Al-Fadhli R, Kabli N, Forman R, Hitkari J, et al. Congenital malformations among 911 newborns conceived after infertility treatment with Letrozole or clomiphene citrate. Fertil Steril 2006;85:1761-5.

Addition of Luteinizing Hormone in Controlled Ovarian Stimulation Protocols using Recombinant FSH

Maruthini D, Manisha Palep-Singh

OVERVIEW

Designing controlled ovarian stimulation protocols for appropriate ovarian folliculogenesis is a challenging task. Having said that, the understanding and management of controlled ovarian hyperstimulation (COH) has evolved tremendously in the recent past. Lately, there is a lot of enthusiasm to prove the benefits of adding luteinizing hormone (LH) to recombinant follicle-stimulating hormone (rFSH) to improve the cycle response and also to potentially improve implantation rates. This chapter highlights the physiological considerations as well as the pros and cons of adding LH on the final outcome of a treatment cycle.

INTRODUCTION

Luteinizing hormone (LH) activity has always been a subject of great ambiguity since the early days of controlled ovarian hyperstimulation (COH). Its role in folliculogenesis is controversial unlike its role in triggering ovulation. It is intriguing to explore the place of LH in various kinds of protocols currently in place for COH. In the initial days of assisted reproduction, ovarian stimulation was carried out using follicle stimulating hormone (FSH) and LH contained in human menopausal urine. When the demand exceeded the supply, recombinant FSH (rFSH) was introduced into the market. At the same time, highly purified FSH (HP-FSH), obtained by purifying urinary gonadotropin to retain the FSH activity and reduce the LH activity came into clinical use. There is no robust evidence to favor one form of gonadotropin over the other in COH, particularly with reference to the LH activity in them. However, studies continue to weigh the benefits against the potential risks of LH in COH. Various views about the addition of LH activity during COH are presented here.

Physiological Role of LH in Folliculogenesis

The "two cell-two gonadotropin model" elucidates the roles of FSH and LH in granulosa and theca cells, respectively. Luteinizing hormone receptors are present in theca cells from fetal life. Luteinizing hormone stimulates theca cells (TCs) to produce androgen. In the early follicular phase, FSH induces follicular development and the granulosa cells (GCs) convert androgens to estrogen under the influence of the enzyme aromatase, the expression of which is induced only by FSH in the GCs of small antral follicles. However, the larger follicles grow and attain dominance over the smaller follicles and also become independent of FSH.[1] Granulosa cells from small preovulatory follicles do not express LH receptors. The GCs from bigger follicles also begin to express LH receptors and become responsive to LH, which can potentially exert all physiological functions of FSH.[2] Hillier et al.[3] revisited the two cell-two gonadotropin theory and highlighted the changing roles of FSH and LH at various time points in an ovarian cycle.[3] Thus, there is a possible overlap of gonadotropin responsiveness by the growing follicles to FSH and LH. However, there is a difference in opinion with regard to whether at least a minimal degree of LH activity is indispensable for folliculogenesis.

Gonadotropin Preparations

Traditional human menopausal gonadotropin (hMG) contains a mixture of FSH and LH activity in a ratio of 50:50 or less. Highly purified forms of hMG (HP-hMG) are available with predominant FSH and negligible LH activity. Currently, some pharmaceutical products add LH activity to

Table 19.1: Types, contents and examples of gonadotropins

Type of gonadotropin	FSH activity	LH activity	Examples
Human derived			
HP FSH	75 IU	<0.1 IU	Metrodin HP, Bravelle
hFSH	75 IU	<1 IU	Metrodin, Fostimon
hMG	75 IU	25–35 IU	Normegon Pergogreen
hMG	75 IU	75 IU	Pergonal, Humegon, Menogon, Repronex
HP-hMG	75 IU	75 IU	Menopur
Recombinants			
rFSH-α	37.5–1200 IU	0	Gonal F
rFSH-β	50–200 IU	0	Puregon, Follistim
rLH	0	75 IU	Luveris
Chorionic gonadotropins			
hCG	0	250–5000 IU	Profasi, Gonasi, Novarel, Choragon
rCG	0	250 ug	Ovitrelle

highly purified hMG. There are recombinant gonadotropin preparations with pure FSH activity, derived from Chinese hamster ovarian cell lines by genetic recombination. They are presented in alfa and beta forms.

Luteinizing hormone activity is available as recombinant LH, human chorionic gonadotropin (hCG) or recombinant hCG. Table 19.1 shows a list of various gonadotropins presently used in the clinical practice.

Use of Gonadotropins in Ovarian Stimulation

Initial experiments on ovarian stimulation were carried out using purified pregnant mare serum followed by human pituitary extracts.[4,5] Subsequently, human menopausal urinary gonadotropin (hMG) was introduced in 1960s.[6] This has both FSH and LH activity. The purification process of FSH evolved with an aim to develop pure FSH activity (HP FSH), as FSH was believed to be the primary folliculogenic factor. However, FSH if used alone for ovarian stimulation in hypogonadotropic-hypogonadism (HH), was required in higher doses and resulted in fewer preovulatory follicles, lower estradiol levels with reduced endometrial thickness and incidence of ovulation.[7-9] In HH patients, folliculogenesis and

serum estrogen levels were found to be positively correlated with the amount of recombinant LH given along with the rFSH.[10] When low dose human chorionic gonadotropin (hCG) or recombinant chorionic gonadotropin (rCG) were combined in the treatment of HH patients, ovarian stimulation was shortened and the HP FSH dose was reduced.[11] Thus, ovulation induction studies in HH women appear to improve the understanding of the importance and support the positive effects of LH activity in ovarian stimulation of patients who are FSH-LH deficient.[10-12] However, there are other studies claiming superiority of recombinant FSH preparations in the same group of women. The advantages of recombinant FSH preparations seem to be the consistency between different batches, purity and comparable efficacy.[13-16]

CLINICAL DISCUSSION

LH Threshold and Ceiling Activity

During folliculogenesis, LH exerts a positive effect through androgen production, which in turn, enhances follicular/granulosa cell proliferation. Nevertheless, excessive LH suppresses granulosa cell proliferation, initiates atresia and premature luteinization. A review by Shonam[17] on selected research papers, addressed the concept of therapeutic window of LH (75 IU) in stimulating follicular growth in hypogonadotropic hypogonadism patients undergoing ovarian stimulation. He also emphasized the detrimental effects when higher doses of recombinant LH (250 IU) were used in patients with PCOS and hypogonadotrophic hypogonadism undergoing ovarian stimulation.[17]

Theoretically this ceiling effect could be used in mono-follicular ovarian induction.[18] In some countries, where there is a limitation in the number of eggs that can be fertilized, there is increasing research on the advantages of the ceiling effect of LH activity in reducing ovarian hyperstimulation and multiple pregnancies while safe-guarding the physical and emotional well-being of women during *in vitro* fertilization (IVF) treatment.[19] The addition of LH at a ceiling level seems to preferentially enhance the growth of a few dominant follicles.

Controlled Ovarian Stimulation Protocols

Several protocols, using a range of doses of various types of gonadotropins, exist for COS during *in vitro* fertilization (IVF). There is no universal opinion either on the best single type of gonadotropin nor on the optimum FSH/LH activity required for COS. A few retrospective systematic meta-analyses have produced conflicting conclusions.[20-23] Some initial studies in the mid-1990s showed better pregnancy rates with rFSH but other randomized controlled trials disproved this finding.[13,24,25] Recently, a randomized controlled trial compared the efficacy of HP-hMG and recombinant FSH in IVF cycles. A total of 731 women were recruited. The results showed more number of oocytes with rFSH but top quality of embryos with the HP-hMG. There was a significant reduction in the serum estradiol levels and increased progesterone concentrations in the rFSH group. The study established that HP-hMG is comparable to rFSH in IVF cycles.[26] Another randomized trial comparing HP-hMG with hMG in intracytoplasmic sperm injection (ICSI) cycles demonstrated increased number of mature oocytes and comparable pregnancy rates with HP-hMG.[27]

Addition of LH to rFSH

There is no convincing, robust, randomized controlled trial to prove the efficacy of adding LH activity to COH protocols. GnRH agonists and antagonists not only inhibit premature LH surge but also endogenous LH activity, which would have been present in a natural cycle. The idea of using LH in an antagonist cycle is further complicated by the possibility of this having a negative effect on the antagonists. It is essential to have thorough understanding and strong evidence to prove the efficacy of using LH in both agonist and antagonist cycles.

The measurement of serum LH concentrations in several women undergoing ovarian stimulation laid a base for the reference range of serum LH in pituitary suppressed women during COH. Different studies showed that the endogenous LH level should be 0.5 to 1.5 IU in long protocols in order to achieve optimum results with COH.

Several revisits have provided reasonable assurance to support the comparable efficacy of urinary hMG and recombinant FSH, thus indirectly supporting the LH activity in COH. However, attempts to guarantee the effectiveness of LH activity when directly added to rFSH in COH, have shown conflicting results. A randomized trial used varying doses of LH in four different groups of patients undergoing COH. The groups were, recombinant FSH, urinary hMG with <1 IU LH activity, urinary hMG with 25 IU LH activity and the last group of urinary hMG with 75 IU LH activity. The authors concluded that there was a trend for better implantation rate with increasing LH activity.[28] Researchers from Denmark evaluated the ovarian response and pregnancy outcome in a prospective randomized study in 231 assisted reproductive technique (ART) cycles. The women were stimulated either with rFSH or a combination of rFSH and rLH in a ratio of 2:1. LH was supplemented from day 8 of the cycle. Overall, the pregnancy rate did not differ in the two groups. It appeared that women aged 35 years and above responded with significantly increased implantation rates and reduced FSH consumption.[29] Ludwig[30] showed that patients treated with the ultra-long antagonist protocol and older patients with a low response to gonadotropins may be benefited by the addition of exogenous LH.[30] Another small study randomized 68 IVF cycles down regulated with GnRH agonists into three

groups based on the stimulation regimens; pure rFSH, hMG and the third group in which recombinant LH was added. Although a better outcome was reported in the two groups where LH activity was present during COH, the results were not statistically significant.[31] Martin et al.[32] added low dose rhCG (300 IU of LH activity) to rFSH in COH cycles of women undergoing oocyte donation. This resulted in higher preovulatory E2 levels and a significantly greater number of oocytes and embryos available for cryopreservation.[32] Filicori et al.[33] tested the effectiveness of a low dose of hCG when added to the COH protocol at a later stage. In this study, on intracytoplasmic sperm injection (ICSI) cycles, hMG was used in the first eight days followed by a low dose of hCG alone for five days. Although pregnancies were reported, no significant improvement was observed in the hCG arm.[32-34]

Balasch et al.[35] on the other hand, expressed concerns over the addition of LH to pituitary suppressed patients undergoing COH. They assessed the effects of recombinant LH in a randomized fashion, where the study group received rFSH along with 75 IU of rLH (n = 13) whereas the control group received rFSH alone (n = 15). The results showed that the addition of recombinant LH to recombinant FSH in pituitary suppressed women did not improve the ovarian response and could potentially impair oocyte maturation and fertilization.[35]

COH in Polycystic Ovary Syndrome

Polycystic ovary syndrome (PCOS) is associated with high endogenous LH secretion, hyperandrogenism, infertility and a high incidence of miscarriages. Women with PCOS have always been a special focus group when undergoing IVF treatment. This is because of their higher risk of ovarian hyperstimulation syndrome (OHSS), cycle cancellation rate, reduced oocyte quality and reduced fertilization rates. However, the pregnancy rate is believed to be similar to non-PCOS women, albeit the risk of OHSS.

Theoretically, PCOS women should have better outcomes with ovarian stimulation protocols that use pure FSH preparations rather than FSH/LH combinations due to the potential detrimental effects of underlying LH hypersecretion. However, a small scale randomized trial and two Cochrane meta-analyses of randomized controlled trials confirmed similar pregnancy rates with rFSH and hMG for ovulation induction in women with PCOS.[36-38] Thus, the LH activity in hMG does not appear to have a negative impact during ovulation induction in women with PCOS. Moreover, LH hypersecretion is not encountered in downregulated IVF cycles or in antagonist cycles as the endogenous LH activity is suppressed. The addition of small doses of hCG to rFSH in antagonist cycles has been shown to yield similar pregnancy rates compared to agonist as well as antagonist cycles without added hCG. However, stimulation protocols with low dose hCG in antagonist cycles favor improved oocyte quality, day 3 embryos and frozen embryos.[39]

CONCLUSION

Manipulation of ovarian folliculogenesis is a challenging task. The understanding and management of COH has evolved tremendously over the past few years. Lately, there is a lot of enthusiasm to prove the benefits of adding LH to recombinant FSH. However, the application of this idea in clinical practice requires further large scale research to guarantee its efficacy and safety.

REFERENCES

1. Campbell BK, Dobson H, Baird DT, Scaramuzzi RJ. Examination of the relative role of FSH and LH in the mechanism of ovulatory follicle selection in sheep. J Reprod Fertil 1999;117:355-67.
2. Zeleznik AJ, Hillier SG. The role of gonadotropins in the selection of the preovulatory follicle. Clin Obstet Gynecol 1984; 27:927-40.
3. Hillier SG, Whitelaw PF, Smyth CD. Follicular oestrogen synthesis: the 'two-cell, two-gonadotrophin' model revisited. Mol Cell Endocrinol 1994;100:51-4.
4. Hamblen E. Endocrine therapy of functional ovarian failure. Am J Obstet Gynaecol 1940;40:615-62.
5. Gemzell CA. Induction of ovulation with human pituitary gonadotrophins. Fertil Steril 1962;13:153-68.
6. Lunenfeld B. Historical perspectives in gonadotrophin therapy. Hum Reprod Update 2004;10:453-67.
7. Shoham Z, Balen A, Patel A, Jacobs HS. Results of ovulation induction using human menopausal gonadotropin or purified follicle-stimulating hormone in hypogonadotropic hypogonadism patients. Fertil Steril 1991;56:1048-53.
8. Schoot DC, Coelingh Bennink HJ, Mannaerts BM, Lamberts SW, Bouchard P, Fauser BC. Human recombinant follicle-stimulating hormone induces growth of preovulatory follicles without concomitant increase in androgen and estrogen biosynthesis in a woman with isolated gonadotropin deficiency. J Clin Endocrinol Metab 1992;74:1471-3.
9. Schoot DC, Harlin J, Shoham Z, Mannaerts BM, Lahlou N, Bouchard P, et al. Recombinant human follicle-stimulating hormone and ovarian response in gonadotrophin-deficient women. Hum Reprod 1994;9:1237-42.
10. Group TERHLS. Recombinant human luteinizing hormone (LH) to support recombinant human follicle-stimulating hormone (FSH)-induced follicular development in LH- and FSH-deficient anovulatory women: a dose-finding study. The European Recombinant Human LH Study Group. J Clin Endocrinol Metab 1998;83:1507-14.
11. Filicori M, Cognigni GE, Taraborrelli S, Spettoli D, Ciampaglia W, de Fatis CT. Low-dose human chorionic gonadotropin therapy can improve sensitivity to exogenous follicle-stimulating hormone in patients with secondary amenorrhea. Fertil Steril 1999;72:1118-20.
12. Balasch J, Miro F, Burzaco I, Casamitjana R, Civico S, Ballesca JL, et al. The role of luteinizing hormone in human follicle development and oocyte fertility: evidence from in vitro fertilization in a woman with long-standing hypogonadotrophic hypogonadism and using recombinant human follicle stimulating hormone. Hum Reprod 1995;10:1678-83.
13. Lispi M, Bassett R, Crisci C, Mancinelli M, Martelli F, Ceccarelli D, et al. Comparative assessment of the consistency and quality of a highly purified FSH extracted from human urine (urofollitropin) and a recombinant human FSH (follitropin alpha). Reprod Biomed Online 2006;13:179-93.
14. Caccia P. Comparative analysis of quality and consistency of urinary and recombinant FSH: comments on a recent article. Reprod Biomed Online 2007;14:127-8.
15. Bassett RM, Driebergen R. Continued improvements in the quality and consistency of follitropin alfa, recombinant human FSH. Reprod Biomed Online 2005;10:169-77.
16. Lenton E, Soltan A, Hewitt J, Thomson A, Davies W, Ashraf N, et al. Induction of ovulation in women undergoing assisted reproductive techniques: recombinant human FSH (follitropin alpha) versus highly purified urinary FSH (urofollitropin HP). Hum Reprod 2000;15:1021-7.
17. Shoham Z. The clinical therapeutic window for luteinizing hormone in controlled ovarian stimulation. Fertil Steril 2002; 77:1170-77.
18. Hillier S. The respective roles of gonadotrophins on follicular growth and oocyte maturation. J Gynecol Obstet Biol Reprod (Paris) 2004;33(6 Pt 2):3S11-4.
19. Vegetti W, Alagna F. FSH and folliculogenesis: from physiology to ovarian stimulation. Reprod Biomed Online 2006;12:684-94.
20. Daya S. Follicle-stimulating hormone and human menopausal gonadotropin for ovarian stimulation in assisted reproduction cycles. Cochrane Database Syst Rev 2000:CD000061.
21. Agrawal R, Holmes J, Jacobs HS. Follicle-stimulating hormone or human menopausal gonadotropin for ovarian stimulation in in vitro fertilization cycles: a meta-analysis. Fertil Steril 2000;73:338-43.
22. Al-Inany H, Aboulghar M, Mansour R, Serour G. Meta-analysis of recombinant versus urinary-derived FSH: an update. Hum Reprod 2003;18:305-13.
23. Oliveira JB, Mauri AL, Petersen CG, Martins AM, Cornicelli J, Cavanha M, et al. Recombinant luteinizing hormone supplementation to recombinant follicle-stimulation hormone during induced ovarian stimulation in the GnRH-agonist protocol: A meta-analysis. J Assist Reprod Genet 2007;24:67-75.
24. Griesinger G, Schultze-Mosgau A, Dafopoulos K, Schroeder A, Schroer A, von Otte S, et al. Recombinant luteinizing hormone supplementation to recombinant follicle-stimulating hormone induced ovarian hyperstimulation in the GnRH-antagonist multiple-dose protocol. Hum Reprod 2005;20:1200-6.
25. De Placido G, Alviggi C, Perino A, Strina I, Lisi F, Fasolino A, et al. Recombinant human LH supplementation versus recombinant human FSH (rFSH) step-up protocol during controlled ovarian stimulation in normogonadotrophic women with initial inadequate ovarian response to rFSH. A multicenter, prospective, randomized controlled trial. Hum Reprod 2005;20:390-96.
26. Andersen AN, Devroey P, Arce JC. Clinical outcome following stimulation with highly purified hMG or recombinant FSH in patients undergoing IVF: a randomized assessor-blind controlled trial. Hum Reprod 2006;21:3217-27.

27. Foutouh IA, Khattab S, Mohesn IA, Moaz M, Al-Inany H. Clinical outcome following stimulation with HMG versus highly purified HMG in patients undergoing ICSI. Reprod Biomed Online 2007;14:145-7.

28. Gordon UD, Harrison RF, Fawzy M, Hennelly B, Gordon AC. A randomized prospective assessor-blind evaluation of luteinizing hormone dosage and *in vitro* fertilization outcome. Fertil Steril 2001;75:324-31.

29. Humaidan P, Bungum M, Bungum L, Yding Andersen C. Effects of recombinant LH supplementation in women undergoing assisted reproduction with GnRH agonist down-regulation and stimulation with recombinant FSH: an opening study. Reprod Biomed Online 2004;8:635-43.

30. Ludwig M. Does the addition of luteinizing hormone in ovarian stimulation protocols improve the outcome? Treat Endocrinol 2003;2:305-13.

31. Toporcerova S, Hredzak R, Ostro A, Zdilova V, Potocekova D. [Influence of exogenous supplementation with luteinizing hormone during controlled ovarian hyperstimulation on the results of IVF cycle]. Ceska Gynekol 2005;70:187-91.

32. Filicori M, Fazleabas AT, Huhtaniemi I, Licht P, Rao Ch V, Tesarik J, et al. Novel concepts of human chorionic gonadotropin: reproductive system interactions and potential in the management of infertility. Fertil Steril 2005;84:275-84.

33. Filicori M, Cognigni GE, Taraborrelli S, Parmegiani L, Bernardi S, Ciampaglia W. Intracytoplasmic sperm injection pregnancy after low-dose human chorionic gonadotropin alone to support ovarian folliculogenesis. Fertil Steril. 2002;78:414-6.

34. Filicori M, Cognigni GE. Clinical review 126: Roles and novel regimens of luteinizing hormone and follicle-stimulating hormone in ovulation induction. J Clin Endocrinol Metab 2001;86:1437-41.

35. Balasch J, Creus M, Fabregues F, Civico S, Carmona F, Puerto B, et al. The effect of exogenous luteinizing hormone (LH) on oocyte viability: evidence from a comparative study using recombinant human follicle-stimulating hormone (FSH) alone or in combination with recombinant LH for ovarian stimulation in pituitary-suppressed women undergoing assisted reproduction. J Assist Reprod Genet 2001;18:250-6.

36. Daya S. Follicle-stimulating hormone and human menopausal gonadotropin for ovarian stimulation in assisted reproduction cycles. Cochrane Database of Systematic Reviews. 2000(2): CD000061.

37. Hughes EG. The effectiveness of ovulation induction and intra-uterine insemination in the treatment of persistent infertility: a meta-analysis. Human Reproduction 1997;12:1865-72.

38. Sagle MA, Hamilton-Fairley D, Kiddy DS, Franks S. A comparative, randomized study of low-dose human menopausal gonadotropin and follicle-stimulating hormone in women with polycystic ovarian syndrome. Fertil Steril 1991;55:56-60.

39. Koichi K, Yukiko N, Shima K, Sachiko S. Efficacy of low-dose human chorionic gonadotropin (hCG) in a GnRH antagonist protocol. J Assist Reprod Genet 2006;23:223-8.

Gonadotropin-releasing Hormone Antagonists: An Unfulfilled Expectation?

Kalyani Patel, Gautam N Allahbadia, Akanksha Allahbadia

OVERVIEW

Ever since their appearance in the market since the early 1990s, gonadotropin-releasing hormone (GnRH) antagonists have proved to be an effective alternative to GnRH agonists to prevent luteinizing hormone (LH) surges during controlled ovarian hyperstimulation (COH) in *in vitro* fertilization (IVF) patients. GnRH antagonists represent a more physiologic mechanism of LH suppression and have provided the basis for the development of innovative stimulation protocols.

Advantages of GnRH antagonists include a short duration of stimulation, decreased total gonadotropin requirements, reduced patient costs, shorter interval between successive treatment cycles, treatment simplicity in that, initiation of gonadotropins can easily be timed to cycles with a more favorable baseline antral follicle count (AFC). They have also proved to be beneficial in specific patient groups, such as women with polycystic ovary syndrome (PCOS), poor responders and in minimal stimulation or natural cycle IVF treatment protocols. However, a significant reduction in pregnancy rates was observed, which had a negative influence on the acceptance and diffusion of GnRH antagonists.

INTRODUCTION

Native GnRH is a small, 10-amino acid peptide, which is intermittently secreted by the hypothalamus, inducing pulsatile secretions of follicle-stimulating hormone (FSH) and LH from the anterior pituitary, by binding to a specific receptor in the pituitary cells to regulate the secretion and synthesis of LH and FSH. After binding with the receptor, the GnRH receptor complex elicits several (calcium-dependent) reactions to release the pituitary hormones (LH and FSH). In addition, the number of GnRH receptors undergoes changes during certain physiological states such as lactation and old age.[1]

Gonadotropin-releasing hormone antagonists, available for clinical use, are GnRH molecules with amino acid modifications in positions 1, 2, 3, 6 and 10.[2] The amino acids at the position number 6 are involved in enzymatic splicing, those in position numbers 2 and 3 are involved in gonadotropin release, while residues 1, 6 and 10 are important for three-dimensional structure and receptor binding.[3]

The first-generation of GnRH antagonists are characterized by a modification on position numbers 1, 2 and 6 of the sequence of human GnRH.

The third-generation GnRH antagonists are characterized by modification on position numbers 1, 2, 3, 6 and 10 of the sequence of human GnRH; two of these compounds, Cetrorelix and Ganirelix, are devoid of the histamine-release property and these two drugs are now widely used in clinical medicine.

Mode of Action

The GnRH antagonists were originally developed as a non-steroid contraceptive drug.[4] These compounds immediately block the GnRH receptor in a competitive fashion.[5] They decrease the LH and FSH secretion within a period of eight hours. Following their action, there is a rapid recovery of normal secretion of endogenous LH and FSH.[6] The inhibition of LH secretion is more pronounced than that of FSH, this being most likely due to the different forms of gonadotropin regulation and the prolonged FSH half-life, or the immunoactive and bioactive forms of FSH.[7]

CLINICAL DISCUSSION

GnRH Antagonists for *In Vitro* Fertilization

Cetrorelix

Cetrorelix is a stable, soluble third-generation GnRH antagonist with minimal histamine-releasing properties. Cetrorelix is available as a 0.25 mg preparation for daily injections, and as a 3 mg depot preparation. After administration of this drug, a rapid reversible suppression of the pituitary-gonadal axis is obtained.

Recent studies have shown that Cetrorelix, either as a single or multiple doses, is effective in preventing the premature LH rise during ovarian stimulation for IVF.[8-11] Pregnancies were reported in all trials. The minimal effective dose of Cetrorelix was 0.25 mg[12] and 3 mg[13] for multiple and single dose, respectively. Cerorelix has no negative influence on the luteal phase,[14,15] although a shortening of the luteal phase and an impairment of corpus luteum function have been reported.[16]

Ganirelix

Ganirelix is a stable, soluble potent third-generation GnRH-antagonist with minimal histamine-releasing properties.[17,18] This compound is characterized by immediate reversible suppression of pituitary gonadotropin release within several hours of administration.[17] Ganirelix is effective in preventing a premature LH rise during ovarian stimulation for IVF.[11] Ganirelix was produced and marketed in a dose of 0.25 mg for use in assisted reproduction.[19]

GnRH Antagonists and Pregnancy Outcomes

Gonadotropin-releasing hormone antagonists have consistently been associated with a trend towards lower clinical pregnancy rates (PRs) compared to GnRH agonists.[20-27] Moreover, a meta-analysis in the Cochrane database reported a significantly lower PR with GnRH antagonists compared to GnRH agonist (odds ratio, 0.79; 95% confidence interval, 0.63–0.99).[28]

It is unclear whether the etiology of this decline is due to a learning curve with the introduction of GnRH antagonists, or if it is due to an intrinsic adverse effect on folliculogenesis or endometrial receptivity.[29-32] Saadat et al.[33] reported decreased follicular fluid estradiol (E2)/testosterone (T) ratios in women who received a GnRH antagonist compared to women who received a GnRH agonist. With regard to the endometrium, the authors found no difference in endometrial histology between GnRH agonist and antagonist cycles.[33]

In contrast, Mirkin et al.[34] reported differences in endometrial gene expression between the two types of protocols.[34] Much attention has focused around the decline in serum E2 levels that occur in approximately one-third of patients when a GnRH antagonist is commenced. It is uncertain whether the decline in E2 levels is exclusively mediated by the pituitary, or if ovarian GnRH receptors also play a role.[35] A recent pharmacologic study found no significant change in serum FSH concentrations after the introduction of 0.25 mg of Cetrotide in seven women on stimulation day 6 of 150 to 300 IU of recombinant FSH, suggesting that there is no need for supplemental FSH with the introduction of the antagonist.[36]

To compensate for the potential decline in serum E2 levels, many programs routinely increase the dose of FSH and LH stimulation when GnRH antagonists are commenced. Aboulghar et al.[37] randomized 151 women stimulated with 150 to 300 IU of gonadotropins to either an increase in the daily dose of hMG by 75 IU when GnRH antagonists were commenced, or a continuation with the same dose. This group found no evidence that increasing the daily dose of gonadotropins with the commencement of a GnRH antagonist improved oocyte yield, number of embryos, implantation rates, or clinical PRs.

Need for LH Supplementation

Improved fertilization and implantation rates were reported with LH supplementation in donor cycles utilizing GnRH antagonists.[38] However, a number of prospective, randomized trials in normal responders failed to demonstrate an advantage of the addition of LH when using GnRH antagonists.

Griesinger et al.[39] randomized 127 women undergoing COH with GnRH antagonists to either recombinant FSH, or a combination of recombinant FSH and LH.[39] Luteinizing hormone supplementation significantly increased serum E2 levels, but had no significant effect on fertilization or implantation rates. In fact, in that study, both implantation rates (13.8% vs 8.1%, respectively) and clinical PRs per cycle (18.4% vs 12.9%, respectively) trended higher in the women stimulated only with recombinant FSH.[39]

Recently, a prospective, randomized trial suggested that there were benefits to LH supplementation in women >35 years of age undergoing COH and using a long protocol with a GnRH agonist for pituitary suppression.[40] In that study, recombinant LH was commenced on cycle day 8, and in women ≥35 years of age, this supplementation was associated with reduced FSH consumption and significantly increased implantation rates. To date, there have been no prospective studies evaluating the role of LH supplementation in poor responders who used GnRH antagonists. However, a recent retrospective analysis of 240 poor responders treated with a GnRH antagonist found comparable outcomes, whether stimulation was achieved with or without supplemental LH.[41] In women ≥40 years of age, exogenous LH was associated with fewer oocytes at retrieval, and fewer embryos available for transfer. Thus, at present, the data are not in favor of LH supplementation in women treated with a GnRH antagonist.[42]

GnRH Antagonists in Poor Responders

The first publication to describe the use of GnRH antagonists in poor responders appeared in 1999.[43] Eighteen poor responders were stimulated with a combination of gonadotropins and Clomiphene citrate (CC), and were started on Cetrorelix 0.25 mg per day once the lead follicle reached at least 14 mm in diameter. Compared to their response in a previous GnRH agonist (GnRHa) cycle, modest improvements in cycle cancellation rates (29% vs 57%), oocyte yield (6.4 vs 4.7), and gonadotropin requirements (4,506 IU vs 5,468 IU) were realized with the GnRH antagonist. More recently, Mohamed et al.[44] compared 57 poor responders treated with a GnRH antagonist to 77 poor responders who received a GnRH agonist flare protocol. The choice of antagonist versus flare was based solely on physician preference. In the antagonist group, Cetrorelix 0.25 mg was started on stimulation day 6. In the flare group, Buserelin, 500 mcg per day, was started with the onset of menstrual bleed. Both the groups were stimulated with 225 to 375 IU of gonadotropin per day. Similar numbers of oocytes (5.4 vs 5.2) and similar implantation rates (12.8% vs 12.8%) were reported in each group, despite the fact that women treated with the GnRH antagonist required, on average, 1 day less of gonadotropin stimulation. There were no significant differences in the clinical PR per cycle or the clinical PR per ET, but there was a higher cycle cancellation rate (7% vs 0%, P < 0.03) in the group of women treated with the GnRH antagonist.

Benefits of the Use of GnRH Antagonists for IVF

- Simplicity of administration.
- *Shorter duration of stimulation*: An IVF regimen with the GnRH antagonist reduces the duration of treatment by two to three weeks, leading to an increase in patients convenience.
- *Reduced consumption of gonadotropins*: An IVF treatment cycle can commence with an undisturbed menstrual cycle and recruitment of a normal cohort of follicles, allowing normal pituitary function in early to mid-follicular phase. In addition to the endogeneous FSH release, exogeneous FSH is administered, which could lead to a reduction in gonadotropin consumption of patients in comparison to the long protocol.
- Reduced patient costs.
- Ability to determine the ovarian reserve immediately prior to initiating gonadotropins. Gonadotropin-releasing hormone antagonist protocols do not require pretreatment with an estrogen-progestin contraceptive or a GnRH agonist. Thus, both an antral follicle count and day 3 serum markers may be obtained immediately prior to deciding whether to initiate gonadotropins, and in a

setting where these values have not been influenced by exogenous hormones.[35]

- *Luteal phase support*: The pituitary has shown to recover rapidly after cessation of GnRH antagonist treatment.[45]
- *Ovarian hyperstimulation syndrome (OHSS) incidence*: It has been reported that the incidence of OHSS with GnRH antagonists is lower compared to GnRH agonist protocols.[46]

Coasting can be used to prevent OHSS in antagonist cycles, however, prolongation of the follicular phase by delaying hCG administration results in higher incidence of endometrial advancement on the day of oocyte retrieval in GnRH antagonist cycles.[47]

The GnRH antagonist was also used to prevent OHSS in high risk cycles stimulated by with the long GnRHa protocol. In a prospective randomized study on GnRHa long protocol cycles, comparing coasting (group A) and GnRH antagonists (group B) in patients at risk of OHSS, there were significantly more high quality embryos and more oocytes in group B compared to group A. In conclusion, GnRH antagonists were superior to coasting in producing more good quality embryos and oocytes as well as in reducing the time until hCG administration. There was no significant difference in pregnancy rate between two groups. No OHSS developed in either group.[48]

Three patients with severe early OHSS, as diagnosed by a hematocrit analysis, white blood cells (WBC) count, serum urea and ultrasonographic assessment of ovarian size and ascitic fluid, were treated with daily GnRH antagonist administration for one week, while the resulting blastocysts were cryopreserved. The progression of severe early OHSS was inhibited in all three patients.[49]

GnRH agonist for triggering final oocyte maturation in the GnRH antagonist protocol.

GnRH antagonist protocols allow the possibility of triggering oocyte maturation by a single bolus of GnRHa, which reduces the incidence of OHSS.[50]

A systematic review of 3 out of 23 publications fulfilled the inclusion criteria for meta-analysis. No OHSS occurred in two of the studies, whereas in one study, the OHSS incidence was not reported. In comparison with hCG, GnRH agonist administration was associated with a slightly reduced rate of clinical pregnancy. The odds of a first trimester pregnancy loss are increased after GnRH agonist triggering; however, the confidence interval crosses unity.[51]

CONCLUSION

The manifold advantages of the use of GnRH antagonists, significantly, a shorter treatment protocol due to a rapid suppression of gonadotropin production, avoidance of prolonged daily injections of GnRH agonists and the initial flare-up of gonadotropins that might cause cyst formation and OHSS, makes it a favorable treatment choice.

However, it seems that the GnRH agonist long protocol is still the most widely used protocol worldwide, possibly because of the higher pregnancy rates. The stress of prolonged daily injections could be markedly diminished if the GnRHa nasal spray were used to replace injections.

REFERENCES

1. Clayton RN, Catt KJ. Gonadotropin-relasing hormone receptors: characterization, physiological regulation, and relationship to reproductive function. Endocr Rev 1981;2:186-209.
2. Karten MJ, Hoeger CA, Hooh WA. The development of safer antagonists: strategy and status. In: Bouchard P, Haour F, Franchimont P, Schatz B, (Eds). Recent progress on LH-RH and Gonadal Pptides. Paris: Elsevier 1990.pp.147-58.
3. Clayton RN, Catt KJ. Receptor-binding affinity of gonadotropin-releasing hormone analogs: analysis by radioligand-receptor assay. Endocrinology 1980;106:1154-9.
4. Kenigsberg D, Hodgen GD. Ovulation inhibition by administration of weekly gonadotropin-releasing hormone antagonist. J Clin Endocrinol Metab 1986;62:734-8.
5. Reissmann T, Felberbaum R, Diedrich K, Engel J, Comaru-Schally AM, Schally AV. Development and applications of luteinizing hormone-releasing antagonists in the treatment of infertility: an overview. Hum Reprod 1995;10:1974-81.
6. Ditkoff EC, Cassidenti DL, Paulson RJ, et al. The gonadotropin-releasing hormone antagonist (Nal-Glu) acutely blocks the luteinizing hormone surge but allows for resumption of folliculogenesis in normal women. Am J Obstet Gynecol 1991; 165:1811-7.
7. Matikainen T, Ding YQ, Vergars M, Huhtaniemi I, Couzinet B, Schaison G. Differing responses of plasma bioactive and immunoreactive follicle-stimulating hormone and luteinizing hormone to gonadotropin-releasing hormone antagonist and agonist treatments in postmenopausal women. J Clin Endocrinol Metab 1992;75:820-5.
8. Olivennes F, Fanchin R, Bouchard P, Taieb J, Selva J, Frydman R. Scheduled administration of a gonadotropin-releasing hormone antagonist (cetrorelix) on day 8 of *in vitro* fertilization cycles: a pilot study. Hum Reprod 1995;10:1382-6.
9. Olivennes F, Fanchin R, Bouchard P, de Ziegler D, Taieb J, Selva J, et al. The single or dual administration of gonadotropin-releasing hormone antagonist cetrorelix in an *in vitro* fertilization-embryo transfer program. Fertil Steril 1994;62:468-76.
10. Diedrich K, Diedrich C, Santos E, Zoll C, al-Hasani S, Reissmann T, et al. Suppression of endogeneous luteinizing hormone surge by gonadotropin-releasing hormone cetrorelix during ovarian stimulation. Hum Reprod 1994;9:788-91.
11. Griesinger G, Felberbaum RE, Schultze-Mosgau A, Diedrich K. Gonadotropin-releasing hormone antagonists for assisted reproductive techniques:are there clinical differences between agents? Drugs 2004;64:563-75.
12. Albano C, Smitz J, Camus M, Reithmuller-Winzen H, Van Steirtegham A, Devroey P. Comparison of different doses of gonadotropin-releasing hormone cetrorelix during controlled ovarian hyperstimulation. Fertil Steril 1997;67:917-22.
13. Olivennes F, Alvarez S, Bouchard P, Fanchin R, Salat Baroux J, Frydman R. The use of a GnRH antagonist (cetrorelix) in a single dose protocol in IVF-embryo Transfer: a dose finding study of 3 versus 2 mg. Hum Reprod 1998;13:2411-4.
14. Albano C, Smitz J, Camus M, Reithmuller-Winzen H, Siebert-Weigel M, Diedrich K, et al. Hormonal profile during the follicular phase in cycles stimulated with a combination of human menopausal gonadotropin and gonadotropin-releasing hormone cetrorelix. Hum Reprod 1996;11:2114-8.
15. Lin Y, Kahn JA, Hillensjo T. Is there a difference in function of granulosa-luteal cells in patients undergoing *in vitro* fertilization either with gonadotropin-releasing hormone agonist or gonadotropin-releasing hormone antagonists? Hum Reprod 1999;14:885-8.
16. Albano C, Grimbizis G, Smitz J, Reithmuller-Winzen H, Reissmann T, Van Steirteghem A, et al. The luteal phase of non-supplemented cycles after ovarian superovulation with human menopausal gonadotropin and the gonadotropin releasing antagonist Cetrorelix. Fertil Streil 1998;70:357-9.
17. Nelson LR, Fujimoto VY, Jaffe RB, Monroe SE. Suppression follicular phase pituitary-gonadal function by a potent new gonadotropin-releasing antagonist with reduced histamine-releasing properties(ganirelix). Fertil Streil 1995;63:963-9.
18. Nestor JJJ, Tahilramani R, Ho TL, Goodpasture JC, Vickery BH, Ferrandon P. Potent gonadotropin-releasing hormone antagonists with low histamine-releasing activity. J Med Chem 1992;35:3942-8.
19. The Ganirelix dose finding study group. A double-blind, randomized, dose finding study to assess the efficacy of the gonadotropin-releasing hormone antagonist ganirelix (Org 37462) to prevent premature luteinizing hormone surges in women undergoing ovarian stimulation with recombinant follicle-stimulating hormone (Puregon). Hum Reprod 1998; 13:3023-31.
20. Borm G, Mannaerts B. Treatment with the gonadotropin-releasing hormone antagonist ganirelix in women undergoing ovarian stimulation with recombinant follicle stimulating hormone is effective, safe and convenient: results of a controlled, randomized, multicenter trial. The European Orgalutran Study Group. Hum Reprod 2000;15:1490-8.
21. Olivennes F, Belaisch-Allart J, Emperaire JC, Dechaud H, Alvarez S, Moreau L, et al. Prospective, randomized, controlled study of *in vitro* fertilization-embryo transfer with a single dose of a luteinizing hormone-releasing hormone (LH-RH) antagonist (cetrorelix) or a depot formula of an LH-RH agonist (triptorelin). Fertil Steril 2000; 73:314-20.
22. European and Middle East Orgalutran Study Group. Comparable clinical outcome using the GnRH antagonist ganirelix or a long protocol of the GnRH agonist triptorelin for the prevention of premature LH surges in women undergoing ovarian stimulation. Hum Reprod 2001;16:644-51.
23. Ludwig M, Felberbaum RE, Devroey P, Albano C, Riethmuller-Winzen H, Schuler A, et al. Significant reduction of the incidence of ovarian hyperstimulation syndrome (OHSS) by using the LHRH antagonist cetrorelix (cetrotide) in controlled ovarian stimulation for assisted reproduction. Arch Gynecol Obstet 2000;264:29-32.

24. Olivennes F, Cunha-Filho JS, Fanchin R, Bouchard P, Frydman R. The use of GnRH antagonists in ovarian stimulation. Hum Reprod Update 2002;8:279-90.

25. Vlaisavljevic V, Reljic M, Lovrec VG, Kovacic B. Comparable effectiveness using flexible single-dose GnRH antagonist (cetrorelix) and single-dose long GnRH agonist (goserelin) protocol for IVF cycles—a prospective, randomized study. Reprod Biomed Online 2003;7:301-8.

26. Loutradis D, Stefanidis K, Drakakis P, Milingos S, Antsaklis A, Michalas S. A modified gonadotropin-releasing hormone (GnRH) antagonist protocol failed to increase clinical pregnancy rates in comparison with the long GnRH protocol. Fertil Steril 2004;82:1446-8.

27. Xavier P, Gamboa C, Calejo L, Silva J, Stevenson D, Nunes A, et al. A randomised study of GnRH antagonist (cetrorelix) versus agonist (busereline) for controlled ovarian stimulation: effect on safety and efficacy. Eur J Obstet Gynecol Reprod Biol 2005;120:185-9.

28. Al-Inany H, Aboulghar M. GnRH antagonist in assisted reproduction: a Cochrane review. Hum Reprod 2002;17:874-85.

29. Hernandez ER. Embryo implantation and GnRH antagonists: embryo implantation: the Rubicon for GnRH antagonists. Hum Reprod 2000;15:1211-6.

30. Ortmann O, Weiss JM, Diedrich K. Embryo implantation and GnRII antagonists: ovarian actions of GnRH antagonists. Hum Reprod 2001;16:608-11.

31. Gordon K. Gonadotropin-releasing hormone antagonists implications for oocyte quality and uterine receptivity. Ann NY Acad Sci 2001;943:49-54.

32. Garcia-Velasco JA, Isaza V, Vidal C, Landazabal A, Remohi J, Simon C, et al. Human ovarian steroid secretion *in vivo*: effects of GnRH agonist versus antagonist (cetrorelix). Hum Reprod 2001;16:2533-9.

33. Saadat P, Boostanfar R, Slater CC, Tourgeman DE, Stanczyk FZ, Paulson RJ. Accelerated endometrial maturation in the luteal phase of cycles utilizing controlled ovarian hyperstimulation: impact of gonadotropin-releasing hormone agonists versus antagonists. Fertil Steril 2004;82:167-71.

34. Mirkin S, Nikas G, Hsiu JG, Diaz J, Oehninger S. Gene expression profiles and structural/functional features of the peri-implantation endometrium in natural and gonadotropin-stimulated cycles. J Clin Endocrinol Metab 2004;89:5742-52.

35. Mahutte NG, Arici A. Role of gonadotropin-releasing hormone antagonists in poor responders. Fertil Steril 2007;87(2):241-9.

36. Griesinger G, Finas D, Alisch A, Roiha K, Schultze-Mosgau A, Schroder AK, et al. FSH time-concentration profiles before and after administration of 0.25 mg cetrorelix in the GnRH-antagonist multiple-dose protocol for ovarian hyperstimulation. J Assist Reprod Genet 2004;21:279-82.

37. Aboulghar MA, Mansour RT, Serour GI, Al-Inany HG, Amin YM, Aboulghar MM. Increasing the dose of human menopausal gonadotrophins on day of GnRH antagonist administration: randomized controlled trial. Reprod Biomed Online 2004;8:524-7.

38. Acevedo B, Sanchez M, Gomez JL, Cuadros J, Ricciarelli E, Hernandez ER. Luteinizing hormone supplementation increases pregnancy rates in gonadotropin-releasing hormone antagonist donor cycles. Fertil Steril 2004;82:343-7.

39. Griesinger G, Schultze-Mosgau A, Dafopoulos K, Schroeder A, Schroer A, von Otte S, et al. Recombinant luteinizing hormone supplementation to recombinant follicle-stimulating hormone induced ovarian hyperstimulation in the GnRH-antagonist multiple-dose protocol. Hum Reprod 2005;83:452-4.

40. Humaidan P, Bungum M, Bungum L, Yding Andersen C. Effects of recombinant LH supplementation in women undergoing assisted reproduction with GnRH agonist down-regulation and stimulation with recombinant FSH: an opening study. Reprod Biomed Online 2004;8:635-43.

41. Chung K, Krey L, Katz J, Noyes N. Evaluating the role of exogenous luteinizing hormone in poor responders undergoing *in vitro* fertilization with gonadotropin-releasing hormone antagonists. Fertil Steril 2005;84:313-8.

42. Kolibianakis EM, Tarlatzis B, Devroey P. GnRH antagonists in IVF. Reprod Biomed Online 2005;10:705-12.

43. Craft I, Gorgy A, Hill J, Menon D, Podsiadly B. Will GnRH antagonists provide new hope for patients considered "difficult responders" to GnRH agonist protocols? Hum Reprod 1999;14:2959-62.

44. Mohamed KA, Davies WA, Allsopp J, Lashen H. Agonist "flare-up" versus antagonist in the management of poor responders undergoing *in vitro* fertilization treatment. Fertil Steril 2005;83:331-5.

45. Ditkoff EC, Cassidenti DL, Paulson RJ, Sauer MV, Paul WL, Rivier J, et al. The gonadotropin releasing hormone antagonist (Nal-Glu) actively blocks the luteinizing hormone surge but allows for resumption of folliculogenesis in normal women. Am J Obstet Gynecol 1991;165:1811-7.

46. Al-Inany HG, Abou-Setta AM, Aboulghar M. Gonadotropin-releasing hormone antagonists for assisted conception. Cochrane database Syst rev 2006;19;3:CD001750.

47. Kolibianakis EM, Bourgain C, Papanikolaou EG, Camus M, Tournaye H, Van Steirteghem AC, Devroey P. Prolongation of follicular phase by delaying hCG administration results in a higher incidence of endometrial advancement on the day of oocyte retrieval in GnRH antagonist cycles. Hum Reprod 2005;20:2453-6.

48. Aboulghar MA, Mansour RT, Amin YM, Al-Inany HG, Aboulghar MM, Serour GI. A prospective randomized study comparing coasting with GnRH antagonist administration in patients at risk for severe OHSS. Reprod Biomed Online 2007;15:271-9.

49. Lainas TG, Sfontouris IA, Zorzovilis IZ, Petsas GK, Lainas GT, Iliadis GS, Kolibianakis EM. Management of severe OHSS using GnRH antagonist and blastocyst cryopreservation in PCOS patients treated with long protocol. Reprod Biomed Online 2009;18:15-20.

50. Aboulghar MA, Rizk B. Role of GnRH antagonist in assisted reproduction. Ovarian Stimulation 2011;6:49-60.

51. Griesinger G, Diedrich K, Devroey P, Kolibianakis EM. GnRH agonist for triggering final oocyte maturation in the GnRH antagonist ovarian hyperstimulation protocol: a systematic review and meta-analysis. Hum Reprod Update 2006;12:159-68.

Rationale for the Use of Insulin Sensitizing Drugs in Polycystic Ovary Syndrome

Meena Chimote, Natachandra Chimote

INTRODUCTION

Polycystic ovary syndrome (PCOS) is a common disease that affects up to 10 percent of women of reproductive age, and one in which hyperandrogenism, enlarged cystic ovaries, and chronic anovulation often coexist with obesity, hyperinsulinemia, and insulin resistance.[1] Furthermore, recent data provide evidence that the metabolic disturbances associated with the syndrome may have important consequences for long-term health, such as an increased risk of developing cardiovascular disease and diabetes.[2] Obesity in women with PCOS is rather high, ranging from 30 to 60 percent,[3] whereas hyperinsulinemia is present in more than 50 percent of patients with PCOS.[4] Moreover, although about 70 percent of obese women with PCOS exhibit an exaggerated insulin secretion, this feature is also present in 20 to 40 percent of lean PCOS subjects.

The degree of insulin resistance is modest in women with PCOS and may arise from either "natural" (genetic defects) or "acquired" (exogenous obesity) causes.[5] This metabolic defect accounts for the 35 to 40 percent decrease in insulin-stimulated glucose utilization found in PCOS independent of obesity.[6] *In vitro* studies have suggested that adipocytes, a classic insulin target cell, in women with PCOS may be deficient in the glucose transporter-Glut 4, which is essential for the passage of glucose into the cell and is a determinant of insulin sensitivity.[7] Although hyperinsulinemia alone does not have an obvious effect on steroidogenesis, it may act in genetically predisposed women to unmask latent abnormalities in steroid production. For instance, in PCOS, hyperinsulinemia may be thought to promote or facilitate excess androgen production.[8]

The mechanism of insulin resistance in at least some women with PCOS appears to be a specific postreceptor defect in which autophosphorylation of tyrosine residues on the insulin receptor (an essential component of insulin action) is decreased, while phosphorylation of serine residues on the receptor is increased.[9] Serine phosphorylation selectively increases 17, 20-lyase enzyme activity, which is necessary for androgen biosynthesis.[10] Thus, in PCOS, activation of a common metabolic pathway results in excessive serine phosphorylation of the insulin receptor in the ovary which results in both decreased insulin sensitivity and increased androgen secretion. A subset of patients appears to have not only insulin resistance but also beta cell secretory dysfunction, which may enhance the risk of development of non-insulin dependant diabetes mellitus (NIDDM) in PCOS.[9]

Given the strong evidence that hyperinsulinemia plays a pivotal pathogenic role in the development of PCOS, it is reasonable to assume that interventions that reduce circulating insulin levels in women with PCOS may restore normal reproductive endocrine function. The improvement in insulin resistance and the decrease in insulin concentration and action can be achieved in different ways:

- By reducing body weight with lifestyle modifications, if the patient is overweight or obese.
- By using insulin-sensitizing agents.
- By using antiandrogens.

Traditionally, non-pharmacologic methods, such as weight loss, nutrition, and exercise, have clearly led to reduced hyperinsulinemia with resolution of hyperandrogenism and, in some cases, resumption of ovulatory function in overweight women with PCOS.[11] However, these regimens are at risk for poor compliance and, over time, the benefit of weight loss is rarely maintained.

CLINICAL DISCUSSION

Insulin Sensitizers

Insulin-sensitizing agents improve insulin action by increasing insulin sensitivity, thereby decreasing hyperinsulinemia.

Recently, a new class of antidiabetic compounds, insulin-sensitizing agents, have been developed, which in early studies, show promise in the treatment of PCOS.[12,13] When administered to insulin resistant patients, these compounds act to increase target tissue responsiveness to insulin, thereby reducing the need for compensatory hyperinsulinemia.[14] Current insulin sensitizing agents include the biguanides and thiazolidenediones.[15-17] Metformin, a second-generation biguanide, was introduced into the market in 1995. The drug works by activating glucose transporters, which allows passage of glucose into hepatic and muscle cells. Peripheral insulin resistance is decreased and serum glucose levels are lowered. Metformin does not stimulate insulin release and, when given alone, does not cause hypoglycemia.

Metformin

Metformin is the oldest and worldwide, still the most used insulin sensitizer in the treatment of states of glucose intolerance, particularly type 2 DM. Metformin is also the most common insulin sensitizer used in PCOS, either alone or in combination with lifestyle intervention.[19] It is considered an insulin sensitizer because it lowers glucose levels without increasing insulin secretion. In fact, it lowers hepatic glucose production by reducing gluconeogenesis and by decreasing glycogenolysis, increases peripheral glucose uptake by skeletal muscle and adipose tissue, and reduces intestinal glucose absorption. It is also possible that Metformin acts, at least in the presence of diabetes, by improving the effect of glucose toxicity and/or lipotoxicity and insulin secretion by pancreatic cells.[20] Metformin use in PCOS has been associated with a reduction in serum androgen levels and gonadotropins, and with an improvement in metabolic derangements, including hyperinsulinemia, altered lipid profile, and prothrombotic factor plasminogen-activator inhibitor type 1. This therapy has also been associated with a decrease in hirsutism and acne, with an improvement or normalization of hypertension, and with a regulation of menses.[21,22] Interestingly, there is increasing evidence that the ovulation and fertility rate can also be significantly improved with Metformin, often regardless of changes in circulating insulin levels.[19] This raises the intriguing possibility that Metformin can exert a direct action at the ovarian level and introduces new routes in the treatment of infertility in PCOS.

In general, clinical studies have shown that Metformin (Glucophage®, 500 mg three times per day or 850 g twice daily with meals) administration to women with PCOS increased the frequency of spontaneous ovulation, menstrual cyclicity, and ovulatory response to Clomiphene.[23-25] Successful pregnancy with the delivery of healthy infants has also been reported.[26] However, a recent study of very obese PCOS women treated with Metformin for three months failed to show improvement in insulin secretion, insulin action, or ovarian steroidogenesis.[27]

Side Effects of Metformin

Side effects of Metformin include gastrointestinal symptoms, which are dose-related and tend to resolve after several weeks. A rare adverse effect of Metformin therapy is lactic acidosis. Therefore, Metformin should not be prescribed to patients with renal, hepatic, or major cardiovascular disease or hypoxia because these patients have a predisposition to elevated lactate levels. Precautionary temporal withdrawal of Metformin is advised in patients undergoing radiological procedures involving intravascular iodinated contrast materials and surgery.

Thiazolidinediones

The second type of new antidiabetic agents, the thiazolidinediones, is under active investigation for PCOS.[28] To date, the available drugs in the market include Rosiglitazone and Pioglitazone. Thiazolidinediones appear to act by binding to peroxisome proliferation activator receptor gamma (PPAR-γ), which decreases peripheral insulin resistance.[29] Short-term treatment with these compounds has resulted in a decrease in androgen levels associated with an attenuation of insulin resistance and reduction of insulin secretion in obese patients with PCOS.[30,31] In some of these women, ovulation also occurred during the period of drug therapy.

The insulin-sensitizing thiazolidinediones are selective ligands of the nuclear transcription factor peroxisome proliferator activated receptor γ.[32] Thiazolidinediones exert their insulin-sensitizing actions through two mechanisms: directly by promoting fatty acid uptake and storage in adipose tissue; and indirectly by increasing the expression of adiponectin, an adipocytokine with an insulin-sensitivity effect, and probably, by decreasing the expression of 11 β-hydroxysteroid dehydrogenase type 1, an enzyme which catalyzes the conversion of inactive cortisone to active cortisol.[18] Most clinical studies, evaluating the effect of thiazolidinediones in PCOS, have demonstrated that these drugs improve insulin resistance, glucose tolerance and hyperandrogenemia.[33-35] Ovulation was also positively influenced by the administration of thiazolidinediones. In addition, treatment with these drugs was associated with a reduction in levels of the prothrombotic factor plasminogen activator inhibitor type 1 and with a relative improvement in endothelium-dependent vasodilation, which correlated with the reduction in insulin levels.[33]

Side Effects of Thiazolidinediones

The primary concern with thiazolidinediones has been liver toxicity. This was particularly true for Roglitazone (Rezulin®), as a significant number of cases of hepatic necrosis were reported. In some instances, liver failure led to death. As a result, the Food and Drug Administration (FDA) recommended that Troglitazone be withdrawn from the market, and it is no longer available for the treatment of type II diabetes mellitus. Both Rosiglitazone and Pioglitazone are approved for use. Patients receiving these drugs should be monitored at regular intervals. Serum alanine aminotransferase (ALT) levels should be measured every two months for the first year and periodically thereafter. Thiazolidenediones should not be initiated in patients with any evidence of liver disease or in patients with elevated ALT levels.[36]

Since there are no well-controlled studies of safety during pregnancy, Metformin has been administered to a small number of women with diabetes throughout their pregnancies, and no fetal abnormalities have been described.[37] Both Metformin and thiazolidenediones are Category B drugs. There is insufficient available human data, but no teratogenic effects have been demonstrated in controlled animal studies. Until more data are available, administration of Rosiglitazone, Pioglitazone, or Metformin during pregnancy is not recommended.

The advantage of insulin-sensitizing agents over traditional therapies for the treatment of PCOS is that the metabolic and hormonal derangements that characterize this disorder are directly addressed. Further, preliminary data suggest that these agents are associated with the resumption of spontaneous ovulatory function, with little or no risk of ovarian hyperstimulation or multiple gestations. It is important to recognize that more clinical studies are necessary to determine the effects of these agents on hyperandrogenic women with insulin resistance. Moreover, conclusive data regarding outcome, patient risks, and complications, while currently being collected, are not yet available. Based on the clinical evidence to date, the use of novel insulin sensitizers, such as the biguanides and thiazolidenediones, promise new treatment options for polycystic ovary syndrome for both fertility and long-term disease prevention.

α-Glucosidase Inhibitors (Acarbose)

Acarbose, the only drug of this class used in clinical practice, reversibly prevents α-glucosidase activity in the brush-border of the intestinal mucosa, decreasing disaccharide digestion, and hence, consequently, reducing enteral monosaccharide absorption.[38] Acarbose has been shown to flatten the post-prandial glucose and insulin increase and to decrease the serum androgen concentrations in hyperinsulinaemic pre-menopausal women with hyperandrogenemia.[39] Since this drug is well-tolerated and has few side effects, it may be used for the treatment of hyperandrogenic women with hyperinsulinemia.

The α-glucosidase inhibitors act by slowing the absorption of carbohydrates from the intestine and thereby, minimize the postprandial rise in blood glucose.[40] Acarbose is a synthetic disaccharide that reversibly inhibits α-glucosidase in the brush-border of the intestinal mucosa.

The inhibition of α-glucosidase is followed by a decrease in disaccharide digestion and by a subsequent decline of enteral monosaccharide absorption.[38] This results in a flattening of postprandial circulating concentrations of both glucose and insulin. Enteral absorption of Acarbose is extremely low (about 0.5 to 1.7%) and its clinical use as an antihyperglycemic compound is well established in patients with non-insulin-dependent diabetes mellitus (NIDDM).[41]

Because of its mechanism of action and safety, Acarbose may represent a good therapeutic approach to patients with PCOS and hyperinsulinemia. Accordingly, Geisthovel et al.[39] reported a decline of ovarian hyperestrogenemia in association with a flattening of the postprandial glucose and insulin increase in seven hyperinsulinemic, hyperandrogenemic pre-menopausal women treated with Acarbose.

Side Effects of Acarbose

The side effects are dose-dependent and limited to abdominal distension, flatulence and diarrhea.[41] Gastrointestinal side effects require gradual dosage increments over weeks or months after therapy is initiated. Serious adverse reactions are rare, and hypoglycemia and lactacidosis are not associated with the use of Acarbose. Therefore, this drug is regarded as the first choice medical treatment of diabetes mellitus in many countries.[42]

Some studies[43] found that Acarbose was able to reduce androgen levels and increase serum sex hormone binding globulin (SHBG) concentrations. These effects were associated with a decreased insulin response to oral glucose tolerance test (OGTT). The observed reduction in androgen concentrations during treatment with Acarbose was probably related to a decreased ovarian cytochrome P450c17 α activity. This effect seems to be limited to ovarian C19-steroids since dehydroepiandrosterone sulfate (DHEAS), the major adrenal androgen, was not affected by Acarbose therapy. The study has confirmed the presence of an abnormal increase in early phase insulin secretion response to OGTT in hyperinsulinemic PCOS patients and the pathogenetic role of hyperinsulinemia in these patients.[43]

D-Chiro Inositol (DCI)

Some actions of insulin may be effected by putative inositol-phosphoglycan (IPG) mediators of insulin action,[44,45] and evidence suggests that a deficiency in a specific DCI-containing IPG (DCI-IPG) may contribute to insulin resistance in individuals with impaired glucose tolerance or type 2 diabetes.[46,47] In support of this idea, oral administration of DCI has been demonstrated to improve glucose tolerance while reducing insulin in both obese and lean[48,49] women with PCOS and also to decrease serum androgens levels and improve ovulatory function.

A deficiency of the D-Chiro-inositol phosphoglycan mediator of the action of insulin may result in resistance to insulin. Insulin resistance has been linked to decreased urinary excretion of Chiro-inositol (a component of the putative D-Chiro-inositol phosphoglycan mediator) in primates[50] in humans with impaired glucose tolerance[51] or type 2 diabetes mellitus,[52] and in non-diabetic first degree relatives of persons with diabetes. The administration of D-Chiro-inositol, which is then presumably used in the formation of the active D-Chiro-inositol phosphoglycan mediator, may increase insulin sensitivity and improve the action of insulin in insulin-resistant subjects. D-Chiro-inositol improves ovulatory function and several metabolic abnormalities related to insulin resistance in women with the PCOS. These observations also suggest that D-Chiro-inositol could be used to treat the PCOS and that D-Chiro-inositol may prove useful in the treatment of other disorders that are pathophysiologically related to insulin resistance.

In obese women with PCOS, Metformin therapy significantly decreased serum insulin concentrations without changing the release of DCI-IPG during OGTT. Therefore, the release of bioactive DCI-IPG per unit of insulin was much higher after Metformin than after placebo, and the correlation between the release of DCI-IPG and insulin also seemed to improve after Metformin.[25] Collectively, these findings suggest that Metformin may enhance the action of insulin in PCOS in part, by improving insulin-mediated release of the DCI-IPG mediator, as evidenced by increased serum DCI-IPG bioactivity released per unit insulin after a glucose load.[26]

Herbal Medicine (Hyponidd) Containing Acarbose and DCI

We carried out a comparative study of the effects of Metformin with an Indian drug—Hyponidd (manufactured by Charak Pharmaceuticals Ltd., India), prepared using plants containing Acarbose (*Source: Gymnema sylvestre* or Gurmar) and D-Chiro-inositol (*Source: Pterocarpus marsupium*). The gas chromatography peaks of Pterocarpus marsupium and Gymnema sylvestre have been shown to correlate with peaks of Acarbose and D-chiro-inositol, respectively (Fig. 21.1).

Acarbose

Acarbose (present in a plant of Gurmar) is an α-glycosidase inhibitor, a drug used in the treatment of NIDDM, with minimal side effects and high clinical efficiency as an anti-hyperglycemic agent.[40]

DCI

An inositol phosphoglycan molecule containing D-Chiro-inositol and galactosamine is known to have a role in activating key enzymes that control the oxidative and non-oxidative metabolism of glucose (*Source: Pterocarpus marsupium*).

A comparative study to determine the efficacy of Hyponidd as an insulin sensitizing drug with Metformin was carried out at our center. The results, presented in Tables 21.1 to 21.4, were as follows:

PCOS subjects (n = 185) were randomly divided into two groups. Metformin group (n = 141) received Metformin (Glycomet 750 mg twice a day) and the Hyponidd group (n = 144) received a herbal medicine containing *Gymnema sylvestre* (112.5 mg per tablet) and *Pterocarpus marsupium* (75 mg per tablet), respectively, 2 BID for 3 months with the objective to compare the efficacy and safety of these drugs in the management of women with PCOS. A comparative difference in pre and posttreatment anthropometric and clinical features of randomly distributed infertile PCOS women are given in Table 21.1.

Though pretreatment hyperandrogenism in both the groups reduced significantly after treatment, the body mass

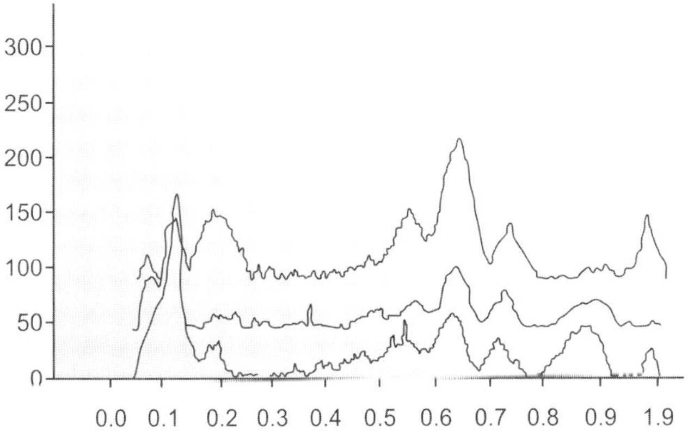
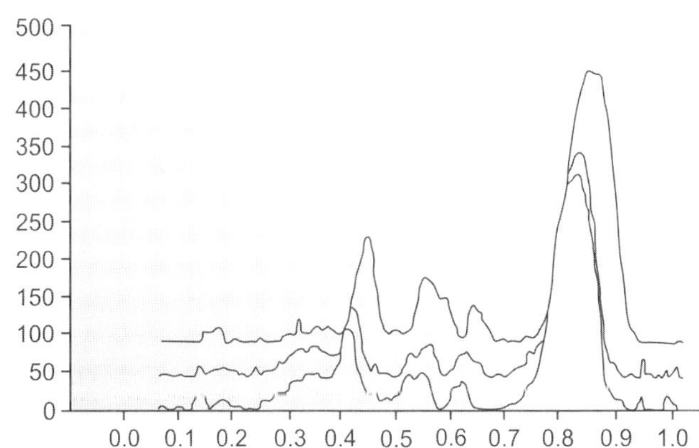

Fig. 21.1: Gas chromatography peaks of *Pterocarpus marsupium* and *Gymnema sylvestre* correlated with peaks of Acarbose and D-Chiro-inositol respectively

Table 21.1: Anthropometric and clinical characteristics of the PCOS subjects

Parameter	Metformin group (n =141)			Hyponidd group (n =144)			Difference in groups
	Pretreatment	Post-treatment	P	Pretreatment	Post-treatment	P	P
Age (yrs)		28.7 ± 0.7			29.0 ± 0.7		NS
Waist girth (cm)	79.8 ± 2.3	79.4 ± 1.8	NS	81.1 ± 1.8	76.1 ± 1.0	< 0.05	< 0.05
BMI (kg/m^2)	24.0 ± 0.5	23.9 ± 0.7	NS	23.9 ± 0.85	22.1 ± 0.4	< 0.05	< 0.05
W/H ratio	0.856 ± 0.004	0.855 ± 0.001	NS	0.858 ± 0.009	0.836 ± 0.005	< 0.005	< 0.005
Clinical hyperandrogenism	10.7 ± 0.35	9.6 ± 0.2	< 0.006	10.5 ± 0.37	9.5 ± 0.2	< 0.05	NS

Table 21.2: Metabolic parameters of the PCOS subjects before and after treatment

Parameters	Metformin group			Hyponidd group			Difference in groups
	Pretreatment	Post-treatment	P	Pretreatment	Post-treatment	P	P
Fasting insulin (µU/mL)	25.6 ± 0.74	15.8 ± 0.6	< 0.0001	25.5 ± 0.5	16.4 ± 0.6	< 0.0001	NS
Fasting glucose (mg/dL)	86.0 ± 1.2	86.3 ± 1.1	NS	89.7 ± 2.6	89.5 ± 2.1	NS	NS
Fasting glucose: insulin ratio	3.4 ± 0.07	5.8 ± 0.19	< 0.0001	3.55 ± 0.1	5.7 ± 0.2	< 0.0001	NS
HOMA - IR	5.4 ± 0.2	3.5 ± 0.3	< 0.0001	5.7 ± 0.2	3.7 ± 0.2	< 0.0001	NS
β-cell function index	457.5 ± 30.9	219.6 ± 11.9	< 0.0001	462.4 ± 63.7	202.4 ± 15.1	0.0002	NS

Table 21.3: Hormone parameters of the subjects before and after treatment

Parameters	Metformin group			Hyponidd group			Difference in groups
	Pretreatment	Post-treatment	P	Pretreatment	Post-treatment	P	P
LH (mIU/mL)	8.6 ± 0.7	7.0 ± 0.4	< 0.05	8.7 ± 0.5	6.97 ± 0.3	< 0.005	NS
FSH (mIU/mL)	3.96 ± 0.3	4.4 ± 0.2	NS	3.8 ± 0.2	4.1 ± 0.2	NS	NS
LH: FSH ratio	2.45 ± 0.2	1.66 ± 0.1	< 0.005	2.46 ± 0.2	1.75 ± 0.04	0.0006	NS
SHBG (nmol/L)	15.3 ± 0.8	45.1 ± 1.2	< 0.0001	15.3 ± 1.2	42.97 ± 1.2	< 0.0001	NS
FEI	18.85 ± 1.7	4.66 ± 0.3	< 0.0001	18.6 ± 2.2	4.4 ± 0.2	< 0.0001	NS
FTI	20.46 ± 2.2	3.88 ± 0.2	< 0.0001	21.97 ± 2.7	4.2 ± 0.2	< 0.0001	NS
Serum estradiol (pg/mL)	68.6 ± 5.4	54.6 ± 3.8	< 0.05	62.4 ± 6.6	43.4 ± 2.1	< 0.005	< 0.05
Serum testosterone (ng/dL)	79.8 ± 6.8	48.2 ± 2.1	< 0.0001	79.4 ± 5.1	51.0 ± 1.4	< 0.0001	NS

Table 21.4: Changes in laboratory and clinical parameters following treatment with Metformin V/s test medicine group

Parameters	Metformin group (n = 141)		Hyponidd group (n=144)		Difference in groups P value
	Pretreatment	Post-treatment	Pretreatment	Post-treatment	
Menstrual irregularity	31/41 (75.6%)	12/41 (29.3%)	30/41 (73.2%)	11/41 (26.8%)	> 0.05
Obesity (BMI >25 kg/m^2)	14/41 (34.1%)	14/41 (34.1%)	14/41 (34.1%)	11/41 (26.8%)	< 0.05
Insulin resistance (FG: FI < 4.5)	40/41 (100%)	6/41 (14.6%)	39/41 (95.1%)	5/41 (12.2%)	> 0.05
Hyperandrogenemia	18/41 (43.9%)	6/41 (14.6%)	15/41 (36.6%)	0/41 (0.0%)	< 0.0001
Hirsutism and Acne	24/41 (58.5%)	11/41 (26.8%)	28/41 (68.3%)	14/41 (34.1%)	> 0.05
LH: FSH ratio	21/41 (51.2%)	8/41 (19.5%)	26/41 (63.4%)	3/41 (7.3%)	< 0.05

index (BMI) and waist girth in obese subjects in the Metformin group did not show any reduction as compared to Hyponidd group.

Hyperinsulinemia in both post-treatment groups was found to be reduced significantly, as evidenced by results given in Table 21.2. Thus, Hyponidd treatment showed an efficacy similar to that of Metformin.

Even the hormone profile in both the post-treatment groups demonstrated an improvement in the luteinizing hormone (LH): follicle-stimulating hormone (FSH) ratio, increased SHBG levels and decreased testosterone levels. However, estradiol levels in the post-treatment Hyponidd group were significantly lowered as compared to those in the Metformin group. This could be accounted to a probable lowering of peripheral aromatization of androgens to estrogens due to a reduction in centroid obesity owing to the decrease in waist girth in Hyponidd group (Table 21.1).

The results in Table 21.4 showed an almost similar improvement in menstrual aberrations, hirsutism and acne occurrence in both the post-treatment groups. However, as compared to the Metformin group, improvement in obesity, hyperandrogenemia and LH: FSH ratio was more evident in the post-treatment Hyponidd group.

Side Effects

Nine out of forty-one (21.9%) subjects in the Metformin group, however, complained about gastrointestinal disturbances such as nausea, vomiting, abdominal pain and diarrhea. Interestingly, none of the subjects in the Hyponidd group complained about any such gastric disturbances.

CONCLUSION

The findings in our study suggested that herbal medicine containing *Gymnema sylvestre* and *Pterocarpus marsupium* effectively reduce insulin resistance, LH: FSH ratio, hyperandrogenemia, acne and hirsutism similar to Metformin. However, the reduction in BMI and waist girth as well as the decrease in the incidence of hyperandrogenemia with *Gymnema sylvestre* and *Pterocarpus marsupium* treatment was more perceptible as compared to Metformin treatment. However, further studies are required to endorse the efficacy of these herbal medicines in obese PCOS anovulatory women as compared to modern medicines like Metformin.

REFERENCES

1. Ciampelli M, Lanzone A. Insulin and polycystic ovary syndrome: a new look at an old subject. Gynecol Endocrinol 1998;12:277-92.
2. Franks S. Polycystic ovary syndrome. N Engl J Med 1995;333: 853-86.
3. Franks S. Polycystic ovary syndrome: a changing perspective. Clin Endocrinol 1989;31:87-120.
4. Lanzone A, Fulghesu AM, Andreani CL, Apa R, Fortini A, Caruso A, et al. Insulin secretion in polycystic ovarian disease: effect of ovarian suppression by GnRH agonist. Hum Reprod 1990;5:143-9.
5. Legro RS, Finegood D, Dunaif A. A fasting glucose to insulin ratio is a useful measure of insulin sensitivity in women with polycystic ovary syndrome. J Clin Endocrinol Metab 1998;83:2694-8.
6. Nestler JE. Role of hyperinsulinemia in the pathogenesis of the polycystic ovary syndrome and its clinical implications. Semin Reprod Endocrinol 1997;15:111-22.
7. Ehrmann DA. Relation of functional hyperandrogenism to noninsulin dependent diabetes mellitus. Baillere's Clin Obstet Gynaecol 1997;11:335-47.
8. Nestler JE. Insulin regulation of human ovarian androgens. Hum Reprod 1997;(Suppl 1):53-62.
9. Dunaif A, Segal KR, Futterweit W, Dobrjansky A. Profound peripheral insulin resistance, independent of obesity, in polycystic ovary syndrome. Diabetes 1989;38:1165-74.
10. Nestler JE, Jakubowicz DJ. Decreases in ovarian cytochrome P450c17 alpha activity and serum-free testosterone after reduction of insulin secretion in polycystic ovary syndrome. N Engl J Med 1996;335:617-23.
11. Huber-Buchholz MM, Carey DG, Norman RJ. Restoration of reproductive potential by lifestyle modification in obese polycystic ovary syndrome: role of insulin sensitivity and luteinizing hormone. J Clin Endocrinol Metab 1999;84:1470-4.
12. Davison RM. New approaches to insulin resistance in polycystic ovarian syndrome. Curr Opin Obstet Gynecol 1998;10:193-8.
13. Sattar N, Hopkinson ZE, Greer IA. Insulin-sensitizing agents in polycystic-ovary syndrome. Lancet 1998;351:305-7.
14. Antonucci T, Whitcomb R, McLain R, Lockwood D, Norris RM. Impaired glucose tolerance is normalized by treatment with the thiazolidinedione troglitazone. Diabetes Care 1998;20:188-93.
15. Henry RR. Thiazolidinediones. Endocrinol Metab Clin North Am 1997; 26:553-73.
16. Nolan JJ, Ludvik B, Beerdsen P, Joyce M, Olefsky J. Improvement in glucose tolerance and insulin resistance in obese subjects treated with troglitazone. N Engl J Med 1994;331:1188-93.
17. Saltiel AR, Olefsky JM. Thiazolidinediones in the treatment of insulin resistance and type II diabetes. Diabetes 1996;45: 1661-9.
18. Yki-Jarvinen H. Thiazolidinediones. N Engl J Med 2004;351: 1106-18.
19. De Leo V, La Marca A, Petraglia F. Insulin lowering agents in the management of the polycystic ovary syndrome. Endocr Rev 2003;24: 633-67.
20. Hundal RS, Inzucchi SE. Metformin: new understanding, new uses. Drugs 2003;63:1879-94.
21. Lord JM, Flight IH, Norman RJ. Metformin in polycystic ovary syndrome: systematic review and meta-analysis. BMJ 2003;327:951-7.
22. Kashyap S, Wells GA, Rosenwaks Z. Insulin-sensitizing agents as primary therapy for patients with polycystic ovary syndrome. Hum Reprod 2004;19:2474-83.
23. Diamanti-Kandarakis E, Kouli C, Tsianateli T, Bergiele A. Therapeutic effects of metformin on insulin resistance and hyperandrogenism in polycystic ovary syndrome. Eur J Endocrinol 1998;138:269-74.

24. Velazquez E, Acosta A, Mendoza SG. Menstrual cyclicity after metformin in polycystic ovary syndrome. Obstet Gynecol 1997;90:392-5.

25. Nestler JE, Jakubowicz DJ, Evans WS, Pasquali R. Effects of metformin on spontaneous and clomiphene-induced ovulation in the polycystic ovary syndrome. N Engl J Med 1998;338:1876-80.

26. Velazquez E, Mendoza S, Hamer T, Sosa F, Glueck CJ. Metformin therapy in polycystic ovary syndrome reduces hyperinsulinemia, insulin resistance, hyperandrogenemia, and systolic blood pressure, while facilitating normal menses and pregnancy. Metabolism 1994;43:647-54.

27. Ehrmann DA, Cavaghan MK, Imperial J, Sturis J, Rosenfield RL, Polonsky KS. Effects of metformin on insulin secretion, insulin action, and ovarian steroidogenesis in women with polycystic ovary syndrome. J Clin Endocrinol Metab 1997;82:524-30.

28. Chen C, Frazier J. Troglitazone: an antidiabetic agent. Am J Health Syst Pharm 1998;55:905-25.

29. Spiegelman BM. PPAR-gamma: adipogenic regulator and thiazolidinedione receptor. Diabetes 1998;47:507-14.

30. Dunaif A, Scott D, Finegood D, Quintana B, Whitcomb R. The insulinsensitizing agent troglitazone improves metabolic and reproductive abnormalities in the polycystic ovary syndrome. J Clin Endocrinol Metab 1996;81:3299-306.

31. Ehrmann DA, Schneider DJ, Sobel BE, Cavaghan MK, Imperial J, Rosen-field RL, et al. Troglitazone improves defects in insulin action, insulin secretion, ovarian steroidogenesis, and fibrinolysis in women with polycystic ovary syndrome. J Clin Endocrinol Metab 1997;82:2108-16.

32. Lehmann JM, Moore LB, Smith-Oliver TA, Wilkison WO, Willson TM, Kliewer SA. An antidiabetic thiazolidinedione is a high affinity ligand for peroxisome proliferator activated receptor gamma (PPAR gamma). J Biol Chem 1995;270:12953-6.

33. Azziz R, Ehrmann D, Legro RS, Whitcomb RW, Hanley R, Fereshetian AG. PCOS/Troglitazone Study Group. Troglitazone improves ovulation and hirsutism in the polycystic ovary syndrome: a multicenter, double blind, placebo-controlled trial. J Clin Endocrinol Metab 2001; 86:1626-32.

34. Belli SH, Graffigna MN, Oneto A, Otero P, Schurman L, Levalle OA. Effect of rosiglitazone on insulin resistance, growth factors, and reproductive disturbances in women with polycystic ovary syndrome. Fertil Steril 2004;81:624-9.

35. Brettenthaler N, De Geyter C, Huber PR, Keller U. Effect of the insulin sensitizer pioglitazone on insulin resistance, hyperandrogenism, and ovulatory dysfunction in women with polycystic ovary syndrome. J Clin Endocrinol Metab 2004;89:3835-40.

36. Chen C, Frazier J. Troglitazone: an antidiabetic agent. Am J Health Syst Pharm 1998;55:905-25.

37. Coetzee EJ, Jackson WP. Metformin in management of pregnant insulin-dependent diabetics. Diabetologia 1979;16:241-5.

38. Toeller, M. Modulation of intestinal glucose absorption: postponement of glucose absorption by alpha-glucosidase inhibitors. In Mogensen CE, Standl E (Eds). Pharmacology of Diabetes 1991. Walter de Gruyter, Berlin, New York.

39. Geisthovel F, Frorath B, Brabant G. Acarbose reduces elevated testosterone serum concentrations in hyperinsulinaemic premenopausal women: a pilot study. Hum Reprod 1996;11:2377-81.

40. Coniff RF, Seaton TB, Shapiro JA, Kleinfield R, Seaton TB, Beisswenger P, McGill JB. Reduction of glycosylated hemoglobin and postprandial hyperglycemia by acarbose in patients with NIDDM. Diabetes Care 1995;18:817-24.

41. Mahler RJ, Adler ML. Type 2 diabetes mellitus: update on diagnosis, pathophysiology, and treatment. J Clin Endocrinol Metab 1999;84:1165-71.

42. Lebovitz HE. Alpha-Glucosidase inhibitors. Endocrinol Metab Clin North Am 1997;26:539-51.

43. Ciotta L, Calogero AE, Farina M, De Leo V, Marca AL, Cianci A. Clinical, endocrine and metabolic effects of acarbose, an α-glucosidase inhibitor, in PCOS patients with increased insulin response and normal glucose tolerance. Hum Reprod 2001;16:2066-72.

44. Romero G, Larner J. Insulin mediators and the mechanism of insulin action. Adv Pharmacol 1993;24:21-50.

45. Saltiel AR. Second messengers of insulin action. Diabetes Care 1990;13:244-56.

46. Asplin I, Galasko G, Larner J. Chiro-inositol deficiency and insulin resistance: a comparison of the chiro-inositol- and the myo-inositol-containing insulin mediators isolated from urine, hemodialysate, and muscle of control and type II diabetic subjects. Proc Natl Acad Sci USA 1993;90:5924-8.

47. Kennington AS, Hill CR, Craig J, Bogardus C, Raz I, Ortmeyer HK, Hansen BC, Romero G, Larner J. Low urinary chiro-inositol excretion in noninsulin-dependent diabetes mellitus. N Engl J Med 1990;323:373-8.

48. Nestler JE, Jakubowicz DJ, Reamer P, Gunn RD, Allan G. Ovulatory and metabolic effects of d-chiro-inositol in the polycystic ovary syndrome. N Engl J Med 1999;340:1314-20.

49. Iuorno MJ, Jakubowicz DJ, Baillargeon JP, Dillon P, Gunn RD, Allan G, Nestler JE. Effects of d-chiro-inositol in lean women with the polycystic ovary syndrome. Endocr Pract 2002;8:417-23.

50. Ortmeyer HK, Bodkin NL, Lilley K, Larner J, Hansen BC. Chiroinositol deficiency and insulin resistance. I. Urinary excretion rate of chiro-inositol is directly associated with insulin resistance in spontaneously diabetic rhesus monkeys. Endocrinology 1993;132:640-5.

51. Suzuki S, Kawasaki H, Satoh Y, et al. Urinary chiro-inositol excretion is an index marker of insulin sensitivity in Japanese type II diabetes. Diabetes Care 1994;17:1465-8.

52. Craig JW, Larner J, Asplin CM. Chiro-inositol deficiency and insulin resistance. In: Draznin B, LeRoith D (Eds). Molecular biology of diabetes. Part 2. Totowa NJ. Humana Press 1994:343-62.

Does Natural Cycle IVF or Minimal Stimulation have a Role in Clinical Practice Today?

Daniel Humberto Méndez Lozano, René Frydman

OVERVIEW

Ovarian aging is one of the most difficult challenges in assisted reproduction technique (ART). Lack of response to traditional ovarian stimulation converts it into an expensive, heavy, in tolerated and inadequate treatment. However, even when the incidence of poor response is 9 to 24 percent, the importance of a homogeneous consensus to define it has been delayed with the consequent multitherapy proposed and the difficulty in making a comparison. The objective of this chapter is to analyze, in a practical sense, the effectiveness of monodominant follicle *in vitro* fertilization (IVF) in the treatment of patients with ovarian aging as compared with the most important alternative trials.

INTRODUCTION

Ovarian aging is actually the most difficult challenge in IVF. During reproductive life, follicle depletion occurs principally by the mechanisms of atresia in younger women or predominantly, by their entry into the growing follicular phase in older women.[1] Moreover, this depletion rate has an important increment after the age of 37 years or when the follicular pool, by virtue of disappearance, has reached less than 25,000 follicles.[2] This weakening of the oocyte quantity and its wide variation determine the outcome of ART.

Conversely, in order to optimize the reproductive capacity of growing antral follicular waves, one of the most important contributions to increase the outcome of IVF has been controlled ovarian hyperstimulation (COH).[3] COH enables multiple oocyte retrieval that allows selective embryo transfer,[4] the key to improve pregnancy rates. Even though COH remains an expensive and complex therapy, the augmented pregnancy rates justify its application. However, embryo selection is not possible when only a few oocytes are collected and embryo transfer is often performed with only the viable embryos with a consequently lower result. For this population, with a reduced response to COH, a different approach seems to be necessary to obtain a better outcome or the same results with a simplified protocol.

DEFINITION

Ovarian aging can be clinically expressed as a poor response to COH and measurable on the basis of the growing follicles,[5-7] the serum estradiol levels[7-9] and/or the retrieved oocytes.[10-12] Even when the poor responder population represents 9 to 24 percent[13] of the entire IVF population, the lack of a precise definition has been one of the principal obstructive factors in the study of management of poor responders, because its conclusions vary depending on the variations in the patients treated.

Although a consensus is still necessary,[14] we believe that growing follicles are amongst the most adequate parameters to study the poor responders and also the most utilized. Since there is no factor capable of absolutely predicting the ovarian response, patients who exhibit negative predictive factors should be considered in a different subgroup in the category of low ovarian reserve even when their behavior could often be similar following COH. Moreover, the serum estradiol level has been used as one of the earliest factors to define the poor responder population, even though one of the most imprecise because of the wide variation in estradiol production by follicle,[15] seen even in the monodominant follicle. However, the definition of poor response should have not only a study objective but also a practical sense, since these cycles could be benefited by a cycle cancellation, follicular flushing or other approaches according to the center, patients and health protection conditions. Similarly, the retrieved oocytes is a recent term that can additionally vary with regard to the immature follicles aspirated.

Even when the most practical and methodological definition for poor response seems to be the number of dominant follicles, the cut-off still varies from 3 to 5 follicles.[5,7,16] One of the most important factors to establish a universal cut-off, in order to be able to compare the different treatment propositions, is to include in the analysis the subsequent therapy for these patients. Thus, the practical sense of cut-off supposes that the poor responder patients to COH will not be included afterwards in a traditional COH or will not be stimulated yet again. On this basis, the definition of poor response should consider the lower limit in which a COH is not justified or moreover, the limit within which another simplified treatment offers the possibility of obtaining the same results.[17]

In addition, a careful difference should be established between the cycles with a poor response due to a low ovarian reserve from the cycles presenting an uncoordinated follicular size before COH, expressed as a reduced quantity of dominant follicles at the end of COH.[18] These two different conditions in the ovarian reproductive potential are of higher importance to determine the subsequent treatment. Like this, the inadequate conditions in COH should not be included in the definition of poor responders. Finally, once the definition of poor responders is established, a consensus is also necessary to determine a classification of this population according to the most predictive factor as age and the presence or absence of a low ovarian reserve.

CLINICAL DISCUSSION

Proposed Approaches

Several alternatives of assisted reproductive technique (ART) treatment have been proposed for patients with ovarian stimulation failure and a careful study of these therapies is highly important as is the selection of patients that can be really treated. The study of these approaches must include the poor responder definition and the time in which the study was completed.

Land et al.[5] studied the effect of proposing a double dose of gonadotropins for ovarian stimulation in poor responder patients. In this study, the poor response population was defined as patients who had less than 5 developing follicles. Even when the number of follicles and oocytes were incremented, the pregnancy rate presented remained unchanged, 4.4 percent per oocyte pick-up (OPU).[5]

In 1997, the flare-up effect was proposed to improve the ovarian response.[19] For this observation, the definition of poor responders was patients with less than 5 preovulatory follicles or serum estradiol levels less than 500 pg/mL. The study was carried out on 80 patients and they underwent COH only if the treatment cycle presented a low basal follicle stimulating hormone (FSH). In this study, 23.8 percent of

cycles were canceled and the pregnancy rate/OPU observed in 43 patients less than 40 years old was 4.7 percent.[19]

Additionally, the technique of intracytoplasmic sperm injection (ICSI) has been proposed for poor responder patients.[20] In this study, 104 cycles were randomized into two groups: *in vitro* fertilization (IVF) and IVF plus ICSI. In this study, 6 or less oocytes retrieved were considered as poor response. A similar pregnancy rate was observed between both the groups (17% vs 21% respectively).[20]

In addition, as an effort to increase the response to ovarian stimulation, the use of dexamethasone as an adjuvant has been proposed.[21] This study compared two populations of candidates undergoing ovarian stimulation—one group treated with dexamethasone (n = 145) and a second with placebo (n = 145). Even when the population treated was not a prescreened poor responder population, they showed a reduced incidence of poor response when dexamethasone was adjusted (12.4% vs 2.8%, respectively). The poor response definition for this study was considered as less than three preovulatory follicles. In this study, the pregnancy rate/OPU was 28.8 percent in the patients treated with dexamethasone as compared with 20.1 percent in patients who underwent traditional stimulation.[21]

The use of aromatase inhibitors has also been proposed as an adjuvant to treat the FSH-stimulated poor responder patients.[22] This study included 12 patients with a previous poor response, defined as less than 3 follicles of 18 mm at the end of ovarian stimulation. The aromatase inhibitor, Letrozole, plus FSH was administered and an increase of 1.4 mature follicles was observed. Four pregnancies were achieved with a 28.5 percent of pregnancy rate/OPU.[22]

Additionally, Aspirin has been tested as an adjuvant to improve the ovarian response to gonadotropins.[23] In this study, the definition of poor response was less than three mature follicles at the end of ovarian stimulation. Sixty patients with a previous poor response were randomized in a classical treatment protocol, and in a second group, with 80 mg of Aspirin as an adjuvant. Similar response and pregnancy rates were found in both the groups. The pregnancy rate/OPU was 4.5 percent for the Aspirin group versus 10 percent for placebo group.[23]

Another alternative proposed for the treatment of poor responders is *in vitro* maturation (IVM).[24] In this case report, three pregnancies in 8 cycles were described using the IVM technique. In this study, poor response was defined as a normal number of immature follicles but an unsuccessful ovarian stimulation observed without dominant follicles and a low serum estradiol level.[24]

Lastly, the administration of testosterone prior to ovarian stimulation was studied recently in poor responder patients.[25] The definition of poor responders was five or less retrieved oocytes and a serum estradiol level lesser than 1200 pg/mL. In this study, two groups were randomized to receive testosterone (n = 24) or placebo (n = 25) 15 days before COH. There was no difference observed between the testosterone and placebo groups with regard to the clinical pregnancy rates/OPU (25% and 5%, respectively) or the implantation rates, which were low (15% and 9%, respectively).[25]

Natural Cycle IVF with Controlled LH Surge Ovulation

An alternative that remains simple, efficient, inexpensive and short-term in the treatment of poor responders is *in vitro* fertilization following a natural cycle (IVF Nat). However, the efficacy of IVF Nat varies from 0 to 23 percent in terms of clinical pregnancy rate per OPU.[17,26-33] These irreproducible results are explained by the lack of standardization in the practice of natural cycle IVF from one center to another.

One of the factors limiting the success of IVF Nat is the OPU failure. In this sense, the semi-natural cycle, based most of all on the utilization of gonadotropin-releasing hormone (GnRH) antagonists, seems to improve the recovery rate by preventing the premature luteinizing hormone (LH) surge.[34-36] Thus, follicular flushing seems to be an adequate method in the semi-natural cycle IVF and it can even duplicate the pregnancy rate/OPU.[37]

A critical point in favor of the semi-natural cycles is the lower cost in terms of clinical pregnancy, as has been previously described by Ubaldi et al.[32] in their analysis, the cost of a clinical pregnancy obtained by classical ovarian stimulation was 72,050 Euros versus 12,300 Euros with semi-natural cycles IVF. The lower cost of the IVF Nat has also been reported by several studies,[26,29,32] and with the non-requirement of anesthesia, the efficacy of semi-natural cycles over classical ovarian stimulation has been established[17] for poor responders patients. In this well-conducted study, 129 patients with a previous response, defined as 3 or fewer mature follicles following ovarian hyperstimulation, were randomized for treatment with the conventional ovarian stimulation (n = 70) or with semi-natural cycle IVF (n = 59). A similar pregnancy rate/cycle was observed between both the groups (15% and 14.3%, respectively, for patients aged lesser than 36 years). Conversely, an elevated implantation rate was observed in patients treated with semi-natural cycle IVF (33.3% vs 12.5%), as has been observed previously by others.[33,35,38]

However, the optimal treatment for poor responder patients depends on the age and the number of cycles offered. Others studies have shown a reduction in the implantation rate with female ageing,[39] possibly linked to an increase in aneuploidy.[40] Hence, semi-natural cycle IVF should not be proposed for patients aged more than 36 to 38 years and the total number of attempts must be restricted to 3 because of the very low results in this subpopulation.[17,33,35] In fact, these studies confirm that for poor responder patients, more than the deficit in ovarian reserve, age is the most important predictive factor.

On the basis of this evidence, seminatural cycle IVF seems to be the most appropriate therapy in patients with a previous poor response as it is cheaper, simpler and at least as effective as the traditional complex protocols. However, it is not indicated in older women and the practice must include the use of antagonists and follicular flushing.

CONCLUSION

The lack of consensus on the definition of poor responder patients obstructs their optimal study and the finding of an adequate treatment. The definition has to have not only a study objective but a practical sense also. Hence, the number of growing follicles seems to be the most reproducible, adequate and practical definition rather than serum estradiol levels or the number of collected oocytes. However, the cut-off for this definition must be based on the previous experience in which case, another protocol could be more useful. In addition, the definition of poor responders must be subclassified according to their age and the presence or absence of a low ovarian reserve, observed by ultrasound or hormonal measurements.

Moreover, semi-natural cycle IVF seems to be the most adequate treatment for poor responder patients. This protocol is the simplest, cheapest and as effective as the classical protocol. However, this protocol must be indicated only in women aged lesser than 36 years and their practice must be include the use of antagonists and follicular flushing. The results after three attempts are very low.

REFERENCES

1. Gougeon A, Ecochard R, Thalabard JC. Age-related changes of the population of human ovarian follicles: increase in the disappearance rate of nongrowing and early-growing follicles in aging women. Biol Reprod 1994;50:653-63.
2. Faddy MJ, Gosden RG, Gougeon A, Richardson SJ, Nelson JF. Accelerated disappearance of ovarian follicles in mid-life: implications for forecasting menopause. Hum Reprod 1992;7:1342-6.
3. Laufer N, DeCherney AH, Haseltine FP, Polan ML, Mezer HC, Dlugi AM, et al. The use of high dose human menopausal gonadotropin in an *in vitro* fertilization program. Fertil Steril 1983;40:734-41.
4. Van Royen E, Mangelschots K, De Neubourg D, Valkenburg M, Van de Meerssche M, Ryckaert G, Eestermans W, Gerris J. Characterization of a top quality embryo, a step towards single-embryo transfer. Hum Reprod 1999;14:2345-9.
5. Land JA, Yarmolinskaya MI, Dumoulin JC, Evers JL. High-dose human menopausal gonadotropin stimulation in poor responders does not improve *in vitro* fertilization outcome. Fertil Steril 1996;65:961-5.
6. Fridstrom M, Akerlof E, Sjoblom P, Hillensjo T. Serum levels of luteinizing and follicle-stimulating hormones in normal and poor-responding patients undergoing ovarian stimulation with urofollitropin after pituitary downregulation. Gynecol Endocrinol 1997;11:25-8.
7. Raga F, Bonilla-Musoles F, Casan EM, Bonilla F. Recombinant follicle-stimulating hormone stimulation in poor responders with normal basal concentrations of follicle stimulating hormone and oestradiol: improved reproductive outcome. Hum Reprod 1999;14:1431-4.
8. Garcia JE, Jones GS, Acosta AA, Wright G Jr. Human menopausal gonadotropin/human chorionic gonadotropin follicular maturation for oocyte aspiration: phase II, 1981. Fertil Steril 1983;39:174-9.

9. Schoolcraft W, Schlenker T, Gee M, Stevens J, Wagley L. Improved controlled ovarian hyperstimulation in poor responder *in vitro* fertilization patients with a microdose follicle-stimulating hormone flare, growth hormone protocol. Fertil Steril 1997;67:93-7.

10. Chong AP, Rafael RW, Forte CC. Influence of weight in the induction of ovulation with human menopausal gonadotropin and human chorionic gonadotropin. Fertil Steril 1986;46:599-603.

11. Rombauts L, Suikkari AM, MacLachlan V, Trounson AO, Healy DL. Recruitment of follicles by recombinant human follicle-stimulating hormone commencing in the luteal phase of the ovarian cycle. Fertil Steril 1998;69:665-9.

12. Surrey ES, Bower J, Hill DM, Ramsey J, Surrey MW. Clinical and endocrine effects of a microdose GnRH agonist flare regimen administered to poor responders who are undergoing *in vitro* fertilization. Fertil Steril 1998;69:419-24.

13. Keay SD, Liversedge NH, Mathur RS, Jenkins JM. Assisted conception following poor ovarian response to gonadotrophin stimulation. Br J Obstet Gynaecol 1997;104:521-7.

14. Hellberg D, Waldenström U, Nilsson S. Defining a poor responder in *in vitro* fertilization. Fertil Steril 2004;82:488-90.

15. Baird DT, Fraser IS. Blood production and ovarian secretion rates of estradiol-17 beta and estrone in women throughout the menstrual cycle. J Clin Endocrinol Metab 1974;38:1009-17.

16. Roest J, van Heusden AM, Mous H, Zeilmaker GH, Verhoeff A. The ovarian response as a predictor for successful *in vitro* fertilization treatment after the age of 40 years. Fertil Steril 1996;66:969-73.

17. Morgia F, Sbracia M, Schimberni M, Giallonardo A, Piscitelli C, Giannini P, Aragona C. A controlled trial of natural cycle versus microdose gonadotropin-releasing hormone analog flare cycles in poor responders undergoing *in vitro* fertilization. Fertil Steril 2004;81:1542-7.

18. Fanchin R, Mendez Lozano DH, Schonauer LM, Cunha-Filho JS, Frydman R. Hormonal manipulations in the luteal phase to coordinate subsequent antral follicle growth during ovarian stimulation. Reprod Biomed Online 2005a;10:721-8.

19. Karande V, Morris R, Rinehart J, Miller C, Rao R, Gleicher N. Limited success using the "flare" protocol in poor responders in cycles with low basal follicle-stimulating hormone levels during *in vitro* fertilization. Fertil Steril 1997;67:900-3.

20. Moreno C, Ruiz A, Simon C, Pellicer A, Remohi J. Intracytoplasmic sperm injection as a routine indication in low responder patients. Hum Reprod 1998;13:2126-9.

21. Keay SD, Lenton EA, Cooke ID, Hull MG, Jenkins JM. Low-dose dexamethasone augments the ovarian response to exogenous gonadotrophins leading to a reduction in cycle cancellation rate in a standard IVF programme. Hum Reprod 2001;16:1861-5.

22. Mitwally MF, Casper RF. Aromatase inhibition improves ovarian response to follicle-stimulating hormone in poor responders. Fertil Steril 2002;77:776-80.

23. Lok IH, Yip SK, Cheung LP, Yin Leung PH, Haines CJ. Adjuvant low-dose aspirin therapy in poor responders undergoing *in vitro* fertilization: a prospective, randomized, double-blind, placebo-controlled trial. Fertil Steril 2004;81:556-61.

24. Liu J, Lu G, Qian Y, Mao Y, Ding W. Pregnancies and births achieved from *in vitro* matured oocytes retrieved from poor responders undergoing stimulation in *in vitro* fertilization cycles. Fertil Steril 2003;80:447-9.

25. Massin N, Cedrin-Durnerin I, Coussieu C, Galey-Fontaine J, Wolf JP, Hugues JN. Effects of transdermal testosterone application on the ovarian response to FSH in poor responders undergoing assisted reproduction technique: a prospective, randomized, double-blind study. Hum Reprod 2006;21:1204-11.

26. Daya S, Gunby J, Hughes EG, Collins JA, Sagle MA, YoungLai EV. Natural cycles for *in vitro* fertilization: cost-effectiveness analysis and factors influencing outcome. Hum Reprod 1995;10:1719-24.

27. Zayed F, Lenton EA, Cooke ID. Natural cycle *in vitro* fertilization in couples with unexplained infertility: impact of various factors on outcome. Hum Reprod 1997;12:2402-7.

28. Bassil S, Godin PA, Donnez J. Outcome of *in vitro* fertilization through natural cycles in poor responders. Hum Reprod 1999;14:1262-5.

29. Janssens RM, Lambalk CB, Vermeiden JP, Schats R, Schoemaker J. *In vitro* fertilization in a spontaneous cycle: easy, cheap and realistic. Hum Reprod 2000;15:314-8.

30. Nargund G, Waterstone J, Bland J, Philips Z, Parsons J, Campbell S. Cumulative conception and live birth rates in natural (unstimulated) IVF cycles. Hum Reprod 2001;16:259-62.

31. Kolibianakis E, Zikopoulos K, Camus M, Tournaye H, Van Steirteghem A, Devroey P. Modified natural cycle for IVF does not offer a realistic chance of parenthood in poor responders with high day 3 FSH levels, as a last resort prior to oocyte donation. Hum Reprod 2004;19:2545-9.

32. Ubaldi FM, Rienzi L, Ferrero S, Baroni E, Sapienza F, Cobellis L, Greco E. Management of poor responders in IVF. Reprod Biomed Online 2005;10:235-46.

33. Castelo Branco A, Achour-Frydman N, Kadoch J, Fanchin R, Tachdjian G, Frydman R. *In vitro* fertilization and embryo transfer in seminatural cycles for patients with ovarian aging. Fertil Steril 2005;84:875-80.

34. Olivenne F, Ayoubi JM, Fanchin R, Rongières-Bertrand C, Hamamah S. GnRH antagonist in single-dose applications. Hum Reprod Update 2000;6:313-7.

35. Castelo-Branco A, Frydman N, Kadoch J, Le Du A, Fernandez H, Fanchin R, Frydman R. The role of the semi-natural cycle as option of treatment of patients with a poor prognosis for successful *in vitro* fertilization. J Gynecol Obstet Biol Reprod 2004;(6 Pt 1):518-24.

36. Frydman R. GnRH antagonists in natural cycles. J Gynecol Obstet Biol Reprod 2004;(6 Pt 2):3S46-9.

37. Méndez Lozano DH, Fanchin R, Chevalier N, Feyereisen E, Hesters L, Frydman N, Frydman R. [The follicular flushing duplicate the pregnancy rate on semi-natural cycle IVF]. J Gynecol Obstet Biol Reprod (Paris) 2007;36:36-41.

38. Rongieres-Bertrand C, Olivennes F, Righini C, Fanchin R, Taïeb J, Hamamah S, et al. Revival of the natural cycles in *in vitro* fertilization with the use of a new gonadotropin-releasing hormone antagonist (cetrorelix): a pilot study with minimal stimulation. Hum Reprod 1999;14:683-8.

39. Cohen MA, Lindheim SR, Sauer MV. Donor age is paramount to success in oocyte donation. Hum Reprod 1999;14:2755-8.

40. Battaglia DE, Goodwin P, Klein NA, Soules MR. Influence of maternal age on meiotic spindle assembly in oocytes from naturally cycling women. Hum Reprod 1996;11:2217-22.

Minimal Monitoring of Ovarian Stimulation: Is it Safe?

Padma Rekha Jirge

OVERVIEW

Ovarian stimulation is an integral part of treatment for all forms of subfertility. However, the type of ovarian stimulation varies depending the treatment strategy planned. Any form of stimulation, including ovarian stimulation with Clomiphene, is fraught with the risks of inadequate or excessive response and multiple pregnancy. Some of these complications, such as severe ovarian hyperstimulation syndrome (OHSS) and antenatal problems, associated with high order multiple pregnancy, in fact necessitate frequent visits to the hospital and/or prolonged hospital admission. Hence, appropriate monitoring should be considered as the minimum required monitoring for the stimulation strategy planned.

INTRODUCTION

Ovarian stimulation encompasses diverse protocols using either chemical or hormonal ovulation induction. It is universally accepted that such treatment cycles should be monitored to ensure both success and patient safety. However, there is no agreement amongst clinicians as to the importance of different modalities of monitoring. The issue of frequency of monitoring is rarely debated. Consequently, it is not possible to define what constitutes optimal monitoring. However, minimal monitoring often implies almost no monitoring of Clomiphene-treated cycles and ultrasound monitoring alone in cycles treated with exogenous gonadotropins.

CLINICAL DISCUSSION

With 10 to 15 percent of the population being infertile at any given time, its management constitutes an important aspect of health care in any country. In the last three decades, enormous progress has been made, both in the pharmacological and laboratory aspects of male and female infertility management. However, actual treatment complexities, such as duration, painful injections, cost of treatment, loss of productivity, inaccessibility of speciality centers and, in addition, perceived misconceptions, often lead to treatment dropouts.[1] Over the years, efforts have been aimed at making these treatments more patient-friendly by introducing self-injections and modifying the monitoring protocols with a resultant decrease in the time spent in traveling and the hospital visits and an increase in cost-effectiveness.[2] Decentralization and setting up of transport and satellite clinics have added to patient-convenience in some countries without adversely affecting the success rate or the patient safety.[3] It is to be remembered that minimizing the monitoring during treatment does not mean any less aggressive selection criteria for choosing the appropriate treatment modality.

Aims of Monitoring

Ovarian stimulation is not a single entity as the stimulants used vary according to the endpoint to be achieved, i.e. mono-follicular ovulation/ovulation of 1 to 3 eggs or indeed, multi-follicular ovulation. The role of monitoring any stimulation protocol is to ascertain adequate response, time any further interventions, such as natural intercourse, administration of human chorionic gonadotropin (hCG), intrauterine insemination (IUI) or oocyte retrieval, identify any factor contributing to failure and maximize the success. In addition, it should ensure patient convenience and safety. Certain factors, such as ongoing research activity, may necessitate more intensive monitoring. Hence, it is understandable that a single protocol or a single modality is unlikely to fulfill all the criteria of adequate monitoring. It is also understandable that the frequency with which any monitoring is required is governed by the intricacies of the treatment itself. Transvaginal ultrasonography and hormonal evaluation of ovulation induction cycles have been invaluable in understanding the follicular and endocrine dynamics during various treatment modalities. Briefly described below is an overview of different scenarios of ovarian stimulation necessitating monitoring.

Monofollicular Ovulation

Clomiphene citrate (CC) is the most widely used stimulant in anovulatory infertility and because of the ease of administration, it is vastly misused as well. Majority of the cycles are not monitored at all. Often, very little importance is given to such treatment cycles and CC has gained the reputation of an orphan drug.[4] However, treatment without appropriate monitoring results in delayed recognition of ineffective doses or of excessive response, leading to potentially life-threatening OHSS and equally worrying higher order multiple pregnancy[5,6] with increased maternal and fetal risk. These consequences have an adverse impact on the treatment, increase the frequency of hospital visits or even necessitate stay in the hospital and have negative psychological and financial implications for the patient. Though not discussed often, failure of CC therapy in some women is due to its antagonistic effect on the endometrium, which goes undetected without monitoring.

Ovarian Stimulation for Intrauterine Insemination

In intrauterine insemination (IUI) cycles, ovarian stimulation consists of Clomiphene alone, gonadotropins alone or a combination of the two. The aim is to achieve ovulation of 1 to 3 follicles. Monitoring is necessary to time the administration of hCG and IUI, to identify multiple follicle development and minimize multifollicular ovulation leading to multiple pregnancies[7,8] or OHSS.

Controlled Ovarian Hyperstimulation for IVF/ICSI

When the stimulation is for *in vitro* fertilization (IVF) or intracytoplasmic sperm injection (ICSI), the scenario is complex. Knowledge gained in the past two decades and its incorporation into routine practice has simplified the management and made it patient-friendly to a large extent.[2] The trend is to provide individualized treatment rather than a standard protocol. Hence, to argue that a single modality of monitoring can provide all the necessary insights into the treatment cycles is to take a simplistic view of the follicular dynamics. The multiple variables involved, such as hormonal manipulation in the pretreatment cycle (oral contraceptive pill or progesterones), protocols used (long or short), type of agonist (depot or daily), route of administration (subcutaneous or intranasal spray), use of antagonist, type of stimulant used, human menopausal gonadotropin (hMG), purified urinary follicle stimulating hormone (FSH) or recombinant FSH (rFSH), all influence the endocrine dynamics to a varying extent.

Conventional monitoring of IVF/ICSI cycles includes both ultrasound and hormonal assays. Over the years, the efforts to make the treatment less complex and patient-friendly have included self injections and development of satellite and transport clinics. Decentralizing the treatment has the advantage of minimizing patient inconvenience without reducing the success.[9] Several studies have questioned the need for endocrine evaluation. It is known that pregnancies have been achieved across all concentrations of serum estradiol (E2) and repeated tests add very little to the understanding of these cycles.[10,11] However, the data on the effect of all the different protocols on the endocrine environment is far from complete. The degree of pituitary suppression, absence of exogenous luteinizing hormone (LH) in stimulation and the occurrence of premature luteinization may influence the treatment outcome. Normal response to a particular protocol does not necessarily ensure a similar response to a different protocol.

A high basal E2 level at the beginning of stimulation may be associated with a high cancellation rate and poor oocyte yield.[12] Profound suppression of LH is seen in 3 to 23 percent of women undergoing IVF depending on the protocol used. Though recent studies have questioned its significance,[13,14] there is evidence to suggest its detrimental effect on the dose of FSH, duration of stimulation, oocyte and embryo yield[15,16] and association with an increased early pregnancy loss.[17] Premature luteinization with raised progesterone levels at the time of hCG administration can result in reduced implantation and pregnancy rates.[18,19]

These conditions do occur in a small proportion of women undergoing assisted reproductive technique (ART) cycles. The adverse consequences may not have any impact on the program success rate, but are nonetheless important for the individuals. In addition, depending on the age of the woman and the protocol used, the follicular recruitment pattern differs.[20] This knowledge should help in deciding the frequency of monitoring.

Proposed Monitoring of Ovarian Stimulation

During treatment with CC, it is important to monitor the first cycle to establish an adequate response or to effect an appropriate change in the dose. Monitoring would recognize any excessive response which, with appropriate precautions, should minimize the risk of multiple pregnancy and OHSS.[5] Previously, basal body temperature, endometrial biopsy and mid-luteal serum progesterone levels have all been used for monitoring.[21] However, these tests provide limited information or are invasive. A single transvaginal ultrasonography performed on the 12th day of the first cycle will confirm adequate, excess or no response and will identify any untoward effect on the endometrium. It is non-invasive and involves a single visit to the hospital. Once the adequate response is confirmed, no further monitoring is required, or one additional ultrasound at the beginning of the following cycle will rule out the presence of any functional ovarian cyst.

In women undergoing IUI, whether the stimulant is CC, low dose gonadotropin or a combination of the two, monitoring by transvaginal ultrasonography alone suffices in a large majority of the women.[22,23] Additional monitoring to detect a spontaneous LH surge, or hormone assays, does not add to the treatment success and certainly adds to the patient inconvenience.[24] In a CC-stimulated cycle, an ultrasound examination on the tenth day of the cycle will determine the response, the frequency of further monitoring and the time of hCG administration. In cycles where gonadotropins are used, ultrasound examination on the seventh or eighth day of the cycle will serve the above purpose and help in any necessary dose adjustments.

In IVF/ICSI cycles, an effort to reduce the number of ultrasound scans does not appear to adversely affect the results or the patient safety.[9] Hence, one visit prior to stimulation for a baseline ultrasound and a blood sample for serum LH and estradiol concentration to confirm adequate downregulation and a second visit for the same monitoring in the mid-follicular phase (stimulation day 7 to 8) to identify the need for any change in dose and the type of stimulant, are mandatory. This visit would also determine the frequency of further ultrasound scans. One more blood sample on the day of hCG will give information about any premature LH surge, premature luteinization, estradiol and progesterone concentrations in the serum.

Highly sensitive and specific markers of ovarian reserve, such as anti-Müllerian hormone (AMH)[25] and antral follicle count (AFC),[26] have been increasingly used in the past decade to choose appropriate ovarian stimulation protocols for individuals. AMH and AFC-based protocols increase the safety and efficacy of stimulation regimes. However, they have not obviated the need for both endocrine and ultrasound monitoring of IVF cycles.

Judicious use of both the modalities of monitoring gives a more complete understanding of individual response than relying on any one modality. Extension of the knowledge gained from the first cycle can help reduce the monitoring further in subsequent cycles.[2]

CONCLUSION

Ovarian stimulation encompasses an array of protocols to result in a single or multiple follicular ovulation. It is understandable that these protocols influence the follicular and endocrine dynamics variably. Monitoring should ensure patient convenience, and safety. However, it is equally important that we gain adequate knowledge of the response, which is necessary to achieve the ultimate endpoint of pregnancy. Simple forms

of ovarian stimulation can be monitored successfully with a minimum number of ultrasound examinations alone. However, IVF/ICSI cycles require the judicious use of both ultrasound and endocrine evaluation to gain a more complete understanding of the response without necessarily increasing the hospital visits or patient discomfort. These tests can also be carried out in some easily accessible satellite centers with suitably trained staff, minimizing the visits to a distant tertiary center where the final part of the treatment is completed. Optimal monitoring, rather than minimal monitoring, is what we should be aiming for.

REFERENCES

1. Gleicher N, Vanderlaan B, Karande V, Morris R, Nadherney K, Pratt D. Infertility treatment dropout and insurance coverage. Obstet Gynecol 1996;88:283-93.
2. Penzias AS. Improving results with assisted reproductive technologies: individualized patient-tailored strategies for ovulation induction. Reprod Biomed Online 2004;9:43-6.
3. Roest J, Verhoeff A, van Lent M, Huisman GJ, Zeilmaker GH. Results of decentralized *in vitro* fertilization treatment with transport and satellite clinics. Hum Reprod 1995;10:563-7.
4. Rostami-Hodjcgan A, Lennard MS, Tucker GT, Ledger WL. Monitoring plasma concentrations to individualize treatment with clomiphene citrate. Fertil Steril 2004;81:1187-93.
5. Nasseri S, Ledger WL. Clomiphene citrate in the twenty-first century. Hum Fertil (Camb) 2001;4:145-51.
6. Derom C, Leroy F, Vlietinck R, Fryns JP, Derom R. High frequency of iatrogenic monozygotic twins with administration of clomiphene citrate and a change in chorionicity. Fertil Steril 2006;85:75-7.
7. Goverde AJ, Lambalk CB, McDonnell J, Schats R, Homburg R, Vermeiden JP. Further considerations on natural or mild hyperstimulation cycles for intrauterine insemination treatment: effects on pregnancy and multiple pregnancy rates. Hum Reprod 2005;20:3141-6.
8. Dickey RP, Taylor SN, Lu PY, Sartor BM, Rye PH, Pyrzak R. Risk factors for high-order multiple pregnancy and multiple birth after controlled ovarian hyperstimulation: results of 4,062 intrauterine insemination cycles. Fertil Steril 2005;83:671-83.
9. Roest J, Verhoeff A, van Heusden AM, Zeilmaker GH. Minimal monitoring of ovarian hyperstimulation: a useful simplification of the clinical phase of *in vitro* fertilization treatment. Fertil Steril 1995;64:552-6.
10. Leerentveld RA, Janssen-Caspers HAB, van Os HC, Wladimiroff JW, Zeilmaker GH, et al. The value and role of plasma 17-estradiol measurements during ovarian hyperstimulation for *in vitro* fertilization. Hum Reprod 1988;3:53-8.
11. Lass A. UK Timing of hCG Group. Monitoring of *in vitro* fertilization embryo transfer cycles by ultrasound versus by ultrasound and hormonal levels: a prospective, multicenter, randomized study. Fertil Steril 2003;80:80-5.
12. Evers JL, Slaats P, Land JA, Dumoulin JC, Dunslman GA. Elevated levels of basal estradiol-17beta predict poor response in patients with normal basal levels of follicle-stimulating hormone undergoing *in vitro* fertilization. Fertil Steril 1998;69:1010-4.

13. Balasch J, Vidal E, Penarrubia J, Casamitjana R, Carmona F, Creus M, Fa'bregues F, Vanrell JA. Suppression of LH during ovarian stimulation: analysing threshold values and effects on ovarian response and the outcome of assisted reproduction in down-regulated women stimulated with recombinant FSH. Hum Reprod 2001;16:1636-43.

14. Kolibianakis EM, Zikopoulos K, Schiettecatte J, Smitz J, Tournave H, Camus M, et al. Profound LH suppression after GnRH antagonist administration is associated with a significantly higher ongoing pregnancy rate in IVF. Hum Reprod 2004;19:2490-6.

15. Fleming R, Rekha P, Deshpand N, Jameison ME, Yates RWS, Lyall H. Suppression of LH during ovarian stimulation: effects differ in cycles stimulated with purified urinary FSH and recombinant FSH. Hum Reprod 2000;15:1440-5.

16. Filicori M, Cognigni GE, Taraborrelli S, Spettoli D, Ciampaglia W, de Fatis CT, et al. Luteinzing hormone activity in menotropins optimizes folliculogenesis and treatment in controlled ovarian stimulation. J. Clin Endocrinol. Metab 2001;86:337-43.

17. Westergaard LG, Laursen SB, Andersen CY. Increased risk of early pregnancy loss by profound suppression of luteinizing hormone during ovarian stimulation in normogonadotrophic women undergoing assisted reproduction. Hum Reprod 2000;15:1003-8.

18. Bosch E, Valencia I, Escudero E, Crespo J, Simon C, Remohi J, Pellicer A. Premature luteinization during gonadotropin-releasing hormone antagonist cycles and its relationship with *in vitro* fertilization outcome. Fertil Steril 2003;80:1444-9.

19. Moreno L, Diaz I, Pacheco A, Zuniga A, Requena A, Garcia-Velasco JA. Extended coasting duration exerts a negative impact on IVF cycle outcome due to premature luteinization. Reprod Biomed Online 2004;9:500-4.

20. Fleming R, Deshpande N, Traynor I, Yates RW. Dynamics of FSH-induced follicular growth in subfertile women: relationship with age, insulin resistance, oocyte yield and anti-Mullerian hormone. Hum Reprod 2006;21:1436-41.

21. Hammond MG. Monitoring techniques for improved pregnancy rates during clomiphene ovulation induction. Fertil Steril 1984;42:499-509.

22. Williams RS, Kipersztok S, Hills D, Dattilo M. A novel, simplified and cost effective protocol for superovulation and intrauterine insemination. J Fla Med Assoc 1997;84:316-9.

23. Lewis V, Queenan J Jr, Hoeger K, Stevens J, Guzick DS. Clomiphene citrate monitoring for intrauterine insemination timing: a randomized trial. Fertil Steril 2006;85:401-6.

24. Awonuga A, Govindbhai J. Is waiting for an endogenous luteinizing hormone surge and/or administration of human chorionic gonadotropin of benefit in intrauterine insemination? Hum Reprod 1999;14:1765-70.

25. Nelson SM, Yates RW, Lyall H, Jameison M, Tainor I, Gaudoin M, et al. Anti-Mullerian Hormone based approach to controlled ovarian stimulation for assisted conception. Hum Reprod 2009; 24:867-75.

26. Broer SL, Dolleman M, Opmeer BC, Fauser BC, Mol BW, Broekmans FJ. AMH and AFC as predictors of excessive response in controlled ovarian hyperstimulation:a meta-analysis. Human Reprod Update 2011;17:46-54.

Contemporary Clinical Management

Do We Need HSG in the Era of 3D/4D Ultrasonography?

Madhusree Ghosh, Shelly Tse, Kamal Ojha

OVERVIEW

Subfertility affects one in ten couples worldwide with global prevalence rates varying from approximately 5 percent in developed countries to 30 percent in certain developing countries. Tubal assessment forms an integral part of the subfertility work-up. Historically, hysterosalpingography (HSG) has been advocated as the first line of investigation to diagnose tubal pathology. However, HSG is associated with risks of radiation and exposure to iodine. Laparoscopy and dye test is the gold standard for diagnosing tubal pathology. Laparoscopy however, involves cost issues and it is not free of complications. With recent developments in ultrasonography and with the introduction of three-dimensional ultrasonography, various ultrasonographic techniques, which involve visualization of the uterine cavity with the use of a contrast agent, have now been devised. Any ultrasound technique that uses fluid as a contrast agent in the evaluation of tubal patency is called hysterosalpingo-contrast-sonography (HyCoSy). The most commonly used dye for HyCoSy is an agent called Sono Vue. HyCoSy is an outpatient procedure. The patient has a transvaginal scan (TVS), and the contrast dye, which is inserted through the cervix, should be observed filling the uterine cavity and spilling out of the tubes through the fimbrial end. Coded contrast imaging (CCI) is a new software that optimizes the use of the ultrasound contrast media and enhances the visualization of the Fallopian tube. CCI can emit an ultrasound beam at a selected frequency, thereby preventing overlap of tissue and contrast responses. Some authors feel that HSG is an outdated investigation and has no place in current day evidence-based medicine. However, in developing countries, it is still the investigation of choice in evaluating women with subfertility and suspected tubal pathology. Expertise and funds are required to perform three-dimensional ultrasonographic procedures.

INTRODUCTION

The appropriateness of many investigations for subfertility continues to be a debate amongst many clinicians. For the concerned couple, an ideal test should be diagnostically accurate, involve the least amount of delay, be minimally invasive and most reliable. Tubal assessment is an integral part of female fertility evaluation and accounts for up to 30 percent of female subfertility.[1] Further investigations should be carried out to screen for and diagnose tubal pathology. Hysterosalpingography (HSG) has been advocated as the first line investigation historically. HSG is a radiographic examination of the uterine cavity and Fallopian tube that involves the use of a radiographic contrast medium. It has been suggested that HSG has a therapeutic role in enhancing subfertility.[2] Laparoscopy and dye test remains the gold standard in diagnosing tubal patency. However, it is an invasive and expensive procedure requiring general anesthesia with a 0.13 percent risk of surgical complications.[3] With advances in diagnostics, more tests, such as those with the use of ultrasound, have been advocated. Various ultrasonographic contrast media have been developed for tubal visualization and have been used in the diagnosis of tubal patency or blockage.[4] Any ultrasound-based technique that uses fluid as a contrast agent in the evaluation of tubal patency is called hysterosalpingo-contrast-sonography (HyCoSy). In an attempt to overcome the limitations with conventional HyCoSy, a newer software called coded contrast imaging (CCI) technology during HyCoSy, with the help of 3-dimensional (3D) ultrasonography (USG), has been studied. The aim of this chapter is to look into the advantages and disadvantages of HSG and 3D USG in the investigation of a subfertile couple, with a brief mention of laparoscopy and fertiloscopy as a part of the same investigative work-up.

CLINICAL DISCUSSION

Hysterosalpingography (HSG)

Hysterosalpingography is an X-ray examination of the uterine cavity and Fallopian tubes that involves the use of a radiographic contrast medium.

Procedure

Hysterosalpingography is performed in the Radiology Department. It is performed between days 7 to 10 of the menstrual cycle to avoid interfering with a possible pregnancy. Table 24.1 presents the indications to perform a hysterosalpingography. The patient is counseled about the actual process and may receive anti-inflammatory agents prior to the procedure as it may involve some pelvic discomfort and pain. The patient is placed in the dorsal position and the posterior vaginal wall is

---

Table 24.1: Indications for hysterosalpingography

- To assess tubal patency
- To identify tubal blockage and dilatation (hydrosalpinx)
- To detect uterine malformations, like uterine septa, in recurrent miscarriages
- To identify translocated intrauterine contraceptive device
- May indicate endometrial polyps, submucous fibroids
- To diagnose uterine synechiae

---

retracted with a Sim's speculum. The cervix may be held with a tenaculum. A hysterosalpingographic cannula is fitted with a syringe containing radio-opaque dye, Urograffin (water soluble iodine). The cannula is passed through the cervix and 5 to 10 mL of dye is slowly introduced. An immediate X-ray plate in the anteroposterior view is taken under fluoroscopic control and another plate is taken 10 to 15 mins later. Tubal patency is assessed by peritoneal spillage, visualized on the X-ray plate (Figs 24.1A and B).

Antibiotic prophylaxis is given with Doxycycline (100 mg twice daily for 5 days) after the procedure. For those allergic to Doxycycline, Azithromycin or Erythromycin may be prescribed. Table 24.2 presents the advantages and disadvantages of HSG.

Three-dimensional Ultrasonography (3D USG)

To overcome the limitations of HSG, newer modalities for testing tubal patency and infertility investigations have been studied. With the advent of high resolution vaginal probes, transvaginal sonography (TVS) has assumed an important role in assessing the myometrium and the endometrial echo complex. The diagnostic value of 3D ultrasound in the detection of intrauterine lesions is superior to 2 dimensional (2D) ultrasound.[9]

Hysterosalpingo-contrast-sonography (HyCoSy)

Recently, various ultrasonographic contrast media have been developed for tubal visualization and have been used in the diagnosis of tubal patency or blockage.[10] Any ultrasound-based technique that uses fluid as a contrast agent in the

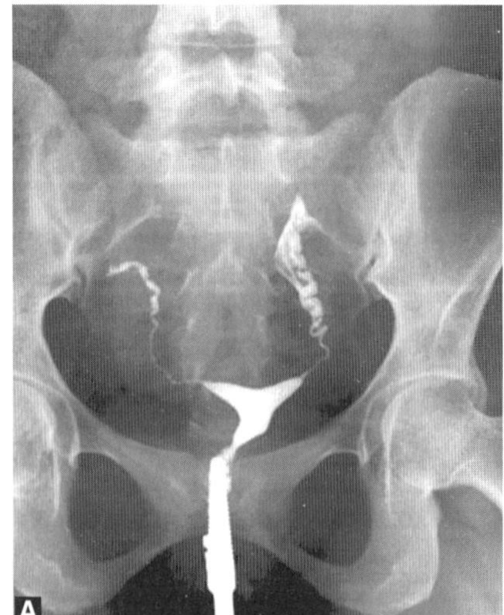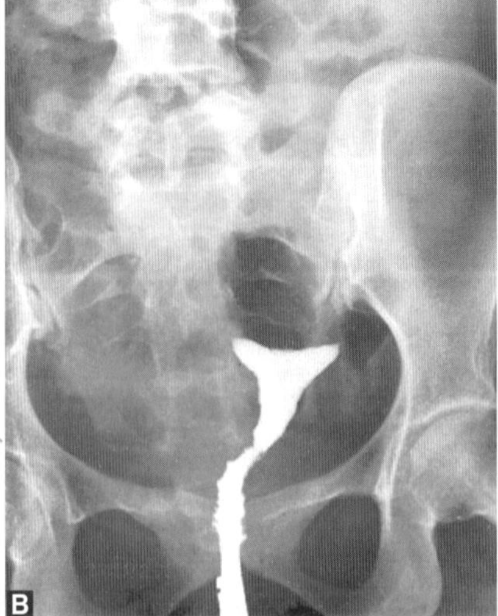

Figs 24.1A and B: (A) A radiograph showing a normal hysterosalpingogram (HSG), with free flow of radio-opaque dye into the abdominal cavity indicating bilateral patency of the Fallopian tubes; (B) Another radiograph showing the outline of the uterus without spillage of dye, indicating bilateral tubal obstruction

Table 24.2: Advantages and disadvantages of hysterosalpingography

Advantages	Disadvantages
• Identifies uterine cavity abnormalities	• Sixty-five percent sensitivity and 83 percent specificity for diagnosing tubal obstruction[5]
• Does not require much expertise	• Pelvic pain and discomfort
• Can be therapeutic-forcing dye through the tube may unblock a blocked tube	• Oil-soluble contrast media may be associated with oil embolism and granulomatous inflammation in blocked or inflamed Fallopian tubes[6]
• Can be performed in low resource settings	• Water-soluble contrast media (more commonly used) have been linked with increased frequency and duration of bleeding post-HSG and higher post-HSG miscarriage rates[7]
	• Overall, 10 percent risk of post-HSG complications
	• Exposure to radiation—the mean dose area product (DAP) for a complete HSG examination is 2.05 Gy cm^2 compared to 0.09 Gy cm^2 for a single posterior anterior chest X-ray examination[8]
	• Involvement of the Radiology department is required

evaluation of tubal patency is called hysterosalpingo-contrast-sonography (HyCoSy). This technique was introduced in the 1990's.

Procedure

It is performed as an outpatient procedure. A speculum is inserted into the vagina to visualize the cervix and a fine tube with a balloon is inserted into the cervix. The speculum is then removed and a TVS probe is inserted. This procedure is traditionally performed using ultrasound contrast media, which is injected through the cervix. The dye should be observed filling the uterine cavity, passing through the tubes and spilling out at the fimbrial end. Figure 24.2 depicts a 3D HyCoSy image of the uterine cavity in a patient with a uterine septum.

Similar to HSG, prophylactic antibiotics need to be prescribed for the HyCoSy procedure.

Different dyes used for HyCoSy
1. Echovist is a suspension of galactose microparticles in aqueous galactose solution and is an echogenic contrast medium. This is no longer available as the manufacturer has withdrawn the dye due to lack of availability of ingredients for the dye. The dye was well-established and quoted in publications.
2. Currently, we are using Sono-Vue, which is a dye for cardiac Doppler. Sono-Vue is a second-generation agent, which provides a substantial harmonic response at low acoustic pressures. It was recently introduced for sonographic tubal patency evaluation.
3. Recently, ExEm gel—hydroxyethylcellulose; glycerol has shown to be very useful for HyCoSy.
4. In places where dye is not available, water can be used for HyCoSy. Rapid movement of water between syringes

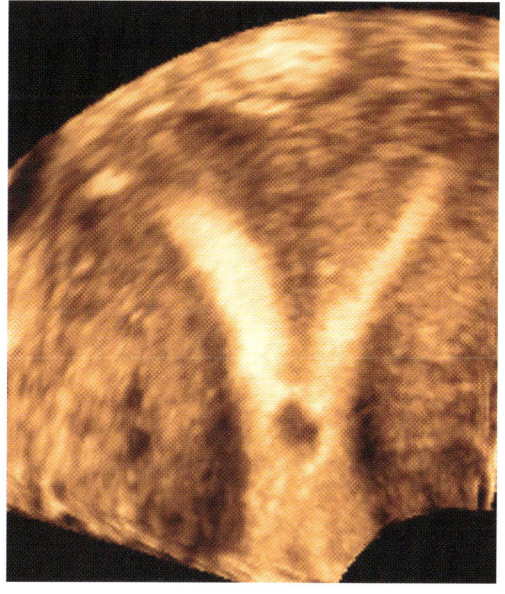

Fig. 24.2: 3D-image of the uterine cavity. The lower-third of the cavity shows the inflated HyCoSy catheter used to insert Echovist dye to outline the uterine cavity and the right Fallopian tube. This is a case of uterine septum with dye on either side of the uterine septum

with a three-way cannula can help to create a bubbling effect and obtain good quality image during HyCoSy examination.

A number of difficulties are encountered with the standard 2D gray-scale HyCoSy technique. Firstly, the Fallopian tube cannot be visualized completely in any scanning plane. Secondly, spill of echo-positive medium from the fimbrial end of the tube is difficult to distinguish from the bowel

Table 24.3: Advantages and disadvantages of Hysterosalpingo-Contrast-Sonography (HyCoSy)

Advantages	Disadvantages
• As accurate as HSG in terms of establishing tubal patency[11]	• Physician learning curve is longer
• Additional advantage of ultrasound assessment of the pelvis at the same time	• Spill of dye from the distal end of the tube may be difficult to visualize because of similar echogenecity with the surrounding bowel
• Superior in detection of intrauterine abnormalities such as endometrial polyps, submucus fibroids, synechiae, hydrosalpinx and abnormal ovaries	• Exact site of blockage may be difficult to ascertain
• Does not require the use of iodine	
• No exposure to radiation	
• Input from other specialties are not required	
• Although the costs of HSG and HyCoSy are similar, costs of HyCoSy can be further reduced by using air/saline as a medium	
• Less painful and better tolerated than HSG	
• Combined with the initial sonographic examination, it is believed to reduce the necessity for laparoscopy, and accelerates the whole investigation process	
• Complication rate (fever, pelvic inflammatory disease) is 4 percent	

Table 24.4: Advantages and disadvantages of 3-Dimensional Power Doppler Imaging (3D PDI)[4]

Advantages	Disadvantages
• Ultrasound assessment of the pelvic organs can be done in the same sitting	Resulting image obtained is not always clear enough to draw a conclusion about tubal patency
• 3D volumes, which include that of the Fallopian tube, can be stored and analyzed later, reducing the examination time of the patient	
• Less contrast agent is required	
• 3D ultrasound helps in diagnosing uterine malformations like bicornuate uterus and uterine septum	

surrounding the tube, which is of similar echogenecity. Thirdly, the procedure needs expertise and training. Table 24.3 presents the advantages and disadvantages of HyCoSy. This procedure has been modified and the feasibility of 3D power Doppler imaging (3D-PDI) in the assessment of tubal patency during HyCoSy has been studied. Table 24.4 presents the advantages and disadvantages of 3D power Doppler imaging.

Three-dimensional Coded Contrast Imaging (3D CCI) During HyCoSy

Coded contrast imaging (CCI) is a new software that optimizes the use of ultrasound contrast medium by means of low acoustic pressure and enhances the visualization of the Fallopian tubes. The image displayed is therefore based on harmonic signals produced by the contrast medium microspheres and broadband ultrasound signals from the surrounding tissue are completely filtered out. In principle, the bubbles reflect ultrasound waves to give the bright image observed during ultrasound examination. CCI is able to

Table 24.5: Advantages of 3D CCI[12]

• 3D volume acquisition of the entire Fallopian tube easily shows the course of the tube
• Allows distinction of contrast medium in the tubes and ovaries from surrounding tissues and organs due to clearly detectable differences between the harmonic response of the contrast medium micro-bubbles and the broadband ultrasonic signals from surrounding tissue
• 3D volume acquisition is static, therefore less dependent on the experience and skill of the operator
• 3D volumes of the uterus and tubes can be stored and analyzed later, thereby reducing examination time for patients

emit an ultrasound beam at a selected frequency, thereby preventing overlap of tissue and contrast responses.[12] Table 24.5 presents the advantages and disadvantages of 3D coded contrast imaging.

Procedure

Coded contrast imaging technology during HyCoSy involves the intrauterine injection of ultrasound contrast medium, which in a completely anechoic pelvis is visualized as hyperechoic fluid. This fluid is first seen in the uterus, in the tube proximally if patent, and finally spills into the abdominal cavity if the distal end of the tube is patent. As the contrast medium is hyperechoic, its course along the uterus and tubes can be studied for several minutes and 3D volume acquisitions can be done. The dye used for this is Sono-Vue solution, which contains sulfur hexafluoride bubbles.

Laparoscopy

Laparoscopy and dye test is the gold standard method to check the Fallopian tubes, particularly in high-risk patients (women with a past history of pelvic infection or abdominal surgery). Laparoscopy allows direct visualization of the internal organs of the abdomen and pelvis and excludes other pathologies such as endometriosis, fibroids, ovarian cysts and adhesions. Most infertile couples require a diagnostic laparoscopy for complete evaluation of their infertility. Among women whose tubes were found to be unobstructed using HSG, 18 percent were found to have tubal obstruction or peritubal adhesions using laparoscopy and a further 34 percent were found to have endometriosis or fibroids.

The laparoscopy procedure is usually done as a day care surgery under general anesthesia. It takes about 15 to 30 minutes.

When performing the laparoscopy procedure, a fine Verres needle is inserted into the abdomen and gas (carbon dioxide) is pumped into the abdomen to push the intestines away. A second incision might also be made so that a probe can be inserted in order to move pelvic organs, such as the ovaries, into clear view. A colored dye (methylene blue) is then injected through the cervix. If the tubes are not blocked the dye should pass along them and spill into the abdomen. If an abnormality is found during laparoscopy, this may be dealt with at the same time, thus avoiding another operation. Diagnostic laparoscopy is associated with approximately 3 percent risk of minor complications, such as nausea and shoulder tip pain. The risk of major complications, such as bowel injury and injury to blood vessels, is about 0.6 to 2/1000.[3]

Fertiloscopy

Fertiloscopy is a new minimally invasive method for the exploration of the posterior cul-de-sacm which allows a complete work up of the mechanical factors of female infertility.

When the indications are correct, fertiloscopy can be considered as a valid alternative to diagnostic laparoscopy. In fact, it uses the vaginal approach and requires relatively simple equipment. Moreover, it can be performed under local anesthesia or under sedation.

Fertiloscopy currently, is mostly a diagnostic procedure with restricted operative possibilities limited to biopsies, minimal adhesiolysis and ovarian drilling; nevertheless, operative fertiloscopy is an emerging technique, which will probably develop in the near future.

Fertiloscopy is the combination of different procedures, which include the following:
- Transvaginal hydrolaparoscopy
- Dye test
- Salpingoscopy
- Microsalpingoscopy
- Hysteroscopy.

CONCLUSION

Tubal damage can be due to various reasons, including pelvic infection, endometriosis and fibroids. A detailed history and physical examination of the patient at the initial visit should be carried out. The main organism causing pelvic inflammatory disease is Chlamydia trachomatis. Microimmunofluorescence (MIF) is widely used for Chlamydia antibody titer (CAT) testing. Although CAT testing does not provide any detail on the anatomy of the uterus and tubes, it should be able to identify women who need further tubal or pelvic evaluation. Historically, HSG has remained the first line of investigation in the diagnosis of tubal patency. However, HSG is associated with risks of exposure to iodine and radiation. With advances in technology, 3D ultrasonography and HyCoSy procedures have gained popularity in the investigation of such patients. 3D ultrasonography gives us the additional advantage of an initial sonographic assessment of the pelvic organs during the same sitting. Complete visualization of the uterine cavity to the fimbrial end of the tube is now possible with the 3D CCI technology during HyCoSy. However, laparoscopy remains the gold standard in diagnosing tubal pathology. Many author's question—whether HSG should be performed as a part of modern fertility investigations? Proponents of HSG would argue that HSG can be performed in low resource settings and does not need the availability of an ultrasound. However, X-ray, fluoroscopic equipment and liason with the Radiology department are required as a bare minimum. Studies have shown that HyCoSy and HSG procedures bear the same cost and accuracy. With the use of 3D USG we can also avoid radiation exposure. Most fertility clinics in the developed world have access to ultrasound as a part of their very basic infertility work-up. Some authors feel that HSG is out of date and has no place in modern evidence-based fertility investigations,[6] however, in developing parts of the world, it is still the investigation of choice, especially because greater training, expertise and funds are required to perform 3D USG procedures.

REFERENCES

1. Cates W, Wasserheit JN. Genital chlamydial infections: epidemiology and reproductive sequelae. Am J Obstet Gynaecol 1991;164:1771-81.
2. Yaegashi N, Kuramoto M, Nakayama C, Nakano M, Hoshai H. Pregnancy rates after hysterosalpingography comparing water soluble contrast medium with oily contrast medium. Nippon Sanka Fujinka Gakkai Zasshi 1987;39:1812-4.
3. Chapron C, Querleu D, Bruhat MA, Madelenat P, Fernandez H, Pierre F, Dubuisson JB. Surgical complications of diagnostic and operative gynaecological laparoscopy: a series of 29,966 cases. Hum Reprod 1998;13:867-72.
4. Sladkevicius P, Ojha K, Campbell S, Nargund G. Three-dimensional power Doppler imaging in the assessment of fallopian tube patency. Ultrasound Obstet Gynecol 2000;16:644-7.
5. Swart P Mol, BWJ van der Veen F, van Beurden M, Redekop WK, Bossuyt PM. The accuracy of hysterosalpingography and the diagnosis of tubal pathology : a meta-analysis. Fertil Steril 1995;64:486-91.
6. Lim CP, Hasafa Z, Bhattacharya S, Maheswari A. Should a hysterosalpingogram be a first-line investigation to diagnose female tubal subfertility in the modern subfertility work-up? Hum Reprod 2011;26:967-71.
7. Spring DB, Barkhan HE, Pruyn SC. Potential effects of contrast materials in hysterosalpingography: a prospective randomized clinical trial. Kaiser Permanente Infertility Work Group. Radiology 200;214:53-7.
8. Hart D, Hillier MC, Wall BF. HPA-RPD-029 – doses to patients from radiographic and fluoroscopic X-ray imaging procedures in the UK-2005. Review 2009;2010:95.
9. El – Shirbiny W, Nasr AS. Value of 3- dimensional sonohysterography in infertility work-up. J Minim Invasive Gynaecol 2011; 18:54-8.
10. Deishert U, Schlief R, Van de Sandt M, Juhnke I. Transvaginal hysterosalpingo-contrast-sonography (HyCoSy) compared with conventional tubal diagnosis. Human Reprod 1989;4:418-24.
11. Heikkinen H, Tekay A, Volpi E, Martikainen H, Jouppila P. Transvaginal salpingosonography for the assessment of tubal patency in infertile women: methodological and clinical experiences. Fertil Steril 1995;64:293-8.
12. Exacoustos C, Di Giovanni A, Szabolcs B, Binder-Reisinger H, Gabardi C, Arduini D. Automated sonographic tubal patency evaluation with three-dimensional coded contrast imaging (CCI) during hysterosalpigo-contrast sonography (HyCoSy). Ultrasound Obstet Gynecol 2009;34:609-12.

How to Approach Submucous Myomas in Infertile Women?

Sunita Tandulwadkar, Anil Chittake, Vineeta Kharb

OVERVIEW

Submucous myomas have a causal relationship with infertility. Submucous myomas are classified on the basis of intramural extension. Preoperatively, transvaginal sonography (TVS) is used to assess size, number, location, the extent of the intramural extension, and the free margin.

Type 0 myomas are systematically shaved off with a resectoscope loop until the pedicle is reached. Dislodging the myoma from the base may pose problem in resecting further.

For Type 1 and 2 myomas, minimal pressure is applied to prevent pushing the fibroid deep in the wall and intravasation of fluid. Following removal of the portion protruding in the cavity, the part vested deep in the myometrium is removed by either controlled endocavitary pressure variation or the cold knife technique. It is recommended that large Type 2 myomas (> 4 cm) be removed laparoscopically.

Intraoperative fluid balance is to be maintained and the duration of the surgery plays a major role. The Versapoint bipolar resectoscope causes a reduced risk of hyponatremia as normal saline is used as the distension media. It causes vaporization and desiccation of tissues so the specimen is not available for histopathological examination (HPE).

INTRODUCTION

Leiomyomas of the uterus are the commonest solid pelvic tumors in women, present in 20 to 25 percent of women aged more than 35 years. Leiomyomas are associated with infertility, the causal relationship in this regard appearing to be more evident for submucosal myomas. Of all the myomata, 5 percent are submucosal,[1] although in selected groups, this may be as high as 18 percent.[2]

Several hypotheses have been suggested to explain how submucosal myomas cause infertility or repeated abortions, but none are definitive. Submucous or intramural myomata may cause dysfunctional uterine contractility, which may interfere with sperm migration, ovum transport or nidation.[3-5] In addition, uterine myomata may be associated with preconceptional (implantation) failure or gestational discontinuation due to focal endometrial vascular disturbance as well as endometrial inflammation, secretion of vasoactive substances, or an enhanced endometrial androgen environment.[4,6] In another study that examined the ultrastructure of the host myometrium of fibromyomatas uteri,[7] the sacrolemmal dense bands of host myometrial myocytes were found to be of significantly greater length than that of normal myometria with a corresponding decrease in the number of caveolae, making the host myometria structurally abnormal. This specific abnormality may affect calcium metabolism in these tissues, which in turn, may cause abnormal contractions leading to reproductive wastage or infertility.

CLASSIFICATION OF SUBMUCOSAL FIBROIDS (TABLE 25.1)

The European Society of Hysteroscopy has agreed on a classification for submucous fibroids.[8]

A submucous fibroid is the one that distorts the uterine cavity. It is further divided into three subtypes:

Type 0: Pedunculated fibroid without intramural extension.

Type 1: Sessile with intramural extension of fibroid of <50 percent.

Type 2: Sessile with intramural extension of fibroid of >50 percent.

Table 25.1: Classification of intrauterine myomas by the European Society of Hysteroscopy

Grade 0 (G0)	Myoma with development limited to the uterine cavity, pedunculated or with limited implant base	
Grade 1 (G1)	Myoma with partial intramural development, intramural component < 50 percent. Angle of protrusion between the myoma and the uterine wall <90°	
Grade 2 (G2)	Myoma with predominantly intramural development. Intramural component >50 percent. Angle of protrusion between the myoma and the uterine wall >90°	

The degree of intramural extension can be assessed by transvaginal ultrasonography or by hysteroscopy by observing the angle between the fibroid and the endometrium at the attachment to the uterine wall.

CLINICAL DISCUSSION

Impact of Fibroids on Assisted Conception (Table 25.2)

A few retrospective cohort studies have examined the impact of fibroids on the results of assisted conception. Results for each type of fibroid are separately analyzed in Table 25.2. The pregnancy rate per embryo transfer in submucous, intramural and subserosal fibroids were 9, 16 and 37 percent respectively, compared with an average of 30 percent in control subjects. The miscarriage rates in various types of fibroids were: submucous 40 percent, intramural 33 percent and subserosal 33 percent compared with the total of 16.4 percent among all the control subjects.

From the data in Table 25.2, it appears that patients should be advised to have submucous and possibly intramural fibroids removed prior to *in vitro* fertilization (IVF).

Preoperative Diagnostic Assessment

Preoperative diagnostic assessment consists of transvaginal ultrasound (TVS). TVS is useful to confirm the diagnosis and to assess the number, size and location of myomas. Ultrasonography must indicate the extent of myomal intramural extension and particularly, the free margin. Three-dimensional (3D) and four-dimensional (4D) USG has almost replaced the need for preoperative magnetic resonance imaging (MRI).

Author	Total cases	ET	PR	IR	FR	LB	On going PR	MR	Control subjects (n)	ET	PR	LB	MR	IR	FR	On going PR
Table 25.2: Outcome of assisted conception treatment in women with fibroids [9-16]																
Subjects with submucosal fibroids																
Farhi et al. (1995)	18	55	5\55 (9)	-	-	3/5 (60)	-	2/5 (40)	50	127	32\127 (25)	24/32 (75)	8/32 (25)	-	-	-
Eldar Geva et al. (1998)	9	10	1\10 (10)	-	-	NS	-	NS	249	318	98/318 (30)	78/h98 (80)	20/98 (20)	-	-	-
Subjects with subserosal fibroids																
Eldar Geva et al. (1998)	46	55	9\55* (16)	-	-	6/9 (67)	-	3/9 (33)	249	318	98/31 (30)	78/98 (80)	20/98 (20)	-	-	-
Flavio Garcia Oliveria et al. 2004	117	-	45/110	-	-	78/245 (32)	-	28/110	110	-	78	77/245 (31.5)	39	-	-	-
Subjects with intramural fibroids																
Seoud et al. (1992)	11	24	10/24 (42)	-	-	5/10 (50)	-	5/10 (50)	1357	2018	586/2018 (29)	484/586 (83)	102/586 (17)	-	-	-
Eldar Geva et al. (1998)	33	41	14/41 (34)	-	-	11/14 (79)	-	3/14 (21)	249	318	98/318 (30)	78/98 (80)	20/98 (20)	-	-	-
R Hart and Yanoub (2001)	106	-	23.3	11.9	-	-	15.1	-	-	-	34.1	-	-	20.9	-	28.3
Z Rafael Tel Aviv	94	-	21.2	-	57.8	-	-	9.09	184	-	22.8	-	8.69	-	58.3	-
Subjects with intramural subserosal fibroids																
Ramzy et al. (1998)	39	39	15/39 (39)	-	-	9/15 (60)	-	6/15 (40)	367	367	123/367 (34)	104/123 (85)	19/123 (15)	-	-	-
Stovali et al. (1998)	91	91	34/91 (37)	-	-	30/34 (88)	-	4/34 (12)	91	91	48/91 (53)	44/48 (92)	4/91 (4.4)	-	-	-
Farhi et al. (1995)	28	86	25/86 (29)	-	-	15/25 (60)	-	10/25 (40)	50	127	32/127 (25)	24/32 (75)	8/32 `(25)	-	-	-

Abbreviations: ET: embryo transfer; PR: pregnancy rate; IR: implantation rate; LB: live births; MR: miscarriage rate

Role of Preoperative GnRH Agonist

There are several publications to support preoperative gonadotropin-releasing hormone (GnRH) treatment.[17-20] Owing to their transient effect, analogs can be used as a preoperative treatment. This therapy results in substantial reduction in the tumor size and control of symptoms, such as menorrhagia and abnormal uterine bleeding. The reduction in volume significantly promotes the hysteroscopic management of larger or multiple myomas. It also controls intravascular intravasation of distension media. It also gives us time to correct anemia. Gonadotropin-releasing hormone (GnRH) analogs can also be used when an initial hysteroscopic attempt fails to completely remove the myoma. Shrinking of a persistent tumor, which is partially intramural, combined with the contractile activity of uterine fibers, provokes protrusion in the uterine cavity. This helps the surgeon to remove the remaining segment in a second hysteroscopic intervention.

Preparation of the patient

It is preferable to do the procedure in the immediate postmenstrual period as this does not require any particular preparation of the patient. It is advisable to take a detailed case history and perform an in depth gynecological work-up. In addition, it is always wise to perform hysteroscopic myomectomy in a fully equipped operating room, where any complications can be dealt with and where simultaneous laparoscopy can be performed in the most complicated cases or when intraoperative complications have occurred.

As regards to the hysteroscopic operability of myoma dimensions and site, the classification proposed by the European Society of Hysteroscopy is currently the best guide for identifying the type of leiomyoma by the degree of intramural development.

Obviously, while even an inexperienced surgeon can handle myomas of Grade 0, myomas of Grade 2 require a great deal of experience in hysteroscopic surgery. It is interesting to note that this classification makes no mention of myoma dimensions, which plays an important role in decision-making regarding the operability. The dimensions of the myoma have a marked effect on the angle. Indeed, despite an open angle of protrusion, small myomas can be easily removed because of their smaller intramural mass; the opposite holds true for large myomas with relatively acute angles and even those reaching the myometrial serous membrane because of their very large size. However, the operability also depends on the intra-mural component of the myoma itself and, in particular, the free margin, i.e. the thickness of the myometrium remaining between the deep edge of the myoma and serous peritoneum of the uterus. Various authors set this safety margin at 0.5 to 1.0 cm.

Anesthesia

Operative hysteroscopy can be performed both, with local anesthesia, administered by a paracervical block, or under general anesthesia. We routinely operate Grade 0 myomas with size less than 2 cm with an office hysteroscope and Versapoint and without any anesthesia.

Surgical Technique

Myomas with a submucosal localization can be treated exclusively using an operative hysteroscope, the standard surgical approach. Neuwirth and Amin[21] first suggested that hysteroscopic myomectomy may be the procedure of choice for treating submucosal myomas.[21] Several retrospective studies of small case series were published during the 1990s,[14,22-25] demonstrating successful reproductive outcomes after hysteroscopic removal of submucosal myomas in infertile women.

The size and number of fibroids to be removed depends upon the individual surgical skill and experience. It is advisable not to remove big anterior and posterior fibroids in the same sitting to avoid intrauterine adhesions or synechiae formation. It is very important to know ahead of time if we are dealing with a type 0, type I or type II, not only because the type II myomas may require more than one sitting, but there is also a slightly different technique when a type 0, type I and type II is resected.

For leiomyoma resection, a 26 Fr resectoscope is normally used with 30 degree telescope. A smaller resectoscope (22 Fr) is used if the uterine cavity and/or cervical canal is narrow. After cervical dilatation upto 10 mm, the resectoscope with the electrosurgical working element for control of the 900 cutting loop is introduced. Distension of the uterine cavity is obtained with glycine or a sorbitol/mannitol solution. Irrigation is controlled with an electronic suction and an irrigation pump, which automatically controls both intrauterine pressure and the flow rate. The system also ensures constant suction.

The following settings are generally used: Flow rate of approximately 250 mL/min, pressure of 80 to 100 mm Hg, monopolar electricity generator at 60 to 100 Watts and suction pressure of 0.25 Bar. The fluid balance is recorded by measuring the infused and drained fluid from the continuous flow resectoscope.

Basic
1. Hold the camera in your left hand (if you are right-handed)
2. Hold the scope with your right hand
3. Know which is the inflow and outflow.

Main Techniques of Resection

Resection is performed by placing the electrical loop behind the myoma to be resected and retracting it towards the distal lens of the hysteroscope (Fig. 25.1).

Type 0: It is systematically shaved off with the resectoscope loop until the pedicle is reached (Figs 25.2A to D). Type 0 myoma should never be dislodged at the base first, which is the most tempting thing to do. One should avoid this as removal of floating myoma from uterine cavity creates a great problem. Once it is separated, resection and slicing down to smaller pieces is not possible.

Type 1 and Type 2: If the myoma is smaller in size, one can give a semicircular incision on the inferior margin at the angle between the myoma and uterine wall. The myoma can be enucleated in toto from its capsule by giving simple mechanical pressure with the loop at the lower edge. One should not attempt this technique for larger myomas, as again, removal of the enucleated myoma will be a great problem.

While resecting Type 1 and Type 2 myomas, particular care should be taken with regard to the intrauterine pressure.

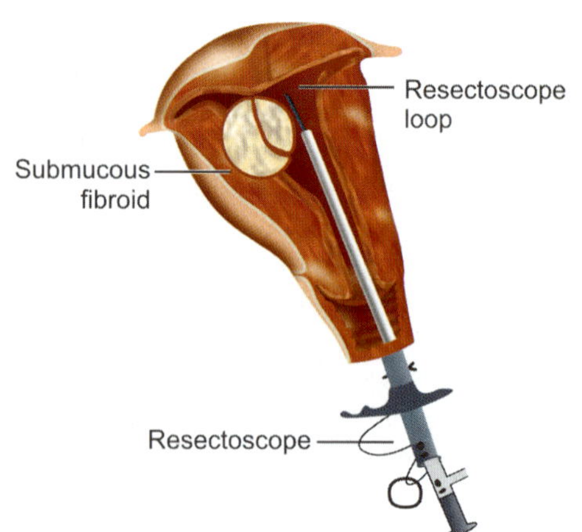

Fig. 25.1: Electrical loop behind the myoma

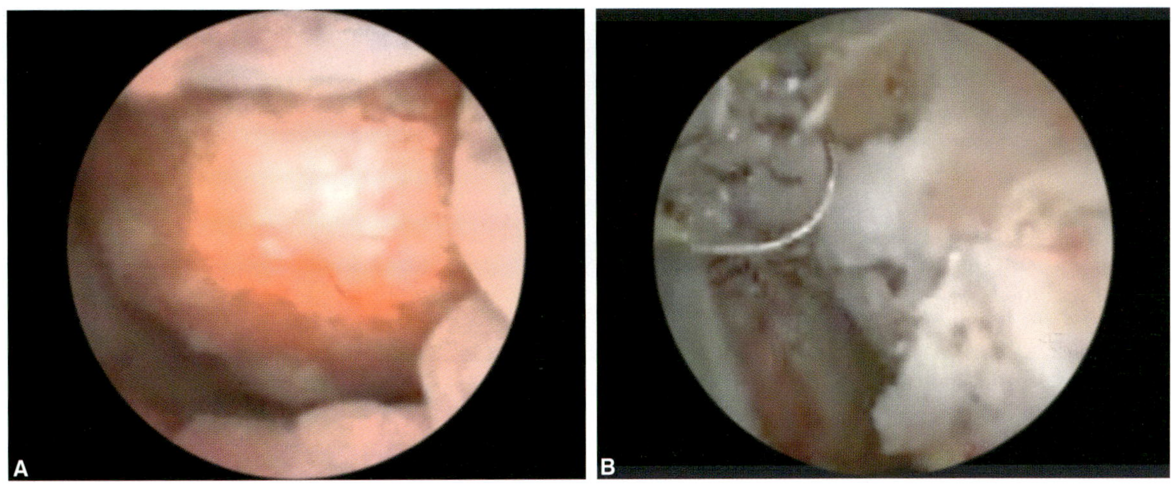

Figs 25.2A and B: (A) Type 0 myoma; (B) Resection of myoma

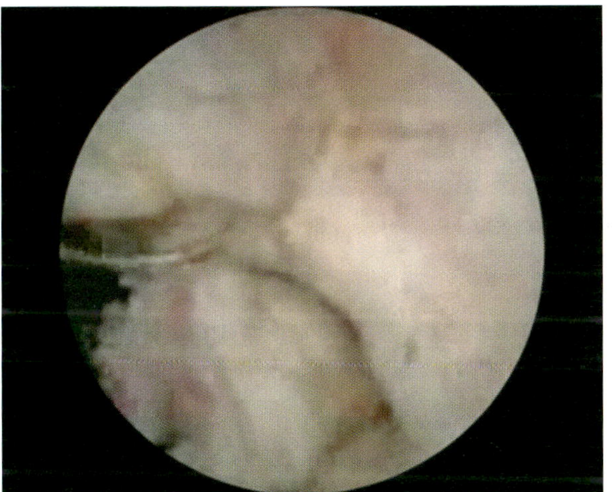

Fig. 25.2C: Resection till pedicle base

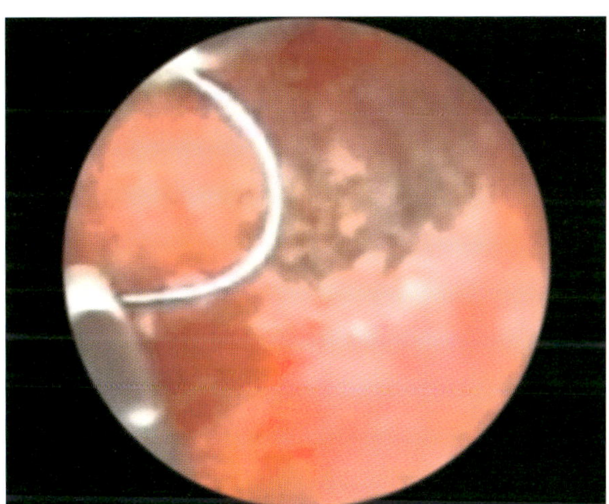

Fig. 25.2D: End result

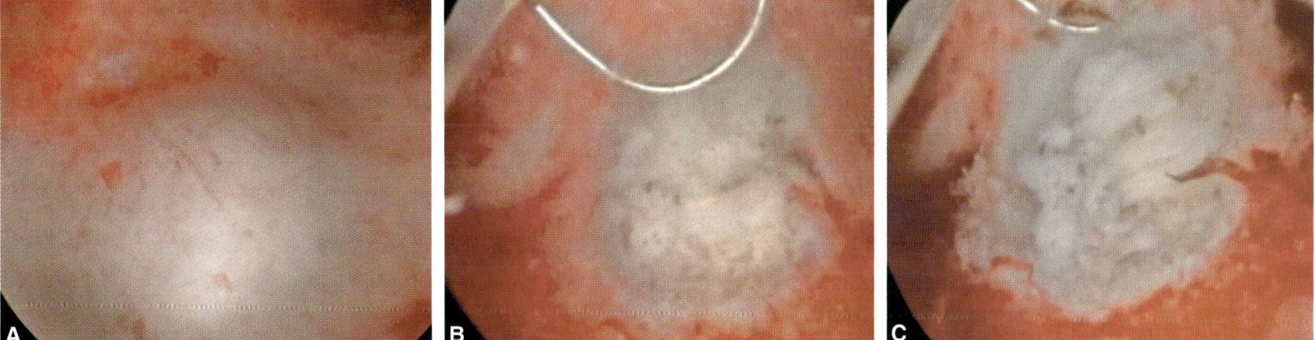

Figs 25.3A to C: (A) Type 2 myoma; (B) Resection with loop; (C) Resection till myoma becomes flat

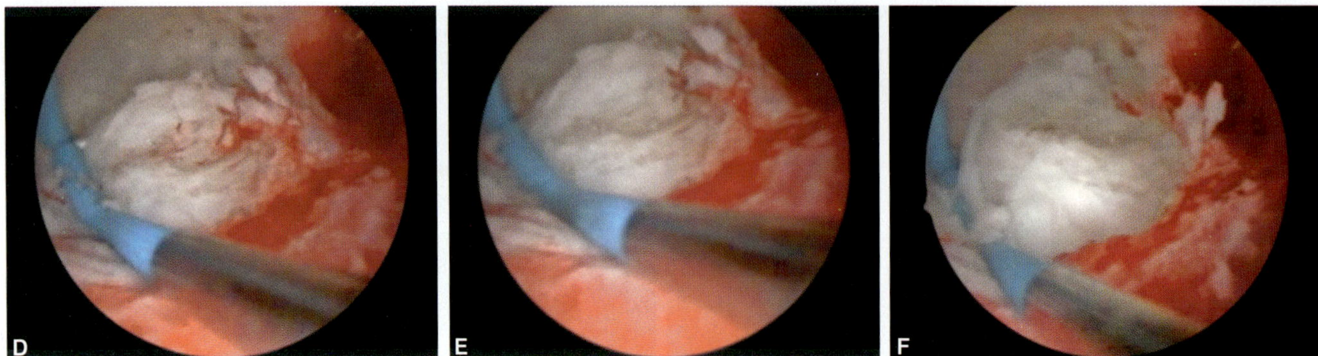

Figs 25.3D to F: (D) Grade II myoma nested deep; (E) Cold knife enucleation; (F) Cold knife enucleation

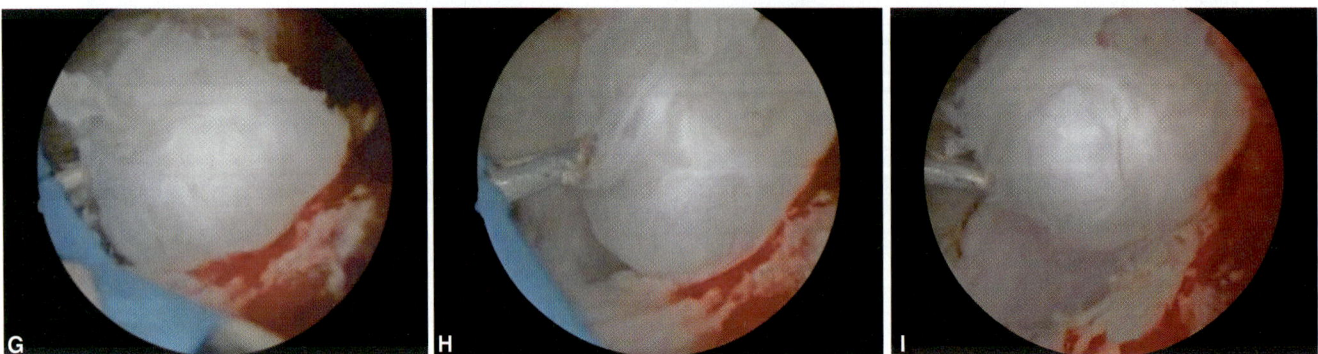

Figs 25.3G to I: (G) Enucleation; (H) Completely enucleated; (I) Completely enucleated with crater in the background

If the pressure is very high, fibroids will be pushed deep into the wall making resection difficult and also, it may increase the intravasation of fluid. To prevent this, the minimal pressure that gives adequate distension and clear vision is used. Resection is done by placing the loop behind the myoma and retracting it towards the scope. The myoma is shaved down with a slicing technique, with the cutting loop to the level of myometrium till the myoma becomes flat (Figs 25.3A to C). After having dissected the portion of myoma protruding into the cavity, an attempt is made to remove the part nested deep in the myometrial wall.

This can be achieved by two techniques:

1. By giving hydromassage by controlled variation of the endocavitary pressure (opening and closing the endo-uterine aspiration system)
2. Cold knife technique, which consists of simple, mechanical passage of the resectoscope loop or Colin's knife along the capsule lining of the myoma, detaching it from the fibrous bridges that anchors it to the uterine wall, without any electrocoagulation (Figs 25.3D to I).

The operation can be considered complete when only the myometrium can be seen throughout the entire surgical area. Utmost care should be taken to prevent damaging the smooth muscle fiber bundles. If it is impossible to totally remove the intramural fibroid in one sitting, despite the above techniques, if it is too deep or because of technical difficulties, the remaining myoma can be coagulated until dry. This effect is achieved by placing the loop in direct contact with the remaining wall of the myoma and applying a high coagulation current for approximately 30 seconds. The fibroid can then be treated at a later date (2–3 months later) as over this period, the intramural component of myoma migrates into the uterine cavity.

When the surgery is complete, very rarely is it necessary to perform selective coagulation of any bleeding myometrial vessels. In the vast majority of the cases, myometrial contractions are sufficient to stop bleeding.

Complications, such as uterine perforation or bleeding, are related more to the surgeon's skills than to the technique used. Intrauterine pressure and duration of surgery are the main factors that can affect the safety of hysteroscopic surgery.

The following intraoperative precautions are recommended:

1. Meticulous attention to intraoperative fluid balance is imperative if a fluid deficit more than 1 to 1.5 liters is detected. Serum sodium is measured and hyponatremia, if present, should be treated. For every liter of electrolyte-free fluid that is absorbed the sodium level will decrease

by approximately 10 mEq/L. This helps the surgeon to determine when to stop a case. If the deficit is approximately 1500 cc, it is advisable to put in a Foley's catheter and give a diuretic.

2. Continuous suction, using a multichannel hysteroscope with wide outflow, is recommended to avoid increased intrauterine pressure above safe levels (70–100 mm Hg). This also facilitates clear field of vision.

3. For surgeons with less experience it is advisable to avoid prolonged operative time and excess fluid use for irrigation in cases of large or multiple myomas. In fact, they should avoid operating grade 2 myomas.

4. Less absorption should occur if resection takes place when the endometrium is relatively avascular in the mid-proliferative phase of menstrual cycle.

5. It is important to diagnose patients who are at great risk of absorbing excessive volumes of fluids: those who have patent Fallopian tubes, no endometrial preparation, large uterine fibroids and poor cardiovascular reserve.

6. Absorption of large volumes of electrolyte-free, low viscosity fluid, especially with large myomas, triggers some systemic changes during the operation. Myomectomy of large myomas is liable to hyponatremia, hypo-osmolality, increased cardiovascular pressure (CVP), increased prothrombin time (PT) and partial thromboplastin time (PTT) and increases most of the cardiodynamic parameters.[26-29] These changes demand that the procedure be performed by an experienced hysteroscopic surgeon using a quick technique with the least possible glycine volume and minimal intrauterine pressure to achieve the goal of a safe minimal access surgery.

Postoperative Care and Follow-up

1. Intraoperative antibiotics are administered to all patients. Most of the time, the patient is discharged on the day of surgery.

2. Routine transvaginal sonography is sufficient to know the optimum results of surgery. Follow-up diagnostic hysteroscopy is generally performed only if multiple myomas are removed in one sitting.

Gynecare Versapoint

Versapoint is a bipolar electrosurgical unit (Figs 25.4A and B). It consists of:
1. Dedicated generators
2. Three 5 Fr electrodes
3. Bipolar resectoscope.

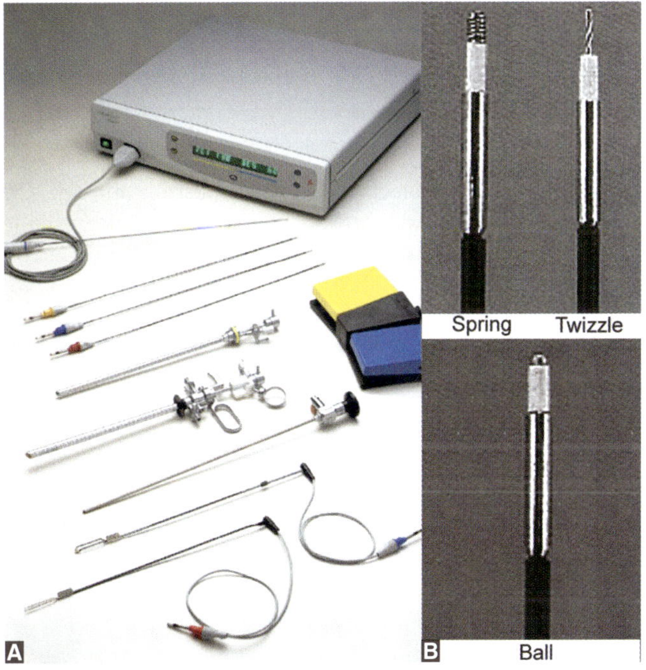

Figs 25.4A and B: (A) Generators; (B) 5 Fr electrodes

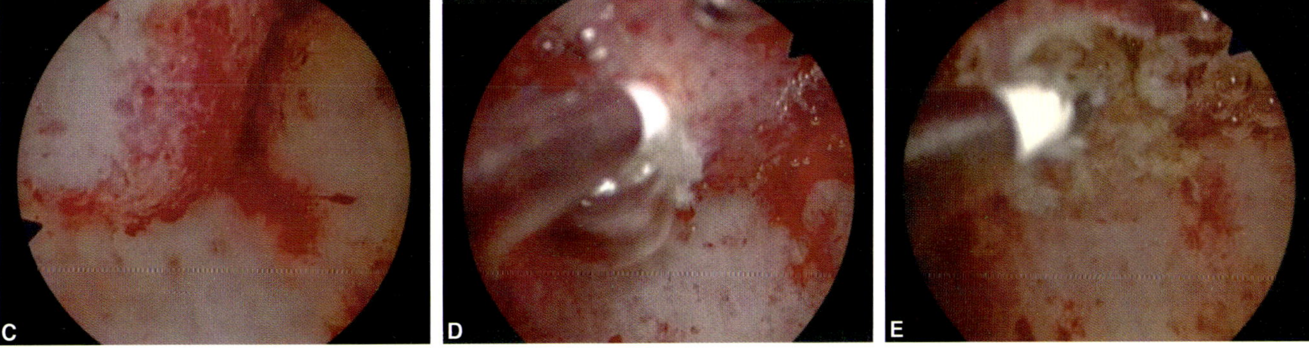

Figs 25.4C to E: (C) Myoma; (D) Versapoint electrode in action; (E) Vaporization of myoma with Versapoint

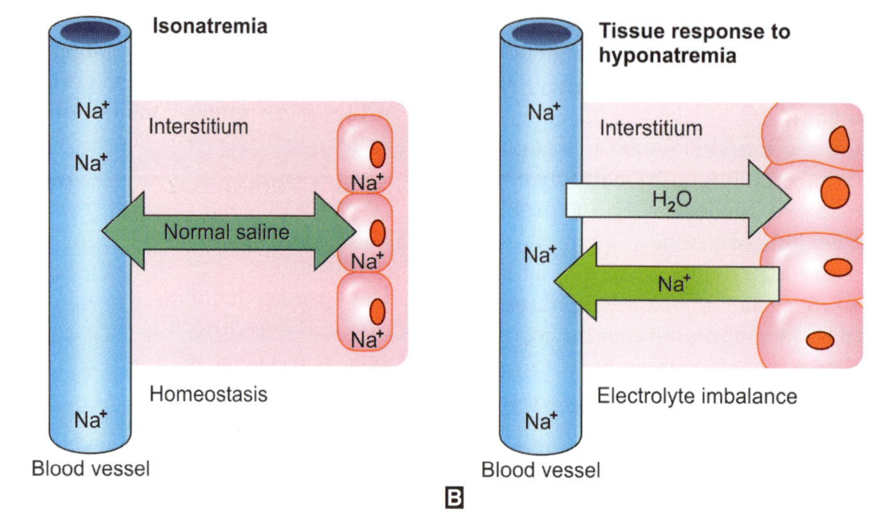

Figs 25.5A and B: Tissue response to hyponatremia

The Versapoint electrode can be passed through the operative channel of therapeutic sheath of the hysteroscope and small myomas (<2 cm) can be dealt with (Figs 25.4C to E).

The advantage of bipolar electrosurgery:

1. It can be used in saline as distention media.
2. Allows for a larger volume of fluid infusion with minimum risk of fluid overload.
3. Reduced risk of hyponatremia compared to non-physiologic solutions.[30-31] Intravascular absorption of non-physiologic solutions may cause hyponatremia, which can result in cerebral and pulmonary edema or cardiac arrhythmia. Normal saline contains physiologic levels of sodium and, therefore, does not disrupt homeostasis (Figs 25.5A and B).
4. Controlled predictable tissue effects.
5. No stray current through patient's body.

Mechanism of Versapoint (Fig. 25.6)

The bipolar system of Gynecare Versapoint functions as follows:

Saline acts as a "safety valve", pulling the electrosurgical current through the path of least resistance and back in the return electrode to the generator.

Vaporization creates a vapor pocket or steam bubble that causes instantaneous cellular rupture upon contact with tissue.

Desiccation dehydrates the cells and leads to hemostasis. Energy returns through the return electrode to prevent over treatment or carbonization.

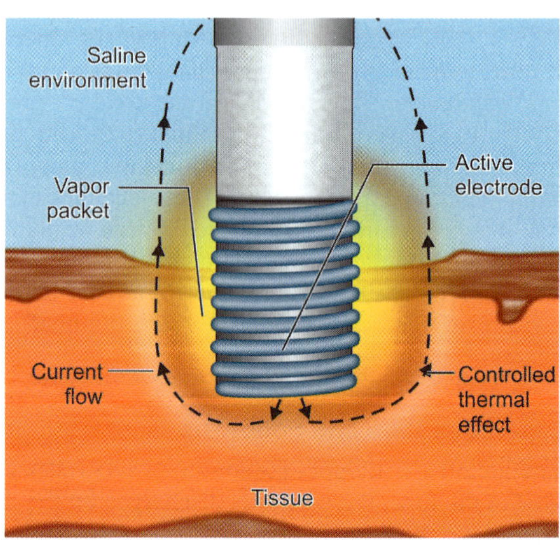

Fig. 25.6: Mechanism of Versapoint

Limitatons with Versapoint

1. Electrodes cannot be used for large myomas but with the bipolar resectoscope, large myomas can be dealt with.
2. Cost of equipment and disposables is the major concern.
3. Since it works with the principle of vaporization, the specimen is not available for histopathological examination.

Complications with Versapoint

Complications as such, only with Versapoint, are rare but air embolism can be a possibility.

Versapoint functions by creating a vapor bubble. These vapor bubbles have been shown to be carbon dioxide, carbon monoxide and hydrogen ions. These vapor bubbles are rapidly absorbed in the bloodstream. They diffuse in the bloodstream and are washed off through respiration. However, if the rate of accumulation of bubbles is faster than the rate of dispersion, signs of air embolism or gas embolism sets in, in the form of a drop in the end tidal CO_2. If, while using this system, signs of gas embolism are noticed, it is advisable to wait for about 15 seconds to allow the body to get rid of it following which, the procedure can be continued. It is a very safe system to use as long as one is aware of its potential complications.

CONCLUSION

Several hypotheses have been suggested to explain how the submucous myoma causes infertility. Retrospective cohort studies have shown that the pregnancy rate and take home baby rate has definitely improved after hysteroscopic myomectomy. Preoperative assessment by transvaginal sonography plays an important role. We do not advise preoperative GnRH preparations. The size and number of fibroids to be removed in one sitting depends upon the grade of myoma, individual skill and expertise. An expert endoscopic surgeon can even remove type 2 myomas in one sitting. Though the Versapoint works on the principle of bipolar energy, its advantage over the monopolar electrosurgical unit has not been proven in any study. One needs to know that utmost care should be taken to prevent damage to the smooth muscle fiber bundles of the myometrium, hence, the cold knife technique may be superior for deep-seated myomas. Intrauterine pressure and duration of surgery are the main factors that can affect the safety of hysteroscopic surgery.

REFERENCES

1. Novak ER, Woodruff JD. Myoma and other benign tumors of the uterus. In Gynecologic and Obstetrics pathology, 8th Edition. WB Saunders, Philadelphia: 1979.pp.260-78.
2. Fedele L, Bianchi S, Dorta M, Brioschi D, Zanotti F, Vercellini P. Transvaginal ultrasonography versus hysteroscopy in the diagnosis of uterine submucous myomas. Obstet Gynecol 1991;77:745-8.
3. Hunt JE, Wallach EE. Uterine factor in infertility and overview. Clin Gynaecol 1974;17:44-64.
4. Buttram VC Jr, Reiter RC. Uterine lieomyoata etiology, symptomatology and management. Fertil Steril 1981;36:433-45.
5. Vollenhoven BJ, Lowrence AS, Hely DL. Uterine fibroids: a clinical review. Br J Obstet Gynaecol 1990;97:285-98.
6. Deligdish L, Lowenthal M. Endometrial changes associated with myomates of the uterus. J Clin Pathol 1970;23:676-80.
7. Richards PA, Richards PD, Tiltman AJ. The ultrastructure of fibromyomatas myometrium and its relationship to infertility. Hum. Reprod. Update 1998;4:520-5.
8. Wamsteker K, Emanuel MH, de Kruif JH. Transcervical hysteroscopic resection of submucous fibroids for abnormal uterine bleeding: results regarding the degrees of intramural extension. Obstet. Gynaecol 1993;82:736-40.
9. Farhi J, Ashkenazi J, Feldberg D, Dicker D, Orvieto R, Ben Rafael Z. Effect of uterine leiomyomata on the results of *in vitro* fertilization treatment. Hum Reprod 1995;10:2576-8.
10. Eldar-Geva T, Meagher S, Healy DL, MacLachlan V, Breheny S, Wood C. Effect of intramural, subserosal, and submucosal uterine fibroids on the outcome of assisted reproductive technology treatment. Fertil Steril 1998;70:687-91.
11. Seoud MA, Patterson R, Muasher SJ, Coddington CC. 3rd. Effects of myomas or prior myomectomy on *in vitro* fertilization (IVF) performance. J Assist Reprod Genet 1992; 9:217-21.
12. Ramzy AM, Sattar M, Amin Y, Mansour RT, Serour GI, Aboulghar MA. Uterine myomata and outcome of assisted reproduction. Hum Reprod 1998;13:198-202.
13. Stovall DW, Parrish SB, Van Voorhis BJ, Hahn SJ, Sparks AE, Syrop CH. Uterine leiomyomas reduce the efficacy of assisted reproduction cycles: results of a matched follow-up study. Hum Reprod 1998;13:192-7.
14. Donnez J, Gillerot S. Bourgonjon D, Clerckx F, Nisolle M. Neodymium: YAG laser hysteroscopy in large submucous fibroids. Fertil Steril 1990;54:999-1003.
15. Oliveira FG, Abdelmassih VG, Diamond MP, Dozortsev D, Melo NR, Abdelmassih R. Impact of subserosal and intramural uterine fibroids that do not distort the endometrial cavity on the outcome of *in vitro* fertilization intracytoplasmic sperm injection. Fertil Steril. 2004;81: 582-7.
16. Ben-Rafael Z. Treatment of intramural fibroids before IVF—the new dilemma Tel Aviv University, Tel Aviv, Israel Myomectomy or art: which comes first?
17. Lethaby A, Vollenhoven B, Sowter M. Preoperative GnRH analogue therapy before hysterectomy or myomectomy for uterine fibroids. Cochrane Database Syst Rev. 2001;(2): CD000547.
18. Mencaglia L, Tantini C. GnRH agonist analogs and hysteroscopic resection of myomas. Int J Gynaecol Obstet 1993;43:285-8.
19. Romer T. Benefit of GnRH analogue pretreatment for hysteroscopic surgery in patients with bleeding disorders. Gynecol Obstet Invest 1998;45 (Suppl 1):12-20.
20. Crosignani PG, Vercellini P, Meschia M, Oldani S, Bramante T. GnRH agonists before surgery for uterine leiomyomas. A review. J Reprod Med 1996;41:415-21.
21. Neuwirth RS, Amin, HK. Excision of submucous fibroids with hysteroscopic control. Am J Obstet. Gynaecol 1970;126:95-9.
22. Goldenberg M, Sivan E, Sharabi Z, Bider D, Rabinovici J, Seidman DS. Outcome of hysteroscopic resection of submucous myomas for infertility. Fertil Steril 1995;64: 714-6.
23. Giatras K, Berkeley AS, Noyes N, Licciardi F, Lolis D, Grifo JA. Fertility after hysteroscopic resection of submucous myomas. J Am Assoc Gynecol Laparosc 1999;6:155-8.
24. Varasteh NN, Neuwirth RS, Levin B, Keltz MD. Pregnancy rate after hysteroscopic polypectomy and myomectomy in fertile women. Obstet Gynaecol 1999;94:168-71.

25. Vercellini P, Zàina B, Yaylayan L, Pisacreta A, De Giorgi O, Crosignani PG. Hysteroscopic myomectomy: long-term effects on menstrual pattern and fertility. Obstet Gynaecol 1999;94:341-7.
26. Goldenberg M, Zolti M, Seidman DS, Bider D, Mashiach S, Etchin A. Transient blood oxygen desaturation, hypercapnia, and coagulopathy after operative hysteroscopy with glycine used as the distending medium. Am J Obstet Gynecol 1994;170:25-9.
27. Whitehouse MM, Kazmers A. Heart and circulation. In: Borlett, JG, Whitehouse, WM, Turcotte, JG, Harper (Eds). Life support systems in intensive care, 2nd edition. Ch. 5, Year book medical publisher, Inc. Chicago 1984;253.
28. Morgan GF, Mikhail M. Management of patients with fluid and electrolyte disturbance. In: Clinical Anaesthetiology, 2nd edition Chap 28, Lang Medical book publishers, USA, 1996;523-31.
29. Istre O, Skajaa K, Schjoensby AP, Forman A. Changes in serum electrolytes after transcervical resection of endometrium and submucous fibroids with use of glycine 1.5 percent for uterine irrigation. Obstet Gynaecol 1992;80:218-22.
30. Loffer FD, Bradley LD, Brill Al, Brooks PG, Cooper JM. Hysteroscopic fluid monitoring guidelines. The ad hoc committee on hysteroscopic training guidelines of the American Association of Gynecologic Laparoscopists. J Am Assoc Gynecol Laparosc 2000;7:167-8.
31. Davis JA, Miller CD. Fluid infusion during hysteroscopic surgery. In: Lewis BV, Magos AL (Eds). Endometrial Ablation. London, UK: Churchill Livingstone 1993.pp.41-56.

Alternatives to Myomectomy

Roy Mashiach

OVERVIEW

Uterine fibroids are benign tumors arising from the myometrial compartment of the uterus. They are clinically apparent in about 25 percent of women, but can be found in 77 percent of women. Fibroids can cause abnormal uterine bleeding (usually hypermenorrhea, abortions, pelvic pain, pregnancy complications and other symptoms. Fibroids are the primary indication for 200,000 to 300,000 hysterectomies performed each year among women in the United States Several factors determine treatment, including the size and location of the fibroids, the presenting symptoms, the age and reproductive desires of the patient, and the skill of the surgeon. As indicated by its name, this chapter will describe the nonsurgical treatment modalities available for treating uterine fibroids. Oral contraceptives, progestins (local and systemic) and androgens are usually the first-line of treatment. They all work by manipulating the endometrial hormonal environment in order to reduce bleeding. Gonadotropin-releasing hormone (GnRH) agonists competitively down-regulate the GnRH receptor activity at the level of the pituitary and create a hypogonadotropic hypogonadal state clinically resembling menopause. Administration of GnRH analogs results in amenorrhea in most women. A reduction in uterine size, of up to 35 to 65 percent usually occurs. The benefits of GnRH analogs are shadowed by symptoms of severe hypoestrogenism, and by the fibroid's tendency to grow back to Its original size or larger over several months after treatment is discontinued. Myolysis by uterine artery embolization or magnetic resonance imaging (MRI)-guided focused ultrasound are new and effective minimally invasive treatments that are extensively discussed in this chapter. Their main benefits are short treatment duration, safety and low rate of side effects. They are considered safe for women who wish to conceive although concern regarding ovarian function and Asherman's syndrome prevents them from becoming the first line of treatment for patients suffering from infertility.

INTRODUCTION

Uterine fibroids are benign tumors arising from the myometrial compartment of the uterus. They are typically well-differentiated have a relatively low mitotic index, and retain their smooth muscle phenotype. They are clinically apparent in about 25 percent of women, but can be found in 77 percent of pathological specimens.[1] Fibroids are responsible for abnormal uterine bleeding (usually hypermenorrhea) infertility, abortions, pelvic pain, and other symptoms. During pregnancy, fibroids may increase the risk of spontaneous abortions, pain, preterm labor and intrauterine growth retardatlon (IUGR). Fetal deformation, pclvic outlet obstruction, postpartum hemorrhage and puerperal sepsis have been described.

Fibroids are the primary indication for 200,000 to 300,000 hysterectomies performed each year among women in the United States.[2] The pathophysiology of fibroids is not well-understood. The growth of these tumors is associated with steroid hormone concentrations, genetic and racial predisposition.

Uterine fibroids, as benign tumors, can generally be managed expectantly unless they cause symptoms. Several factors determine treatment, including the size and location of the fibroids, the presenting symptoms, the age and reproductive desires of the patient, and the skill of the surgeon.

This chapter will describe the nonsurgical treatment modalities for uterine fibroids.

CLINICAL DISCUSSION

Medical Therapy

Several medical therapies are available for the treatment of uterine fibroids; all of them act by manipulating the hormonal environment. Uterine fibroids are hormonally responsive. Their growth was shown to be dependent on estrogen and progesterone,[3,4] they rarely are observed before puberty, are most prevalent and tend to grow during the reproductive years, can grow during times of elevated steroid levels, such as in pregnancy, and typically regress during menopause.[3] Risk factors for fibroid development, such as obesity, early age of first menarche and infertility, as well as protective factors, like—smoking, exercise, oral contraceptive use, and parity,[5-7] are estrogen-dependent. Estrogen and progesterone receptors were found in higher concentrations in fibroids than in the surrounding myometrium. DNA synthesis in fibroid cells, can be stimulated by estrogen and progesterone and inhibited by their antagonists. Mitotic activity counts of fibroid cells were found to be higher during the secretory phase and during progestin therapy.[8]

Oral Contraceptives

Oral contraceptives, whether in the form of combined or progesterone only pills, are often the first-line of treatment for patients with uterine fibroids and abnormal uterine bleeding. These agents can decrease bleeding by producing endometrial atrophy and stabilization, but do not reduce the size of the fibroids.[3,9] Moreover, *in vitro* evidence suggests that estrogens and progestins can stimulate fibroid growth and should therefore, be used carefully in patients with symptomatic fibroids.[10]

Marshall et al.[7] used data from the Nurses' Health Study II to investigate the association between oral contraceptive use and incidence of fibroids. The only notable association with any aspect of oral contraceptive use was a significantly elevated risk among women who first used oral contraceptives between the ages 13 to 16 years compared with those who had never used oral contraceptives.

Progestin Therapy

Progestin studies have shown mixed results in the treatment of fibroids. On one hand, early small studies and case reports showed a marked enlargement of fibroids during progestin therapy, an effect that was reversed after the therapy was discontinued.[11,12] Furthermore, significant fibroid growth occurred with the use of progestins as add-back therapy after gonadotropin-releasing hormone (GnRH) analog treatment.[13,14] *In vitro*, the mitotic activity in fibroids was significantly greater with progestin therapy, whereas mitotic activity with estrogen-progestin therapy and in controls was

the same.[8] On the other hand, several studies documented a decrease in the size of a myomatous uterus during progestin therapy.[15] Venkatachalam et al.[16] administered medroxyprogesterone acetate (MPA) (Depo-Provera), 150 mg/months for 6 months, to 20 premenopausal (average age 35 years) South African women who had symptomatic multifibroid uteri of the size of 14 to 22 weeks.[16] Amenorrhea was achieved in six participants (30%) within 3 months of initiation of MPA. Fourteen of 20 participants (70%) experienced resolution or improvement in their bleeding, 15 percent had a mean increase in hemoglobin levels (from 9.35 g/dL to 10.78 g/dL), and a reduction in mean uterine (48%) and mean fibroid volumes (33%).[16] Although larger randomized studies are indicated, this therapy may be valuable in regions of the world where other therapies are not available.[16]

Progestin-containing Intrauterine Contraceptive Devices

The Levonorgestrel intrauterine system (LNG-IUS) has been studied extensively; it is a proven, effective, reversible treatment for menorrhagia, which functions by inducing endometrial atrophy and inactivity.[17,18] Studies showed a reduction in menstrual blood loss by up to 90 percent after 3 to 12 months of use with few side effects and high patient satisfaction.[17,18] Side effects included irregular bleeding, headache, nausea, mastalgia, acne, functional ovarian cysts, depression, weight gain, and lower abdominal pain.[18] Enlarged or distorted uterine cavity or a submucosal fibroid are contraindications for LNG-IUS use.

Grigorieva and colleagues[19] studied 67 premenopausal women with mildly enlarged (<12 weeks) uteri, 39 percent of whom had menorrhagia. A significant reduction in menstrual blood loss was noted after 3 months and persisted for 12 months; 40 percent of the patients had amenorrhea at 12 months. Reduction in fibroid size was not significant.[19] In a study by Inki et al.[20] there was no change in uterine in fibroid size but a decrease in endometrial thickness was noted.[20]

Androgen Therapy

Danazol and Gestrinone have been extensively studied for the treatment of uterine fibroids. Danazol inhibits pituitary gonadotropin secretion and ovarian steroid production and suppresses endometrial growth. Danazol's main effect is androgenic, but it also has moderate progestogenic, anti-progestogenic and anti-estrogenic properties.[21,22] Danazol effectively decreased fibroid volume when given at 400 mg/day for 4 months (24% decrease in fibroid volume).[21]

Gestrinone has anti-estrogenic and anti-progestogenic properties. It induces amenorrhea and decreases fibroid volume. Gestrinone is not available in the United States.

The androgenic side effects of these treatments including weight gain, edema, decreased breast size, acne, oily skin, hirsutism, a deepened voice, headache, hot flushes, altered libido and muscle cramps, and more serious but rare side effects, such as hepatocellular damage, marked fluid retention and spontaneous pregnancy loss, prevent them from being true alternatives for women with fibroids.

Steroid Synthesis Inhibitors

Gonadotropin-releasing hormone (GnRH) agonists

Treatment with GnRH agonists is the mainstay of medical therapy for fibroids. These agents act by competitive inhibition of the GnRH receptor at the level of the pituitary. They first increase the release of luteinizing hormone (LH) and follicle-stimulating hormone (FSH) ("flare-up effect") and then, by receptor down regulation, create a hypogonadotropic hypogonadal state, clinically resembling menopause. Administration of GnRH analogs results in amenorrhea in most women.

These agents produce a significant reduction in uterine size, generally 35 to 65 percent.[15] The decrease in size is most pronounced within three months of treatment.[23] This volume reduction probably accounts for the reduction in symptoms such as bleeding, pelvic pressure and pain and distortion of adjacent organs observed.[24]

The benefits of GnRH analogs are shadowed by the symptoms of severe hypoestrogenism: hot flushes, headaches, vaginal dryness, depression, and bone demineralization that leads to osteoporosis.[3,4,25,26] Furthermore, after discontinuation of therapy, fibroids tend to grow back to their original size or larger over several months.[21,23,24,27] Although the side effects of GnRH analogs can be alleviated by add-back therapy using estrogen, progestin, or both, the addition of hormones can limit the effectiveness of this therapy in reducing uterine and fibroid size.

GnRH agonists are not appropriate for prolonged use and are primarily used to allow a woman to prepare for surgery and for perimenopausal women.[23-25,27]

GnRH antagonists

These medications block pituitary GnRH receptors and produce an immediate decline in FSH and LH without the "flare-up" effect of the analogs. They have been shown to reduce fibroid and uterine volume.[28-30] Flierman et al.[29] have studied the effect of daily treatment with 2 mg of the GnRH antagonist Ganirelix in 20 women with symptomatic fibroids requiring surgery. They performed weekly ultrasounds and hormonal studies. The median change in fibroid volume was 42.7 percent when measured by ultrasonography (USG) and 29.2 percent when assessed by magnetic resonance imaging (MRI). The median number of days of treatment to achieve maximal fibroid size reduction was 19 (1 to 65). Seventeen patients (85%) reported at least one adverse event. Hot flushes and headaches were reported most frequently in 75 percent and 45 percent of the cases, respectively. These results are comparable to those obtained following treatment with GnRH analogs, but were achieved sooner. Larger studies are needed to investigate how fibroids behave after treatment is discontinued.

Future Directions for Treatment

The biology of uterine fibroids has been explained in terms of steroid hormones. All current medical therapies manipulate these hormones. Innovative ways to modulate the actions of these hormones are the basis for future treatment directions.

Aromatase inhibitors

Aromatase inhibitors inhibit ovarian estrogen synthesis in the ovary. Fibroids over express aromatase, which synthesizes estrogen, and may produce their own estrogen.[31] Adrozole, an aromatase inhibitor, was used to treat a 53 year old woman with a 20 weeks pregnant size myomatous uterus that caused acute urinary retention[32] Fibroid volume declined by 61 percent at 4 weeks and 71 percent at 8 weeks, and the urinary retention resolved by 14 days.[32] The main advantage of aromatase inhibitors is their rapid hypoestrogenic effect and lack of "flare-up" effect that allows the initiation of therapy at any time in the menstrual cycle. Aromatase inhibitors could be developed to inflict a differential effect on ovarian and fibroid estrogen production, and thus, act preferentially to cause fibroid shrinkage without causing hypoestrogenism and the related adverse effects.[31] Further research is necessary in the reproductive-age population.

Steroid antagonists

Mifepristone: High concentrations of progesterone receptors have been identified in fibroids compared with the surrounding myometrium.[7] Studies have shown marked enlargement of fibroids during progestin therapy.[11,12] Furthermore, significant fibroid growth occurred with the use of progestins as add-back therapy after GnRH analog treatment.[13,14] *In vitro*, the mitotic activity in fibroids was significantly greater with progestin therapy, whereas mitotic activity with estrogen-progestin therapy and in controls was the same.[8]

Mifepristone, or RU-486, targets and reduces the number of progesterone receptors and effectively produces amenorrhea and fibroid suppression.[24,33,34] Mifepristone also inhibits ovarian cyclicity, maintains a hormonal state similar to the early follicular phase, and affects the vascular supply of fibroids.[33-35] Small studies that used Mifepristone, 12.5 mg to 50 mg/day, noted a 40 to 50 percent reduction in fibroid volume and a high prevalence of amenorrhea; vasomotor symptoms were the most common side effects. Mifepristone achieves fibroid regression through a direct antiprogesterone effect.[34] Daily doses of 5, 25 and 50 mg RU-486 were used in a small number of patients.[35] All three doses induced ovarian acyclicity. Fibroid volume decreased to 44 to 78.1 percent of the baseline. Mifepristone, 25 mg daily, appears to be the effective dose to cause a clinically significant 50 percent decrease in fibroid volume.

Eisinger et al.[36] used Mifepristone 5 to 10 mg/day for 6 months to treat premenopausal women with symptomatic fibroids.[36] Overall, there was a similar prevalence of hot flushes and simple endometrial hyperplasia without atypia (28% of subjects overall). Fibroid volume decrease was comparable (48% vs 49%, respectively). Fibroid symptoms were reduced in both groups, and amenorrhea was prevalent in 60 to 65 percent of the patients.[36]

Steinauer and colleagues[33] reviewed six clinical trials from 1985 to 2002. Overall, 166 premenopausal women with symptomatic fibroids were treated with 5 to 50 mg/day of Mifepristone for 3 to 6 months. Although these studies had many methodological flaws, they consistently demonstrated that daily administration of Mifepristone resulted in significantly decreased mean fibroid volume (26–74%) and uterine volume (27–49%); up to a 75 percent reduction in fibroid related symptoms, such as menorrhagia, dysmenorrhea, and pelvic pressure, and a 91 percent rate of amenorrhea. There was no correlation between dosage and response. Significant side effects included hot flushes (38%), elevated hepatic enzymes, and endometrial hyperplasia (found in 14% of the patients that received 10 mg of the drug).

We can conclude that Mifepristone therapy effectively achieves reduction of fibroid related symptoms and fibroid regression while maintaining stable bone density. Endometrial hyperplasia may limit the long-term use of this medication. Further studies are warranted, including direct comparisons with GnRH analogs.

Selective estrogen receptor modulators (SERMs)

Selective estrogen receptor modulators (SERMs) are non-steroidal agents that bind to estrogen receptors and exhibit estrogen agonist or antagonist effects depending on the target tissue. Tamoxifen acts as an antagonist in breast tissue and as agonist in bone, cardiovascular, and endometrial tissue. Tamoxifen was linked to an increased risk for endometrial hyperplasia and cancer.[37] A small retrospective study of the use of Tamoxifen in women with symptomatic fibroid uterus[38] found that after 6 months of treatment, although there was no change in the fibroid size, the blood loss and pelvic pain did improve. Side effects, such as ovarian cyst formation, hot flushes, dizziness, and endometrial thickening, were noted. The investigators concluded that this therapy had marginal benefit for treating symptomatic fibroids, but unacceptable side effects.

Raloxifene, another SERM, has no agonist activity on the endometrium and subtle general antiestrogenic effects.[39]

Palomba and colleagues[39] compared the use of 60 mg/day Raloxifene for 12 months in postmenopausal women with placebo. Raloxifene induced significant size reduction and seemed to target the fibroids with less effect on a normal myometrium.

A following study by the same group[40] noted that dosages up to 180 mg/day did not affect uterine or fibroid size significantly, disrupt normal ovarian cycling, or affect the length or severity of bleeding.[40] While new fibroids were noted in the first study, it seemed that 180 mg effectively prevents the formation of new fibroids. A similar but smaller study noted a nonsignificant decrease in fibroid size in the study group (Raloxifene, 180 mg/day for 3 months) compared with the "no treatment" control group, and the control group in which the fibroid size increased.[41]

In an effort to decrease endogenous estrogen levels, Palomba and colleagues treated 100 premenopausal women with symptomatic fibroids with GnRH analog plus Raloxifene, 60 mg/day, for 6 months, and compared them to treatment with GnRH analog alone.[40] Both the groups demonstrated a significant decrease in uterine and fibroid sizes, as well as in the symptoms. A significantly greater decrease in fibroid size occurred in the group that received Raloxifene compared with the placebo group.[40] No further decrease was seen when treatment was extended.[42] Raloxifene was well-tolerated in all the studies.

Selective progesterone receptor modulators

Selective progesterone receptor modulators (SPRMs) act on the endometrium to create amenorrhea by suppressing proliferation without affecting basal estrogen concentration or ovulation (and thus, no symptoms of estrogen deprivation or breakthrough bleeding). Treatment with Asoprisnil (given in doses of 5, 10 and 25 mg/day) decreased fibroid size, reduced pressure symptoms, suppressed uterine bleeding, and increased hemoglobin levels. Eighty percent of the women, treated with 25 mg/day, had amenorrhea. All the doses were well-tolerated.[43] Further studies of this novel therapy are indicated.

Regulation of growth factor pathways

Pirfenidone is an antifibrotic agent investigated for use in patients with pulmonary fibrosis. It inhibits production of transforming growth factor-β and collagen, and decreases fibroid cell proliferation *in vitro*. However, cell death is not achieved.[44] There are no published clinical data on the use of Pirfenidone in women with fibroids. Interferons can reverse the proliferative effects of bFGF on fibroid cells in culture.

Gene therapy

Preliminary studies have begun on both identification of genes through a genome-wide scan and sib-pair analysis and elucidation of possible mechanisms of gene therapy that take advantage of the physiology of fibroids.

Myolysis

Uterine Artery Embolization (UAE)

In the early 1990s, Jacques H Ravina first applied the technique of embolization of uterine arteries that has been used successfully for pelvic bleeding (after labor, surgery or pelvic trauma) to treat uterine fibroids in women at high risk for complications during surgery.[45] They then expanded the treatment in order to reduce complications during surgery.[46] In the next step, they treated 16 patients, aged 34 to 48 years, with symptomatic uterine fibroids, for which a major surgical procedure was planned after failure of medical treatment, by selective-free flow arterial embolization as the primary treatment.[47] Symptoms resolved in 11 patients; menstrual cycles returned to normal in 10 of these. Three patients had partial improvement and two failures required surgery. In 14 cases, embolization caused pelvic pain requiring analgesia.[47] Today, interventional radiologists worldwide perform uterine-artery embolization.

Technical aspects

Uterine artery embolization is achieved by delivering particulate material, typically polyvinyl alcohol (PVA) particles, PVA microspheres, or gelatin-coated tris-acryl polymer microspheres into one or both uterine arteries to produce ischemic change to fibroids without causing permanent damage to the uterus. UAE can be performed under conscious sedation or epidural anesthesia. A single femoral artery, typically, is catheterized and pelvic arteriography is performed to define the vascular tree and preclude vascular anomalies. Initially, complete occlusion of both uterine arteries was the goal of UAE. Recent data with PVA or gelatin-coated tris-acryl polymer microspheres suggest that incomplete embolization of both arteries may produce effective infarction of fibroids with less severe pain.[48] The procedure requires approximately 1 hour to perform (typically 45–135 min[49]) and the ovaries are exposed to approximately 20 rads (20 cGy) of ionizing radiation.[49] Women are observed for up to 24 hours postprocedure and treated with regional anesthesia or narcotics for pain. Uterine cramping may be severe, but usually, is reduced by nonsteroidal antiinflammatory drugs.[50] The normal myometrium rapidly establishes a new blood supply through collateral vessels from the ovarian and the vaginal circulations. However, fibroids appear to be supplied by end arteries without the collateral flow found in normal myometrium and therefore, are preferentially affected by the reduction in flow. The reduction in blood supply results in a decrease in fibroid volume of between 30 to 50 percent,[49] however, symptomatic improvement may be achieved without a remarkable change in fibroid size.

Clinical outcome

Table 26.1 outlines the outcome of the first study by Ravina et al.[46] and of the 8 largest articles that investigated clinical outcomes after UAE for symptomatic fibroids. As seen in the table, uterine fibroid size was reduced in 35 to 73 percent of the patients and menorrhagia was reduced by 80 percent or more in all studies.

Risks and complications

Major complications are estimated to occur in 1 to 5 percent of women undergoing the procedure for the treatment of uterine fibroids.[51] Chronic vaginal discharge affects 4 to 7 percent of patients. This resolves spontaneously in 94 percent of patients. In some patients, hysteroscopy or dilation and curettage was required after embolization to remove degenerating submucus fibroids.

Ovarian failure is experienced in 1 to 2 percent of subjects after this procedure. Most of these cases occur in perimenopausal patients, but loss of ovarian function was reported for some women younger than 40 years old. This complication could be devastating in young women who have not yet completed childbearing. Tissue ischemia arising from embolization of the ovaries through the collateral utero-ovarian artery is suspected. Serious infectious complications affect 1 to 2 percent of cases, more frequently with embolization of larger fibroids.

Postembolization syndrome

Postembolization fever and leukocytosis, that are the result of fibroid infarction and necrosis, develop in 15 to 33 percent of all patients, and may be associated with nausea and vomiting, malaise and anorexia. This syndrome is troubling because it is difficult to distinguish it from postembolization infection.

Hysterectomy after UAE is necessary in approximately 1 percent of patients. Three deaths have been reported after an estimated 15,000 UAE procedures worldwide. The cause of death was sepsis in one case and massive pulmonary embolism in another. The need and efficacy of preventive measures is questionable.[50]

Pregnancy outcome after UAE

According to the American College of Obstetricians and Gynecologists (ACOG) committee,[52] there is insufficient data to conclude that UAE is a safe option for women who wish to retain their fertility. Overall, fewer than 150 pregnancies have been reported after UAE for fibroids.[45] Marshburn et al.[50] reviewed 93 pregnancies reported after UAE for fibroids.[50] Delivery outcome was provided for 52 of those pregnancies. Overall, most pregnancies were delivered full term without complications. Despite these encouraging results, no randomized controlled trials (RCTs) have compared the effects of UAE and myomectomy on future fertility.[50] One retrospective study that assessed pregnancy outcome indicated an increased risk for preterm delivery and malpresentation after UAE compared with laparoscopic myomectomy.[53]

Table 26.1: Outcome of uterine artery embolization for symptomatic fibroids					
Reference	*No*	*Uterine volume reduction (%)*	*Menorrhagia reduction (%)*	*Follow-up*	*Serious complications*
Ravina 1997	88	69	89%	2–6 m	1 hysterectomy d/t necrosis
					7 failures (req. hysterectomy or myomectomy)
					2 req. D and C
Spies 1999	169	35	88%	12 m	1 delayed fibroid passage
					1 hysteroscopic resection
					1 D and C req.
					4 irregular cycles
					2 treatment failures req. hysterectomy
					2 ovarian failures
Hutchins 1999	305	48%	86% 3 m	2 m	1 hysterectomy
			85% 6 m		4 puncture site hematomas
			92% 12 m		2 readmissions d/t pain
Ravina 1999	184	87% of patients 6 m	90%	29 m	1 hysterectomy d/t bowel obstruction
					6 fibroid expulsions
McLucas 2001	167	49% 6 m	82% 6 m	6 m	8 fibroid passages
		52% 12 m			1 hysterectomy d/t infection
Spies 2001	200	42% 3 m	86% 3 m	21 m	2 endometrial infections
		60% 12 m	88% 6 m		1 fibroid expulsions
			90% 12 m		1 pulmonary embolus
					1 DVT
Walker and Pelage 2002	400	64% by MRI 73% by U/S	84	17 m	3 hysterectomy d/t infection 26 amenorrhea
					9 fibroid expulsions
					13 chronic vaginal discharge
Pron 2003	538	42	83	3 m	21 amenorrhea

Abbreviations: d/t: due to; req: requiring; U/S: Ultrasound.

Randomized trial of embolization versus surgical treatment for fibroids (REST)

In January 2007, the REST study, a randomized, multicenter trial comparing uterine-artery embolization with abdominal surgery in women with symptomatic uterine fibroids was published in the New England Journal of Medicine.[54] The investigators randomly assigned 106 women to undergo embolization and 51 women to undergo surgery (43 for hysterectomy and 8 for myomectomy). They found no significant differences in the quality of life scores between the two groups at 1 year, although symptom scores were better in the surgical group at that follow-up assessment. Complication rates were similar at 1 year in the two groups, although the study was not powered to detect differences in these rates or to detect rare complications. The embolization group had the advantages of a significantly shorter hospital stay and a more rapid resumption of normal activities.

We can conclude that currently available data suggest that UAE is safe and that, short-term results of UAE are similar to those of myomectomy, and long-term outcomes are to be investigated. Safe implementation of UAE requires close cooperation between gynecologists and radiologists. One of the possible advantages of UAE, namely, preservation and improvement of fertility, was not examined enough to offer this treatment to women who might wish future pregnancies.

MRI-guided Focused Ultrasound (MRgFUS)

Heat can cause cell damage and death. When the cell reaches temperatures between 60 and 100°C, there is near instantaneous induction of protein coagulation, which irreversibly damages key enzymes, as well as nucleic acid-histone protein complexes.

Technical aspects

Focused ultrasound uses an externally generated, high-frequency, alternating pressure wave, which propagates through the body, causing the tissue under focus to vibrate. This act is termed "sonication". The amount of heat differs by orders of magnitude with a very sharp transition from focus to the areas outside where the temperature is raised by a few degrees or less, creating no damage. During treatment, a small "bean-shaped" volume of focused ultrasound energy is directed into the target for approximately 15 seconds and heats the tissue between 60°C and 90°C to induce thermal coagulation, as seen in Figure 26.1.

Heating tissue to a temperature of above 60°C, for 1 second causes cell death in that designated tissue volume. Figure 26.2 shows a tissue before, during and after sonication. In 1926, the first study that showed that focused ultrasound could have a biologic effect on tissue was conducted. Over the past eight decades, research has been conducted to evaluate the potential use and safety of this technology. In the 1950s, focused ultrasound was evaluated primarily for Parkinson's disease and other brain-related disorders. The technique provides an approach for destroying diseased brain tissue, obviating the need for invasive surgery in treating these diseases. The lack of methods to visualize and control the process became the major set back to development. The success in using magnetic resonance imaging (MRI) for monitoring and guiding treatment gave the needed breakthrough, and in October 2004, ExAblate® 2000 was approved by the Food and Drug Administration (FDA) for the treatment of uterine fibroids. Magnetic resonance images taken during sonication provide a real time loop monitoring of the target tissue and a quantitative, realtime temperature map overlay as function of time to confirm the therapeutic effect of the treatment. The transducer is then automatically moved to the succeeding treatment point and the process is repeated until the entire volume has been treated.

Prior to the delivery of any treatment sonications, the patient received analgesia and sedation (e.g. fentanyl and versed) to reduce pain and prevent any unnecessary motion, as well as to help alleviate anxiety and any feelings of

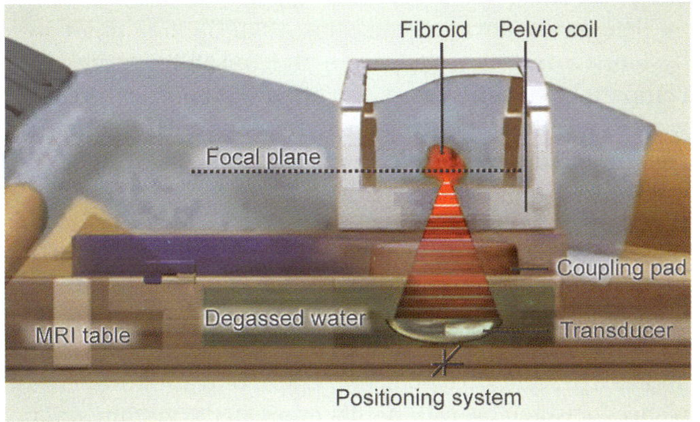

Fig. 26.1: The principle of focused ultrasound

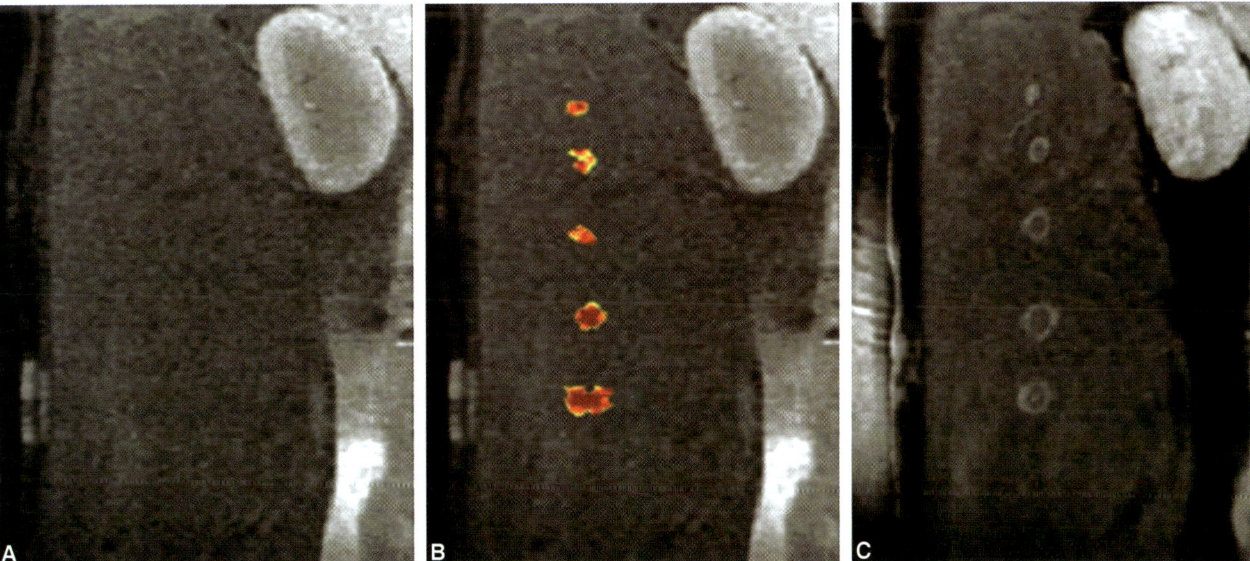

Figs 26.2A to C: Thermal dose verification using MRI: (A) Before sonication; (B) During sonication; (C) After sonication

claustrophobia. Typically, 20 to 50 individual sonications are delivered over a 2-hour period to complete the treatment.

Clinical outcome

The initial feasibility study employed 55 women who were treated with MRgFUS prior to a planned hysterectomy. The average age and BMI were 43.3 years and 26 kg/m³, respectively. Women weighing over 250 pounds (113 kg) were excluded because they could not fit into the MRI machine. The median treatment time was approximately 105 minutes. Postoperative pain and discomfort were encouraging. Seventy-two hours after the treatment, only 10 percent of the patients needed analgesics, approximately 25 percent had general discomfort, 5 percent were complaining of pain or abdominal tenderness, and 10 percent of women had nausea. Pathological examination revealed a nonperfused area that was approximately three-fold greater than the treatment volume.

In a following pivotal study,[55] 109 women treated with MRgFUS were compared to 83 women undergoing abdominal hysterectomy. The primary outcome measure was the uterine fibroid symptomatology, using Uterine Fibroid Symptom and Health-Related Quality of Life questionnaire (UFS-QOL). Other outcome measures were symptom severity and quality-of-life scale (QOL) with six dimensions (concern, activities, energy/mood, control, self consciousness, and sexual function). Patients' general health status and recovery were assessed using the Medical Outcomes Study Short Form-36® (SF-36).

The two groups were similar in terms of age, BMI and hormonal status. They were slightly different in terms of race. The control treatment arm also showed lower values in each pretreatment SF-36 subscale, indicating that the control arm was in better condition.

Results: Patients treated with MRgFUS suffered fewer adverse events: 19 percent of the patients in the MRgFUS group had no adverse effect (compared to only 1% in the control group). Twenty-seven percent of the patients had one adverse effect compared to 5 percent of the patients who underwent hysterectomy. The number of patients with more than seven adverse events per patient was much higher in the hysterectomy group (22%) compared to the MRgFUS group (3%).

Immediately after the treatment with MRgFUS the majority of patients reported no pain (75%) or only mild pain (18%) and no discomfort (68%) or mild discomfort (25%). One week after the procedure, more MRgFUS patients than hysterectomy patients reported no pain (79% versus 23%, respectively), no bowel symptoms (88% versus 67%, respectively) and no nausea (89% versus 73%, respectively). Depending on the pain, the differences diminished within six months but were still apparent. The appraisal of efficacy after 6 months was performed using the UFS-QOL, as seen in Figure 26.3. Seventy percent of the patients reported an

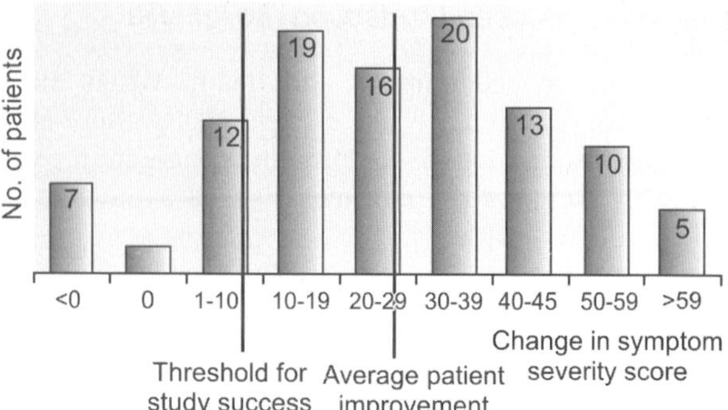

Fig. 26.3: Number of patients per 10-point cluster of change in symptom severity score

improvement of 10 points or greater, which is considered significant. In most cases, the improvement was much higher, giving an average of almost 27.3 points of improvement on a 100-point scale.

The main advantage of the MRgFUS treatment over hysterectomy was noted when the "disability days" were compared. Women treated with MRgFUS reported 1.4 days of worked missed and 1.5 days in bed as opposed to 18.9 and 9.7 after hysterectomy (data from the UF002 pivotal study).

Results from other studies

An expanded treatment with an optional second session was investigated (Fennessy et al. personal communication) at 3, 6, 12 and 24 months, 89 percent, 88 percent, 87 percent and 85 percent of patients respectively achieved improvement, and 79.2 percent, 78.6 percent, 77.4 percent and 79.4 percent, respectively achieved 10 points or greater symptom severity improvement. A study among 73 African American patients followed for 36 months showed improvement in 95 percent of the patients. Furthermore, 90.5 percent of the patients achieved 10 points or greater improvement in their fibroid symptom severity score.

In another study, MRgFUS treatment following administration of GnRH agonist in 50 patients with fibroids >10 cm was investigated. 45 percent of the patients demonstrated a reduction in median symptom severity score at 6 months and 48 percent at 12 months.[56]

Risks and Complications

The initial feasibility study has demonstrated a high safety profile: 4 percent of women had minor skin burns and 4 percent had increased bleeding following the treatment. One patient was hospitalized following the procedure for nausea. In one case, non-targeted sonication of the uterine serosa with no clinical sequelae was noted. Technical aspects learnt in this study, like avoiding clips and scars, shaving pubic hair and voiding the bladder during treatment (to prevent the uterus from changing place), were implemented in order to reduce adverse effects.

Table 26.2: Pregnancy results after MRgFUS	
Total number of pregnancies	23 (21 patients)
Mean age (range)	36.8 (28–44) years
Mean months to conception	9.9
Mean fibroid volume (mL)	268
Pregnancies carried to 3rd trimester	48% (11)
Term vaginal deliveries	64% (7)
Term c-section	36% (4)
Spontaneous abortions	13% (3)
Miscarriages	30% (7)
Ongoing pregnancies	9% (2)
Average baby weight at term delivery (kg)	3.307 kg

It is estimated that up to date, 2500 patients have been treated. Severe adverse events reported included one case of bowel perforation, thermal nerve damage causing leg weakness and pain, several cases of third degree skin burns, and a few cases of severe vaginal bleeding. Moderate and mild adverse events reported include skin burn, abdominal pain, fever, heavy menses and abnormal vaginal discharge, urinary symptoms following usage of a urinary catheter, fatigue, and gastrointestinal symptoms.

The current labeling for the focused ultrasound device is that it is indicated for the treatment of premenopausal women who have symptomatic uterine fibroids and no desire for future fertility.

Pregnancy after MRgFUS

Although the FDA has limited treatment for women who do not wish to deliver, 23 pregnancies were recorded in 21 patients after treatment. Table 26.2 describes the characteristics and outcome of those pregnancies. No uterine rupture, preterm labor, placental abruption or abnormal placentation leading to fetal growth restriction was noted. The FDA reviewer has agreed that "these data may support revisions to the current labeling regarding pregnancy following ExAblate".

CONCLUSION

Albeit the small number of patients we can conclude that MRgFUS treatment has the potential to deliver safe and effective treatment for uterine fibroid symptoms without damaging patient fertility or creating additional pregnancy related risks. Moreover, this treatment has the potential to become the preferred treatment in those women who would like to preserve their fertility potential and also where the fibroids are suspected to be the cause of infertility.

REFERENCES

1. Buttram Jr VC, Reiter RC. Uterine leiomyomata: etiology, symptomatology, and management. Fertil Steril 1981;36:433-45.
2. Keshavarz H, Hillis SD, Kieke BA, et al. Hysterectomy surveillance—United States, 1994–1999. MMWR Surveill Summ 2002;51(SS-5):1-8.
3. Chwalisz K, DeManno D, Garg R, Larsen L, Mattia-Goldberg C, Stickler T. Therapeutic potential for the selective progesterone receptor modulator asoprisnil in the treatment of leiomyomata. Semin Reprod Med 2004;22:113-9.
4. De Leo V, Morgante G, La Marca A, Musacchio MC, Sorace M, Cavicchioli C, Petraglia F. A benefit-risk assessment of medical treatment for uterine leiomyomas. Drug Saf 2002;25:759-79.
5. Stewart EA. Uterine fibroids. Lancet 2001;357:293-8.
6. Cook JD Walker CL. Treatment strategies for uterine leiomyoma: the role of hormonal modulation. Semin Reprod Med 2004;22:105-11.
7. Marshall LM, Spiegelman D, Goldman MB, Manson JE, Colditz GA, Barbieri RL, Stampfer MJ, Hunter DJ. A prospective study of reproductive factors and oral contraceptive use in relation to the risk of uterine leiomyomata. Fertil Steril 1998;70:432-9.
8. Tiltman AJ. The effect of progestins on the mitotic activity of uterine fibromyomas. Int J Gynecol Pathol 1985;4:89-96.
9. Stewart EA, Nowak RA. Leiomyoma-related bleeding: a classic hypothesis updated for the molecular era. Hum Reprod Update 1996;2:295-306.
10. Stewart EA. Treatment of uterine leiomyomas. In: Rose BD, editor. UpToDate. Waltham, Massachusetts 7 UpToDate; 2005.
11. Mixson WT, Hammond DO. Response of fibromyomas to a progestin. Am J Obstet Gynecol 1961;82:754-60.
12. Harrison-Woolrych M, Robinson R. Fibroid growth in response to high-dose progestogen. Fertil Steril 1995;64:191-2.
13. Carr BR, Marshburn PB, Weatherall PT, Bradshaw KD, Breslau NA, Byrd W, Roark M, Steinkampf MP. An evaluation of the effect of gonadotropin-releasing hormone analogs and medroxyprogesterone acetate on uterine leiomyomata volume by magnetic resonance imaging: a prospective, randomized, double blind, placebo-controlled, crossover trial. J Clin Endocrinol Metab 1993;76:1217-23.
14. Friedman AJ, Daly M, Juneau-Norcross M, Gleason R, Rein MS, LeBoff M. Long-term medical therapy for leiomyomata uteri: a prospective, randomized study of leuprolide acetate depot plus either oestrogen-progestin or progestin add-back therapy for 2 years. Hum Reprod 1994;9:1618-25.
15. Rackow B, Arici A. Options for Medical Treatment of Myomas Obstet Gynecol Clin N Am. 2006;33: 97-113.
16. Venkatachalam S, Bagratee JS, Moodley J. Medical management of uterine fibroids with medroxyprogesterone acetate (Depo Provera): a pilot study. J Obstet Gynaecol 2004;24:798-800.
17. Hurskainen R, Paavonen J. Levonorgestrel-releasing intra-uterine system in the treatment of heavy menstrual bleeding. Curr Opin Obstet Gynecol 2004;16:487-90.
18. Stewart A, Cummins C, Gold L, Jordan R, Phillips W. The effectiveness of the levonorgestrel-releasing intrauterine system in menorrhagia: a systematic review. BJOG 2001;108:74-86.
19. Grigorieva V, Chen-Mok M, Tarasova M, et al. Use of a levonorgestrel-releasing intrauterine system to treat bleeding related to uterine leiomyomas. Fertil Steril 2003;79:1194-8.
20. Inki P, Hurskainen R, Palo P, Ekholm E, Grenman S, Kivelä A, Kujansuu E, Teperi J, Yliskoski M, Paavonen J. Comparison of ovarian cyst formation in women using the levonorgestrel-

releasing intrauterine system vs hysterectomy. Ultrasound Obstet Gynecol 2002;20:381-5.

21. De Leo V, la Marca A, Morgante G. Short-term treatment of uterine fibromyomas with danazol. Gynecol Obstet Invest 1999;47:258-62.

22. La Marca A, Musacchio MC, Morgante G, Petraglia F, De Leo V. Hemodynamic effect of danazol therapy in women with uterine leiomyomata. Fertil Steril 2003;79:1240-42.

23. Olive DL, Lindheim SR, Pritts EA. Nonsurgical management of leiomyoma: impact on fertility. Curr Opin Obstet Gynecol 2004;16:239-43.

24. The Practice Committee of the American Society for Reproductive Medicine. Myomas and reproductive function. Fertil Steril 2004;82(Suppl 1):S111-6.

25. Wallach EE, Vlahos NF. Uterine myomas: an overview of development, clinical features, and management. Obstet Gynecol 2004;104:393-406.

26. Nowak RA. Fibroids: pathophysiology and current medical treatment. Baillieres Best Pract Res Clin Obstet Gynecol 1999; 13:223-38.

27. Manyonda I, Sinthamoney E, Belli AM. Controversies and challenges in the modern management of uterine fibroids. BJOG 2004;111:95-102.

28. Felberbaum RE, Germer U, Ludwig M, Riethmüller-Winzen H, Heise S, Buttge I, et al. Treatment of uterine fibroids with a slow-release formulation of the gonadotrophin-releasing hormone antagonist Cetrorelix. Hum Reprod 1998;13:1660-8.

29. Flierman PA, Oberye JJ, van der Hulst VP, de Blok S. Rapid reduction of leiomyoma volume during treatment with the GnRH antagonist ganirelix. BJOG 2005;112:638-42.

30. Gonzalez-Barcena D, Alvarez RB, Ochoa EP, Cornejo IC, Comaru-Schally AM, Schally AV, et al. Treatment of uterine leiomyomas with luteinizing hormone-releasing hormone antagonist Cetrorelix. Hum Reprod 1997;12:2028-35.

31. Shozu M, Murakami K, Inoue M. Aromatase and leiomyoma of the uterus. Semin Reprod Med 2004;22:51-60.

32. Shozu M, Murakami K, Segawa T, Kasai T, Inoue M. Successful treatment of a symptomatic uterine leiomyoma in a perimenopausal woman with a nonsteroidal aromatase inhibitor. Fertil Steril 2003;79:628-31.

33. Steinauer J, Pritts EA, Jackson R, Jacoby AF. Systematic review of mifepristone for the treatment of uterine leiomyomata. Obstet Gynecol 2004;103:1331-6.

34. Murphy AA, Kettel LM, Morales AJ, Roberts VJ, Yen SS. Regression of uterine leiomyomata in response to the antiprogesterone RU 486. J Clin Endocrinol Metab 1993;76:513-7.

35. Murphy AA, Morales AJ, Kettel LM, Yen SS. Regression of uterine leiomyomata to the antiprogesterone RU486: dose-response effect. Fertil Steril 1995;64:187-90.

36. Eisinger SH, Meldrum S, Fiscella K, le Roux HD, Guzick DS. Low-dose mifepristone for uterine leiomyomata. Obstet Gynecol 2003;101:243-50.

37. Cook JD, Walker CL. Treatment strategies for uterine leiomyoma: the role of hormonal modulation. Semin Reprod Med 2004;22:105-11.

38. Sadan O, Ginath S, Sofer D, Rotmensch S, Debby A, Glezerman M, Zakut H. The role of tamoxifen in the treatment of symptomatic uterine leiomyomata—a pilot study. Eur J Obstet Gynecol Reprod Biol 2001;96:183-6.

39. Palomba S, Sammartino A, Di Carlo C, Affinito P, Zullo F, Nappi C. Effects of raloxifene treatment on uterine leiomyomas in postmenopausal women. Fertil Steril 2001;76:38-43.

40. Palomba S, Orio Jr F, Morelli M, Russo T, Pellicano M, Zupi E, et al. Raloxifene administration in premenopausal women with uterine leiomyomas: a pilot study. J Clin Endocrinol Metab 2002;87:3603-8.

41. Jirecek S, Lee A, Pavo I, Crans G, Eppel W, Wenzl R. Raloxifene prevents the growth of uterine leiomyomas in premenopausal women. Fertil Steril 2004;81:132-6.

42. Palomba S, Orio Jr F, Russo T, Falbo A, Cascella T, Doldo P, et al. Long-term effectiveness and safety of GnRH agonist plus raloxifene administration in women with uterine leiomyomas. Hum Reprod 2004;19:1308-14.

43. Chwalisz K, Parker RL, Williamson S, et al. Treatment of uterine leiomyomas with the novel selective progesterone receptor modulator (SPRM). J Soc Gynecol Investig 2003;10(2 Suppl).

44. Lee BS, Margolin SB, Nowak RA. Pirfenidone: a novel pharmacological agent that inhibits leiomyoma cell proliferation and collagen production. J Clin Endocrinol Metab 1998;83:219-23.

45. Tulandi T. Treatment of uterine fibroids—is surgery obsolete? N. Engl. J Med. 2007;25;356:411-3.

46. Ravina JH, Merland JJ, Herbreteau D, Houdart E, Bouret JM, Madelenat P. Preoperative embolization of uterine fibroma. Preliminary results (10 cases. Presse Med. 1994;23:1540.

47. Ravina JH, Herbreteau D, Ciraru-Vigneron N, Bouret JM, Houdart E, Aymard A, Merland JJ. Arterial embolisation to treat uterine myomata. Lancet 1995;346:671-2.

48. Spies JB. Recovery after uterine artery embolization: understanding and managing short-term outcomes. J Vasc Interv Radiol 2003;14:1219-22.

49. Gupta JK, Sinha AS, Lumsden MA, Hickey M. Uterine artery embolization for symptomatic uterine fibroids. Cochrane Database Syst Rev. 2006;CD005073.

50. Marshburn PB, Matthews ML, Hurst BS. Uterine artery embolization as a treatment option for uterine myomas. Obstet Gynecol Clin North Am. 2006;33:125-44.

51. Spies JB, Spector A, Roth AR, Baker CM, Mauro L, Murphy-Skrynarz K. Complications after uterine artery embolization for leiomyomas. Obstet Gynecol 2002;100:873-80.

52. Committee Opinion of the American College of Obstetricians and Gynecologists. Uterine artery embolization. ACOG Committee on Gynecologic Practice 2004;293:403-04.

53. Goldberg J, Pereira L, Berghella V, Diamond J, Daraï E, Seinera P, Seracchioli R. Pregnancy outcomes after treatment for fibromyomata: uterine artery embolization versus laparoscopic myomectomy. Am J Obstet Gynecol 2004;191:18-21.

54. The REST Investigators. Uterine-artery embolization versus surgery for symptomatic uterine fibroids. N Engl J Med 2007; 356:360-70.

55. Stewart EA, Rabinovici J, Tempany CM, Inbar Y, Regan L, Gostout B, Hesley G, Kim HS, Hengst S, Gedroyc WM. Clinical outcomes of focused ultrasound surgery for the treatment of uterine fibroids. Fertil Steril 2006;85:22-9.

56. Smart OC, Hindley JT, Regan L, Gedroyc WG. Gonadotrophin-releasing hormone and magnetic-resonance-guided ultrasound surgery for uterine leiomyomata. Obstet Gynecol. 2006; 108:49-54.

Diagnosis of Genital Tuberculosis: Newer Techniques for an Old Disease

Lakhbir Dhaliwal, Shalini Gainder

OVERVIEW

Confirmation of diagnosis of genital tuberculosis is a challenging problem even when clinical suspicion exists. Demonstration of acid fast bacilli and isolation of *Mycobacterium tuberculosis* by conventional methods have limitations of speed, sensitivity and specificity.

During the last two decades, several new rapid tests have been introduced for the early diagnosis of this disease. Tests that are prominent are BACTEC, mycobacterial growth indicator tube (MGIT), polymerase chain reaction-restriction fragment length polymorphisms (PCR-RFLP) methods. Better understanding of the genetic structure of the *Mycobacterium* has led to the development of various gene probes and gene amplification methods. These gene probes and gene amplification methods are demonstrably highly sensitive and offer unparalleled capability to enhance the diagnosis of tuberculosis in future.

The recently introduced Xpert MTB/RIF assay simultaneously detects the presence of *M. tuberculosis* and its susceptibility to the important first-line drug Rifampicin (RIF). This test detects by PCR amplification of the Rifampicin resistance-determining region (RRDR) of the *M. tuberculosis* rpoB gene and subsequent probing of this region for mutations that are associated with RIF resistance.

In addition to these, there are tests that test the presence of antigen or are based on the antibody response to *M. tuberculosis*. Interferon gamma release assay (IGRAs) detects sensitization to *M. tuberculosis* by measuring interferon gamma (IFN-γ) release in response to antigens representing *M. tuberculosis*. Three IGRAs (QuantiFERON-TB Gold test, QuantiFERON-TB Gold in Tube, T-Spot test) have been approved by the FDA for the detection of active and latent tuberculosis.

However, these newer tests are under evaluation and the literature does not ascertain which new test can best be used for the confirmation of diagnosis based on which treatment can be started.

INTRODUCTION

Genital tuberculosis often remains asymptomatic or presents only as infertility, therefore, a thorough history and clinical examination, keeping a high index of suspicion, may give some clue to the presence of genital tuberculosis. In developing countries like India, where the incidence of tuberculosis is high, it becomes mandatory to screen women for tuberculosis before proceeding with treatment for infertility. Early confirmation of the diagnosis of genital tuberculosis is a challenging problem, especially when it exists silently, causing irreversible damage to the tubes and endometrium. While treating a woman with infertility, it is mandatory to rule out tuberculosis causing endometritis before performing any invasive evaluation or else it may spread from the endometrium to the tubes. A routine endometrial biopsy, as a screening method, has been a useful tool to diagnose genital tuberculosis. Therefore, it is a must to rule out tuberculosis in the endometrial biopsy; should the biopsy be positive for tuberculosis it becomes important to treat it before laparoscopy or hysterosalpingography (HSG).

Endometrial Biopsy

Endometrial biopsy is a simple office procedure, performed in the premenstrual phase of the cycle (day 21 onwards) or it can be done on the first day of the cycle. Using an endometrial curette, and complete aseptic precautions, an adequate sample of endometrium is retrieved and forwarded to the laboratory without delay in normal saline for microbiological tests and in formalin for the histopathology test. Some tests will require special transport medium for transportation to the laboratory.

Laboratory Evaluation

Isolation of mycobacteria poses a special problem for the laboratory. Mycobacteria require a prolonged time for replication (approximately 15 to 22 hours), whereas other bacteria replicate in a short time of 20 to 30 minutes. This may therefore lead to disproportionate growth between contaminant bacteria and mycobacteria and also accumulation of their metabolic acids that liquefy the culture making it unsatisfactory for recovery of mycobacteria. Therefore, successful isolation of mycobacteria depends on selective suppression of contaminating bacteria. Smear microscopy and conventional culture methods have been frequently used for the diagnosis of tuberculosis. Histopathology is characteristic, however, there could be problems in getting a representative specimen and non-specific features.

There are no definite guidelines available as of date as to how to optimally use the number of diagnostic tests, which have become available over a period, to establish or rule out the diagnosis of tuberculosis in a given patient. The diagnostic modalities should have certain desirable features like sensitivity, specificity, predictive value, speed, reproducibility and cost effectiveness.

There are two basic approaches for the diagnosis of tuberculosis. The direct approach includes detection of mycobacteria or its products and indirect approach includes measurement of humoral and cellular responses of the host against tuberculosis.

CLINICAL DISCUSSION

Direct Approach

Microscopy

It is the simplest and most rapid procedure available to detect acid fast bacilli in clinical specimens by Ziehl-Neelsen staining methods that requires at least 5000 bacilli/mL for detection.[1,2] Smear microscopy has the advantage of being inexpensive and simple.

Culture

Culture is presently the yardstick for diagnosis. The pretreatment procedure has tremendous influence on the sensitivity of results. The positivity of culture depends on proper transportation, decontamination and centrifugation method adopted for processing the specimen. At present, the mycobacterial culture can be performed in conventional Lowenstein Jensen medium or an agar-based medium, such as Middle Brook 7H10 or 7H11, and liquid media such as Kirchner's or Middle Brook 7H9 broth. The culture takes about three to six weeks to show results. A few modern rapid methods are also available. These include:

Microcolony Detection on Solid Media

This method involves pouring of a thin layer of Middle Brook 7H11 agar medium on plates which are incubated.[3] In less than 7 days, microcolonies of slow growing mycobacteria can be detected. This is a less expensive and faster method for the detection of tubercle bacilli. The problem is that it is labor-intensive.

Septi-chek AFB Method

This is a biphasic medium system consisting of enriched selective broth and a slide with nonselective Middle Brook agar on one side with two sections on the other side—one with NAP (beta nitroalpha acetylamine beta hydroxyl propiophenone) and egg containing agar and the second with chocolate agar for detection of contamination. This method requires three weeks for incubation. This method gives better culture results compared to BACTEC 460 TB system.[4]

Radiometric BACTEC 460 TB Method

This method is based on generation of radioactive carbon dioxide from the substrate palmitic acid. This method has been extensively used all over the world and growth can be detected within 5 to 10 days with this system. The inclusion of NAP helps in distinguishing *M. tuberculosis* from other mycobacteria. This system has been widely used as a comparative standard.[5]

Mycobacteria Growth Indicator Tube

In this method, the growth of mycobacteria is detected by a non-radioactive detection system using fluorochromes for detection.[5,6] This system helps in early detection (7–12 days) of mycobacterial growth and has been reported to be useful for drug susceptibility testing.

MB/Bac T

This system is based on colorimetric detection of CO_2. The mean detection time of *M. tuberculosis* with this method is 13.7 days.[7]

ESP Culture System II

This diagnostic system detects the pressure changes within head space above the broth culture medium in the sealed bottle, i.e. either gas production or consumption due to microbial growth.

Rapid Identification of Mycobacterial Isolates

Traditionally, biochemical methods were used for the identification of mycobacterial isolates from cultures. To overcome these limitations, chemical methods based on lipid profiles, hybridization with specific gene probes, polymerase chain reaction—restriction fragment length polymorphism (PCR – RFLP) methods have been described:

- *Analysis of lipid profiles:* Mycobacteria have characteristics lipid profiles. These lipid profiles can be used to identify the mycobacterial isolates.[8]
- *DNA probes:* Well-defined oligonucleotide probes identify specific gene sequences for the identification of various clinically relevant mycobacteria. The identity can be established in 1 to 2 days.[9,10]
- *Ribosomal rRNA based probes:* These targeting probes have been found to be 10 to 100 fold more sensitive than DNA targeting.[11] They can detect as low as 100 organisms.
- *Gene amplification methods for identification:* Amplification of specific gene regions followed by hybridization with species specific probes.[12]
  Sequencing and RFLP analysis such as hsp 65kDa gene,[13] katG 22[14] rRNA gene[15] have been described. This approach can easily be practised in clinical mycobacterial laboratories for the identification of isolates from cultures and also from clinical specimens.
- *Gene amplification methods for direct detection of M. tuberculosis sequences from clinical specimens:* These can be polymerase chain reaction (PCR) and others based on isothermal amplification reactions.[16] Gene amplification is highly sensitive and can detect up to 1 to 10 organisms in the specimen.[16,17]

PCR Method

The PCR method allows sequences of DNA present in only a few copies of mycobacteria to be amplified *in vitro* such that the amount of amplified DNA can be visualized and identified. Even 10 to 1000 organisms present in a specimen can be identified.[1] A number of target genes have been evaluated for diagnosis.[18-20] The most common target used in PCR is IS 6110. This sequence is specific for the *M. tuberculosis* complex and is present up to 20 times in the genome, therefore offering multiple targets for identification.

A variety of PCR methods have been developed which may target either DNA or RNA and these could be based on conventional DNA-based PCR, nested PCR and RT-PCR. Indian laboratories have been active in development of PCR methods using separate gene targets like—MPB 64, devR, 38Kd, IS 1081.

Polymerase chain reaction is now widely being used to confirm the diagnosis of tuberculosis. The gene amplification methods have been found to be highly sensitive (ranging between 70 to 100%) whereas a specificity of 80 to 100 percent has been reported by different investigators. With the PCR

methodology, rapid results are available within a day of DNA extraction from the sample.

It can also be applied to sterile fluids, like peritoneal fluid, where the culture is difficult due to a low bacterial load. However, the PCR test has its own share of false negative results, which are largely due to contamination of the sample with heparin, which is a known PCR inhibitor, absence of even a single AFB in the sample collected, and high salt concentration of a specimen which interferes with the PCR results.

Other methods are transcription mediated amplification and nucleic acid amplification. The ligase chain reaction, nucleic acid amplification, strand displacement amplification, nucleic acid sequence-based amplification and transcription-mediated amplification are others variants of the PCR test.

Xpert MTB/RIF Test

To develop a faster and easier-to-use test, researchers developed a DNA-based test called Xpert MTB/RIF.[21] The test detects *M. tuberculosis* and also resistance to Rifampicin. RIF resistance is a good indicator of multidrug resistance. Drug-resistant TB requires different treatment than drug-susceptible TB. As described in the 2010 issue of the New England Journal of Medicine, the researchers assessed the performance of the new automated test on 1,730 patients with suspected TB in four countries. The new automated test successfully identified 98 percent of all confirmed TB cases and 98 percent of patients with RIF-resistant bacteria in less than 2 hours. In addition, a single MTB/RIF analysis detected TB in over 72 percent of patients who did not appear to have TB according to smear microscopy but who were later found to have TB in culture tests. When the automated test was repeated, the sensitivity increased by about 13 percent. When the test was run a third time, it detected about 90 percent of TB cases that were missed by smear microscopy. The Xpert MTB/RIF assay detects *M. tuberculosis* and RIF resistance by PCR amplification of the Rifampicin resistance-determining region (RRDR) of the *M. tuberculosis* rpoB gene and subsequent probing of this region for mutations that are associated with RIF resistance. Approximately 95 percent of RIF-resistant tuberculosis cases contain mutations in this 81-bp region.

Histopathology

A histological diagnosis is made with traditional hematoxylin and eosin (HE) staining as well as with Ziehl-Neelsen staining with a basic Fuschin dye. The classic features are caseous necrosis, giant cells, epithelial cell clusters and lymphocyte infiltration. Lesions are highly indicative of but not exclusive to TB unless tubercle bacilli are seen. A similar picture may also be seen in fungal or sarcoid disease.

Serological Diagnosis of Tuberculosis

These tests are widely being used to detect tuberculosis because they have a high negative predictive value and are useful screening tests. Various methods are:

Antigen Detection in Body Fluids

These are polyclonal antibodies raised against crude mycobacterial antigen. The sensitivity of the test ranges from 40 to 50 percent and specificity of from 80 to 95 percent.

The most commonly used antigens include PPD, Ag5 (38 kDa), AgA60, 45/47 kDaAg, Agkp90, 30kDaAg, P32 Ag, cord factor and LAM. The methods used are sandwich ELISA, inhibition ELISA, latex agglutination and reverse passive hemagglutination tests.

Antigen 5 (38 kDa Antigen)

This test shows reasonable sensitivity and high specificity. In a study from China, the test was 89 percent sensitive and 94 to 100 percent specific for patients with active pulmonary TB. Cole, et al.[22] also used antigen 5 in a serological test but modified it by using a rapid membrane-based antibody assay and found the sensitivity to be 89 percent in patients with smear positive, culture positive TB. In a group of 91 patients, who were both smear and culture negative, the sensitivity was 74 percent while they were on antituberculous therapy. The specificity was 93 percent.

A-60 Antigen

This is a thermostable component of PPD and has been used in the serodiagnosis of tuberculosis. An ELISA revealed a sensitivity of 76.2 percent for patients with active pulmonary TB and 59 percent for patients with extrapulmonary TB,[23] in 153 individuals with inactive tuberculous infection, the specificity was only 81.7 percent. In a study of 560 Chinese patients with pulmonary and extrapulmonary TB[24] and over 700 controls, measurement of IgM appeared to be sensitive (80%) for active primary TB and specific (100%) for latent TB. IgG against the A-60 antigen was predictive of active post-primary TB (sensitivity of 89%). Among 529 healthy persons, most of whom were vaccinated with BCG, including 287 of whom were PPD positive, there were less than 1 percent false positives.

30 kDa Antigen

The specificity of 30 kDa antigen using Dot enzyme immunoassay and standard ELISA assay were 92 and 97 percent, respectively. Where active TB patients were compared to the ones who had no disease, the sensitivity was 69 and 78 percent, respectively. It was also seen that the group with active disease had a strong humoral response to the 30 kDa antigen. Thus, humoral response in a patient to the 30 kDa antigen suggests active infection and also indicates non-protective immune response.

These tests have a few limitations and therefore, cannot replace the conventional tests. Suboptimal sensitivity in smear negative and immunocompromised patients will miss these cases. These tests fail to distinguish between active and latent TB infection. They do not suggest whether the patient has pulmonary or extrapulmonary tuberculosis, making interpretation of results difficult for the gynecologist. The other disadvantages are the high cost and requirement for greater personnel training.

Tuberculosis Skin Testing (TST)

The diagnosis of asymptomatic tuberculous infection tests principally upon delayed type hypersensitivity (DTH) reaction to a purified protein derivative. Tuberculin skin testing is virtually the only means of identifying latent TB infection since by definition, all culture material must be negative to qualify as latent infection. False negative results may occur as a result of waning of DTH, which commonly occurs with prolonged intervals between the infection and testing seen in the elderly or in immunocompromised patients. Active TB itself may suppress cell-mediated immunity such that the PPD is negative. The PPD skin test has a false-negative result of 25 percent. This appears to be due to poor nutrition, acute illness or immunosuppression.

A valid TST requires proper administration by the Mantoux method with intradermal injection of 0.1 mL of tuberculin-purified protein derivative (PPD) into the volar surface of the forearm. In addition, patients must return to a health-care provider for test reading, however, inaccuracies and bias exist in reading the test. Additionally, false-positive TSTs can result from contact with non-tuberculous mycobacteria or vaccination with Bacille-Calmette-Guerin (BCG) because the TST test material (PPD) contains antigens that are also in BCG and certain non-tuberculous mycobacteria.

Previous Vaccination with BCG

Immunization with the BCG vaccine causes a tuberculin reaction <10 mm. A reaction greater than 10 mm is considered a positive reaction and indicates infection with *M. tuberculosis.*

The various reasons are: (i) Tuberculin test conversion rates after vaccination may be less than 100 percent (ii) tuberculin sensitivity tends to wane after BCG vaccination over time. Therefore, it is important that vaccinated persons, who have positive reaction to the tuberculin skin test, be evaluated for tuberculosis.[25]

MPB 64 Patch Test

To overcome poor specificity of the existing skin test based on tuberculin, well-defined antigens are needed to distinguish between infected individuals and those with active disease. The latest of these is the MPB 64 patch test.

MPB 64 is a specific mycobacterial antigen for the *M. tuberculosis* complex. This patch test becomes positive 3 to 4 days after application of the patch and lasts for a week. The test has a specificity of 100 percent and a sensitivity of 98.1 percent.[26]

Interferon Gamma Release Assay

Recognition that interferon gamma (IFN-γ) plays a critical role in regulating cell-mediated immune responses to *M. tuberculosis* infection led to the development of IFN-γ release assays (IGRAs) for the detection of *M. tuberculosis* infection.[27] IGRAs detect sensitization to *M. tuberculosis* by measuring IFN-γ release (from sensitized lymphocytes in whole blood) in response to antigens representing *M. tuberculosis*. IGRAs assess the response to synthetic overlapping peptides that represent specific *M. tuberculosis* proteins, such as early secretory antigenic target-6 (ESAT-6) and culture filtrate protein 10 (CFP-10). These proteins are present in all *M. tuberculosis* strains and they stimulate a measurable release of IFN-γ in most infected persons, but they are absent from BCG vaccine strains and from most non-tuberculous mycobacteria.

QuantiFERON-TB Gold

According to the US Center for Disease Control, the QuantiFERON-TB Gold (QFT-G) test is a whole-blood test for use as an aid in diagnosing *M. tuberculosis* infection, including latent tuberculosis infection (LTBI) and active tuberculosis (TB) disease. This test was approved by the US Food and Drug Administration (FDA) in 2005.[28]

Blood samples are mixed with antigens (substances that can produce an immune response) immediately after phlebotomy and controls. For QFT-G, the antigens include mixtures of synthetic peptides representing two *M. tuberculosis* proteins, ESAT-6 and CFP-10. After incubation of blood with the antigens for 16 to 24 hours, the amount of IFN-γ is measured. If the patient is infected with *M. tuberculosis*, their white blood cells will release IFN-γ in response to contact with the TB antigens. The QFT-G results are based on the amount of IFN-γ that is released in response to the antigens.

Advantages of the test are:
- Requires a single patient visit to draw a blood sample.
- Results can be available within 24 hours.
- Does not boost responses measured by subsequent tests, which can happen with tuberculin skin tests (TST).

- It is not subject to reader bias that can occur with TST.
- It is not affected by prior BCG vaccination.

Disadvantages and limitations of the test are:
- Blood samples must be processed within 12 hours after collection while white blood cells are still viable.
- There are limited data on the use of QFT-G in children younger than 17 years of age, among persons recently exposed to *M. tuberculosis*, and in immunocompromised persons (e.g. impaired immune function caused by HIV infection or acquired immunodeficiency syndrome [AIDS], current treatment with immunosuppressive drugs, selected hematological disorders, specific malignancies, diabetes, silicosis, and chronic renal failure).
- Errors in collecting or transporting blood specimens or in running and interpreting the assay can decrease the accuracy of QFT-G.
- Limited data on the use of QFT-G to determine who is at risk for developing TB disease.
- False positive results can occur with *M. szulgai, M. kansasii,* and *M. marinum.*

QuantiFERON-TB Gold In-tube

Following FDA approval for a modification of the QuantiFERON-TB Gold to an in-tube collection system that consists of three blood collection tubes—Nil, TB antigen, and mitogen, the modified device is marketed under the trade name QuantiFERON-TB Gold in-tube and is indicated for use as an *in vitro* diagnostic test. It uses a peptide cocktail simulating ESAT-6, CFP-10 and TB 7. 7(p4) proteins to stimulate cells in heparinized whole blood drawn directly into specialized blood collection tubes. Detection of interferon-γ by enzyme-linked immunosorbent assay (ELISA) is used to identify *in vitro* responses to these peptide antigens that are associated with *M. tuberculosis* infection.

According to the FDA approved package insert, Quanti-FERON TB Gold in-tube has a consistent specificity of >99 percent in low risk individuals and a sensitivity as high as 92 percent in individuals with active disease, depending on the setting and extent of disease. The specificity in two studies of a few hundred people is 96 to 98 percent in a health-immunized population.

T-Spot IGRA Test

T-Spot became the fourth IGRA to be approved by FDA.[29] For this test, peripheral blood mononuclear cells (PBMCs) are incubated with control materials and two mixtures of peptides, one representing the entire amino acid sequence of ESAT-6 and the other representing the entire amino acid sequence of CFP-10. The test uses an enzyme-linked immunospot assay (ELISpot) to detect increases in the number of cells that secrete IFN-γ (represented as spots in each test well) after stimulation with antigen as compared to the media control (Nil).

Indirect Approach

Detection of Antibodies for Diagnosis of TB

Antibodies to the mycobacterial antigen in the sera of patients are detected either by using monoclonal or polyclonal antibodies. The newer approaches are as follows:

TB STAT–PAK: Immunochromatographic test to detect antibodies to differentiate active from dormant TB infection is under research.[30]

Enzyme immunoassay for detection of anti-mycobacterial superoxide dismutase antibody: Superoxide dismutase is a secretory protein of *M. tuberculosis* and is being used for the serodiagnosis of tuberculosis.[31]

Insta test TB: It is used for the detection of antibodies in active disease using the patient's serum, antibody-binding protein conjugated to a colloidal gold particle, and a unique combination of TB antigens immobilized on the membrane.[32]

Adenosine deaminase: Estimation of adenosine deaminase (ADA) in pleural fluid, as well as peritoneal fluid has shown that the activity of this enzyme is increased in patients with tuberculous effusions as compared to its levels in conditions like parapneumonic effusions or malignancy.

Hysterosalpingography: Hysterosalpingography (HSG) is routinely performed for the evaluation of the Fallopian tubes and the uterine cavity in infertile women. Since tuberculosis often affects the genital tract in these women, it can lead to certain characteristic findings that can point to the presence of this disease. Fallopian tubes may show terminal (tobacco pouch appearance) or complete hydrosalpinx, a beaded appearance, or a straight lead pipe-like appearance, and sometimes, no dye fills the tube due to a cornual block. The uterine cavity shows an irregular outline with filling defects suggestive of synechiae. There is extravasation of the dye into venous and lymphatic vessels, cavity may appear T-shaped at times, and scarring towards one side may give the false appearance of a unicornuate cavity.

Ultrasonography: Sometimes, a routine ultrasonography of the pelvis may suggest the presence of tuberculosis. The finding of elongated tubular structures along the ovary may be suggestive of hydrosalpinx. Fluid with thin septa around pelvic organs and cysts with low level echoes suggest the presence of ovarian or adnexal masses containing pus. The endometrium may be thin or irregular suggesting the presence of intrauterine adhesions.

Magnetic resonance imaging (MRI)/computed tomography (CT) scan: These tests are not indicated unless adnexal masses of unknown etiology are evaluated.

Laparoscopy: Laparoscopy is performed only when active tuberculosis is not present based on a preoperative endometrial biopsy. However, we may still encounter evidence of this disease in the pelvis, suggested by the presence of serous fluid collections with thin septations. Tubercles may be present on the uterus, Fallopian tubes or the peritoneum. The Fallopian tubes may show hydrosalpinges or terminal dilatations due to fimbrial agglutination. Tubes may be blocked and appear shortened, thickened, rigid, inflamed, beaded or buried in adhesions. On attempting tuboplasty or fimbrioplasty, caseous material may be seen. Tubo-ovarian abscesses may rarely be present.

Hysteroscopy: Tuberculosis, involving the uterine cavity, may lead to the formation of synechiae or adhesions. It may be difficult to performing hysteroscopy as the cervix is often difficult to dilate and the cavity may be shrunken or obliterated. Sometimes, the endometrium appears pale or in active endometritis, may appear reddened, ulcerated or with white patches suggestive of caseation. Even when all the tests and evaluation are negative for tuberculosis, the disease may still be missed and AFB can be demonstrated in the wound discharge from the non-healing scar of laparoscopy or any surgical scar. Definite clinical suspicion can surely lead to the diagnosis of tuberculosis.

CONCLUSION

To treat or not to treat is a great dilemma for the physician, especially when there is either a clinical suspicion or investigations suggest but do not confirm the diagnosis of tuberculosis. Further research is needed to establish clear criteria for diagnosing genital tuberculosis.

REFERENCES

1. Katoch VM. Newer diagnostic techniques for TB. Indian J Med Res 2004;120:418-28.
2. Smithwick RW. Laboratory manual of acid-fast microscopy (2nd edition). Centre for Disease Control, Altants, 1975.
3. Mejia GI, Castrillon L, Trijilo H, Robledo JA. Micro colony detection on 7H 11 thin layer culture as an alternative for rapid diagnosis of *Mycobacterium tuberculosis* infection. Int J Tuberc Lung Dis 1999;3:138-42.
4. Isenberg HD, D' Amato RF, Heifets L, Murray PR, Scardamaglia M, Jacobs MC, et al. Collaborative feasibility study of a biphasic system (Roche Septi-chek AFB) for rapid detection and isolation of Mycobacteria. J Clin Microbiol 1991;29:1719-22.
5. Bemer P, Palicova F, Rusch-Gerdes S, Drugeon HB, Pfyffer GE. Multicenter evaluation of fully automatic BALTEC mycobacteria growth indicator tube 960 system for susceptibility testing of *Mycobacterium tuberculosis*. J Clin Microbiol 2002; 40:150-54.
6. Tortoli E, Mandler F, Tronci M, Penti V, Sbaraglia G, Costa D, et al. Multicenter evaluation of mycobacteria growth indicator

tube (MGIT) compared with the BACTEC radiometric method, BBL biphasic growth medium and Lowenstein-Jensen medium. Clin Microbiol Infect 1997;3:468-9.

7. Rohner P, Ninel B, Metral C, Emler S, Auckenthaler R. Evalution of MB/Bac T system and comparison with BACTEC 460 system and solid media for isolation of mycobacteria from clinical specimens. J Clin Microbiol 1997;35:3127-31.

8. Duffey PS, Gutherrtz LS, Evans GC. Improved rapid identification of mycobacteria by combining solid-phase extraction with high-performance liquid chromatography analysis of BACTEC cultures. J Clin Microbiol 1996;34:1939-43.

9. Kaminski DA, Hardy DJ. Selective utilization of DNA probes for identification of *Mycobacterium* species on the basis of cord formation in primary BACTEC 12B cultures. J Clin Microbiol 1995;33:1548-50.

10. Ruiz P, Gulierrez J, Zerolo FJ, Casal M. Geno Type *Mycobacterium* assay for identification of mycobacterial species isolated from human clinical samples by using liquid medium. J Clin Microbiol 2002;40:3076-8.

11. Sharma RK, Katoch K, Shiva Nnavar, et al. Comparisons of sensitivity of probs targeting RNA vs DNA in leprosy cases. Indian J Med microbial 1996;14:99-104.

12. Brunello F, Fontana R. Reliability of the MB-bact T system for testing susceptibility of *Mycobacterium tuberculosis* complex slrains of anti-tuberculous drugs. J Clin Microbiol 2000;38:872-3.

13. Telenti A, Marchesi F, Balz M, Bally F, Böttger EC, Bodmer T. Rapid identification of mycobacteria to the species level by polymerase chain reaction and restriction enzyme analysis. J Clin Microbiol 1993;31:175-8.

14. Goyal M, Young D, Zhang V, Jenkins PA, Shaw RJ. PCR amplification of variable sequence upstream of katG gene to subdivide strains of *Mycobacterium tuberculosis* complex. J Clin Microbiol 1994;32:3070-9.

15. Roth A, Reischl U, Streubel A, Naumann L, Kroppenstedt RM, Habicht M, et al. Novel diagnostic algorithm for indetification of mycobacteria using genes specific amplification of 165–235 rRNA gene spacer and restriction endonucleases. J Clin Microbiol 2000;38:1094-6.

16. Forbes BA, Hicks KES. Direct detection of *Mycobacterium tuberculosis* in respiratory specimens in a clinical laboratory by polymerase chain reaction. J Clin Microbiol 1993;31:1688-94.

17. Verma A, Rattan A, Tyagi JS. Development of a 235 rRNA based PCR assay for the detection of mycobactria. Indian J Biochem Biophys 1994;31:288-94.

18. Shankar P, Manju Nath N, Mohan KK, Prasad K, Behari M, Sriniwas, et al. Rapid diagnosis of tuberculosis meningitis by polymerase chain reaction. Mancet 1991:337:3-7.

19. Verma A, Dasgupta N, Agarwal AN, Pande JN, Tyagi JS. Utility of a *Mycobacterium tuberculosis* GC-rich repetitive sequence in the diagnosis of tuberculosis pleural effusion by PCR. Indian J Biochem Biophys 1995;32:429-36.

20. Singh KK, Nair MD, Radhakrishnan K, Tyagi JS. Utility of PCR assay in diagnosis of en-plaque tuberculoma of the brain. J Clin Microbiol 1999;37:467-70.

21. Blakemore R, Story E, Helb D, Kop J, Banada P, Owens MR, et al. Evaluation of the analytical performance of the Xpert MTB/RIF assay. J Clin Microbiol 2010;48:2495-501.

22. Cole RA, Lu HM, Shi YZ, Wang J, De-Hna T, Zhow AT. Clinical evaluation of a rapid immunochromatographic assay based on the 38 kDa antigen of *Mycobacterium tuberculosis* on patients with pulmonary tuberculosis in China. Tuber Lung Dis 1996; 77:363-8.

23. Luh KT, Yu CJ, Yang PC, Lee LN. Tuberculosis antigen A60 serodiagnosis in tuberculous infection: application in extra-pulmonary and smear-negative pulmonary tuberculosis. Respirology 1996;1:145-51.

24. Zou YL, Zhang JD, Chen MH, Shi GQ Prignot J, Cocito C. Serological analysis of pulmonary and extrapulmonary tuberculosis with enzyme-linked immunosorbent assays for anti-A60 immunoglobulins. Clin Infect Dis 1994;19:1084-91.

25. Bowerman RJ. Tuberculin skin testing in BCG-vaccinated populations of adults and children at high risk for tuberculosis in Taiwan. Int J Tuberc Lung Dis 2004;8:1228-33.

26. Nakamura RM, Velmonte MA, Kawajiri K et al. MPB64 mycobacterial antigen: A new skin test reagent through patch method for rapid diagnosis of active tuberculosis. Int J Tuberc Lung Dis 1998;2:541-6.

27. Updated Guidelines for Using Interferon Gamma Release Assays to Detect *Mycobacterium tuberculosis* Infection - United States, 2010, June 25, 2010 / Vol. 59 / No. RR-5.

28. Marra F, Marra CA, Sadatsafavi M, Morán-Mendoza O, Cook V, Elwood RK, et al. Cost-effectiveness of a new interferon-based blood assay, QuantiFERON (R)-TB Gold, in screening tuberculosis contacts. Int J Tuberc Lung Dis 2008;12:1414-24.

29. Oxford Immunotec Limited. T-Spot.TB [U.S. package insert]. Available at http://www.oxfordimmunotec.com/ USpageInsert. Accessed June 16, 2010.

30. Bothamley GH. Serological diagnosis of tuberculosis. Eur Resp J 1995;8:676-9.

31. Ahmad A, Afghan S, Raykundlia C, Catty D. Diagnosis of tuberculosis by using enzyme-linked immunosorbent assay to detect antimycobacterial superoxide dismutase in the patients. J Islamic Acad of Sci 1998;11:1-3.

32. Chan ED, Heifets L, Iseman MD. Immunologic diagnosis of tuberculosis: A review. Tuberc Lung Dis 2000;80:131-3.

Management of Polycystic Ovary Syndrome

Kamala Selvaraj, Priya Selvaraj, Deepu Rajkamal Selvaraj

OVERVIEW

We conducted a retrospective study on clinical and surgical practices at our Fertility Research Center, during the period 2004 to 2005 on 3584 infertile cases to expound the clinical and surgical management of polycystic ovary syndrome (PCOS). The incidence of PCOS was 29.66 percent (1063/3584). The pregnancy rate was 20.88 percent (222/1063). Among 142 patients on whom laparoscopic electrocoagulation of ovarian surface (LEOS) was performed, we achieved a pregnancy rate of 28.17 percent (40/142). Letrozole did not prove better than Clomiphene citrate (CC) or gonadotropins except in few PCOS cases. Hence, patients with PCOS should be identified for preventive treatment. Lifestyle modifications should be suggested prior to considering the use of pharmacological therapy or assisted reproductive technique (ART). While CC is accepted as the first-line treatment, CC+ gonadotropins gives good results in CC-resistant cases. Insulin sensitizing agents are most effective as an adjuvant therapy. *In vitro* fertilization (IVF) is best instituted in patients with persistent elevated luteinizing hormone (LH) levels. The treatment protocol should be tailored to meet individual requirements.

INTRODUCTION

The prevalence of PCOS in the general population is about 20 to 33 percent and in infertile patients, it is about 30 percent. At our center (FRC, GG Hospital), the incidence is about 20 to 35.38 percent among the infertile group.

The management strategies of PCOS address issues like menstrual disturbances, obesity, infertility, hirsutism and long-term sequelae. The strategies involve regularizing the menstrual cycle, weight reduction, ovulation induction, ovarian drilling, assisted reproductive technique (ART) and individualized therapy for the management of long-term sequelae like diabetes, hypertension, endometrial and ovarian cancer.

CLINICAL DISCUSSION

Menstrual Disturbances/Disorders

The most common presentation among the menstrual disorders is oligomenorrhea (87%). These patients spontaneously menstruate and have either normal or profuse bleeding. Amenorrhea is found in about 26 percent of cases and these cases need induction of menstrual cycles with pills. They have no estrogen deficiency and therefore, have no risk of osteoporosis but may be at risk for developing endometrial hyperplasia. Regular cycles were seen in patients with body mass index (BMI) <30 kg/m^2 (around 32% cases) and BMI > 30 kg/m^2 (around 22% cases).

Management here involves weight reduction to at least 5 to 10 percent. Low dose oral contraceptive (OC) pills help in regularizing the cycles. The other way to regularize the cycle is by substituting with progestogens with low androgenic potential (Medroxyprogesterone acetate/Dydrogesterone) for 10 days from day 16 to induce withdrawal bleeding. Sometimes progesterone-releasing intrauterine devices (IUDs), like Mirena systems, can be used.

Polycystic Ovary Syndrome in Adolescents

Low birth weight (LBW) predisposes adolescents to PCOS with genetic forms of insulin resistance, type 1 diabetes, precocious puberty (PP) and childhood obesity. The preventive approach to adolescent' PCOS involves lifestyle modifications, diet-induced weight loss, insulin-sensitizing agents, antiandrogens and oral contraceptives.[1] Early recognition of the syndrome and treatment may prevent and possibly, ameliorate all the symptoms and the later potential development of metabolic and cardiovascular complications.

Obesity[2]

A BMI $\geq$ 30 kg/m^2 and more metabolically active visceral adipose tissue is an indication of obesity. Study on the amount of visceral fat correlated with insulin resistance and the distribution of fat is important. Android (central) obesity more of a risk factor than gynecoid obesity. A weight reduction of 5 to 10 percent leads to a 30 percent loss of visceral adipose tissue. A waist circumference more than 88 cm is a better indicator of an increased metabolic risk than the conventional waist:hip ratio.

The high-risk indicators of PCOS are abdominal obesity with a waist circumference > 88 cm, triglycerides $\geq$ 150 mg/dL, high density lipoprotein (HDL)-c < 50 mg/dL, blood pressure $\geq$ 130/90 mm Hg and an abnormal oral glucose tolerance test (OGTT).

The ideal mission for weight reduction is a cardiovascular workout and stretching exercises for a minimum of three times a week or brisk walking for one hour everyday combined with yoga thrice a week. Additionally, aerobic exercises can burn calories, lower blood pressure, raise HDL cholesterol and improve insulin resistance. The dietary recommendation for nonobese/obese women with PCOS is a balanced diet with a moderate intake of carbohydrates (approximately 40–50% calories), select complex unrefined carbohydrates, select low glycemic index foods, green vegetables (leafy and nonleafy) and no tubers.

For PCOS with hypothyroidism—avoid, cauliflower, turnip, cabbage and asparagus are best avoided while the carbohydrate intake must be spaced. The diet should be tailored to fit the individual person.[3]

Hirsutism

Hirsutism is associated with menstrual disturbances, leading to excess hair growth on the body. Hirsutism can be managed by administering ethinyl estradiol (35 μgm), Cyproterone acetate (Diane-35, Krimson 35), 2 mg or Drosperinone 5 mg (yasmin). Other therapeutic methods use combined oral contraceptive pills (OCPs), progestogens, spironolactone, flutamide, finasteride, gonadotropin-releasing hormone (GnRH) agonists and metformin. Depilatory creams that uproot hair, electrolysis and laser therapy are useful adjuncts to medical therapy. A reliable contraception should be used while on antiandrogen therapy. At least 6 months of treatment is needed for significant improvement. Most therapies are palliative than curative.

Infertility

The management of PCOS-associated infertility may be involve a medical and/or surgical approach. The basic

pathophysiology of hyperinsulinemia leads to anovulation, elevated LH and miscarriages, resulting in infertility. Both obese and non-obese individuals are more insulin-resistant and hyperinsulinemic than age and weight-matched controls.

Elevated LH levels in the early follicular phase decrease follicular maturation and increase the incidence of unruptured follicle syndrome (UFS) and miscarriages. High day 2 LH concentrations can be expected in cases of PCOS, bad obstetric history (BOH), in the perimenopausal group and also in infertility of anovulatory origin. The mean normal value of LH on day 2 should be preferably less than 6 IU/L. According to our study, fetal wastage was observed in 5.17 percent (55/1063) of the patients (Table 28.1).

Ovulation induction strategies can be divided into medical, surgical and ART. The medical strategies are:
- Clomiphene citrate (CC) + corticosteroids + estrogen
- CC step-up regimen and CC + gonadotropins [low dose follicle-stimulating hormone (FSH) + human menopausal gonadotropin (hMG)] + metformin.
- Surgically, ovarian drilling can be done.
- The long protocol, short protocol or ultrashort protocol may be used when ART is the management of choice.

Clomiphene citrate (CC), administered in a dosage of 50 to100 mg over a period of 5 to 7 days. Its dose can be increased by 50 mg up to 250 mg over the same period. Estradiol (2 mg) valerate should be used for 10 days to combat the antiestrogenic effect of Clomiphene at the level of endometrium. Following stimulation with CC, an 80 percent ovulatory rate, 40 percent cumulative pregnancy rate and a 40 percent miscarriage rate has been reported. The use of CC for more than 1 year may increase the risk of ovarian cancer.

About 20 to 25 percent of anovulatory women with PCOS are Clomiphene-resistant. These cases can be treated with an

Table 28.1: PCOS—statistics (2004–2005)

• Infertile patients (%)	:	3584
• PCOS patients (%)	:	1063/3584 (29.66%)
• Pregnancies (%)	:	222/1063 (20.88%)
• Total fetal wastage (%)	:	55/1063 (5.17%)
– ART	:	93
- Fetal wastages	:	31
- Delivered	:	44
- Lost in follow-up	:	2
- Ongoing	:	16
– IUI	:	68
- Fetal wastages	:	18
- Delivered	:	26
- Lost in follow-up	:	13
- Ongoing	:	11
– Natural	:	61
- Fetal wastages	:	6
- Delivered	:	28
- Lost in follow-up	:	16
- Ongoing	:	11

Table 28.2: Letrozole vs CC or gonadotropins					
Drug	*Cases*	*Pregnancies*	*Outcome*		
			Ongoing	*Wastage*	*Delivered*
Letrozole	118	8 (6.7)	6	2	–
Letrozole + GnRH	60	8 (13.3)	4	3	1
Letrozole + FSH + CC	56	6 (10.7)	2	–	4
Letrozole + CC	16	9 (56.2)	9	–	–
Total	**250**	**31**	**21**	**5**	**5**

increase in the CC dosage, or CC step-up and gonadotropin supplementation. Decreased cervical mucus found in about 15 percent of cases can be overcome by performing intra-uterine insemination (IUI). Dexamethasone (0.5 mg) at bedtime, which suppresses the adrenal androgen secretion and induces responsiveness to Clomiphene in previous nonresponders, may be used as an adjunct to Clomiphene therapy.

Metformin is an oral biguanide with multifactorial action. It primarily acts at the post receptor level to improve insulin sensitivity, enhances peripheral glucose uptake and inhibits hepatic glucose production. Metformin is a useful adjunctive therapy in infertile patients with CC-resistant PCOS and markedly improves ovulation and pregnancy rates. It enhances the follicular response to ovulation induction with exogenous gonadotropins. The dosage is 500 mg once daily for patients with a BMI 19 to 24 kg/m^2, 500 mg twice daily for patients with a BMI 25 to 28 kg/m^2, and 850 mg twice daily for patients with a BMI 29 to 35 kg/m^2.

According to our study,[4] Letrozole did not prove better than CC or gonadotropins, except in few cases of PCOS[4] (Table 28.2).

Parental gonadotropins were added to CC in cases with inadequate response to induce ovulation. Cumulative conception and live birth rates were reported to be 62 percent and 54 percent, respectively after 6 months and 73 percent and 62 percent, respectively after 12 months.[5] PCOS patients are very sensitive to the use of gonadotropins, so it is best to start with low dose injections. Failure to conceive following the administration of CC or CC + GnRH within 6 to 12 ovulatory cycles, warrants ART using the step-up, low dose step-up, or step-down protocol.

The Impact of PCOS on ART

- Patients with PCOS have an explosive response to conventional ovarian stimulation.
- Though ovarian stimulation increases follicle numbers, it results in poor quality oocytes, increased estrogen levels and decreased fertilization rates.
- Compared to PCOS, the pregnancy rate per embryo transfer in normal patients was 28.65 percent.
- A small group of poor responder PCOS patients may benefit from the use of growth hormone.
- The incidence of miscarriages were more in PCOS when compared to normal patients.
- We prefer the long protocol, using the conventional agonist rather than the antagonist in PCOS patients.

Surgical Management

The indications for surgical management at our center are:
- Obese/lean with or without hirsutism.
- Previous failure of response to CC.
- Ovarian volume >10 cm^3.

Laparoscopic electrocoagulation of ovarian surface (LEOS) was described by Gjönnaess[6] in 1984. Destruction of follicles and stroma results in reduction of ovarian androgen levels. The procedure uses unipolar coagulating current, with 2 to 4 mm deep penetration and 3 to 5 mm diameter for about 2 to 4 seconds depending on the size of

Table 28.3: LEOS statistics (2004–2005)		
• Total no of LEOS cases done	:	142
• Pregnancies	:	40 (28.17%)
– Natural	:	15
- Fetal wastages	:	1
- Delivered	:	7
- Lost in follow-up	:	5
- Ongoing	:	2
– IUI	:	13
- Fetal wastages	:	5
- Delivered	:	5
- Lost in follow-up	:	2
- Ongoing	:	1
– ART	:	12
- Fetal wastages	:	3
- Delivered	:	6
- Ongoing	:	3

the ovary and number of microcysts (5–20 punctures). This procedure ensures minimal morbidity, decreases ovarian hyperstimulation syndrome (OHSS) and multiple pregnancy rates and decreases the spontaneous abortion rate. The rate of adhesions at second-look diagnostic laparoscopy is between 19.3 to 26.9 percent. Using this procedure, best results can be obtained within 6 to 12 months. The pregnancy rate with LEOS at our center was 28.17 percent (40/142) (Table 28.3).

The procedure is not performed for the treatment of hirsutism, PCOS patients without infertility and in unmarried PCOS patients. Ovarian drilling should not be done in regularly menstruating women when polycystic ovaries are diagnosed by ultrasound only. Though these patients are anovulatory, they are responsive to ovulation induction (OI) protocols.

The indications for ART in PCOS patients are tubal factor, 4 to 6 failed IUI cycles, persistent elevated LH on day 2/3, resistance to or failure of Clomiphene therapy, poor response to CC and gonadotropin therapy, severe male factor, and for patients demanding ART.

New Trends in PCOS: *In vitro* Maturation

Minimal stimulation with the retrieval of immature oocytes combined with *in vitro* maturation (IVM) could potentially replace standard stimulation protocols, which provoke OHSS and reduce the cost and duration of treatment. Although immature oocytes retrieved from untreated ovaries can be matured, fertilized and developed *in vitro*, the rate of implantation of the cleaved embryo is low.[6]

CONCLUSION

- Girls at risk for PCOS should be identified early and appropriate treatment given to prevent progression and long-term sequelae.

- Lifestyle modifications (eucaloric diet and physical activity) should be advised ideally prior to initiating the use of any drug or ART.

- Clomiphene citrate is accepted as a first-line of treatment. In CC-resistant cases, a combination of CC with gonadotropins gives good results.

- Insulin sensitizing agents are best effective as adjuvant therapy.

- *In vitro* fertilization is best instituted in patients with persistent elevated LH levels.

- Cases should be individualized and treatment protocols should be tailored to meet individual requirements.

REFERENCES

1. IBANEZ Lourdes, FERRER Angela, ONG Ken, et al. Insulin sensitization early after menarche prevents progression from precocious pubarche to polycystic ovary syndrome. J Pediatric 2004;144:23-9.
2. Tang T, Glanville J, Hayden CJ, White D, Barth JH, Balen AH. Combined lifestyle modification and metformin in obese patients with polycystic ovary syndrome. A randomized, placebo-controlled, double-blind multicenter study. Hum Reprod 2006; 21:80-9.
3. Douglas CC, Gower BA, Darnell BE, Ovalle F, Oster RA, Azziz R. Role of diet in the treatment of polycystic ovary syndrome. Fertil Steril 2006;85:679-88.
4. Selvaraj K, Selvaraj P. Comparison of clomiphene citrate and letrozole for ovulation induction and resultant pregnancy outcome. J Obstet Gynecol Ind 2004;54:579-82.
5. Adam H Balen, Catherine J Hayden, Anthony J. Rutherford. Clinical efficiency of recombinant gonadotrophins. Hum Reprod 1999;14·1411-7.
6. Gjönnaess H. Polycystic ovarian syndrome treated by ovarian electrocautery through the laparoscope. Fertil Steril 1984;41: 20-5.

Recurrent Endometriosis: Physiopathology, Epidemiology, Prevention and Treatment

Céline Lefebvre Lacoeuille, Catala Laurent, Boussion F, Philippe Descamps

OVERVIEW

Although endometriosis appears to yield to current medical and surgical treatment, the rate of recurrence is alarmingly high. This article reviews recent work on the physiopathology, epidemiology, prevention and treatment of recurrent post-therapeutic endometriosis. The precise mechanisms involved in the development of recurrent endometriosis are not fully understood but it is now clear that the post therapeutic formation of new lesions is closely associated with the reactivation of residual lesions. Surgery, whatever the technique used, has proved to be the best method of preventing recurrences so far. However, none of the treatments available at present, including iterative conservative surgery and even radical surgery, which is considered particularly effective, eliminate the risk of further recurrence. The improved management of recurrent endometriosis will require a better understanding of the physiopathology of the disease. Recent progress in fundamental research promises the development of novel treatments, based on aromatase and metalloproteinase inhibitors as well as various antiangiogenic substances, now undergoing clinical tests.

INTRODUCTION

Endometriosis is one of the most common gynecological pathologies, estimated to affect about 10 percent of women.[1] The physiopathology of the disease is poorly understood but it is known to involve various genetic, hormonal, immunological and anatomical factors.[1,2] In contrast, the recurrence of the disease, despite apparently effective surgical or medical treatment, is very frequent.[3-10] Recurrent endometriosis is basically a benign disorder but the accompanying pain, the incidence of fertility and the therapeutic constraints on patients may be highly invalidating. The aim of this work is to review the literature to collate current information concerning the physiopathology, the epidemiology, the prevention and the treatment of recurrent endometriosis.

CLINICAL DISCUSSION

Physiopathology of Recurrent Endometriosis

The precise mechanisms behind the development of recurrent endometriosis are not yet fully understood but the disorder may be secondary, either to the post-therapeutic development of endometriotic lesions or to the persistence and the reactivation of existing post-therapeutic lesions.

Recurrent Endometriosis due to the Development of New Lesions

The theory most commonly put forward to explain the development of pelvic endometriosis involves retrograde menstruation, i.e. the tubal reflux of menstrual fluid accompanied by the dissemination and implantation of endometrial cells in the pelvis.[1,2,11-14] While it is generally admitted that peritoneal endometriotic implants are secondary to this mode of dissemination, the physiopathology of ovarian endometriosis and endometriosis of the rectovaginal septum is still a matter of debate. Some authors favor the hypothesis of metaplasia,[15] whereas others believe that peritoneal endometriosis, ovarian endometriosis and endometriosis of the rectovaginal septum are merely different expressions of a disorder caused by the same mechanism, i.e. the tubal reflux.[1,16]

Several elements favor the theory of menstrual dissemination. The greater risk of endometriosis observed in patients presenting precocious menarche or abundant periods may be explained by the increased risk of contamination of the peritoneal cavity due to the tubal reflux of endometrial matter.[1] Several authors have observed the asymmetry of peritoneal and ovarian endometriotic lesions. These are more frequently located to the left than to the right of the pelvis.[13,14] This lateralization may be explained by the close anatomical relationship between the sigmoid colon and the left appendage, which creates an isolated zone favoring the implantation of endometrial cells carried by the tubal reflux into the peritoneal cavity. Incidentally, an investigation of premenstrual uterine contractility has shown that the basic tonus of the uterus, the frequency of uterine contractions, and the amplitude and incidence of retrograde uterine contractions are higher in patients presenting endometriosis than in those free from the disease.[11] The authors therefore hypothesize that the genesis of endometriosis may be favored by anomalies of uterine contraction leading to menstrual reflux.

Endometriosis and endometriotic recurrences probably develop along the same lines. After treatment by conservative surgery, ensuring the complete ablation of the endometriotic lesions, or after medical treatment designed to block ovarian activity, the menstrual reflux may persist or reappear. The subsequent dissemination of endometrial cells in the peritoneal cavity may trigger recurrent endometriosis.[12,17]

The menstrual reflux occurs roughly each month in the vast majority of women during normal genital activity, but only a fraction are likely to suffer from endometriosis. The genesis of the disease clearly involves other etiological factors. The development of peritoneal endometriotic lesions appears to be directly related to the mechanism of tubal transport, but the process also depends on the survival, adhesion, proliferation, invasive activity and vascularization of endometrial cells.[1,2] These steps in the development of the lesions, implicating various genetic, immunological and hormonal factors, are but little known.[1,18] The surgical treatment of endometriosis allows the resection of the lesions without addressing the etiologic factors of the disease. The main action of the medical treatment of endometriosis relies on the reversible induction of hypoestrogenicity. Thus, current medical and surgical treatments offer only a palliative to recurrent endometriosis since they do not bring into play the physiopathological mechanisms that would prevent the formation of post-therapeutic endometriotic lesions.

Recurrent Endometriosis due to the Reactivation of Existing Lesions

Diagnostic laparoscopy has revealed a significant reduction in the number and size of endometriotic lesions in patients treated with Danazol, a synthetic steroid hormone; however, the lesions reappeared with the resumption of ovarian activity after the cessation of treatment.[19] Similarly, after cessation of treatment with gonadotropin-releasing hormone (GnRH) agonists, persistent histological lesions of endometriosis were observed.[20] Thus, medical treatment fails to eradicate endometriosis.

According to some authors, the drugs used in the treatment of endometriosis increase the apoptotic index and decrease the proliferative activity of endometrial cells.[21,22] However, a study of biopsies of ovarian endometriosis showed comparable lesions whether the patients had received medical treatment or not.[23] Thus, the drugs used do not seem to lead to the complete suppression of the proliferative activity of the endometriotic lesions. This may be due to several factors: the ovarian secretion of estrogens, temporarily suppressed by the administration of the drugs, may resume, stimulating the development of residual endometrotic lesions, or the drugs may act exclusively on the ovarian secretion without affecting the other mechanisms of the biosynthesis of estrogens. One such mechanism involves aromatase, an enzyme that mediates the transformation of the adrenal androgens, androstenedione and testosterone, into estrone and estradiol. Aromatase, which is not found in normal endometrial tissue, is found in several other tissues such as the fatty tissue, the skin and bone tissues.[24,25] However, high levels of aromatase have been detected in the endometrotic lesions and the endometrium of patients with endometriosis.[2,24,25] Thus, despite the drug-induced suppression of ovarian activity, the biosynthesis of estrogens may continue in peripheral tissues as well as within the endometriotic implants. Taken together, these findings indicate that recurrent endometriosis, arising after medical treatment, can be attributed in most cases to the persistence and reactivation of residual endometriotic lesions.

The surgical treatment of endometriosis is based on the ablation of all the endometriotic lesions. However, laparotomy may overlook the smaller or more atypical lesions, thereby exposing the patient to recurrent endometriosis. Studies on biopsies of apparently normal peritoneum have revealed the presence of microscopic endometriotic lesions. Thus, in patients suffering from infertility or presenting with pelvic pain, microscopic lesions were detected in 11 to 13 percent of the patients with microscopic endometriosis and in 6 percent of the patients without the disease.[23,26] However, a prospective study using diagnostic laparoscopy for pelvic pain in 44 patients revealed microscopic lesions in apparently healthy peritoneum in only 0.5 percent of the cases.[27] In spite of the variability of the results, the existence of microscopic endometriosis is now admitted. The persistence and development of this infra-clinical infection may explain the appearance of recurrent endometriosis after surgical treatment.

Epidemiology of Recurrent Endometriosis

Frequency of Recurrent Post-therapeutic Endometriosis

Several clinical studies mention the frequency of recurrent endometriosis in the evaluation of the efficacy of the treatments used. However, the criteria used to define recurrence differ widely. They may be based on the resurgence of pelvic pain, the detection of endometriotic lesions by medical imaging or during clinical examination, the discovery of the lesions during a laparoscopic check-up and, sometimes, on positive histological findings.

The frequency of recurrence reported after conservative surgical treatment of endometriosis varies from one study to another (Table 29.1). Thus, the frequency of the resurgence of pelvic pain fluctuated between 25 and 45 percent.[4,6,28,29] With conservative laparotomy, in cases of stage III or IV endometriosis, according to the revised American Fertility Society (rAFS) classification, the frequency of recurrence, detected by clinical or ultrasound examination, was 15 percent at 12 months, and 9 percent at 18 months of follow-up.[4,6] A retrospective study on 423 patients, treated with conservative surgery for minimum, moderate or severe endometriosis, reported histologically documented recurrence in 9 percent of the cases at 1 year, 13.5 percent at 3 years, and 40.3 percent at 5 years of postoperative follow-up.[10] Two years after conservative laparotomy for stage I or II endometriosis (rAFS), histological evidence of recurrence was found in 9.6 percent of the patients.[30] A prospective study reported a much higher frequency of postoperative recurrence (64% at 1 year of follow-up) but it was based on a rather small number of patients.[17] The reported frequency of reoperation after primary conservative surgery also varied considerably, being estimated at 33 percent[3] and at 63.6 percent[10] at 5 years of follow-up. The frequency of recurrent endometrioma after conservative laparotomy is presented in Table 29.2.

The two main techniques of laparotomy, proposed for the conservative treatment of endometriosis, are cystectomy, which consists of the excision of the cystic sacs, and the drainage followed by the destruction of the cystic sacs by laser vaporization or by bipolar coagulation. The frequency of endometriotic recurrence accompanied by pelvic pain has been reported to vary from 10 to 20 percent after laparoscopic cystectomy,[5,31-38] and from 52.9 to 75 percent after cystic drainage and bipolar coagulation of the cystic sacs.[32,37] The frequency of endometriotic recurrence, detected by ultrasound, has been reported to vary from 2.9 to 11.1 percent after laparoscopic cystectomy, from 12.0 to 20.8 percent after cystic drainage and bipolar coagulation of the cystic sacs, and from 8.0 to 14.3 percent after cystic drainage and laser vaporization of the cystic sacs.[5,32,33-37,39] The frequency of reoperation for the recurrence of endometrioma is estimated at 7.0 to 23.6 percent after cystectomy, and at 57.8 percent after drainage of the endometrioma and the destruction of the cystic sacs.[5,31,38,40]

Three years after conservative surgery of the rectovaginal septum in 83 patients with endometriosis, recurrence accompanied by pelvic pain occurred in 28 percent, clinical or ultrasound examination revealed endometriotic recurrence in 34.2 percent, and reoperation for recurrence was required in 27 percent of the cases.[40] In another group of 169 patients with endometriosis, 36 percent suffered from recurrence

<table>
<tr><td colspan="9" align="center">Table 29.1: Frequency of recurrent endometriosis after conservative surgery</td></tr>
<tr><td>Authors</td><td>Year</td><td>N</td><td>Follow-up (months)</td><td>rAFS stage</td><td>Pelvic pain</td><td>Recurrence (%) clinical or ultrasound examination</td><td>Histology</td><td>Reoperation (%)</td></tr>
<tr><td>Wheeler</td><td>1983</td><td>423</td><td>12</td><td>NI</td><td>/</td><td>/</td><td>0.9</td><td>1.4</td></tr>
<tr><td></td><td></td><td></td><td>36</td><td>NI</td><td>/</td><td>/</td><td>13.5</td><td>19.4</td></tr>
<tr><td></td><td></td><td></td><td>60</td><td>NI</td><td>/</td><td>/</td><td>40.3</td><td>63.6</td></tr>
<tr><td>Bianchi</td><td>1999</td><td>41</td><td>12</td><td>III–IV</td><td>34</td><td>15</td><td>/</td><td>/</td></tr>
<tr><td>Busacca</td><td>2001</td><td>44</td><td>18</td><td>III–IV</td><td>29</td><td>9</td><td>/</td><td>/</td></tr>
<tr><td>Bulletti</td><td>2001</td><td>14</td><td>12</td><td>I–IV</td><td>/</td><td>/</td><td>64</td><td>/</td></tr>
<tr><td>Schweppe</td><td>2002</td><td>220</td><td>24</td><td>I–II</td><td>/</td><td>/</td><td>9.2</td><td>/</td></tr>
<tr><td>Zullo</td><td>2003</td><td>63</td><td>12</td><td>I–IV</td><td>33</td><td>/</td><td>/</td><td>/</td></tr>
<tr><td>Vercellini</td><td>2003</td><td>90</td><td>12</td><td>I–IV</td><td>25</td><td>/</td><td>/</td><td>/</td></tr>
<tr><td></td><td></td><td></td><td>36</td><td>I–IV</td><td>36</td><td>/</td><td>/</td><td>/</td></tr>
<tr><td>Vercellini</td><td>2003</td><td>20</td><td>12</td><td>I–IV</td><td>45</td><td>/</td><td>/</td><td>/</td></tr>
<tr><td>Abott</td><td>2003</td><td>135</td><td>60</td><td>I–IV</td><td>/</td><td>/</td><td>/</td><td>33</td></tr>
</table>

N: Number of patients included in the study
rAFS stage: Stage of endometriosis (revised classification of the American Fertility Society, 1985)
NI: Stage of endometriosis not indicated in the study

Table 29.2: Frequency of recurrent endometrioma after conservative laparotomy						
Authors	*Year*	*N*	*Follow-up (months)*	*Pelvic pain*	*Recurrence (%)* *Ultrasound* *examination*	*Reoperation (%)*
Laparoscopic cystectomy						
Canis	1992	42	6	/	/	7.6
Bateman	1994	36	12	/	11.1	/
Muzii	1996	21	12	/	4.8	/
Ahmed	1997	104	32	/	/	7
Hemming	1998	23	36	/	8	/
Beretta	1998	32	24	DM 15.8 DP 20 CPP 10	6.2	/
Saleh	1999	161	18	/	/	6.1
			42		/	23.6
Muzii	2000	35	22	17.1	2.9	/
Drainage and bipolar coagulation of the cystic sac						
Beretta	1998	32	24	DM 52.9 DP 75 CPP 52.9	18.8	/
Hemmings	1998	80	36	/	12	/
Jones	2002	23	12	/	20.8	/
Drainage and laser vaporization of the cystic sac						
Donnez	1996	814	2–11*	/	8	/
Jones	2002	50	12	/	14.3	/
Drainage and bipolar coagulation or laser vaporization of the cystic sac						
Saleh	1999	70	18	/	/	21.9
			42	/	/	57.8

* Years
N: Number of patients included in the study
DM: Dysmenorrhea; DP: Dyspareunia; CPP: Chronic pelvic pain

with pelvic pain necessitating iterative surgery; however, endometriotic recurrences were histologically documented in only 15 percent of the cases.[42] The frequency of recurrent endometriosis of the rectovaginal wall after surgical or medical treatment is presented in Table 29.3.

Various medical treatments may be proposed for the management of endometriosis, including progestational and estroprogestational drugs, Danazol and GnRH agonists. The action of the drugs, based on the estrogen-dependent nature of the endometriotic implants, inhibits the ovarian biosynthesis of estrogens by reducing or suppressing ovarian stimulation, by altering ovarian steroidogenesis, or by reducing the fraction of free estrogen. All these drugs produce similar results in cases of endometriosis, leading to the regression of endometriotic lesions while alleviating pelvic pain and ameliorating the quality of life of the patients.[43-45] Nevertheless, the frequency of recurrence after administration of medical treatment alone is greater than 50 percent.[7-9,46,47] The frequency of recurrent endometriosis after exclusively medical treatment is presented in Table 29.4.

Some authors have estimated the frequency of recurrent endometriosis following combined conservative surgery

Table 29.3: Frequency of recurrent endometriosis of the rectovaginal wall after surgical or medical treatment

Authors	Year	N	Follow-up (months)	Pelvic pain	Recurrence (%) clinical or ultrasound examination	Histology	Reoperation (%)
Surgical treatment							
Varol	2003	169	36	/	/	15	36
Ford	2004	60	12	/	/	/	13
Fedele	2004	83	36	28	34.2	/	27
Medical treatment: GnRHa during 6 months							
Fedele	2000	15	12	87	/	/	/

N: Number of patients included in the study
GnRHa: GnRH agonist

Table 29.4: Frequency of recurrent endometriosis after exclusive medical treatment

Authors	Year	N	Follow-up (months)	Medical treatment (6-month course)	Recurrence* (%)
Waller	1993	130	60	GnRHa	53.4
Vercellini	1997	70	6	Progestational or estroprogestational	50
Franke	2000	23	6	GnRHa	73.9

N: Number of patients included in the study
*Frequency of recurrence accompanied by pelvic pain
GnRHa: GnRH agonist

Table 29.5: Frequency of recurrent endometriosis after conservative surgery followed by postoperative medical treatment

Authors	Year	N	Follow-up (months)	rAFS stage	Treatment	Pelvic pain	Recurrence (%) Clinical or ultrasound examination
Regidor	1997	42	78	I - IV	GnRHa (6 months)	66.7	/
Bianchi	1999	36	12	III - IV	Danazol (6 months)	26	8.3
Busacca	2001	45	18	III - IV	GnRHa (3 months)	23	9

N: Number of patients included in the study
rAFS Stage: Stage of endometriosis (Revised Classification of the American Fertility Society, 1985)
GnRHa: GnRH agonist

and postoperative medical treatment (Table 29.5). Thus, in a group of 42 patients presenting with minimum to severe endometriosis treated by conservative surgery followed by a 6-month course of Buserelin acetate, a nasally administered GnRH agonist, the frequency of recurrence accompanied by pelvic pain was 66.7 percent.[48] Two studies on patients with stage III or IV endometriosis (rAFS), treated with conservative surgery followed by a 3-month postoperative course of intramuscular injections of slow-release leuprorelin [a luteinizing hormone-releasing hormone (LHRH) analog],[6] or by a 6-month course of Danazol,[4] respectively reported recurrence of pelvic pain in 23 and 26 percent of the patients, respectively, and the recurrence of lesions detected by clinical or ultrasound examination in 8.3 and 9.0 percent of the patients, respectively.

Risk Factors Associated with Recurrent Endometriosis (Table 29.6)

The hypothesis according to which the severity of endometriosis is predictive of the appearance of post-therapeutic recurrence has been contested. A retrospective evaluation 5 years after conservative surgery for endometriosis found no significant relationship between the frequency of the recurrence and the severity of the primary infection.[10]

Table 29.6: Characteristics and results of the various studies evaluating the risk factors for recurrent endometriosis

Authors	Year	N	Treatment	Variable studied	p
Risk factors for recurrent endometriosis					
Wheeler	1983	423	Surgical	rAFS stage	NS
Waller	1993	130	Medical	rAFS stage	< 0.05
Redigor	1997	42	Medical and surgical	rAFS score	NS
Abott	2003	135	Surgical	rAFS score > 70	0.03
				Age	NS
Risk factors for recurrent endometrioma					
Busacca	1999	366	Laparoscopic intraperitoneal cystectomy	rAFS score	< 0.05
				Diameter > 4 cm	< 0.05
				Number of cysts	NS
				Age	NS
Saleh	1999	161	Laparoscopic IPC	Diameter > 4 cm	< 0.05
		70	D + CB or laparoscopic IPC	Diameter > 4 cm	NS
Jones	2002	73	Laparoscopic IPC + D + CB or VP	Bilateral cysts	0.032
Ghezzi	2001	121	Laparoscopy or laparotomy	Left lateralization of lesions	< 0.05
Vercellini	2002	1407	Laparoscopy or laparotomy	Left lateralization of lesions	NS
Risk factors for recurrent endometriosis of the rectovaginal wall					
Fedele	2004	83	Surgery	Age	< 0.01

N: Number of patients included in the study
rAFS stage or score: Stage or score of endometriosis (Revised Classification of the American Fertility Society, 1985)
IPC: Intraperitoneal cystectomy
D + CB: Drainage and destruction of the cystic sac of the endometrioma by bipolar coagulation
D + VP: Drainage and destruction of the cystic sac of the endometrioma by laser vaporization
p: Statistically significant difference with p < 0.05; NS: Difference not statistically significant

Similarly, a retrospective study of 42 cases of endometriosis, treated by conservative surgery followed by a 6-month course of a GnRH agonist found no significant relationship between the pretherapeutic staging of the disease based on the rAFS classification and the resurgence of pelvic pain.[48] In contrast, the results of a long-term follow-up of 130 patients with endometriosis, treated with a GnRH agonist, showed that the frequency of recurrence accompanied by pelvic pain was significantly higher in cases of initially serious disease.[47] Another report indicates that severe endometriosis with an rAFS score greater than 70 is a risk factor for recurrence after conservative laparotomy.[3]

An investigation of the risk factors for the recurrence of endometrioma following laparoscopic cystectomy showed that the rAFS staging and the rAFS score were both significantly correlated with the risk of clinical recurrence, whereas the rAFS score alone showed a correlation with the risk of

reoperation.[5] Thus, the rAFS staging of the disease seems to be less satisfactory than the rAFS score for evaluating the risk of recurrence. Independent of the total rAFS score, the size of the endometrioma, if greater than 4 cm, has been described as a risk factor for recurrence after laparoscopic cystectomy, though not after drainage followed by bipolar coagulation or laser vaporization of the cystic sacs.[5,38] After cystectomy for endometrioma, the frequency of recurrence did not appear to vary with the number of the tumors treated.[5] However, in a study of 63 patients suffering from endometrioma, after drainage followed by bipolar coagulation or by laser vaporization of the cystic sacs, the frequency of recurrence was significantly greater in patients with bilateral cysts than in patients with a single cyst.

Only a few authors have examined the relationship between the age of the patients and the frequency of recurrent endometriosis. A study of 135 patients treated by conservative laparotomy revealed no significant variation in the frequency of recurrence with age.[3] Similarly, after conservative laparotomy for endometrioma, the risk of recurrence appeared to be independent of the age of the patients.[5,35] However, in a study of 83 patients with endometriosis of the rectovaginal septum, treated by conservative surgery, the frequency of recurrence accompanied by pelvic pain or revealed by clinical or ultrasound examination, and requiring particularly drastic treatment, was significantly greater in patients younger than 25 years than in the others.[41]

The relationship between the localization of the primary endometriotic lesions and the risk of recurrence has also been investigated. One study on recurrent endometriosis following conservative laparotomy reported that the risk was significantly higher when the left hemipelvis was affected than the right.[49] However, this finding has not been substantiated. Thus, in 148 patients treated for recurrent endometrioma, no relationship was found between the lateralization of the first endometriotic cyst treated and the risk of recurrence.[50] As we have already observed, the anatomical configuration may favor the left lateralization of endometriotic lesions. However, it remains to be established whether this constitutes a factor of risk for recurrent endometriosis.

Prevention of Recurrent Endometriosis

Prevention of Recurrence by Conservative Surgical Management

Since the late 1980s, the development of endoscopic surgery has revolutionized the treatment of endometriosis. The efficacy of the technique is widely recognized in the conservative treatment of endometriosis.[3,39,51-55] However, only a few studies have compared the frequency of recurrent endometriosis after conservative surgery by laparotomy and laparoscopy. A retrospective study 2 years after surgery on 67 patients treated by laparoscopy and 149 patients treated by laparotomy showed no significant difference between the two groups in terms of the frequency of recurrence accompanied by pelvic pain.[53] Similarly, in a group of patients treated for moderate to severe endometriosis, the risk of recurrence, evaluated during a second-look laparoscopy, was roughly the same for patients treated with laparoscopy and those treated with laparotomy.[55] Several other reports indicate that the results of surgical treatment of endometrioma, particularly with respect to the risk of recurrence, are similar whether the operation is done by laparoscopy or by laparotomy.[39,51] Since the risk of recurrence appears to be the same with laparoscopy and laparotomy, the choice of the surgical technique should be conditioned only by the experience of the surgeon and the nature of the lesions.

A retrospective study has compared the frequency of postoperative recurrence in patients treated for stage I or II endometriosis (rAFS) according to the phase of the menstrual cycle during which the laparotomy was performed.[30] Two years after surgery, the frequency of recurrence was twice as high and the remission significantly shorter after treatment during the luteal phase than during the follicular or periovulatory phase of the menstrual cycle. These results have a biological explanation. As we have mentioned, endometriosis is generally attributed to the dissemination of endometrial cells by tubal reflux during menses into the peritoneal cavity, followed by implantation on the peritoneum or the pelvic organs. Some *in vitro* studies have suggested that an intact peritoneal epithelium might prevent the adhesion of endometrial cells.[1,56] If this is indeed the case, a damaged peritoneal epithelium would favor the development of endometriotic lesions. Thus, the surgical treatment of endometriosis, involving the excision, coagulation and vaporization of peritoneal implants, may produce traumatic lesions. If such lesions are not fully cicatrized before the menstrual tubal reflux occurs, the adhesion of the endometrial cells may be facilitated, thereby increasing the risk of recurrence. Thus, conservative surgical treatment of endometriosis during the first part of the menstrual cycle should contribute to the prevention of recurrent endometriosis.

The hypothesis that the menstrual reflux participates in the development of endometriosis has suggested a therapeutic strategy to prevent recurrence by associating laparotomy with endometrectomy. In a prospective randomized study, two groups of 14 patients presenting with invalidating dysmenorrhea were treated by conservative laparotomy for stage II to IV endometriosis (rAFS), and one of the groups underwent complementary endometrectomy.[17] Two years after treatment, a second-look laparoscopy of the patients revealed that 9 of the patients treated with exclusively laparoscopic surgery suffered from recurrences, whereas there were no recurrences in any of the patients who had undergone complementary endometrectomy. The authors therefore recommend the extirpation of the uterine mucosa in cases of endometriosis when the patients do not envisage any further pregnancy.

Conservative surgical treatment of endometrioma may be based on different techniques. A comparative study of the techniques should help to determine the surgical management consistent with the prevention of the cysts. Transvaginal, ultrasound-guided puncture and laparoscopic drainage of endometriomas has failed to prevent recurrence (Table 29.7). Several studies have indicated a very high frequency of recurrence: between 80 and 100 percent, six months after drainage alone or associated with postoperative medical treatment.[38,57,58] Some authors have compared the results of conservative laparoscopic treatment of endometrioma by cystectomy and drainage followed by destruction of the cystic sacs either by laser vaporization

Table 29.7: Frequency of recurrence of endometrioma after simple laparoscopic or ultrasound-guided transvaginal drainage of the cyst

Authors	Year	N	Follow-up (months)	Postoperative medical treatment	Recurrence* (%)
Vercellini	1992	18	6	/	100
		15	6	GnRH (3 months)	100
Zanetta	1995	18	6	/	100
Saleh	1999	15	6	/	80

N: Number of patients included in the study
GnRHa: GnRH agonist
* Recurrence of endometrioma revealed by ultrasound examination

or by bipolar coagulation.[32,34,35,38] Only one of these studies compared the risk of recurrence after drainage and destruction of the cystic sacs by laser vaporization with the risk of recurrence after drainage and destruction of the cystic sacs by bipolar coagulation.[35] This prospective study on 73 patients revealed no significant difference in the frequency of recurrence of endometriomas between the two techniques. Some studies have compared the results obtained by cystectomy and those obtained by drainage followed by destruction of the cystic sacs, independently of the technique. In a 3-year retrospective study, the frequency of recurrence after cystectomy was similar to that after cystic drainage followed by bipolar coagulation of the cystic sacs.[34] The only randomized, comparative study performed showed that two years after surgery, the frequency of recurrence accompanied by chronic pelvic pain, dysmenhorrea or dyspareunia was lower in patients treated by cystectomy.[32] The authors also found that the remission from pelvic pain before recurrence was significantly longer after cystectomy. Similarly, a retrospective study of 231 premenopausal women treated for endometriomas by laparotomy showed that the frequency of reoperation was significantly higher after cystic drainage and destruction of the cystic sacs than after cystectomy.[38] The frequencies of reoperation at 18 and 42 months of follow-up were 6.1 percent and 23.6 percent, respectively after cystectomy, and 21.9 and 57.8 percent after cystic drainage and destruction of the cystic sacs. Although there have been only a few comparative studies, each describing a small number of patients, the results indicate that cystectomy appears to prevent the recurrence of endometriomas at least as effectively as cystic drainage followed by destruction of the cystic sacs.

The prevention of recurrence in the surgical management of endometriosis of the rectovaginal septum has received little attention. One evaluation of the results of surgery in a group of 60 patients suffering from endometriosis of the rectovaginal septum reported greater relief from pelvic pain and a better quality of life in patients who had undergone a rectal resection.[59] Another study on 83 premenopausal women with endometriosis of the rectovaginal septum, treated by surgery conserving the uterus and at least one ovary, showed that the recurrence could be predicted by whether or not a rectal resection had been performed.[41,58] At 36 months of follow-up, the frequency of recurrence with the presence of pelvic pain, lesions detected clinically or by ultrasound, and lesions requiring new treatment, was greater in patients who had not had rectal resection than in those who had. The decreased risk of secondary recurrence following rectal resection is due to a better local control of the disease. Histological analysis of 50 tissue samples taken during radical surgery, including rectosigmoidal resection, for endometriosis of the rectovaginal septum showed that in each case, the endometriosis had invaded the digestive wall at least as far as the muscle layer, with multifocal lesions in 62 percent of the cases, and multicentric lesions in 38 percent.[60] Thus, the total exeresis of the lesions, necessary for the prevention of recurrence, would seem difficult to realize by means of a simple excision of a portion of the digestive wall. Effective surgical treatment calls for a digestive resection extirpating the main endometriotic lesions with a safety margin extending 2 cm into the surrounding tissue.

Prevention of Endometriosis by Medical Management

The current medical treatment of endometriosis does not completely eradicate the disease. The use of drugs fails to prevent recurrence of the symptoms in more than half the cases.[9,46,47] A retrospective study of 264 patients, presenting with mild to severe endometriosis, evaluated the risk of recurrence after a 6-month course of Danazol or a GnRH agonist.[8] The mean remission from pelvic pain was 6.1 months with Danazol, and 5.2 months with the GnRH agonist. Although the remission varied with the severity of the disease, it was disappointingly short in all cases.

Combined medical and surgical treatment is proposed for better management of endometriosis. This may be associated with conservative surgery and pre or postoperative medical treatment. The preoperative medical treatment aims at inactivating the endometriotic centers so as to facilitate the surgical excision and allow better control of the disease. A prospective multicentric study compared the results of a six-month course of a GnRH agonist in patients treated for stage III or IV endometriosis (rAFS) before and after surgery.[61]

The decrease in the rAFS score, evaluated during a second-look laparoscopy, was significantly higher with preoperative than with postoperative administration of the GnRH agonist. Thus, the results failed to confirm the hypothesis that preoperative medical treatment facilitates the surgery in cases of endometriosis.[61] Moreover, the use of a GnRH agonist seems to offer no special advantage in the surgical treatment of endometrioma in terms of operating time or ease of cystectomy.[36] To date, there is no proof of the usefulness of preoperative medical treatment in the prevention of recurrent endometriosis.

The postoperative medical treatment is aimed at preventing the development of the microscopic endometriotic centers that may have escaped surgery, thereby eliminating the risk of the iatrogenic dissemination of endometriotic cells. However, the efficacy of the treatment needs to be confirmed. Several prospective randomized studies have attempted to evaluate the risk of recurrent endometriosis after conservative surgery followed by a medical treatment but the results are contradictory (Table 29.8). Thus, in two studies of patients with endometriosis treated by conservative surgery, a 3-month postoperative course of Danazol or a GnRH agonist failed to prevent recurrence of the disease.[4,6] In contrast, a 6-month course of postoperative administration of a GnRH agonist compared to the administration of a placebo, led not only to a significantly lower risk of recurrence but also a longer period free from pelvic pain before further treatment was required.[62] Another study comparing conservative surgery for endometriosis with combined medical and surgical treatment of the disease found that the mean remission before the recurrence of endometriosis was significantly greater in patients who had received a 6-month postoperative course of a GnRH agonist than those who had been treated exclusively by surgery.[63] Thus, although it has not been proved that the postoperative administration of a GnRH agonist actually reduces the overall risk, it may retard the appearance of recurrent endometriosis. Recently, a novel combination of a GnRH agonist and an aromatase inhibitor, which suppresses the ovarian and extraovarian biosynthesis of estrogens, has been used in the postoperative medical treatment of endometriosis. In a group of patients with severe endometriosis, a 6-month postoperative course of a GnRH agonist associated with an aromatase inhibitor, compared to the administration of the GnRH agonist alone, led to a reduction of recurrence (7% vs 35%, respectively), as well as a longer remission before recurrence of the disease (>24 months vs 17 months, respectively), with no modification in the therapeutic tolerance and without any long-term accentuation of bone loss.[64] However, the absence of deleterious short and long-term effects of this therapeutic association remains to be confirmed. A prospective randomized study of 40 patients under treatment for symptomatic endometriosis has reported that the postoperative use of a Levonorgestrel-releasing intrauterine device significantly reduced the risk of recurrence

Table 29.8: Comparison of the frequencies of recurrent endometriosis according to whether postoperative medical treatment is administered or not

Authors	Year	Follow-up (months)	N	Postoperative treatment	Recurrence (%)		p
					Pelvic pain	Clinical examination	
Hornstein	1997	18	49	GnRHa (6-months)	25	/	< 0.001
			44	Placebo	47	/	
Bianchi	1999	12	36	Danazol (3-months)	26	8.3	NS
			36	No treatment	34	15	
Vercellini	1999	12	107	GnRHa (6-months)	13.1	/	NS
		24			23.5	/	
		12	103	No treatment	21.4	/	
		24			36.5	/	
Busacca	2001	18	45	GnRHa (3-months)	23	9	NS
			45	No treatment	29	9	
Vercellini	2003	13	20	LNgIUD	10	/	0.03
				No treatment			

N: Number of patients included in the study
GnRHa: GnRH agonist
LNgIUD: Levonorgestrel-releasing intrauterine device
p: Statistically significant difference with p < 0.05; NS: Difference not statistically significant

during a one-year follow-up.[65] This treatment, presenting very few secondary effects and constraints, appears to offer an interesting alternative in the combined surgical and medical management of endometriosis. However, the efficacy of the method will need to be confirmed by further studies on larger numbers of patients and longer follow-up periods.

Treatment of Recurrent Endometriosis

Iterative Conservative Surgery

Iterative conservative surgery is the treatment of choice for endometriosis patients seeking to ameliorate or preserve their fertility. Several studies have described the techniques used and indicated the results obtained in terms of the changes in fertility and the risks of recurrence of the disease.

Only one study had compared the results of laparotomy and laparoscopy in the conservative treatment of recurrent endometriosis. During a 2-year follow-up, no significant difference was observed in the frequency of pregnancy or recurrence of the disease with respect to the surgical technique used.[66] The frequency of pregnancy after iterative conservative surgery for recurrent endometriosis varied between 20.7 percent and 54 percent.[10,12,67–69] This is comparable to the 40 to 59 percent frequency of pregnancy observed after primary conservative surgery for endometriosis.[3,4,6] Although the use of conservative surgery in stage I and II endometriosis (rAFS) has been contested, some authors consider it the treatment of choice for endometriosis associated with infertility.[70,71] One study, reporting a frequency of spontaneous pregnancy in 54 percent patients 2 years after a second conservative laparotomy for endometriosis, claims that iterative conservative surgery is best indicated for recurrent endometriosis in infertile patients.[66] Table 29.9 presents the frequency of spontaneous pregnancy following iterative conservative surgery for recurrent endometriosis in infertile patients. Nevertheless, some authors recommend the use of assisted reproductive techniques for such patients. A retrospective study of patients who had remained infertile after primary conservative surgery for stage III or IV endometriosis (rAFS) reported a significantly higher frequency of pregnancy after two cycles of in vitro fertilization than after reoperation.[69] However, another study making the same comparison found no significant difference between the frequencies of pregnancy secondary to an *in vitro* fertilization cycle and a reoperation for endometriosis.[68] Table 29.10 presents the frequency of pregnancy in infertile patients with recurrent endometriosis receiving surgical treatment compared with that of patients resorting to *in vitro* fertilization.

Iterative conservative surgery may not always ensure a definite cure for endometriosis but it does offer certain patients a period free from recurrence of the disease, thus favoring fertility. A post-therapeutic study after iterative conservative surgery, with a follow-up of greater than 24 months, reported recurrent endometriosis accompanied by pain in 25 to 34 percent of the patients, and about 20 percent cases detected by clinical or ultrasound examination.[66] Another study of 42 patients treated by iterative conservative laparotomy for recurrent endometriosis, with a follow-up of 3 years, reported recurrence with pelvic pain in 12.5 percent, and recurrence requiring a third surgical intervention in 14 percent of the patients.[67]

Medical Treatment of Recurrent Endometriosis

Hormone therapy offers an alternative treatment for patients with recurrent endometriosis, who do not envisage further pregnancies. Several therapeutic plans have been proposed for the long-term treatment of recurrent endometriosis to ensure better control of the disease.

<table>
<tr><td colspan="7" align="center">Table 29.9: Frequency of spontaneous pregnancy following iterative conservative surgery for recurrent endometriosis in infertile patients</td></tr>
<tr><td>Authors</td><td>Year</td><td>N</td><td>Follow-up (months)</td><td>rAFS Stage</td><td>Surgery as main treatment</td><td>Pregnancy (%)</td></tr>
<tr><td>Wheeler</td><td>1983</td><td>15</td><td>18</td><td>NI</td><td>Laparotomy</td><td>47</td></tr>
<tr><td>Candiani</td><td>1991</td><td>42</td><td>36</td><td>III – IV</td><td>Laparotomy</td><td>35</td></tr>
<tr><td>Evers</td><td>1993</td><td>8</td><td>18</td><td>NI</td><td>Laparotomy</td><td>38</td></tr>
<tr><td>Pagidas</td><td>1996</td><td>18</td><td>9</td><td>III – IV</td><td>Laparotomy/Laparoscopy</td><td>24.4</td></tr>
<tr><td>Busacca</td><td>1999</td><td>41</td><td>24</td><td>I – IV</td><td>Laparotomy</td><td>45</td></tr>
<tr><td></td><td></td><td>40</td><td>24</td><td>I – IV</td><td>Laparoscopy</td><td>54</td></tr>
<tr><td>Cheewadhanaraks</td><td>2004</td><td>32</td><td>12</td><td>III – IV</td><td>Laparotomy</td><td>20.5</td></tr>
</table>

N: Number of patients included in the study
rAFS Stage: Stage of endometriosis following the revised classification of theAmerican Fertility Society (1985)
NI: Stages of endometriosis not indicated

Table 29.10: Frequency of pregnancy in infertile patients with recurrent endometriosis receiving surgical treatment compared with that of patients resorting to *in vitro* fertilization

Authors	Year	N	Follow-up (months)	Treatment	Pregnancy (%)	p
Pagidas	1996	18	9	Iterative surgery	24.4	< 0.05
		23	/	IVF – 2 cycles	69.6	
Cheewadhanaraks	2004	32	12	Iterative surgery	20.5	NS
		24	/	IVF – 1 cycle	12.5	

N: Number of patients included in the study
IVF: *In vitro* fertilization
p: Statistically significant difference with p < 0.05; NS: Difference not statistically significant

Thus, low doses of progestational drugs, such as C proterone acetate (12.5 mg), and estroprogestational drug associations, such as ethinyl estradiol (0.02 mg) and desogestrel (0.15 mg), administered daily so as to provoke amenorrhea, significantly reduce recurrent endometriosis accompanied by pelvic pain.[72,73] The good clinical tolerance of these treatments allows prolonged use.

The efficacy of a Levonorgestrel-releasing intrauterine device was prospectively evaluated in 20 patients suffering from recurrent dysmenorrhea after conservative surgery for endometriosis. At one year follow-up, there was a significant reduction in pelvic pain. This amelioration has been attributed to the amenorrhea induced by the local action of the progestational drug on one hand, and the possible systemic action of Levonorgestrel on the other.[74]

A significant clinical improvement was reported after a 3-month follow-up of patients with recurrent endometriosis treated for 3 months with a GnRH agonist.[75] However, although GnRH agonists or other hormonal treatments of endometriosis may allow a control of the disease, they expose the patients to a high-risk of recurrence on cessation of medication.[46,47] Moreover, the secondary effects, including bone loss inherent to the drug-induced hypoestrogenia, make the prolonged use of this type of treatment rather difficult. To reduce these secondary effects and avoid bone loss, some authors suggest an add-back therapy, i.e. the association of progestational and estroprogestational drugs, such as Tibolone, in the treatment of endometriosis with a GnRH agonist. This therapeutic association, after a 6-month or even a 12-month course, did not affect the efficacy of the action of the GnRH agonist on endometriosis and maintained the bone density.[46,76] The add-back therapy may therefore allow prolonged treatment of endometriosis with GnRH agonists.

Aromatase inhibitors have been used in the management of recurrent endometriosis in patients having already received multiple medical and surgical treatments. A 6-month course of an aromatase inhibitor administered to a menopausal patient is reported to have produced significant relief of pelvic pain and regression of the endometriotic lesions. Bone loss, secondary to the hypoestrogenia provoked by the treatment, was offset by the addition of a progestational drug or a biphosphonate, and calcium and vitamin D supplements.[77,78] A study of 10 menopausal patients reported the efficacy and good tolerance of a 6-month administration of Letrozole (2.5 mg/day) and norethisterone acetate (2.5 mg/day) associated with calcium and vitamin D supplements. This rapidly relieved pelvic pain and a second-look laparoscopic examination 2-months after cessation of treatment showed significant regression of the endometriotic lesions.[79] In premenopausal patients, aromatase inhibitors may prevent the negative hypothalamic retro-control of estradiol, thus inducing ovarian stimulation or hyperstimulation. However, the monthly ultrasound and biological check-up during and after treatment detected no development of ovarian cysts and no increase in plasma FSH and LH levels. In addition, there was no significant bone loss during the treatment. The use of aromatase inhibitors associated with the administration of a progestational drug therefore seems to be a safe treatment for recurrent endometriosis in premenopausal women. The results obtained with aromatase inhibitors appear promising but need to be confirmed by further randomized comparative studies.

Radical Surgery in Recurrent Endometriosis

After repeated recourse to medical treatment and conservative surgery for recurrent endometriosis, some patients with no plans for further pregnancies may opt for radical surgery.

The question of the conservation of the uterine appendages arises when radical surgery is proposed for severe endometriosis in premenopausal patients. A retrospective study compared two groups of premenopausal patients treated for endometriosis either by radical surgery with adnexal conservation or by surgical castration followed by hormone replacement therapy. Compared to bilateral ovariectomy followed by hormone replacement therapy, the risk of recurrent endometriosis accompanied by pelvic pain was 6 times greater in cases of hysterectomy with adnexal conservation (62% vs. 10%, respectively), while the risk of reoperation for the disease was 8 times higher (31% vs. 3%, respectively).[80]

In younger patients, hormone replacement therapy after total non-conservative hysterectomy for endometriosis prevents the consequences of menopause. A prospective, randomized study compared the results of non-conservative surgery for endometriosis with and without hormone replacement therapy. Although no statistically significant difference could be established, recurrence occurred in 3.5 percent of the patients receiving hormone replacement therapy, whereas there were no cases of recurrence among patients without hormone therapy, and among the patients receiving hormone treatment, there appeared to be a higher recurrence of the disease in those having been treated with radical surgery than the others.[81]

CONCLUSION

Endometriosis tends to recur frequently in patients treated for the disease, and surgery appears to be the treatment of choice for the prevention of recurrence. The association of surgery with the administration of postoperative medical treatment increases the duration of remission. Exclusive medical treatment is associated with a high-risk of recurrence and should not be considered as the prime therapy for endometriosis.

The management of recurrent endometriosis may require several successive surgical and medical treatments, imposing constraints that patients may find difficult to bear, particularly when the long-term efficacy of the therapy proves to be unsatisfactory. Improved management of the disease calls for greater insights into the physiopathology of endometriosis.

Fundamental research, especially at the molecular level, has recently revealed new therapeutic targets. Thus, the discovery of the role of aromatase in the extraovarian biosynthesis of estrogens, particularly within the endometriotic lesions, has suggested the use of aromatase inhibitors in the treatment of endometrioisis. The first clinical trials of these new drugs have produced encouraging results.[64,77-79]

The survival and development of endometriotic implants depend on the neovascularization induced by the action of angiogenic factors.[1,82] These factors, among which, the best-known is the vascular endothelial growth factor (VEGF), are potential targets in the treatment of endometriosis. A study on a murine model of endometriosis has shown that inhibitors of angiogenesis significantly reduce the number and size of the endometriotic lesions.[82] These results now await confirmation by clinical tests on patients with endometriosis.

The inhibition of metalloproteinases, the enzymes involved in the mechanisms of cell adhesion and tissue invasion that are active in endometriosis, is currently being investigated.[83]

Thus, the inhibition of the enzymatic activity of aromatase and metalloproteinase, and the inhibition of angiogenesis appear to offer promising new treatments in the near future for the better prevention of recurrent endometriosis.

REFERENCES

1. Vigano P, Parazzini F, Somigliana E, Vercellini P. Endometriosis: Epidemiology and aetiological factors. Best Pract Res Clin Obstet Gynecol 2004;18:177-200.
2. Nap AW, Griffioen AW, Dunselman GA, et al. Antiangiogenesis therapy for endometriosis. J Clin Endocrinol Metab 2004;89: 1089-95.
3. Abbott JA, Hawe J, Clayton RD, Garry R. The effects and effectiveness of laparoscopic excision of endometriosis: A prospective study with 2-5 year follow-up. Hum Reprod. 2003; 18:1922-7.
4. Bianchi S, Busacca M, Agnoli B, Candiani M, Calia C, Vignali M. Effects of 3 month therapy with danazol after laparoscopic surgery for stage III/IV endometriosis: A randomized study. Hum Reprod. 1999;14:1335-7.
5. Busacca M, Marana R, Caruana P, et al. Recurrence of ovarian endometrioma after laparoscopic excision. Am J Obstet Gynecol 1999;180:519-23.
6. Busacca M, Somigliana E, Bianchi S, et al. Postoperative GnRH analogue treatment after conservative surgery for symptomatic endometriosis stage III-IV: A randomized controlled trial. Hum Reprod 2001;16:2399-2402.
7. Fedele L, Bianchi S, Zanconato G, Tozzi L, Raffaelli R. Gonadotropin-releasing hormone agonist treatment for endo-metriosis of the rectovaginal septum. Am J Obstet Gynecol 2000;183:1462-7.
8. Miller JD, Shaw RW, Casper RF, Rock JA, Thomas EJ, Dmowski WP, et al. Historical prospective cohort study of the recurrence of pain after discontinuation of treatment with danazol or a gonadotropin-releasing hormone agonist. Fertil Steril 1998;70:293-6.
9. Vercellini P, Cortesi I, Crosignani PG. Progestins for symptomatic endometriosis: A critical analysis of the evidence. Fertil Steril 1997;68:393-401.
10. Wheeler JM, Malinak LR. Recurrent endometriosis: Incidence, management, and prognosis. Am J Obstet Gynecol 1983;146:247-53.
11. Bulletti C, De Ziegler D, Polli V, Del Ferro E, Palini S, Flamigni C. Characteristics of uterine contractility during menses in women with mild to moderate endometriosis. Fertil Steril 2002;77:1156-61.
12. Evers HL, Dunselman GA, Land JA, Bouckaert PX, van der Linden EP. Diagnostic d'endométriose après un traitement apparemment efficace: Formation *de novo*, réapparition ou persistance? Réf Gyn Obstet 1993;1:434-9.
13. Parazzini F. Left-right side ratio of endometriotic implants in the pelvis. Eur J Obstet Gynecol Reprod Biol 2003;111:65-7.
14. Vercellini P, Aimi G, De Giorgi O, Maddalena S, Carinelli S, Crosignani PG. Is cystic ovarian endometriosis an asymmetric disease? Br J Obstet Gynaecol 1998;105:1018-21.

15. Nisolle M, Donnez J. Peritoneal endometriosis, ovarian endometriosis, and adenomyotic nodules of the rectovaginal septum are three different entities. Fertil Steril 1997;68:585-96.

16. Somigliana E, Infantino M, Candiani M, Vignali M, Chiodini A, Busacca M. Association rate between deep peritoneal endometriosis and other forms of the disease: Pathogenetic implications. Hum Reprod 2004;19:168-71.

17. Bulletti C, DeZiegler D, Stefanetti M, Cicinelli E, Pelosi E, Flamigni C. Endometriosis: Absence of recurrence in patients after endometrial ablation. Hum Reprod 2001;16:2676-9.

18. Yang WC, Chen HW, Au HK, Chang CW, Huang CT, Yen YH, Tzeng CR. Serum and endometrial markers. Best Pract Res Clin Obstet Gynaecol 2004;18:305-18.

19. Evers JL. The second-look laparoscopy for evaluation of the result of medical treatment of endometriosis should not be performed during ovarian suppression. Fertil Steril 1987;47: 502-4.

20. Donnez J, Nisolle-Pochet M, Clerckx-Braun F, Sandow J, Casanas-Roux F. Administration of nasal Buserelin as compared with subcutaneous Buserelin implant for endometriosis. Fertil Steril 1989;52:27-30.

21. Meresman GF, Auge L, Baranao RI, Lombardi E, Tesone M, Sueldo C. Oral contraceptives suppress cell proliferation and enhance apoptosis of eutopic endometrial tissue from patients with endometriosis. Fertil Steril 2002;77:1141-7.

22. Meresman GF, Bilotas M, Buquet RA, Baranao RI, Sueldo C, Tesone M. Gonadotropin-releasing hormone agonist induces apoptosis and reduces cell proliferation in eutopic endometrial cultures from women with endometriosis. Fertil Steril 2003; 80:702-7.

23. Nisolle-Pochet M, Casanas-Roux F, Donnez J. Histologic study of ovarian endometriosis after hormonal therapy. Fertil Steril 1988;49:423-6.

24. Karaer O, Oruc S, Koyuncu FM. Aromatase inhibitors: Possible future applications. Acta Obstet Gynecol Scand 2004;83:699-706.

25. Zeitoun KM, Bulun SE. Aromatase: A key molecule in the pathophysiology of endometriosis and a therapeutic target. Fertil Steril 1999;72:961-9.

26. Balasch J, Creus M, Fabregues F, Carmona F, Ordi J, Martinez-Román S, Vanrell JA. Visible and non-visible endometriosis at laparoscopy in fertile and infertile women and in patients with chronic pelvic pain: A prospective study. Hum Reprod 1996;11:387-91.

27. Walter AJ, Hentz JG, Magtibay PM, Cornella JL, Magrina JF. Endometriosis: Correlation between histologic and visual findings at laparoscopy. Am J Obstet Gynecol 2001;184: 1407-13.

28. Vercellini P, Aimi G, Busacca M, Apolone G, Uglietti A, Crosignani PG. Laparoscopic uterosacral ligament resection for dysmenorrhea associated with endometriosis: Results of a randomized, controlled trial. Fertil Steril 2003;80:310-19.

29. Zullo F, Palomba S, Zupi E, Russo T, Morelli M, Sena T, et al. Effectiveness of presacral neurectomy in women with severe dysmenorrhea caused by endometriosis who were treated with laparoscopic conservative surgery: A 1-year prospective randomized double-blind controlled trial. Am J Obstet Gynecol 2003;189:5-10.

30. Schweppe KW, Ring D. Peritoneal defects and the development of endometriosis in relation to the timing of endoscopic surgery during the menstrual cycle. Fertil Steril 2002;78:763-6.

31. Ahmed MS, Barbieri RL. Reoperation rates for recurrent ovarian endometriomas after surgical excision. Gynecol Obstet Invest 1997;43:53-4.

32. Beretta P, Franchi M, Ghezzi F, Busacca M, Zupi E, Bolis P. Randomized clinical trial of two laparoscopic treatments of endometriomas: Cystectomy versus drainage and coagulation. Fertil Steril 1998;70:1176-80.

33. Donnez J, Nisolle M, Gillet N, Smets M, Bassil S, Casanas-Roux F. Large ovarian endometriomas. Hum Reprod 1996;11:641-6.

34. Hemmings R, Bissonnette F, Bouzayen R. Results of laparoscopic treatments of ovarian endometriomas: Laparoscopic ovarian fenestration and coagulation. Fertil Steril 1998;70:527-9.

35. Jones KD, Sutton CJ. Recurrence of chocolate cysts after laparoscopic ablation. J Am Assoc Gynecol Laparosc 2002;9: 315-20.

36. Muzii L, Marana R, Caruana P, Mancuso S. The impact of preoperative gonadotropin-releasing hormone agonist treatment on laparoscopic excision of ovarian endometriotic cysts. Fertil Steril 1996;65:1235-7.

37. Muzii L, Marana R, Caruana P, Catalano GF, Margutti F, Panici PB. Postoperative administration of monophasic combined oral contraceptives after laparoscopic treatment of ovarian endometriomas: A prospective, randomized trial. Am J Obstet Gynecol 2000;183:588-92.

38. Saleh A, Tulandi T. Reoperation after laparoscopic treatment of ovarian endometriomas by excision and by fenestration. Fertil Steril 1999;72:322-4.

39. Bateman BG, Kolp LA, Mills S. Endoscopic versus laparotomy management of endometriomas. Fertil Steril 1994;62:690-95.

40. Canis M, Mage G, Wattiez A, Chapron C, Pouly JL, Bassil S. Second-look laparoscopy after laparoscopic cystectomy of large ovarian endometriomas. Fertil Steril 1992;58:617-9.

41. Fedele L, Bianchi S, Zanconato G, Bettoni G, Gotsch F. Long-term follow-up after conservative surgery for rectovaginal endometriosis. Am J Obstet Gynecol 2004;190:1020-24.

42. Varol N, Maher P, Healey M, Woods R, Wood C, Hill D, Lolatgis N, et al. Rectal surgery for endometriosis—should we be aggressive? J Am Assoc Gynecol Laparosc 2003;10:182-9.

43. Shaw RW. An open randomized comparative study of the effect of goserelin depot and danazol in the treatment of endometriosis. Zoladex Endometriosis Study Team. Fertil Steril 1992;58:265-72.

44. Telimaa S, Puolakka J, Ronnberg L, Kauppila A. Placebo-controlled comparison of danazol and high-dose medroxy-progesterone acetate in the treatment of endometriosis. Gynecol Endocrinol 1987;1:13-23.

45. Trabant H, Widdra W, de Looze S. Efficacy and safety of intranasal buserelin acetate in the treatment of endometriosis: A review of six clinical trials and comparison with danazol. Prog Clin Biol Res 1990;323:357-82.

46. Franke HR, van de Weijer PH, Pennings TM, van der Mooren MJ. Gonadotropin-releasing hormone agonist plus "add-back" hormone replacement therapy for treatment of endometriosis: A prospective, randomized, placebo-controlled, double-blind trial. Fertil Steril 2000;74:534-9.

47. Waller KG, Shaw RW. Gonadotropin-releasing hormone analogues for the treatment of endometriosis: Long-term follow-up. Fertil Steril 1993;59:511-5.

48. Regidor PA, Regidor M, Kato K, Bier UW, Buhler K, Schindler AE. Long-term follow-up on the treatment of endometriosis with the GnRH-agonist buserelinacetate. Long-term follow-up data (upto 98 months) of 42 patients with endometriosis who were treated with GnRH-agonist buserelinacetate (Suprecur), were evaluated in respect of recurrence of pain symptoms and pregnancy outcome. Eur J Obstet Gynecol Reprod Biol 73: 153-60.

49. Ghezzi F, Beretta P, Franchi M, Parissis M, Bolis P. Recurrence of ovarian endometriosis and anatomical location of the primary lesion. Fertil Steril 2001;75:136-40.

50. Vercellini P, Busacca M, Aimi G, Bianchi S, Frontino G, Crosignani PG. Lateral distribution of recurrent ovarian endometriotic cysts. Fertil Steril 2002;77:848-9.

51. Catalano GF, Marana R, Caruana P, Muzii L, Mancuso S. Laparoscopy versus microsurgery by laparotomy for excision of ovarian cysts in patients with moderate or severe endometriosis. J Am Assoc Gynecol Laparosc 1996;3:267-70.

52. Chapron C, Jacob S, Dubuisson JB, Vieira M, Liaras E, Fauconnier A. Acta Obstet Gynecol Scand 2001;80:349-54.

53. Crosignani PG, Vercellini P, Biffignandi F, Costantini W, Cortesi I, Imparato E. Laparoscopy versus laparotomy in conservative surgical treatment for severe endometriosis. Fertil Steril 1996;66:706-11.

54. Donnez J, Pirard C, Smets M, Jadoul P, Squifflet J. Surgical management of endometriosis. Best Pract Res Clin Obstet Gynaecol 2004;18:329-48.

55. Fayez JA, Collazo LM. Comparison between laparotomy and operative laparoscopy in the treatment of moderate and severe stages of endometriosis. Int J Fertil 1990;35:272-9.

56. Groothuis PG, Koks CA, De Goeij AF, Dunselman GA, Arends JW, Evers HL. Adhesion of human endometrial fragments to peritoneum in vitro. Fertil Steril 1999;70:1119-24.

57. Vercellini P, Vendola N, Bocciolone L, Colombo A, Rognoni MT, Bolis G. Laparoscopic aspiration of ovarian endometriomas. Effect with postoperative gonadotropin, releasing hormone agonist treatment. J Reprod Med 1992;37:577-80.

58. Zanetta G, Lissoni A, Dalla Valle C, Trio D, Pittelli M, Rangoni G. Ultrasound-guided aspiration of endometriomas: Possible applications and limitations. Fertil Steril 1995;64:709-13.

59. Ford J, English J, Miles WA, Giannopoulos T. Pain, quality of life and complications following the radical resection of rectovaginal endometriosis. Br J Obstet Gynecol 2004;111: 353-6.

60. Kavallaris A, Kohler C, Kuhne-Heid R, Schneider A. Histopathological extent of rectal invasion by rectovaginal endometriosis. Hum Reprod 2003;18:1323-7.

61. Audebert A, Descamps P, Marret H, Ory-Lavollee L, Bailleul F, Hamamah S. Pre or postoperative medical treatment with nafarelin in stage III-IV endometriosis: A French multicenter study. Eur J Obstet Gynecol Reprod Biol 1998;79:145-8.

62. Hornstein MD, Hemmings R, Yuzpe AA, Heinrichs WL. Use of nafarelin versus placebo after reductive laparoscopic surgery for endometriosis. Fertil Steril 1997;68:860-64.

63. Vercellini P, Crosignani PG, Fadini R, Radici E, Belloni C, Sismondi P. A gonadotropin-releasing hormone agonist compared with expectant management after conservative surgery for symptomatic endometriosis. Br J Obstet Gynaecol 1999;106, 672-7.

64. Soysal S, Soysal ME, Ozer S, Gul N, Gezgin T. The effects of post-surgical administration of goserelin plus anastrozole compared to goserelin alone in patients with severe endometriosis: A prospective randomized trial. Hum Reprod 2004;19:160-67.

65. Vercellini P, Frontino G, De Giorgi O, Aimi G, Zaina B, Crosignani PG. Comparison of a levonorgestrel-releasing intrauterine device versus expectant management after conservative surgery for symptomatic endometriosis: A pilot study. Fertil Steril 2003; 80:305-9.

66. Busacca M, Fedele L, Bianchi S, et al. Surgical treatment of recurrent endometriosis: Laparotomy versus laparoscopy. Hum Reprod 1998;13:2271-4.

67. Candiani GB, Fedele L, Vercellini P, Bianchi S, Di Nola G. Repetitive conservative surgery for recurrence of endometriosis. Obstet Gynecol 1991;77:421-4.

68. Cheewadhanaraks S. Comparison of fecundity after second laparotomy for endometriosis to *in vitro* fertilization and embryo transfer. J Med Assoc Thai 2004;87:361-6.

69. Pagidas K, Falcone T, Hemmings R, Miron P. Comparison of reoperation for moderate (stage III) and severe (stage IV) endometriosis-related infertility with *in vitro* fertilization-embryo transfer. Fertil Steril 1996;65:791-5.

70. Donnez J, Squifflet J, Pirard C, Jadoul P, Wyns C, Smets M. The efficacy of medical and surgical treatment of endometriosis-associated infertility and pelvic pain. Gynecol Obstet Invest 2002;54:2-10.

71. Gordts S, Campo R, Brosens I, Puttemans P. Endometriosis: Modern surgical management to improve fertility. Best Pract Res Clin Obstet Gynaecol 2003;17:275-87.

72. Vercellini P, De Giorgi O, Mosconi P, Stellato G, Vicentini S, Crosignani PG. Cyproterone acetate versus a continuous monophasic oral contraceptive in the treatment of recurrent pelvic pain after conservative surgery for symptomatic endometriosis. Fertil Steril 2002;77:52-61.

73. Vercellini P, Frontino G, De Giorgi O, Pietropaolo G, Pasin R, Crosignani PG. Continuous use of an oral contraceptive for endometriosis-associated recurrent dysmenorrhea that does not respond to a cyclic pill regimen. Fertil Steril 2003;80:560-3.

74. Vercellini P, Aimi G, Panazza S, De Giorgi O, Pesole A, Crosignani PG. A levonorgestrel-releasing intrauterine system for the treatment of dysmenorrhea associated with endometriosis: A pilot study. Fertil Steril 1999;72:505-8.

75. Hornstein MD, Yuzpe AA, Burry K, Buttram VC Jr, Heinrichs LR, Soderstrom RM, et al. Retreatment with nafarelin for recurrent endometriosis symptoms: efficacy, safety, and bone mineral density. Fertil Steril 1997;67:1013-8.

76. Surrey ES, Hornstein MD. Prolonged GnRH agonist and add-back therapy for symptomatic endometriosis: Long-term follow-up. Obstet Gynecol 2002;99:709-19.

77. Razzi S, Fava A, Sartini A, De Simone S, Cobellis L, Petraglia F. Treatment of severe recurrent endometriosis with an

aromatase inhibitor in a young ovariectomised woman. Br J Obstet Gynecol 2004;111:182-4.

78. Takayama K, Zeitoun K, Gunby RT, Sasano H, Carr BR, Bulun SE. Treatment of severe postmenopausal endometriosis with an aromatase inhibitor. Fertil Steril 1998;69:709-13.

79. Ailawadi RK, Jobanputra S, Kataria M, Gurates B, Bulun SE. Treatment of endometriosis and chronic pelvic pain with letrozole and norethindrone acetate: A pilot study. Fertil Steril 2004;81:290-96.

80. Namnoum AB, Hickman TN, Goodman SB, Gehlbach DL, Rock JA. Incidence of symptom recurrence after hysterectomy for endometriosis. Fertil Steril 1995;64:898-902.

81. Matorras R, Elorriaga MA, Pijoan JI, Ramon O, Rodriguez-Escudero FJ. Recurrence of endometriosis in women with bilateral adnexectomy (with or without total hysterectomy) who received hormone replacement therapy. Fertil Steril 2002;77:303-8.

82. Nap AW, Griffioen AW, Dunselman GA, Bouma-Ter Steege JC, Thijssen VL, Evers JL, et al. Antiangiogenesis therapy for endometriosis. J Clin Endocrinol Metab 2004;89:1089-95.

83. Olive DL, Lindheim SR, Pritts EA. New medical treatments for endometriosis. Best Pract Res Clin Obstet Gynaecol 2004;18:319-28.

Treatment of Deep Rectovaginal Endometriosis

Elizabeth Ball, Charles Koh

OVERVIEW

Rectovaginal endometriosis is the most challenging variety of intestinal endometriosis and is often undertreated because of a lack of understanding of the extent of disease or the inability to treat the concomitant bowel, bladder and ureteric involvement. It can cause chronic pain, acute and chronic obstruction and contribute to infertility. With an increasing number of specialist endometriosis centers developing worldwide, appropriate surgical treatment is becoming more available. There is little doubt about the efficacy of complete resection of uterosacral or vaginal deep disease to disease-free margins, however, this requires advanced laparoscopic skills. Expectant management may be indicated for rectosigmoid disease in asymptomatic patients. In our practice, partial thickness resection is reserved only for endometriosis that involves the outer longitudinal muscularis, where it can be completely removed. 'Shaving' deeper disease is often incomplete, may lead to repeated surgeries and does not reduce complications. Full thickness disk resection is indicated when the disease has invaded the inner muscularis or if the mucosa is involved. Segmental bowel resection is indicated for the larger (>4 cm) or multifocal lesions. The safety and efficacy of laparoscopic segmental resection is well-established in many centers, including our own. At present, deep disease can only be identified by radical microdissection, but new developments in preoperative imaging are promising. Rectovaginal endometriosis is best managed laparoscopically and with an established multi-specialty team of an expert gynecologist, surgeon, urologist and a good operating theater team. Until the supporting specialists become capable of identifying endometriosis and the extent of resection needed, gynecologic endometriosis surgeons have to take the lead. In order to do so, they must be able to independently perform urinary tract and bowel surgery.

INTRODUCTION

Recent publications confirm the safety and efficacy of radical fertility-sparing surgery in deep endometriosis involving the rectum[1-3] when performed with appropriate training and in a multidisciplinary center of excellence. In contrast, medical suppressive therapy is either ineffective,[4] associated with high recurrence[5] or incompatible with fertility plans.[6]

With regard to advanced endometriosis surgery, there is a discrepancy between demand and supply. Currently, less than a dozen gynecologists perform advanced laparoscopic surgery for severe endometriosis in the UK, but 5000 women per year with severe disease require treatment.[7]

Hence, this chapter aims to highlight the advantages of laparoscopic treatment of rectovaginal endometriosis, discuss preoperative examinations and describe the required laparoscopic techniques.

There is a lack of consensus on the extent of excision required; this will depend on the disease location, the patient's symptoms and surgical resources. However, we strongly believe that hysterectomy and bilateral salpingo-oopherectomy, which is often the mainstay in patients with advanced endometriosis, is indiscriminate, leads to unnecessary iatrogenic infertility and is likely to leave behind endometriotic lesions, especially when technical limitations necessitate a subtotal approach. However, concomitant adenomyosis is an indication for hysterectomy at the time of excision of endometriosis when fertility is not desired because pain may persist otherwise.[8]

Laparoscopy has a clear advantage over open surgery of improved access to the retroperitoneal space and magnification, a prerequisite for microsurgery, which is required to achieve radical excision of endometriosis and when unraveling the frozen pelvis. Conversions are rare in expert units and account for less than one percent in our center.

CLINICAL DISCUSSION

Definition and Topography of Rectovaginal Endometriosis

The sigmoid is the most common section of the gastrointestinal tract affected by endometriosis (37%) followed by the rectosigmoid junction (20%), appendix (20%), and rectum (10%).[9] The depth of lesions correlates with an increase in pain;[10] deep endometriosis includes endometriotic glands, stroma and fibromuscular tissue and has previously been described as lesions of more than 5 mm below the surface of the peritoneum.[11] However, in our experience, endometriosis of the pelvic peritoneum is always superficial except when it involves the uterosacral-cardinal ligaments, bladder, periureteric and rectovaginal area. The cut-off of 5 mm, defined before complete dissection, was commonly achieved. Cul-de-sac obliteration does not equal infiltrative bowel or vaginal disease; the latter can only be diagnosed after radical dissection. In contrast, cul-de-sac obliteration can be caused simply by adhesions.

Rectovaginal and Rectal Endometriosis

Endometriosis of the rectovaginal septum is a misnomer, as the septum is not the origin of the lesion as previously postulated. It may be infiltrated when a bulky lesion in the cul-de-sac has invaded the muscularis of the vagina (Figs 30.1 to 30.4), rectum or both, but the most likely origin is the peritoneum of the cul-de-sac;[11] lesions then infiltrate the proximal rectum and vagina and extend deep into the rectovaginal space. Complete cul-de-sac obliteration does not always imply rectal involvement.[12] Treatment is indicated for obstructive symptoms or when imaging suggests stenosis.

Understanding the common sites and the nature of progression of deep endometriosis is the prerequisite to a logical and consistent approach and to successful and complete resection. The most common area of involvement of deep endometriosis is the uterosacral ligament.

With increasing lateral extension of the disease, the cardinal ligament and the periureteric tissue become infiltrated, leading to external constriction of the ureter (Figs 30.1, 30.2 and 30.5). Whilst this rarely involves the ureteric muscularis, hydroureter and hydronephrosis with renal failure can occur with severe stenosis or obstruction.

With medial extension, the serosa and later, the external muscularis of the adjacent rectum may become involved, but the rectal mucosa is rarely affected. In a series of colectomies for endometriosis, endometriotic lesions were identified in the serosa and muscularis propria in 100 percent, in the submucosa in 34 percent and in the mucosa in only 10 percent.[13]

Anterior extension of the disease can infiltrate the posterior cervix and vagina (Figs 30.1 to 30.4 and 30.6 to 30.10).

Central lesions occur in the cul-de-sac between the rectum and the vagina (Figs 30.6, 30.7 and 30.10 to 30.12). There is debate whether these lesions arise from the rectovaginal septum or represent cul-de-sac lesions covered by the rectum.[14,15] We favor the infiltration theory, as we have never seen an early septal lesion below the level of the cul-de-sac in a patient who has not been operated on before. In the coronal plane, these lesions extend laterally and may merge with the uterosacral lesion described above. When this occurs bilaterally, there is true cul-de-sac obliteration by a confluent sheet of fibrotic endometriosis.

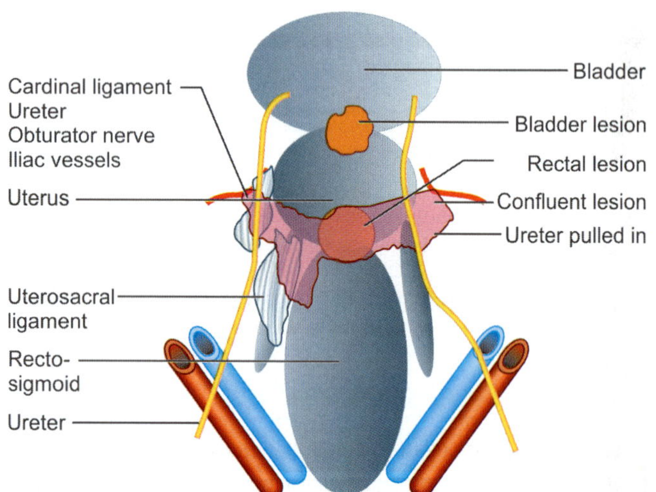

Fig. 30.1: Location and spread of deep endometriosis

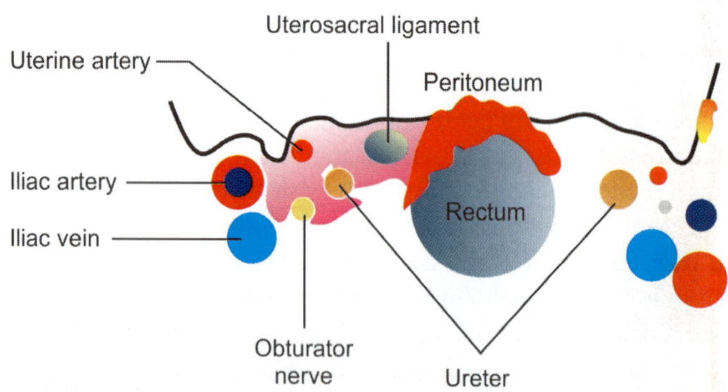

Fig. 30.2: Superficial and deep endometriosis in relation to ureter, rectum and pelvic sidewall

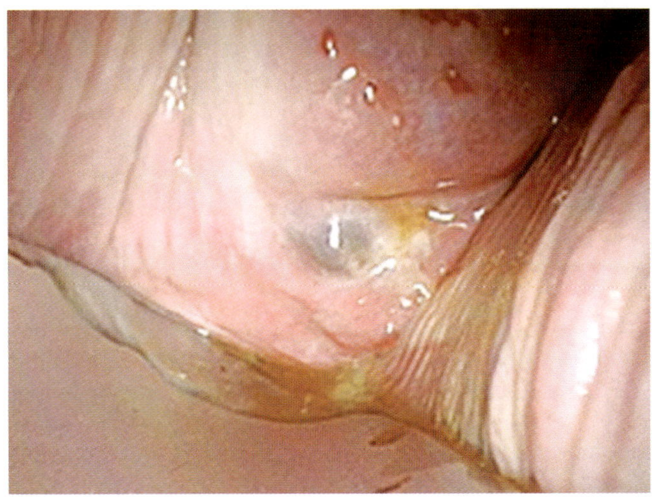

Fig. 30.3: Retrocervical endometriotic nodule

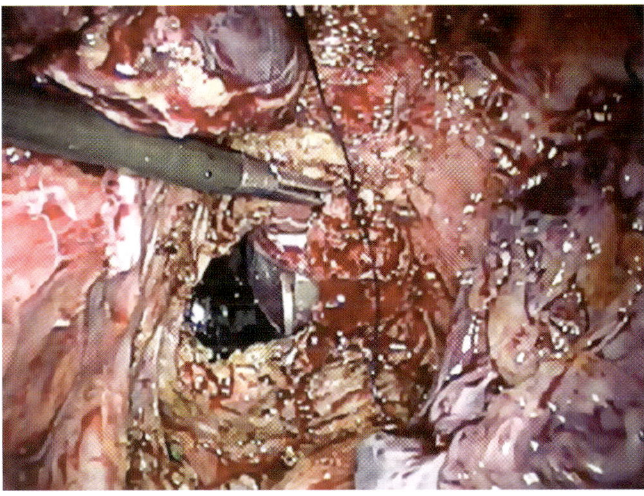

Fig. 30.4: Vaginal repair after excision of retrocervical and vaginal endometriosis

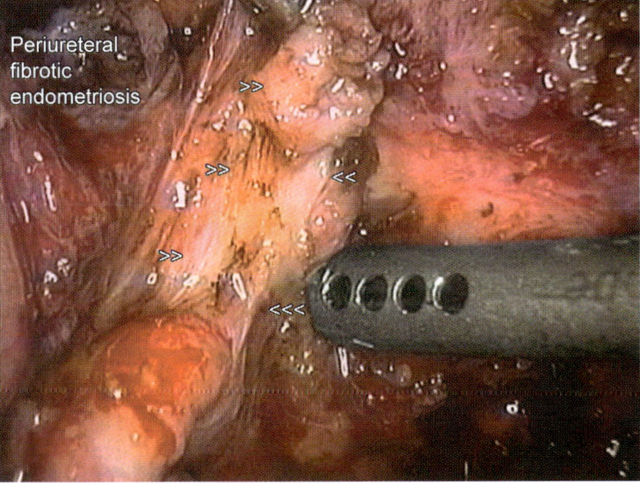

Fig. 30.5: Endometriosis leading to external constriction of the ureter

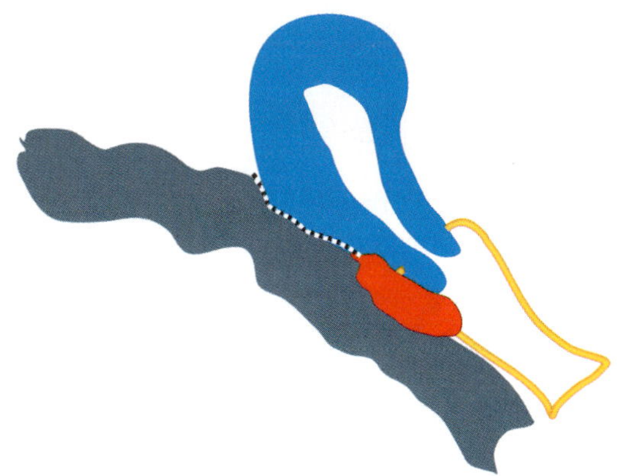

Fig. 30.6: Sagittal view of rectovaginal endometriosis

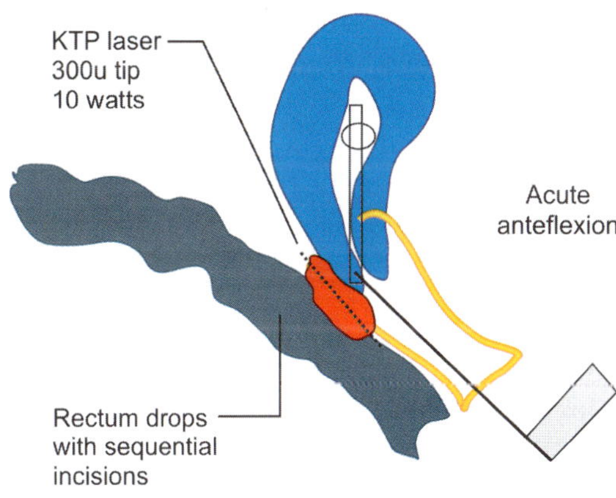

Fig. 30.7: Direction of incision into the rectovaginal lesion towards the rectovaginal space. The key movement is acute anteversion of the uterus with a RUMI manipulator

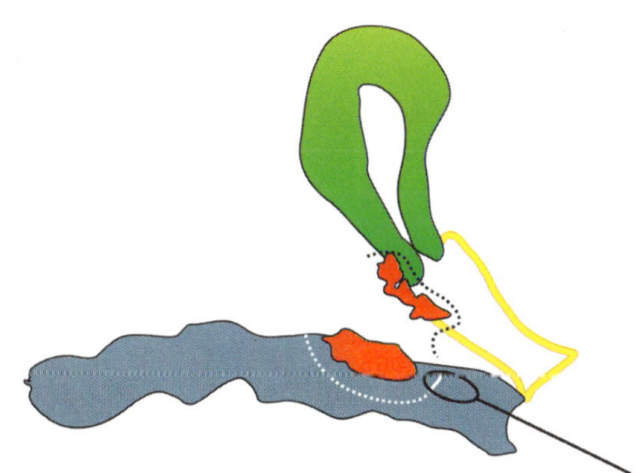

Fig. 30.8: White dotted line shows the extent of rectal and vaginal resection that is needed to achieve disease-free margins

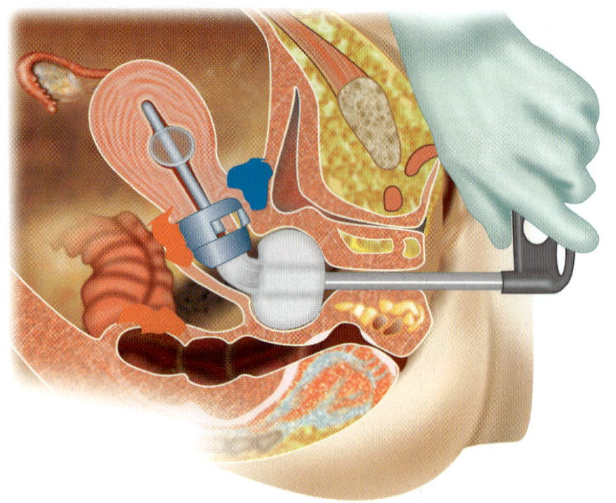

Fig. 30.9: KOH cup and pneumo-occluder with RUMI uterine manipulator. This set-up is required for acute uterine anteversion

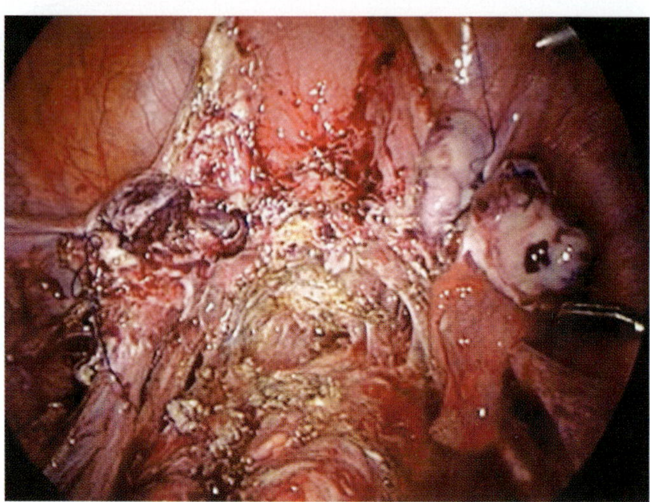

Fig. 30.12: Ovary and Fallopian tube lateralized, rectum medialized

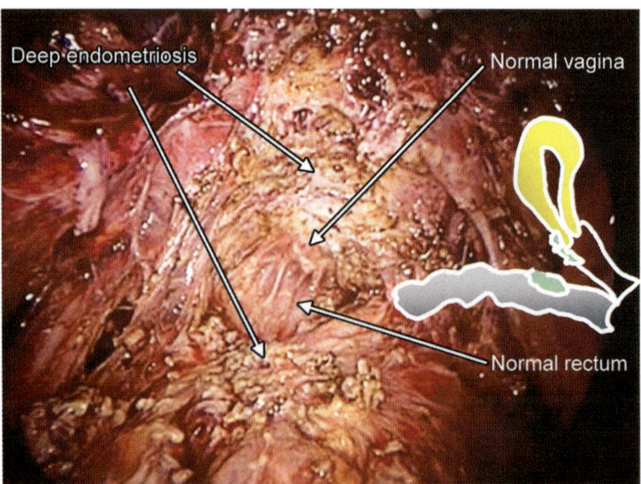

Fig. 30.10: Dissection down to normal rectovaginal space

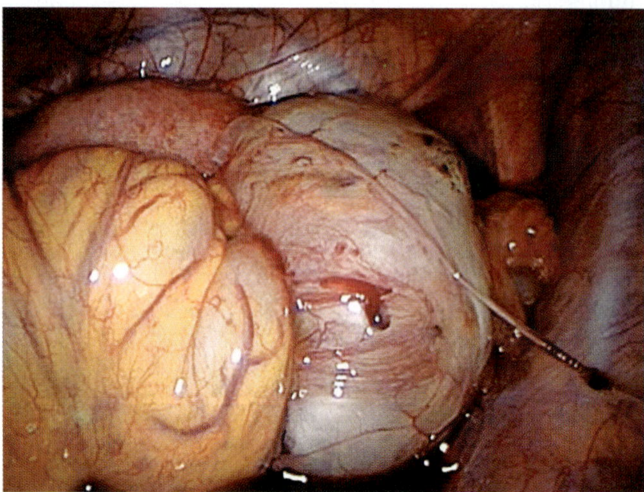

Fig. 30.13: Sigmoid-ovarian-uterine adhesion. Cul-de-sac obliteration presumed. Gel MRI shows rectosigmoid thickening and posterior fornix endometriosis

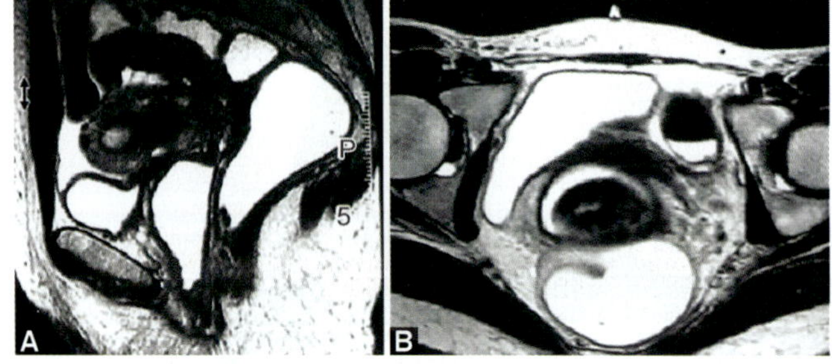

Figs 30.11A and B: Gel MRI showing endometriosis involving sigmoid, posterior vagina and fornix

Endometriosis of the Sigmoid

Endometriosis is more common at the junction of the rectum and sigmoid than in the remaining sigmoid.[16] Sigmoid endometriosis begins on the serosal surface and later tends to invaginate and thicken the intestinal wall[17,18] causing adhesions (Fig. 30.13); histologically, fibromuscular hypertrophy interspersed with glands and stroma can be detected. There is no 'benign' fibrosis without glands or stroma in these lesions. Superficial disease may cause no symptoms or be responsible for disproportionately severe dyschezia, which is completely cured by excision. Bulky, deeply invasive lesions often result in symptoms of subacute obstruction, constipation alternating with diarrhea and intestinal bloating and cramping. The sigmoid is attached to the sidewall by congenital adhesions, which usually require division in order to improve laparoscopic access to the pelvis and ureter.

Preoperative Evaluation

The preoperative diagnosis of sigmoid or rectal wall involvement helps with surgical planning, such as triaging patients to centers capable of radical endometriosis surgery, predicting operating times and liaising with bowel surgeons. In units like ours, where surgeons experienced in laparoscopic colectomy are available at any time and partial and full thickness resections of rectum are performed without the general surgeon, precise preoperative triaging is less important.

Currently, none of the preoperative investigations are perfect and many depend on the expertise of the user. At present, the only definitive method of diagnosing intestinal endometriosis is by thorough exploration at the time of surgery, when sigmoid lesions are usually evident on inspection and palpation. The bowel segment affected by endometriosis may show fibrosis, black or red endometriotic lesions and may be adherent, extremely distorted or even obstructed; bowel cancer is a differential diagnosis. Conversely, when the cul-de-sac is obliterated, the diagnosis of rectal endometriosis is only possible after skilled dissection of the rectovaginal space, which is rarely practised outside specialized endometriosis centers.

Digital Examination

Low rectovaginal endometriosis can be readily palpated by rectovaginal digital examination. In rare cases, vaginal speculum examination may reveal obvious posterior fornix endometriosis as part of a large infiltrating mass extending between the vaginal and the rectal mucosa. A rectovaginal nodule of more than 3 cm will involve the ureter, causing stenosis and hydronephrosis in 11.2 percent of the cases.[19] Pelvic examination for nodules often misses lesions in the upper uterosacral ligament and rectum[20] and other sites of intestinal endometriosis are not amenable to digital examination.

Colonoscopy

Occasionally, endometriosis can be diagnosed with colonoscopy, but it has a poor specificity because endometriotic lesions are usually submucosal. In 77 consecutive colonoscopies of patients with bowel endometriosis undergoing colon resection, only two of 74 proctosigmoidoscopic biopsies were positive.[21] Therefore, colonoscopy should not be used to rule out the presence

of, or determine whether surgery is indicated in bowel endometriosis.

Vaginal and Rectal Ultrasound

Endometriotic lesions below the rectosigmoid junction can be detected sonographically as a hypoechoic mass penetrating into the intestinal wall, but neither depth nor distance from the anal margin can be assessed. Bazot et al.[22] reported a sensitivity of 95 percent and a specificity of 100 percent in diagnosing colorectal involvement.

Transrectal ultrasound can identify involvement of the muscularis, lesion size and distance from the anus. The sensitivity for detecting colorectal endometriosis has been reported as 100 percent with a specificity of 95 percent.[22] However, this technique is operator-dependent and requires analgesia in some cases. Lesions in the upper colon cannot be assessed with transrectal ultrasound.

Magnetic Resonance Imaging

All disease requiring significant surgery or bowel resection involves thickening of the bowel wall with luminal stenosis, which can be detected on magnetic resonance imaging

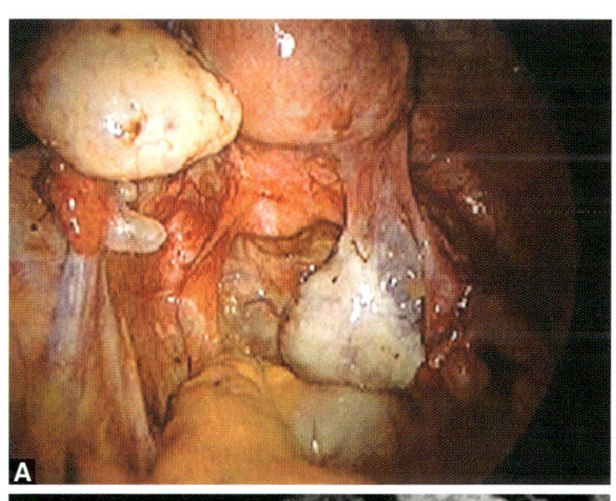

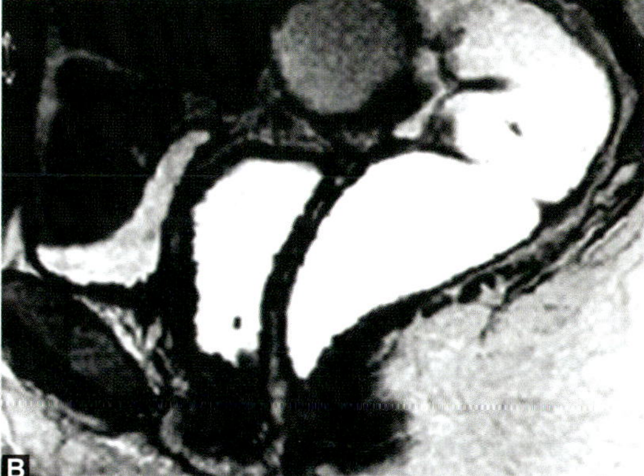

Figs 30.14A and B: Gel MRI of normal cul-de-sac

(MRI). T2 weighted imaging facilitates this diagnosis. For lower sigmoid and rectal lesions, the use of ultrasound gel placed into the vagina and rectum delineates the lesion and is highly specific (Figs 30.11A and B, 30.14A and B). In contrast to vaginal and rectal ultrasound, endometriosis of the entire intestine can be imaged, however, it is not always possible to identify the degree of infiltration of the muscularis.[16] MRI diagnosis of rectosigmoid involvement varies with studies (sensitivity 83–88%, specificity 76–93%).[16,23] The comparatively high inter- and intraobserver agreement in the identification of rectosigmoid endometriosis[24] is an advantage of MRI.

Clinical Management

Expectant Management

Expectant management can be warranted in the absence of symptoms, when bowel endometriosis is an incidental finding. It is unclear how fast endometriosis of the sigmoid and colon progresses and which factors predict future obstruction. However, the patient should be informed that she might require surgery in the future.

Medical Management

Currently, there is no evidence for effective medical treatment of intestinal endometriosis, as these therapies only temporarily suppress the pain and eliminate neither superficial nor deep disease. Estrogenic suppression with gonadotropin-releasing hormone (GnRH) agonists is often followed by relapse in superficial endometriosis and is rarely effective in symptomatic deep rectovaginal disease; for the same reason, oopherectomy is futile and indeed, doctors are doing more harm than good by removing the ovaries in this context.

Interestingly, recent results from a small study on the use of Levonorgestrel intrauterine system in persistent rectovaginal endometriosis have been encouraging,[4] but larger trials[25] and studies with a focus on intestinal endometriosis are needed.

Surgical Management

Though there is a trend towards less radical surgery in many areas of oncology, in endometriotic surgery, we observe a shift towards organ-sparing and thus, fertility-preserving but more radical excision of disease. Our group focuses on the complete resection of deep endometriosis until normal tissue margins can be seen or palpated, even if this requires disk excision of the rectosigmoid or reanastomosis. Reasons for inadequate surgery include ignorance of the nature of deep endometriosis, fear of operative complications, future infertility and a lack of centers specializing in radical excision.

All patients should undergo mechanical bowel preparation prior to surgery when intestinal endometriosis is anticipated. Regimes for bowel preparation include:

- Magnesium citrate, either the day before surgery or in combination with two days of liquid diet and one day of clear liquids.
- Sodium chloride, sodium bicarbonate and potassium chloride for oral solution (Golytely®, Nulytely®,).
- Sodium phosphate enema (Fleet®) in the morning on the day before surgery.

2 mg Cefoxitim IV is recommended intraoperatively, and if bowel is entered, this should be repeated after six and 12 hours.

In expert centers, all endometriotic bowel surgery is performed laparoscopically, either totally or assisted, together with resection of peritoneal, deep or ovarian endometriosis as indicated.

The advantages of laparoscopic bowel resection include elimination of postoperative nasogastric suction, early return of bowel sounds within 29 h (mean), reduced hospital stay (3–6 days) and an early return to work. Primary anastomosis without defunctioning colostomy is the standard treatment in our center.

Endometriosis of the Rectovaginal Septum and Rectum

Bowel endometriosis is rarely found in isolation[26] (Fig. 30.13) and although rectovaginal endometriosis often spares the rectum, dissection of the rectovaginal space is the initial step towards full assessment and complete removal of the endometriotic lesions.

The treatment of rectal endometriosis is technically challenging because it is usually associated with cul-de-sac obliteration, deep infiltration of uterosacral and cardinal ligaments and the periureteric area (Figs 30.1, 30.2 and 30.5). In order to cure the symptoms, these areas of deep endometriosis have to be excised (Figs 30.10, 30.12 and 30.15)

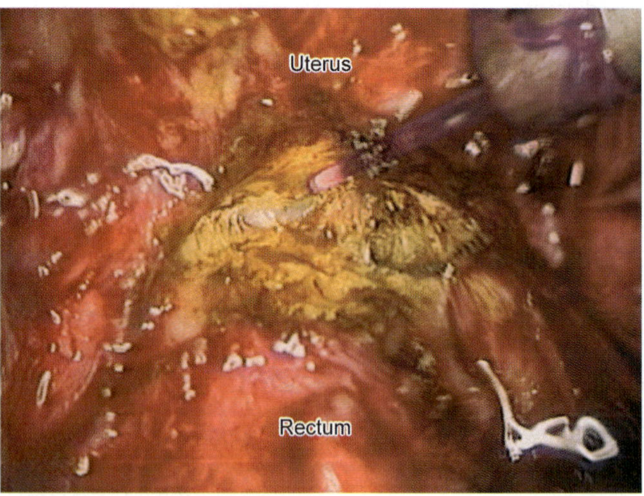

Fig. 30.15: A sculpted laser tip is used to release the rectum from the vagina in cul-de-sac obliteration

in addition to complete removal of the rectal endometriosis. Following dissection of the cul-de-sac obliteration down to the normal rectovaginal space beyond the disease, all deep disease of the ureter, uterosacral cardinals and posterior vagina is excised to normal margins (Fig. 30.10). The extent of rectal disease is then assessed and treated as described below. The surgical tools required for the dissection of the rectovaginal space include:

- RUMI uterine manipulator®, KOH cup®, pneumo-occluder® (Cooper Surgical, Figure 30.9).
- Ring forceps and rectal probe to outline, splint and reflect the rectum.
- Ring forceps for posterior vaginal fornix placed under the RUMI uterine manipulator handle.
- KTP laser with 300 μm sculpted tip.
- Laparoscopic ureteric grasper, bowel grasper, dissecting forceps, micro-jaw and macro-jaw disposable bipolar, monopolar hook, serrated straight reusable scissors, 3 mm ultra micrograspers, Storz macro- and microneedle holders.
- 3-0 PDS on an SH needle for intracorporeal suturing.
- 3 chip camera (microdissection is achieved by employing × 20 magnification).

We approach dissection with a systematic routine so that all rectovaginal disease can be identified and successfully resected laparoscopically.

- *Mapping of peritoneal disease*: We use laser to map the total outline of the bladder, cul-de-sac and lateral pelvic wall peritoneal disease at the start of surgery so that later ecchymoses do not distort the boundaries of peritoneal resection. If an ovarian endometrioma is adherent to the posterior uterus, it is first drained and the content aspirated in order to create space for further dissection.
- *Sigmoid mobilization and ureterolysis*: This step is carried out to expose the left common iliac artery. Medial dissection will reveal the ureter crossing over. All investing layers of the ureter down to the adventitia are divided using a 3 mm ultra micrograsper as a backstop. This approach allows for the microdissection of the overlying fibrosis from the ureter in the cardinal uterosacral area (Fig. 30.5). In the case of a left ovarian endometrioma adherent to the ureteric peritoneum, this step allows the safe mobilization of the ovary away from the ureter including mobilization of diseased peritoneum of the ovarian fossa. Dissection of the ovary from its adhesions to the rectum may also be necessary and superficial rectal serosa or muscularis should be resected in order to avoid ovarian tissue remaining attached to the rectum, causing future ovarian remnant syndrome. After mobilization of the ovarian cyst, the ureter can be exposed down to its ureteric tunnel.
- *En bloc excision of anterior rectal, posterior cul-de-sac, and uterosacral disease*: If the uterosacral ligaments are thickened, we lateralize the ureters and divide the uterosacral ligaments medial to the ureter towards the central rectovaginal mass. With maximum anteflexion of the uterus afforded by the RUMI® manipulator and with slight traction on the rectum, the KTP laser is used to release the rectum from the posterior uterus and vagina (Figs 30.7 to 30.9, 30.12, 30.15 and 30.16). A grasper is then inserted into the lateral rectovaginal space behind the central mass and the overlying thick endometriotic tissue is incised towards the grasper. This results in bi-section of rectovaginal disease, leaving a half of it attached to the rectum and the other half to the posterior vagina, which will be resected later (Fig. 30.8).

After further dissection with the laser and dissector, the unaffected distal rectovaginal space is entered (Fig. 30.10) where a ring forceps in the rectum helps to identify normal rectal muscularis. Thus, before proceeding further to resect the rectal disease, the normal boundary is identified. At this point, a laser incision is made along the initial outline to include the uterosacral ligament pararectal tissue bilaterally in the dissection. Using laparoscopic palpation with a bowel grasper, the depth of rectal infiltration is assessed.

Partial thickness resection ('shaving') should only be performed when the outer longitudinal muscularis is involved and can be peeled mechanically from the inner circular muscularis.

If the inner muscularis (with its circular fibers) is affected, a full thickness disk resection is required because the inner muscularis cannot be separated and any attempted resection will be incomplete, causing recurrence and postoperative complications. In our experience, multifocal lesions or those larger than 4 cm in diameter require laparoscopically-assisted colectomy regardless of mucosal involvement.

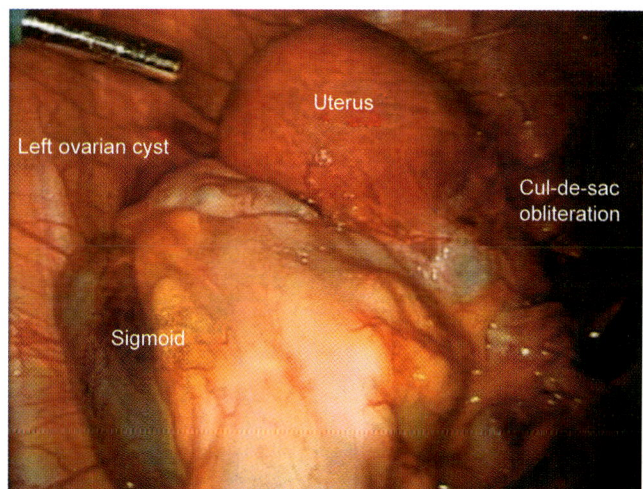

Fig. 30.16: Patient with cul-de-sac obliteration and rectal bleeding

With partial or full thickness anterior rectal resection, 3-0 PDS on an SH needle is used to approximate the outer longitudinal muscularis in one or two layers continuously with the first comprising of mucosa and muscularis and the second of muscularis with or without serosa. The initial knot is tied at the starting angle; the second layer is completed with the same suture running back towards the starting angle and tied intracorporeally to the tail of the initial knot. A third, serosal layer is optional.

To confirm integrity of the suture, air is insufflated into the rectum via a 30 cc Foley's. Leakage can be excluded if no bubbles are observed laparoscopically in the fluid-filled pelvis. Alternatively, a Betadine® solution can be instilled into the rectum via a blocked 30 cc Foley's catheter under laparoscopic vision.

Sigmoid Endometriosis

Sigmoid endometriosis requires laparoscopically-assisted bowel resection unless lesions are small, isolated and amenable to full or partial thickness disk resection; the upper limit is 3 cm. With larger or multifocal lesions, a general surgeon carries out a laparoscopically-assisted colectomy with end-to-end stapled anastomosis (Figs 30.17 to 30.21). Multifocal lesions can be diagnosed by laparoscopic palpation using a bowel grasper (Fig. 30.17).

Briefly, after resection of nonintestinal endometriosis, the sigmoid mesentery is opened and the inferior mesenteric artery is skeletonized. A linear laparoscopic stapler is introduced to transect the colon below the lesion and to seal the lumen (Fig. 30.18).

Following this, the colon is exteriorized, transected above the lesion with a linear stapler, the diseased segment is removed through a 4 cm incision in the left iliac fossa, a purse string suture is introduced (Fig. 30.20) and the superior bowel segment is tightened over an anvil, which is part of a circular cutting stapler. The counterpart of the stapler is introduced through the rectum and the colon stump is loaded onto it. Anvil and counterpart (Fig. 30.20) are connected and circular cutting and stapling carried out. The suture line (Fig. 30.21) is checked for integrity as described above.

Results and Follow-up

Laparoscopic radical bowel resection is now established in specialized centers and there is an accumulating

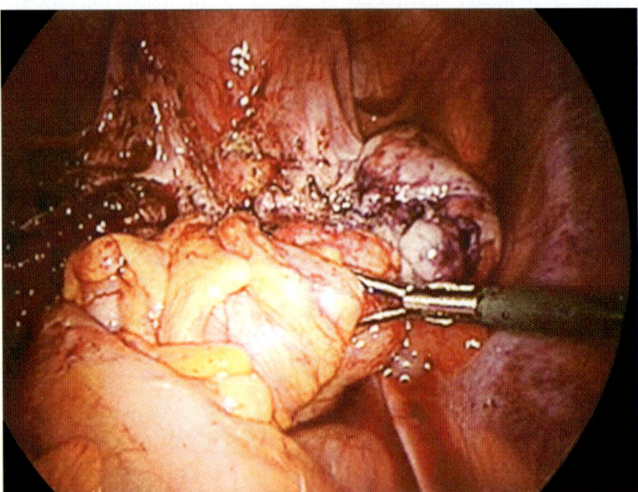

Fig. 30.17: A grasper is used to palpate the rectosigmoid thickening

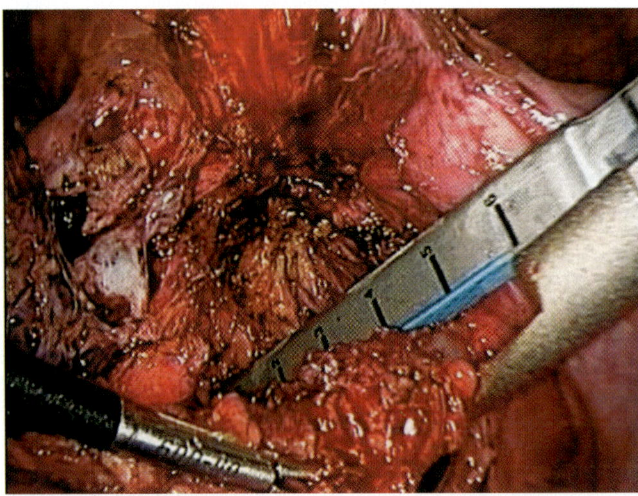

Fig. 30.18: A linear stapler is introduced to transect the colon below the lesion

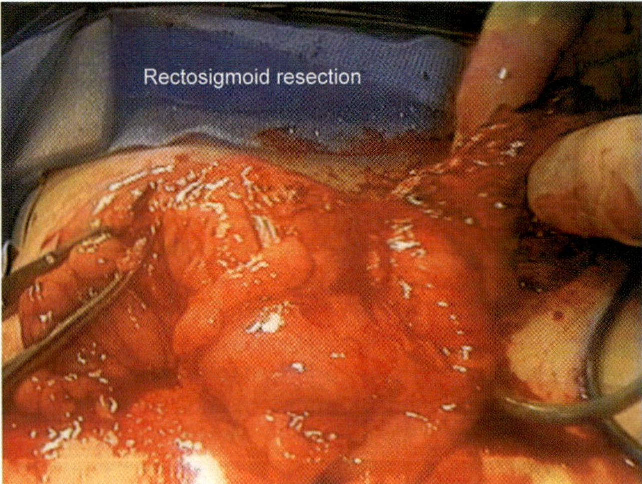

Fig. 30.19: The superior bowel segment is exteriorized and closed with a purse string suture

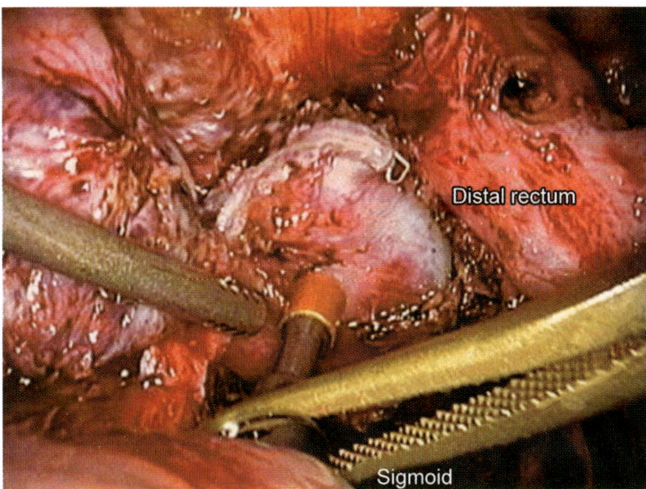

Fig. 30.20: Anvil and counterpart of circular stapler are connected laparoscopically prior to cutting and stapling

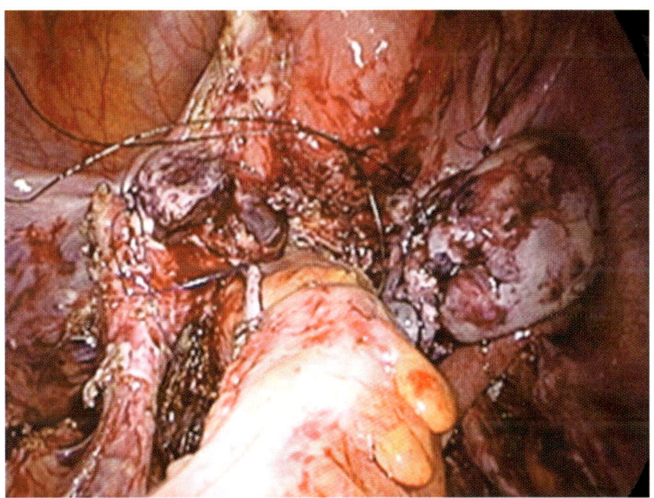

Fig. 30.21: Completed end-to-end anastomosis

Table 30.1: Experience of laparoscopic bowel resection for endometriosis with the range of complication rates		
Author	*Year*	*Number treated*
Riberio	2006	125
Lyons	2006	7
Keckstein	2005	202
Dubenard	2006	58
Darai	2005	34
Landi	2006	20+25
Fleisch	2005	23
Mohr	2005	48
Campagnacci	2005	29
Koh, Janik	2002	22
Pereira	2009	168
Ruffo	2010	436
Stricture	3–6%	
Anastomosis leak	0.6–3%	
Fistula, including rectovaginal	2–10%	
Abscess	1%	

There is no doubt that radical excision of endometriosis improves quality of life, provides effective long-term pain relief and that, ovarian preservation does not impair fertility outcomes.[1,12,39,42-44] However, functional problems affecting sexual function, bladder and bowel have been reported, albeit rarely (2% for persistent bowel dysfunction).[40] Problems are more common after a low rectum than after a sigmoid resection, which should be taken into account when choosing the type of resection.[45]

Rectosigmoid Endometriosis and Fertility

Multiple factors contribute to the reduction of fertility in endometriosis, including reduced ovarian responsiveness to controlled ovarian hyperstimulation with ovarian endometriomata[46] and lower implantation rates, particularly in severe disease.[47] In addition to this, distortion of the pelvic anatomy impairs the pick-up and transport of oocytes by reducing tubal motility or causing blockage. Finally, pelvic pain caused by endometriosis may lead to dyspareunia and apareunia.

The contribution of intestinal endometriosis to infertility is not known, in fact, asymptomatic intestinal endometriosis may be ignored and fertility treatment, including *in vitro* fertilization, can be commenced. Where stimulation with gonadotropins causes exacerbation of intestinal symptoms, prolonged down regulation with a gonadotropin-releasing hormone agonist for 3 to 6 months prior to stimulation with gonadotropins has been effective in assisted reproduction.[48]

body of literature available[27-37] with acceptably low rates of complications (Table 30.1) and different modes of resection[27,29,30,32,34,38-41] (Table 30.2). We have evaluated over 400 cases of deep infiltrating endometriosis of the cul-de-sac. Of these, 105 had rectal disease, 22 required laparoscopic colectomy, 17 had full thickness anterior rectosigmoid resection, and 56 had partial thickness resection. All, apart from one early case, were performed laparoscopically. After surgery, only one serious complication occurred, a rectal perforation, which was treated with diverting temporary colostomy. Of the 22 patients, who were followed-up between 2 to 9 years, 19 were pain-free and none required additional hormonal suppression or later bilateral oophorectomy.

Table 30.2: Treatment spectrum of rectosigmoid endometriosis					
Author	*Year*	*Total*	*Shaving*	*Full thickness disk resection*	*Colectomy*
Koh, Janik	2002	95	56	10	24
Duepree	2002	51	26	5	18
Ford	2004	60	48	2	10
Keckstein	2005	142	-	-	142
Darai	2005	36	-	-	36
Mohr	2005	187	100	39	48
Riberio	2006	125	8	2	125
Pereira	2009	172	22	52	92
Pandis	2010	177	56	7	15

However, this may not be feasible in older patients; furthermore, severe symptoms of bowel obstruction have occurred despite prolonged down regulation.[49] Hall et al.[50] reported a case of endometriosis flare-up caused by using a GnRH agonist, which led to bowel obstruction and an emergency total abdominal hysterectomy with bilateral salpingo-oophorectomy. Such an unfortunate outcome could have been prevented by prior excision of the intestinal endometriosis before commencing assisted reproduction. We have treated many similar cases of intestinal endometriotic exacerbation following up-regulation (despite prolonged down regulation) for *in vitro* fertilization. Following laparoscopic colorectal resection, these patients were subsequently able to undergo successful assisted reproduction, and good pregnancy rates have been reported after radical endometriosis excision, including bowel resection[1,12,27,29,30,32,35,51] (Table 30.3).

Another compelling danger to fertility in intestinal endometriosis is iatrogenic; recommending total abdominal hysterectomy and bilateral salpingo-oophorectomy at the time of bowel resection is without merit or supporting data. Moreover, with adequate excision of deep endometriosis and laparoscopic bowel resection, symptoms can be ameliorated without the need for performing hysterectomy or salpingo-oophorectomy.[12,27] Predictive criteria for successful fertility treatment after colorectal resection include young age, a low American Society of Reproductive Medicine score and the laparoscopic surgical route. Adverse outcomes appear to be linked to the presence of adenomyosis.[52]

RECENT ADVANCES

Fortunately, the last few years have seen an increased uptake and growth in the expertise of fertility sparing excision of intestinal endometriosis. Recent advances focus on cosmetic improvements by avoiding an abdominal incision for removal of the excised bowel segment, but suggest transantral removal.[53]

Table 30.3: Pregnancy rates after radical endometriosis excision including segmental bowel resection		
Author	*Year*	*Pregnancy rate*
Koh, Janik	2002	40%
Possover	2004	53%
Keckstein	2005	54%
Redwine	2001	43%
Chopin	2005	54%
Darai	2005	45%
Mohr	2005	18%
Lyons	2006	100%
Kavallaris	2010	37%
Darai	2010	44%
Stepniewska	2010	45-58%

CONCLUSION

Intestinal endometriosis is readily diagnosed at laparoscopy by careful exploration. Laparoscopic bowel resection is increasingly being employed in specialized centers and provides the patient with the advantages of minimally invasive surgery.

The safety and efficacy of laparoscopically-assisted segmental bowel resection is well-established. The most difficult surgical cases are those that involve cul-de-sac obliteration and rectal endometriosis. Adequate and complete resection of the bowel lesion cures intestinal endometriosis and does not depend on hysterectomy or oophorectomy for remission. It is imperative that concomitant deep pelvic endometriosis is excised for good symptom relief. It is always possible to preserve the uterus and ovary when treating intestinal or rectovaginal endometriosis, and there is no contraindication to future childbearing. Hysterectomy may be indicated when there is severe adenomyosis and fertility is no longer desired. A subtotal hysterectomy is contraindicated for cul-de-sac obliteration as further surgery will often become necessary. The need for colorectal resection is determined by the symptoms and extent of intestinal distortion and does not depend on the involvement of bowel mucosa.

With greater awareness of intestinal endometriosis and its implications, afflicted patients can look forward to effective treatment with reduced morbidity and without sacrificing fertility.

REFERENCES

1. Kavallaris A, Chalvatzas N, Hornemann A, Banz C, Diedrich K, Agic A. 94 months follow-up after laparoscopic-assisted vaginal resection of septum rectovaginale and rectosigmoid in women with deep infiltrating endometriosis. Arch Gynecol Obstet 2011;283:1059-64.
2. Tarjanne S, Sjoberg J, Heikinheimo O. Radical excision of rectovaginal endometriosis results in high rate of pain relief - results of a long-term follow-up study. Acta Obstet Gynecol Scand 2010;89:71-7.
3. Brouwer R, Woods RJ. Rectal endometriosis: results of radical excision and review of published work. ANZ J Surg 2007;77: 562-71.
4. Fedele L, Bianchi S, Zanconato G, Tozzi L, Raffaelli R. Gonadotropin-releasing hormone agonist treatment for endometriosis of the rectovaginal septum. Am J Obstet Gynecol 2000;183:1462-7.
5. Shaw RW. Treatment of endometriosis. Lancet 1992;340: 1267-71.
6. Kemp S. Endometriosis, Investigation and Management. In: London: Royal College of Obstetricians and Gynaecologists; 2006.
7. Blott M. The Future Role of the Consultant. In: London: Royal College of Obstetricians and Gynaecologists; 2005.
8. Ferrero S, Camerini G, Menada MV, Biscaldi E, Ragni N, Remorgida V. Uterine adenomyosis in persistence of dysmenorrhea after surgical excision of pelvic endometriosis and colorectal resection. J Reprod Med 2009;54:366-72.
9. Weed JC, Ray JE. Endometriosis of the bowel. Obstet Gynecol 1987;69:727-30.
10. Koninckx PR, Meuleman C, Demeyere S, Lesaffre E, Cornillie FJ. Suggestive evidence that pelvic endometriosis is a progressive disease, whereas deeply infiltrating endometriosis is associated with pelvic pain. Fertil Steril 1991;55:759-65.
11. Cornillie FJ, Oosterlynck D, Lauweryns JM, Koninckx PR. Deeply infiltrating pelvic endometriosis: Histology and clinical significance. Fertil Steril 1990;53:978-83.
12. Redwine DB, Wright JT. Laparoscopic treatment of complete obliteration of the cul-de-sac associated with endometriosis: Long-term follow-up of en bloc resection. Fertil Steril 2001;76: 358-65.
13. Kavallaris A, Kohler C, Kuhne-Heid R, Schneider A. Histopathological extent of rectal invasion by rectovaginal endometriosis. Hum Reprod 2003;18:1323-7.
14. Donnez J, Nisolle M, Gillerot S, Smets M, Bassil S, Casanas-Roux F. Rectovaginal septum adenomyotic nodules: A series of 500 cases. Br J Obstet Gynaecol 1997;104:1014-8.
15. Vercellini P, Aimi G, Panazza S, Vicentini S, Pisacreta A, Crosignani PG. Deep endometriosis conundrum: Evidence in favor of a peritoneal origin. Fertil Steril 2000;73:1043-6.
16. Bazot M, Darai E, Hourani R, Thomassin I, Cortez A, Uzan S, et al. Deep pelvic endometriosis: MR imaging for diagnosis and prediction of extension of disease. Radiology 2004;232:379-89.
17. Johnson CG, Coppola AF, Moll CF. Complications of endometriosis of the sigmoid colon. South Med J 1957;50:893-7.
18. Vercellini P, Frontino G, Pietropaolo G, Gattei U, Daguati R, Crosignani PG. Deep endometriosis: Definition, pathogenesis, and clinical management. J Am Assoc Gynecol Laparosc 2004;11:153-61.
19. Donnez J, Nisolle M, Squifflet J. Ureteral endometriosis: A complication of rectovaginal endometriotic (adenomyotic) nodules. Fertil Steril 2002;77:32-7.
20. Chapron C, Dubuisson JB, Pansini V, Vieira M, Fauconnier A, Barakat H, et al. Routine clinical examination is not sufficient for diagnosing and locating deeply infiltrating endometriosis. J Am Assoc Gynecol Laparosc 2002;9:115-9.
21. Coronado C, Franklin RR, Lotze EC, Bailey HR, Valdes CT. Surgical treatment of symptomatic colorectal endometriosis. Fertil Steril 1990;53:411-6.
22. Bazot M, Detchev R, Cortez A, Amouyal P, Uzan S, Darai E. Transvaginal sonography and rectal endoscopic sonography for the assessment of pelvic endometriosis: A preliminary comparison. Hum Reprod 2003;18:1686-92.
23. Abrao MS, Goncalves MO, Dias JA, Jr., Podgaec S, Chamie LP, Blasbalg R. Comparison between clinical examination, transvaginal sonography and magnetic resonance imaging for the diagnosis of deep endometriosis. Hum Reprod 2007;22:3092 7.
24. Saba L, Guerriero S, Sulcis R, Ajossa S, Melis G, Mallarini G. Agreement and reproducibility in identification of endometriosis using magnetic resonance imaging. Acta Radiol 2010;51:573-80.
25. Abou-Setta AM, Al-Inany HG, Farquhar CM. Levonorgestrel-releasing intrauterine device (LNG-IUD) for symptomatic endometriosis following surgery. Cochrane Database Syst Rev 2006:CD005072.
26. Redwine DB. Ovarian endometriosis: A marker for more extensive pelvic and intestinal disease. Fertil Steril 1999;72: 310-15.
27. Koh CH, Janik GM. The surgical management of deep rectovaginal endometriosis. Curr Opin Obstet Gynecol 2002;14:357-64.
28. Campagnacci R, Perretta S, Guerrieri M, Paganini AM, De Sanctis A, Ciavattini A, et al. Laparoscopic colorectal resection for endometriosis. Surg Endosc 2005;19:662-4.
29. Keckstein J, Wiesinger H. Deep endometriosis, including intestinal involvement: The interdisciplinary approach. Minim Invasive Ther Allied Technol 2005;14:160-66.
30. Mohr C, Nezhat FR, Nezhat CH, Seidman DS, Nezhat CR. Fertility considerations in laparoscopic treatment of infiltrative bowel endometriosis. JSLS 2005;9:16-24.

31. Fleisch MC, Xafis D, De Bruyne F, Hucke J, Bender HG, Dall P. Radical resection of invasive endometriosis with bowel or bladder involvement; Long-term results. Eur J Obstet Gynecol Reprod Biol 2005;123:224-9.

32. Darai E, Thomassin I, Barranger E, Detchev R, Cortez A, Houry S, et al. Feasibility and clinical outcome of laparoscopic colorectal resection for endometriosis. Am J Obstet Gynecol 2005;192(2):394-400.

33. Landi S, Ceccaroni M, Perutelli A, Allodi C, Barbieri F, Fiaccavento A, et al. Laparoscopic nerve-sparing complete excision of deep endometriosis: Is it feasible? Hum Reprod 2006;21:774-81.

34. Ribeiro PA, Rodrigues FC, Kehdi IP, Rossini L, Abdalla HS, Donadio N, et al. Laparoscopic resection of intestinal endometriosis: A 5-year experience. J Minim Invasive Gynecol 2006;13:442-6.

35. Lyons SD, Chew SS, Thomson AJ, Lenart M, Camaris C, Vancaillie TG, et al. Clinical and quality-of-life outcomes after fertility-sparing laparoscopic surgery with bowel resection for severe endometriosis. J Minim Invasive Gynecol 2006;13: 436-41.

36. Dubernard G, Piketty M, Rouzier R, Houry S, Bazot M, Darai E. Quality of life after laparoscopic colorectal resection for endometriosis. Hum Reprod 2006;21:1243-7.

37. Ruffo G, Scopelliti F, Scioscia M, Ceccaroni M, Mainardi P, Minelli L. Laparoscopic colorectal resection for deep infiltrating endometriosis: analysis of 436 cases. Surg Endosc 2010;24:63-7.

38. Duepree HJ, Senagore AJ, Delaney CP, Marcello PW, Brady KM, Falcone T. Laparoscopic resection of deep pelvic endometriosis with rectosigmoid involvement. J Am Coll Surg 2002;195: 754-8.

39. Ford J, English J, Miles WA, Giannopoulos T. Pain, quality of life and complications following the radical resection of rectovaginal endometriosis. BJOG 2004;111:353-6.

40. Pereira RM, Zanatta A, Preti CD, de Paula FJ, da Motta EL, Serafini PC. Should the gynecologist perform laparoscopic bowel resection to treat endometriosis? Results over 7 years in 168 patients. J Minim Invasive Gynecol 2009;16:472-9.

41. Pandis GK, Saridogan E, Windsor AC, Gulumser C, Cohen CR, Cutner AS. Short-term outcome of fertility-sparing laparoscopic excision of deeply infiltrating pelvic endometriosis performed in a tertiary referral center. Fertil Steril 2010;93:39-45.

42. Garry R, Clayton R, Hawe J. The effect of endometriosis and its radical laparoscopic excision on quality of life indicators. BJOG 2000;107:44-54.

43. Darai E, Carbonnel M, Dubernard G, Lavoue V, Coutant C, Bazot M, et al. Determinant factors of fertility outcomes after laparoscopic colorectal resection for endometriosis. Eur J Obstet Gynecol Reprod Biol 149:210-4.

44. Stepniewska A, Pomini P, Scioscia M, Mereu L, Ruffo G, Minelli L. Fertility and clinical outcome after bowel resection in infertile women with endometriosis. Reprod Biomed Online 2010;20:602-9.

45. Ret Davalos ML, De Cicco C, D'Hoore A, De Decker B, Koninckx PR. Outcome after rectum or sigmoid resection: A review for gynecologists. J Minim Invasive Gynecol 2007;14:33-8.

46. Gupta S, Agarwal A, Agarwal R, Loret de Mola JR. Impact of ovarian endometrioma on assisted reproduction outcomes. Reprod Biomed Online 2006;13:349-60.

47. Kuivasaari P, Hippelainen M, Anttila M, Heinonen S. Effect of endometriosis on IVF/ICSI outcome: Stage III/IV endometriosis worsens cumulative pregnancy and live-born rates. Hum Reprod 2005;20:3130-5.

48. Marcus SF, Edwards RG. High rates of pregnancy after long-term down-regulation of women with severe endometriosis. Am J Obstet Gynecol 1994;171:812-7.

49. Anaf V, El Nakadi I, Simon P, Englert Y, Peny MO, Fayt I, et al. Sigmoid endometriosis and ovarian stimulation. Hum Reprod 2000;15:790-4.

50. Hall LL, Malone JM, Ginsburg KA. Flare-up of endometriosis induced by gonadotropin-releasing hormone agonist leading to bowel obstruction. Fertil Steril 1995;64:1204-6.

51. Chopin N, Vieira M, Borghese B, Foulot H, Dousset B, Coste J, et al. Operative management of deeply infiltrating endometriosis: results on pelvic pain symptoms according to a surgical classification. J Minim Invasive Gynecol 2005;12: 106-12.

52. Darai E, Bazot M, Rouzier R, Coutant C, Ballester M. [Colorectal endometriosis and fertility]. Gynecol Obstet Fertil 2008;36: 1214-7.

53. Knol J, D'Hondt M, Dozois EJ, Vanden Boer J, Malisse P. Laparoscopic-assisted sigmoidectomy with transanal specimen extraction: A bridge to NOTES? Tech Coloproctol 2009;13: 65-8.

Management Practices for Endometriotic Cysts Associated with Infertility

Alain Audebert

OVERVIEW

Endometriotic cyst is a frequent lesion found in patients with infertility. Despite lack of specific epidemiological studies, it seems that an ovarian endometrioma is présent in more than 20 percent of patients with endometriosis-associated infertility, with a left side predominance. The causal relationship between this lesion and infertility and the mechanisms involved still remains debated, especially for unilateral cysts without other associated endometriotic lesions. In the absence of significant adhesions impairing tubal function, altered folliculogenesis and poor oocyte quality have been suggested.

For a long-time, surgical excision of the cyst, preferably with a laparoscopic approach, was recommended as the first-line treatment, when the diameter was 3 to 4 centimeters or more. Nowadays, the management of ovarian endometrioma associated with infertility is more versatile and individualized in light of recent studies:

- Suggesting the risk of surgery with regard to ovarian reserve, mainly in case of bilateral endometrioma or iterative surgery. When surgery is performed, great technical care should be taken in order to reduce impairment of healthy ovarian tissue
- Showing a limited and controversial impact of ovarian endometrioma on pregnancy rates after *in vitro* fertilization (IVF), and
- Indicating a possible role for transvaginal aspiration of an ovarian endometrioma, usually a simple ultrasound-guided procedure, performed without general anesthesia.

Clear recommendations cannot presently be proposed due to the lack of controlled studies and contradictory results of available series.

After adequate laparoscopic excision, or fenestration, about 50 percent of patients will conceive, thus surgery is an acceptable procedure for many patients.

The results of ultrasonographic endometrioma aspiration are still limited. This procedure bears a high-risk of adhesion formation and recurrence. For these reasons, no conclusion can presently be drawn.

A wait-and-watch approach can be proposed for small diameter ovarian endometriomas, IVF is required when no pregnancy has occurred after surgery or after a period of observation. The option of IVF versus surgery should be discussed when facing recurrent endometriomas.

INTRODUCTION

The ovary is one of the more frequent sites of pelvic endometriotic lesions.[1] Management of ovarian endometriosis is thus, a frequent clinical issue in routine practice.

Nevertheless, various aspects of ovarian endometriosis are still uncertain or debated. Its pathophysiology, the correlation with attributed symptoms (pain and subfertility) and the optimal therapeutic strategy to apply, are still controversial. Removal of lesions is usually considered as the gold standard, for endometriomas of at least 3 centimeter size, especially more when there is associated pain. According to a meta-analysis of 170 patients with a mean age of 46 years, this is the only way to obtain histologic proof of the exact nature of the cyst and also to eliminate the rare cases of malignancy, usually affecting older patients. Malignant transformation in endometriosis may be associated with presumed estrogenic stimulation. Tumors arising in endometriosis are predominantly low grade and confined to the site of origin, either confined to the ovary, the extragonadal site of origin, or spread throughout the peritoneal cavity.[2] In case of associated infertility, the optimal strategy is even more controversial. Some questions that do not have any clear answers include:

- The real impact of a unilateral endometrioma, without extensive adhesions impairing tubal function, on fecundity
- The impact of iterative surgery on the ovarian reserve
- The role of alternative therapeutic and therapeutic abstention.

Epidemiology of Ovarian Endometriomas

In most of the epidemiolgical studies on endometriosis, ovarian endometriomas are rarely specifically assessed. It is however, usually assumed that ovarian endometriomas are identified in around 22 percent of patients with endometriosis, associated with subfertility or pelvic pain.[3] The left side is more frequently affected with unilateral lesions than the right side (60% vs. 40%, respectively).[4] A left side predominance is also found for recurrent endometriomas.[5] In a personal unpublished series of 414 ovarian endometriomas, of at least 3 centimeters diameter, the mean age of patients was 35 years. Ovarian endometriomas are rarely identified in adolescent girls. On the contrary, during postmenopause, ovarian endometriomas are more frequently reported.

Ovarian Endometriomas and Infertility

For unilateral endometriomas, as previously evoked, the causal relationship with infertility is uncertain. According to the revised American Fertility Society (AFS) classification (1995), the presence of an ovarian endometrioma, of 3 centimeters size, leads to such a score, that the resulting stage is inevitably III, or moderate endometriosis. Moderate endometriosis is associated with an impairment of fecundity, with a spontaneous conception rate of 2.3 percent according to a literature analysis.[6] Indeed, the predictive value of this classification is still very controversial. An observational study indicates that infertility is more prevalent among peritoneal endometriosis cases than among those with ovarian or peritoneal and ovarian involvement (P = 0.008).[7]

After surgical treatment of ovarian endometriomas the reported conception rates are in the range of 50 percent. These findings suggest that an ovarian endometrioma might impair fertility. However this negative effect is not always demonstrated.[8] The impact of endometriomas on the results of IVF are also controversial.

If this assumption is accepted, the question of which mechanisms are involved is raised for endometriomas not associated with moderate or severe adhesions impairing the adnexal function. Abnormalities of folliculogenesis, oocyte or sperm transport have been hypothetized for peritoneal implants, eventually asssociated with ovarian endometriomas.[9,10] No specific study, experimental or clinical, is devoted specifically to ovarian endometriomas.

Therapeutic Tools

In case of infertility, as the main symptom, the main objective of the treatment is to improve the fecundity and the conception rate. An accessory objective is to have a histologic proof of the type of the cyst and its benign nature, as well as to eliminate the presence of atypias.[11] For this latter purpose, surgical removal of the whole cyst is mandatory.[12] However other therapeutic options have been proposed (Table 31.1).

Abstention

Theoreticallly, abstention should be limited to the cases where a definitive diagnosis has been established. However, for ovarian endometriomas of less than 3 centimeters size, the advances in imaging techniques provide a high probability on the nature of the cyst.

The impact of these endometriomas on fertility is mostly minimal. For young women, the probability of a malignant lesion is very low. Thus, abstention can legitimately be offered to these patients, as well as in cases of recurrence of an ovarian endometrioma after surgery.

A regular imaging control of the cyst is however recommended. Futhermore, magnetic resonance imaging (MRI) is now able to detect cases of malignant transformation.[13]

Hormonal Suppression

It is usually assumed that medical treatment, whichever drug used, has little impact on ovarian endometriomas larger than 3 centimeters size. Hormonal treatment should not be recommended in such situations.

Observational studies have however, demonstrated a decrease in size of the cyst after medical treatment, reaching in some cases 50 percent.[14,15] Medical treatment has been also associated with surgery, but no beneficial effect on fertility has been demonstrated.

Donnez et al.[16] demonstrated, in a series of 814 cases, that laparoscopic fenestration of the ovarian endometrioma completed by a postsurgical medical treatment, with GnRH analog, is able to decrease the size of the cyst (50%), as observed at the second-look laparoscopy.[16] Medical treatment has also been associated with ultrasound-guided cyst aspiration, especially before performing an IVF.

Ultrasound-guided Cyst Aspiration

Transvaginal aspiration of an ovarian endometrioma is usually a simple procedure, performed without general anesthesia

Table 31.1: Therapeutic tools

1. Abstention
2. Hormonal suppression
3. Ultrasound-guided cyst aspiration
4. Surgery
5. IVF

under ultrasound guidance. Two specific complications of this procedure are however associated with endometriomas:

- If a leakage of chocolate cyst liquid occurs, the risk of adhesion formation is high, because this liquid bears a strong adhesiogenic capacity. A study has compared adhesion scores, determined by laparoscopy, in two groups of patients: 13 patients with previous ultrasonographic aspiration were compared to 42 others without such a previous procedure.[17] Occasonial cases of severe adhesions occuring after ultrasonographic aspiration have been reproted.[18]
- The second risk, unexpected and more recently highlighted, is secondary infection. A study, published more than 25 years ago,[19] has found that 11 endometriomas, in a series of 510 cysts, showed histologic signs of infection. In a more recent series of 218 endometriomas, 7 cases of adnexal abscess have been observed, including two after a surgical procedure or an ultrasound-guided aspiration.[20] A recent analysis of 83 cases of tubal or ovarian abscess indicates that endometriosis stages III and IV were a significant risk factor, with an odds ratio (OR) of 2.95.[21] Several cases of ovarian abscess, complicating an ultrasound-guided ovum pick-up for IVF have been reported,[22] sometimes with delay, when an antibiotic prophylaxis was used.[23]

If endometrioma aspiration is associated with an improvement in symptoms, the reported rates of recurrences vary from 28 to 100 percent. In order to reduce this risk of recurrence, aspiration has been completed by injection of various sclerosing or cytotoxic agents, such as methotrexate,[24] ethanol[25] or tetracycline[26] within the empty cyst. Small series have been published, the main outcomes of which are listed in Table 31.2.

Several cases of spontaneous or post-IVF pregnancies, occuring after cyst aspiration, have been reported. These interesting findings should be confirmed by larger series, as well as the real rate of recurrence according to the procedure performed. From a practical point of view, counseling should be clear on the risk of infection, when an aspiration is offered to a patient. Futhermore, ultrasound-guided cyst aspiration should be perfomed only in infertile patients with a recurrence and before IVF.[34]

Surgical Treatment

Surgical treatment is still considered as the gold standard. Three major issues have to be assessed, in addition to technical aspects and results:

1. Postoperative adhesions
2. Recurrence after surgery
3. Impact of surgery on ovarian function and ovarian reserve.

Technical aspects: The laparoscopic approach is feasible in most instances. Operative laparoscopy leads to results similar to those formerly obtained with laparotomy, including microsurgery.[35-39] Thus, owing to the well-known advantages of laparoscopy, such as cost, morbidity, and short period of hospitalization, this procedure should be recommended. Schematically, two main procedures are presently used:

- Cystectomy, with complete removal of the cyst wall,
- Fenestration and medical treatment, followed 3 months later, by a second laparoscopy, in order to destroy the remaining cyst wall (or three step treatment), as described by Donnez et al.[16]

According to the size of the cyst, this later procedure might be easier to perform. The cleavage of the cyst wall might also be difficult to complete without clear reason, but most probably, depending upon the invasiveness of the disease and the inflammatory reaction of the surrounding ovarian tissue, than upon the use of a preoperative medical treatment.

Each technique has advantages and disavadvantages, to be discussed later in this review.

Postsurgical Adhesions: The ovary is known as an organ at high risk of postoperative adhesions. Recurrence of adhesions can reach 82 percent, and *de novo* adhesions can occur in 21 percent of the cases.[40] Preoperative hormonal suppression appears to be a rational tool to use, however, no clinical study has presently demonstrated its beneficial effect on postoperative adhesion rates.

Today, optimization of the operative procedure (applying microsurgical principles) is the main measure

Table 31.2: Recurrence rates after ultrasound-guided ovarain endometrioma aspiration				
Author	*Year*	*Number*	*Recurrence (%)*	*Follow-up*
Simple aspiration				
Giorlandino et al.[27]	1993	34	57	6-20 months
Messali et al.[28]	2003	10	10	Mean 21 months
Chan et al.[29]	2003	8	83.3	12 months
Aspiration + methotrexate				
Agostini et al.[30]	2004	14	14.3	Mean 8 months (3–13)
Aspiration + ethanol				
Noma and Yoshida[25]	2001	74	14.9	At least 6 months
Koike et al.[31]	2202	45	13.3	Delay for recurrence 5.2 months
Aspiration + tetracycline				
Chang et al.[26]	1997	32	46.9	12 months
Fisch et al.[32]	2004	32	25	Several months
Aspiration + medical treatment				
Troiano and Taylor[33]	1998	9	66.6	–
Mittal et al.[34]	1999	22	31.8	Mean 20 months

to ensure a reduced rate of adhesions. The use of adjuvant preventive methods (Interceed, Adept, Spraygel, Oxiplex, etc.) has demonstrated some beneficial effects in preventing postoperative adhesions after gynecological surgery. None of these methods, except Interceed,[41] have been specifically evaluated for ovarian endometrioma surgery. The results of a large randomized multicentric study with Adept should soon be disclosed.

Recurrence: Reported recurrence rates are very variable, ranging from 0 to 30 percent.[42] Numerous factors may interact with the risk of recurrence:

- Severity of lesions
- Theoretically, the host characteristics (predispositons due to a genetic abbnormality).
- Quality of surgical procedure.
- Methodological factors—definition of a recurrence, length of follow-up, etc.

The latter factor is probably one of the most frequent variables.[43] Stage IV and iterative surgery are unfavorable factors.[41]

An ovarian cyst on the operated ovary (cystectomy) was ultrasonographically identified in 10.6 percent of the 47 cases evaluated.[44] A more recent retrospective study found an overall recurrence (presence of a cyst of at least 2 cm in size at ultrasound evaluation) rate of 30.4 percent at two years in a series of 224 patients after excision.[45] Previous medical treatment of endometriosis or a large cyst size was a significant factor associated with a higher recurrence of the disease.[45]

Cystectomy appears to reduce the risk of recurrence in comparison with a three-step treatment, according to one observational study[46] and two prospective randomized series[47,48] as listed in Table 31.3.

Preservation of healthy ovarian tissue: The necessity to optimally preserve healthy ovarian tissue is a major issue that has recently been addressed.[49] This challenge is even more crucial in case of voluminous bilateral endometriomas or iterative surgery. Ovarian stripping (cystectomy) is associated with a significant decrease in residual ovarian volume, which may result in diminished ovarian reserve and function.[50] Theoretically, the three-step treatment should lead to a better response to ovarian preservation.[51,52] However, cystectomy, when performed meticulously, appears to adequately fulfill this requirement.[53,54]

Results: Many factors, unrelated to lesions, act upon the results of any treatment for infertility, such as age, eventual sperm alterations, associated lesions, length of follow-up, and method of assessement of results. With regard to lesions, the main factor is the severity of lesions and associated adhesions.

Numerous observational series have evaluated the results of ovarian endometrioma surgery in infertile patients. A recent review[55] and a meta-analysis[56] provided similar findings, with a conception rate close to 50 percent at five years follow-up. Several studies, including at least 50 cases, are listed in Table 31.3.

Two comparative studies indicate that conception rates are superior after cystectomy in comparison with the three-step treatment (fenestration, medical treatment for 3 months and *in situ* wall destruction).[48,57] The main studies are listed in Table 31.4.

Table 31.3: Incidence of reoperation after surgery for ovarian endometrioma

Author	Technique	N	Cumulative reoperation	
			Months	*%*
Busacca et al.[43]	Cystectomy	366	12	3.3
			48	8.2
Saleh and Tulandi[46]	Cystectomy	71	18	6.1
			42	23.6
	Fenestration+ablation	161	18	21.9
			42	57.8
Jones and Sutton[47]	KTP/coagulation/ablation	73	12	24.6
Alborzi et al.[48]	Cystectomy	52	12	5.8
	Fenestration+ablation	48	12	22.9

Note: These findings explain why consensus statements usually favor cystectomy.

Table 31.4: Cumulative pregnancy rates after surgery for ovarian endometrioma

Author	Technique	N	Follow-up (months)	Cumulative pregnancy %
Donnez et al.[16]	Vaporization	814	12	51
Sutton et al.[59]	Vaporization	66	36	45
Beretta et al.[57]	Cystectomy	32	24	66.7
	Coagulation	32	24	23.5
Hemmings et al.[60]	Coagulation	67	36	60
Busacca et al.[43]	Cystectomy	57	24	53
Yoshida et al.[61]	Cystectomy	92	37.5	43
Alborzi et al.[48]	Cystectomy	52	12	59.4
	Coagulation	48	12	23.3

Note: These findings explain why consensus statements favor cystectomy.

One study compared the results of primary surgical excision (359 cases) versus reoperation (54 cases) and found that the recurrence of pain and the reproductive outcome were comparable.[58]

In Vitro Fertilization

In vitro fertilization (IVF) is indeed, immediately indicated after an incomplete surgical excision of severe endometriotic lesions, or if a marked male factor is associated. This is also the ultimate resort for the 50 percent of patients who have not conceived after surgery. Several issues have to be addressed.

Impact of Ovarian Endometriomas on IVF Results

During the last two decades, many studies evaluated the impact of endometriosis on IVF results. Various abnormalities, some still controversial, have successfully been reported: decreased ovarian reserve, decreased ovarian response to stimulation, antisperm effects, decreased oocyte quality, decreased fecundity rate, decreased embryo quality, decreased implantation rate and increased spontaneous abortion rate. For some of them, fundamental research has provided some explanation for the observed abnormalities. In routine clinical practice, the most documented consequences are an increased cancelation rate, a small decrease in the fecundity rate and embryo quality, but the impact of these disturbances on pregnancy rates are in fact, limited. Pregnancy rates are comparable to those obtained in other indications, such as tubal occlusions, usually selected as the control group. The only exceptions are severe endometriosis, where results are significantly decreased.[62] A Cochrane Library meta-analysis of three randomized controlled trials concluded that the administration of gonadotropin-releasing hormone (GnRH) agonists for a period of three to six months prior to IVF or intracytoplasmic sperm injection (ICSI) in women with endometriosis increases the odds of clinical pregnancy four-fold. Data regarding the adverse effects of this therapy on the mother or fetus are not available at present.[63]

Data on the impact of ovarian endometriomas on IVF results are more limited. The results of 4 studies are listed in Table 31.5. They are however, difficult to compare because the number of cases reported are limited and the selected control groups are different. No difference in pregnancy and delivery rates have been observed in comparison with the results of the various control groups. Increased cancelation rate,[52] probably due to a reduced responsiveness to gonadotropins,[68] and spontaneous abortion rate,[65] are the most frequently reported negative impacts of ovarian endometriomas. Finally, the impact of an ovarian endometriomas on the results of IVF does appear very limited, and the presence of an ovarian endometrioma is not a contraindication to perform an IVF, with or without ICSI.

The impact of ovarian stimulation on endometriosis, including ovarian endometriomas, is a concern frequently questioned. As of the date of writing this article no clinical data demonstrates that temporary exposure to a very high level of estradiol induces an immediate negative effect on endometriotic lesions. A retrospective cohort study evaluated the effect of ovarian hyperstimulation (OH) on the recurrence rate of stages III and IV endometriosis.[69] The recurrence rate was lower after ovarian hyperstimulation for IVF than after low dose ovarian stimulation for IUI, suggesting that temporary exposure to very high estradiol levels in women during OH for IVF is not a major risk factor for the recurrence of endometriosis in women treated with assisted reproductive technique (ART).[69]

Aspiration of an ovarian endometrioma, incidentally identified during OH or ovum pick-up for IVF, does not appear to be required, except in cases of large size cysts or associated pain. One should be aware of the infectious risk associated with this procedure, and at least 15 cases of abscess have been reported after ovum pick-up in these patients. Unexpected puncture of an ovarian endometrioma during ovum pick-

Author	Endometrioma			Control group		
	N	*Pregnancies*	*Delivery*	*N*	*Pregnancies*	*Delivery*
Isaac et al.[64]				Endometriosis		
	24	17.2%	-	84	10.9%	-
Yanushopolski et al.[65]				Other indications		
	37	46%	24%/cycle	56	38%	32%/cycle
Tinkanen and Kujansuu[66]				No endometriosis		
	45	38%/cycle	27%/cycle	55	22%/cycle	20%/cycle
Pouly[67]				Endometriosis		
	52	-	23%/cycle	252	-	20%/cycle

Table 31.5: Results of IVF in patients with an ovarian endometrioma

up has no impact on the results of IVF, but bears the risks of infection.[70]

Impact of Previous Surgical Treatment of Ovarian Endometrioma on IVF Results

Several issues have already been addressed, such as the ovarian reserve and the responsiveness to OH. A decreased responsiveness to ovarian stimulation by gonadotropins has been reported for iterative surgery and severe endometrioses with large sized bilateral ovarian endometriomas.

A comparative study comparing endometriosis patients, with or without endometriomas, with tubal infertility patients, indicates a trend to obtain a reduced number of oocytes during ovum pick-up patients with ovarian endometriomas.[53] In contrast, a recent study indicates that for women aged below 35 years, the responsiveness to OH with Clomiphene citrate was altered, but responsiveness to OH with gonadotropins was unaffected.[71]

There is no marked difference concerning the type of surgical technique performed.[51] In this study, the size of the endometrioma was the only factor affecting the number of oocytes obtained.

Laparoscopic endometrioma cystectomy does reduce the ovarian reserve. However, diminished ovarian reserve does not translate into impaired pregnancy outcome.[72] According to one study, ultrasound-guided aspiration of the endometrioma leads to an increase number of oocytes obtained and a better fecundity rate in comparison with patients with previous surgical treatment of the endometrioma.[73]

Finally, a recommendation on whether or not surgery is advisable before performing an IVF, is still difficult to establish. A study supporting this recommendation[74] is in contrast to another study advising against surgery prior to IVF,[75] while the latest published report concludes that removal of the ovarian endometrioma does not improve the results of IVF.[76]

CONCLUSION

Clear recommendations cannot be presently proposed. The present available data, including too few controlled studies and contradictory results of observational studies, does not allow the proposal of any clear recommendations.

Role of Surgery, IVF and Ultrasound-guided Aspiration

For endometriomas larger than 3 cm in size, without an additional infertility factor (male), laparoscopic surgery should be offered as the first-line treatment, especially if pain is associated with infertility. Cystectomy (or excision), sometimes difficult to perform, appears to offer better results in term of spontaneous pregnancy and recurrence rates. Fenestration, with secondary ablation, should be considered

for difficult cystectomies or, perhaps, when large size bilateral endometriomas are encountered.

In the 50 percent of women who fail to conceive, or in women with an associated marked male factor, IVF should be performed, and the results (pregnancy and delivery) are minimally affected, except after iterative surgery or in case of severe endometriosis lesions, provided the surgical procedure has been adequately perfomed.

The results of ultrasonographic endometrioma aspiration are still limited. This procedure bears a high risk of adhesions formation and recurrence. For these reasons, no conclusion can presently be drawn.

Role of Abstention

Ovarian endometriomas, with a size below 3 cm, appear to have little impact on fertility. Thus, surgery is not an obligatory treatment, provided ultrasonographic supervision can be conducted. When IVF becomes necessary the results are not impaired by the presence of the ovarian endometrioma. The results are not impaired even if the endometrioma is accidently punctured during ovum pick-up. One should however, be aware of secondary ovarian abscesses, that occur in some occasions after a few weeks.[75]

Recurring ovarian endometriomas should not be systematically removed before performing an IVF. Iterative surgery may impair the ovarian reserve, in contrast, the presence of the ovarian endometrioma does not impair the expected results of IVF. Ovarian endometrioma, identified during the COH phase of the IVF, should not lead to any specific treatment. Beneficial effects of ultrasonographic aspiration prior to performing IVF are insufficiently demonstrated at present to recommend such a procedure.

REFERENCES

1. Jenkins S, Olive DL, Haney AF. Endometriosis: Pathogenic implications of the anatomic distribution. Obstet Gynecol 1986;67:335-8.
2. Heaps JM, Nieberg RK, Jonathan SB. Malignant neoplasms arising in endometriosis. Obstet Gynecol 1990;75:1023-8.
3. Koninckx PR, Meuleman C, Demeyere S, Lesaffre E, Cornillie FJ. Suggestive evidence that pelvic endometriosis is a progressive disease, whereas deeply infiltrating endometriosis is associtaed with pelvic pain. Fertil Steril 1991;55:759-5.
4. Vercellini P, Aimi G, De Giorgi O, Maddalena S, Carinelli S, Crosignani PG. Is cystic ovarian endometriosis an asymmetric disease? Br J Obstet Gynaecol 1998;105:1018-21.
5. Vercellini P, Busacca M, Aimi G, Bianchi S, Frontino G, Crosignani PG. Lateral distribution of recurrent ovarian endometriotic cysts. Fertil Steril 2002;77:848-9.
6. Adamson GD. Treatment of endometriosis-associated infertility. Sem Reprod Endocrinol 1997;15:263-71.
7. Hassa H, Tanir HM, Uray M. Symptom distribution among infertile and fertile endometriosis cases with different stages

and localisations. Eur J Obstet Gynecol Reprod Biol 2005;119: 82-6.

8. Fujishita A, Khan KN, Masuzaki H, Ishimaru T. Influence of pelvic endometriosis and ovarian endometrioma on fertility. Gynecol Obstet Invest 2002;53(Suppl 1):40-5.

9. Mamhood TA, Templeton A. Pathophysiology of mild endometriosis: Review of litterature. Hum Reprod 1990;5:765-4.

10. Rock JA, Markham SM. Pathogenesis of endometriosis. Lancet 1992;340:1264-7.

11. Ballouk F, Ross JS, Wolf BC. Ovarian endometriotic cysts. An analysis of cytologic atypia and DNA ploidy patterns. Am J Clin Pathol 1994;102:415-9.

12. Busacca M, Vignali M. Ovarian endometriosis: from pathogenesis to surgical treatment. Curr Opin Obstet Gynecol 2003;15:321-6.

13. Wu TT, Coakley FV, Qayyum A, Yeh BM, Joe BN, Chen LM. Magnetic resonance imaging of ovarian cancer arising in endometriomas. J Comput Assist Tomogr 2004;28:836-8.

14. Batioglu S, Celikkanat H, Ugur M, Mollamahmutoglu L, Yesilyurt H, Kundakci M. The use of GnRH agonists in the treatment of endometriomas with or without drainage. J Pak Med Assoc 1996;46:30-2.

15. Rana N, Thomas S, Rotman C, Dmowski WP. Decrease in the size of ovarian endometriomas during ovarian suppression in stage IV endometriosis. Role of preoperative medical treatment. J Reprod Med 1996;41:384-92.

16. Donnez J, Nisolle M, Gillet N, Smets M, Bassil S, Casanas-Roux F. Large ovarian endometriomas. Hum Reprod 1996;11:641-6.

17. Muzii L, Marana R, Caruana P, Catalano GF, Mancuso S. Laparoscopic findings after transvaginal ultrasound-guided aspiration of ovarian endometriomas. Hum Reprod 1995;10: 2902-3.

18. Garvey TS, Kazer RR, Milad MP. Severe pelvic adhesions following attempted ultrasound guided drainage of bilateral ovarian endometriomas: case report. Hum Reprod 1999;14: 2748-50.

19. Schmidt CL, Demopoulos RI, Weiss G. Infected endometriotic cysts: Clinical charactérization and pathogenesis. Fertil Steril 1981;36:27-30.

20. Kutoba T, Ishi K, Takeuchi H. A study of tubo-ovarian abscess and ovarian abscess, with a focus on cases with endometriois. J Obstet Gynaecol Res 1997;23:421-6.

21. Chen MJ, Yang JS, Yang YS, Ho HN. Increased occurrence of tubo-ovarian abscesses in women with stage III and IV endometriosis. Fertil Steril 2004;82:498-9.

22. Padilla SL. Ovarian abscess following puncture of an endometrioma during ultrasound-guided oocyte retrieval. Hum Reprod 1993;8:1282-3.

23. Younis JS, Ezra Y, Laufer N, Ohel G. Late manifestation of pelvic abscess following oocyte retrieval, for *in vitro* fertilization, in patients with severe endometriosis and ovarian endometriomata. J Assist Reprod Genet 1997;14:343-6.

24. Mesogitis S, Antsaklis A, Daskalakis G, Papantoniou N, Michalas S. Combined ultrasonographically guided drainage and methotrexate administration for treatment of endometriotic cysts. Lancet 2000;355:1160.

25. Noma J, Yoshida N. Efficacy of ethanol sclerotherapy for ovarian endometriomas. Int J Gynaecol Obstet 2001;72:35-9.

26. Chang CC, Lee HF, Tsai HD, Lo HY. Sclerotherapy—an adjuvant therapy to endometriosis. Int J Gynaecol Obstet 1997;59:31-4.

27. Giorlandino C, Taramanni C, Muzii L, Santillo E, Nanni C, Vizzone A. Ultrasound-guided aspiration of ovarian endometriotic cysts. Int J Gynaecol Obstet 1993;43:41-4.

28. Messalli EM, Cobellis G, Pecori E, Pierno G, Scaffa C, Stradella L, Cobellis L. Alcohol sclerosis of endometriomas after ultrasound-guided aspiration. Minerva Ginecol 2003;5:359-62.

29. Chan LY, So WW, Lao TT. Rapid recurrence of endometrioma after transvaginal ultrasound-guided aspiration. Eur J Obstet Gynecol Reprod Biol 2003;109:196-8.

30. Agostini A, Cravello L, Roger V, Bretelle F, Blanc B. Lee traitement des kystes endométriosiques de l'ovaire par injection échoguidée de méthotrexate. La Lettre Gynécol 2004;289:16-7.

31. Koike T, Minakami H, Motoyama M, Ogawa S, Fujiwara H, Sato I. Reproductive performance after ultrasound-guided transvaginal ethanol sclerotherapy for ovarian endometriotic cysts. Eur J Obstet Gynecol Reprod Biol 2002;105:39-43.

32. Fisch JD, Sher G. Sclerotherapy with 5 percent tetracycline is a simple alternative to potentially complex surgical treatment of ovarian endometriomas before *in vitro* fertilization. Fertil Steril 2004;82:437-41.

33. Troiano RN, Taylor KJ. Sonographically guided therapeutic aspiration of benign-appearing ovarian cysts and endometriomas. Am J Roentgenol 1998;171:1601-5.

34. Mittal S, Kumar S, Kumar A, Verma A. Ultrasound guided aspiration of endometrioma-a new therapeutic modality to improve reproductive outcome. Int J Gynaecol Obstet 1999;65:17–23.

35. Audebert A. Ovarian endometrioma and infertility: when not to treat? Gynecol Obstet Fertil 2005;33:416-22.

36. Tardif D, Benifla JL, Batallan A, Madelenat P. Treatment of a case of ovarian cysts in a patient known to have endometriosis. Gynecol Obstet Fertil 2002;30:231-5.

37. Bateman BG, Kolp LA, Mills S. Endoscopic versus laparotomy management of endometriomas. Fertil Steril 1994;62:690-5.

38. Mais V, Ajossa S, Marongiu D, Guerriero S, Piras B, Floris M, Palomba M, Melis GB. Treatment of Laparoscopic management of endometriomas: A randomized trial versus laparotomy. J Gynecol Surg 1996;12:41-6.

39. Catalano GF, Marana R, Caruana P, Muzii L, Mancuso S. Laparoscopy versus microsurgery by laparotomy for excision of ovarian cysts in patients with moderate or severe endometriosis. J Am Assoc Gynecol Laparosc 1996;3:267-70.

40. Canis M, Mage G, Wattiez A, Chapron C, Pouly JL, Bassil S. Second-look laparoscopy after laparoscopic cystectomy of large ovarian endometriomas. Fertil Steril 1992;58:617-9.

41. Sekiba K. Use of Interceed (TC7) absorbable adhesion barrier to reduce postoperative adhesion reformation in infertility and endometriosis surgery. The Obstetrics and Gynecology Adhesion Prevention Committee. Obstet Gynecol 1992;79:518-22.

42. Chapron C, Dubuisson JB, Fauconnier A, Vieira M. Management of endometriosis ovarian cysts. J Gynecol Obstet Biol Reprod 2001;30 (Suppl 1):S78-85.

43. Busacca M, Marana R, Caruana P, Candiani M, Muzii L, Calia C, Bianchi S. Recurrence of ovarian endometrioma after laparoscopic excision. Am J Obstet Gynecol 1999;180:519-23.

44. Muzii L, Bellati F, Plotti F, Manci N, Palaia I, Zullo MA, Angioli R, Panici PB. Ultrasonographic evaluation of postoperative

ovarian cyst formation after laparoscopic excision of endometriomas. J Am Assoc Gynecol Laparosc 2004;11:457-61.

45. Koga K, Takemura Y, Osuga Y, Yoshino O, Hirota Y, Hirata T, Morimoto C, Harada M, Yano T, Taketani Y. Recurrence of ovarian endometrioma after laparoscopic excision. Hum Reprod 2006;2171-4.

46. Saleh A, Tulandi T. Reoperation after laparoscopic treatment of ovarian endometriomas by excision and by fenestration. Fertil Steril 1999;72:322-4.

47. Jones KD, Sutton CJ. Recurrence of chocolate cysts after laparoscopic ablation. J Am Assoc Gynecol Laparosc 2002;9:315-20.

48. Alborzi S, Momtahan M, Parsanezhad ME, Dehbashi S, Zolghadri J, Alborzi S. A prospective, randomized study comparing laparoscopic ovarian cystectomy versus fenestration and coagulation in patients with endometriomas. Fertil Steril 2004;82:1633-7.

49. Hock DL, Sharafi K, Dagostino L, Kemmann E, Seifer DB. Contribution of diminished ovarian reserve to hypofertility associated with endometriosis. J Reprod Med 2001;46:7-10.

50. Exacoustos C, Zupi E, Amadio A, Amoroso C, Szabolcs B, Romanini ME, Arduini D. Recurrence of endometriomas after laparoscopic removal: sonographic and clinical follow-up and indication for second surgery. J Minim Invasive Gynecol 2006; 13:281-8.

51. Donnez J, Wyns C, Nisolle M. Does ovarian surgery for endometriomas impair the ovarian response to gonadotropin? Fertil Steril 2001;76:662-5.

52. Wyns C, Donnez J. Laser vaporization of ovarian endometriomas: the impact on the response to gonadotrophin stimulation. Gynecol Obstet Fertil 2003;31:337-42.

53. Canis M, Pouly JL, Tamburro S, Mage G, Wattiez A, Bruhat MA. Ovarian response during IVF-embryo transfer cycles after laparoscopic ovarian cystectomy for endometriotic cysts of >3 cm in diameter. Hum Reprod 2001;16:2583-6.

54. Marconi G, Vilela M, Quintana R, Sueldo C. Laparoscopic ovarian cystectomy of endometriomas does not affect the ovarian response to gonadotropin stimulation. Fertil Steril 2002;78:876-8.

55. Jones KD, Sutton C. Fertility after laparoscopic surgery for endometriomas. Hum Fertil (Camb) 2002;5:117–22.

56. Adamson DG, Pasta DJ. Surgical treatment of endometriosis-associated infertility: Meta-analysis compared with survival analysis. Am J Obstet Gynecol 1994;171:1488-505.

57. Beretta P, Franchi M, Ghezzi F, Busacca M, Zupi E, Bolis P. Randomized clinical trial of two laparoscopic treatments of endometriomas: cystectomy versus drainage and coagulation. Fertil Steril 1998;70:1176-80.

58. Fedele L, Bianchi S, Zanconato G, Berlanda N, Raffaelli R, Fontana E. Laparoscopic excision of recurrent endometriomas: long-term outcome and comparison with primary surgery. Fertil Steril 2006;85:694-9.

59. Sutton CJ, Ewen SP, Jacobs SA, Whitelaw NL. Laser laparoscopic surgery in the treatment of ovarian endometriomas. J Am Assoc Gynecol Laparosc 1997;4:319-23.

60. Hemmings R, Bissonnette F, Bouzayen R. Results of laparoscopic treatments of ovarian endometriomas: laparoscopic ovarian fenestration and coagulation. Fertil Steril 1998;70:527-9.

61. Yoshida S, Harada T, Iwabe T, Terakawa N. Laparoscopic surgery for the management of ovarian endometrioma. Gynecol Obstet Invest 2002;54(Suppl 1):24-7.

62. Kuivasaari P, Hippelainen M, Anttila M, Heinonen S. Effect of endometriosis on IVF/ICSI outcome: stage III/IV endometriosis worsens cumulative pregnancy and live-born rates. Hum Reprod 2005;20:3130-5.

63. Sallam HN, Garcia-Velasco JA, Dias S, Arici A. Long-term pituitary down-regulation before in vitro fertilization (IVF) for women with endometriosis. Cochrane Database Syst Rev. 2006; 1: CD004635.

64. Isaacs JD Jr, Hines RS, Sopelak VM, Cowan BD. Ovarian endometriomas do not adversely affect pregnancy success following treatment with in vitro fertilization. J Assist Reprod Genet 1997;14:551-3.

65. Yanushpolsky EH, Best CL, Jackson KV, Clarke RN, Barbieri RL, Hornstein MD. Effects of endometriomas on ooccyte quality, embryo quality, and pregnancy rates in in vitro fertilization cycles: a prospective, case-controlled study. J Assist Reprod Genet 1998;15:193-7.

66. Tinkanen H, Kujansuu E. *In vitro* fertilization in patients with ovarian endometriomas. Acta Obstet Gynecol Scand 2000;79: 119-22.

67. Pouly JL. Endométriome et fécondation *in vitro*. J Gynecol Obstet Biol Reprod 2003;32:4S37-4S41.

68. Somigliana E, Infantino M, Benedetti F, Arnoldi M, Calanna G, Ragni G. The presence of ovarian endometriomas is associated with a reduced responsiveness to gonadotropins. Fertil Steril 2006;86:192-6.

69. D'Hooghe TM, Denys B, Spiessens C, Meuleman C, Debrock S. Is the endometriosis recurrence rate increased after ovarian hyperstimulation? Fertil Steril 2006;86:283-2.

70. Loh FH, Tan Tan A, Kumar J, Ng SC. Ovarian response after laparoscopic ovarian cystectomy for endometriotic cysts in 132 monitored cycles. Fertil Steril 1999;72:316-21.

71. Donnez J, Wyns C, Nisolle M. Does ovarian surgery for endometriomas impair the ovarian response to gonadotropin? Fertil Steril 2001;76:662-5.

72. Esinler I, Bozdag G, Aybar F, Bayar U, Yarali H. Outcome of *in vitro* fertilization/intracytoplasmic sperm injection after laparoscopic cystectomy for endometriomas. Fertil Steril 2006; 85:1730-5.

73. Suganuma N, Wakahara Y, Ishida D, Asano M, Kitagawa T, Katsumata Y, Moriwaki T, Furuhashi M. Pretreatment for ovarian endometrial cyst before *in vitro* fertilization. Gynecol Obstet Invest 2002;54 (Suppl 1):36-40.

74. Dlugi AM, Loy RA, Dieterle S, Bayer SR, Seibel MM. The effect of endometriomas on *in vitro* fertilization outcome. J *In Vitro* Fert Embryo Transf 1989;6:338-41.

75. Garcia-Velasco JA, Mahutte NG, Corona J, Zuniga V, Giles J, Arici A, Pellicer A. Removal of endometriomas before *in vitro* fertilization does not improve fertility outcomes: A matched, case-control study. Fertil Steril 2004;81:1194-7.

76. Chen MJ, Yang JH, Yang YS, Ho HN. Increased occurrence of tubo-ovarian abcess in women with stage III and IV endometriosis. Fertil Steril 2004;82:498-9.

Management of Mild to Moderate Endometriosis in the Infertile Patient

Surveen Ghumman

OVERVIEW

Endometriosis is an important cause of infertility. It may lead to dysmenorrhea and dysparunia. Diagnosis is usually surgical. Treatment can be expectant where the disease is mild. Medical treatment is given if pain is the only symptom. Surgical treatment is preferred in patients who are infertile. This is usually followed by controlled ovarian stimulation (COH) and intrauterine insemination (IUI). Endometriomas more than 3 cm are removed laparoscopically. Cystectomy is preferred to ablation. However, ovarian surgery may cause adhesions or a decrease in ovarian reserve. Management of infertility after surgery depends on the age of the patient, duration of infertility and stage of endometriosis. Younger patients may be taken-up for 4 cycles of COH-IUI. Older patients, those with long-standing infertility or with severe endometriosis, where there is adnexal involvement, should be taken-up for *in vitro* fertilization (IVF) directly. Prior suppression for three months has shown increased success rates. Endometriosis affects the results of IVF as the oocyte and embryo quality is affected. However, ovarian stimulation does not affect endometriosis.

INTRODUCTION

Endometriosis has remained an enigma with its etiology still not clearly defined. It affects 10 to 15 percent of women during the reproductive years. The ovary is a common site leading to the formation of endometriotic cysts. The classic triad of dysmenorrhea, dyspareunia and infertility is characteristic of the disease. Endometriosis can be classified as mild, moderate or severe according to the American Fertility Society classification. Treatment of endometriosis causes a dilemma in an infertile patient because of variability in the presenting symptoms, lack of good randomized controlled trials, unpredictability of the outcome of surgery, numerous treatment options available for decision-making and other associated factors. The first step towards managing a patient is assessing the extent of the disease.

Assessment of the Disease

Since endometriosis is usually a surgical diagnosis made during laparoscopy, it is accompanied by a concomitant surgery. Hence, an accurate evaluation of the disease during the endoscopy along with maintenance of objective records is a must. There should be a detailed description of the pelvis, record of the outcome after the surgery and an assessment by the surgeon as to the chances of achieving a pregnancy. Evaluation should include details such as the energy source used, type of approach (laparoscopy or laparotomy) and the type of techniques used, such as ablation, resection, cystectomy, etc.

Prognostic Factors

A number of factors affect the probability that the patient will conceive. An endometriosis fertility index has been devised to predict postsurgical prognosis in an infertile patient and includes age, duration of infertility, number of prior operations and other associated causes of infertility like anovulation and oligozoospermia.[1] Younger patients with a short duration of infertility are more likely to conceive with treatment.[2] Patients with associated infertility factors have a poor prognosis and should be counseled for assisted reproductive techniques (ART) initially. Patients with pain may want immediate relief without the consideration of fertility and may be unable to tolerate prolonged fertility treatment. All the above factors should be considered keeping in mind the need of the patient.

CLINICAL DISCUSSION

Expectant Management

The monthly fecundity was found to be 2 to 10 percent in untreated patients in comparison to the 15 to 20 percent fecundity of normal young couples.[3] The expectant line of treatment evolved when it was realized that in mild to moderate endometriosis, hormonal therapy did not give better results than expectant management in infertility patients.[4] Usually, endometriosis is diagnosed on laparoscopy and operative intervention must be done while performing the diagnostic laparoscopy. Laparoscopic laser ablation of minor disease of endometriosis appears to lessen the interval to conception although the cumulative pregnancy rate remains nearly the same as that of women managed conservatively. In advanced disease, surgical therapy is more successful in comparison to expectant or medical treatment as it removes mechanical factors causing infertility. The potential benefit of cytoreductive therapy must be weighed against the risk of adhesion formation through surgical devitalization of peritoneal surfaces.

Surgical Treatment of Early Stage Endometriosis

Surgery should be undertaken with the objective of removing the maximum amount of disease tissue and restoring pelvic anatomy and function. In a meta-analysis, surgical treatment of early stage disease showed a pregnancy rate of 58 percent compared to 45 percent in expectant management.[5,6] Similar results were seen with another randomized controlled study, where pregnancy rates were 29 percent compared to 19 percent when expectant treatment was used.[7] Whether this benefit was because of removal of adhesions or removal of disease is debatable. In stage III/IV endometriosis with invasive adhesive endometriotic disease, surgery has shown beneficial results.[5]

Surgical Approach—Laparoscopy vs Laparotomy

In patients where endometriosis was the only cause of infertility, the results of laparoscopy and laparotomy were similar in mild/minimal disease but were better with laparoscopy in moderate to severe disease. Laparoscopy was superior because there was less reformation of adhesions and the magnified view provided by the laparoscope was an advantage while dissecting the diseased tissue.[8] Laparoscopy may provide better visualization of the cul-de-sac. Hence, the laparoscopic approach is preferred while treating a patient with endometriosis-related infertility as results are equivalent if not better.

Conservative Surgery

Conservative surgery, like ablation of endometriotic implants, adhesiolysis or ovarian cystectomy is indicated in all cases of infertility. Conservative procedures are carried out to remove all implants, resect adhesions, relieve pain, restore normal anatomy of involved organs and reduce the risk of disease recurrence and postoperative adhesion formation. Restoration of the normal tubo-ovarian relationship is necessary to enhance fertility. The basic techniques available are excision, coagulation and vaporization. The extent of tissue penetration is related to the power and type of current, duration of application and size of electrode. These surgeries are cytoreductive and recurrence may actually be progression of microscopic residual disease and not a true recurrence.

Peritoneal Implants

Implants should be destroyed in the most effective and least traumatic manner so as to minimize postoperative adhesion formation. Small lesions less than 5 mm in diameter on the peritoneum are treated with laser or bipolar coagulation or are excised. Deep lesions or lesions more than 5 mm in diameter must be excised with a tissue margin of 2 to 4 mm as microscopic lesions are commonly found close to the visible implant. Ablation leads to greater tissue destruction and subsequent adhesion formation. Additionally, there may be inadequate tissue resection. Ablation may further create difficulty due to the proximity of vital structures like ureters, bladder or vessels. The deep lesions need to be assessed by rectovaginal palpation preoperatively and laparoscopic blunt probe palpation. Excision is preferable to ablation in an infertile patient as it leaves less chance of deep residual disease, there is lesser tissue destruction and a lower chance of subsequent adhesion formation. All peritoneal defects should be ablated as they often have microscopic disease.

Outcome

Pregnancy rates, 2 years after follow-up, were 60 percent for minimal to mild endometriosis, 50 percent for moderate disease and 40 percent for extensive disease. Pregnancy rates decrease to half after 15 months.[9] Crude pregnancy rates were 38 percent higher with surgical treatment as compared to medical treatment, where there was delay in initiating treatment for infertility.[5] Medical treatment before or after surgery does not improve success rate.

Ovarian Suppression

Ovarian suppression can be achieved with drugs such as oral contraceptives, progesterone, Danazol and gonadotropin releasing hormone (GnRH) agonists or antagonists. There was no difference in pregnancy rate in patients who took no treatment and those who took medical treatment with ovarian suppression.[5] Ovarian suppression delays fertility, has side effects and is an additional cost without improved results. There appears to be no role of primary ovarian suppression in the treatment of minimal to mild endometriosis-associated infertility.[10]

Preoperative ovarian suppression: Presurgical ovulation suppression has been suggested to improve technical results by reducing adhesions and decreasing blood flow and inflammation, but data is still inconclusive.

Postoperative ovarian suppression: Medical therapy following surgery does not improve results.[11]

Management of Endometriotic Cysts Associated with Infertility

The ovary is one of the more frequent sites of pelvic endometriotic lesions. Management of ovarian endometriosis, though a frequent problem, still has many gray areas with unresolved debates. Its pathophysiology, correlation with symptoms, staging and the optimal treatment remain controversial. Ovarian endometriomas are identified in around 20 percent of patients with endometriosis, associated with subfertility or pelvic pain.

Controversies exist regarding the correlation of AFS classification with fertility outcomes. An ovarian endometrioma of 3 centimeters in size leads to an AFS score of stage III, or moderate endometriosis. A spontaneous conception rate of 22 percent is associated with this stage. After surgical treatment of ovarian endometriomas, the reported conception rates are in the range of 50 percent. These findings suggest that an ovarian endometrioma might impair fertility. However, this effect has not been backed by any randomized controlled trial.

Treatment

Medical treatment is not recommended for endometriomas as it is not effective.[12] Removal of lesions is usually done for endometriomas of at least 3 centimeter in size, especially when pain is an associated factor. In case of infertility, the main objective of the treatment is to improve the fecundity. Removal of the cyst also provides a histological proof of the nature of the whole cyst. There are many treatment options (Flow chart 32.1).

Expectant

Endometriomas less than 3 cm in size do not have a significant effect on fertility. These young women can be treated expectantly with regular ultrasound monitoring of the cyst size.

Hormonal Suppression

As medical treatment has little impact on ovarian endometriomas larger than 3 centimeters in size, it should not be recommended in such situations. A 50 percent decrease in size

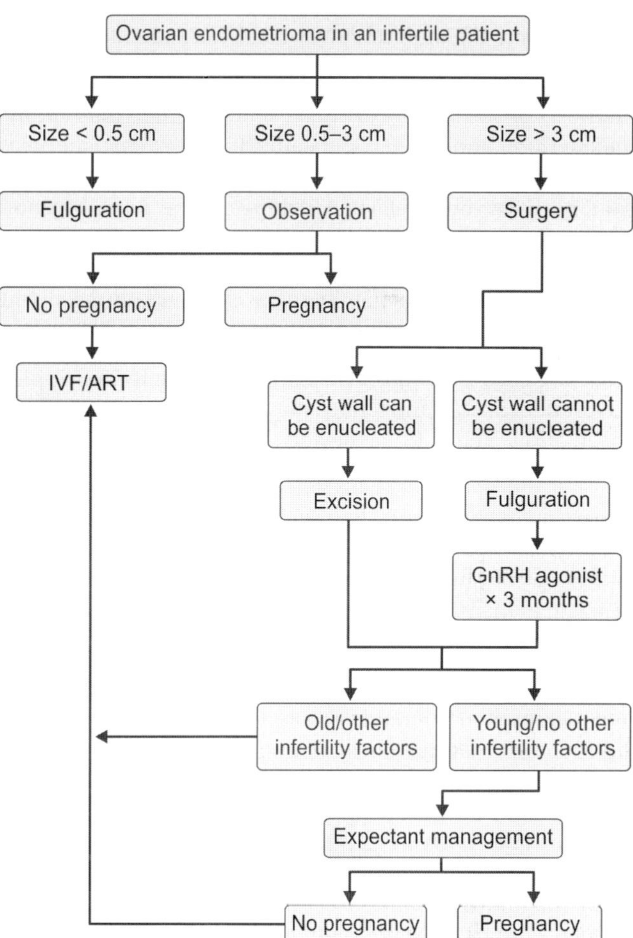

Flow chart 32.1: Treatment of ovarian endometrioma in infertility

of the cyst has been observed after medical treatment but with a high recurrence rate at 6 to 12 months. Medical treatment prior to and after surgery showed no benefit.

Ultrasound-guided Cyst Aspiration

Transvaginal ultrasonographic aspiration of an ovarian endometrioma is usually a simple procedure, performed without general anesthesia. There are risks of adhesions in case of spillage of the cyst contents and ovarian abscess formation. It is associated with recurrence, which can be reduced by injecting the empty cyst with various sclerosing or cytotoxic agents, such as methotrexate, ethanol or tetracycline.[13] Beneficial effects of ultrasonographic aspiration prior to performing IVF are inadequately established to presently recommend such a procedure.

Surgical Treatment

Surgery is the treatment of choice for a large endometrioma. The laparoscopic approach is preferred. Two main techniques are used: cystectomy or aspiration and ablation. It is important to avoid excessive destruction of ovarian tissue in the infertile patient, justifying undertreatment of these patients.

Superficial small ovarian endometriomas: Superficial endometriosis of the ovary usually presents as small dark, punctuate lesions immediately beneath the cortical surface. Tiny surface lesions can be vaporized or coagulated by bipolar cautery. Layer by layer vaporization can be done by short bursts of laser. Occasionally, the visible lesion may be a tip of a larger deeper lesion. If a deeper lesion is suspected with a superficial endometrioma, the implant should always be excised and the ovary explored.

Moderate endometriomas: There may be difficulty in stripping the pseudocapsule and it may often have to be excised. Laser coagulation helps in achieving hemostasis. The ovarian wound is left open.

Large endometriomas: Large endometriomas may be adherent to the adjoining tissues. They are difficult to remove endoscopically because of extensive adhesions and care must be taken in identifying the ureters.

Three major postoperative problems need to be tackled.
1. *Postoperative adhesions*: Postoperative adhesions are frequently encountered after surgery.
2. *Recurrence*: Recurrence after surgery may occur in upto 30 percent depending on the surgical procedure, the definition and the length of follow-up. The cumulative recurrence rate was 11.7 percent with a reoperation rate of 8.2 percent after 48 months in a recent study.[14] Cystectomy seems to lead to fewer recurrences, as demonstrated by randomized controlled studies.
3. *Impact of surgery on ovarian function and ovarian reserve*: Raised FSH levels have been found in patients after surgery as there may be removal of healthy tissue leading to a decreased ovarian reserve. On histopathological analysis 54 percent of patients had ovarian tissue on the cyst wall.[15] However, none of the tissues had follicles. Most endometriotic cysts are not true cysts. They are formed by invagination of the ovarian cortex. Oocytes may be lost by the removal of the ovarian cortex that forms the pseudocyst. CO_2 laser vaporizes the cyst wall layer by layer with superficial depth and prevents excessive destruction of the cortex. With cautery, damage may be more widespread as there is scattering. Scissor excision may have a role as it gives a tissue feel. However, it can be argued that since the ovarian cortex invaginates, it is unavailable for external ovulation and removal causes no harm. Ovarian response was reduced during IVF-ET cycles in patients with history of severe endometriosis and laparoscopic excision of endometriomas compared to women with mild or minimal endometriosis without ovarian surgery.[16]

Cystectomy vs Ablation

A recent randomized control trial showed lower reoperative rates (6% vs 23%) and higher pregnancy rates (59% vs 23%) with laparoscopic ovarian cystectomy in comparison with fenestration and coagulation.[17] Cystectomy was found to be superior in terms of risk of recurrent symptoms, cyst reoperations and pregnancy rates. It was strongly recommended especially in infertile patients. A similar conclusion was drawn by a recent Cochrane review.[18] Another randomized controlled trial showed a pregnancy rate of 18.8 percent vs 6.2 percent for cystectomy in comparison to ablation, respectively in a 24-month follow-up.[19] With a 42-month follow-up, a recurrence rate of 26.3 percent vs 57.8 percent was seen with cystectomy and ablation, respectively.[20] The number and size of the endometriomas did not affect the pregnancy rate.[21] Intracystic vaporization offers a better chance of preserving the oocyte stock. The difference in the two techniques in terms of ovarian function is a 10 percent higher oocyte retrieval rate after stimulation for IVF, with cyst vaporization.[22] Cystectomy is preferred if feasible and intracystic vaporization or coagulation is done if cystectomy is not possible.

In Vitro Fertilization (IVF)

About 50 percent of patients do not conceive after surgery and need IVF. An ovarian endometrioma does not affect results of IVF and its presence is not a contraindication to perform an IVF. Aspiration of an ovarian endometrioma, incidentally identified during ovarian hyperstimulation or ovum pick-up for IVF, is not required and may lead to infection and abscess formation. If found accidentally during IVF cycle stimulation, it should be ignored and the cycle continued. It is not necessary to operate on endometriomas before IVF. Unexpected puncture of an ovarian endometrioma during ovum pick-up has no impact on the results of IVF, but bears a risk of infection. Presence of chocolate fluid (hemosiderin) in follicular puncture does not impair the quality of oocytes.[23,24] Patients with prior ovarian surgery may require a higher dose of gonadotropins because of an effect on the ovarian reserve but no difference has been observed in the pregnancy rates. Endometriomas do not cause any complications in pregnancies resulting from IVF.

Rectovaginal Endometriosis in an Infertile Patient

The prognosis for an infertile patient with rectovaginal nodules depends on tubal adhesions. If tubal adhesions are absent there is a high chance of spontaneous pregnancy. If adhesions are present, IVF should be the primary treatment. Conservative surgery for rectovaginal endometriosis in infertile women does not modify the reproductive prognosis although it does increase the pain-free time.[25]

If there is recurrence with severe pain, either repeat surgery or IVF should be considered. However, it should be kept in mind that surgery may not enhance fertility, and IVF should be attempted prior to radical surgery. Radical surgery is the last option in an infertile patient and care should be taken to preserve the ovarian tissue.

Frozen Pelvis with Extensive Endometriosis

Since there are extensive adhesions, surgery has a poor prognosis for fertility and IVF is the treatment of choice.

Recurrence—Repeat Surgery vs IVF

About 50 to 70 percent patients are infertile after surgery and have to make a choice between ART and repeat surgery. There are no randomized controlled trials. A retrospective analysis showed cumulative pregnancy rates of 5.9 percent, 18.1 percent and 24.4 percent 3, 7 and 9 months, respectively. The cumulative pregnancy rate was 33 percent and 70 percent for the first and second cycle of ART, respectively. Hence, ART would be the recommended as the second line of treatment following recurrence.[26] For stage III and IV endometriosis, IVF is considered a better option.[27] Postsurgical prognosis may not be the same in all situations. The AFS staging has no relation to fertility prognosis in the absence of adnexal adhesions irrespective of the presence of endometriomas. The presence of adnexal adhesions, mainly tubal, would decrease the fertility rate from 52 percent to 15 percent.[28] Other factors should also be taken into consideration such as age (more than 38 years), duration of infertility and male factor. When the duration of infertility is more than 8 years, a decrease in pregnancy rate of 15 percent is reported. Male factor (oligoasthenozoospermia) may decrease the pregnancy rate to 18 percent. Hence, it is justified that patients in whom adnexal adhesions are present and a poor postsurgical prognosis is expected, be directly referred for ART. Intrauterine insemination (IUI) and controlled ovarian stimulation (COS) should be the second line of therapy after laparoscopic treatment failure unless there is an absolute indication for IVF like older women, male factor infertility, long standing infertility or tubal adhesions. IVF results are superior to COS and IUI.[29]

ART in Endometriosis

Assisted reproductive techniques (ART) form an important treatment option for patients with endometriosis-related infertility and 50 percent of patients may require it. COS and IUI should be tried before IVF. It is self-evident that IVF will be of value in advanced disease due to its low background pregnancy rate and the known success rate with IVF. The value of IVF in early stage disease is unproven.

Choice of ART procedure: There is a wide range of procedures that can be attempted like IUI IVF, gamete intrafallopian insemination (GIFT) and intracytoplasmic sperm injection (ICSI). In case of tubal blocks or adhesions, IVF is recommended. ICSI is performed in cases of male factor infertility and where women experience repeated fertilization failure. Altered secretion of inhibin in the late follicular phase in patients with endometriosis causes an impaired secretion of gonadotropins leading to poor quality oocytes. This occurs because of the effect of cytokines on granulosa cells. Sperm immobilization is observed, with peritoneal fluid from these patients causing impaired fertilization. IVF avoids these effects. It removes the critical step of fertilization and early embryo development from an *in vivo* environment that is perceived to be hostile.

Treatment strategies are based on specific situations. Younger patients with minimal endometriosis can be managed expectantly. In patients more than 35 years of age with minimal endometriosis, COS and IUI or IVF is the treatment of choice. IVF at an earlier stage is the preferred option in patients with severe endometriosis, tubal disease, male factor or a combination of etiologies (Flow chart 32.2).

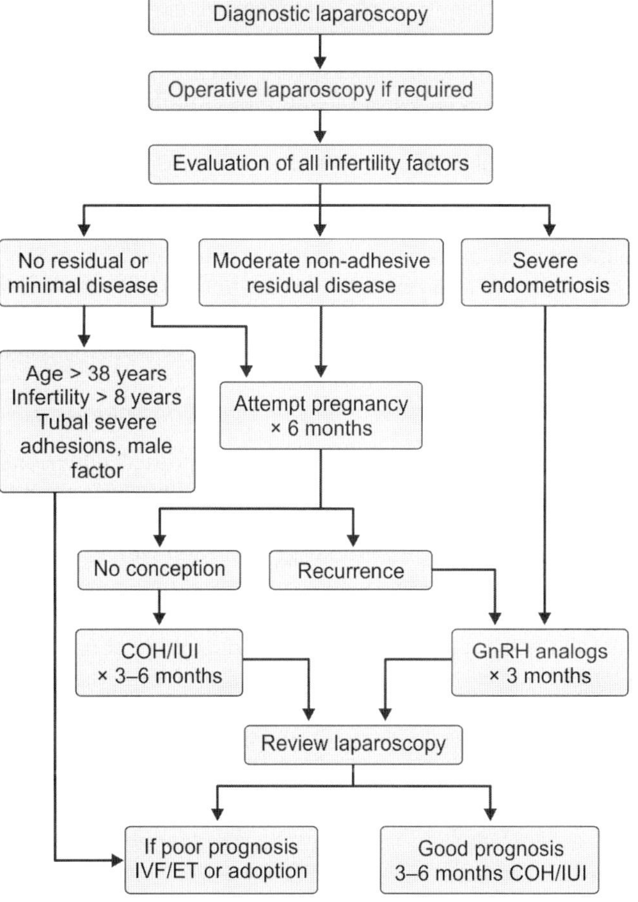

Flow chart 32.2: Postsurgical management of an infertility patient

Controlled Ovarian Stimulation

Contolled ovarian stimulation (COS) and IUI increased the fecundity rate from 2 to 4 percent to 5 to 18 percent in unexplained infertility. Pregnancy rates in unexplained infertility are thought to be similar to those seen in minimal to mild endometriosis after initial laparoscopy.[30]

Controlled ovarian stimulation increases pregnancy rates in minimal and mild endometriosis. Gonadotropins have a higher success rate than Clomiphene citrate. With severe endometriosis, because of anatomical distortion, the results are not good. Usually, 3 to 4 cycles can be tried and in selected cases, up to 3 to 6 cycles with gonadotropins can be tried along with IUI. Single insemination per cycle is adequate.[31]

Impact of Endometriosis on IVF

Deleterious effects on IVF outcome have been reported in patients with endometriosis. Increased human menopausal gonadotropin (hMG) dose and decreased number of oocytes in these patients support the theory of reduced ovarian reserve. However, this has not been supported by all studies.[32]

There is a reduced oocyte yield in such patients, not only because of impaired folliculogenesis but because of difficulties in oocyte retrieval. There may be difficulty in monitoring these patients. Fertilization and implantation rates are impaired. Poor oocyte and embryo quality have been reported, which can affect early embryonic development. There is a lower cleavage rate and fewer embryos reach the 4-cell and blastomere stages hampering the ART process. The incidence of aberrant nuclear and cytoplasmic morphology is higher in these embryos.[33] Poor pregnancy rates were observed when oocytes were donated from endometriosis patients.[34] No difference in results was found in patients with mild endometriosis due to the disease but patients with severe disease had lower pregnancy rates.[35] Some studies do not support this difference.[36] Hence, the evidence is inconclusive.

Precautions During IVF in Patients of Endometriosis

In patients with small endometriomas or peritubal adhesions, a baseline transvaginal sonography should be performed to evaluate the periovarian pouches, and the site and size of endometriomas in order to avoid confusion with follicles at a later stage. In patients with symptoms of pain, ovum pick-up should not be done under local anesthesia. Puncturing of endometriomas should be avoided as there is danger of abscess formation. If it is unavoidable, an informed consent, explaining the risk to the patient, should be taken.

The cost-effectiveness of IVF and its optimal use in endometriosis needs to be evaluated, although, it is definitely a satisfactory option.

Ovarian Stimulation and IUI vs IVF

The crude delivery rate was 15 percent per cycle with a cumulative pregnancy rate of 41 percent after 3 cycles of COS and IUI. This is attributed to adhesions in severe endometriosis. A 12 percent multiple pregnancy rate was seen. With IVF, the success rate was 26 percent in the first cycle and increased to 58 percent after 3 cycles. The multiple pregnancy rate was 23 percent.[37] The financial and psychological strain is significantly more with IVF. COS and IUI should be the second line of treatment after surgery in the absence of specific indications for IVF. Attempts of IUI should be limited to 3 to 6 cycles as success rates decrease thereafter.

Ovarian Suppression Prior to IVF

Some support the use of ovarian suppression for long periods of 6 months in severe endometriosis before IVF.[38] Medical treatment with GnRH analogs for 3 to 6 months, known as the 'ultra-long agonist protocol', followed by controlled COS with hMG and IVF towards the end of the treatment has been tried. In a randomized trial, the ultra-long protocol showed a pregnancy rate of 63 percent versus 21 percent for the standard protocol.[39] This conclusion has not been supported by other studies.[40] It is expensive, has side effects and in older women, precious time is lost.

Surgical Treatment Prior to IVF

Surgical treatment would be justified in these cases with the view that endometriosis causes adverse effects on embryo and oocyte quality. However, it has not shown an effect on pregnancy rates. Surgery on the ovary may result in a decreased ovarian reserve, which may lead to an unpredictable response to gonadotropins.[41] Treatment of clinically or ultrasono-graphically evident endometriosis before ART is not required. Although there are no substantial evidence-based studies, it has been seen that it does not change the prognosis even in cases where IVF is being done for other reasons like male infertility or tubal factors.[42]

Impact of ART on Endometriosis

High estrogen levels do not exacerbate the disease as would be expected.

CONCLUSION

Endometriosis remains a difficult clinical problem. The treatment of endometriosis focuses upon amelioration of two symptoms: pain and infertility. The treatment of endometriosis-associated pain can be well-treated medically and all medical treatments are equally effective. In the treatment of endometriosis-associated infertility, surgical treatment improves fertility, probably for all stages of the disease. Assisted reproduction is an effective treatment option for these patients.

REFERENCES

1. Adamson GD, Pasta DJ. Pregnancy rates can be predicted by validated endometriosis fertility index (EFI). Fertil Steril 2002;77:S48.
2. Practice Committee of American Society for Reproductive Medicine. Aging and infertility in women. Fertil Steril 2004;82: S102-6.
3. Hughes EG, Federkow DM, Collins JA. A quantitative overview of controlled trials in endometriosis –associated infertility. Fertil Steril 1993;59:963-70.
4. Hull ME, Moghissi KS, Magyar DF, Hayes MF. Comparison of different treatment modalities of endometriosis in infertile women. Fertil Steril 1987;47:40.
5. Adamson GD, Pasta DJ. Surgical Treatment of endometriosis associated infertility. A meta analysis compared with survival analysis. Am J Obstet Gynecol 1994;171:1488-1505.
6. Olive DJ, Schwartz LB. Endometriosis. N Eng J Med 1993;328: 1759-69.
7. Marcoux S, Maheux R, Besule S. Laparoscopic surgery in infertile women with minimal or mild endometriosis. N Engl J Med 1997;337:217-22.
8. Diamond MP, Danielle JF, Festa J, Surrey MW, McLaughlin DS, Friedman S, Vaughn WK, Martin DC. Adhesion reformation and denovo adhesion formation following reparative pelvic surgery. Fertil Steril 1987;47:864-6.
9. Adamson GD, Hurd SJ, Pasta DJ. Laparoscopic endometriosis treatment: Is it better ? Fertil Steril 1993;59:35-44.
10. Olive DL, Lindheim SR, Pritts EA. Endometriosis and Infertility: What we do for each stage? Curr Womens Health Rep 2003;3: 389-94.
11. Yap C, Furness S, Farquhar C. Pre- and Postoperative medical therapy for endometriosis surgery. Cochrane Database Rev 2004;(3):CD 003678.
12. Chapron C, Vercellini P, Barakal H, Vieira M, Dubuisson JB. Management of ovarian endometriomas. Hum Reprod Update. 2002;8:591–7.
13. Fisch JD, Sher G. Scelerotherapy with 5 percent Tetracycline is a simple alternative to potentially complex surgical treatment of ovarian endometriosis before *in vitro* fertilization. Fertil Steril 2004;82:437-41.
14. Bucassa M, Marana M, Caruana P, Candiani M, Muzii L, Calia C, Bianchi S. Recurrence of endometrioma after laparoscopic excision. Am J Obstet Gynecol 1999;180:519-23.
15. Muzii L, Biandu A, Croce C, Manci N, Panici PB. Laparoscopic examination of ovarian cyst: Is stripping technique a tissue sparing procedure? Fertil Steril 2002;77:609-14.
16. Yazbeck C, Madelenat P, Sifer C, Hazout A, Poncelet C. Ovarian endometriomas: Effect of laparoscopic cystectomy on ovarian response in IVF-ET cycles. Gynecol Obstet Fertil 2006;34(9):808-12.
17. Alborzi S, Zarei A, Alborzi S, Alborzi M. Management of ovarian endometrioma. Clin Obstet Gynecol 2006;49:480-91.
18. Hart RJ, Hickey M, Maouris P, Buckett W, Garry R. Excisional surgery versus ablative surgery for ovarian endometriomata. Cochrane Database Syst Rev 2005;(3):CD004992.
19. Berreta P, Franchi M, Ghezzi F, Busacca M, Zupi E, Bolis P. Randomized controlled trials of two laparoscopic treatment of endometrioma Cystectomy vs drainage and coagulation. Fertil Steril 1998;70: 1176-80.
20. Sutton CSG, Ewen SP, Jacob SA, et al. Laser laparoscopic surgery in treatment of ovarian endometriomas. J Am Assoc Gynecol Laparoscopy 1997;4:319-23.
21. Adamson GD, Subak LL, Pasta DJ. Comparison of CO_2 laser laparoscopy with laparotomy for treatment of endometrioma. Fertil Steril 1992;57:965-73.
22. Cannes M, Pouly JL, Tamburro S, et al. Ovarian response during IVF embryo transfer cycles after laparoscopic ovarian cystectomy for endometriotic cysts of more than 3 cm in diameter. Hum Reprod 2001;16:2583-6.
23. Khamsi F, Yavas Y, Lacanna IC, Roberge S, Endman M, Wong JC. Exposure of human oocytes to endometrioma fluid does not alter fertilization or an early embryonic development. J Assist Reprod Genet 2001;18:106-9.
24. Survey ES, School craft WB. Does surgical management of endometriosis within 6 months of an IVF ET cycle improves outcome? J Assist Reprod 2003;20:365-70.
25. Vercellini P, Pietropaolo G, De Giorgi O, Daguati R, Pasin R, Crosignani PG. Reproductive performance in infertile women with rectovaginal endometriosis: Is surgery worthwhile? Am J Obstet Gynecol 2006;195:1303-10.
26. Pagidas K, Falcone T, Hemmings R, Miron P. Comparison for reoperations for moderate (Stage III) and severe (Stage IV) endometriosis related infertility with *in vitro* fertilization and embryo transfer. Fertil Steril 1996;65:791-5.
27. The Practice Committee of American Society of Reproductive Medicine. Endometriosis and infertility. Fertil Steril 2004;81: 1441-6.
28. Pouly JL, Kamble M, Canis M, Janny L, Botroschiriti R, Piekrischvili R, Schubert B. Endometriosis and assisted reproduction. In: Sutton C, Jones K, Adamson GD (Eds). Modern Management of endometriosis. Taylor and Francis Group Oxon UK 2006;307-16.
29. Dmowski WP, Pri M, Ding J, Rana N. Cycle specific and cumulative fecundity in patients with endometriosis who are undergoing controlled ovarian stimulation with intrauterine insemination or *in vitro* fertilization with embryo transfer. Fertil Steril 2002;78:750-6.
30. Werbrouck E, Spiessens C, Meuleman C, D'Hooghe T. No difference in cycle pregnancy rate and in cumulative live-birth rate between women with surgically treated minimal to mild endometriosis and women with unexplained infertility after controlled ovarian hyperstimulation and intrauterine insemination. Fertil Steril 2006;86:566-71.
31. Glizick DS. For now one well timed IUI is the way to go. Fertil Steril 2004;82:17-24.
32. Marhutte NG, Arici A. New advances in understanding and regulating infertility. J Reprod Immunol 2002;55:73-83.

33. Pellicon A, Oliviera N, Ruiz A, Remohí J, Simón C. Exploring the mechanism of endometriosis related infertility: An analysis of embryo development and implantation in assisted reproduction. Hum Reprod 1995;10:91-7.

34. Diaz I, Navarro J, Blasco L, Simón C, Pellicer A, Remohí J. Impact of stage III-IV endometriosis on recipients of sibling oocytes: Matched case-control study. Fertil Steril 2000; 74:31-4.

35. Dokras SA, Olive DL. Endometriosis and assisted reproductive technologies. Clin Obstet Gynecol 1999;42:687-8.

36. Sung L, Mukherjee T, Takeshige T, Bustillo M, Copperman AB. Endometriosis is not detrimental to embryo implantation in oocyte recipients. J Assist Reprod Genet 1997;14:152-6.

37. Prado Perez J, Navarro Martinez C, Lopez Rivadeneira E, et al. The impact of endometriosis on the rate of pregnancy of patients submitted to intrauterine insemination. Fertil Steril 2002;78: 750-6.

38. Zikopanulos K, Kolibianakis EM, Derroey P. Ovarian stimulation for IVF in patients with endometriosis. Acta Obstet Gynecol Scand 2004;83:651-5.

39. Nakamura K, Oosawa M, Kondou I, Inagaki S, Shibata H, Narita O, Suganuma N, Tomoda Y. Menotropin stimulation after prolonged gonadotropin-releasing hormone agonist pretreatment for *in vitro* fertilization in patients with endometriosis. Assist Reprod Genet 1992;9:113-7.

40. Chadid S, Camus M, Smitz J, Van Steirteghem AC, Devroey P. Comparison among different ovarian stimulation regimens for assisted procreation procedures in patients with endometriosis. Hum Reprod 1995;10:2406-11.

41. Donnez J, Wynes C, Nisolle M. Does ovarian surgery for endometriomas impair the ovarian response to gonadotropins? Fertil Steril 2001;76:662-5.

42. Garcia—Velasco JA, Mahutte NG, Corona J, et al. Removal of endometrioma before *in vitro* fertilization does not improve fertility outcomes: A matched case-control study. Obstet Gynecol Surv 2004;59:661-2.

Hydrosalpinx and ART:
Options and Rationale for Treatment

Daniel B Williams

OVERVIEW

A thorough evaluation of the Fallopian tubes plays an important role in the diagnosis and treatment of women with infertility. In women found to have severe distal tubal disease with hydrosalpinx, the literature clearly favors *in vitro* fertilization (IVF) over tuboplasty. It is well-recognized that the presence of hydrosalpinges will adversely affect IVF success rates. It is also evident that treatment of hydrosalpinges (salpingectomy or proximal tubal occlusion) prior to IVF will significantly increase chances for success. Therefore, patients with hydrosalpinges should be offered treatment prior to starting IVF. In patients who are not good candidates for surgery, hysteroscopic placement of a microinsert (Essure) to occlude the ostia may be a reasonable alternative.

INTRODUCTION

A thorough evaluation of the Fallopian tubes plays an important role in the diagnosis and treatment of women with infertility. The easiest aspect of tubal function to assess is tubal patency. In addition, the presence or absence of adhesions, as well as the prevalence of other factors that affect tubal function (e.g. endometriosis and pelvic inflammatory disease) are of important consideration in the infertility work-up.[1] A variety of factors can adversely affect the physiologic functions of the oviduct, such as fertilization and embryo transport. However, it is more difficult to accurately determine actual tubal function. Although reconstructive tubal surgery for women with tubal factor infertility has largely been replaced by *in vitro* fertilization (IVF), the presence of hydrosalpinx poses additional challenges for the treatment of infertility with assisted reproductive techniques (ART).

It is now well-recognized that the presence of distal tubal disease adversely affects fertility outcomes in patients undergoing IVF treatment.[2] While laparoscopy with tubal evaluation and patency assessment with chromotubation is considered by some to be the gold standard in tubal evaluation,[3] there are other methods to evaluate the Fallopian tubes that are less invasive. This chapter will provide an insight into the detection of hydrosalpinx, as well as the rationale and methods for treatment prior to IVF.

CLINICAL DISCUSSION

Non-surgical Evaluation of the Fallopian Tubes

Proper evaluation of the infertile couple would not be complete without assessment of tubal patency and morphology. Patent tubes are required for oocyte transport, fertilization, and embryo transport to the uterus. Although laparoscopy and chromotubation is the gold standard by which to evaluate the Fallopian tubes, laparoscopy is not typically utilized as a first-line diagnostic tool in patients with unexplained infertility. A variety of methods that do not require general anesthesia and do not have the potential for surgical complications, inherent in performing laparoscopy, are available for tubal evaluation and ultimately, for diagnosis of hydrosalpinges. These include hysterosalpingography (HSG), selective salpingography (SSG), and hystero-contrast-sonography (HyCoSy). Therefore, in patients who do not require initial laparoscopy, less invasive testing can be used to aid in determining which patients would benefit from laparoscopy for further evaluation and treatment.

Hysterosalpingography (HSG)

Hysterosalpingography utilizes contrast dye and fluoroscopy for the evaluation of the uterine cavity and uterine tubes. Following injection of contrast dye into the uterine cervix, serial fluoroscopic images are taken with the assessment of the passage of dye through the cavity and out from the proximal aspect of each uterine tube. The procedure is best performed early in the follicular phase of the menstrual cycle to reduce the risk of interruption of an early pregnancy and to decrease the risk of infection.[3] In addition to tubal assessment, HSG also provides valuable information regarding the presence or absence of mechanical factors, which may distort the endometrial cavity (endometrial polyps, submucosal myomas and adhesions).

The ability of HSG to accurately evaluate tubal patency in women with unexplained infertility has been investigated by comparing HSG findings with those at time of laparoscopy and chromotubation. As a diagnostic tool, HSG has been determined to have a relatively low sensitivity (0.65) and high specificity (0.83) when evaluating tubal patency.[4] If proximal tubal occlusion is identified on HSG, there is a relatively high likelihood that the tube is actually patent at the time of laparoscopy. If, however, tubal patency is demonstrated on HSG, the false negative rate is low and there is a low likelihood that tubal occlusion is present.[3] In addition to proximal tubal occlusion, HSG can also demonstrate findings associated with distal tubal disease, such as loculated spill or hydrosalpinges. Findings suggestive of distal tubal disease would require further evaluation, usually in the form of laparoscopy, as will be discussed later.

Few studies have evaluated the prognostic value of HSG in predicting fecundability, which is the ability to conceive during one menstrual cycle. In a retrospective cohort study of 359 patients, evaluated for subfertility, the presence of unilateral tubal occlusion did not appear to significantly alter the pregnancy rates. However, the pregnancy rates were decreased in those in whom bilateral tubal occlusion was diagnosed on HSG.[5] At the present time, it is generally recommended that patients with evidence of proximal tubal occlusion on HSG have additional testing to exclude non-pathologic causes (tubal spasm, mucus plug).[1]

Selective Salpingography

An additional method by which tubal patency and morphology can be assessed is selective salpingography (SSG). This procedure is generally performed to evaluate abnormalities of the proximal Fallopian tube, detected on an HSG examination. SSG employs cannulation of the tubal ostia with injection of contrast dye directly into the Fallopian tube. This is generally performed under fluoroscopy, and is especially valuable in the evaluation of proximal tubal occlusion.[6] SSG can also be used therapeutically by using a thin wire to perform recanalization of the proximal tube in cases where the dye does not easily pass after initial tubal catheterization.

Hystero-contrast-sonography (HyCoSy)

Hystero-contrast-sonography (HyCoSy) is an additional modality, which is used to assess patency of the Fallopian tubes. Mechanistically similar to saline infusion sonography (SIS), HyCoSy utilizes transvaginal ultrasonography and injection of ultrasound contrast media (air filled albumin microspheres) through the uterine cervix for the evaluation of uterine architecture and tubal morphology.[6,7] Several studies have evaluated the accuracy of HyCoSy in determining Fallopian tube patency. In one small study of forty-four patients, HyCoSy was found to have a specificity of 0.85 and a sensitivity of 0.85 when compared to results obtained at the time of laparoscopy and chromotubation.[8] In this study, HyCoSy was thought to be better than saline infusion sonography in determining tubal patency. HyCoSy confers the benefit of not requiring radiation exposure as does HSG. Furthermore, HyCoSy is thought to potentially provide a better evaluation of the uterine cavity compared to HSG.[7] Limitations of the procedure include lack of adequate image documentation and limited availability of the procedure itself.

Transvaginal Ultrasound

While not useful for evaluating tubal patency by itself, transvaginal ultrasound (TVS) is generally performed during the evaluation of the infertile patient. When large hydrosalpinges are found, this would lead to discussion with the patient about surgical evaluation/treatment. In one large study (n = 414), TVS identified only 34 percent of hydrosalpinges later found on HSG, suggesting a lower sensitivity of TVS in the detection of hydrosalpinges.[9] However, a recent study did find that the sensitivity and specificity of TVS diagnosis of hydrosalpinx was 84.6 percent and 99.7 percent, respectively. The addition of Doppler flow did not provide any additional benefit.[10] Thus, TVS is a useful evaluation tool, particularly in patients who are planning to undergo IVF and do not require tubal evaluation.

CLINICAL DISCUSSION

Hydrosalpinx and Fertility

In the event that hydrosalpinx is demonstrated during evaluation of the Fallopian tubes, care must be taken to thoroughly evaluate the extent of disease as well as to properly plan for therapeutic intervention. Although it is generally well accepted that hydrosalpinges adversely affect IVF outcomes,[2,11] there has previously been some controversy regarding the specific role of salpingectomy for treating different forms of hydrosalpinx (thin vs thick-walled, small vs large, visible on transvaginal ultrasound, etc.) on embryo implantation rates and subsequent pregnancy rates.[12] The following sections will address the current data regarding the impact of hydrosalpinx as well as the recommended intervention.

Surgical Management of Hydrosalpinges

If hydrosalpinges are present, current recommendations are to perform bilateral salpingectomy in preparation for IVF. It is thought that hydrosalpingeal fluid is embryotoxic, and can contain reactive oxygen species and endotoxins, while causing an impairment in endometrial receptivity and possible 'washout' of embryos following embryo transfer.[13] A recent study demonstrated that a transcription factor, HOXA 10, which is up-regulated around the time of implantation is decreased in patients with hydrosalpinges but that, salpingectomy resulted in significantly increased levels of HOXA 10.[14] Similarly, leukemia inhibitory factor (LIF), a cytokine that is expressed during implantation, was found to be significantly lower in infertile women with hydrosalpinges compared with fertile controls. However, salpingectomy resulted in significant increases in LIF, again suggesting a role for this procedure in women with hydrosalpinges who are planning to undergo IVF.[15] A recent review of five randomized controlled trials, involving 646 women, reported an increase in the odds of ongoing pregnancy (Peto OR 2.14, 95% CI 1.23 to 3.73) and of clinical pregnancy (Peto OR 2.31, 95% CI 1.48 to 3.62) with laparoscopic salpingectomy for hydrosalpinges prior to IVF compared to no treatment before IVF. Laparoscopic occlusion of the Fallopian tube versus no intervention did not increase the odds of ongoing pregnancy significantly (Peto OR 7.24, 95% CI 0.87 to 59.57) but the odds of clinical pregnancy (Peto OR 4.66, 95%CI 2.47 to 10.01) had sufficient power to show a significant increase. The authors concluded that laparoscopic tubal occlusion is an alternative to laparoscopic salpingectomy in improving IVF pregnancy rates in women with hydrosalpinges. Further research is required to assess the value of aspiration of hydrosalpinges prior to or during IVF procedures and also the value of tubal restorative surgery as an alternative (or as a preliminary) to IVF.[11] However, in a recent study of 115 patients with hydrosalpinges, proximal tubal occlusion, performed by bipolar diathermy prior to IVF treatment, was found to significantly increase the ongoing pregnancy rates compared to those with no surgical intervention, and was comparable to those who underwent salpingectomy.[16] In this study, a similar effect was seen whether the patients had bilateral or unilateral hydrosalpinges.

There is some potential concern with regards to a compromise of ovarian blood supply following salpingectomy and subsequent ovarian response. A retrospective study of 168 patients with hydrosalpinges compared gonadotropin response in those who had pretreatment salpingectomy or proximal tubal occlusion to patients without presurgical treatment.[17] While patients who underwent salpingectomy had slightly higher basal follicle-stimulating hormone (FSH) levels post-operatively compared to the other two groups; this was still within the normal range (< 10 mIU/mL). Finally, although the egg yield was slightly lower in the salpingectomy group, pregnancy rates between the groups were not different.

Thus, it appears that patients who are found to have a hydrosalpinx would benefit from salpingectomy prior to IVF treatment. In patients who have moderate to severe adhesive disease, or if the surgeon prefers to be more conservative, proximal tubal ligation appears to give a similar benefit.

Alternative Management of Hydrosalpinges

An interesting dilemma exists for those patients found to have hydrosalpinges, but who have severe pelvic adhesions and/or a frozen pelvis, making surgical intervention more risky if not impossible. Certainly, laparoscopic proximal ligation can be performed in some patients where the distal aspects of the tubes are not accessible. However, in patients who have documented severe adhesions or a frozen pelvis, even simple proximal tubal ligation may not be feasible. The question of whether it is worthwhile to perform laparotomy in such patients has not been answered and is certainly not without a significant risk of intraoperative complications. However, two less invasive methods that have been recently reported may give physicians additional options for dealing with this challenging situation.

One of these is transvaginal aspiration of hydrosalpinx during an IVF cycle at the time of egg retrieval in conjunction with prophylactic antibiotics. Previous small, non-randomized studies have been inconclusive. Recently, a small randomized trial (n = 66) looked at patients who underwent aspiration of hydrosalpinges versus a control group.[18] While clinical pregnancy rates appeared to be higher in the treatment group (31% vs 18%), this did not meet statistical significance, probably due to low numbers. The use of a hysteroscopically placed microinsert (Essure®; Conceptus, Mountain View, CA) to occlude the ostia has been reported to be useful in patients with hydrosalpinx undergoing IVF treatment.[19,20] More recently, a prospective two-center series of 20 patients with either unilateral or bilateral hydrosalpinx underwent Essure placement prior to IVF with reported successful occlusion in 95 percent (19 out of 20 patients) and a live birth rate of 57 percent per embryo transfer.[21]

Laparoscopic Management of Tubal Pathology

Once the decision has been made to proceed with laparoscopy, consideration must be given to potential procedures that would be performed depending on intraoperative findings. For example, although it is important to discuss potential salpingectomy with a patient who has preoperative findings suggestive of severe hydrosalpinx, it is also important to discuss alternatives, and in some cases, more conservative surgical procedures.

Tubal patency should always be assessed in patients who are interested in current or future fertility by injection of indigo carmine or methylene blue dye through an intrauterine manipulator. If recent uterine cavity assessment has not been performed, diagnostic hysteroscopy should also be performed in conjunction with laparoscopy. Laparoscopy is generally considered to be a better modality by which to predict fertility success compared to HSG. In a study of 794 patients, who underwent both HSG and laparoscopy, determination of tubal patency by laparoscopy better predicted spontaneous pregnancy rates compared to HSG.[22]

Distal Tubal Disease

Laparoscopic findings in patients with distal tubal disease can include adhesions (filmy or dense), as well as complete distal occlusion with hydrosalpinx. Use of less invasive methods for tubal evaluation before surgery can help in surgical planning. The possibility of hydrosalpinges can be detected by either ultrasound or HSG. It is also important to discuss possible treatment options with the patient prior to surgery, including the potential for salpingectomy.

Once the laparoscope is placed, the surgeon must first determine whether or not the fimbria are normal. If there is significant fimbrial damage, it is much less likely that the patient will have success without the use of IVF. Adhesiolysis may be required to aid in making this determination. If adhesions are so dense, that they cannot be safely lysed via laparoscopy, there is no evidence to suggest that converting to a laparotomy to complete the procedure would significantly impact pregnancy outcome. The wisest course of action in this scenario would be to perform proximal tubal ligation (if previously discussed with patient) and move directly to IVF.

Surgical Repair of Distal Tubal Disease

Before IVF treatment became successful, the use of neosalpingostomy was widely used to restore fertility in patients with complete distal tubal occlusion. However, with the current success of IVF, with a low risk of ectopic gestation, in addition to data regarding IVF success rates in the presence of hydrosalpinges, it is difficult to advocate tubal surgery for severe distal tubal disease, particularly when the fimbria are absent. In a relatively large study in which the pregnancy outcome was evaluated in 172 patients undergoing neosalpingostomy, the overall live birth rate was 18.0 percent, the ectopic gestation rate was 16.5 percent and the spontaneous abortion rate was 6.5 percent.[23] Interestingly, the mucosal grade by salpingoscopy was not predictive of pregnancy outcome, although pregnancy rates were lower when thick adhesions were present. This study would suggest that while these results are far inferior when compared to IVF, select patients certainly have a chance to conceive. If a 'good-prognosis' patient (small hydrosalpinx, minimal or filmy adhesions, minimal or no mucosal scarring) cannot undergo IVF secondary to cost or religious issues, it may be reasonable to discuss the possibility of neosalpingostomy. However, patients should be extensively counseled on the risk of ectopic gestation and should be reliable for prompt follow-up if menses are missed. It is also important to counsel patients that there is a risk for recurrence of hydrosalpinx, although it is higher in poor prognosis patients.[24]

CONCLUSION

Evaluation of the Fallopian tubes is an important aspect of the infertility work-up. Use of non-invasive testing, particularly HSG, can aid in this evaluation and also help to determine patients who might benefit from laparoscopic evaluation. The pregnancy rates in women with hydrosalpinges undergoing IVF is approximately half the rate of those women without hydrosalpinges. Salpingectomy or proximal tubal occlusion significantly increases the pregnancy rates in those patients with hydrosalpinges. Patients who are poor candidates for laparoscopy may benefit from hysteroscopic occlusion. Therefore, patients who are found to have hydrosalpinges should be counseled on the benefit of salpingectomy versus proximal tubal ligation prior to IVF treatment.

REFERENCES

1. The Practice Committee of the American Society for Reproductive Medicine. Optimal evaluation of the infertile couple. Fertil Steril 2006;86 (Suppl 4):S264-7.
2. Camus E, Poncelet C, Goffinet F, Wainer B, Merlet F, Nisand I, Philippe HJ. Pregnancy rates after *in vitro* fertilization in cases of tubal infertility with and without hydrosalpinx: A meta-analysis of published comparative studies. Hum Reprod 1999;14:1243-9.
3. Speroff L, Fritz MA. Clinical gynecologic endocrinology and infertility (7th edn), Philadelphia: Lippincott Williams and Wilkins; 2005.
4. Evers JLH, Land JA, Mol BW. Evidence-based medicine for diagnostic questions. Semin Reprod Med 2003;21:9-15.
5. Mol BWJ, Swart P, Bossuyt PMM, van der Veen F. Is hysterosalpingography an important tool in predicting fertility outcome? Fertil Steril 1997;67:663-9.
6. Boudghene FP, Bazot M, Robert Y, Perrot N, Rocourt N, Antoine JM, Morris H, et al. Assessment of fallopian tube patency by HyCoSy: Comparison of a positive contrast agent with saline solution. Ultrasound Obstet Gynecol 2001;18:525-30.
7. Cheong YC, Li TC. Evidence-based management of tubal disease and infertility. Curr Obstet Gynaecol 2005;15:306-13.
8. Reis MM, Soares SR, Cancado ML, Camargos AF. Hysterosalpingo contrast sonography (HyCoSy) with SH U 454 (Echovist®) for the assessment of tubal patency. Hum Reprod 1998;13):3049-52.
9. Atri M, CN Tran, PM Bret, AE Aldis, GM Kintzen. Accuracy of endovaginal sonography for the detection of fallopian tube blockage. J Ultrasound Med 1994;13:429-34.

10. Guerriero S, Ajossa SA, Lai MP, Mais V, Paoletti AM, Mells GB. Transvaginal ultrasonography associated with colour Doppler energy in the diagnosis of hydrosalpinx. Hum Reprod 2000;15:1568-72.

11. Johnson N, van Voorst S, Sowter MC, Strandell A, Mol BWJ. Surgical treatment for tubal disease in women due to undergo *in vitro* fertilisation. Cochrane Database Syst Rev 2010 Jan 20;(1):CD002125.

12. Dechaud H. Hydrosalpinx and ART: Hydrosalpinges suitable for salpingectomy before IVF. Hum Reprod 2000;15:2464-5.

13. Strandell A, Lindhard A, Eckerlund I. Cost-effectiveness analysis of salpingectomy prior to IVF, based on a randomized controlled trial. Hum Reprod 2005;20:3284-92.

14. Daftary GS, Kayisli U, Seli E, Bukulmez O, Arici A, Taylor HS. Salpingectomy increases peri-implantation endometrial HOXA10 expression in women with hydrosalpinx. Fertil Stertil 2007;87:367-72.

15. Seli E, Kayisli UA, Cakmak H, Bukulmez O, Bildirici I, Buzeloglu-Kayisli, Arici A. Removal of hydrosalpinges increases endometrial leukaemia inhibitory factor (LIF) expression at the time of the implantation window. Hum Reprod 2005;20: 3012-17.

16. Kontoravdis A, Makrakis E, Pantos K, Botsis D, Deligeoroglou E, Creatsas G. Proximal tubal occlusion and salpingectomy result in similar improvement in *in vitro* fertilization outcome in patients with hydrosalpinx. Fertil Steril 2006;86:1642-9.

17. Gelbaya TA, Nardo LG, Fitzgerald CT, Horne G, Brison DR, Lieberman BA. Ovarian response to gonadotropins after laparoscopic salpingectomy or the division of fallopian tubes for hydrosalpinges. Fertil Steril 2006;85:1464-8.

18. Hammadieh N, CoomarasamyA, Ola B, Papaionno S, Afrian M, Sharif K. Ultrasound-guided hydrosalpinx aspiration during oocyte collection improves pregnancy outcome in IVF: A randomized controlled trial. Hum Reprod 2008;23:1113-7.

19. Rosenfield RB, Stones RE, Coates A, Matteri RK, Hesla JS. Proximal occlusion of hydrosalpinx by hysteroscopic placement of microinsert before *in vitro* fertilization-embryo transfer. Fertil Steril 2005;83:1547-50.

20. Kerin JF, Cattanach S. Successful pregnancy outcome with the use of *in vitro* fertilization after Essure hysteroscopic sterilization. Fertil Steril 2007;87:1212.e1-4.

21. Galen DI, Khan N, Richter KS. Essure multicenter off-label treatment for hydrosalpinx before *in vitro* fertilization. J Minim Invasive Gynecol 2011;18:338-42.

22. Mol BWJ, Collins JA, Burrows EA, van der Veen F, Bossuyt PMM. Comparison of hysterosalpingography and laparoscopy in predicting fertility outcomes. Hum Reprod 1999;14:1237-42.

23. Taylor RC, Berkowitz J, McComb PF. Role of laparoscopic salpingostomy in the treatment of hydrosalpinx. Fertil Steril 2001;75:594-600.

24. Bayrak A, Harp D, Saadat P, Mor E, Paulson RJ. Recurrence of hydrosalpinges after cuff neosalpingostomy in a poor prognosis population. J Assist Reprod Genet 2006;23:285-8.

In Women with Unexplained Infertility, should IVF be the First or Last Treatment Option?

Surveen Ghumman

OVERVIEW

Unexplained infertility is a diagnosis made when a couples fails to establish pregnancy despite there being no obvious cause. The diagnostic protocol should show a normal laboratory assessment of ovulation, evaluation of tubal patency and semen analysis. There is a wide variation in the incidence, which may be due to the differences in definition of unexplained infertility, interpretation of tests and the evaluation process. It is a diagnosis of exclusion. Controversies exist in the inclusion of postcoital test, antisperm antibodies and laparoscopy as essential for diagnosis. Expectant treatment is an option. The therapy consists of two basic management principles—increasing availability of gametes by ovulation induction and intrauterine insemination (IUI) and bringing gametes together by IUI and *in vitro* fertilization (IVF). Gonadotropins may be preferred in older patients or where Clomiphene has failed as it produces greater number of follicles. With IVF and intracytoplasmic sperm injection (ICSI), the ovulation and male factors are enhanced and the cervical and tubal factors are bypassed at the same time, taking care of subtle defects in fertilization. IVF and ICSI have the advantage of assessing fertilization. In many cases of infertility, there may be subtle defects in fertilization for which the treatment would be donor gametes, zona drilling or ICSI. IVF must be performed as a first choice in patients with advanced age and time must not be wasted, or in case of long-standing infertility. Recent evidence has shown that keeping in view the better success rates of IVF, it may be considered as first-line treatment in some.

INTRODUCTION

Unexplained infertility is a diagnosis made when a couple fails to establish pregnancy despite there being no obvious cause. The diagnostic protocol should show a normal laboratory assessment of ovulation, evaluation of tubal patency and semen analysis. Delayed conception in apparently normal couples can be because of three reasons—the couple may be completely normal and may have not conceived because of a chance factor, they may be subfertile because of a subtle defect in fertilization, embryo transport and/or implantation, which remain undetected by routine diagnostic tests, or they may be truly sterile, where the defect present has remained undetected and cannot be remedied. Unexplained infertility is diagnosed in 15 percent of the couples.[1]

Since these patients have reduced reproductive capacity, it may take longer for them to conceive. Their monthly fecundity is 3 percent compared to 20 percent for normal fertile couples. Thus, most couples with unexplained infertility will conceive given time. Their chance of successful pregnancy without any intervention is as high as 60 percent in 3 years.[2] Viewed from this aspect, the rationale of treatment in unexplained infertility is to increase the monthly probability of pregnancy, hence reducing the time interval for conception and identifying early couples who would not respond to treatment. Superovulation with intrauterine insemination or *in vitro* fertilization (with or without intracytoplasmic sperm injection) has been shown to increase the chance of pregnancy.[3,4] However, there are no standard protocols for treatment of unexplained infertility as the etiology remains unknown.

Diagnosis

There is a wide variation in the incidence, which may be due to the differences in definition of unexplained infertility, interpretation of tests and the evaluation process. It is a diagnosis of exclusion. There are multiple tests but no consensus on which is necessary for diagnosis. When the diagnosis of 'unexplained infertility' is made, a careful review of their entire infertility evaluation is conducted. It is ensured that each test was performed correctly and is technically sound. The interpretation drawn from the results is reassessed. Tests that are inconclusive are repeated. Further investigation may be done to evaluate processes necessary for conception like fertilization and implantation. It must be kept in mind that values of tests can alter during the course of investigation.

Controversies in Diagnosis

Controversies exist in the inclusion of postcoital test, antisperm antibody and laparoscopy as essential for diagnosis. In a study, laparoscopy revealed abnormalities that resulted in changed treatment decisions in 25 percent of the patients who would normally have been scheduled for IUI if laparoscopy had not been performed.[5] More advanced tests, like evaluation of endometrial function and tests for ovarian reserve, have been suggested but there is no consensus whether they contribute to effective diagnosis. The controversy arises when the cause of infertility is attributed to abnormal testing without ensuring its reliability in impairing fertility. The American Society of Reproductive Medicine (ASRM) recommended five important diagnostic criteria for unexplained infertility, which include evidence of ovulation by basal body temperature/mid luteal serum progesterone level, normal semen parameters, normal postcoital test, normal uterus and tubes, as demonstrated by hysterosalpingography, and a normal pelvic anatomy on laparoscopy.

The European Society of Human Reproduction and Embryology (ESHRE) grouped the basic infertility tests into three categories (Table 34.1). These tests are grouped according to the prognosis.[6,7] Category 1 would imply that an abnormal test impairs fertility without therapy. Category 2 includes abnormal results, frequently associated with subsequent fertility without therapy. Hysteroscopy is

included in this category, as even with an abnormal finding, patients conceive, and the presence of an intrauterine lesion alone is not an indication for surgery as the effectiveness of surgical treatment of uterine abnormalities on improving pregnancy rates has not been established. Category 3 data shows that abnormal tests have a lack of correlation with pregnancy. Assessment of tubal function and falloposcopy would come under this category. Similarly, women should not be offered an endometrial biopsy to evaluate the luteal phase as part of the investigation of fertility problems because there is no evidence that medical treatment of luteal phase defect improves pregnancy rates.

Evaluation of Fertilizing Capacity of Sperm

These tests are not included in the routine work-up because they are not easily available and there is no evidence that they help to improve the pregnancy rates. There is no correlation between hamster egg penetration assay and fertilization or pregnancy rates.[8] Screening for antisperm antibodies should not be offered because there is no evidence of effective treatment to improve fertility.

Tests for Ovarian Reserve

Tests of ovarian reserve currently have limited sensitivity and specificity in predicting fertility. However, women who have high levels of gonadotropins should be informed that they are likely to have reduced fertility but the value of assessing ovarian reserve using Inhibin B is uncertain and is therefore, not recommended routinely. Diminished ovarian response to controlled ovarian hyperstimulation (COH) in *in vitro* fertilization (IVF) may be the very first sign of ovarian aging in young women diagnosed with idiopathic and mild male subfertility.[9]

Gonadotropin antibodies: It may represent an independent marker of ovarian autoimmunity in unexplained infertility as they are correlated with ovarian antibodies and are present in patients not treated with gonadotropins.[10] Their presence may precede changes in regulatory hormones.[11]

Uterine Receptivity

Cytokines, integrins, trophonins and heat shock protein are important for endometrial receptivity. Markers of uterine receptivity, like integrins, are now increasing in importance. Deficiency of these factors may cause unexplained infertility.

CLINICAL DISCUSSION

Management

Decisions about treatment can be made when each therapy has a scientific rationale and known effectiveness. In

Table 34.1: Basic tests for unexplained infertility (ESHRE)

Category I: Tests established with correlation to pregnancy

1. Semen analysis
2. Documentation of tubal patency (HSG or laparoscopy)
3. Mid luteal phase progesterone to document ovulation

Category 2: Tests not consistently correlated with pregnancy

1. Zona-free hamster egg penetration assay
2. Postcoital test
3. Antisperm antibody testing

Category 3: Tests that do not correlate with pregnancy

1. Endometrial biopsy for dating
2. Varicocele assessment
3. Chlamydia testing

unexplained infertility, as the cause remains unknown, there can be no rationale for therapy. No standard protocol for management is present. The problem is that the definition and inclusion criteria for unexplained infertility vary in each trial. Hence, the treatment ranges from expectant management to varied empirical treatment. The knowledge of effectiveness of therapy is lacking due to the absence of sufficient randomized controlled trials. It is known that in this condition, the natural course may take the path of spontaneous cure. Hence, randomized trials between treatment and no treatment are essential. Analysis of data is also dependent on the period of follow-up. In the natural course of the condition and its treatment, fecundity decreases with time, hence altering the likelihood of pregnancy with time. A group of patients followed up for 3 months cannot be compared to a group with a longer follow-up. An average pregnancy rate of 4.1 percent per month after 6 months but 1.9 percent after 24 months has been reported.[12]

Counseling

Providing information and helping patients to make the right choice in unexplained infertility is the most demanding role for the infertility specialist. Couples with unexplained infertility should be explained that they have a reasonable chance for conception but may take longer than normal fertile couples. Treatment is costly, inconvenient and emotionally trying. They should be aware of the benefits, risks and limitations of all the options.

The therapy consists of two basic management principles:
1. Increasing the availability of gametes by ovulation induction and IUI.
2. Bringing gametes together by IUI and IVF.

Expectant treatment: It has been seen that spontaneous conception occurs in patients with unexplained infertility without treatment. However, the pregnancy rates vary with the age of the female and the duration of infertility.[13] Cumulative pregnancy rate was 31 percent in women more than 30 years of age and 42 percent in women less than 30 years of age. The pregnancy rate decreased from 46 percent to 27 percent when the duration of infertility was more than 3 years. Patients with secondary infertility had a higher conception rate than those with primary infertility.[14]

Empirical therapy: Defects in folliculogenesis, gamete development, fertilization and/or embryo implantation may be responsible for unexplained infertility. The rationale of empirical therapy is to enhance or bypass as many causative factors as possible. Assisted reproductive techniques (ART) are used to overcome known deficiencies, such as using IVF to circumvent damaged Fallopian tubes. Because these techniques are based upon enhancement and/or substitution, they can be applied to unexplained infertility

patients with the hope that what is being enhanced or substituted is the element responsible for the infertility. To enhance the decreased reproductive capacity in couples with unexplained infertility, the number of gametes can be increased. Ovulation induction besides increasing number of gametes helps in removing subtle defects of ovulation, which may be responsible for unexplained infertility. Increasing the density of motile sperms in semen prepared for IUI might increase the probability of pregnancy. The empirical treatment can be divided into different levels. The success rates and cost increase with each level. One can go on to the last level directly. Each level involves treatments, which enhance certain factors while bypassing other factors.

1. *Controlled ovarian hyperstimulation (COH) with Clomiphene citrate (CC) and intrauterine insemination (IUI)*: COH with Clomiphene combined with IUI is attempted in cases of unexplained infertility. The ovulatory and male factors are enhanced while the cervical factor is bypassed. Since Clomiphene is a safe drug, a 3-month trial with Clomiphene is recommended. *Efficacy of IUI:* COH without IUI gives success but rates are improved when combined with IUI. In a retrospective analysis, adding IUI to COH with human menopausal gonadotropin (hMG) increased the pregnancy rate from 2.4 percent to 19.3 percent.[15]

   In the six trials, where IUI was compared with timed intercourse (TI), both in stimulated and natural cycles, there was evidence of an increased chance of pregnancy. A significant increase in pregnancy rate was also found for women where IUI with COH was compared with IUI in a natural cycle.[16] IUI does not alter the frequency of antisperm antibodies and is reasonably safe. Based on the results of pregnancy rate per couple of two trials, double intrauterine IUI showed no significant benefit over single IUI in the treatment of subfertile couples with husband's semen.[17] Where IUI is used to manage unexplained fertility problems, Fallopian tube sperm perfusion for insemination should be offered because it improves pregnancy rates compared with standard insemination techniques.

   In a retrospective analysis of 45 published reports, success rates were analyzed as pregnancy rate per initiated cycle (Table 34.2).

2. *Controlled ovarian hyperstimulation (COH) with gonadotropins*: Gonadotropins may be preferred in older patients or where Clomiphene has failed as it produces greater number of follicles. It is also free from the antiestrogenic effect of Clomiphene. Three cycles of gonadotropins combined with IUI may be tried. Here again, the ovulatory and male factors are being enhanced while the cervical factor is being bypassed. A combined pregnancy rate per initiated cycle of 17.1 percent has been quoted.[18] However, a recent randomized clinical trial of

Table 34.2: Success rates of treatments for unexplained infertility[18]	
Treatment	*Combined pregnancy rates per initiated cycle*
No treatment	1.3–4.1%
IUI	3.8%
CC + IUI	8.3%
hMG	7.7%
hMG + IUI	17.1%
IVF	20.7%
GIFT	27%

CC versus low dose recombinant follicle stimulating hormone (rFSH) for ovarian hyperstimulation in IUI cycles in 68 couples with unexplained infertility showed no significant difference in live birth rates between CC and rFSH. They concluded that since CC seems the more cost-effective drug, it can be offered as the drug of first choice.[19]

3. *Danazol*: Danazol has been used for patients with unexplained infertility. A recent Cochrane review analyzed two trials involving 71 women.[20] There was no statistically significant difference in the live birth/ongoing pregnancy rate between Danazol and placebo at the end of treatment. However, there were significantly more clinical pregnancies during the follow-up period in the Danazol group compared with the placebo group. Available data demonstrate no evidence of the benefit of Danazol for unexplained subfertility. The need for contraception during treatment, the adverse effects and costs of Danazol, make its use for this problem unwarranted. The increased pregnancy rate in the long-term follow-up data may be attributed to additional therapies and do not influence the live birth/ongoing pregnancy data.

4. *IVF*: With IVF and ICSI, the ovulation and male factors are enhanced and the cervical and tubal factors are bypassed at the same time, while taking care of subtle defects in fertilization. IVF provides further diagnostic information like fertilization efficiency of the sperm and embryo development prior to transfer. This information may provide clues to a prior undiagnosed infertility factor. A 26 percent success rate has been reported following IVF compared to controlled ovarian stimulation and IUI, where 15 percent achieved a clinical pregnancy.[21] Three cycles of IVF are recommended. IVF is now a widely accepted treatment for unexplained infertility. With increasing awareness of the role of expectant management and less invasive procedures, such as IUI, and concerns about multiple complications and costs associated with IVF, it is extremely important to evaluate the effectiveness of IVF against other treatment options in couples with unexplained infertility. IVF has not been rigorously evaluated in comparison with other fertility treatments, making evidence-based decisions difficult.

5. *Gamete intrafallopian transfer (GIFT)*: Gamete intrafallopian transfer has also been used in couples with unexplained infertility. However, IVF has the advantage of assessing fertilization. In many cases of infertility, there may be subtle defects in fertilization for which the treatment would be donor gametes, zona drilling or ICSI.

COH and IUI versus IVF

When comparing IVF to COH and IUI, it was seen that the cycle fecundity falls with COH and IUI after 3 cycles. In a study on 594 couples with unexplained infertility, COH and IUI showed a cycle fecundity of 16.4 percent and a cumulative pregnancy rate (PR) of 39.2 percent after the first 3 cycles. However, following cycles 4 to 6 of COH and IUI, the cumulative PR rose to 48.5 percent by cycle 6, a further increase of only 9.3 percent. In the women undergoing IVF and ICSI, a cycle fecundity of 36.6 percent per cycle was obtained. In unexplained infertility, the cycle fecundity in the first three trials of COH and IUI was higher than in cycles 4 to 6, with a statistically significant difference. Since cycle fecundity was low in cycle 4 to 6 patients should be offered IVF or ICSI if they fail to conceive after three trials of COH and IUI.[22]

Should IVF be Recommended as the First-line of Treatment?

Current evidence shows that any effect of IVF relative to other treatment options in terms of live birth rates for couples with unexplained subfertility is unknown and requires larger trials to give a definite opinion. IVF may have a better clinical pregnancy rate but the live birth rate was not significantly different. What we do know with surety is that IVF does cost much more and has some definite risks. However, IVF may be the first choice in cases where time may be a consideration. A number of factors like age, cost, patient's choice, risks and efficacy of treatments contribute to the final decision and each case needs to be individualized.

Age

The chance of a live birth following *in vitro* fertilization treatment decreases with increasing age of the female, being only 10 to 15 percent for women aged 36 to 40 years and 6 percent for women older than 40 years. Hence, patients who are older may not like to waste time on a stepwise protocol when IVF and ICSI may solve undetected fertilization defects.

Cost

In vitro fertilization is costly and often not covered by insurance. However, consideration must be given to the fact that with many years of unexplained infertility, such costly treatment may be justified. For couples with unexplained and mild male factor subfertility, the primary offer of a full IVF cycle is less costly and more cost-effective than providing IUI (of any modality) followed by IVF.[23]

Risk

Risks of IVF include psychological stress, multiple gestations, operative risks and ovarian hyperstimulation syndrome (OHSS). Besides psychological stress, there are rigorous treatment schedules and financial concerns. Multiple gestations occur in 25 percent of IVF pregnancies and carry an increased risk of premature delivery, low birth weight, spontaneous abortion, and congenital abnormalities. Although complications with egg retrieval are rare, the procedure carries operative risks such as bleeding and infection as well as the risks associated with general anesthesia. Ovarian hyperstimulation syndrome is a potentially fatal effect of the use of gonadotropins and gonadotropin agonists, with an incidence of 6 to 14 percent. Any therapy with such significant risks should benefit from a rigorous evaluation of its effectiveness before making it the first choice.

Counseling and Choice of the Couple

The factors affecting treatment decisions among couples with unexplained infertility include issues other than efficacy of therapy. Since no study has proved that IVF is less effective than any other treatment, it still remains the final treatment, which would be offered after all others have failed. There may be couples, who after a prolonged period of infertility, may not want to go stepwise from a less costly to more costly protocol. The lack of a proven rationale and efficacy of therapy brings to light the fact the patient's wishes must be an important factor in choosing therapy.

Efficacy of Treatments

An important aspect to decision making is the success rates of various treatments. These success rates differ depending on whether the outcome was taken as clinical pregnancy rate or live birth rate. A recent Cochrane review, updated in 2005, examined in the context of unexplained infertility, randomized controlled studies (RCTs) that variously compared IVF with expectant management, IUI with or without ovarian stimulation, GIFT, and CC, using live birth rate per woman as the primary outcome.[24] Ten randomized controlled trials were identified but only four were eligible for inclusion. There was no evidence of a difference in live birth rates between IVF and IUI either with or without ovarian stimulation. Clinical pregnancy rates with IVF in comparison to expectant management were significantly higher. There was no significant difference between IVF and GIFT for the one RCT that reported live birth rates but clinical pregnancy

rates were significantly higher for IVF than GIFT. There was no evidence of a difference in the multiple pregnancy rates between IVF and IUI with ovarian stimulation, however, IVF had a higher multiple pregnancy rate than GIFT. The review concluded that any effect of IVF relative to expectant management, CC, IUI with or without ovarian stimulation and GIFT in terms of live birth rates for couples with unexplained subfertility remains unknown. The studies were limited by their small sample size and inadequate with unequal periods of follow-up. Live birth rates and adverse effects, such as multiple pregnancy and OHSS have also not been reported in most studies. Larger trials with adequate power are warranted to establish the effectiveness of IVF in these women and should include adverse effects and costs of the treatments as outcomes. Factors that have a major effect on these outcomes, such as fertility treatment, female partner's age, duration of infertility and previous pregnancy history, should also be considered.

The debate on what the initial treatment for idiopathic infertility should be has been re-ignited with recent recommendations of ovarian stimulation with IUI being proposed as an effective treatment option for couples with unexplained infertility.[25] When conventional treatment of unexplained infertility has not been successful, the next choice lies between either gonadotropin treatment with intrauterine insemination (FSH/IUI) and IVF. Although IVF is superior to FSH/IUI treatment in terms of clinical pregnancy, this benefit is achieved only at a considerable cost. Similar benefits are not seen when the outcome is evaluated as live births.[26] The relevant evidence should come from randomized controlled trials, and the results need to be recalculated for the outcome of greatest interest, a singleton live birth. With the current available evidence, progress should be made from less costly to more costly and advanced technology treatment. Although IVF is used routinely for the treatment of unexplained infertility, it has certain risks and there is insufficient evidence to recommend it as an alternative to other therapies such as, CC, IUI or GIFT. There are however, exceptions in cases where age may be advanced and any wastage of time may lead to poor results with IVF, or where couples choose not to waste time on a stepwise protocol after the risks and benefits have been explained. Another issue is the duration of infertility, which if longer, may be suggestive of a direct recommendation to IVF as failure rates are higher with other treatments. The benefits of treatments are associated with side effects hence, each treatment protocol needs to be individualized. A large multicenter trial is needed to evaluate the relative value of existing empirical treatments for unexplained infertility.

IVF versus ICSI

Another question, which needs to be discussed, is whether ICSI would be better than IVF for these couples with unexplained infertility as they may have subtle defects in fertilization, which could be overcome with ICSI. In a recent study, sixty women with unexplained infertility were randomized to IVF or ICSI. There was no statistically significant difference in the fertilization rate (77.2% IVF vs. 82.4% ICSI), implantation rate (38.2% IVF vs. 44.4% ICSI), clinical pregnancy rate (50% in each group), or live birth rate (46.7% IVF vs. 50% ICSI). There were two cases of failed fertilization in the IVF group. There was no significant difference in embryo quality or clinical outcomes between the two groups.[27] However, in another study, the ICSI fertilization rate of 61 percent per allocated oocyte was higher than the IVF fertilization rate of 51.6 percent. Complete fertilization failure occurred in 19.2 and 0.8 percent of the IVF and ICSI cycles, respectively.[28] Patients with disordered zona pellucida-induced acrosome reaction have a low or zero fertilization rate with standard IVF but high fertilization and pregnancy rates with ICSI. Up to 29 percent of patients with unexplained infertility with normal semen analysis may have this condition, which should be diagnosed and treated with ICSI rather than standard IVF. [29] In a prospective study, conventional IVF and ICSI were performed on sibling oocytes of 22 patients with unexplained infertility.[30] The study showed that 22.7 percent of patients with unexplained infertility would have lost their chance of embryo transfer completely because of total failure of fertilization if ICSI had not been performed on some oocytes in this cycle. The policy of splitting the sibling oocytes can effectively minimize complete fertilization failure while maintaining high chances of achieving a pregnancy. At the same time, the optimal fertilization method for subsequent treatment cycles can be determined.[30]

Treatment by ICSI should be considered for couples in whom a previous IVF treatment cycle has resulted in failed or very poor fertilization, in cases with disordered zona pellucida-induced acrosome reaction, or where there have been failures with direct intraperitoneal insemination. IVF may be more effective than IUI+COS as suggested by a recent Cochrane review.[31]

Repeated IVF Failure in Unexplained Infertility

If one is faced with repeated IVF failures, the next option depends on a number of factors (Flow chart 34.1):

1. The IVF cycles, the response to stimulation, and the embryology records should be evaluated.
2. For various reasons (severe male factor infertility, recurrent abortion), genetic testing is becoming more and more common during infertility evaluation. Genetic abnormalities have been found more commonly among couples with repeated IVF failure, and testing should be considered in these cases.[32]
3. The ovarian reserve should be evaluated. Often, women with unexplained infertility have elevated baseline hormone levels, suggesting a diminished ovarian reserve. The IVF outcome is usually poor in such cases.

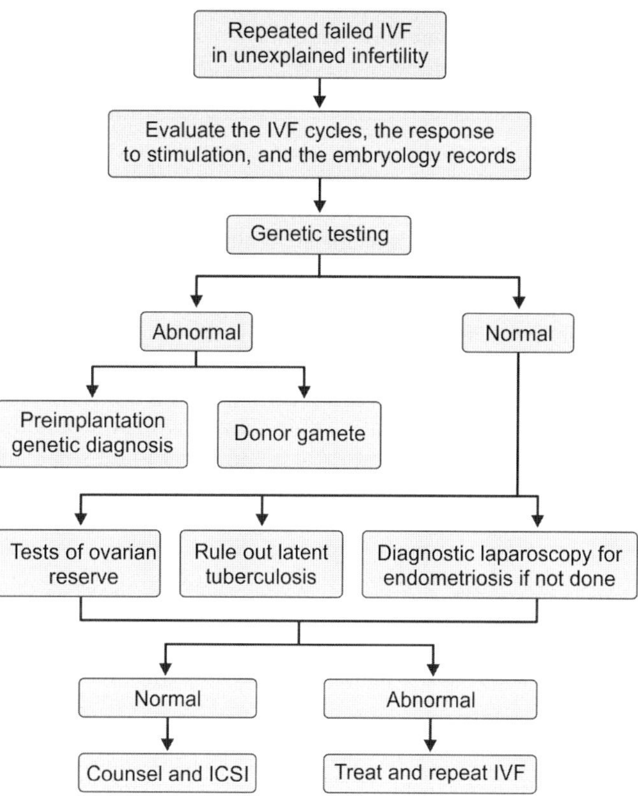

Flow chart 34.1: Management of repeated IVF failure in unexplained infertility

4. Other conditions in association with unexplained infertility need to be ruled out. Endometriosis occurs in about 10 percent of women, the incidence is about 35 percent among infertile women.
5. Implantation failure has been attributed to immunologic abnormalities. Implantation is an active process between the blastocyst and the endometrium. Both secrete cytokines that affect the other and ultimately determine whether or not implantation occurs. If this signaling process is abnormal, endometrial development will be affected and implantation will fail. Many trials have evaluated the effects of immunotherapy (intravenous immunoglobulin) on pregnancy outcome, but the results are very controversial.[33] Currently, the use of intravenous immunoglobulin to manage infertility is only recommended as part of a research protocol.
6. Tuberculosis has been found to be an important cause of unexplained infertility and repeated IVF failures. A study conducted on 81 women with unexplained infertility, who had repeated IVF failures, showed them to be positive for tuberculosis. The amount of gonadotropin required required was lesser and the number of oocytes recovered and endometrial thickness was greater after treatment for

tuberculosis. The study indicates that latent tuberculosis should be considered in young patients presenting with unexplained infertility with apparently normal pelvic factors and repeated IVF failure.[34]

CONCLUSION

Despite improvements in diagnostic assessment of infertile couples, many couples still have no explanation for their infertility. The treatment options for unexplained infertility are several. When counseling patients regarding treatment options, both the expected increase in cycle fecundity and treatment expense should be considered. Expectant management can be recommended if the woman is under 28 to 30 years of age and if the infertility duration is lesser than 2 to 3 years. *In vitro* fertilization can be used as both, a diagnostic and a therapeutic tool in couples with unexplained infertility. The existing empirical treatments for unexplained infertility, like IUI, superovulation, GIFT and IVF require appropriately designed trials to evaluate their relative value.

REFERENCES

1. Templeton P. The incidence, characteristics, and prognosis of patients whose infertility is unexplained. Fertil Steril 1982;37:175-82.
2. Lobo RA. Unexplained infertility. J Reprod Med 1993;38:241-9.
3. Adashi EY, Rock JA, Rosenwaks Z. Reproductive Endocrinology, Surgery, and Technology. Philadelphia, Pa: Lippincott-Raven 1996:1909-11.
4. Aboulghar MA, Mansour RT, Serour GI, Amin Y, Ramzy AM, Sattar MA, Kamal A. Management of long-standing infertility: A prospective study. Am J Obstet Gynecol 1999;181:371-5.
5. Tanahatoe SJ, Hompes PG, Lambalk CB. Investigation of the infertile couple: Should diagnostic laparoscopy be performed in the infertility work-up programme in patients undergoing intrauterine insemination? Hum Reprod 2003;18:8-11.
6. Crosignani PG, Collin J, Cooke ID, Diczfalusy E, Rubin B. Recommendations of ESHRE workshop on unexplained infertility. Hum Reprod 1992;8:977.
7. Crosignani PG, Rubin BL. Optimal use of infertility diagnostic tests and treatments. The ESHRE Capri Workshop Group. Hum Reprod 2000;15:723-32.
8. Leto S, Frensilli FJ. Changing parameters of donor semen. Fertil Steril 1981;36:766.
9. Goverde AJ, McDonnell J, Schats R, Vermeiden JP, Homburg R, Lambalk CB. Ovarian response to standard gonadotropin stimulation for IVF is decreased not only in older but also in younger women in couples with idiopathic and male subfertility. Hum Reprod 2005;20:1573-7.
10. Shatavi SV, Llanes B, Luborsky JL. Association of unexplained infertility with gonadotropin and ovarian antibodies. Am J Reprod Immunol 2006;56:286-91.
11. Luborsky J, Llanes B, Roussev R, Coulam C. Ovarian antibodies, FSH and inhibin B: Independent markers associated with unexplained infertility. Hum Reprod 2000;15:1046-51.
12. Collins JA, Enkin M. Is GIFT (gamete intrafallopian transfer) the best treatment for unexplained infertility. Br J Obstet Gynecol 1992;99:169-70.
13. Collins J, Rowe T. Age of female partner is a prognostic factor in prolonged unexplained infertility. A multicenter study. Fertil Steril 1989;52:15.
14. Lenton E, Weston G, Cook I. Lomg term follow-up of apparently normal couple with complaints of infertility. Fertil Steril 1977;28:913.
15. Nulsen JC, Walsh S, Dumez S, Metzger DA. A randomized and longitudinal study of human menopausal gonadotropin with intrauterine insemination in treatment of infertility. Obstet Gynecol 1993;82:780.
16. Verhulst SM, Cohlen BJ, Hughes E, Te Velde E, Heineman MJ. Intra-uterine insemination for unexplained subfertility. Cochrane Database Syst Rev 2006;(4):CD001838.
17. Cantineau AE, Heineman MJ, Cohlen BJ. Single versus double intrauterine insemination (IUI) in stimulated cycles for subfertile couples. Cochrane Database Syst Rev 2003;(1):CD003854.
18. Guzick DS, Sullivan MW, Adamson GD, Cedars MI, Falk RJ, Peterson EP, Steinkampf MP. Efficacy of treatment for unexplained infertility. Fertil Steril 1998;70:207-13.
19. Dankert T, Kremer JA, Cohlen BJ, Hamilton CJ, Pasker-de Jong PC, Straatman H, van Dop PA. A randomized clinical trial of clomiphene citrate versus low dose recombinant FSH for ovarian hyperstimulation in intrauterine insemination cycles for unexplained and male subfertility. Hum Reprod 2007;22:792-7.
20. Hughes E, Brown J, Tiffin G, Vandekerckhove P. Danazol for unexplained subfertility. Cochrane Database Syst Rev. 2007;(1):CD000069.
21. Peterson CM, Hatasaka HH, Jones, Poulson AM Jr, Carrell DT, Urry RL. Ovulation induction with gonadotropins and intrauterine insemination compared with *in vitro* fertilization and no therapy – a prospective randomized controlled cohort study and meta analysis. Fertil Steril 1994;62:535.
22. Aboulghar M, Mansour R, Serour G, Abdrazek A, Amin Y, Rhodes C. Controlled ovarian hyperstimulation and intrauterine insemination for treatment of unexplained infertility should be limited to a maximum of three trials. Fertil Steril 2001;75:88-91.
23. Pashayan N, Lyratzopoulos G, Mathur R. Cost-effectiveness of primary offer of IVF vs. primary offer of IUI followed by IVF (for IUI failures) in couples with unexplained or mild male factor subfertility. BMC Health Serv Res 2006;6:80.
24. Pandian Z, Bhattacharya S, Vale L, Templeton A. *In vitro* fertilization for unexplained subfertility. Cochrane Database Syst Rev. 2005;(2):CD003357.
25. Homburg R. The case for initial treatment with intrauterine insemination as opposed to *in vitro* fertilization for idiopathic infertility. Hum Fertil (Camb) 2003;6:122-4.
26. Collins J. Stimulated intra-uterine insemination is not a natural choice for the treatment of unexplained subfertility. Current best evidence for the advanced treatment of unexplained subfertility. Hum Reprod 2003;18:907-12.
27. Foong SC, Fleetham JA, O'Keane JA, Scott SG, Tough SC, Greene CA. A prospective randomized trial of conventional *in*

vitro fertilization versus intracytoplasmic sperm injection in unexplained infertility. J Assist Reprod Genet 2006;23:137-40.

28. Jaroudi K, Al-Hassan S, Al-Sufayan H, Al-Mayman H, Qeba M, Coskun S. Intracytoplasmic sperm injection and conventional *in vitro* fertilization are complementary techniques in management of unexplained infertility. J Assist Reprod Genet 2003;20: 377-81.

29. Liu DY, Baker HW. Disordered zona pellucida-induced acrosome reaction and failure of *in vitro* fertilization in patients with unexplained infertility. Fertil Steril 2003;79:74-80.

30. Aboulghar MA, Mansour RT, Serour GI, Sattar MA, Amin YM. Intracytoplasmic sperm injection and conventional *in vitro* fertilization for sibling oocytes in cases of unexplained infertility and borderline semen. J Assist Reprod Genet 1996;13:38-42.

31. Pandian Z, Gibreel A, Bhattacharya S. *In vitro* fertilisation for unexplained subfertility. Cochrane Database Syst Rev 2012;4: CD003357.

32. Raziel A, Friedler S, Schachter M, Kasterstein E, Strassburger D, Ron-El R. Increased frequency of female partner chromosomal abnormalities in patients with high-order implantation failure after *in vitro* fertilization. Fertil Steril 2002;78:515-19.

33. Stephenson MD, Fluker MR. Treatment of repeated unexplained *in vitro* fertilization failure with intravenous immunoglobulin: A randomized, placebo-controlled Canadian trial. Fertil Steril 2000;74:1108-13.

34. Dam P, Shirazee HH, Goswami SK, Ghosh S, Ganesh A, Chaudhury, Chakravarty B. Role of latent genital tuberculosis in repeated IVF failure in the Indian clinical setting. Gynecol Obstet Invest 2006;61:223-27.

Management of the Obese Infertile Patient

Kulvinder Kochar Kaur, Gautam N Allahbadia, Mandeep Singh

OVERVIEW

Obesity, particularly the abdominal phenotype is associated with a diverse set of metabolic disorders and reproductive consequences that are complex and not well-understood. An important role appears to be played by the presence of a condition of functional hyperandrogenism and hyperinsulinemia, which accompanies the insulin-resistant state. In women with polycystic ovary syndrome (PCOS), abdominal obesity may be co-responsible.

The development of hyperandrogenism and associated chronic anovulation is mediated through mechanisms primarily involving the insulin-mediated overstimulation of ovarian steroidogenesis and decreased sex hormone binding globulin (SHBG) blood concentrations. By these mechanisms, obesity may also favor resistance to Clomiphene and gonadotropins-induced ovulation, thus reducing outcomes of *in vitro* fertilization (IVF) and intracytoplasmic sperm injection (ICSI) procedures. Leptin, produced by the adipose tissue, has dominated the literature with regard to complications in female fertility, however, other adipokines, namely adiponectin and resistin, may also play a likely role. Also, the cannabinoid receptor (CB1) and peroxisome proliferator-activated receptors (PPARs) have recently been found in reproductive tissue and their influence on obesity and fertility has been discussed. Due to the beneficial effects of weight loss, lifestyle intervention programs should be adopted as the first-line approach in the treatment of infertile obese women. Insulin sensitizing agents may add further benefits, particularly if administered in combination with a hypocaloric diet. Therefore, individualized pharmacological support, aimed at favoring weight loss and improving insulin resistance, should be widely extended in clinical practice in obese infertile patients. This may be beneficial even during pregnancy, thereby permitting favorable physiological delivery and healthy babies.

INTRODUCTION

The worldwide incidence of obesity continues to escalate despite increased awareness and global efforts to understand and confront its origins. The World Health Organization (WHO) estimates that 9 to 25 percent of women in developed countries are severely obese.[1] In essence, dysregulated energy homeostasis stems from a societal reduction in physical activity, an increase in accessibility and overindulgence in energy-rich foods combined with a myriad of genetic, social and economic factors, including drug addiction and adulteration[2] all over the world. The mechanisms that control energy metabolism and body fat mass are inherently linked to those that govern fertility and stem back to the evolutionary drive to survive in times of limited food supply. The rising incidence of obesity and associated metabolic disturbances highlights a loss of control in this homeostatic system, which remains ill-defined but in desperate need of understanding.

Overweight (BMI > 25 kg/m^2) and obesity (BMI > 30 kg/m^2) are associated with an increased risk of anovulatory infertility.[3] Reduced fecundity of overweight women is probably related to multiple endocrine and metabolic alterations, which include but are not limited to effects on steroid metabolism and altered secretion and actions of insulin and other hormones such as resistin, ghrelin, or adiponectin. These alterations can affect follicle growth, embryo development and implantation.[4,5]

It has been reported that obese women are at an increased risk of miscarriages after IVF or ICSI, an association not fully explained by the high prevalence of PCOS, which by itself, is related to miscarriages among obese infertile women,[6] confirming the harmful effects of obesity. Weight loss was found to improve the outcome of assisted reproduction treatment in obese women.[7,8] Fedorcsac et al.[9] found that obesity is associated with an impaired response to ovarian stimulation and with lower chances for live birth after IVF and ICSI.[9]

CLINICAL DISCUSSION

Before understanding how to manage an obese infertile patient, it is important to understand the pathophysiology by which obesity with or without associated PCOS affects fertility.

Mechanisms by which Obesity may Affect Fertility in Women

Fertility involves complex factors and mechanisms of both ovarian and extraovarian origin. Obesity may interfere with many neuroendocrine and ovarian functions, thereby reducing both, ovulatory and fertility rates in otherwise healthy women.

As previously reported, obesity affects reproductive function early in life, both before and during pubertal development. Moreover, it clearly appears that it is associated with an increased risk of hyperandrogenism and anovulation in women of reproductive age, as supported by the strong association between obesity and the PCOS, the most common androgenic disorder.[10] The mechanisms underlying the relationship between hyperandrogenism and obesity are multifactorial.[11] Available data support the concept that simple obesity, particularly the abdominal phenotype, may be associated with several alterations in the balance of sex hormones, particularly, androgens, leading to a condition of 'functional hyperandrogenism'.

Obesity as a Condition of Sex Hormone Imbalance in Women

It is well-known that an increase in body weight and fat tissue is associated with several abnormalities in the sex steroid balance, especially in fertile women. Such alterations involve both androgens and estrogens and overall, their carrier protein, sex hormone-binding globulin (SHBG). Changes in SHBG concentrations lead to alterations in androgen and estrogen delivery to the target tissues. SHBG levels are regulated by a complex of factors, including stimulating agents, such as estrogens, iodothyronines and growth hormone and inhibiting factors, such as androgens and insulin as inhibiting factors.[12] The net balance of this regulation is probably responsible for the decrement in SHBG concentration observed in obesity. Body fat distribution has also been shown to affect SHBG concentrations.[13] In fact, women with central obesity usually have lower SHBG concentrations in comparison with their age and weight-matched counterparts

with peripheral obesity.[12] This seems to be dependent on higher circulating insulin in abdominally obese women and on the inhibiting capacity of insulin on SHBG liver synthesis. Reduction of circulating SHBG determines an increase in the metabolic clearance rate of circulating SHBG-bound steroids, specifically testosterone, dihydrotestosterone and androstenediol, which is the principal active metabolite of dihydrotestosterone.[14] However, this effect is compensated by a consequent elevation of production rates. Obesity also affects the metabolism of the androgens not bound to SHBG. In fact, both the production rates and metabolic clearance rates of dehydroepiandrostenedione (DHEA) and androstenedione are equally increased in obesity.[15] The role of adipose tissue is crucial in controlling the balance of sex hormone availability in the target nonfat tissues, indeed, adipose tissue is able to store various lipid soluble steroids, including androgens. Most sex hormones appear to be preferentially concentrated within the adipose tissue rather than in the blood. As a consequence, since the amounts of fat in obesity are larger than their intravascular space, and the steroid tissue concentration is much higher than in plasma, the steroid pool in obese individuals is greater than that found in normal weight individuals.[16] Fat also represents a site of intensive sex hormone metabolism and interconversion due to the presence of several steroidogenic enzymes, such as 3β-dehydrogenase,[17] β-hydroxydehydrogenase and the aromatase system. The pattern of body fat distribution can regulate androgen production and metabolism to a significant extent. In fact, women with central obesity have higher testosterone production rates than those with peripheral obesity.[15] Accordingly, the metabolic clearance rates of testosterone and dihydrotestosterone are significantly higher in women with central than peripheral obesity. The maintenance of normal circulating levels of these hormones in obesity may lead to the prediction of the presence of a sophisticated regulation that can adjust both, the production rate and metabolic clearance rate of these hormones to the body size. Due to a greater reduction in SHBG concentrations, the percentage of free testosterone fraction tends to be higher in women with central obesity than in those with peripheral obesity.[17] An inverse correlation exists between waist-to-hip ratio (or other indices of body fat distribution) and testosterone or SHBG concentrations regardless of the body mass index (BMI) values.[17] Therefore, a condition of 'relative functional hyperandrogenism' seems to be associated with the central obese phenotype in women. Due to their action in the adipose tissue, it has been argued that this endocrine milieu may play a crucial role in favoring the development of visceral fat enlargement in women.

Obesity can also be considered a condition of increased estrogen production, the rate of which correlates significantly with body weight and the amount of body fat.[15] Reduced SHBG concentrations may in turn, lead to an increased exposure of target tissues to free estrogens. In addition, obesity is associated with a decreased formation of inactive 17 β-estradiol metabolites (e.g. 2-hydroxyestrogens), which are virtually devoid of peripheral estrogen activity, and a higher production of estrone sulfate, an important reservoir of active estrogens. Altogether, these alterations lead to an increased ratio of active to inactive estrogen as a final result. However, in spite of these changes, blood estrogen levels are usually normal or only slightly elevated in both premenopausal and postmenopausal obese women.[18] This finding may be attributed to the ability of enlarged body fat to act as a storage for the excess formed estrogen, contributing in this way to maintain normal levels of circulating hormone. In addition, there are no systematic differences in the blood estrogen levels in women with different obesity phenotypes, although estrogen production rates have been found to be particularly increased in women with peripheral obesity.[18] Increased estrogenization in simple obese women may be important in protecting against the development of the abdominal obesity phenotype, which may, as previously reported, be a sign of tissue-specific androgenization in both fertile and postmenopausal women. The dichotomy of fat distribution according to sex is under the control (among other hormones) of both androgens and estrogens.[19] In the adipose tissue of women, the androgen receptors seem to have the same characteristics as those found in male adipose tissue. However, estrogens downregulate the density of these receptors (whereas testosterone upregulates them), and this may be a mechanism whereby estrogens protect the adipose tissue from androgen effects. In addition, estrogen receptors are expressed in human adipose tissue and show a regional variation of density, though the quantity of these receptors appears to be of physiological importance, this has not been clearly established.[19]

The Obesity-PCOS Link: Pathophysiological Aspects

As cited above, PCOS, the most common cause of anovulatory infertility in young women, is frequently associated with obesity (50%)[10] and the history of weight gain frequently precedes the onset of clinical manifestations of the syndrome, suggesting a pathogenetic role of obesity in the development of PCOS and related infertility. Moreover, there are numerous studies indicating that obese women have a higher likelihood of PCOS and related infertility. Moreover, there are numerous studies indicating that obese women with PCOS (notably those with an abdominal body fat distribution phenotype) have a more severe insulin resistance,[20,21] dyslipidemia[20,21] and hyperandrogenic state[22] along with more frequent menstrual abnormalities[22] and a lower incidence of spontaneous and stimulated ovulations and pregnancy rates[23] than their 'normal weight' counterparts. Mechanisms

by which obesity interferes with the pathophysiology and clinical expression of PCOS are complex and not completely understood. As reported in the previous section, obesity *per se* represents a condition of functional hyperandrogenism. In women with PCOS, however, obesity is believed to play a distinct pathophysiological role in the development of hyperandrogenism. In an obese PCOS woman, the former presence of obesity in the mother during pregnancy appears to influence susceptibility to develop hyperandrogenism and the PCOS phenotype later in time, although pathophysiological mechanisms for this have not been defined.[4] By contrast, it has been hypothesized recently that *in-utero* androgen excess may be an important factor programming subsequent PCOS development during puberty.[24] By these mechanisms, it has been suggested that a primary ovarian disorder may even occur early in the woman's life, leading to the development of a hyperandrogenized ovary later in life.[24] Along with this line of thinking, it is also possible that the early onset of overweight or obesity during the peripubertal age, may play a role in the development of hyperandrogenism by the intervention of multiple inter-related mechanisms, which primarily involve inappropriate signals from different hormones and/or alterations of specific regulatory pathways. These include insulin, the insulin-growth factor system, the opioid system, estrogens and several newly discovered cytokines.

It is well-known that obesity, particularly the abdominal phenotype, is a condition of insulin resistance and compensatory hyperinsulinemia. Contrary to what occurs in the classical target tissues of insulin action (muscle, liver, adipose tissue) that have become resistant to insulin, the ovaries remain responsive to insulin throughout the interaction with their own receptor. During the past two decades, a large number of *in vitro* studies have shown that, in the ovaries of PCOS women, excess insulin is capable of stimulating steroidogenesis and excessive androgen production from the theca cell system.[5] In addition, by inhibiting SHBG synthesis by the liver proportionally to its blood levels, excess insulin may further increase the delivery of free androgens to target tissues.[5] *In vivo*, numerous studies have subsequently shown that both acute and chronic hyperinsulinemia can stimulate testosterone production and that, suppression of insulin levels can conversely decrease both androgen concentrations.[5,11] The excess local ovarian androgen production induced by excess circulating insulin may also cause premature follicular atresia and then favor anovulation.[5] It can therefore be speculated that insulin-resistance and hyperinsulinemia, which develop together with the obese state, may play a dominant role in favoring hyperandrogenism in women susceptible to the development of PCOS, particularly during the pubertal age. The same dangerous insulin-dependent process on both, ovarian steroidogenesis and androgen metabolism may obviously also occur in women who had PCOS before becoming obese, and this worsens both hyperandrogenism and associated clinical features, including anovulation.

The influence of obesity on hyperandrogenism can also be mediated by other factors and mechanisms. As in simple obesity, a hyperestrogenic state is also present in obese PCOS women. Excess estrogens may exert a positive feedback regulation on gonadotropin release, triggering in turn, a rise in ovarian androgen production, according to a still valid theory proposed many years ago.[10]

An additional factor involved in the dysregulation of this complex circuit may be an increased tone of the opioid system, which has been demonstrated in the presence of obesity, as well as in women having PCOS.[25,26] Several studies have shown that β-endorphin is able to stimulate insulin secretion.[27] The possibility that increased opioid activity may favor the development of hyperinsulinemia and in turn, of hyperandrogenemia, is further supported by the finding that both acute and chronic administration of opioid antagonists (e.g. naloxone, naltrexone) suppresses basal and glucose-stimulated insulin blood concentrations.[28] Whether alterations of the opioidergic system play a role in determining infertility in women is still undefined, however, several studies have shown that opioid antagonists given to obese PCOS women may improve menses.

Finally, several peptide adipokines (leptin, adiponectin, resistin and ghrelin) are currently emerging as potential candidates involved in the pathogenesis of hyperandrogenism and related infertility in PCOS women. Leptin is considered to be one of the main peripheral signals that affects food intake and energy balance, and obesity is a classic condition of circulating leptin excess.[29] Leptin has been found to decrease appetite and food intake and reduce the massive obesity in leptin-deficient ob/ob mice, and the concentrations of leptin in the blood, during the feeding state, vary with the amount of adipose tissue in the body.[30] Leptin production and secretion by adipocytes is under complex regulation by many stimulating hormones, particularly insulin, glucocorticoids, cytokines (including tumor necrosis factor α and interleukin-1) and inhibiting hormones and factors such as catecholamines, testosterone and peroxisome proliferator activated receptor (PPARα) agonists.[31] Under physiological conditions, the amount of leptin produced by fat tissue is directly correlated with both adipose tissue mass and local mRNA expression. In humans, leptin blood levels are 2-fold higher in females than in males, and are also affected by growth and energy consumption. The discrepancy between high leptin blood levels and its central effects represents the basis to support the concept that most forms of obesity may represent a condition of leptin-resistance. On the other hand, many tissues besides fat mass have been shown to express leptin and its receptors. Several lines of evidence indicate that leptin acts directly on the ovary. In particular, functional leptin receptors have been detected on the surface of ovarian follicular cells, including granulosa, theca and interstitial cells,[32] and recent *in vivo* data indicate that leptin may exert a direct inhibitory effect on ovarian function, by inhibiting both granulosa and theca cell steroidogenesis, probably through antagonism of stimulatory factors such as insulin-like growth factor,[1] transforming growth factor-β, insulin and LH.[33] Moreover, high leptin concentrations in the ovary may interfere with the development of dominant follicles and oocyte maturation, as demonstrated by both *in vitro* and *in vivo* studies.[34] Finally exogenous leptin infusion has been shown to significantly decrease the ovulation rate in female rats.[34] Taking into account the involvement of leptin in the control of ovulation and reproduction, interest focused on leptin levels in PCOS women, who are generally obese, have reported contradictory results on leptin levels in PCOS to date. Whether high leptin levels in the peripheral circulation and/or in the ovarian tissues may play a role in determining anovulation in obese PCOS women is presently unknown, although it cannot be excluded that this may somehow be involved in the processes leading to the development of infertile ovaries.

Another newly discovered peptide, ghrelin, may be involved in the pathophysiology of hyperandrogenism and infertility in obese PCOS women. This acylated 28 amino acid peptide, a natural ligand of the growth hormone (GH) secretagogue receptor, G-protein-coupled receptor, primarily expressed in the pituitary and the hypothalamus that has been shown to be a potent stimulant of GH secretion.[35] Ghrelin is mainly produced in the stomach, although several other tissues may express ghrelin and its receptors. Ghrelin has also attracted attention for its involvement in the control of food intake and energy balance. When administered centrally or peripherally to rodents and humans, ghrelin has been shown to enhance appetite, reduce fat utilization, and cause adiposity.[36] Moreover a putative regulation of ghrelin secretion by nutrients or related factor, such as insulin, has also been hypothesized, since circulating levels of ghrelin increase on fasting and decrease following food intake.[37] Plasma ghrelin concentrations have been shown to be lower in obese patients than in normal subjects,[38] though mechanisms responsible for this situation has not yet been defined. Interestingly, however, data are available, which suggest that obese women with PCOS may have lower plasma ghrelin levels, compared with age and weight-matched controls.[39]

A highly significant negative correlation has also been demonstrated between ghrelin and androgen levels, which is in line with in recent *in vitro* data indicating that gonads may be an Important target of ghrelin action. In fact, ghrelin's binding sites have been detected in both, the human ovary and testis.[40] On the other hand, it also appears that androgens may be involved in the regulation of ghrelin secretion and/

or metabolism. It has been shown recently that when androgen levels in obese PCOS women were suppressed by flutamide (a pure antiandrogenic compound, which acts at the androgen receptor level and also inhibits androgen secretion from the gonads), there was a significant increase in plasma ghrelin concentrations to values within the normal range. In addition, it has been shown that ghrelin levels in hypogonadal men were significantly lower with respect to weight-matched obese and normal-weight individuals, and significantly increased to expected values based on their BMI values after long-term testosterone replacement therapy (unpublished data). Taken together, these data point to an important role of androgens on ghrelin levels in humans. Since ghrelin concentrations are negatively correlated with insulin resistance,[36,39] it might be speculated that this peptide represents a link between hyperandrogenism and the insulin system in conditions such as obesity and PCOS. It therefore appears that ghrelin, like leptin, may represent a further endocrine factor that is related not only to energy balance and metabolism, but also to the gonadal function. Whether alterations in ghrelin secretion and action are involved in the infertility associated with obesity and PCOS remain to be elucidated, however.

Management

After a thorough general physical examination, following investigations are done:
- Hemogram
- Routine urine analysis
- Serum follicle stimulating hormone (FSH)/luteinizing hormone (LH)/Prolactin/thyroid stimulating hormone (TSH)/Dehydroepiandrosterone sulfate (DHEAS).
- Sex hormone-binding globulin (SHBG)/fasting serum insulin/oral glucose tolerance test (OGTT), leptin if possible.

Treatment

With regard to treatment, weight loss by diet, exercise or pharmacotherapy, remains one of the major goals:
1. *Lifestyle interventions:* Lifestyle interventions, particularly with a hypocaloric diet, with or without associated increased physical activity have shown to be effective (Fig. 35.1 and Flow chart 35.1). It is important to try and treat every patient as a whole rather than prioritizing for fertility treatment alone. In New Zealand, clinical priority access criteria (CPAC) have been made to define which patients need priority for treatment according to

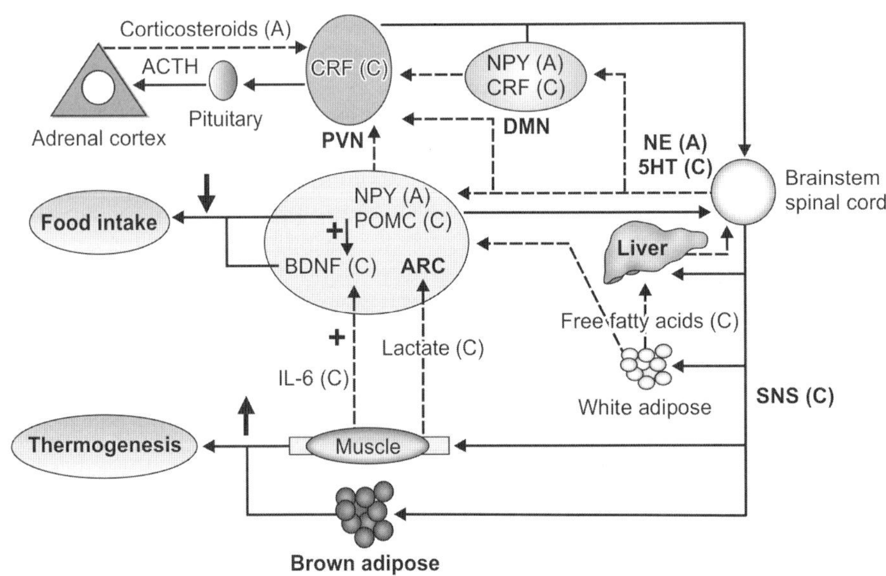

Fig. 35.1: Hypothetical model of potential exercise-induced peripheral signals that alter central pathways involved in energy homeostasis. Catabolic factors (C) decrease food intake (downward arrow) and/or increase thermogenesis (upward arrow). Anabolic factors (A) increase intake and/or decrease thermogenesis. Both IL-6 and -MSH, released from arcuate nucleus proopiomelanocortin neurons increase (+) BDNF production. Dotted arrows represent afferent signals from the periphery, whereas solid arrows represent efferent outputs from brain sites to other brain areas or peripheral organs involved in energy homeostasis. *Abbreviations:* ACTH: adrenocorticotropic hormone; CRF: corticotropin-releasing factor; NPY: neuropeptide Y; DMN: dorsomedial nucleus; PVN: paraventricular hypothalamic nucleus; POMC: pro-opiomelanocortin; BDNF: brain-derived neurotrophic factor; ARC: arcuate nucleus; IL-6: interleukin 6; SNS: sympathetic nervous system; 5HT: 5-hydroxytryptamine; NE: norepinephrine

Flow chart 35.1: Mechanism underlying the beneficial effects of dietary restriction, and physical and mental exercise on neurons. All three environmental factors impose a mild stress on neurons, which results from increased activity in neuronal circuits and/or metabolic stress. The cellular stress involves increased levels of intracellular calcium and reactive oxygen species which, in turn, activate kinases and transcription factors. The transcription factors induce the expression of genes that encode stress resistance proteins (SRPs), neurotrophic factors such as BDNF, and antiapoptotic genes such as Bcl-2. Kinases may phosphorylate substrate proteins involved in maintenance of ion homeostasis, energy metabolism, and stress resistance

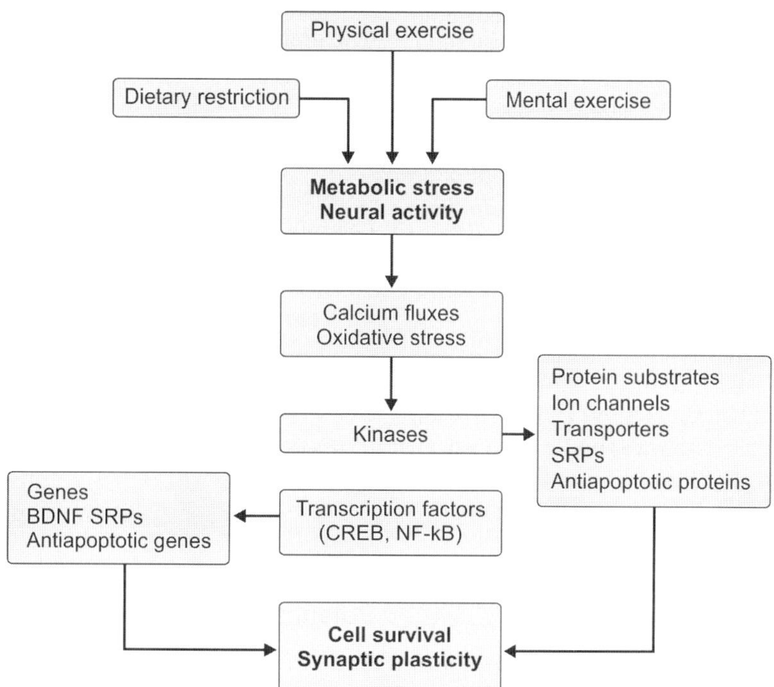

BMI.[41] This is highlighted in the case report presented subsequently.

2. *Insulin sensitizers*:
   - *Metformin:* In women with PCOS, Metformin, administered at doses of up to 1500 mg/day decreases insulin, testosterone and LH levels and it also appears to favor some weight loss.[42]
   - *In cases of obese PCOS women with hirsutism:* Drugs such as Flutamide, Finasteride, Spironolactone and Cyproterone acetate are prescribed with the idea of reducing androgen levels and related clinical manifestations such as hirsutism and menstrual abnormalities. Ovulation induction should be avoided in these cycles as antiandrogens can prove teratogenic.[42]
   - *Metformin and Flutamide:* Flutamide (250 mg/day) with Metformin is effective in an additive manner in affecting menses and improving lipid profile.[42]
   - *Thiazolidinediones:* They are selective ligands of the nuclear transcription factor peroxisome-proliferator activated receptor γ (PPARγ), which is expressed most abundantly in adipose tissue, but recently has also

been demonstrated in the reproductive organs the testes and the ovaries. In the latter, PPARγ is involved in both folliculogenesis and in the corpus luteum. Several studies suggest a role of PPARγ in steroidogenesis and prostaglandin production, angiogenesis by regulating vascular endothelial growth factor (VEGF), secreted by lutein cells.[43] The two currently available PPARγ agonists are Pioglitazone and Rosiglitazone.[42]
   - *Metformin and Thiazolidinediones:* Only two studies have been conducted so far, and the results show that combined therapy is helpful only in a subset of women.[42]
   - *New potential drug-somatostatin analogs:* Somatostatin is a 14-amino acid endogenous hypothalamic peptide with a short half-life, that, besides blunting the LH responses to gonadotropin-releasing hormone (GnRH) and decreasing GH pituitary secretion, inhibits pancreatic insulin release.[42]
   - *Ovulation induction with*:
     i. Clomiphene citrate
     ii. Gonadotropins[42]
     iii. Pulsatile GnRH.

Most of the patients will respond by the formation of a dominant follicle (DF), but some patients may be so grossly obese that even without downregulation, no DF may form with as high as 300 to 375 IU of gonadotropins and ovaries may also not be accessible on transvaginal ultrasonography. In that case, it is better to first attempt weight loss as is highlighted in the following case report. If the patient does not conceive spontaneously after 20 to 30 percent weight loss, Topiramate,[44] has been found to be very effective in achieving weight loss even in the presence of leptin resistance, in contrast to conventional Sibutramine. Once weight loss has been initiated by dieting and exercise, ovulation induction should be re-attempted with clomiphene citrate and gonadotropins.

Case Report

A 26-year-old non-resident Indian attended our Center with three years secondary infertility. She was extremely obese with a weight of 125 kg and height 5′4″. Her BMI was 48 kg/m². She was mildly hypertensive and was on Envas, 5 mg for the same. She had a missed abortion at six months for which, a dilatation and curettage was done in 2006. Examination revealed extreme obesity with a blood pressure (BP) of— 126/80 mm Hg. Ultrasonography (USG) revealed bilateral polycystic ovarian disease. Her blood work-up was as follows (normal ranges are given in brackets): Serum FSH 5.78 μIU/L (2.9–9.0), LH 6.47 μIU/L (1.5–8.0), TSH 2.49 μIU/L (0.25–7.0), prolactin 17.5 ng/mL (1.9–25), DHEAS 398.4 μg/dL (35–430), testosterone (total) 68.8 ng/dL (15–81), free testosterone 1.7 pg/mL (0.45–3.17) and serum insulin 31.03 μIU/L (6.0–27). Her oral glucose tolerance test (OGTT) showed values of 167, 171, 151 and 153. Her growth hormone values were 0.05 ng/mL (0.06–5.0), 8-am serum cortisol 78.1 ng/mL (60–285), 4-pm cortisol 71.6 ng/mL (30–150), adrenocorticotropic hormone (ACTH) 26.4 (0–46) and leptin 45.9 ng/mL (18–25). Her husband's routine semen analysis showed a count of 42 mill/mL, 66 percent motility with 65 percent having normal morphology. Her complete blood count (CBC) showed a hemoglobin (Hb) value of 11g percent, total lymphocyte count (TLC) of 8700/cmm, differential count of 67 percent neutrophils, 28 percent lymphocytes, 2 percent monocytes and 3 percent eosinophils. Her platelet count was 2.5 lakhs.

Since the serum insulin level was raised, the patient was put on Metformin 850 mg TDS and induced with Clomiphene citrate (CC) and pure-FSH (Fostine-Zydus Cadilla) 225 IU/day along with 100 IU human chorionic gonadotropin (hCG) for LH activity for 9 days, but no DF formed. During that time, she developed overtly abnormal sugars precipitated by an infection of the big toe hence, she was put on Pioglitazone, 15 mg BD as well to control her blood sugar [fasting blood sugar (FBS) 181 mg, postprandial (PP) 220 mg], after getting the baseline liver function test (LFT) and Topiramate to achieve weight loss. Envas was replaced by Lobet, 50 mg OD, and in the subsequent cycle she was stimulated with 300 IU FSH+100 IU hCG for 9 days but by the 12th day no dominant follicle appeared. The dose of 300 IU was continued for 4 days when a 9 mm follicle formed on the right side, hence she was given the same dose for another 3 days when 2 follicles 16 mm and 14 mm formed on the right side and ovulation induction was done with hCG but the patient did not conceive. At this time, she lost 7 kg despite the leptin resistance on Topiramate and since she was a NRI and had to return back. She was sent back on Topiramate 25 mg, Pioglitazone 15 mg BD, and Metformin 850 mg TDS with the idea that she loses weight and after control of the insulin resistance to return back after 3 months for repeat ovulation induction but luckily the patient conceived spontaneously on that regimen. When she informed us, we then omitted the Topiramate and Pioglitazone as the safety of these is not established in pregnancy (Pioglitazone being a category C drug and the safety of Topiramate has yet to be established). However, Metformin was continued as Metformin is known to prevent abortions in obese PCOS patients.[45] Her weight finally decreased to 92 kg with a total weight loss of 32 kg.

RECENT ADVANCES

Potential Role of Endocannabinoid System

The identification of the endocannabinoids (EC), the enzymatic machinery for their synthesis and degradation and the specific cannabinoid receptors type 1 (CB1) and type II (CB2) is the result of scientific research performed in the last decade. Endocannabinoids, Anandamide (AEA) and 2 Arachidonoyl glycerol (2-AG) are deeply involved in the dynamic and homeostatic regulation of feeding and energy metabolism. They act as orexigenic compounds, by contrast, antagonists of the CB1 receptors reduce food intake. The regulation of metabolic processes includes both central and peripheral actions at the hypothalamic levels and in the adipose tissue and the liver, respectively. The peripheral action of the endocannabinoids have been documented in animal models treated with a selective CB1 antagonist, Rimonabant.[46] While endogenous cannabinoids AEA and 2-AG promote lipogenesis, CB1 antagonists have been found to increase energy expenditure through activation of futile cycles, enhance lipolysis and stimulate glucose metabolism by increasing glucose transporter-4 recruitment and activation.[47] By these mechanisms, the CB1 antagonist Rimonabant has been proposed as a new pharmacological treatment for tackling obesity. Indeed, it has been clearly documented that the endocannabinoid system may be overactivated in dietary-induced and genetic animal models, therefore favoring increased adipocyte enlargement. Interestingly, however the endocannabinoid system has been found to regulate multiple endocrine functions, including the hypothalamic-pituitary-gonadal (HPG) axis–the study of which is still in the re-experimental stage.[48]

However, although phase-III clinical trials showed the ability to regulate intra-abdominal fat tissue levels, lipedemic, glycemic and inflammatory parameters, and safety concerns have led to its withdrawal in the USA by the Food and Drugs Administration (FDA) mainly because of depressive side effects, including suicidal tendencies. The EC system in mammalian reproduction is an emerging research area, given its implication in fertilization, preimplantation embryos and spermatogenesis. Hence, relevant preclinical data on EC signaling opens up new perspectives as a target to improve reproductive health in humans.[49] However, controversy still exists regarding the use of Rimonabant in humans with use allowed in Europe. For a more complete evaluation on the safety of this drug, additional studies are in progress.[50]

Role of Other Adipokines

The role of adiponectin and resistin has been described in Figures 35.2 and 35.3.[48]

Role of Topiramate

Topiramate (Tp) is an anticonvulsant, incidentally discovered to cause weight loss. In contrast to other anticonvulsants, it is a sulfamate-substituted monosaccharide, related to fructose, a rather unusual chemical structure.

With regard to weight loss, Tp has been shown to be insulin sensitizing *in vivo* with direct effects on adipocytes and enhanced insulin sensitivity at the level of tissue. Glucose disposal, [insulin-stimulated glucose disposal rate (ISGDR)], liver inhibition of hepatic glucose output (HGO) and adipose tissue suppression of lipolysis also causes skeletal muscle insulin sensitization, increased high molecular weight adiponectin {A Crp 30(3–4)},[51] and increase in phospho 5′-AMP-activated protein kinase (AMPK) in skeletal muscle. Additionally, Topiramate has been found effective for weight reduction and improvement in glycemic control in obese subjects with type 2 diabetes mellitus (DM) treated with Metformin monotherapy[52] and hence, should prove effective in controlling hyperinsulinemia in obese PCOS patients. The authors are conducting a study on the same.

CONCLUSION

With the incidence of obesity being on the rise globally, assisted reproductive techniques (ART) specialists are likely to encounter more and more cases of obesity of greater severity along with mainly PCOS-associated infertility. In the last decade, insulin sesitizers have revolutionized the management of obese PCOS. However, since one is likely to encounter cases with a greater severity of obesity in those cases, even insulin sensitizers may not work. Hence, the next decade is waiting for a trial of drugs like Rimonabant-A, a CB1 receptor antagonist, which has finished phase 4 trials for

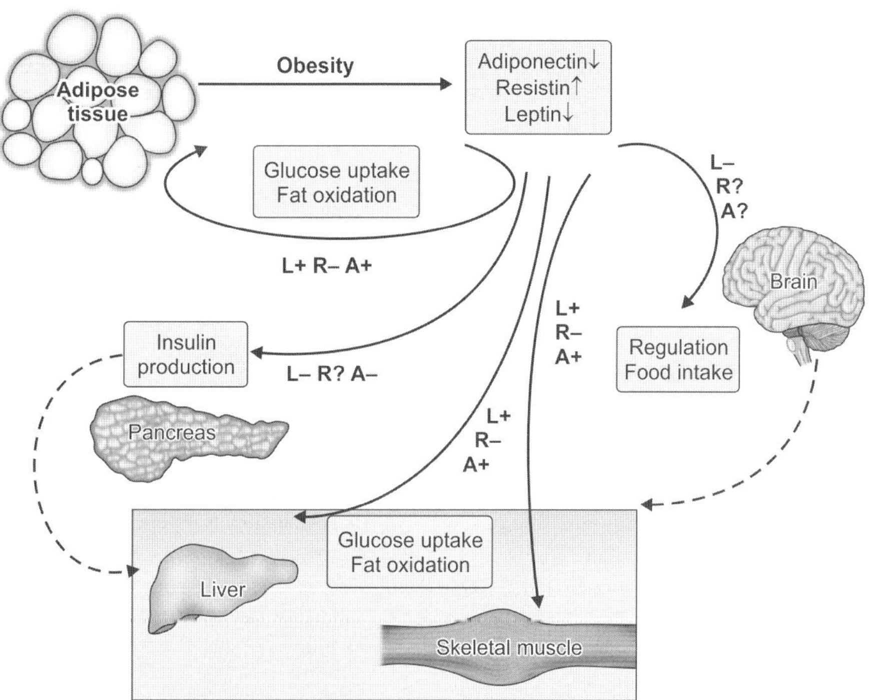

Fig. 35.2: The role of leptin, adiponectin and resistin. *Abbreviations:* L: leptin; A: adiponectin; R: resistin

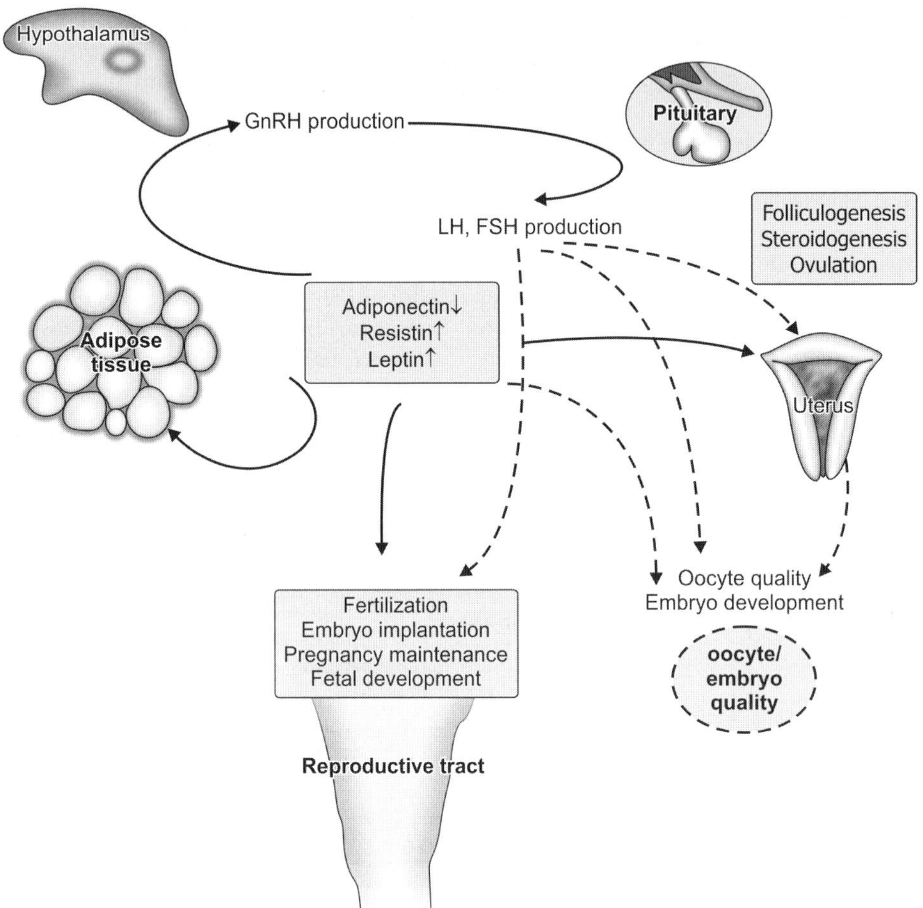

Fig. 35.3: Mechanism underlying beneficial effects of dietary restriction, and physical and mental exercise on neurons. All three environmental factors impose a mild stress on the neurons, which results from increased activity in neuronal circuits and/or metabolic stress. The cellular stress involves increased levels of intracellular calcium and reactive oxygen species which, in turn, activate kinases and transcription factors. The transcription factors induce the expression of genes that encode stress resistance proteins (SRPs), neurotrophic factors such as BDNF, and antiapoptotic genes such as Bcl-2. Kinases may phosphorylate substrate proteins involved in maintenance of ion homeostasis energy metabolism, and stress resistance

obesity and since CB1 receptors are expressed in reproductive organs, and reward circuitry, it is possible that they may work in PCOS also. Topiramate has already been found to be highly effective in severe PCOS and has been used to treat obesity with type 2 DM but its safety in pregnancy needs to be established. Flow chart 35.2 summarizes the management of an obese PCOS patient according to BMI.

ACKNOWLEDGMENT

I would like to acknowledge the help extended by Mr Ajay Katyal C/o Solvay Pharma India Ltd. in preparing this manuscript prepared.

REFERENCES

1. ESHRE Capri Workshop Nutrition and reproduction in women. Group Hum Reprod 2006;12:193-207.
2. Kaur KK. Confused hypothalamus–A cause for obesity world wide. Gynaecological Endocrinology Abstract (Book of Abstract for the 12th world congress of Endocrinology) 2006;132(Suppl 1)22:239.
3. Rich-Edwards JW, Spiegelamn D, Garland M, Hertzmark E, Hunter DJ, Colditz GA, Willett WC, Wand H, Manson JE. Physical activity, body mass index, and ovulatory disorder infertility. Epidemology 2002;13:184-90.
4. Pasquali R, Pelusi C, Genghini S, Cacciari M, Gambineri A. Obesity and reproductive disorders in women. Hum Reprod Update 2003;9:539-72.

Flow chart 35.2: Flow diagram for the management of an obese PCOS patient according to BMI

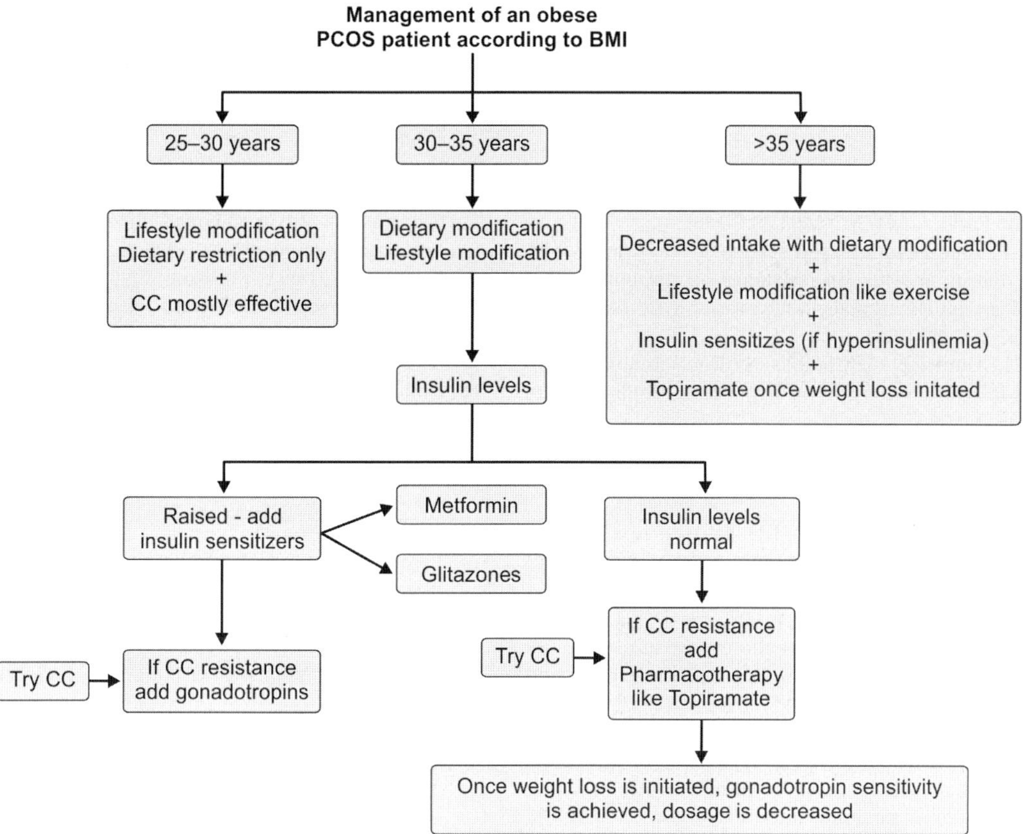

5. Poretsky L, Cataldo NA, Rosenwaks Z and Giudice LC. The insulin related ovarian regulatory system in health and disease. Endocr Rev 1999;200:535-82.

6. Wang JX, Davies MJ and Norman RJ. Obesity increases the risk of spontaneous abortion during infertility treatment. Obes Res 2002;10:551-54.

7. Clark AM, Thormley B, Tomlinson L, Galletely C, Norman RJ. Weight loss in obese infertile women results in improvement in reproductive outcomes for all forms of fertility treatment. Hum Reprod 1999;13:1502-5.

8. Norman RJ, Noakes M, Wu R, Davies MJ, Moran L, Wang JX. Improving reproductive performance in overweight/obese women with effective weight management.Hum Reprod Update 2004;10:267-80.

9. Dale OP, Storeng R, Ertzeid G, Bjercke S, Omland KA, Abyholm T, Tanbo T. Impact of overweight and uderweight on assisted reproduction treatment P. Fedorcask. Hum Reproduction 2004; 19:2523-28.

10. Yen SSC. The polycystic ovary syndrome. Clin Endocrinol 1980;(Oxf.)12:177-208.

11. Gambineri A, Pelusi C, Vicennati V, Pagotto U, Pasquali R. Obesity and the poycystic ovary syndrome. Int J Obesity 2002a;26:883-96.

12. Von Shoultz B, Calstrom KJ. On the regulation of sex-hormone-binding globulin. A challenge of old dogma and outlines of an alternative mechanism. Steroid Biochem 1989;32:327-34.

13. Pasquali R, Casimirri F, Plate L, Capelli M. Characterization of obese women with reduced sex-hormone-binding globulin concentrations. Horm Metab Res 1990;22:303-6.

14. Samojlik E, Kirschner MA, Silber D, Scneider G, Ertel NH. Elevated production and metabolic clearance rates of androgens in morbidly obese women. J Clin Endocrinol Metab 1984;59:949-54.

15. Kirschner MA. Obesity, androgens, oestrogens, and cancer risk. Cancer Res 1982;42:3281-85.

16. Azziz R. Reproductive endocrinologic alterations in female asymptomatic obesity. Fertil Steril 1989;52:703-25.

17. Evans DJ, Hoffman RG, Kalkoff RK, Kissebah AH. Relationship of androgenic activity to body fat topography, fat cell morphology and metabolic aberrations in premenopausal women. Clin Endocrinol Metab 1990;57:304-10.

18. Pasquali R, Casimirri F, Cantobelli S, Labate AM, Venturoli S, Paradisi R, Zannarini L. Insulin and androgen relationships with abdominal body fat distribution in women with and without hyperandrogenism. Horm Res 1993;39:179-87.

19. Wajchenberg BL. Subcutaneous and visceral adipose tissue: their relation to the metabolic syndrome. Endocr Rev 2000;21:697-38.

20. Conway GS, Agarwal R, Beeteridge DJ, et al. Risk factors for coronary artery disease in lean and obese women with the polycystic ovary syndrome. Clin Endocrinol 1992;37:119-25.

21. Holte J, Bergh T, Gennarelli G, et al. The independent effects of polycystic ovary syndrome and obesity on serum concentrations of gonadotrophins and sex steroids in premenopausal women. Clin Endrocrinol 1994;41:473-81.

22. Pasquali R, Casimirri F. The impact of obesity on hyperandrogenism and polycystic ovary syndrome in premenopausal women. Clin Endocrinol (Oxf.) 1993;39:1-16.

23. Fedoresak P, Dale PO, Storeng R, Tanbo T, Abyholm T. The impact of obesity and insulin resistance on the outcome of IVF or ICSI in women with polycystic ovarian syndrome. Hum Reprod 2001;16:1086-91.

24. Abbott DH, Dumesic DA, Franks S. Development origin of polycystic ovary syndrome–A hypothesis. J Endrocrinol 2002;174:1-5.

25. Genazzani AR, Facchinetti F, Petraglia F, Pintor C, Corda RJ. Hyperendorphinemia in obese children and adolescents. Clin Endocrinol Metab 1986;62:36-40.

26. Giuliano D, Salvatore T, Cozzolino D, Ceriello A, Torella R, D'Onofrio F. Sensitivity to endorphins as a cause of human obesity. Metabolism 1987;36:974-78.

27. Giuliano D, Cozzolino D, Torella R. Arguments for a role of opioid peptides in some pathogenetic events of obesity. In: Lardy H, Stratmen F. (Eds). Hormones, Thermogenesis, and Obesity. Elsevier Science, New York; 1989. pp. 209–18.

28. Pasquali R, Cantobelli S, Casimirri F, Bortoluzzi L, Boschi S, Carpelli M, Melchionda K, Barbara L. The role of the opioid peptides in the development of hyperinsulinemia in obese women with abdominal body fat distribution. Metabolism 1992;41:763-67.

29. Considine RV, Sinha MK, Heiman ML, Kriauciunas A, Stephens TW, Nyce MR. Serum immunoreactive leptin concentrations in normal-weight and obese humans. N Engl J Med 1996; 334:292-5.

30. Campfied LA, Smith FJ, Burn P. The Ob protein (leptin) pathway-a link between adipose tissue mass and central neutral networks. Horm Metab Res 1996;28:619-32.

31. Friedman JM, Halaas JL. Leptin and the regulation of body weight in mammals. Nature 1998;395:763-70.

32. Wiesner G, Vaz M, Collier G, Seals D, Kaye D, Jennings G, et al. Leptin is released from the human brain: influence of adiposity and gender. J Clin Endocrinol Metab 1999;84:2270-74.

33. Aggarwal SK, Vogel K, Weitsmen SR, Magoffin DA. Leptin antagonizes the insulin-like growth factor-I augmentation of steroidogenesis in granulosa and theca cells of the human ovary. J Clin Endocrinal Metab 1999;84:1072-6.

34. Duggal PS, Van Der Hoek KH, Milner CR, et al. The *in vivo* and *in-vitro* effects of exogenous leptin on ovulation in rat. Endocrinology 2000;141:1971-6.

35. Aravat E, Di Vito L, Broglio F, Papotti M, Muccioli G, Dieguez C, et al. Preliminary evidence that ghrelin, the natural GH secretagogue (GHS)-receptor ligand, stronly stimulates GH secretion in humans. J Endocrinol Invest 2000;23:493-5.

36. Tschop M, Smiley DL, Heiman ML. Ghrelin induces adiposity in rodents. Nature 2000;407:908-13.

37. Ariyashu H, Takaya K, Tagami T, Ogawa Y, Hosoda K, Akamizu T, et al. Stomach is a major source of circulating ghrelin, and feeding state determines plasma ghrelin-like immunoreactivity levels in humans. J Clin Endocrinol. Metab 2001;86:4753-8.

38. Weyer CC, Tataranni AP, Devanarayan V, Ravussin E, Heiman ML. Circulating ghrelin levels are decreased in human obesity. Diabetes 2002;50:707-9.

39. Pagotto U, Gambineri A, Vicennati V, Heiman ML, Tschop M, Pasquali R. Obesity and the polycystic ovary syndrome: Correlations with insulin resistance and andorgen levels. J Clin Endocrinol Metab 2002;87:5625-9.

40. Papotti M, Ghe C, Cassoni P, Catapano F, Deghenghi R, Ghigo E, Muccioli G. Growth hormone secretagogue binding sites in peripheral human tissues. J Clin Endocrinol Metab 2000;85:3803-7.

41. Gillett WR, Putt T, Farquhar CM. Prioritising for fertility treatments—the effect of excluding women with a high body mass index BJOG 2006;113:1218-21.

42. Pasquali R, Gambineri A. Insulin-sensitizing agents in polycystic ovary syndrome. Eur J Endocrinol 2006;154:763-75.

43. Froment P, Gizard F, Defever D, Staels B, Dupont J, Monget P. Peroxisome proliferator-activated receptors in reproductive tissues: from gametogenesis to parturition. J Endocrinol 2006;189:199-209.

44. Astrup A, Caterson I, Zelissen P, Guy-Grand B, Carruba M, Levy B, et al. Topiramate: Long-term maintenance of weight loss induced by a low-calorie diet in obese subjects. Obes Res 2004;12(10):1658-69.

45. Khattab S, Mohsen IA, Ramdaan A, Moaz M, ALInany H. metformin reduces abortion in women with polycystic ovary syndrome. Gynecol Endocrinol 2006;22:608-84.

46. Cota D, Marsicano G, Lutz B, Vicennati V, Stalla GK, Pasquali R, et al. Endogenous cannabinoid system as a modulator of food intake. Int J Obes Relat Metab Disord 2003;27:289-301.

47. Pasquali R, Gambineri A, Pagotto U. The impact of obesity on reproduction in women with polycystic ovary syndrome. BJOG 2006;113:1148-60.

48. Mitchell M, Armstrong DT, Robker RL, Norman RJ. Adipokines: implications for female fertility and obesity. Reproduction 2005;130:583-97.

49. Mouslech Z, Valla V. Endocannabinoid system: An overview of its potential in current medical practice. Neuro Endocrinol Lett 2009;30:153-79.

50. Leite CE, Mocelin CA, Petersen GO, Leal MB, Thiesen FV. Rimonabant: An antagonist drug of the endocannabinoid system for the treatment of obesity. Review. Pharmacological Reports 2009;61:217-24.

51. Jason J, Wilkes MT, Audry Nguyen, Gautam K Bandyopadhyay, Elizabeth Nelson, Jerrold M. Olefsky. Topiramate treatment causes skeletal muscle insulin sensitization and increased Acrp 30 secretion in high-fat-fed male Wistar rats. Am J Physiol Endocrinol Metab 2005;289:E1015-E1022.

52. Astrup A, Caterson I, Zelissen P, Guygrand B, Carruba M, Levy B, Sun X, Fitcher M for the OBES 004 Study Group. Topiramate: Long-term management of weight loss induced by a low calorie diet in obese subjects. Obes Rese 2004;12:1658-69.

The Endometrium

What can Clinicians do to Improve Implantation?

Arpita Ray, Amit Shah, Anil Gudi

OVERVIEW

Implantation of an embryo is the most important part of assisted reproductive treatment. Co-ordination of a properly matured endometrium with a well-developed embryo is the key to a successful outcome. However, clear evidence is lacking in various fields of implantation and research is ongoing. Various pharmacological agents have been used but no definitive answer has been found. Identification of a uterine receptive phase for a particular embryo is still unclear. Improvement in the embryo transfer technique is the only aspect that has contributed to a definite improvement in implantation.

INTRODUCTION

Successful implantation is the result of correct orchestration between a hatched blastocyst capable of implantation and the simultaneous development of an endometrium that is receptive to the embryo. It is very difficult to achieve this correct balance in assisted reproductive techniques (ART). Even with the transfer of a high-grade embryo, the implantation rate has remained low over the years. In the natural cycle, successful implantation involves a complex interaction between the stromal cells overlying the endometrial epithelium and the embryo itself. Most of the classical embryo transfer experiments have confirmed the existence of a receptive phase that extends from day 5 to day 10 after the leutinizing hormone (LH) surge, although the exact duration of this receptive phase is less well-defined in humans than in rodents.[1] As research is ongoing in different fields to improve implantation, various clinical strategies have been adopted by the clinicians before clear evidence for their efficacy and safety has been established.

In this chapter, various clinical methods will be reviewed and appraised to assess their efficacy to increase the chance of implantation.

CLINICAL DISCUSSION

Preconceptual Care

Preconceptional interventions, aimed to optimize factors related to lifestyle and nutrition, may improve outcomes of fertility treatment. Body mass index (BMI) and smoking both have a negative impact on ovarian response to *in vitro* fertilization (IVF) stimulation. Smoking was observed to have a premature aging effect as a result of which, twice the number of cycles are required to achieve conception in smokers than in non-smokers.[2]

Nutritional supplements also play an important role in improving the microenvironment of the oocyte and seminal fluid. Folic acid supplement alters the oocyte microenvironment.[3] A high intake of caffeine has been showed to increase the risk of spontaneous miscarriage and lower the live birth rate after IVF treatment.[4] It is likely that increased preconceptual counseling on lifestyle and nutritional factors could contribute to improved implantation rate and pregnancy outcome following IVF.

Adjuvant Pharmaceutical Therapies

Adjuvant drug therapy required for ovarian stimulation is often applied in an empirical manner with a view to improve implantation. Aspirin, nitric oxide donors, ascorbic acid, aromatase inhibitors, glucocorticoids, insulin sensitizing drugs, gonadotropin-releasing hormone (GnRH) agonist and prolonged progesterone are different pharmacological products, which have been used from time to time.

Aspirin

Aspirin is used as a vasodilator and anticoagulant. The aim of Aspirin use in the context of IVF is to improve blood perfusion to the ovaries and endometrium. Randomized controlled trials (RCTs), investigating the use of Aspirin as an empirical therapy in a non-selected IVF population have shown conflicting results. Aspirin along with heparin has shown to be effective in treating recurrent miscarriage in women with antiphospholipid syndrome. A randomized, double-blind, placebo-controlled trial of heparin and Aspirin for women with implantation failure following IVF and antiphospholipid or antinuclear antibodies reported that Aspirin and heparin neither improved the implantation rate or the pregnancy rate when compared with placebo.[5] A very recent meta-analysis showed no statistically significant improvement in the clinical pregnancy rate (OR1.18, 95% CI 0.86–1.61) following the use of Aspirin in women undergoing IVF treatment. However, the noted trend of improvement in clinical pregnancy and the lack of power even when the studies were pooled highlight the need for a definitive trial.[6]

Nitric Oxide Donors

Nitric oxide donors might improve endometrial receptivity by stimulating uterine vasodilatation. Initial studies suggested a beneficial effect on implantation,[7] but more recent studies have highlighted their detrimental effect on implantation.[8] Present available data suggest the use of nitric oxide donors with caution only with the perspective of well-designed studies.

Aromatase Inhibitors

Aromatase inhibitors (AIs) help to increase gonadotropin secretion and stimulate follicular growth[9] by inhibiting endogenous estradiol synthesis. Oral administration of the aromatase inhibitor. Letrozole is effective for ovulation induction in anovulatory infertility and for increased follicle recruitment in ovulatory infertility. Letrozole appears to avoid the unfavorable effects on the endometrium, frequently seen with antiestrogen use for ovulation induction.[9] AIs have been shown to be as effective as Clomiphene in inducing ovulation, with the major advantage of absence of any antiestrogenic adverse effects, lower serum estrogen production per developing follicle resulting in more physiological estrogen levels around the time of ovulation, and good pregnancy rates with a lower incidence of multiple pregnancy than with Clomiphene. When combined with gonadotropins for assisted reproductive techniques (ART), AIs reduce the dose of gonadotropins required for optimal follicle recruitment and improve the response to gonadotropin stimulation in poor responders.[10] However, further studies are required to establish the value of aromatase inhibitors in IVF.

Ascorbic Acid

Ascorbic acid appears to play a part in normal folliculogenesis,[11] ovulation[12] and corpus luteum formation and regression.[13] High dose ascorbic acid can stimulate anti-inflammatory and immunostimulant effects that may improve embryo implantation. However, Griesinger et al.[14] demonstrated no clinical evidence of any beneficial effect (as defined by main outcome measures) of ascorbic acid on IVF-ET compared with placebo, suggesting no obvious value of high dose intake of vitamin C during luteal phase in infertility treatment.[14]

Glucocorticoids

Uterine natural killer (NK) cells and locally acting growth factors, and cytokines play an important role in controlling uterine receptivity. Ledde–Bataille et al.[15] reported a higher number of NK cells in the endometrial biopsies from women with implantation failure versus fertile controls.[15] Therefore, glucocorticoids can improve the uterine environment by acting as immunomodulators. Nevertheless, a meta-analysis reported no clear evidence that administration of peri-implantation glucocorticoids in ART cycles significantly improves clinical outcome in a routine IVF/intracytoplasmic sperm injection (ICSI) population. Further, well-designed randomized studies are required to elucidate the possible role of this therapy in well-defined patient groups.[16] However, studies on women with autoantibodies, or treatment cycles where assisted hatching is performed, showed improvement with glucocorticoids. There are conflicting results following the use of glucocorticoids to improve ovarian response therefore, they should be used only within the context of randomized controlled trials.

Progesterone

Progesterone generally plays a role in uterine receptivity. In a natural cycle, after ovulation, the progesterone level increases. Following ovarian stimulation for IVF, the luteal phase is abnormal with a characteristic rise in progesterone levels in the early luteal phase and then a dramatic and premature fall in the unsupported midluteal phase.[17] The luteal phase can be restored by stimulating the corpora lutea with human chorionic gonadotropin (hCG) as luteal phase support or supplementation with progesterone. The optimal duration of progesterone administration is not very clear yet. Fanchin et al.[18] showed a significant decrease in the uterine contraction frequency when progesterone was started on the day of egg collection compared to that started on the day of the embryo transfer.[18] Progesterone has also shown to have potentially beneficial immunomodulatory properties.[19] Although progesterone supplementation is widely used to improve implantation rates, the role of estradiol supplementation remains controversial. A meta-analysis of three RCTs[20-22] reported no difference in the pregnancy rate when estrogen was added to progesterone in the luteal phase.[23] In contrast, Lukaszuk et al.[24] showed significantly higher pregnancy and implantation rates after estradiol supplementation. However, more substantive research is needed to obtain a concrete conclusion.[24]

Insulin Sensitizing Drugs

Metformin is an insulin sensitizing drug used in the treatment of anovulation, that has been shown to be effective in achieving ovulation in women with polycystic ovary syndrome (PCOS).[25] However, although the risk of ovarian hyperstimulation syndrome (OHSS) is significantly reduced following Metformin use, a meta-analysis of randomized controlled trials on Metformin co-administration during gonadotropin ovulation induction or IVF in women with PCOS concluded that it is difficult to comment about the clinical pregnancy rate as it was not considered as a primary outcome measure in the studies.[26]

GnRH Agonist

Higher hormone concentrations compared to the physiological levels are observed among GnRH-treated women in the early stages of implantation. The increased hormone levels may affect embryonic development rather than improve corpus luteal function.[27] GnRH agonist has an LH-releasing property, therefore, the use of intranasal GnRH spray can replace the use of hCG and be followed up by progesterone supplementation. However, there is conflicting evidence from two different studies about the benefit of using GnRH. A study by Pirard et al.[28] showed that the use of GnRH nasal spray three times a day along with progesterone supplementation is compatible with normal implantation and pregnancy and is as effective as hCG administration followed by progesterone. However, Hugues et al.[27] showed that administration of a GnRH analog and progesterone on the day of embryo transfer and 3 days after embryo replacement versus no GnRH did not show any benefit.

Ovarian Stimulation Regimen

The first IVF pregnancy was ectopic and the first child was conceived in a natural cycle IVF.[29] The aim of the superovulation technique is to enable women to produce a large number of oocytes so that more embryos can be created, giving the best chance of implantation to the

Table 36.1: Evolution of the superovulation regime over the years	
1970s	Natural cycle, Clomiphene
1980s	Clomiphene and u-hMG
	Analog and u-hMG, flare, ultra short and short protocols
1990s	Analogs + u-FSH (im)
	Analogs + HP-FSH (sc)
	Analogs + r-FSH (sc)
Late 1990s-2000+	Antagonists + r-hFSH
	+ r-hLH
	+ r-hCG

highest grade of embryo. However, this technique has its own disadvantages as well. Ovarian stimulation and the resultant supraphysiological estradiol concentrations have a negative impact on endometrial receptivity.[30,31] This impact is probably due to the advanced endometrial maturation and defective induction of progesterone receptors. Therefore, over the years, ovarian stimulation regimes have been modified to improve and achieve the best outcome. Table 36.1 shows the evolution of the superovulation regime over the years.

Urinary FSH has been largely replaced by recombinant FSH (r-FSH). The American Society for Reproductive Medicine (ASRM) stated in their Practice Committee report in June, 1998 that 'recombinant FSH was more effective for IVF than urinary FSH in stimulating multiple follicular development, and when results from cryopreserved embryos were included, was associated with higher pregnancy rates.' Guidelines from the Royal College of Obstetricians and Gynaecologists (RCOG) commented that ovulation induction with recombinant FSH and human menopausal gonadotropin (hMG) yield similar pregnancy and ovarian hyperstimulation rates. Benefit should be assessed following a comparison of the cost of the medication (Grade A recommendation). For women with hypogonadotropic hypogonadism (WHO group I), treatment with hMG was reported to be more effective than FSH alone.[32] A systematic review of 14 RCTs found no significant difference between hMG and u-FSH with regard to pregnancy rate per cycle, miscarriage rate, multiple pregnancy rate, ovulation rate per cycle or ovarian hyperstimulation rate per cycle.[33] There was also no significant difference between recombinant FSH and urinary FSH in patients with polycystic ovary syndrome.[34] Table 36.2 summarizes the advantages of r-FSH.

Basir et al.[35] showed that ovarian stimulation either has no effect on endometrial maturation several days after ovulation or it causes endometrial delay. However, Ma et al.[36] showed that high levels of estrogen affect the duration of uterine

Table 36.2: Advantages of r-FSH
• Logical pharmaceutical process
• Controlled manufacture
• More homogeneous effect
• Potentially unlimited supply, independent of urinary supply
• Greater purity and specificity, hence no risk of contamination or infection
• Less traumatic subcutaneous injection
• Smaller doses needed
• More predictable cost
• Reduced batch to batch variability

Table 36.3: The relative significance of factors that influence the success of embryo transfer[50-51]	
Factors	*Score/10*
Removal of hydrosalpinges	6.8
Absence of blood/mucus	6.6
Type of catheter	6.1
Not touching fundus	5.8
Avoiding tenaculum	5.7
Removal of cervical mucus	5.2
Prior ultrasound of the cavity	4.3
Leave catheter in place for 1 min	4.2
Bed rest for 30 min	3.8
Trial ET	3.1
Ultrasound monitoring of ET	2.6
Antiprostaglandin treatment	1.9

receptive phase.[36] Increasing awareness about the possible adverse effect of standard stimulation protocol has helped to develop a milder approach to ovarian hyperstimulation. A randomized comparison of two ovarian stimulation protocols with GnRH antagonist co-treatment for IVF, commencing recombinant FSH on cycle day 2 or 5 and the standard GnRH agonist protocol showed that delay in starting FSH as late as day 5 results in a similar clinical IVF outcome. The quality of embryos in the mild stimulation group was shown to be better than that in the conventional protocol and with better outcomes in patients with a poor oocyte yield.[37] Individualizing the dose of r-FSH is another approach to obtain higher pregnancy rate. A model developed by Popovic-Todrovic et al.[38,39] used screening methods like number of antral follicles, ovarian volume and smoking habits. They showed that using this model, the individualized dose could help to obtain higher pregnancy rates than the standard 150 IU/day dose.[38,39]

Though the conventional long protocol achieves a higher number of oocytes, mild stimulation helps to develop a higher number of euploid embryos per oocyte obtained.[40] This may be attributed to natural selection during follicular development, which may be suppressed in the conventional maximal stimulation group.

Embryo Transfer Technique

Depth of transfer: The technique of embryo transfer has been reviewed in various studies as a way of improving the ART outcome. Traditionally, embryo transfer has been performed blindly with the aim of placing the embryo 1 cm below the fundus.[41] However, later studies showed that transferring the embryo lower in the uterine cavity improves the implantation rate. Better results were obtained when the catheter tip was placed in the middle of the uterine cavity.[42] Another randomized study showed higher implantation rates when the embryos were deposited 2 cm from fundus.[43] Pope et al.[44] suggested that for every additional decrease in the distance of embryo transfer by 1 cm from fundus, the odds of clinical pregnancy rate increased by 11 percent. It also lowers the ectopic pregnancy rate.[44] The postulated disadvantage of embryo transfer in the uterine segment is the increased risk of placenta previa. There is a six-fold higher risk of placenta previa in pregnancies conceived by assisted fertilization.[45]

Ultrasound-guided embryo transfer: Ultrasound-guided embryo transfer can also improve the chance of implantation compared to blind transfer. A meta-analysis of four RCTs comparing ultrasound-guided embryo transfer versus clinical touch showed a significantly higher pregnancy rate and implantation rate (1.38, 95%CI 1.20–1.60) following ultrasound-guided embryo transfer compared to clinical touch.[46]

Effect of infection: The role of bacterial vaginosis (BV), as a cause of reduced implantation rate in assisted reproduction, has been questioned over the years. Salim et al.[47] reported a significantly higher pregnancy rate among women without cervical colonization (37%) versus women with BV (16.3%).[47]

Choice of catheter: Softer catheters, such as the Wallace and Cook catheters, are more effective than hard catheters. Wood and associates[48] have shown that the pregnancy rate with soft catheters is higher than that obtained with hard catheters (36% vs 19%, respectively). Table 36.3 shows the relative significance of techniques and variables affecting the success of embryo transfer on a score of 10.[49,50]

Selecting the Optimal Embryo and Endometrium

Improved selection of the embryo and the optimum endometrial environment remains the key to improve implantation. In recent years, embryologists have made progress in improving embryo quality and selection for transfer. Preimplantation genetic diagnosis and screening for embryo aneuploidy has improved the selection of the best embryo.[51] Assisted hatching,[52] *in vitro* maturation,[53] and the use of sequential media[54] help to improve the implantation rate.

Parallel to these methods, preconception assessment of endometrial receptivity offers the potential of correcting and optimizing receptivity prior to embryo transfer. No single highly sensitive, specific and non-invasive marker has so far been identified, which will detect endometrial receptivity. So far, integrins, glycodelin and leukemia inhibitory factor have been proposed as mediators that can alter endometrial receptivity.[55,56] There is also evidence that the development of functional receptivity depends in part upon signals from the embryo. In experimental animals, the ability of the embryo to modulate endometrial receptivity has been demonstrated.[57,58] Microarray analysis of endometrial gene expression may allow classification of the endometrium into receptive and non-receptive.[59] However, there are no appropriate clinical studies so far to provide the evidence base for practical use.

A Japanese study[60] has suggested that stimulation of endometrium embryo transfer (SEET) by injecting the embryo culture supernatant into the uterus before blastocyst transfer can improve the implantation and pregnancy rate for patients undergoing ART for the first time.

CONCLUSION

Over the last 30 years, there have been revolutionary changes in Reproductive Medicine and the treatment of infertile patients. However, improving the implantation rate is still the biggest challenge for clinicians. The increasing legal trend for single embryo transfer has also highlighted the need for improving the implantation rate and a successful pregnancy outcome. Possible methods have been discussed and reviewed in this chapter. The technique of embryo transfer and choosing the optimal dose of ovarian stimulation carries the highest importance in achieving a higher implantation rate. The type of catheter and embryo transfer position have a role in obtaining better success rates. Adjuvant pharmacological therapies have been reviewed in the light of available evidence but their efficacy and safety profile is limited so these agents should be used only in a research set-up. Preconceptual counseling about optimal health status should be discussed with the couple before embarking on fertility treatment. Simple methods, like weight loss, can help to improve the pregnancy rate, therefore, patient awareness about this matter is important. Multiple factors are responsible for implantation failure. A better understanding of uterine receptivity and physiological chemical agents controlling it is needed.

REFERENCES

1. Bergh PA, Navot D. The impact of embryonic development and endometrial maturity on the timing of implantion. Fertil Steril 1992;57:537-42.

2. Lintsen AM, Pasker-de Jong PC, de Boer EJ, Burger CW, Jansen CA, Braat DD, van Leeuwen FE. Effects of subfertility cause, smoking and body weight on the success rate of IVF. Hum Reprod 2005;20:1867-75.

3. Boxmeer JC, Brouns RM, Lindemans J, Steegers EA, Martini E, Macklon NS, et al. Preconception folic acid treatment affects the microenvironment of the maturing oocyte in humans. Fertil Steril 2008;89:1766-70.

4. Klontoff-Cohen H, Bleha J, Lam-Kruglick P. A prospective study of the effect of female and male caffeine consumption on the reproductive endpoint of IVF and gamete intra-fallopian transfer. Hum Reprod 2002;17:1746-54.

5. Stern C, Chamley L, Norris H, Hale L, Baker HW. A randomized, double-blind, placebo-controlled trial of heparin and aspirin for women with *in vitro* fertilization implantation failure and antiphospholipid or antinuclear antibodies. Fertil Steril 2003;80:376-83.

6. Khairy M, Banerjee K, El-Toukhy T, Coomarasamy A, Khalaf Y. Aspirin in women undergoing *in vitro* fertilization treatment: a systematic review and meta-analysis. Fertil Steril 2007;88:822-31.

7. Battaglia C, Salvatori M, Maxia N, Petraglia F, Facchinetti F, Volpe A. Adjuvant L-arginine treatment for *in vitro* fertilization in poor responder patients. Hum Reprod 1999;14:1690-7.

8. Battaglia C, Regnani G, Marsella T, Facchinetti F, Volpe A, Venturoli S, Flamigni C. Adjuvant L-arginine treatment in controlled ovarian hyperstimulation: A double-blind, randomized study. Hum Reprod 2002;17:659-65.

9. Mitwally MF, Casper RF. Use of an aromatase inhibitor for induction of ovulation in patients with an inadequate response to clomiphene citrate. Fertil Steril 2001;75:305-9.

10. Mitwally MF, Casper RF. Potential of aromatase inhibitors for ovulation and superovulation induction in infertile women. Drugs 2006;66:2149-60.

11. Luck MR, Jeyaseelan I, Scholes RA. Ascorbic acid and fertility. Biol Reprod 1995;52:262-6. Review.

12. Igarashi M. Augmentative effect of ascorbic acid upon induction of human ovulation in clomiphene-ineffective anovulatory women. Int J Fertil 1977;22:168-73.

13. Luck MR, Zhao Y. Identification and measurement of collagen in the bovine corpus luteum and its relationship with ascorbic acid and tissue development. J Reprod Fertil 1993;99:647-52.

14. Griesinger G, Franke K, Kinast C, Kutzelnigg A, Riedinger S, Kulin S, Kaali SG, Feichtinger W. Ascorbic acid supplement during luteal phase in IVF. J Assist Reprod Genet 2002;19:164-8.

15. Lédée-Bataille N, Bonnet-Chea K, Hosny G, Dubanchet S, Frydman R, Chaouat G. Role of the endometrial tripod interleukin-18, -15, and -12 in inadequate uterine receptivity in patients with a history of repeated *in vitro* fertilization-embryo transfer failure. Fertil Steril 2005;83:598–605.

16. Boomsma CM, Keay SD, Macklon NS. Peri-implantation glucocorticoid administration for assisted reproductive technology cycles. Cochrane Database Syst Rev. 2007;(1): CD005996. Review.

17. Jones HW Jr. What has happened? Where are we? Hum Reprod. 1996;11 Suppl 1:7-24.

18. Fanchin R, Righini C, de Ziegler D, Olivennes F, Ledée N, Frydman R. Effects of vaginal progesterone administration on uterine contractility at the time of embryo transfer. Fertil Steril 2001;75:1136-40.

19. Blois SM, Joachim R, Kandil J, Margni R, Tometten M, Klapp BF, Arck PC. Depletion of CD8 + cells abolishes the pregnancy protective effect of progesterone substitution with dydrogesterone in mice by altering the T H 1/T H 2 cytokine profile. J Immunol 2004;172:5893-9.

20. Smitz J, Bourgain C, Van Waesberghe L, Camus M, Devroey P, Van Steirteghem AC. A prospective randomized study on oestradiol valerate supplementation in addition to intravaginal micronized progesterone in buserelin and HMG induced superovulation. Hum Reprod 1993;8:40-5.

21. Lewin A, Benshushan A, Mezker E, Yanai N, Schenker JG, Goshen R. The role of estrogen support during the luteal phase of *in vitro* fertilization-embryo transplant cycles: A comparative study between progesterone alone and estrogen and progesterone support. Fertil Steril 1994;62:121-5.

22. Farhi J, Weissman A, Steinfeld Z, Shorer M, Nahum H, Levran D. Estradiol supplementation during the luteal phase may improve the pregnancy rate in patients undergoing *in vitro* fertilization-embryo transfer cycles. Fertil Steril 2000;73:761-6.

23. Pritts EA, Atwood AK. Luteal phase support in infertility treatment: A meta-analysis of the randomized trials. Hum Reprod 2002;17:2287-99. Review.

24. Lukaszuk K, Liss J, Lukaszuk M, Maj B. Optimization of estradiol supplementation during the luteal phase improves the pregnancy rate in women undergoing *in vitro* fertilization-embryo transfer cycles. Fertil Steril 2005;83:1372-6.

25. Lord JM, Flight IH, Norman RJ. Insulin sensitizing drugs (Metformin, troglitazone, rosiglitazone, pioglitazone, d-chiroinositol) for polycystic ovary syndrome. Cochrane Database of Systematic Reviews 2003, CD003053.

26. Costello MF, Chapman M, Conway U. A systematic review and meta-analysis of randomized controlled trials on metformin co-administration during gonadotrophin ovulation induction or IVF in women with polycystic ovary syndrome. Hum Reprod 2006;21:1387-99.

27. Hugues JN, Cedrin-Durnerin I, Bstanding B, et al. Administration of gonadotrophin releasing hormone agonist during the luteal phase of GnRH – antagonist IVF cycles, 22nd annual meeting of the ESHRE. Hum Reprod 2006; 21.i3 Abstract no 1.0–007.

28. Pirard C, Donnez J, Loumaye E. GnRH agonist as novel luteal support: results of a randomized, parallel group, feasibility study using intranasal administration of buserelin. Hum Reprod 2005;20:1798-1804.

29. Steptoe PC, Edwards RG. Birth after the reimplantation of a human embryo. Lancet 1978;2:366.

30. Simón C, Cano F, Valbuena D, Remohí J, Pellicer A. Clinical evidence for a detrimental effect on uterine receptivity of high serum oestradiol concentrations in high and normal responder patients. Hum Reprod 1995;10:2432-7.

31. Macklon NS, Fauser BC. Impact of ovarian hyperstimulation on the luteal phase. J Reprod Fertil Suppl 2000;55:101-8.

32. Shoham Z, Balen A, Patel A, Jacobs HS. Results of ovulation induction using human menopausal gonadotropin or purified follicle-stimulating hormone in hypogonadotropic hypogonadism patients. Fertil Steril 1991;56:1048-53.

33. Nugent D, Vandekerckhove P, Hughes E, Arnot M, Lilford R. Gonadotrophin therapy for ovulation induction in subfertility associated with polycystic ovary syndrome. Cochrane Database Syst Rev. 2000;(4):CD000410.

34. Bayram N, van Wely M, van Der Veen F. Recombinant FSH versus urinary gonadotrophins or recombinant FSH for ovulation induction in subfertility associated with polycystic ovary syndrome. Cochrane Database Syst Rev 2001;(2):CD002121.

35. Basir GS, O WS, Ng EH, Ho PC. Morphometric analysis of peri-implantation endometrium in patients having excessively high oestradiol concentrations after ovarian stimulation. Hum Reprod 2001;16:435-40.

36. Ma WG, Song H, Das SK, Paria BC, Dey SK. Estrogen is a critical determinant that specifies the duration of the window of uterine receptivity for implantation. Proc Natl Acad Sci USA 2003;100:2963-8.

37. Hohmann FP, Macklon NS, Fauser BC. A randomized comparison of two ovarian stimulation protocols with gonadotropin-releasing hormone (GnRH) antagonist cotreatment for *in vitro* fertilization commencing recombinant follicle-stimulating hormone on cycle day 2 or 5 with the standard long GnRH agonist protocol. J Clin Endocrinol Metab 2003;88:166-73.

38. Popovic-Todorovic B, Loft A, Bredkjaeer HE, Bangsbøll S, Nielsen IK, Andersen AN. A prospective randomized clinical trial comparing an individual dose of recombinant FSH based on predictive factors versus a 'standard' dose of 150 IU/day in 'standard' patients undergoing IVF/ICSI treatment. Hum Reprod 2003;18:2275-82.

39. Popovic-Todorovic B, Loft A, Lindhard A, Bangsbøll S, Andersson AM, Andersen AN. A prospective study of predictive factors of ovarian response in 'standard' IVF/ICSI patients treated with recombinant FSH. A suggestion for a recombinant FSH dosage normogram. Hum Reprod 2003;18:781-7.

40. Baart EB, Van Opstal D, Eijkemans MJ, et al. Does the magnitude of ovarian stimulation for IVF affect chromosomal competence of embryos as assesses by PGS? 21st Annual Meeting of the ESHRE. Hum Reprod 2005;0–246: I 91-i92.

41. Schoolcraft W. Embryo transfer. In: Gardner D, Weissman A, Howles CM, Sholam K (Eds). Text book of assisted reproductive techniques; Laboratory and clinical perspectives 2001(2nd edn). Taylor and Francis, London p.751.

42. Oliveira JB, Martins AM, Baruffi RL, Mauri AL, Petersen CG, Felipe V, et al. Increased implantation and pregnancy rates obtained by placing the tip of the transfer catheter in the central area of the endometrial cavity. Reprod Biomed Online 2004;9:435-41.

43. Coroleu B, Barri PN, Carreras O, Martínez F, Parriego M, Hereter L, Parera, et al. The influence of the depth of embryo replacement into the uterine cavity on implantation rates after IVF: a controlled, ultrasound-guided study. Hum Reprod 2002;17:341-6.

44. Pope CS, Cook EK, Arny M, Novak A, Grow DR. Influence of embryo transfer depth on *in vitro* fertilization and embryo transfer outcomes. Fertil Steril 2004;81:51-8.

45. Romundstad LB, Romundstad PR, Sunde A, von Düring V, Skjaerven R, Vatten LJ. Increased risk of placenta previa in

pregnancies following IVF/ICSI; a comparison of ART and non-ART pregnancies in the same mother. Hum Reprod 2006;21:2353-8.

46. Buckett WM. A review and meta-analysis of prospective trials comparing different catheters used for embryo transfer. Fertil Steril 2006;85:728-34.

47. Salim R, Ben-Shlomo I, Colodner R, Keness Y, Shalev E. Bacterial colonization of the uterine cervix and success rate in assisted reproduction: Results of a prospective survey. Hum Reprod 2002;17:337-40.

48. Wood EG, Batzer FR, Go KJ, Gutmann JN, Corson SL. Ultrasound-guided soft catheter embryo transfers will improve pregnancy rates in *in vitro* fertilization. Hum Reprod 2000;15: 107-12.

49. Kovacs GT. What factors are important for successful embryo transfer after *in vitro* fertilization? Hum Reprod 1999 r;14:590-2.

50. Schoolcraft WB, Surrey ES, Gardner DK. Embryo transfer: Techniques and variables affecting success. Fertil Steril 2001;76: 863-70.

51. Rubio C, Rodrigo L, Pérez-Cano I, Mercader A, Mateu E, Buendía P, Remohí J, Simón C, Pellicer A. FISH screening of aneuploidies in preimplantation embryos to improve IVF outcome. Reprod Biomed Online 2005;11:497-506.

52. Seif MM, Edi-Osagie EC, Farquhar C, Hooper L, Blake D, McGinlay P. Assisted hatching on assisted conception (IVF and ICSI). Cochrane Database Syst Rev 2005;(4):CD001894.

53. Mikkelsen AL. Strategies in human *in vitro* maturation and their clinical outcome. Reprod Biomed Online 2005;10:593-9.

54. Macklon NS, Pieters MH, Hassan MA, Jeucken PH, Eijkemans MJ, Fauser BC. A prospective randomized comparison of sequential versus monoculture systems for *in vitro* human blastocyst development. Hum Reprod 2002;17:2700-5.

55. Thomas K, Thomson A, Wood S, Kingsland C, Vince G, Lewis-Jones I. Endometrial integrin expression in women undergoing *in vitro* fertilization and the association with subsequent treatment outcome. Fertil Steril 2003;80:502-7.

56. Lédée-Bataille N, Laprée-Delage G, Taupin JL, Dubanchet S, Frydman R, Chaouat G. Concentration of leukaemia inhibitory factor (LIF) in uterine flushing fluid is highly predictive of embryo implantation. Hum Reprod 2002;17:213-8.

57. Godkin JD, Bazer FW, Thatcher WW, Roberts RM. Proteins released by cultured Day 15–16 conceptuses prolong luteal maintenance when introduced into the uterine lumen of cyclic ewes. J Reprod Fertil 1984;71:57-64.

58. Shiotani M, Noda Y, Mori T. Embryo-dependent induction of uterine receptivity assessed by an *in vitro* model of implantation in mice. Biol Reprod 1993;49:794-801.

59. Ponnampalam AP, Weston GC, Trajstman AC, Susil B, Rogers PA. Molecular classification of human endometrial cycle stages by transcriptional profiling. Mol Hum Reprod 2004;10:879-93.

60. Goto S, Kadowaki T, Hashimoto H, Kokeguchi S, Shiotani M. Stimulation of endometrium embryo transfer can improve implantation and pregnancy rates for patients undergoing assisted reproductive technology for the first time with a high-grade blastocyst. Fertil Steril 2009;92:1264-8.

Endometrial Receptivity in Infertility

Sujata Kar

OVERVIEW

Endometrial receptivity is an area of intense research in reproductive biology, probably because implantation is the single most important rate limiting step in assisted reproduction. Barely 10 to 15 percent of all embryos transferred ever end up in conception.

Thus, the focus is now shifting to the 'endometrium'. At a cellular and molecular level, the dynamics of the endometrium is very complex as it undergoes cyclic morphological as well as functional changes in preparation for blastocyst implantation. The exact sequence of events that makes the endometrium receptive to the embryo and allows invasion deep into the maternal tissues is poorly understood.

INTRODUCTION

In vitro fertilization and embryo transfer has come a long way in the last 25 years. Pregnancy rates have improved considerably mostly because of highly researched and easily available culture media, advances in gonadotropin preparations and culture conditions. Different kinds of recombinant and urinary gonadotropins with excellent consistency, bioavailability and ease of administration have flooded the markets. Excellent cycle control, ovulation induction, reduced ovarian hyperstimulation syndrome (OHSS), reduced cycle cancellation, and optimal culture conditions have ensured the production of good quality embryos in the laboratory. Yet, majority of the embryos transferred do not get implanted.

With the focus now shifting to the endometrium, the complex dynamics of the endometrium at the cellular and molecular levels are coming to light. While it is known that the human endometrium undergoes cyclic morphological and functional changes in preparation for blastocyst implantation, the exact sequence of events that lead to endometrial receptivity and facilitate embryo implantation are poorly understood. Potentially, molecular biology could find many links leading to failure of implantation. However, infertility related to endometrial causes remains largely undiscovered. A breakthrough in the understanding of these complex events would have the potential to push assisted reproduction to the next higher levels of success.

CLINICAL DISCUSSION

The Implantation Window

Human implantation is a three stage process that involves apposition, adhesion and invasion. This can take place only during a period of uterine receptivity, which normally lasts between day 20 to 24 (longest) or day 21 to 23 (shortest) in a regular 28 day cycle, or day 7 to 11 post-luteinizing hormone (LH) surge.

Approximately 4 days after the LH surge and 3 days after ovulation, a blastocyst (preimplantation embryo with cell numbers varying from 30 to 200) is formed. Implantation begins with the loss of the zona pellucida (hatching) about 1 to 3 days after the embryo enters the uterine cavity.

The endometrium, very grossly speaking, changes histologically from proliferative to secretory to decidual in the process of becoming receptive to the embryo. However, numerous biochemical and molecular events are involved in bringing about these changes. The growth and progress of the embryo needs to synchronize perfectly with the endometrial events so as to establish a successful pregnancy. The embryo–endometrium cross talk is like a finely orchestrated event, where missing a single beat or a single link can throw the entire performance out of synchrony.

Therefore, the implantation window can be defined as "a self limiting period of uterine receptivity that usually lasts between day 20 to 24 of a normal cycle or 7 to 11 days post LH surge." There is now enough evidence to support the existence of "the implantation window". Studies involving endomertrial dating, scanning electron microscopic studies of pinopodes formation, immunohistochemical determinants of integrins alpha 1β3, alpha 4 β1, alpha 5 β1, leukemia inhibitory factor (LIF), interleukin–1 receptor type, the transmembrane mucin (muc-1), P4 receptor expression and so many such biomolecular markers are available that prove the presence of "a nidation/implantation window".

Knowledge concerning implantation has been gained from a number of animal studies. In some species, there is delayed implantation and the embryo can lie dormant in the uterus for long periods of time, even unto one-to-one and half years.[1] Off course, this does not happen in humans, where the embryo has a very short time to act, or else miss the chance!

The Receptive Endometrium

The primary endocrine requirement for the endometrium is luteal phase progesterone, although the preovulatory hormonal milieu is equally important.

Under the influence of progesterone, the endometrium is 10 to 14 mm thick, secretory activity reaches a peak, and the endometrial cells are rich in glycogen and lipids. In fact, the preimplantation embryo is nourished by the glandular secretions until the end of the first trimester of pregnancy, when significant blood flow begins in the fetomaternal unit.[2]

The biochemical signals to herald endometrial receptivity probably comes from the preimplantation embryo. Even before the blastocyst has entered the uterine cavity, a dialog between the mother and the early embryo begins.

Three well-recognized signals are:
- Early pregnancy factor
- Human chorionic gonadotropin (hCG) from the embryo
- Platelet activating factor.

Early pregnancy factor (EPP) is secreted by the ovary and by the early embryo. It can be detected within 1 to 2 days of fertilization.[3] It promotes growth and cell proliferation and has immunosuppressive properties.

Human chorionic gonadotropins are also secreted by the embryo before implantation.[1] This preimplantation signalling maintains the corpus luteum and increases production of estradiol and progesterone.

Platelet-activating factor is another substance secreted by the preimplantation embryo, which also has immunosuppressive functions.

'Implantation', i.e. the embedding of the blastocyst in the endometrial stroma begins with the shedding of the zona pellucida (hatching). Simultaneously, the endometrium enters the receptive phase. Surface epithelial cells undergo changes, various growth factors, cell surface receptors, and cytokines are secreted by the endometrium. These morphological and biochemical tools help to carry out the physical process of trophoblast adhesion and invasion.

The major hurdle the embryo faces as invasion proceeds is the maternal immune system. Although the embryo is in control, the endometrium has to play a facilitatory role. Human decidual natural killer (NK) cells are massively recruited at the site of embryonic implantation. They differ in many ways from peripheral blood NK cells in terms of gene expression, phenotype and functionality. The major subpopulation of decidual NK cells is CD 56(bright), minor subset CD 56(dim), which is in contrast to peripheral blood whose major subpopulation is CD 56(dim).[4] Decidual NK cell have reduced cytolytic activity and produce cytokines different from peripheral blood NK cells.

Human decidual NK cell potential functions at the maternal-fetal interface are not well-delineated but they have a possible role in the control of extra villous invasion, uterine vascular remodeling and local antiviral activity.

RECENT ADVANCES

Markers of Endometrial Receptivity

Morphological Markers

One of the earliest signs of a receptive endometrium is the appearance of pinopodes. Using electron microscopy, several studies have demonstrated the formation of pinopodes, dome-shaped projections at the apical portion of the endometrial surface epithelium, around the window of implantation that are believed to be important markers for endometrial receptivity. Pinopodes are smooth protrusions of cell membrane of the surface epithelial cells. They appear and regress during the implantation window. Their appearance follows the peak in progesterone levels and decrease in progesterone receptor B in the endometrium.

Pinopodes probably help in absorbing the uterine fluid, forcing the blastocyst to stick to the endometrium thereby, promoting adhesion.

Biochemical Markers (Table 37.1)

The lengthy catalog of biochemical markers, linked with endometrial receptivity, matches the ever-increasing number of scientists working in this field. Following is a brief summary:

The endometrium produces at least three cytokines involved in implantation.[5]
- Colony – stimulating factor – 1 (CSF – 1)
- Leukemia – inhibitory factor (LIF)
- Interleukin – 1(IL-1).

Table 37.1: Some biochemical tools involved in implantation

Cytokines	Growth factor (GF)	Lipids
• Interleukin – 1α	• Vascular endothelial GF	• Prostaglandins
• Interleukin – 1β	• Insulin-like growth factor (IGF)	• Thromboxanes
• Interleukin – 6	IGF – I	**Cell surface receptors**
• Interleukin – γ	IGF – II	• Integrins and selectins
• Colony stimulating factor – 1	IGF – 1-6	• Mucins
• Tumor necrosis factor – α	• Epidermal growth factor (EGF) family	• Peptides
• Leukemia inhibiting factor	EGF	• Calcitonin
	• Transforming growth factor-alpha (TGF-α)	• Ephrins
	• Heparin binding EGF	• Matrix metalloproteinases

Their expression peaks in the deciduas during implantation. Studies in mice have shown that inactivating mutation in CSF-1 or the LIF gene can cause infertility by preventing blastocyst implantation.[6]

Growth Factors

• Epidermal growth factor family
• Insulin-like growth factor (IGF) family
• Vascular endothelial growth factor (VEGF).

Angiogenesis, controlled growth, and appropriate regression are the key to implantation.

The next important group is the whole collection of adhesion molecules, integrins and selectins. They are cell surface receptors that are involved in cell to cell and cell to matrix interactions. Implantation starts with adhesion due to binding with endometrial integrins. Lack of expression of these adhesion molecules during the implantation window can cause infertility.

Thus, the human endometrium is an exquisitely hormone-sensitive tissue that undergoes complex structural and biochemical changes during the menstrual cycle. These changes, now appreciable at the molecular level, are essential for embryonic implantation. Biochemical markers with proposed or demonstrated importance include LIF, HOXA–10, HOXA–11, osteopontin and integrins. Receptors for L–selectin ligands and αVβ3 integrins are localized to the cellular apex of the receptive endometrial surface epithelium where the initial interaction with the embryo occurs.

Despite marked advances in the understanding of endometrial physiology, endometrial receptivity is still a biological mystery. What characterizes receptivity and what controls it, will lead us to understand its relationship to fertility. This knowledge can then be used to either treat infertility or to cause antifertility (contraception).

Genetic Regulation of Endometrial Receptivity

HOX genes are transcriptional regulators that play an essential role in determining tissue identity during embryonic development. HOX genes are involved in the development of the Müllerian system and then continue to be expressed in the adult uterus.[12]

As we know, the endometrium undergoes an ordered process of differentiation, leading to receptivity to embryonic implantation. HOXA 10 and HOXA 11 expression increases during the menstrual cycle, with a drastic increase during the mid-luteal phase at the time of implantation. The expression is regulated by sex steroid hormones, mostly progesterone. This expression is necessary for implantation of the blastocyst, as demonstrated by the decreased implantation rates in women with altered HOX expression.[13] HOX genes are therefore, markers of endometrial receptivity. The possibility of augmenting HOX gene expression with gene therapy to improve implantation has promise for the future.

Clinical Applications

Understanding the complex endocrine behavior of the endometrium and the amazing capability of the embryo to invade and establish itself in the maternal tissues, can be applied to understand many clinical situations.
• Recurrent pregnancy loss.
• Implantation failure following *in vitro* fertilization-embryo transfer (IVF-ET).
• Immunology of maternal tolerance of the fetal allograft.
• Luteal phase defect.
• Controlled ovarian hyperstimulation (COH) and endometrial synchrony/development.

We know that in nature, more that 46 percent of pre-implantation embryos are lost, i.e. when the loss of fertilized oocytes before implantation is included, approximately 46 percent of all pregnancies end up being clinically perceived. Pregnancy loss after implantation is around 30 percent.

The etiology of recurrent pregnancy loss cannot be explained in nearly 50 percent of cases. It is possible that a significant proportion of this loss is due to defects in endometrial receptivity.

Poor implantation is a major challenge in assisted reproduction. The largest percentage of IVF/intracytoplasmic sperm injection (ICSI) cycles simply exhibit failure of implantation in spite of excellent embryos and blastocyst transfer.

Maternal tolerance of the fetal allograft is still a mystery. With oocyte donation pregnancies, it has become obvious that even embryos with no common genetic match to the host can implant and grow to a full term pregnancy. Therefore, invasion and survival of the fetus depends on factors that are capable of suppressing the maternal immune response to the embryonic antigens. The endometrial tissues synthesize immuno-suppressing proteins in response to the blastocyst even before implantation.[7] One of the great mysteries associated with implantation is the mechanism by which the mother rejects a genetically abnormal embryo or fetus. It is possible that the abnormal embryo cannot produce a signal in early pregnancy that can be recognized by the mother.

Luteal phase defects, although considered an ovulatory dysfunction, have profound effects on endometrial development, and may be responsible for recurrent implantation failure and recurrent abortion. Luteal phase progesterone (P) is the pregnancy hormone. *In vivo* studies have shown that P is the only steroid hormone necessary to induce decidualization and decidual prolactin synthesis. Progesterone directs specific protein synthesis by the endometrium, which then facilitates implantation, inhibits uterine prostaglandin production, modulates the maternal immune system [progesterone-induced blocking factor (PIBF)]. Luteal phase deficiency and its impact on endometrial receptivity has a lot of scope for research.

Lastly, an area of intense debate in assisted reproduction is controlled ovarian hyperstimulation (COH) and endometrial dysfunction. COH, following downregulation with gonadotropin-releasing hormone analog (GnRHa), profoundly affects the internal hormonal milieu. It results in supraphysiological levels of estradiol, downregulation of luteinizing hormone (LH) receptors, and defective granulosa cell functions following ovarian oocyte collection. Ovarian stimulation for IVF is known to affect luteal phase function. The endometrium in IVF cycles is subject to an altered endocrinological environment possibly due to a direct effect of COH therapy. Factors affecting the endometrial receptivity in such cycles are poorly understood. Studies also demonstrate a modified endometrial steroid receptor regulation, profound antiproliferative effect and premature expression of pinopodes and integrins.[10]

Further unraveling of molecules involved in the implantation mechanisms is needed for a better understanding of the link between altered endometrial development and receptivity in IVF cycles. There are now enough studies to show that COH with GnRHa results in significant luteal phase endometrial defects.[8-11] There is early luteal advancement and mid-luteal delay. Additionally, there is asynchrony between stromal and glandular development. Therefore, a change in concept is required. We need to understand that extreme fine turning between endometrial maturity and embryo development is required. Synchronizing embryo transfer and opening of the implantation window may be much more difficult than we realize.

Clinical Strategies to Assess Endometrial Receptivity

Currently, ultrasonography and Doppler assessment of the endometrium is used to assess the quality and functionality of the endometrium in assisted reproductive techniques (ART) cycles. Endometrial function tests, which assess the presence of biochemical markers of endometrial receptivity are also available now. Following are the various methods to assess endometrial receptivity.

Endometrial Biopsy for Histology

Endometrial biopsy during the luteal phase is the gold standard to evaluate endometrial maturity in relation to ovarian steroid cycle, and is based on the criteria defined by Noyes et al.[14] In 1950, however, with the availability of hormone assays and transvaginal sonography, it has become obsolete. Scanning electron microscopy for the appearance of pinopodes, though a better indicator of endometrial receptivity, is expensive, and not available universally. Additionally, for obvious reasons, it is not practical to carry out a biopsy in a treatment cycle.

Ultrasound and Doppler

This is based on the sonographic changes in the endometrium cyclically, dependant on varying levels of estrogen and progesterone. Additionally, the entire uterine vasculature undergoes marked changes during the menstrual cycle. There is increased vascularity and low impedance to blood flow in the secretory phase. The number of sonographic variables can be combined to formulate endometrial receptivity scoring (Table 37.2), also called uterine biophysical profile or ultrasound scoring system (USS) that have been proposed to positively correlate with pregnancy rates.[15,16]

Endometrial Thickness and Morphology

It is generally accepted that endometrial thickness correlates with endometrial function, although there is insufficient data

Table 37.2: Variables for ultrasound scoring system for uterine receptivity	
• Endometrial thickness	• ≥ 9 vs < 9 mm
• Endometrial morphology	• Trilaminar vs non-layering
• Myometrial echogenicity	• Homogenous vs non-homogenous
• Uterine A Doppler	
• Pulsatility index (PI)	• ≤ 3 vs >3
• Resistance index (RI)	• ≤ 0.9 vs > 0.9
• Telediastolic flow	• Present vs absent
• Protodiastolic notch	• Present vs absent

to prove a linear positive correlation between endometrial thickness and the probability of pregnancy.[17] A trilaminar endometrium is considered morphologically ideal, compared to non-layering or homogeneity. An endometrium, which is homogenous, echogenic and less than 6 mm will probably not support a pregnancy.[18]

Endometrial Volume using 2D or 3D Scan

Three-dimensional (3D) estimation of endometrial volume has recently emerged as a new efficient predictor of endometrial response to hormonal stimulation. An endometrial volume <2 mL signifies low endometrial receptivity. A volume >2 mL on the day of embryo transfer could be a positive indicator of ART outcome.[19,20]

Uterine and Ovarian Doppler

A number of studies provide evidence that there is an association between utero-ovarian perfusion and reproductive outcome following IVF treatment. Uterine artery pulsatality index (PI) ≤ 3 has been associated with a favorable outcome.

The chance of achieving a pregnancy was shown to be low in women where uterine artery Doppler and perifollicular blood flow PI values were higher than 3.26 and RI values were higher than 1.08.[21] Therefore, these blood flow studies can be used to identify women whose pregnancy chances are significantly limited.

Endometrial and Sub-endometrial Blood Flow Assessment using 2D/3D Power Doppler

Recent advances in 3D ultrasonography have made studies of uterine receptivity more accurate. The degree of endometrial perfusion by color Doppler and 3D power Doppler studies on the day of embryo transfer can indicate a favorable endometrial milieu for successful outcome in IVF-ET.[22]

Endometrial visualization, as assessed by color flow mapping and power Doppler, is performed to determine vascularization index (VI), flow index (FI), and vascularization flow index (VFI). Endometrial blood flow is categorized as subendometrial, basal layer, mid-zone, inner layer and cavity. The deeper the vascularization better the outcome. Failure of vascularization into and beyond the basal layer is associated with a uniformly poor outcome.

Endometrial Contractions

Endometrial and myometrial contractions are observed on sonography regularly. The presence or lack of presence of these contractions possibly has some role in the successful establishment of pregnancy, even though this role has not been identified.[18]

Evaluation of Biochemical Markers

Kits for immunohistochemical evaluation of some biomarkers are commercially available now.

β-3 Integrins

The appearance of β-3 integrins on the epithelial lining of the endometrium correlates well with the timing of implantation. There are three typical patterns of integrin expression as assessed by test results

- β-3 integrin positive with an "in phase" endometrium—this is a normal pattern of expression.
- β-3 integrins negative with an "out of phase" endometrium as in the case of luteal phase defect (LPD).
- β-3 integrins negative with a normal 'in phase' endometrium. This is often associated with unexplained infertility, minimal or mild endometriosis or hydrosalpinx.[23-25]

Cyclin E and P_{27}

Glandular cyclin E and P_{27} expression changes in intensity and subcellular localization throughout the menstrual cycle. Thus, they may be clinically useful markers of endometrial development.[26]

For these tests, a carefully timed endometrial biopsy must be planned in a non-ART cycle. Usually, the specimen is collected on cycle days 20 to 24 (7–10 days post LH surge).

CONCLUSION

The Future

Elucidating the functional genomics of the endometrium will dominate research in the future. New molecular tools will allow us to know the gene expression pattern of the endometrium at the time of implantation by comparing receptive versus non-receptive endometrium.

The endometrial genomic profile may be a more reliable and accurate predictor of endometrial receptivity than morphology.

We hope, a time will come when it will be possible to test for onset of "the window of implantation" just as we test for onset of the "LH surge" today.

REFERENCES

1. Leon Speroff, Marc A. Fritz, Clinical Gynaecologic Endocrinology and Infertility, (7th ed). Lippincott Williams and Wilkins 2005.
2. Burton GJ, Watson AL, Hempstock J, Skepper JN, Jauniaux E. Uterine glands provide histiotrophic nutrition for the human fetus during the first trimester of pregnancy. J Clin Endocrinol Metab 2002;87:2954-9.
3. Morton H, Rolfe BE, Cavanagh AC. Pregnancy proteins: basic concepts and clinical applications. Seminars Reprod Endocrinol 1992;10:72.
4. Tabiasco J, Robot M. Human decidual NK cells: Unique phenotype and functional properties—a review. Placenta 2006; 27:1034-5.
5. Simon C, Gimeno MJ, Mercader A, Frences A, Velasco JG, Remohi J, Polan ML, Pellicer A. Cytokines—adhesion molecules- invasive proteinases. The missing paracrine/autocrine link in embryonic implantation? Mol Hum Reprod 1996;2:405-24.
6. Aghajanora l. Leukemia inhibitory factor and human embryo implantation. Ann NY Acad Sci 2004;1034:176-83.
7. Clark DA, Slapsys RM, Croy BA, Kreck J, Rossant J. Local active suppression by suppressor cells in the deciduas: A review. Am J Reprod Immunol 1984;6:78-83.
8. Horcajados JA, Riesewijk A. Effect of controlled ovarian hyperstimulation in IVF on endometrial gene expression profiles. Mol Hum Reprod 2005;11:195-205.
9. Devroey P, Bourgan C, Macklon NS, Fauser BC. Reproductive biology and IVF: Ovarian stimulation and Endometrial receptivity trends. Endocrinol Metab 2004;84-90.
10. Bourgain C, Devroey P. The endometrium in stimulated cycles for IVF. Hum Reprod Update 2003;9:515-22.
11. Fauser BC, Devroey P. Reproductive biology and IVF; ovarian stimulation and luteal phase consequences. Trends Endocrinol Metab 2003;14:236-42.
12. Taylor HS. The role of HOX genes in human implantation. Hum Reprod Update 2000;6:75-9.
13. Eun knon H, Taylor HS. The role of HOX genes in human implantation. Ann NY Acad Sci 2004;1034:1-18.
14. Noyes RW, Hertig AT, Rock J. Dating the endometrial biopsy. Fertil steril 1950;1:3-25.
15. Baruffi RL, Contart P, Mauri AL, Petersen C, Felipe V, Garbellini E, Franco JG. A uterine scoring system as a method for the Prognosis of embryo implantation. J Assit Reprod Genet 2002; 19:99-102.
16. Sepulveda J, Hermandez S, Santos R, Galache P, Flores H, Patrizio P. Predicting Pregnancy in IVF Patients using an ultrasonographic score prognostic system. Fertil Steril 2005;84 (Supp 1):0-282.
17. Friedler S, Schenker JG, Herman A, Lewis A. The role of ultrasonography in the evaluation of endometrial receptivity follow assisted reproductive treatments, a critical review. Hum Reprod Update 1996;2:323-5.
18. Pierson RA. Imaging the endometrium; are there any predictors of uterine receptivity? J Obstet Gynaecol Can 2003;25:360-8.
19. No authors listed. Measurement endometrial volume and endometrial thickness for assessment of endometrial receptivity in ART, Akush Ginecol (saffia); 2005;44(suppl 2);27-33.
20. Raqa F, Bonilla Musoles F, Casan EM, Klein O, Bonilla F. Assessment of endometrial volume by 3D ultrasound prior to embryo transfer: Clues to endometrial receptivity. Hum Reprod 1999;14:2851-4.
21. Ozturk O, Bhattacharya S, Saridogan E, Jauniaux E, Templeton A. Role of utero-ovarian vascular impedance: Predictor of on going pregnancy in an IVF—ET Programme. Reprod Biomed Online 2004;9:299-305.
22. Kupesic S. Three dimensional ultrasonographic uterine vascularization and embryo implantation. J Gynecol Obstet Biol Reprod (Paris) 2004;33:S 18-20.
23. Lessey BA, Castlebaum AJ, Sawin SW, Sun J. Integrins as markers of uterine receptivity in women with primary unexplained infertility. Fertil Steril 1995;63:535-42.
24. Lessey BA, Castlebaum AJ, Sawin SW, Buck CA, Schinnar R, Bilker W, Storm BL. Aberrant integrin expression in the endometrium of women with endometriosis, J Clin Endocrinol Metab. 1994;79:643-9.
25. Meyer WR, Castlebaum AJ, Somkuti S, Sagokin AW, Doyle M, Harris JE, Lessey BA. Hydrosalpinges adveresely affects markers of endometrial receptivity. Human Rep 1997;12:1393-8.
26. Dubowy RL, Feinberg RF, Keefe DL, Doncel GF, Williams SC, McSweet JC, Kliman HJ. Improved endometrial assessment using cyclin E and p 27. Fertil Steril 2003;80:146–56.

Management of a Persistently Thin Endometrium

Murat Berkkanoglu, Kemal Ozgur

OVERVIEW

Establishment of a pregnancy depends upon successful implantation, involving a complex series of interactions between the uterus and the blastocyst. Asynchrony between embryo development and endometrial differentiation is critical,[1] thus delineating a bifactorial, transient, but well-defined, period when implantation can ensue. This is commonly referred to as the 'implantation' or 'nidation window.' Assisted reproductive technique (ART) cycles allow us to understand human biology in detail and to develop some objective clinical parameters to measure and, in turn, to determine successful implantation. An adequate thickness of endometrium is indispensable for a successful pregnancy in ART cycles.[2-7] However, criteria for adequacy of endometrium for a successful pregnancy are still controversial. High-resolution ultrasonography serves as a non-invasive method, using endometrial pattern and thickness as parameters to assess endometrial receptivity. From the infertility point of view, pregnancy does not practically occur if the thickness of the endometrium is below 6 mm.[8] A minimal endometrial thickness of 7 to 8 mm appears to be a prerequisite for successful embryo implantation.[9,10] If Asherman's syndrome is not an underlying cause for a thin endometrium, some clinicians use low-dose Aspirin, vaginal Sildenafil, vaginal administration of micronized estradiol, antifibrotic treatment with pentoxifylline, high-dose vitamin E, or gonadotropin releasing hormone (GnRH) agonist to improve the reproductive outcome. However, the results of these medications are also controversial. Larger cohort studies are needed to evaluate the results efficiently.

RATIONALE

The objective of this chapter is to investigate the relationship between a thin endometrium, measured by ultrasound, and the reproductive outcome of assisted reproductive techniques and to address the widespread discrepancy of outcomes in the literature.

INTRODUCTION

Infertility and recurrent pregnancy losses are an enduring problem to women's health. Establishment of a pregnancy depends upon successful implantation, involving a complex series of interactions between heterogenous cell types of the uterus and the blastocyst. Implantation begins with apposition when the free-floating blastocyst-stage embryo is captured by the uterine luminal epithelium. During this period, it can be easily dislodged.[11] Shortly thereafter, the blastocyst firmly adheres to the uterine wall and the trophoblast transmigrates across the luminal epithelium, burying the embryo beneath the epithelial surface. Trophoblast adhesion to the uterine wall is the requisite first step of implantation and subsequent placentation. A synchrony between embryo development and endometrial differentiation is critical,[1] thus delineating a bifactorial, transient, but well-defined, period when implantation can ensue. This is commonly referred to as the 'implantation' or 'nidation window.' Various architectural, cellular, biochemical, and molecular events in the endometrium are coordinated within the 'implantation window' and constitute essential elements in the repertoire that signifies endometrial receptivity.

Assisted reproductive technique (ART) cycles allow us to understand human biology in detail and to develop some objective clinical parameters to measure and in turn, to determine successful implantation. As endometrial biopsy is invasive and hormonal milieu assessment inaccurate, the need to evaluate endometrial development encouraged the use of high-resolution ultrasonography as an alternative non-invasive method of assessment for uterine receptivity. An adequate thickness of endometrium is indispensable for a successful pregnancy in ART cycles.[2-7] However, criteria for adequacy of the endometrium for a successful pregnancy are still controversial.

The endometrium thickens during the proliferative phase of the menstrual cycle in response to estrogen secretion by maturing follicles. The thickened endometrium provides a site for embryo attachment and is the source of nourishment for an implanting embryo during its first few weeks until the placenta develops. While there is little doubt that a physiologically thickened endometrium is critical to a successful implantation and pregnancy, controversy exists regarding the clinical significance of variation in endometrial thickness observed among patients undergoing assisted reproduction. Previous observational studies reported conflicting results with regard to the association between endometrial thickness and pregnancy rate (PR) after *in vitro* fertilization (IVF) and embryo transfer (ET). Several studies have suggested a correlation between endometrial thickness and receptivity, reporting significantly greater endometrial thickness for pregnancy versus non-pregnancy cycles of either autologous[2,12,13] or donor oocyte[14] IVF, or significantly higher PRs with thicker versus thinner endometrial linings in autologous[5,13,15-18] or donor-oocyte[4,19,20] IVF cycles. Some studies reported no successful pregnancies with an endometrial thickness below a threshold of 6 to 9 mm,[9,21-24] although the number of embryo transfers to patients with linings below these thresholds were very small (n = 5 and 15, respectively),[23,24] or were not reported.[9,21,22] In contrast, many studies reported no correlation between endometrial thickness and PRs with either autologous[9,10,23-28] or donor-oocyte[29,30] IVF. Weissman et al.[31] addressed the question of endometrial thickness and PRs by questioning whether there was a maximal value for endometrial thickness above which pregnancy is unlikely to occur. They found that in their patient population, PRs were significantly lower above a maximum thickness of 14 mm, and they also suggested a possible increase in spontaneous abortion rates. Similarly, Dickey et al.[16] reported increased biochemical pregnancy rates with an endometrial thickness ≥14 mm, and Rashidi et al.[24] reported no pregnancies with an endometrial thickness >12 mm (n = 9). However, other studies refuted these findings, reporting similar PRs with endometrial measurements <14 mm and >14 mm.[32-34]

CLINICAL DISCUSSION

Diagnosis

High-resolution ultrasonography serves as a non-invasive alternative method of diagnosis using endometrial pattern and thickness as parameters to assess endometrial receptivity.[35,36]

Sonographic appearance of the endometrium is known to change during the menstrual cycle, eliciting a hypoechoic texture with a well-defined central echogenic line during the proliferative phase and hyperechogenic texture lacking central echogenic line during the secretory phase.[21,37] Lack of a homogeneous hyperechogenic sonographic echo pattern by the mid-luteal phase has also been found to be associated with decreased fecundity in infertile women not receiving follicle maturing drugs or patients undergoing IVF using controlled ovarian hyperstimulation.[38] There is evidence, however, that ovarian stimulation may have an adverse effect on implantation.[39,40] The fact that 32.5 percent patients undergoing oocyte retrievals had a non-homogeneous hyperechogenic pattern three days post-embryo transfer versus only 12.7 percent undergoing frozen embryo transfer could suggest that at least some individuals with adverse implantation factors following ovarian stimulation can be identified by observing a non-homogeneous hyperechogenic pattern in the luteal phase.[41] Increasing evidence indicates that echogenic patterns of the endometrium reflect histologic processes that are involved in the establishment of receptivity. This constitutes a possible explanation for premature hyperechogenic patterns of the endometrium and poor implantation rates.[42,43] However, a few investigators, studying the relationship between sonographic measurements of the endometrium during the luteal phase and histologic dating of endometrial biopsy, have found no clear correlation.[44-46] Some researchers[47,48] opine that the absence of a hyperechogenic pattern in the luteal phase was an indication for further evaluation. Grunfeld et al.[47] demonstrated that in women where the endometrial histology demonstrated asynchrony of the glands and stroma, the sonographic echo pattern correlated with stromal dating but not with glandular dating, probably due to increased echogenicity because of stromal edema. Hyperechoic endometrial area ratio dating has also been demonstrated to correlate with the histologic dating.[48] It is, however, not known whether a non-homogeneous hyperechogenic mid-luteal phase echo pattern predicts sub-fertility even in women with in-phase endometrial biopsies.

There has also been considerable controversy concerning the value of endometrial thickness in the prediction of endometrial receptivity.[49] Endometrial thickness is the minimal distance between the echogenic interfaces of the myometrium and endometrium, measured in the plane through the central longitudinal axis of the uterine body. Ultrasonographic measurements have showed that the endometrial thickness ranges from 1 to 4 mm in the menstrual phase, 4 to 8 mm in the mid-proliferative phase, 8 to 14 mm in the late follicular phase, and 7 to 14 mm in the secretory phase.[50,51] There is still no consensus on the description of a 'thin endometrium'. Oral contraceptives maintain a very thin, flat endometrium with a thickness of 1–3 mm, even in the late follicular phase.[51]

On the contrary, from the infertility point of view, pregnancy does not practically occur if the thickness of endometrium is below 6 mm.[8] A minimal endometrial thickness of 7 to 8 mm appears to be a prerequisite for successful embryo implantation.[9,10] If the endometrial thickness is increased, it is associated with improved pregnancy rates in *in vitro* fertilization and embryo transfer (IVF-ET) cycles.[5] Several groups have reported significantly higher mean endometrial thickness in conception compared with non-conception cycles.[36,52] According to Kovacs et al.[53] higher pregnancy rates were observed in subjects where endometrial thickness reached at least 10 mm. However, pregnancy outcome in certain studies have found no such association.[26,10] Successful implantation has been reported to occur even when endometrial thickness was <4 mm.[54] According to Remohi et al.[29] cycles with an endometrial thickness of <6 mm yielded implantation and pregnancy rates comparable to those with an endometrial thickness of 7 to 9 mm, 9 to 11 mm or >12 mm at the time of oocyte donation. This is in agreement with the findings of Schild et al.[55] showing lack of relationship between mean endometrial thickness on the day of oocyte retrieval and IVF outcome. However, despite the endometrial thickness and pattern having no influence on the pregnancy rate in an IVF-ET cycle, patients with a triple line endometrial pattern and endometrial thickness of 10 to 14 mm showed better pregnancy outcomes.[56]

Donor oocyte programs suggest that a pregnancy cannot be achieved if the endometrial thickness is below a certain critical cut-off limit. Although some studies show that the thickness of the endometrium for successful implantation can be as thin as 4 mm,[17,41,54] in the majority of the cases, an endometrial thickness of at least 6 mm is required for successful implantation.[8] Some studies have proposed a thickness of 7 mm,[22,55,57] and even 8 mm[4,7,58-60] for successful implantation.

According to Zhang et al.[5] endometrial thickness has predictive value for treatment outcome in young patients, in patients who require prolonged gonadotropin stimulation, or in those who have poor quality embryos. The absence of an association between endometrial thickness and pregnancy rates in the older patients might be due to the dominant impact of age *per se* on pregnancy rates.

The ability to accurately quantify the endometrial volume, using 3D transvaginal ultrasound, has helped to predict endometrial receptivity much more accurately as compared to endometrial thickness.[61] An endometrial volume of >2 mL has been found to be a prerequisite for good endometrial receptivity.[62] While no pregnancy was achieved with an endometrial volume of <1 mL, an increase in volume beyond 2 mL does not necessarily increase the chances of conception.[55] It is conceivable that once minimum endometrial growth has

been attained, factors playing a substantial role in embryo–endometrial interaction during early implantation appear necessary.[63]

Steer et al.[64,65] found a statistically significant difference in blood flow impedance, as expressed by pulsatility index (PI), between pregnant and non-pregnant women and suggested the use of Doppler measurements to predict uterine receptivity in assisted conception programs. Significantly higher implantation rates have been observed following IVF-ET in patients with a PI of < 3.00 compared to those with a high PI (≥3.00).[66] In contrast, however, several investigators did not find any association between uterine blood flow and pregnancy rate in patients undergoing assisted reproductive procedures and have challenged the predictive value of this method.[10,67]

If Asherman's syndrome is present, the thin endometrium is related to the physical obliteration of the cavity by adhesions. If the endocervical canal is blocked by adhesions or there are pockets of residual endometrium with no route for regress, cyclic pelvic pain can ensue. The remaining endometrium, however, may be atrophic due to limited local exposure to circulating hormones, as uterine perfusion is impaired in Asherman's syndrome.[68] This appears to be a consequence of myometrial fibrosis, which is significantly increased in women with intrauterine adhesions (IUA) compared with controls.[69]

Hysteroscopy represents the gold standard for the diagnosis of IUA. Comparatively, sonohysterography and hysterosalpingography have a sensitivity of 75 percent with positive predictive values of about 43 percent and 50 percent, respectively.[70]

Treatment

When Asherman's syndrome is present, the extent and location of IUA are best defined with hysteroscopy and they can simultaneously be treated. Surgical lysis of IUA should be performed hysteroscopically since blind adhesiolysis, for example by curettage, is likely to be less precise.[71] Hysterotomy for IUA is no longer used, except under extenuating circumstances for the most severe of cases.[72] The goal of hysteroscopic lysis of adhesions is to restore the normal anatomy of the uterus.

In other cases of thin endometrium, some clinicians may choose to freeze all the embryos when the endometrium is less than 7 mm and transfer them after stimulation with high-dose estrogens. However, others, to improve the uterine blood flow, which may boost endometrial development, have been using low-dose Aspirin, vaginal Sildenafil, vaginal administration of micronized estradiol, antifibrotic treatment with pentoxifylline, high-dose vitamin E, or gonadotropin releasing hormone (GnRH) agonist.

There are many controversial studies regarding the effect of low-dose Aspirin on pregnancy rates. Although some studies have shown that low-dose Aspirin can improve endometrial thickness, pattern, and endometrial blood flow,[59,73] others have not found Aspirin to have beneficial effects on such parameters influencing the success of implantation.[74,75]

Another option for the treatment of a thin endometrium is estrogen administration. However, most studies come from the frozen embryo transfer cycles. It was found that the mean endometrial thickness in the study group increased significantly from 6.7 to 8.6 mm following extended estrogen therapy for 14 to 82 days. The pregnancy rate in the study group was significantly higher than that in the control group (38.5% vs 4.3%, respectively).[76]

Vaginal Sildenafil citrate has also been used in the treatment of women with a thin endometrium. Sildenafil citrate, a phosphodiesterase-5 inhibitor, potentiates the vasodilatory effects of native nitric oxide, which in turn, may increase the endometrial blood flow. Vaginal Sildenafil citrate suppositories have been shown to be helpful in increasing the endometrial thickness and achieving pregnancy in women with poor endometrial development.[77] Recently, it has been shown that two infertility patients with Asherman's syndrome achieved pregnancy after using vaginal Sildenafil citrate (25 mg), four times a day for 6 to 14 days during the first half of their cycles.[78]

Another treatment option for a thin endometrium is vitamin E because it has been reported to improve capillary blood flow in a variety of organs.[79] Therefore, 25 patients with a thin endometrium were given Vitamin E (600 mg/day) throughout the menstrual cycle. Twenty-three out of 25 patients showed improved radial artery resistance index, 17 patients showed increased endometrial thickness, and 13 patients developed an endometrial thickness more than 8 mm following Vitamin E administration.

Anti-fibrotic treatment, using a combination of pentoxifylline and high-dose Vitamin E (Tocopherol), has been shown to improve pregnancy rates in patients with a thin endometrium by increasing the endometrial thickness and improving ovarian function.[80]

It was also shown that GnRH agonist improves the pregnancy rate when given as luteal phase supplementation in IVF cycles.[81,82] One study[82] evaluated 138 women, who were assigned to receive a single injection of 0.1 mg Triptorelin, six days after intracytoplasmic sperm injection (ICSI), or to receive placebo. Significantly higher implantation and pregnancy rates were reported in the GnRH agonist–treated group compared with placebo. Qublah et al.[83] also did a prospective controlled randomized study to determine the effect of luteal phase supplementation of GnRH agonist on the implantation and pregnancy rates in women with endometrial thickness 7 mm or less at the time of oocyte retrieval. They evaluated 120 IVF patients who were randomly allocated into two groups: group A (n = 60) received Triptorelin (0.1 mg) on the day of ovum pick up (OPU), on the day of embryo transfer and three days thereafter, and group B (n=60) received placebo. The estradiol (E2), progesterone levels and endometrial thickness were significantly higher in the group of patients who received GnRH agonist, with a significant increase in the implantation and pregnancy rates. The authors attributed the improved results to a direct effect of GnRH agonist on the endometrium and corpus luteum. Furthermore, there was a significant increase in the endometrial thickness in the GnRH agonist–treated group compared with the placebo group, even when a single injection of 0.1 mg Triptorelin was administered at the time of OPU, suggestive of a direct effect on the endometrium.[83]

CONCLUSION

The implantation window is the most critical period of time in human reproduction. During this period, the human embryo at the blastocyst stage and the endometrium in the secretory phase come in contact with each other; in turn, apposition, attachment and invasion should come about in order to establish and maintain a healthy pregnancy. High-resolution ultrasonography serves as a non-invasive alternative method to evaluate the endometrial pattern and thickness as parameters to assess endometrial receptivity.[35,36] An adequate endometrial thickness is indispensable for a successful pregnancy in ART cycles.[2-7] However, criteria for adequacy of the endometrium for a successful pregnancy are still controversial.

From the infertility point of view, pregnancy does not practically occur if the thickness of endometrium is below 6 mm.[8] A minimal endometrial thickness of 7 to 8 mm appears to be a prerequisite for successful embryo implantation.[9,10] If Asherman's syndrome is not an underlying cause for a thin endometrium, some clinicians use low-dose Aspirin, vaginal Sildenafil, vaginal administration of micronized estradiol, antifibrotic treatment with pentoxifylline, high-dose Vitamin E, or GnRH agonist to improve the reproductive outcome. However, the results of these medications are also controversial. Larger cohort studies are needed to evaluate the results efficiently.

REFERENCES

1. Wilcox AJ, Baird DD,Weinberg CR. Time of implantation of the conceptus and loss of pregnancy. N Engl J Med. 1999;340:1796-99.
2. Gonen Y, Casper RF, Jacobson W, Blankier J. Endometrial thickness and growth during ovarian stimulation: A possible predictor of implantation in *in vitro* fertilization. Fertil Steril 1989;52:446-50.
3. Hock DL, Bohrer MK, Ananth CV, Kemmann E. Sonographic assessment of endometrial pattern and thickness in patients treated with clomiphene citrate, human menopausal

gonadotropins, and intrauterine insemination. Fertil Steril 1997;68:242-5.

4. Zenke U, Chetkowski RJ. Transfer and uterine factors are the major recipient related determinants of success with donor eggs. Fertil Steril 2004;82:850-6.

5. Zhang X, Chen CH, Confino E, Barnes R, Milad M, Kazer RR. Increased endometrial thickness is associated with improved treatment outcome for selected patients undergoing *in vitro* fertilization-embryo transfer. Fertil Steril 2005;83:336-40.

6. Esmailzadeh S, Faramarzi M. Endometrial thickness and pregnancy outcome after intrauterine insemination. Fertil Steril 2007;88:432-7.

7. McWilliams GD, Frattarelli JL. Changes in measured endometrial thickness predict *in vitro* fertilization success. Fertil Steril 2007;88:74-81.

8. Shapiro H, Cowell C, Casper RF. The use of vaginal ultrasound for monitoring endometrial preparation in a donor oocyte program. Fertil Steril 1993;59:1055-8.

9. Oliveira JB, Baruffi RL, Mauri AL, Petersen CG, Borges MC, Franco JG Jr. Endometrial ultrasonography as a predictor of pregnancy in an *in vitro* fertilization programme after ovarian stimulation and gonadotrophin-releasing hormone and gonadotrophins. Hum Reprod 1997;12:2515-8.

10. Schild RL, Knobloch C, Dorn C, Fimmers R, van der Ven H, Hansmann M. Endometrial receptivity in an *in vitro* fertilization program as assessed by spiral artery blood flow, endometrial thickness, endometrial volume, and uterine artery blood flow. Fertil Steril 2001;75:361-6.

11. Norwitz ER, Schust DJ, Fisher SJ. Implantation and the survival of early pregnancy. N Eng J Med 2001;345:1400-8.

12. Glissant A, de Mouzon J, Frydman R. Ultrasound study of the endometrium during *in vitro* fertilization cycles. Fertil Steril 1985;44:786-90.

13. Kovacs P, Matyas S, Boda K, Kaali SG. The effect of endometrial thickness on IVF/ICSI outcome. Hum Reprod 2003;18:2337-41.

14. Abdalla HI, Brooks AA, Johnson MR, Kirkland A, Thomas A, Studd JW. Endometrial thickness: A predictor of implantation in ovum recipients? Hum Reprod 1994;9:363-5.

15. Check JH, Nowroozi K, Choe J, Dietterich C. Influence of endometrial thickness and echo patterns on pregnancy rates during *in vitro* fertilization. Fertil Steril 1991;56:1173-5.

16. Dickey RP, Olar TT, Curole DN, Taylor SN, Rye PH. Endometrial pattern and thickness associated with pregnancy outcome after assisted reproduction technologies. Hum Reprod 1992;7:418-21.

17. Noyes N, Liu HC, Sultan K, Schattman G, Rosenwaks Z. Endometrial thickness appears to be a significant factor in embryo implantation in *in vitro* fertilization. Hum Reprod 1995;10:919-22.

18. Rinaldi L, Lisi F, Floccari A, Lisi R, Pepe G, Fishel S. Endometrial thickness as a predictor of pregnancy after *in vitro* fertilization but not after intracytoplasmic sperm injection. Hum Reprod 1996;11:1538-41.

19. Check JH, Nowroozi K, Choe J, Lurie D, Dietterich C. The effect of endometrial thickness and echo pattern on *in vitro* fertilization outcome in donor oocyte-embryo transfer cycle. Fertil Steril 1993;59:72-5.

20. Noyes N, Hampton BS, Berkeley A, Licciardi F, Grifo J, Krey L. Factors useful in predicting the success of oocyte donation: a 3-year retrospective analysis. Fertil Steril 2001;76:92-7.

21. Gonen Y, Casper RF. Prediction of implantation by the sonographic appearance of the endometrium during controlled ovarian stimulation for *in vitro* fertilization (IVF). J *In Vitro* Fert Embryo Transfer 1990;7:146-52.

22. Coulam CB, Bustillo M, Soenksen DM, Britten S. Ultrasonographic predictors of implantation after assisted reproduction. Fertil Steril 1994;62:1004-10.

23. Liu HM, Xing FQ, Chen SL, Li H. [Predictive value of endometrial ultrasonography and age for the outcome of *in vitro* fertilization embryo transfer]. Di Yi Jun Yi Da Xue Xue Bao 2005;25:570-2.

24. Rashidi BH, Sadeghi M, Jafarabadi M, Tehrani Nejad ES. Relationships between pregnancy rates following *in vitro* fertilization or intracytoplasmic sperm injection and endometrial thickness and pattern. Eur J Obstet Gynecol Reprod Biol 2005;120:179-84.

25. Yuval Y, Lipitz S, Dor J, Achiron R. The relationships between endometrial thickness, blood flow and pregnancy rates in *in vitro* fertilization. Hum Reprod 1999;14:1067-71.

26. Bassil S. Changes in endometrial thickness, width, length and pattern in predicting pregnancy outcome during ovarian stimulation in *in vitro* fertilization. Ultrasound Obstet Gynecol 2001;18:258-63.

27. Puerto B, Creus M, Carmona F, Civico S, Vanrell JA, Balasch J. Ultrasonography as a predictor of embryo implantation after *in vitro* fertilization: A controlled study. Fertil Steril 2003;79:1015-22.

28. Laasch C, Puscheck E. Cumulative embryo score, not endometrial thickness, is best for pregnancy prediction in IVF. J Assist Reprod Genet 2004;21:47-50.

29. Remohi J, Ardiles G, Garcia-Velasco JA, Gaitan P, Simon C, Pellicer A. Endometrial thickness and serum oestradiol concentrations as predictors of outcome in oocyte donation. Hum Reprod 1997;12:2271-6.

30. Garcia-Velasco JA, Isaza V, Caligara C, Pellicer A, Remohi J, Simon C. Factors that determine discordant outcome from shared oocytes. Fertil Steril 2003;80:54-60.

31. Weissman A, Gotlieb L, Casper RF. The detrimental effect of increased endometrial thickness on implantation and pregnancy rates and outcome in an *in vitro* fertilization program. Fertil Steril 1999;71:147-9.

32. Yakin K, Akarsu C, Kahraman S. Cycle lumping or sampling—a witches' brew? Fertil Steril 2000;73:175.

33. Dietterich C, Check JH, Choe JK, Nazari A, Lurie D. Increased endometrial thickness on the day of human chorionic gonadotropin injection does not adversely affect pregnancy or implantation rates following *in vitro* fertilization-embryo transfer. Fertil Steril 2002;77:781-6.

34. Yoeli R, Ashkenazi J, Orvieto R, Shelef M, Kaplan B, Bar-Hava I. Significance of increased endometrial thickness in assisted reproduction technology treatments. J Assist Reprod Genet 2004;21:285-9.

35. Shoham Z, Dicarlo C, Patel A, Conway GS, Jacobs HS. Is it possible to run a successful ovulation induction programme based solely on ultrasound monitoring? The importance of endometrial measurements. Fertil Steril 1991;56:836-41.

36. Freidler S, Schenker JG, Herman A, Lewin A. The role of ultrasonography in the evaluation of endometrial receptivity following assisted reproductive treatments: a critical review. Hum Reprod Update 1996;2:323-35.

37. Fleisher AC, Harbrt CM, Sacks CA, Wentz AC, Entmann SS, James AE, Jr. Sonography of the endometrium during conception and non-conception cycle of *in vitro* fertilization and embryo transfer. Fertil Steril 1986;46:442-7.

38. Check JH, Gandica R, Dietterich C, Lurie D. Evaluation of a non-homogeneous endometrial echo pattern in the mid-luteal phase as a potential factor associated with unexplained infertility. Fertil Steril 2003;79:590-3.

39. Check JH, O'Shaughnessy A, Lurie D, Fisher C, Adelson HG. Evaluation of the mechanism for higher pregnancy rates in donor oocyte recipients by comparison of fresh with frozen embryo transfer pregnancy rates in shared oocyte programme. Hum Reprod 1995;10:3022-7.

40. Check JH, Choe JK, Katsoff D. Controlled ovarian hyperstimulation adversely affects implantation following *in vitro* fertilization-embryo transfer. J Assist Reprod Genet 1999;16:416-20.

41. Check JH, Dietterich C, Lurie D. Non-homogeneous hyper-echogenic pattern 3 days after embryo transfer is associated with lower pregnancy rates. Hum Reprod 2000;15:1069-74.

42. Fanchin R, Righini C, Ayoubi J-M, Olivennes F, de Ziegler D, Frydman R. New look at endometrial echogenecity objective computer assisted measurements predict endometrial receptivity in *in vitro* fertilization-embryo transfer. Fertil Steril 2000;74:274-81.

43. Fanchin R. Assessing uterine receptivity in 2001. Ann NY Acad Sci 2001;943:185-202.

44. Doherty CM, Siliver B, Binor Z, Molo MW, Radwanska E. Transvaginal ultrasonography and the assessment of luteal phase endometrium. Am J Obstet Gynecol 1993;168:1702-7.

45. Ficicioglu C, Tasdemir S, Arioglu PF, Unlu R, Yorgance C. The use of transvaginal ultrasonography in the evaluation of luteal phase endometrium. Acta Eur Fertil 1995;26:35-40.

46. Sterizik KK, Grab D, Schneider V, Strehler EJ, Gagsteiger F, Rosenbusch BE. Lack of correlation between ultrasonography and histologic staging of the endometrium in *in vitro* fertilization (IVF) patients. Ultrasound Med Biol 1997;23:165-70.

47. Grunfeld L, Walker B, Bergh PA, Sandler B, Hofmann G, Navot D. High resolution endovaginal ultrasonography of the endometrium: A non invasive test for endometrial adequacy. Obstet Gynecol 1991;78:200-4.

48. Tani M. Relationship between sonographic endometrial images and endometrial histology during the secretory phase. Nippon Sanka Fusinka Gokkai Zasshi 1992;44:537-44.

49. Senturk LM, Erel T. Thin endometrium in assisted reproductive technology. Current Opinion in Obstetrics and Gynecology 2008;20:221-8.

50. Bakos O, Lundkvist O, Bergh T. Transvaginal sonographic evaluation of endometrial growth and texture in spontaneous ovulatory cycles – a descriptive study. Hum Reprod 1993;8:799-806.

51. Grow DR, Iromloo K. Oral contraceptives maintain a very thin endometrium before operative hysteroscopy. Fertil Steril 2006;85:204-7.

52. Turnbull LW, Lesney P, Killick SR. Assessment of uterine receptivity prior to embryo transfer: A review of currently available imaging modalities. Hum Reprod Update 1995;1:505-14.

53. Kovacs P, Matyas SZ, Boda K, Kaali SG. The effect of endometrial thickness on IVF/ICSI outcome. Hum Reprod 2003;18:2337-41.

54. Sundstrom P. Establishment of a successful pregnancy following *in vitro* fertilization and an endometrial thickness of no more than 4 mm. Hum Reprod 1998;13:1550-2.

55. Schild RL, Indefrei D, Eschweiler S, Vander Ven H, Fimmers R, Hansmann M. Three dimensional endometrial volume calculation and pregnancy rate in an *in vitro* fertilization programme. Hum Reprod 1999;14:1255-8.

56. Ayustawati HS, Obara H, Hirano Y, Tancichi A, Suzuki T, Takamizawa S, Sato I. Influence of endometrial thickness and pattern on pregnancy rates in *in vitro* fertilization-embryo transfer. Reprod Med Biol 2002;1:17-21.

57. Kupesic S, Bekavac I, Bjelos D, Kurjak A. Assessment of endometrial receptivity by transvaginal color Doppler and three-dimensional power Doppler ultrasonography in patients undergoing *in vitro* fertilization procedures. J Ultrasound Med 2001;20:125-34.

58. Alam V, Bernardini L, Gonzales J, Asch RH, Balmaceda JP. A prospective study of echographic endometrial characteristics and pregnancy rates during hormonal replacement cycles. J Assist Reprod Genet 1993;10:215-9.

59. Weckstein LN, Jacobson A, Galen D, Hampton K, Hammel J. Low-dose aspirin for oocyte donation recipients with a thin endometrium: prospective, randomized study. Fertil Steril 1997;68:927-30.

60. Basir GS, O WS, So WW, Ng EH, Ho PC. Evaluation of cycle-to-cycle variation of endometrial responsiveness using transvaginal sonography in women undergoing assisted reproduction. Ultrasound Obstet Gynecol 2002;19:484-9.

61. Lee A, Sator M, Kratochwil A, Deutinger J, Vytiska-Bisdorfer E, Bernaschek G. Endometrial volume change during spontaneous menstrual cycles: Volumetry by transvaginal three dimensional ultrasound. Fertil Steril 1997;68:831-5.

62. Zollner U, Zollner KP, Blissing S, Pohls U, Steck T, Dietl J, Müller T. Impact of three-dimensionally measured endometrial volume on the pregnancy rate after intrauterine insemination. Zentralbl Gynakol 2003;125:136-41.

63. Raga F, Bonilla-Musoles F, Casan EM, Klein O, Bonilla F. Assessment of endometrial volume by three dimensional ultrasound prior to embryo transfer: Clues to endometrial receptivity. Hum Reprod 1999;14:2851-4.

64. Steer CV, Campbell S, Tan SL, Grayford T, Mills C, Mason BA, Collins WP. The use of transvaginal color flowimaging after *in vitro* fertilization to identify optimum uterine condition before embryo transfer. Fertil Steril 1992;57:372-6.

65. Steer CV, Tan SL, Dhillon D, Mason BA, Campbell S. Vaginal color Doppler assessment of uterine artery impedance correlation with immunohistochemical markers of endometrial receptivity required for the implantation of an embryo. Fertil Steril 1995;63:101-8.

66. Zaidi J, Pittrof R, Shaker A,Kyei-Mensah A, Campbell S, Tan SL. Assessment of uterine artery blood flow on the day of human chorionic gonadotropin administration by transvaginal color

Doppler ultrasound in an *in vitro* fertilization program. Fertil Steril 1996;65:377-81.

67. Salle B, Bied-Damon V, Benchaib M, Desperc S, Gaucherand P, Rudigoz RC. Preliminary report of an ultrasonography and color Doppler uterine score to predict uterine receptivity in an *in vitro* fertilization program. Hum Reprod 1998;13:1669-73.

68. Polishuk WZ, Siew FP, Gordon R, Lebenshart P. Vascular changes in traumatic amenorrhea and hypomenorrhea. Int J Fertil 1977; 22:189-92.

69. Yaffe H, Ron M, Polishuk WZ. Amenorrhea, hypomenorrhea, and uterine fibrosis. Am J Obstet Gynecol 1978;130:599-601.

70. Soares SR, Barbosa dos Reis MM, Camargos AF. Diagnostic accuracy of sonohysterography, transvaginal sonography, and hysterosalpingography in patients with uterine cavity diseases. Fertil Steril 2000;72:406-11.

71. Schenker JG, Margalioth EJ. Intra-uterine adhesions: an updated appraisal. Fertil Steril 1982;37:593-610.

72. Reddy S, Rock JA. Surgical management of complete obliteration of the endometrial cavity. Fertil Steril 1997;67:172-4.

73. Kuo HC, Hsu CC, Wang ST, Huang KE. Aspirin improves uterine blood flow in the peri-implantation period. J Formos Med Assoc 1997;96:253-7.

74. Check JH, Dietterich C, Lurie D, Nazari A, Chuong J. A matched study to determine whether low-dose aspirin without heparin improves pregnancy rates following frozen embryo transfer and/or affects endometrial sonographic parameters. J Assist Reprod Genet 1998;15:579-82.

75. Urman B, Mercan R, Alatas C, Balaban B, Isiklar A, Nuhoglu A. Low-dose aspirin does not increase implantation rates in patients undergoing intracytoplasmic sperm injection: a prospective randomized study. J Assist Reprod Genet 2000; 17:586-90.

76. Chen MJ, Yang JH, Peng FH, Chen SU, Ho HN, Yang YS. Extended estrogen administration for women with thin endometrium in frozen-thawed *in vitro* fertilization programs. J Assist Reprod Genet 2006;23:337-42.

77. Sher G, Fisch JD. Vaginal sildenafil (Viagra): a preliminary report of a novel method to improve uterine artery blood flow and endometrial development in patients undergoing IVF. Hum Reprod 2000;15:806-9.

78. Zinger M, Liu JH, Thomas MA. Successful use of vaginal sildenafil citrate in two infertility patients with Asherman's syndrome. J Womens Health (Larchmt) 2006;15:442-4.

79. Chung TW, Yu JJ, Liu DZ. Reducing lipid peroxidation stress of erythrocyte membrane by alpha-tocopherol nicotinate plays an important role in improving blood rheological properties in type 2 diabetic patients with retinopathy. Diabet Med 1998; 15:380-5.

80. Lédée-Bataille N, Olivennes F, Lefaix JL, Chaouat G, Frydman R, Delanian S. Combined treatment by pentoxifylline and tocopherol for recipient women with a thin endometrium enrolled in an oocyte donation programme. Hum Reprod 2002; 17:1249-53.

81. Tesarik J, Hazout A, Mendoza C. Enhancement of embryo developmental potential by a single administration of GnRH agonist at the time of implantation. Hum Reprod 2004;19: 1176-80.

82. Tesarik J, Hazout A, Mendoza-Tesarik R, Mendoza N, Mendoza C. Beneficial effect of luteal-phase GnRH agonist administration on embryo implantation after ICSI in both GnRH agonist- and antagonist-treated ovarian stimulation cycles. Hum Reprod 2006;21:2572-9.

83. Qublan H, Amarin Z, Al-Qudah M, Diab F, Nawasreh M, Malkawi S, Balawneh M. Luteal phase support with GnRH-a improves implantation and pregnancy rates in IVF cycles with endometrium of <or=7 mm on day of egg retrieval. Hum Fertil (Camb) 2008;11:43-7.

Assisted Reproductive Techniques

Luteal Phase Support in Ovarian Stimulation Cycles

Robab Taheripanah, Mybodi Karimzadeh

OVERVIEW

Luteal phase defect is an iatrogenic adverse effect of ovarian stimulation protocols in assisted reproductive techniques (ART). Gonadotropin-releasing hormone (GnRH) agonist, used in these cycles in order to downregulate the pituitary compromises the corpus luteum function and implantation, if luteal hormonal support is not given. The evidence suggests that luteal support is beneficial but the optimal regimens, length and route of use remain unresolved at present. Although progesterone is the most popular drug that has been used for luteal phase via different routes, there are controversies about the best route and efficacy of progesterone with regard to cost and patient convenience. Although serum progesterone level is higher following intramuscular progesterone, the vaginal route of administration is accompanied with fewer complications and more convenience. Estrogen addition from the early or mid-luteal phase can overcome the adverse effects of hormonal decline in the mid-luteal phase after clearing the human chorionic gonadotropin (hCG) from plasma. hCG supplementation or a single injection of hCG in the mid-luteal phase may be useful and better outcomes may be achieved. Though a meta-analysis was performed, larger series of randomized controlled trials need to resolve this problem.

INTRODUCTION

Since the early days of *in vitro* fertilization (IVF), the 'ideal' scheme of luteal phase in stimulated cycles has been a matter of debate. Edwards and Steptoe in 1980, were the first to postulate luteal phase inadequacy resulting from ovarian stimulation as a cause of IVF failure.[1] As the question of optimal support remains unresolved, some studies have been designed to evaluate this subject. Although different treatments are suggested to overcome this problem, there has not been any accepted standard luteal phase support protocol worldwide.

This chapter addresses the luteal phase characteristics in natural and stimulated cycles. First of all, the physiology, pathology and differences between the fertile and infertile women undergoing assisted reproductive techniques will be explained. Then, by focussing on the consequences of the abnormal luteal phase, and with the aim of providing a sound scientific and clinical basis for the management of luteal phase and optimizing outcomes, different types of drugs and their advantages and disadvantages will be reviewed.

Definition

The luteal phase is defined as the period from the occurrence of ovulation until the establishment of a pregnancy or the resumption of menses two weeks after it. This phase produces a favorable environment for implantation. No event in Reproductive Medicine is an isolated occurrence, but as with all other physiological processes, each event is interdependent on the proper working of the entire reproductive system.

Progesterone is the principal secretory product of the corpus luteum and induces secretory transformation of the endometrium. Progesterone is secreted due to pulsatile secretion of luteinizing hormone (LH) every one to four hours and the LH pattern determines the timing and quantity of progesterone secretion (Fig. 39.1).[2]

Continuous stimulation of LH is necessary for adequate production of steroids by the luteinized granulosa cells and LH stimulation is provided by the effect of human chorionic gonadotropin (hCG), produced by pregnancy, on the LH receptors.[3] In a normal luteal phase of non-pregnant women, peak estrogen and progesterone production occurs four days after ovulation, and wanes about 10 days after ovulation. A

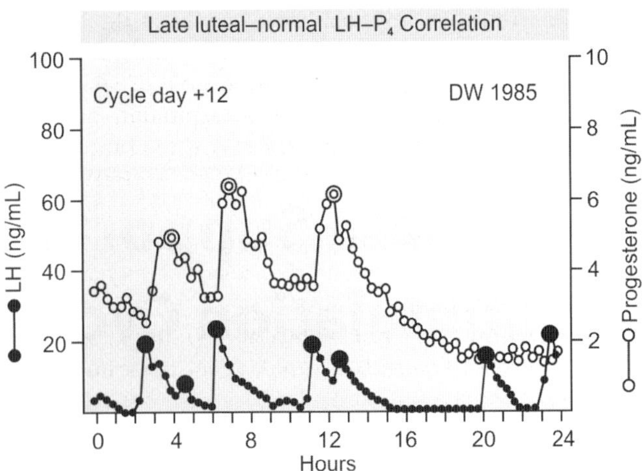

Fig. 39.1: The simultaneous pulsatile LH and pulsatile progesterone levels are illustrated over 24 hours in the late luteal phase of a normal woman's cycle. The points on the LH and progesterone secretion curves indicate secretory events following most but not all, of the LH secretory events. *Adopted from Keye et al.[2]*

dip in ovarian progesterone can occur even during the early days in cycles of pregnancy, but it is quickly reverted by hCG stimulation of the corpus luteum. Before implantation, the embryo will secrete hCG, which stimulates the ovary to respond appropriately by enhancing steroid production. This process is called luteal rescue. If this process happens too late or if pregnancy does not occur, LH stimulation decreases, progesterone levels decrease and uterine prostaglandins are released. Ovarian production of gonadal steroids shifts to placenta over a period of weeks.

CLINICAL DISCUSSION

Physiology

Implantation is a complicated process and a receptive endometrium is necessary for the implantation of a blastocyst as well as for the maintenance of pregnancy. The most important aspect here is that there is a window of implantation, where certain proteins appear on the epithelial cells of the endometrial lining and then disappear. If these factors are not present, implantation will not occur. Many factors affect this window of implantation and uterine receptivity. Both, estrogen and progesterone act as regulatory factors for implantation and growth factors.[4,5]

The concept of a luteal phase defect was first introduced by Jones in 1949, and has been defined as a corpus luteum defective in progesterone production.[6] The incidence of luteal phase defect, based on an out of phase endometrium, was reported in 3 to 20 percent of the infertile population and 23 to 60 percent of women with recurrent abortion.[7] Luteal phase defect is seen in almost all IVF cycles in which LH secretion

was suppressed with GnRH agonist (GnRH-a) administration in the luteal phase. The aspiration of granulosa cells that surround the oocyte can interfere with the production of progesterone.[8]

In the last two decades, there have been great advances in ART, especially in the pharmaceutical aspects, the drug variety, as well as biochemical and technological improvements to enhance success. As we know, the highest rate of failure occurs following embryo transfer. This failure is the reason for much research in this area. What happens in the uterus that is called the 'black box'?

A number of studies have focussed on the mechanisms underlying the luteal phase defect after ovarian stimulation for IVF. The exact mechanism behind this defect remains unclear.[2] There are different multiple corpora lutea in stimulated cycles and the levels of both progesterone and estrogen are supraphysiological in the early luteal phase. There is a theory about the effect of estrogen and progesterone ratio in luteal phase and duration. It seems that high progesterone in the early luteal phase of stimulated cycles has adverse effects on luteolysis. Luteolysis occurs earlier and the duration of ovarian steroid production is usually shorter than normal by 1 to 3 days. Becker, et al.[9] in a study, tried to mimic the characteristics of IVF cycles for volunteers, with the administration of exogenous hormones in the early luteal phase, as in ovarian stimulation. They found that the LH level decreased due to the negative feedback mechanism of high estrogen concentrations.[9] Hence, they could demonstrate that if the progesterone level is higher during 3 days of the early luteal phase, luteolysis will be induced and hormone production will be impaired. Multifollicular growth, by itself, and supraphysiological estrogen and progesterone had an effect on the duration of the luteal phase with or without luteal phase support. It is expected that the corpora lutea are only supported in the early luteal phase but not in the mid-to-late luteal phase by exogenous hCG, which is very important for implantation.

Serum estrogen and progesterone levels decrease very rapidly to low levels on day 6 after oocyte pick-up compared to normal cycles.[10] This decrease is more significant in long protocol cycles downregulated with GnRH agonists.[11,12] The main causes of luteal decline in sex steroid levels are most probably related to the high concentrations of estradiol (E2) in the early luteal phase.[13] E2 is involved in the regulation of LH secretion[10] and might cause extremely low LH concentrations in the luteal phase as a result of a strong negative feedback mechanism.[14]

Second, it seems that the early luteal support is a result of the bolus of exogenous hCG that is injected for triggering the LH surge and inducing ovulation 36 hours before oocyte pick-up. However, the supportive effects of hCG on the corpus luteum cannot produce the hormones after the half-life of hCG and its clearance on the 8th day of injections.

It seems that the ratio of the peak estradiol to mid-luteal estradiol is very important to predict the IVF outcome.[15] Sharara et al.[15] revealed that the magnitude of estradiol concentration declines between the days of hCG injection and 8 days later. They showed a sharp decline in mid-luteal estradiol (ratio > 5) is associated with a significantly lower ongoing implantation rate and pregnancy rate.[15,16] Therefore, it seems that exogenous estrogen in the early and mid-luteal phase will be useful for correction of the estrogen to progesterone ratio.

On the other hand, high estrogen/progesterone ratio, which is associated with an inhibitory effect on embryo implantation, should be considered. The progesterone level also drops when the hCG effects disappear after 8 days in unsupported corpus luteum and the addition of progesterone will be useful to increase the implantation rate.[15]

The last theory is the aspiration and flushing of the follicles that may deplete and damage granulosa cells, which theoretically causes a further insufficiency of luteal progesterone secretion.

With the advent of gonadotropin-releasing hormone (GnRH) agonist use in the late 1980s, the problem of the short luteal phase became more common. The main mechanism of luteal phase deficiency by gonadotropin releasing hormone agonist (GnRH-a) is the result of downregulation and persistent block of the LH output for at least 10 days after discontinuing GnRH-a, which can result in impairment of progesterone secretion by the corpus luteum.[17]

Some years ago, Becker et al.[9] conducted a study to investigate whether the early cessation of the GnRH agonist would prevent early luteolysis.[9] They compared 3 groups. (i) long GnRH-a/hMG + hCG; (ii) early follicular phase cessation of GnRH-a without luteal support; and (iii) a long GnRH-a protocol without luteal support. No premature LH surges were found after early cessation of GnRH-a. Although, the LH levels were extremely low in the early and mid-luteal phase in all of the groups and pituitary recovery occurred during the late luteal phase in some patients who stopped the GnRH-a earlier, but this did not improve the corpus luteum function. Probably, progesterone concentrations were dependent on the preovulatory bolus of hCG and were very low in the mid-luteal phase. Hence, the corpus luteum function will be compromised even by early cessation of GnRH-a due to early luteolysis and a need for hormonal support.

Luteal Support Regimens

Although the exact mechanism with which luteal phase support enhances implantation is not clear, it is well accepted that luteal phase supplementation is crucial during the gap period, that is, the time between the disappearance of exogenous hCG, administered for final oocyte maturation and the rise in endogenous hCG during early implantation.[18]

Luteal support has been routinely used since the late 1980s. Many different protocols have been described but it is unclear which type of luteal phase support is the best and whether the need for luteal support varies according to (a) the type of stimulation regimen, (b) the degree of stimulation achieved, (c) whether or not follicle aspiration has been carried out, and (d) the type of subjects treated (anovulatory versus ovulatory subjects). In addition, for a given type of luteal support, e.g. progesterone or hCG, there is also a lack of agreement among various investigators on how frequently this should be administered, at what dose and at what time(s) during the luteal phase.

With the advent of GnRH antagonists for use in ovulation induction protocols, modern and new luteal phase treatments have been suggested. Recently, authors have been attracted to estradiol supplements in the early or mid-luteal phase and increased improvement was observed in some studies. However, the most important factors that may impact the choice of treatment regimens are the patient condition and improvement in the IVF outcome.

Progesterone

Progesterone is the most common drug that has been used, combined with estrogen for endometrial preparation in egg or embryo donation cycles and freeze-thaw embryo programmed cycles. Since the 1980s, many investigations have been designed for the determination of progesterone efficacy in luteal phase support in ART cycles; the pregnancy rate was found to be significantly higher with progesterone use as compared to unsupported IVF-ET cycles.[19] Although, the administration of progesterone has been established for many years and many practitioners believe that it is the only important hormone in luteal physiology that has a central role in endometrial preparation and pregnancy support, the optimal route of progesterone administration has not yet been established. Different routes of progesterone administration have been used for luteal phase support, including natural oral and vaginal progesterone and intramuscular progesterone. Some authors have suggested intramuscular (IM) progesterone-in-oil as the best method of luteal phase support[20] because serum progesterone levels were above the physiological range and also higher in women who used the intramuscular rather than the vaginal route with adequate secretory endometrial transformation. However, serum progesterone concentrations are not indicative of the local bioavailability, despite being seven times higher after intramuscular administration, but endometrial progesterone concentrations were almost 10 times higher after vaginal administration. As daily intramuscular injection of progesterone is associated with patient discomfort and produces potentially serious adverse effects, such as sterile abscess and acute eosinophilic pneumonia due to accumulation of the oil vehicle in the body,[21] some authors have suggested that intramuscular injections of 341 mg 17-hydroxyprogesterone caproate (Proluton) every 3 days, beginning within 24 hrs of embryo transfer, resulted in a pregnancy rate of 32.5 percent versus 18.3 percent in the control group.[19] Although authors found no differences in the outcome following the use of 17-HPC and intramuscular progesterone for supporting the luteal phase, injection of 17-HPC every 3 days have been considered convenient for the patient.[19,22]

Vaginal administration of progesterone offers a number of advantages in terms of patient convenience and tolerability. Although serum progesterone levels in the vaginal group are lower than the IM administration,[23] the endometrial tissue concentrations of progesterone are higher, which is indicative of the first uterine pass effect and a better bio-availability in the uterus with minimal systemic undesirable effects and similar clinical pregnancy rates.[24,25] Indeed, normal synchronous endometrial development occurred only after vaginal administration, rather than the oral or intramuscular administration despite similar serum concentrations being achieved.[26,27]

In order to enhance patient convenience, prefilled vaginal progesterone gel (Crinone 8%) is now available and its usage is easier than vaginal suppositories. Anserini et al.[28] also reported that vaginal progesterone gel is a good alternative to parental progesterone for luteal phase support in ART cycles with similar clinical pregnancy rates.[28] Abate[19] and Damario[20] demonstrated that implantation efficiency is reduced when Crinone 8 percent vaginal progesterone gel rather than IM progesterone-in-oil is used for luteal phase support after IVF-ET cycles.[19,20] They concluded that IM natural progesterone appears to be the most suitable route of administration for luteal phase support in IVF-ET cycles.[29] However, Friedler et al.[30] compared vaginal and oral progesterone used for luteal phase support and concluded that the clinical pregnancy rate was similar between the two groups, with a significantly higher implantation rate in the vaginal progesterone group. It is recommended that a low dose of micronized progesterone, administered vaginally, is simple, easy and well-tolerated, so it can be the method of choice for luteal support, especially for high responder patients at risk of ovarian hyperstimulation syndrome (OHSS).[30]

Oral progesterone, as luteal phase support, seems appealing as it is easy to use. However, there is concern that progesterone is extensively and rapidly metabolized in the gastrointestinal system after oral administration and circulating concentrations are inadequate for endometrial transformation in IVF cycles.[27] Oral progesterones have been associated with a high rate of progesterone metabolism due to the hepatic first-pass, which is responsible for a bioavailability of <10 percent.[31,32] Increasing the dose to achieve the sufficient circulating levels results in an unacceptable incidence of adverse effects, especially sedation. Therefore, amongst the different routes of progesterone administration, the oral preparation is associated with lower pregnancy rates

and lower efficacy. One study evaluated the clinical efficacy of two routes of progesterone administration, used separately for luteal phase support in IVF-ET cycles, oral Duphaston and vaginal Cyclogest, and compared the associated clinical pregnancy rates with that obtained following the use of IM hCG. The clinical pregnancy rate was found to be similar in all the three groups, which indicates that all the three routes of administration used for luteal support are equally effective. This is supported by the findings of Norman et al.[33] who reported that orally and vaginally administered progesterone have similar bioavailability.[33]

A comparison of the efficacy of different types of luteal phase support, including oral, vaginal and intramuscular progesterone with regard to the clinical pregnancy rates has presented controversial evidence in several studies about the different routes of progesterone use. A systematic review, performed to evaluate the different types of progesterone supplementation in stimulated cycles, failed to conclude preference of a particular route of progesterone administration over the other due to various doses of intramuscular or vaginal progesterone as capsules/suppositories/vaginal cream in various administration regimens.[17] Some practitioners believe that there is no significant difference in the outcome of IVF-ET cycles when different types of vaginal progesterone were used for luteal support, including gel, pessaries and capsules.[17,34-36]

However, the best type of luteal phase support to use with good clinical pregnancy rates is unknown and needs more investigation. We suggest that practitioners should choose the best route and regimen on the basis of the patient condition and her demands.

Finally, it seems that progesterone is the best option for luteal phase support, with better pregnancy results with the use of synthetic progesterone.[37]

Human Chorionic Gonadotropin

There is some debate as to whether human chorionic gonadotropin (hCG) or progesterone provides better luteal support; it is generally accepted that hCG is more beneficial, unless there is a significant risk of ovarian hyperstimulation syndrome, in which case, progesterone support would be preferable. As mentioned before, in long protocols, LH concentrations are suppressed by GnRH-a, and progesterone supplementation alone lacks luteotrophic stimulation apart from the hCG given prior to oocyte retrieval. As a consequence, the corpus luteum may undergo irreversible changes and impaired function ensues. The argument for the use of hCG is that it is a luteotrophic agent, which stimulates the corpus luteum to increase production of all the hormones and factors normally produced by the corpus luteum rather than substituting only one product and it may be associated with a higher endometrial receptivity and better outcomes. Earlier studies showed that treatment with hCG resulted in pregnancy rates between 18.7 to 50 percent versus 9.3 to 17 percent in unsupported cycles.[38,39]

The hCG effects expire in one week and the progesterone and estradiol levels begin to decline. It seems that a low serum estradiol level in the mid-luteal phase is associated with lower pregnancy rates and increased preclinical pregnancy wastage, especially if it is lower than 100 pg/mL. Hence, combined hCG plus progesterone therapy for luteal phase support can increase the pregnancy rate from 13.3 percent in progesterone only to 31.7 percent in hCG plus progesterone regimens.[16] It can be expected the addition of hCG in the mid-luteal period bridges the time gap between exogenous hCG and the beginning of the endogenous gestational hCG and avoids the impairment of corpus luteum function once pregnancy occurs. However, with regard to the corpus luteum function, some authors recommend the routine use of a single mid-luteal injection of 2500 IU hCG in IVF cycles, except in patients with a risk for OHSS.[40]

A meta-analysis of randomized trials by several authors showed that hCG gives better results than progesterone alone.[41-43] hCG in combination with progesterone is an effective immunosuppressive factor that can facilitate the implantation process as a fetal allograft. In another study, hCG was compared with vaginal progesterone for luteal support and it was found that the pregnancy rate was similar between the two groups with equal effectiveness (36.7% vs 35.3%).[43] Although Buvat et al.[44] reported that the pregnancy rate was significantly higher in the luteal phase supported with hCG compared to oral progesterone, it was similar to vaginal progesterone.[44] Daya et al.[45] concluded that while hCG increased the magnitude and duration of the luteal progesterone secretion, it did not clearly improve the pregnancy rate versus progesterone use for luteal support in IVF-ET cycles.[45] Therefore, the available evidence shows that hCG offers no superiority over progesterone for luteal support in IVF cycles, but it increases the chance of OHSS in patients; the odds of OHSS are increased 20-fold when hCG is administered from the early luteal phase.[16] Hence, luteal phase support with hCG should be considered for selective patients especially in stimulated cycles that use GnRH antagonists.

Estrogen

As mentioned before, if the superiority of hCG over progesterone is in fact due to the stimulation of estrogen production, especially in the mid-luteal phase, then simple replacement of estrogen in addition to progesterone might be helpful. However, the role of estrogen in implantation and maintenance during the luteal phase in human is controversial.[46] While estrogen does not directly mediate luteinization, some estrogen is likely to be required to stimulate progesterone receptor replenishment so that progesterone can act. Although estrogen and progesterone are normally secreted from the corpus luteum, both of them fall prematurely in most cases after ovarian stimulation cycles. It was demonstrated that serum estradiol concentrations had a precipitous drop by more than 50 percent over a 48-hour period, 10 days from hCG administration. MicroRNAs (miRNAs) have now been recognized as key players in the process of cell proliferation and differentiation.[47] Ovarian stimulation or altered steroid hormone levels may affect miRNA profiles, and consequently, affect endometrial receptivity.[48, 49] It seems that adding estrogen could be partially reverse the well-known anti-proliferative effect of progesterone on the endometrium and could be possibly exerted by a localized increase in miRNA expression,[49] but their effects on the implantation rate needs further research. Unfortunately, the luteal phase combination support has attracted only limited attention and has not become common practice amongst infertility centers.[50,51] Sabi, et al.[52] evaluated the effect of estrogen supplementation in preclinical pregnancy loss.[52] Authors observed that the pregnancy rate was lower with progesterone only, especially in women with E2 < 100 pg/mL on 11 days after embryo transfer (ET). It indicates the role of estrogen in establishing endometrial receptivity in the late luteal phase. However, it seems that subsequent pregnancy loss may be reduced with luteal estrogen supplementation.[52] On the other hand, the beneficial effects of estradiol addition would correlate with differences between the endometrium receptivity in young and older women. It was observed that endometrial receptivity is higher in older patients in egg donation artificial cycles.[53] It may be due to the relative levels of estradiol and progesterone rather than their absolute levels, and these factors determine the developmental potential of the endometrium.[54] The necessary ratio of these hormones changes with progress in age. It is unclear whether this reflects a change in endometrial hormone receptor activity or a change in ovarian performance with regard to hormone production. Hence, the addition of estradiol to progesterone should be restricted to women younger than 38 years because it may be associated with better pregnancy rates.[55]

The lack of benefit of estrogen supplementation during the luteal phase of GnRHa/hMG stimulated cycles could be explained by the frequency of low E2 concentrations during these cycles.

However, some researchers have investigated the effects of adding estrogen to progesterone in different doses and estradiol starting times, but it is still a matter of debate and none of them have been able to confirm the validity of such a treatment conclusively. For example, Farhi et al.[56] believed that estradiol substitution should be initiated once a precipitous drop in estradiol levels has occurred, e.g. in the mid-luteal phase.[56] He found that the pregnancy rate was 39.6 percent with estrogen and progesterone versus 25.6 percent with progesterone only in long protocol stimulated cycles. It seems that early estrogen supplementation before the estradiol drop would be expected to enhance live birth rates. Smitz et al.[50] evaluated the advantage of adding 6 mg daily of E2 valerate to intravaginal micronized progesterone (600 mg daily) as luteal supplementation in a prospective randomized study.[50] There were no differences in the clinical

Table 39.1: Comparison of the effect of adding estrogen to progesterone for luteal phase support in ART cycles				
Author	*Stimulation protocol*	*No. of cycles*	*Luteal phase support*	*Pregnancy rate (%) (implantation) (%)*
Buvat et al. (1990)[41]	Triptorelin/hMG (short)	32	hCG 3 × 1500IU[a]	62.5[b]
		19	Utrogestan 400 mg/day orally	5
		20	Utrogestan 400 mg/day vaginally	55[c]
	Triptorelin/hMG (long)	47	hCG 3 × 1500IU[a]	40
		41	Utrogestan 400 mg/day orally	27
		35	Utrogestan 400 mg/day vaginally	40
Smithz et al. (1992)[62]	Buserelin/hMG (long)	131	Progesterone 50 mg IM + estradiol valerate 6 mg/day	30.5 (11.6)*
		131	Utrogestan 600 mg vaginally + estradiol valerate 6 mg/day	35.1 (16.3)*
Artini et al. (1995)[63]	Buserelin/pFSH + hMG (long)	44	hCG 3 × 2000IU	13.6
		44	Progesterone 50 mg/day	13.6
		44	Micronized progesterone in vaginal cream 100 mg/day	15.6
Pouly et al. (1996)[64]	Decapeptyl/hMG (long)	139	Crinone 90 mg/day vaginally	28.8 (35.3)
		144	Utrogestan 300 mg/day orally	25 (29.9)
Licciardi et al. (1999)[65]	GnRH/FSH/hMG (long)	19	Progesterone 50 mg IM	57.9 (40.0)**
		24	Micronized progesterone 600 mg/day orally	45.8 (18.1)**
Herman et al. (1996)[66]	Decapeptyl/hMG (long)	85	Progesterone IM 50 mg/day	29
		85	Progesterone IM 50 mg/day + hCG 2500 IU (7th day ET)	31
Farhi et al. (2000)[56]	GnRH/hMG (long)	113	Progesterone IM 150 mg/day	25.6 (10.2)
		101	Progesterone IM 150 mg/day + E2, 2 mg/bid oral (after 7th day ET)	39.6 (15.2)
	GnRH/hMG (short)	36	Progesterone IM 150 mg/day	16.6 (7.5)
		35	Progesterone IM 150 mg/day + E2 2mg/bid oral (after 7th day ET)	17.1 (8.0)
Gorkemli et al. (2004)[58]	GnRH/rFSH/HMG (long)	148	Micronized progesterone 600 mg/day	9.5
		140	Micronized progesterone 600 mg/day + transdermal E2 100 µg/day	31.4
Lukaszuk et al (2005)[57]	GnRH/HMG (long)	78	Utrogestan 600 mg/vaginally	23.1 (9.8)
		70	Utrogestan 600 mg/vaginally + E2, 2 mg /day orally	32.8 (17.8)
		76	Utrogestan 600 mg/vaginally + E2, 6 mg/day orally	51.3 (29.9)

Utrogestan = natural micronized progesterone capsules; Crinone = natural progesterone in vaginal gel
[a]No hCG was given as luteal phase support if the concentration of estradiol was >2700 pg/mL
[b]P < 0.01 versus oral; [c]P < 0.01 versus oral
*P = 0.07; **P = 0.04

pregnancy rates between the two groups. The beneficial effect of E2 might be related to the dose and time in which it is used. Lukaszuk et al.[57] in a prospective randomized study, recently evaluated the effect of addition of different E2 supplementation doses (0, 2 or 6 mg/day) to vaginal progesterone in the luteal phase of stimulated cycles on implantation and pregnancy rates. It was shown that the addition of a high dose of E2 to daily progesterone supplementation significantly improved the probability of pregnancy in women treated with a long GnRH-a protocol.[57] Similarly, Fahri et al.[56] demonstrated that starting 2 mg E2 on day 7 after embryo transfer in progesterone supported cycles, stimulated with the long GnRH-a protocol, has a beneficial effect on pregnancy and implantation rates.[56] Gorkemli et al.[58] demonstrated that other routes of estradiol administration, such as transdermal estradiol 100 µg/day, added to progesterone, is associated with a significantly higher pregnancy rate (31.4% vs 9.5%).[58] However, such an effect could not be shown in the short GnRH-a protocol. A meta-analysis by Pritts and Atwood[60] suggested that progesterone, in combination with E2, is the best luteal support in long and short agonist protocols.[59]

The important problem that will be of concern is the high levels of estradiol in the luteal phase that have also been reported to be embryotoxic and to prevent implantation.[61] It is therefore, important to understand that the dosages utilized here are not in an embryotoxic range and are identical to those used in artificial cycles.[50,61] Moreover, the micronized estradiol utilized here is a natural product (Table 39.1).

GnRH Agonist (GnRH-a)

The mechanism of the possible beneficial effect of GnRH-a is poorly defined. It was suggested that the addition of 0.1 mg GnRH-a on the 6th day after oocyte pick-up can be beneficial in the maintenance of the corpus luteum, acting directly on the endometrium via local receptors, a direct effect on the embryos, or by some combination of these possibilities. It seems that GnRH-a has a direct effect on regulatory activity in the synthesis and secretion of hCG by preimplanted embryos and causes higher beta-hCG concentrations in pregnancies where GnRH-a luteal support was used compared to control groups.[67] In a systematic review, Kyrou et al.[68] showed that GnRH-a in the mid-luteal phase significantly increases the live birth rate in ART cycles, and using GnRH-a for downregulation in long protocols does not change the beneficial effects of agonists in implantation.[68] However, owing to the discrepancy in the research pertaining to luteal GnRH-a support, it is too early to accept its use to obtain higher pregnancy rates.[69]

GnRH Antagonist Stimulated Cycles and the Luteal Phase

Nowadays, GnRH antagonists are used to stimulate the ovaries in ART cycles. With regard to the GnRH antagonist mechanism, that immediately suppresses the LH and FSH secretion, it seems that discontinuing the GnRH antagonist 2 days before oocyte pick-up causes LH secretion to return to the normal pattern. In this case, we do not need progesterone or other drugs for supplementation. But, Fatemi et al.[70] showed that the progesterone supplement is necessary even with GnRH antagonist use.[70]

Hence, it seems that the use of GnRH-a for triggering ovulation instead of hCG can be effective for the prevention of ovarian hyperstimulation syndrome (OHSS) in high risk patients, especially in GnRH antagonist cycles.[71] Low mid-luteal progesterone was reported in about 70 percent of cycles treated with a GnRH-a ovulation trigger with a short luteal phase in 16 to 42 percent of cases.[72] Balasch et al.[73] showed that the luteal phase following GnRH-a triggering of ovulation in gonadotropin-stimulated cycles is characterized by prompt and adequate luteinization of the follicles, but the progesterone production is inadequate in both amount and duration.[73] In fact, a single injection of GnRH-a induces an FSH and LH surge similar to the physiological pattern and it has two advantages. First of all, it induces an FSH surge that is effective for follicular maturation, expansion of cumulus, and ovulation, which is comparable with hCG in both, ovulation induction and IVF cycles. The second potential advantage is a short LH surge (34 hours) that is more similar to the physiological condition than the extended LH surge by hCG that remains for 6 days.[74] This short time of stimulation can trigger the ovulation of fewer follicles compared with hCG under similar conditions, and a lower frequency of multiple pregnancy could be expected in patients undergoing ovulation induction.[75,76] However, progesterone supplementation alone is not enough to compensate for the short luteal phase completely, and it seems that hCG can overcome this problem. This may be explained by the shorter duration of LH activity after GnRH-a, which may reduce the stimulation of the corpus luteum at the time that a new corpus luteum needs the gonadotropin support for repair and synthesis of the cells. In this case, hCG supplementation is better, but may be associated with multiple pregnancy in ovulation induction cycles because the effect of GnRH-a is very short and non-ovulated follicles may continue to grow in the luteal phase. However, 6 and 10 days after the GnRH-a injections seems to be an appropriate time for hCG doses to prevent the effect on growing follicles and additional luteal ovulation.[73]

Duration of Luteal Phase Support

The next question that arises is the duration of luteal supplementation. The duration of progesterone therapy as luteal phase support is controversial. It has been used for as little as 2 weeks and for as long as 12 weeks of gestation. As explained physiologically, the luteoplacental shift, when progesterone production is taken over by the developing placenta, does not take place until about weeks 8 to 10 of pregnancy,[77] and it is recommended that luteal phase support should be continued until this time. In one study, discontinuation of progesterone treatment after 2 weeks of embryo transfer and an established biochemical pregnancy lead to abortion in 20 percent of the biochemically pregnant patients.[8] Although significantly more bleeding episodes were observed in the first trimester after early cessation of progesterone supplementation in 5 weeks, the abortion rate was similar among singleton pregnancies.[78] Although there is no firm evidence to support the continuation of luteal phase support until 10 to 12 weeks' gestation, this practice is used in the majority of IVF cycles worldwide.[79]

CONCLUSION

Considering what has been stated so far, it could be concluded that luteal phase is one of the most important stages in any IVF treatment cycle, ignorance of which will significantly reduce fertility and pregnancy. During the past two decades, in line with the great advancements in assisted reproductive techniques, adequate attention has been paid to the endometrium and uterus as the site of embryo implantation and growth. Moreover, endometrial receptivity has been evaluated both, in the cellular and morphologic aspects. The effects of different modes of progesterone administration, as well as the efficacy of hCG and GnRH-a hormones have been examined. What is clear is that there is a need for luteal phase support in ART cycles. It seems that progesterone is the best and safest drug that can be used both vaginally and muscularly. Although hCG is followed by a better prognosis, yet, due to the risk of developing OHSS, its prescription is limited to those who are not at risk for OHSS. Adequate attention paid to estrogen supplementation in recent years, is an interesting point, though it needs more research to arrive at a definite result, especially with regard to its role in endometrial receptivity.

REFERENCES

1. Edwards R, Steptoe P. Establishing full-term human pregnancies using cleavage embryos grown *in vitro*. Br J Obstet Gynaecol 1980;87:737-56.
2. Keye W, Chang R, Rebar R, Soules M. Infertility: Evaluation and treatment. first edn. Newyork. Sounders 1995. pp. 178-94.
3. Van der Wiele RL, Bagumil J, Dyrenfurth I, Ferin M, Jewelewicz R, Warren M, et al. Mechanisms regulating the menstrual cycles in women. Recent progress in hormone research 1970;6:63-103.
4. Simon C, Cano F, Valbuena D, Rembohj J, Lepicer A. Clinical evidence for detrimental effect on uterine receptivity of high serum estradiol concentrations in high and normal responder patients. Hum Reprod 1995;10:2432-7.
5. Sher G, Zouves C. Optimizing implantation: Diagnostic and Therapeutic considerations; in Brindsen PR (Ed). A textbook of *in vitro* fertilization and assisted reproduction, 2 edn. New York, Parthenon, 1999. pp. 275-83.
6. Jones GES. Some newer aspects of the management of infertility. JAMA 1949;14:1123-9.
7. Bourgain CJ. Endometrial biopsy in the evaluation of endometrial receptivity. IJ Gynecol Obstet Biol Reptod 2004;33:513-7.
8. Gazvani R, Sajjad Y, Russell R, Alfirevic Z. Duration of luteal support (DOLS) with progesterone pessaries to improve the success rates in assisted conception: study protocol for a randomized controlled trial. Trials 2012;13:118.
9. Beckers NJM, Laven JSE, Eijkemans, Fauser BCJM. Follicular and luteal phase characteristics following early cessation of gonadotropin releasing hormone agonist during ovarian stimulation for *in vitro* fertilization. Hum Reprod 2000;15:43-9.
10. Stewart Dr, Overstreet JW, Nakajim ST, Lassey BL. Enhanced ovarian steroid secretion before implantation in early human pregnancy. J Clin Endocrinol Metab 1993;76:1470-6.
11. Nippoldt T, Reame N, Kelch R, Marshall J. The roles of estradiol and progesterone in decreasing luteinizing hormone pulse frequency in the luteal phase of the menstrual cycle. J Clin Endocrinol Metab 1989;69:67-76.
12. Smitz J, Bourgain C, Van Waesberghe L, Camus M, Devroey P, Van Steirteghem A. A prospective randomized study on estradiol valerate supplementation in addition to intravaginal micronized progesterone in buserelin and hMG-induced superovulation. Hum Reprod 1993;8:40-5.
13. De Ziegler D, Bergeron C, Cornel C, Medalie D, Massal M, Milgrom E, et al. Effects of luteal estradiol on the secretory transformation of human endometrium and plasma gonadotropins. J Clin Endocrinol Metab 1992;74:322-31.
14. Beckers NG, Macklon NS, Eijkemans MJ, Ludwig M, Felberbaum RE, Diedrich K, Bustion S, et al. Non–supplemented luteal phase characteristics after the administration of recombinant human chorionic gonadotropin, recombinant luteinizing hormone, or gonadotropin releasing hormone (GnRH) agonist to induce final oocyte maturation in *in vitro* fertilization patients after ovarian stimulation with recombinant follicle stimulating hormone and GnRH antagonist co-treatment. J Clin Endocrinol Metab 2003;88:4186-92.
15. Sharara Fl, Mcclamrock HD. Ratio of estradiol concentration on the day of human chorionic gonadotropin administration to mid-luteal estradiol concentration is predictive of IVF outcomes. Hum Reprod 1999;14:2777-82.
16. Fujimoto A, Osuga Y, Fujiwara T, Yano T, Tsutsumi O, Momoeda M, Kugu K, Koga K, Morita Y, Wada O, Taketani Y. human chorionic gonadotropin combined with progesterone for luteal support improves pregnancy rate in patients with low late-mid-luteal estradiol levels in IVF cycles. J Assisted Reprod Genet 2002;19:550-4.
17. Daya S. Efficacy of progesterone support in the luteal phase following *in vitro* fertilization and embryo transfer: Meta-analysis of clinical trials. Hum Reprod 1988;3:731-4.

18. Nyboe Andersen A, Popovic-Todorovic B, Schmidt KT, Loft A, Lindhard A, Hojgaard A, et al. Progesterone supplementation during early gestations after IVF or ICSI has no effect on the delivery rates: A randomized controlled trial. Hum Reprod 2002;17:357-61.

19. Abate A, Brigandi A, Abate FG, Manti F, Unfer V, Perino M Luteal phase support with 17alpha-hydroxylprogesterone versus unsupported cycles in *in vitro* fertilization: A comparative randomized study. Gynecol Obstet Invest 1999;48:78-80.

20. Damario MA, Goudas VT, Session DR, Hammitt DG, Dumesic DA. Crinone 8 percent vaginal progesterone gel results in lower embryonic implantation efficiency after *in vitro* fertilization-embryo transfer. Fertil Steril 1999;72:829-36.

21. Bouckaert Y, Robert F, Englert Y, et al. Acute eosinophilic pneumonia associated with intramuscular administration of progesterone as luteal phase support after IVF: Case report. Hum Reprod 2004;19:1806-10.

22. Unfer V, Casini ML, Costabile L, Gerli S, Baldini D, Di Renzo GC. 17 alpha-hydroxyprogesterone caproate versus intravaginal progesterone in IVF-embryo transfer cycles: A prospective randomized study. Reprod Biomed Online 2004;9:17-21.

23. Cicinelli E, de Ziegler D, Bulletti C, Matteo MG, Schonauer LM, Galantino P. Direct transport of progesterone from vagina to uterus. Obstet Gynecol 2000;95:403-6.

24. Tavaniotou A, Smilz J, Bourgain C, Devroey P. Comparison between different routes of progesterone administration as luteal phase support in infertility treatment. Hum Reprod Update 2000;6:139-48.

25. Penzias As. Luteal phase support. Fertil Steril 2002;77:318-23.

26. Devroey P, Palermo G, Bourgain C, Van Waesberghe L, Smitz J, Van Steirteghem AC. Progesterone administration in patients with absent ovaries. Int J Fertil 1989;34:188-93.

27. Bourgain C, Devory P, Van Waesberghe L, Smith J, Streingen AC. Effects of natural progesterone on the morphology of the endometrium in patients with primary ovarian failure. Hum Reprod 1990;5:537-43.

28. Anserini P, Costa M, Remorgida V, Sarli R, Guglielminetti E, Ragni N. Luteal phase support in assisted reproductive cycles using either vaginal (Crinone 8%) or intramuscular (Prontogest) progesterone: Results of a prospective randomized study. Minerva Ginecol 2001;53:297-301.

29. Abate A, Perino M, Abate FG, Brigandi A, Costabile L, Manti F. Intramuscular versus vaginal administration of progesterone for luteal phase support after IVF-ET. A comparative randomized study. Clin Exp Obstet Gynecol 1999;26:203-6.

30. Friedler S, Raziel A, Schachter M. Luteal support with micronized progesterone following *in vitro* fertilization using a downregulation protocol with gonadotropins releasing hormone agonist: A comparative study between vaginal and oral administration. Hum Reprod 1999;14:1944-8.

31. Nahoul K, Dehennin L, Scholler R. Radioimmunoassay of plasma progesterone after oral administration of micronized progesterone. J Steroid Biochem 1987;26:241-9.

32. Nahoul K, Dehennin L, Jondet M, Roger M. Profiles of plasma estrogens, progesterone and their metabolites after oral or vaginal administration of estradiol or progesterone. Maturitas 1993;16:185-202.

33. Norman TR, Morse CA, Dennerstein L. Comparative bioavailability of orally and vaginally administered progesterone. Fertil Steril 1991;56:1034-9.

34. Dunstone T, Zosmer A, Hussain S, Tozer A, Paney N, Wilson C, et al. A comparison between cyclogest pessaries and crinone gel as luteal support in IVF-ET cycles. British Fertility Society Annual Meeting Abstract Book 1999;62 (Abstract# Fc21).

35. Ludwig M, Schwartz P, Babahan A, Weiss JM, Felberbaum R, et al. Luteal phase support using either Crinone 8 percent or uterogest: Results of a prospective randomized study. Europ J Obstet Gynaecol 2002;103:48-52.

36. Polyzos NP, Messini CI, Papanikolaou EG, Mauri D, Tzioras S, Badawy A, Messinis IE.Vaginal progesterone gel for luteal phase support in IVF/ICSI cycles: A meta-analysis. Fertil Steril. 2010;94:2083-7.

37. Van der Linden M, Buckingham K, Farquhar C, Kremer JA, Metwally M. Luteal phase support for assisted reproduction cycles. Cochrane Database Syst Rev 2011;(10) CD009154.

38. Smith EM, Anthony FW, Gadd SC, Masson GM. Trials of support treatment with human chorionic gonadotropin in the luteal phase after treatment with buserelin and human menopausal gonadotropin in women taking part *in vitro* fertilization programme. Br Med J 1989;298:1483-6.

39. Bellaisch-Allart J, De Mouzon J, Lapousterle C, Mayer M. The effect of hCG supplementation after combined GnRH agonist/hMG treatment in an IVF programme. Hum Reprod 1990;5:163-6.

40. Herman A, Ron EL R, Golan A. Pregnancy rate and ovarian hyper-stimulation after luteal human chorionic gonadotropin releasing hormone analogue and menotrophins. Fertil Steril 1990;53:92-6.

41. Buvat J, Marcolin G, Guittard C. Luteal support after luteinizing hormone releasing hormone agonist for *in vitro* fertilization: Superiority of human gonadotropins over oral progesterone. Fertil Steril 1990;53:490-4.

42. Soilman S, Daya S, Collins J, Hughes EG. The role of luteal phase support in infertility treatement: A meta-analysis of randomized trials. Fertil Steril 1994;61:1068-76.

43. Nikkanenn V, Kersanov I, Makinen J, Vourento T. The effect of luteal support with hCG or progesterone on the daily progesterone profile after different types of ovarian stimulation. Hum Reprod 1992;7:333-6.

44. Martinez F, Coroleu B, Parera N. Human chorionic gonadotropin and intravaginal natural progesterone are equally effective for luteal phase support in IVF. Gynecol Endorinol 2000;14:316-20.

45. Daya S, Gunby J. Luteal phase support in assisted reproductive cycles. (Cochrane review) In: The Cochrane library, Issue 3, chichester, UK: John Wiley and Sons Ltd. 2004.

46. Ghosh D, Sengupta J, Sengupta PD. Luteal phase ovarian oestrogen is not essential for implantation and maintenance of pregnancy from surrogate embryo transfer in the rhesus monkey. Hum Reprod 1994;9:629-37.

47. Shingara J, Keiger K, Shelton J, Laosinchai-Wolf W, Powers P, Conrad R. et al. An optimized isolation and labeling platform for accurate microRNA expression profiling. RNA. 2005;11:1461-70.

48. Haouzi D, Assou S, Mahmoud K, Tondeur S, Rème T, Hedon B, De Vos J, Hamamah S. Gene expression profile of human endometrial receptivity: comparison between natural and stimulated cycles for the same patients. Hum Reprod 2009;24:1436-45.

49. Yulian Zhao, Howard Zacur, Chris Cheadle, Ning Ning, Jinshui Fan, Nikos F Vlahos. Effect of luteal-phase support on endometrial microRNA expression following controlled ovarian stimulation. Reprod Biol Endocrinol 2012;10:72.

50. Smitz J, Bourgain C, Van Waesberghe L, Camus M, Devroey P, Van Steirteghem A. A prospective randomized study on estradiol valerate supplementation in addition to intravaginal micronized progesterone in buserelin and hMG-induced superovulation. Hum Reprod 1993;8:40-5.

51. Lewin A, Benshushan A, Mezker E, Yanai N, Schenker J, Goshen R. The role of estrogen support during the luteal phase of *in vitro* fertilization-embryo transplant cycles: A comparative study between progesterone alone and estrogen and progesterone support. Fertil Steril 1994;62:212-5.

52. Kaider AS, Coulam CB. Luteal estrogen supplementation in pregnancies associated with low serum estradiol concentrations. Early Pregnancy 2000;4:191-9.

53. Meldrum DR, Marr B, Stubbs C, Wisot A, Yeo L, Hamilton F. Impaired uterine receptivity in the infertile women over age 40 having oocyte donation and correction with increased progesterone replacement. Reprod Fertil Dev 1992;4:689-93.

54. Benadiva CA, Metzger YA. Superovulation with human menopausal gonadotropins in associated with endometrial glandstroma dyssynchrony. Fertil Steril 1994;61:700-4.

55. Gleicher N, Brown T, Dudkiewicz T, Karande V, Rao R, Balin M, Campbell D, Pratt D. Estradiol/Progesterone Substitution In The Luteal Phase Improves Pregnancy Rates In Stimulated Cycles-But Only In Younger Women. Early pregnancy. Biology and Medicine 2000;1:P 064-073.

56. Farhi J, Weissman A, Steinfeld Z, Shorer M, Nahum H, Levran D. Estradiol supplementation during the luteal phase may improve the pregnancy rate in patients undergoing *in vitro* fertilization-embryo transfer cycles. Fertil Steril 2000;73:761-5.

57. Lukaszuk K, Liss J, Lukaszuk M, Maj B. Optimization of estradiol supplementation during the luteal phase improves the pregnancy rate in women undergoing *in vitro* fertilization-embryo transfer cycles. Fertil Steril 2005;83:1372-6.

58. Gorkemli H, AK D, akyurek C, Aktan M, Duman S. comparison of pregnancy outcomes of progesterone or progesterone + estradiol for luteal phase support in ICSI-ET cycles. Obstet Gynecol Invest 2004;58:140-4.

59. Clark DH, Schrader WT, O'Malley BW. Mechanisms of steroid hormone action. In: Wilson JD, Foster DW (Eds) 1985.

60. Pritts E, Atwood A. Luteal phase support in infertility treatment: A meta-analysis of the randomized trials. Hum Reprod 2002;17:2287-99.

61. Li TC, Warren MA, Cooke ID. The artificial cycle as an effective treatment of persistently retarded endometrium in the luteal phase. Human Reprod 1994;9:409-12.

62. Smitz J, Devroy P, Faguer B, Bourgain C, Camus M, Van Steirteghem AC. A prospective randomized comparison of intramuscular or intravaginal natural progesterone as a luteal phase and early pregnancy supplement. Hum Reprod 1992;7:168-75.

63. Artini PG, Volpe A, Angioni S, Galassi MC, Battaglia C, Genazzani AR. A comparative, randomized study of three different progesterone support of the luteal phase following IVF/ET program. J of Endocrinol Invest 1995;18:51-6.

64. Pouly JL, Bassil S, Frydman R, et al. Luteal support after *in vitro* fertilization: Crinone 8 percent a sustained release vaginal progesterone gel versus uterogestan. An oral micronized progesterone. Hum Reprod 1996;11:2085-9.

65. Licciardi F, Kwiatkowski A, Noyes N, et al. Oral versus intramuscular progesterone for *in vitro* fertilization: A prospective randomized study. Fertil Steril 1999;71:614-8.

66. Herman A, Raziel A, Dtrassburger D, soffer Y, Bukovsky I, Ron-EL R. The benefits of mid luteal addition of human chorionic gonadotropin in IVF using a down-regulation protocol and luteal support with progesterone. Hum Reprod 1996;7:1552-7.

67. Tesarik J, Hazout A, Mendoza-Tesarik R, Mendoza N, Mendoza C: Beneficial effect of luteal-phase GnRH agonist administration on embryo implantation after ICSI in both GnRH agonist and antagonist-treated ovarian stimulation cycles. Hum Reprod 2006; 21:2572-9.

68. Kyrou D, Kolibianakis EM, Fatemi HM, Tarlatzi TB, Devroey P, Tarlatzis BC.Increased live birth rates with GnRH agonist addition for luteal support in ICSI/IVF cycles: A systematic review and meta-analysis. Hum Reprod Update 2011;17:734-40.

69. Oliveira JB, Baruffi R, Petersen CG, Mauri AL, Cavagna M, Franco JG Jr.Administration of single-dose GnRH agonist in the luteal phase in ICSI cycles: A meta-analysis. Reprod Biol Endocrinol 2010;8:107.

70. Fatemi H, Kolibianakis M, Camus M, Tournaye H, Donoso P, Papanikolaou E, Devroey P. Addition of estradiol to progesterone for luteal supplementation in patients stimulated with GnRH antagonist/rFSH for IVF: A randomized controlled trial. Hum Reprod 2006;21:2628-32.

71. Balasch J, Tur R. Creus M. Triggering of ovulation by gonadotropin releasing hoemone agonist in gonadotroppin stimulated cycles for prevention of ovarian hyperstimulation syndrome and multiple pregnancy 1994;8:7-12.

72. Penarrubia J, Balasch J, Fabregues F, Creus M, casamitjana R, Ballesca J, Puetro B, Vanrell A. Human chorionic gonadotropin luteal support overcomes luteal phase inadequacy after gonadotropin releasing hormone agonist induced ovulation in gonadotropins stimulated cycles 1998;13.3315-8.

73. Balash J, Fabergues F, Tur R, et al. Further chrachterization of the luteal phase inadequacy after GnRH- agonist induced ovulation in gonadotropin stimulated cycles. Hum Reprod 1995;10:1377-81.

74. Casper RF. Ovarian hyperstimulation: Effects of GnRH analogues. Does triggering ovulation with gonadotrophin-releasing hormone analogue prevent severe ovarian hyperstimulation syndrome? Hum Reprod 1996;11:1144-6.

75. Kol S, Lewit N, Itskovitz-Eldor J. Ovarian hyperstimulation: effects of GnRH analogues. Ovarian hyperstimulation syndrome after using gonadotropin releasing hormone analogue as a

trigger of ovulation: Causes and implications. Hum Reprod 1996;11:1143-4.

76. Itskovitz J. Levron J, Kol S. Use of gonadotropin releasing hormone agonist to cause ovulation and prevent the ovarian hyperstimulation syndrome. Clin Obstet Gynecol 1993;36: 701-10.

77. Ludwig M, Diedrich K. Evaluation of an optimal luteal phase support protocol in IVF. Acta Obstet Gynecol Scand 2001;80: 452-66.

78. Kohls G, Ruiz F, Martínez M, Hauzman E, de la Fuente G, Pellicer A, Garcia-Velasco JA. Early progesterone cessation after in vitro fertilization/intracytoplasmic sperm injection: A randomized, controlled trial. Fertil Steril 2012;98:858-62.

79. Vaisbuch E, Leong M, Shoham Z. Progesterone support in IVF: Is evidence-based medicine translated to clinical practice? A worldwide web-based survey. Reprod Biomed Online. 2012;25:139-45.

Should We Encourage Patients to Try Complementary Therapies as a Means of Improving Well-being and Fertility Success?

Sandra de la Garza, Carmen Martinez Jover

INTRODUCTION

During the 1980s, various studies were published, suggesting that stress, and ways of dealing with stress, are related to the condition of infertility, which in itself may be considered a situation of chronic stress. Studies have also suggested that stress can affect the outcome of infertility treatments. In the 1990s, Newton et al.[1] developed an instrument to evaluate perceived infertility-related stress. The 'Inventory of Problems Associated to Infertility' provided a reliable measure of perceived infertility-related stress and enabled characterization of the responses from individuals. They showed that patterns of infertility-related stress differed depending on gender, fertility history, and infertility diagnosis, and it showed that among patients receiving treatment, social, sexual, and relationship concerns appeared central to current distress, and suggested that counseling interventions targeting these domains appeared likely to offer maximum therapeutic benefit.[1]

Domar et al.[2] demonstrated a positive effect when physiological intervention was applied to a group of infertile women, who were followed for a period of one year. The team showed a statistically significant difference between the cognitive-behavioral group and the controls, concluding that group psychological interventions appear to lead to increased pregnancy rates in infertile women.[2]

The Stress of Infertility: Lack of Control

Infertility support organizations are constantly told by those they support that whereas the treatments generate a physical wear-out, the emotional wear-out that the whole situation produces is greater. The emotional roller coaster, which couples embark upon when they are diagnosed with infertility is driven by disbelief, fear, lack of control, and is often accompanied by a sense of loss and grief.[3]

This lack of control of the situation when faced with fertility problems is as important an issue to address as the process of treatment itself. When in the situation, where 'lack of control' is experienced, the infertile couple, more often than not, takes a passive role in the doctor-patient relationship, subsequently building non-effective relations. The physician has his knowledge and medical techniques under control, but in this relationship, the patient relinquishes all responsibility of success and may be quick to apportion blame and guilt when the result is not what was anticipated or desired.

Infertility is not a terminal illness; it will not kill a body but it can lead to spiritual death.

Addressing Stress and Infertility

The Mexican Infertility Association (AMI) has decided to address the relationship between psychology and infertility, but without pretending to analyze this issue in-depth, nor to come up with definitive answers or magic formulas. Instead, the AMI has chosen to build on existing knowledge and to work with patients to assist them with changing their attitude of how to cope with the infertility process. The authors hypothesize that such assistance could be the key to increasing the percentage of success in infertility treatments.

The pilot program, 'Accompanying', uses a psycho-educative intervention, based on the experience of working with infertile couples, and utilizing an interdisciplinary, individual and integral approach to incorporate into the medical protocol. The goal is to create a supportive environment, where the patient leaves the passive doctor-patient relationship and starts to act as part of the team.

The key component in this program is to accompany people and support them so they can face the entire fertility treatment process emotionally well-balanced, and take responsibility for their own treatment. This change in attitude may result in an increase in the percentage of treatment success.

Accompanying Program

Sixteen participants with different medical problems, age, socioeconomic background, treatments and doctors were enrolled in the pilot Accompanying program. The only common denominator was their infertility. Of those 16, 12 have been successful in obtaining pregnancy, either through intrauterine insemination (IUI) or *in vitro* fertilization (IVF).

The program consists of a six week curriculum, where the AMI representatives accompany the patient during the treatment process and provide tools to control stress. A 24-hour telephone hotline is available exclusively to these patients. The program, just like all of the AMI's events, has been created and carried out by volunteers of this non-profit organization. The help and support come from someone, who at some point in his or her life, was in the same situation as the person(s) they are supporting. This is based on the philosophy that one of the most effective therapies for a patient is to feel the support of a 'survivor'.

Week 1: Informative

Patients are provided with information that enables them to interpret and understand the information provided by infertility clinics. Doubts and erroneous perceptions are identified and addressed, ultimately helping with the decision-making process. Every detail regarding what they will be exposed to during these six weeks and the support that can be provided throughout the process, is explained clearly.

Week 2: Psychological Support

Support is provided on the different ways in which to face infertility and the treatment, enabling patients to channelize all the positive attitudes, which is necessary to keep intact during the treatment process. It is essential that it is identified how each individual presents anxiety and to subsequently identify their own successful ways of facing stress in such situations.

Weeks 3 and 4: Assertiveness Program and Meditation Techniques

During these two weeks, the program concentrates on addressing the expression of feelings and emotions. The participants are encouraged to express everything that worries or concerns them at that very moment in order to identify the source(s) of stress and the subsequent reactions of each participant.

First, the participants are asked to change the names of every event in the process (embryo transfer, oocyte aspiration, ultrasound monitoring, prescriptions, etc.). The purpose is to reduce anxiety during the treatment process. The most popular names have been: Satellite images (for ultrasounds), lovely bugs (sperm), the Titanic treasure (prescriptions), and Eskimos (frozen embryos).

Following these suggestions, the aim is to make the process of assisted fertilization a more accessible situation. It also helps to make it more personalized and reduces uncertainty by allowing the patient to take part in, and to take control of the situation. Meditation techniques are taught to assist with managing how to reach autocontrol and assertiveness. The patient herself is encouraged to identify the technique(s) that works best for her.

Week 5: Reflexology

Reflexology is provided to the woman before *in vitro* or insemination, depending on the case, to help eliminate tension.

Week 6: The Waiting Period

During this part of the program, participants learn how to identify irrational thoughts, eliminate negative anticipation, and how to generate positive thoughts. It has been possible to identify that anxiety levels are lower and depression almost non-existent in those participating in the program.

'Day Zero' is what most people call the day the laboratory results come in to tell them the outcome of the whole process. What worries most patients is the fear that after all they have been through the result might be negative. AMI has achieved through the program to change the attitude towards 'Day Zero' into: 'Every negative result from now on is a step towards our final goal.' Such support provides patients with the emotional tools to continue almost immediately with a new medical option, if treatment has failed. This eliminates the stage known as 'bench warming', which is when the patient does not handle the emotional stress well and then decides to take some time off to recover emotionally before pursuing other fertility treatments. With time often being of the essence, reduction of 'bench warming' is essential for potential future success.

CONCLUSION

In the Accompanying program, 77 percent of participants (n = 16) conceived.

A larger patient population and a longer duration of the program is necessary before it is possible to quantify the efficiency of the program, but early results suggest that accompanying enhances the quality of life for couples, who find themselves in the situation of having to deal with infertility and supports them in addressing the possibility of assisted reproductive technique (ART) failure. The program allows patients to take control during the ART process, reduces uncertainty, and supports couples during a process, which can affect their social function, self-esteem, and their relationship with each other.

Through emotional support, a multidisciplinary approach and the provision of knowledge, the program has demonstrated that most people have the capacity to change the way in which they face stress associated with infertility. Addressing the psychological aspects related to infertility needs to be incorporated into the infertility treatment protocol so that counseling programs and psychological support are available for couples who have to deal with infertility and undergo ART.

REFERENCES

1. Newton CR, Sherrard W, Glavac I. The Fertility Problem Inventory: Measuring infertility perceived stress. Fertil Steril 1999;72:54-62.
2. Domar A, Clapp D, Slawsby EA, Dusek J, Kessel B, Freizinger M. Impact of group psychological interventions on pregnancy rates in infertile women. Fertil Steril 2000;73:805-11.
3. Hummelshoj L, Bush D. Coping with endometriosis-related infertility. In: Allahbadia GN, Mechant R, De Wilde RL, Verhoeven HC (Eds). Gynecological Endoscopy and Infertility. India: Jaypee Brothers 2005. pp. 400-03.

Age and ART Success:
Where do We Draw the Line?

Neri Laufer, Avi Tsafrir

OVERVIEW

The tendency to postpone childbearing in developed countries and the relatively high rate of infertility in older women contribute to an increase in the percentage of women aged 40 years and older opting for infertility treatments. The main factor for infertility in this group is oocyte senescence, but since this process does not have a specific diagnosis, many of these patients will be classified as having 'unexplained infertility'. Since the efficacy of the traditional clinical approach for this condition in older women, such as superovulation and intrauterine insemination (IUI), is low, assisted reproductive techniques (ART) should be considered at an early stage for such patients. Since female age is the most significant factor affecting the *in vitro* fertilization (IVF) outcome, results are, however, quiet disappointing. Delivery rates per started cycle are 10 to 17 percent at the age of 40, with a decline with each additional year of age: 2 to 7 percent between the age 43 to 44 years and no more than 2 percent over 44 years of age. Delivery beyond age 45 years following IVF treatment is extremely rare. Pregnancy loss rates are 30 to 40 percent, contributing to the low delivery rates. Transferring more embryos is associated with a significantly increased delivery rate, with a negligible additional risk of high order multifetal pregnancies. When counseling older women considering ART, we believe the key is providing thorough information regarding her personal chances for live birth based on actual figures, with preference to the IVF unit's own experience. The final decision should be based on the patient's choice considering her personal beliefs and opinions, and other options for parenthood such as oocyte donation and adoption.

INTRODUCTION

Female fertility declines with age, from the mid 4th decade of life. In historical observations in a population in which contraception is condemned, 33 percent of women are found to be infertile at the age of 40 years.[1] This results from the aging processes, involving almost every aspect of the reproductive system, but is mainly caused by a decline in oocyte number and quality.[2-4] In many Western societies, social trends have led to a delay in childbearing, and many women attempt to conceive for the first time in their late 30's and early 40's.[5] Some of these women suffer from infertility, but routine fertility evaluation appears normal, leading to the relatively common diagnosis of 'unexplained infertility'. As a result, the aging women form an increasing portion of patients entering assisted reproductive techniques (ART) programs. For example, the American Society of Reproductive Medicine (ASRM) reported that 22 percent of *in vitro* fertilization (IVF) treatment cycles in 2006 were initiated in patients aged 40 years and older.[6] In Europe, in 2006, the percentage women at age 40 and older was 4 to 27 percent of all IVF patients.[7]

Female age is the single most important determining factor for successful human reproduction. In a similar trend to natural fertility, ART success rates begin to decline from the early 30's. This trend accelerates towards the late 30's, reaching a live birth rate of near zero at age 45. The growing number of infertile aging women faces a natural burden, unresolved by contemporary medical practice, excluding oocyte donation. Since ART is expensive, demanding and not free of risk, the question is, from what age should fertility treatment be limited. In this chapter, we review current knowledge of ART [i.e. IVF and intracytoplasmic sperm injection (ICSI)] success in older patients and discuss some aspects of this complex clinical and ethical dilemma.

ART Success in Patients Aged 40 and Older

The largest data collection on IVF outcome in older patients is derived from multicenter experience and national registries. The British Human Fertilisation and Embryology Authority report for the years 1998–99, demonstrated a birth rate of 7.3 percent per treatment cycle in 1037 cycles in the 41 to 42 age group.[8] This rate decreased to 3 percent in 404 cycles at 43 to 44 years of age, and to 0.5 percent in 210 cycles at 45 years. The ASRM reported on a delivery rate of 8.1 percent in women over 40 years.[6] Single center studies provide additional details important for clinical decision-making, such as results for each year of age after 40. Data from single-center reports of over 500 cycles performed in advanced maternal age (AMA) IVF patients (defined in this text as ≥40 years of age) are summarized in Tables 41.1 and 41.2. Additional information was also reported by Orvieto et al.[9] and Ciray et al.,[10] which do not fit with the tables created here. There is a gradual decline in the number of available oocytes, embryos, and overall success with each year of age after 40 (Table 41.3). Since the rate of miscarriage is 30 to 40 percent, the rate of delivery is approximately 10 to 15 percent at age 40 years, 5 to 8 percent at age 42 to 43 years, and nearly zero after age 44 years.

Table 41.1: Summary of the largest reports on IVF in advanced aged women: ART results at age 40-41 years

Author	No. of IVF cycles	No. of patients	Pregnancy rate (%)	Delivery rate (%)
Klipstein, et al.[11]	1436	760	17.2	12
Tsafrir, et al.[12]	711	183	10	6.6
Lass	305	305	14	10.5
Opsahl	201	144	20	9.4
Grimbizis, et al.[13]	388	NR	15	10.5*

*Approximation based on reported ongoing pregnancy rates after 12 weeks of gestation.
Abbreviation: NR: not reported

Table 41.2: Summary of the largest reports on IVF in advanced aged women: ART results at age 42-43 years

Author	No. of IVF cycles	No. of patients	Pregnancy rate (%)	Delivery rate (%)
Klipstein, et al.[11]	970	383	14	8.5
Tsafrir, et al.[12]	436	115	8	5
Lass	252	106	9	6
Opsahl	136	89	21	6
Grimbizis, et al.[13]	190	NR	9	5*

*Approximation based on reported ongoing pregnancy rates after 12 weeks of gestation.
Abbreviation: NR: not reported

Table 41.3: Outcome of 1217 IVF cycles in 381 women aged 40 years and older, stratified according to year of age[12]

Patient age during IVF cycle	Number of patients (% of all patients)	Number of treatment cycle (% of all cycles)	Cancellation before OPU (%)	Mean number of oocytes retrieved	Mean number of embryos transferred	Pregnancy rate per initiated cycle (%)*	Delivery rate per initiated cycle (%)*	Percent of patients who had a live birth by the end of analysis (%)
40	114 (30)	209 (17)	14.4	6.5	3	13.9	9	17
41	69 (18)	230 (19)	13.5	5.4	2.7	6.1	4.3	15
42	71 (19)	237 (19.5)	17.7	5.8	2.7	8.7	6.3	21
43	44 (11.5)	199 (16)	17	4.8	2.6	7	4	18
44	43 (11.3)	150 (12)	16.7	5.5	3.1	4	2.7	9
45	30 (8)	143 (12)	19.6	4.7	2.5	2.8	0.7	3.3
46-7	10 (2.6)	49 (4)	26.1	3.2	2	0	0	0
Total	381	1217	16.6	5.5	2.7	7.3	4.7	15

*Significant association between age and outcome (P < 0.01), with a significant linear trend (P < 0.001).
Abbreviation: OPU: ovarian pick-up

Predictive Factors for ART Success in AMA Patients

Infertility Diagnosis

Interestingly, both Klipstein et al.[11] and our group[12] did not find a correlation between the specific cause of infertility and ART outcome. The impact of the aging process on female fertility surpasses all the other disorders.

Obstetric History

In our series, a third of the patients had already delivered at least once before treatment at advanced age.[12] These patients did not have higher success rates in ART after age 40 than nulliparas. Again, female aging has a dominant effect on ART success even in patients who were previously fertile or succeeded in ART at a younger age.

Number of Embryos

There is a correlation between the number of embryos transferred as well as embryo quality and ART success in older women.[9] Grimbizis et al.[13] have shown that when four embryos or less were selected from a higher number of embryos, the results were comparable to cycles in which five or more available embryos were transferred.[13] Combelles et al.[14] demonstrated that in women aged 40 years and older, transfer of 5 embryos resulted in higher delivery rates when compared to a smaller number.[14] However, transfer of 6 or more embryos did not contribute to better results. Therefore, they concluded that the transfer of 5 embryos is optimal for AMA IVF patients. In our experience of 1217 cycles in 318 women, there was a positive correlation between treatment success and the number of oocytes retrieved.[12] When >4 oocytes were considered a 'good' ovarian response, it was found that higher pregnancy rates were achieved by younger women (age 40–41 years). In older patients, this effect was blunted. Similarly, in our study group as a whole, both pregnancy and delivery rates increased when more embryos were transferred. The mean number of embryos transferred was 2.7, but in 32 percent of cycles 3 embryos or more were replaced. While the transfer of three embryos or more correlated with a significantly higher pregnancy rate in younger women (40–41 years), this effect was not observed in older women.

Basal FSH

Klipstein et al.[11] found that low follicle-stimulating hormone (FSH) levels on menstrual day 3 were correlated with pregnancy and live birth rates in ART women aged 40 and above.[11] Ciray et al.[10] also reported that patients who had more than 5 oocytes had significantly lower FSH levels.[10] Those patients also had higher delivery rates. However, a multivariate analysis of these results was not performed. In contrast, in our cohort, elevated FSH, defined as higher than either 10 or 15 IU/mL was not associated with the outcome.[12]

How Many Cycles?

Most pregnancies are achieved in the first four treatment cycles. Data on cumulative success rate in AMA patients is limited. Based on 116 patients starting treatment at age 40 to 43, the Brussels group found a delivery rate of 9, 10, 12 and 15 percent in the first to fourth cycle, respectively. However, only 17 patients reached the fourth cycle. In our experience of 1217 cycles in 318 patients aged 40 years and older, pregnancy rates were 3.2, 5.4 and 5.7 percent in the first, second and third treatment cycle, respectively. 75 percent of all pregnancies were achieved in the first two treatment cycles. Only 3 of 88 (3.4%) pregnancies occurred after the 6th cycle of treatment. It seems therefore, that performing over 5 IVF cycles adds almost no deliveries in this age group.

When is there no Chance at All?

Approaching the age of 44 years, the chances of live birth are practically non-existent. Klipstein et al.[11] reported 6 live births out of 230 started cycles at age 44 years (2.6%), and one birth out of 52 started cycles at age 45 years (1.9%).[11] We had 4 deliveries, resulting from 150 initiated cycles at age 44 (2.7%), and one out of 143 at age 45 (0.7%).[12] Ciray, et al.[10] reported one delivery in 149 ICSI cycles, performed on women aged 44 to 45 years (0.7%).[10] In another series of 158 ICSI cycles performed at age 44 to 46 years, one 44 year old woman had an ongoing pregnancy after 12 weeks.[13] Delivery after age 45 in ART using one's own oocytes is such a rare event that it has been published as a case report.[15] The largest published experience on this issue comes from Cornell Medical Center. In a series of 231 cycles started at age 45 years and older, the pregnancy rate per retrieval was 21 percent. However, due to an 85 percent pregnancy loss, the result was 2 percent delivery rate per initiated cycle. Eventually, 5 women, all at age 45 years, had a delivery, but none above that age.[16]

CONCLUSION

Where do we Draw the Line?

The dilemma of limiting fertility treatments from reproductively aging women involves clinical, financial and ethical aspects. ART appears ineffective for women aged 45 years and older. In our opinion, the chances are fairly reasonable up to age 42 years. For all aging patients, we believe the key to this issue is providing the patient with information. Clinicians should supply aged patients, who are considering ART, an estimate of the chance of live birth. The natural tendency for over-optimism may be balanced by informing the patient on the actual figures of a specific unit in her age. For example, some patients base their hopes on various factors, such as having already delivered a child, or specific infertility diagnoses unrelated to age such as male infertility. However, these factors appear not to change the overall poor prognosis. Other alternatives for parenthood, such as oocyte donation and adoption, should be discussed. If the patient is well-informed, we believe that it is her right to choose any treatment, even if it is costly, bares some risks, and has little chance to succeed.

Obviously, ART in aging patients is not cost-effective. Health care policy in this matter varies in different countries, reflecting not only financial resources but cultural and religious priorities. For example, in Israel, national health insurance covers most fertility treatments, including IVF, up to a limit of two children. The age limit of IVF, using a woman's own oocytes is 45 years, but there is no limit on the number of treatment cycles. On the other hand, the number of oocytes available for donation is severely limited. In other countries, such as the US, ART is provided only privately, but oocyte donation is available. Based on data, such as reviewed here, policy makers should decide on the age limit of ART.

REFERENCES

1. Tietze C. Reproductive span and rate of reproduction among Hutterite women. Fertil Steril 1957;8:89.
2. Armstrong DT. Effects of maternal age on oocyte developmental competence. Theriogenology 2001;55:1303-22.
3. Baird DT, Collins J, Egozcue J, Evers LH, Gianaroli L, Leridon H, et al. Fertility and ageing. Hum Reprod Update 2005;11:261-76.
4. te Velde ER, Pearson PL. The variability of female reproductive ageing. Hum Reprod Update 2002;8:141-54.
5. Hewlett SA. Executive women and the myth of having it all. Harvard Business Review 2002;80:66-73.
6. Centers for Disease Control and Prevention, American Society for Reproductive Medicine, Society for Assisted Reproductive Technology. 2006 Assisted Reproductive Technology Success Rates: National Summary and Fertility Clinic Reports, Atlanta: U.S. Department of Health and Human Services, Centers for Disease Control and Prevention; 2008.
7. de Mouzon J, Goossens V, Bhattacharya S, Castilla JA, Ferraretti AP, Korsak V, et al. Assisted reproductive technology in Europe, 2006: Results generated from European registers by ESHRE. Hum Reprod 2010;25:1851-62.
8. Human Fertilisation and Embryology Authority. Ninth annual report. HEFA, London 2000.
9. Orvieto R, Bar-Hava I, Yoeli R, Ashkenazi J, Rabinerson D, Bar J, et al. Results of *in vitro* fertilization cycles in women aged 43–45 years. Gynecol Endocrinol 2004;18:75-8.
10. Ciray HN, Ulug U, Tosun S, Erden HF, Bahceci M. Outcome of 1114 ICSI and embryo transfer cycles of women 40 years of age and over. Reprod Biomed Online 2006;13:516-22.
11. Klipstein S, Regan M, Ryley DA, Goldman MB, Alper MM, Reindollar RH. One last chance for pregnancy: A review of 2,705 *in vitro* fertilization cycles initiated in women age 40 years and above. Fertil Steril 2005;84:435-45.
12. Tsafrir A, Simon A, RA, Reubinoff B, Lewin A, Laufer N. Retrospective analysis of 1217 *in vitro* fertilization (IVF) cycles in women aged 40 and older. Reprod Biomed Online 2007;14: 348-55.
13. Grimbizis G, Vandervorst M, Camus M, Tournaye H, Van Steirteghem A, Devroey P. Intracytoplasmic sperm injection, results in women older than 39, according to age and the number of embryos replaced in selective or nonselective transfers. Hum Reprod 1998;13:884-9.
14. Combelles CM, Orasanu B, Ginsburg ES, Racowsky C. Optimum number of embryos to transfer in women more than 40 years of age undergoing treatment with assisted reproductive technologies. Fertil Steril 2005;84:1637-42.
15. Dal Prato L, Borini A, Cattoli M, Preti MS, Serrao L, Flamigni C. Live birth after IVF in a 46-year-old woman. Reprod Biomed Online 2005;11:452-4.
16. Spandorfer SD, Bendikson K, Dragisic K, Schattman G, Davis OK, Rosenwaks Z. Outcome of *in vitro* fertilization in women 45 years and older who use autologous oocytes. Fertil Steril 2007;87:74-6.

Is There an Ideal Luteal Phase Support Protocol in ART?

Shevach Friedler

OVERVIEW

There is a wide consensus regarding the necessity of luteal support after controlled ovarian hyperstimulation (COH) for *in vitro* fertilization (IVF), involving use of any gonadotropin-releasing hormone (GnRH) analog. Although serial human chorionic gonadotropin (hCG) injections offer the most efficient treatment, it is more prudent to administer progesterone to avoid iatrogenic aggravation of possible ovarian hyperstimulation syndrome (OHSS). Intramuscular or vaginal administration of progesterone are both effective but the choice of any specific progesterone preparation should be individualized considering costs and possible side effects. At present, there is insufficient data in the literature to state that the addition of estradiol to progesterone is also mandatory.

INTRODUCTION

Impairment of the luteal phase in COH cycles preceded by gonadotropin-releasing hormone agonist (GnRHa) down-regulation has long been observed.[1,2] In these cycles, luteal phase insufficiency occurs, caused by prolonged suppression of gonadotropin secretion, leading to insufficient stimulation of the corpora lutea[3-5] combined with an impaired ability of progesterone production of their luteal cells.[6]

Defect of corpus luteum function implies less progesterone (P), estradiol (E2) and 17-hydroxy progesterone (17-OH P), possible lack of other substances and impaired endometrial morphology,[7,8] or asynchrony between stromal and glandular maturation.[5] All the endometrial features in non-supplemented cycles, investigated by Bourgain et al,[9] including endometrial maturation assessed by histology, ultrastructure by electron microscopy and estradiol and progesterone receptor distribution by immunocytochemistry, were consistent with an impaired progesterone bioavailability.

The consequences of luteal phase deficiency are a reduced embryo implantation rate, a lower pregnancy rate and an increased miscarriage rate when pregnancy is established.[10]

Indeed, a wide consensus exists concerning the need for luteal phase progesterone supplementation after oocyte retrieval during IVF cycles, if GnRH analog was incorporated into the controlled ovarian stimulation treatment.[5,11-14]

GnRH antagonists have more recently joined the armamentarium of the medications used for assisted reproductive technique (ART) treatment. Being competitive inhibitors, they are administered for a significantly shorter period of time compared to the agonist, and have a shorter duration of effect. However, luteal phase insufficiency has also been reported in GnRH antagonist-treated cycles,[15-18] thus making luteal support mandatory after COH using both GnRH agonist or antagonist.

CLINICAL DISCUSSION

Methods of Luteal Phase Support

There is no one single method of luteal support. In an attempt to enhance the probability of pregnancy, various studies investigated the best methodology for luteal support using different treatment protocols with varying outcomes.

In general, luteal phase support may be given by:

- Addition of serial doses of human chorionic gonadotropin (hCG), acting similarly as the hCG secreted endogenously by the early conceptus, activating and prolonging the function of the corpus luteum.
- Supplementation of progesterone alone.
- Supplementation of progesterone with estradiol.
- Supplementation of progesterone with the addition of a single injection of hCG.

Examining the several meta-analyses found in the literature regarding luteal phase support after ART, it is evident that both hCG and progesterone support were found to have better pregnancy rates when compared to placebo. An early meta-analysis by Daya[19] did not support the routine use of progesterone in IVF cycles stimulated with Clomiphene citrate and human menopausal gonadotropin (hMG). However, that analysis is irrelevant today because it was performed in cycles which were not downregulated with any GnRH analog. A subsequent meta-analysis by Soliman et al.[20] supported the routine use of hCG in GnRH agonist IVF cycles. Progesterone was also found to be beneficial as luteal phase support in IVF cycles.[20]

In a more recent meta-analysis, Pritts and Atwood[10] found that intramuscular progesterone is the treatment of choice for luteal phase support in IVF cycles. However, Nosarka et al.[21] in a recent meta-analysis, showed again that hCG supplementation provided the highest pregnancy rates. The controversy expressed in the various meta-analyses might be explained by the fact that these analyses include reports covering different time intervals, using variable COH treatment methodologies and variable luteal support treatments.

Furthermore, no definite consensus exists concerning the length of luteal phase support in IVF cycles. Although some studies presented evidence that withdrawal of vaginal progesterone at the time of a positive pregnancy test had no effect on the delivery rate,[22,23] most treatment protocols advocate the use of progesterone throughout the first trimester of pregnancy, based on the findings of the knowledge about the luteoplacental shift, occurring at around 8 to 10 weeks of pregnancy.[24,25]

As there is no uniformity in the various studies conducted, a closer look at the studies upon which some of the meta-analyses were based is necessary to gain a better understanding of the subject matter.

hCG Supplementation

Serial injections of hCG, 2500 IU, on days +3, +6, +9 after the initial hCG given for oocyte maturation prior to oocyte aspiration, has been proposed as an effective method of luteal support.[11,12] Comparing treatment cycles with serial hCG doses to cycles without luteal support or placebo, Smith et al.[11] and Belaisch-Allart et al.[12] have reported a significant improvement in ongoing pregnancy rates following *in vitro* fertilization-embryo transfer (IVF-ET) when COH included a long GnRHa/hMG protocol. Significantly better pregnancy and ongoing pregnancy rates were reported in cycles supported with hCG (1500 IU, in three doses) compared to micronized progesterone administered orally (400 mg/day)[13] or by intramuscular injections (IM).[26]

Meta-analyses of randomized trials of luteal support have found a preference for hCG[20,21] in terms of pregnancy rates achieved.

The main disadvantage of this method is that it may induce or aggravate the development of ovarian hyperstimulation syndrome (OHSS), especially in the high risk group of patients, such as those with polycystic ovary syndrome (PCOS).[13,14,27-33] Comparing luteal support with hCG (38 patients) and intramuscular (IM) progesterone (39 patients), Araujo et al.[29] found no difference in the pregnancy rates (PR) between the two groups, but in the hCG group, 5 patients developed moderate to severe OHSS. Therefore, Araujo et al.[29] suggested avoiding hCG luteal supplementation in patients responding to COH with peak estradiol (E2) levels over 2500 pg/mL and the number of follicles exceeding 10.

Progesterone Supplementation

As progesterone is available in variable preparations, one has to consider the most appropriate method of progesterone administration. The various methods of natural progesterone supplementation available include IM injection of natural progesterone in oil, micronized progesterone ingested orally and direct absorption of micronized progesterone or progesterone gel through the vaginal mucosa.

The early studies from the Free University of Brussels, regarding luteal phase support, were enlightening. Their numerous studies comparing the use of the various routes of progesterone administration in ART cycles supported the advantages of intravaginal administration and demonstrated that this route was at least as good as the intramuscular route and clearly better than the oral route of administration.[5,7,34-37] Serial injections of hCG, given in a regimen of 2000 IU on days +4,+8,+12, were compared to luteal support with natural progesterone given intramuscularly in a regimen of 50 mg/day combined with estradiol valerate, 6 mg/day from day +6. No significant difference in the pregnancy rate (PR) was observed.[5] As the latter method carried no risk of augmenting OHSS, it was recommended as the preferable regimen for luteal support.[5] Regarding endometrial histology, in cycles supplemented with hCG, 50 percent of the endometria were in phase but asynchrony still persisted (stroma being advanced by 3 days). However, in cycles supplemented with natural progesterone (IM or vaginal) 75 to 80 percent of cycles were in phase and no asynchrony was noted.[9,38] Features of impaired progesterone bioavailability improved with luteal support, especially with vaginally administered progesterone, evidencing the strong uterine first-pass effect.[9,38]

Compared to placebo, any kind of luteal phase progesterone supplementation, whether oral, intramuscular or vaginal, is superior.[21]

Progesterone administered orally demonstrated lower bioavailability (<10%) due to the first-liver-pass effect,[39] which calls for the use of higher doses that give rise to a fairly large number of side effects such as dryness, flushing, and nausea[40] somnolence and sedation due to the high rate of various metabolites binding to specific sites within gamma-aminobutyric acid (GABA) receptors.[41] Oral progesterone is also associated with a lower pregnancy rate compared to intramuscular or vaginal administration.[37,42-45] Even the increased dose of oral P (200 or 300 mg daily) failed to induce homogenous secretory endometrial transformation among menopausal women.[35]

A metabolically stable and orally effective stereoisomer of progesterone, dydrogesterone, was reported to be a successful alternative of progesterone administration in cases where oral therapy is preferred. Chakravarty et al.[46] reported no significant difference in pregnancy rates, miscarriage rates or viable delivery rates using oral dydrogesterone (20 mg/day) as luteal support compared with vaginal micronized progesterone (600 mg/day), corroborating previous studies using dydrogesterone for luteal support after ovulation induction,[47] artifical endometrial preparation for donated oocyte recipients[105] and luteal support after IVF-ET.[48,49]

Intramuscular administration provides very high serum levels of progesterone and this route is effective with regard to pregnancy rates. However, the intramuscular injection of progesterone in oil is frequently painful, is not recommended to be self-administered and it may be associated with complications, such as local soreness, abscesses, and inflammatory reactions.[50,31]

However, there is increasing evidence that vaginal and intramuscular progesterone are at least equally effective, considering the rate of biochemical and clinical pregnancies and deliveries.[37,42,44,45]

As vaginal preparations are self-administered and achieve high concentrations of progesterone at the tissue level due to the first uterine pass effect,[51,52] via the effective direct vagina-uterine transport,[38,53-55] homogenous secretory transformation of the endometrium is achieved[56] resulting in good clinical pregnancy rates, hence, vaginal administration has become the method of choice for many IVF units, worldwide.[10,31,57-59] The infrequent major side effects of this mode of treatment carries with is vaginal irritation or pruritus and discharge.

The optimal effective dosage of micronized progesterone has not been established yet. Treatment regimens were based upon the experience learned in cycles where the endogenous ovarian steroid production was insignificant due to the lack of corpus luteum, such as in recipients of oocyte donation or cryopreserved-thawed embryo transfers. Use of 200 to 600 mg/day has been reported.[13,36,60,61] Endometrial preparation for cryopreserved-thawed embryo transfer was successfully performed using a protocol combining estrogen (transdermal and oral preparations) with micronized P given vaginally at a daily dose of 100 mg twice a day.[60] Vaginal administration of a low dose of 200 mg/day of micronized progesterone achieved a significantly better implantation rate compared to a regimen of oral administration of 800 mg/day.[62]

Buvat et al.[13] compared the efficacy of 400 mg/day micronized progesterone, administered orally or vaginally, to hCG injected every third day following embryo transfer (ET) at a dose of 1500 IU. When the peak serum estradiol (E2) level was > 2700 pg/mL, the implantation rate (IR) was 5 to 6 times higher with vaginal administration compared to oral treatment (26% vs 5%). The pregnancy rate (PR) and IR with vaginal treatment were similar to that following hCG injections.

Further studies[36,61] compared natural progesterone, administered IM or vaginally. The daily dosage of natural progesterone used in these studies was 600 mg/day micronized progesterone given vaginally compared with 50 mg/day progesterone in oil given intramuscularly. Vaginal administration resulted in better ongoing PR (30.5% vs 19.1%, respectively) as well as a lower rate of early spontaneous abortions (2.9% vs 9.1%, respectively).[36,61]

Another study compared luteal support with 90 mg progesterone gel administered vaginally to 300 mg/day micronized progesterone taken orally and found no difference regarding PR/ET, rate of spontaneous abortions or number of babies born per embryos replaced.[63]

Simunic et al.[64] recently reported similar rates of clinical pregnancies in a study comprising of a total of 285 women undergoing IVF-ET who were treated with either Crinone 8 percent vaginal progesterone gel (90 mg/day) or Utrogestan vaginal capsules (600 mg/day). The efficacy of the two vaginal progesterone formulations was nearly the same, but the tolerability and acceptability of Crinone 8 percent gel were superior in the opinion of patients. These results corroborate previous studies[59,65] reporting comparable IVF-ET success with the use of both the supplements.

Presently, several pharmacological preparations are used in different countries, including vaginal tablets or suppositories, administered twice or three times a day or vaginal gel, given once daily.

No sufficient randomized controlled trials (RCTs) favoring any specific method of vaginal supplementation have been reported in the literature regarding clinical efficacy, and the appropriate choice should take into consideration individual patient's comfort. In fact, a few studies evaluated patients' convenience and side effects of variable progesterone preparations.

In a randomized study, comparing side effects and patient convenience of Cyclogest suppositories and Endometrin tablets used for luteal phase support in IVF cycles, Ng et al.[66] reported no significant difference in perineal irritation on days 6 and 16 between the two groups. There were no differences in the hormonal profiles in the luteal phase and IVF outcomes between the two groups. Ludwig et al.[59] reported less vaginal discharge and fewer application difficulties after the use of Crinone gel when compared with Utrogestan capsules. Kleinstein[65] demonstrated comparable local irritation or discomfort between patients receiving Utrogestan capsules (6.9%) and Crinone gel (8%). Clearly, due to lack of standardization and great variability in the published studies, it is not possible to arrive at one single recommendation.

Considering that hCG administration for luteal support, although effective, carries the risk of maintaining or enhancing OHSS,[10,31,32,58,67] many fertility units worldwide prefer using progesterone as the treatment of choice for luteal phase support, based on reports about its comparable efficiency.

Mid-luteal Addition of Estradiol

Serum levels of E2 and progesterone begin to decline from the mid-luteal phase in IVF-ET cycles in which pituitary suppression is used to obtain COH.[4,5,68] This decline may be as dramatic as 95 percent compared to their levels on the day of hCG administration.[69]

While the role of estradiol in the follicular phase is well-established, its importance during the luteal phase is controversial in the relevant literature. No obligatory role of estradiol during the luteal phase was confirmed in animals[70] and its role during the luteal phase in humans is believed to be permissive rather than obligatory.[53,71,72] During artificial preparation of the endometrium for oocyte donation in women with no endogenous corpus luteum, pregnancies have been established without luteal estrogenic support.[73-75] In addition, morphologic studies have shown no significant effect of estrogen support during the luteal phase.[76,77]

Controversial results exist regarding the absolute mid-luteal E2 level required for implantation and a specific definition of an ideal luteal E2 level required for implantation is lacking. Several studies have not found any difference in mid-luteal E2 levels between conception and non-conception cycles during various circumstances, including natural cycles in infertile patients,[78] after COH for IVF-ET without pituitary downregulation[79-81] and COH with pituitary downregulation.[69,82,83]

Other studies reported significantly higher mid-luteal E2 levels in conception cycles during various circumstances, such as natural cycles in fertile patients[84-86] or after COH for IVF-ET without pituitary downregulation[78,87-89] or with.[90] The depletion of E2 during the luteal phase had a negative effect on implantation in women undergoing oocyte donation.[91]

Still, there are very few studies addressing the importance of the significant decline in serum E2 levels around the mid-luteal phase in IVF cycles, especially in cycles with high E2 concentrations on the day of hCG administration. Controversial findings, reported in retrospective studies published in the literature, regarding the actual clinical impact of markedly elevated serum E2 levels during the late follicular phase and its mid-luteal decline after COH with pituitary downregulation for IVF-ET, have caused intense debate.[69,82,83]

Whereas Sharara and McClamrock[82] found that an 80 percent decline in estradiol levels from the hCG day to the mid-luteal phase resulted in significantly decreased implantation and PRs,[82] Ng et al.[83] reported no adverse effect on the outcome of 763 ART cycles, despite the observed mid-luteal E2 decline.[83]

According to Friedler et al,[69] in a study comprising 100 patients on a long GnRHa downregulation protocol and vaginal progesterone luteal supplementation, multifactorial analysis refuted the negative role of supraphysiologic levels of E2 on the day of hCG administration or its dramatic decline in the mid-luteal phase on the success rate after embryo transfer. Successful implantations were observed in a wide range of mid-luteal E2 levels.

Based on the notion that significant deviations from the physiologic levels of steroids produced by the ovaries could be detrimental to implantation after ET, affecting endometrial priming and receptivity as well as oocyte maturation and embryo quality, the addition of estradiol was proposed together with the progesterone supplementation, aiming to mimic the corpus luteum function in the normal luteal phase.

However, the value of adding E2 to progesterone[58] to support the luteal phase in GnRH agonist cycles is still controversial.[10] Some well-designed prospective randomized studies reported no benefit in increasing pregnancy rates.[92,93] Comparing micronized progesterone, administered vaginally (600 mg/day), with or without estrogen supplementation (6 mg/day), no difference in endometrial morphology was found, with 75 percent being in phase and no asynchrony noted.[92] There was no difference in the PR/ET and live birth rates comparing 50 mg IM progesterone, administered alone, with 50 mg IM progesterone, administered with 2 mg estradiol valerate supplementation, indicating that estrogen addition to the luteal support regimen showed no clinical advantage.[93]

On the other hand, several reports advocate the supplementation of estradiol during the luteal phase. Farhi et al.[94] found a significant increase in implantation and pregnancy rates using luteal estrogen support, but only in patients on a long protocol of pituitary downregulation with GnRHa depot. They used a daily dose of 4 mg Estradiol valerate.

Another study, comprising 213 patients reported statistically significantly higher a implantation rate, clinical PR, and ongoing pregnancy/delivery rate in patients who underwent GnRH-agonist pituitary downregulation for IVF and who received progesterone plus phytoestrogens (1,500 mg daily) for luteal phase support in comparison with patients receiving progesterone and placebo.[95]

Gorkemli et al.[96] randomized 310 ICSI cycles to use either 600 mg/day micronized progesterone vaginally or transdermal estradiol 100 mg/day + 600 mg/day vaginal micronized progesterone. A significantly higher pregnancy rate was observed in the latter group (13.5% vs 38.5%, respectively), suggesting that the addition of estradiol was beneficial.

In a recent study by Lukaszuk et al[97] a significantly higher implantation and pregnancy rate were recorded in patients who received low-dose (2 mg/day) E2 supplementation compared with no substitution (PR 32.8% vs 23.1%, respectively). Significantly higher implantation and pregnancy rates were found in the group with high-dose E2 supplementation (6 mg/day) (PR 51.3%), indicating that in women treated with a long GnRH analog protocol for COH, the addition of a high-dose of E2 to daily progesterone supplementation was very beneficial.[97]

There is very little information regarding the value of estradiol addition to progesterone for luteal support after COH in GnRH-antagonist cycles. A recent study by Ata et al.[98] conducted in 2012, did not find a beneficial effect of orally administered estrogen as adjunct to progesterone for luteal support, even in a dose of 6 mg/day, when administered to all patients in an unselective manner.[98] However, evaluation of the luteal phase hormone profiles in these patients showed that the addition of 4 mg E2 for luteal support after stimulation with recombinant follicle-stimulating hormone (rFSH) and GnRH-antagonist does not alter significantly the endocrine profile of the luteal phase until day 7 after hCG. On day 10 after hCG, the E2 levels were significantly higher in the E2 supplemented group.[99]

One has to note that the safety of luteal phase E2 supplementation has not been thoroughly investigated yet.[100]

Mid-luteal Addition of hCG in Cycles with Progesterone Supplementation

Mimicking the natural conception cycle, where endogenous hCG stimulates the function of the corpus luteum, mid-luteal addition of hCG was proposed.

No benefit of *in vitro* hCG supplementation in the early lutel phase, up to day +8 (postovulatory hCG), was demonstrated.[101] A single dose of hCG on day 7 may serve as an alternative to late luteal estrogen supplementation, raising late luteal estrogen and progesterone serum levels.[88,102] In two prospective studies, this assumption has not been proven neither in conjunction with vaginal progesterone[30] nor with intramuscular progesterone.[103] Actually, according to Mochtar et al.[30] the mid-luteal addition of hCG resulted in more cases with OHSS, higher day +11 (post hCG) E2 and progesterone but lower pregnancy rates compared to patients treated with progesterone only. However, Fujimoto et al.[104] attempted to make clinical decisions on the basis of mid-luteal E2 levels in unsuccessful IVF first cycles. They achieved a significant improvement in PR (almost 2.5 times higher) in the randomized group, who were given supplemental progesterone and hCG versus the group given supplemental progesterone alone during the luteal phase. In the progesterone + hCG group, the mid-luteal phase E2 concentration was 15 times higher than in the P-only group.

GnRH Agonist as Luteal Phase Support

A pilot study by Pirard et al.[105] demonstrated that repeated administration of a GnRH agonist (Buserelin) during the luteal phase of GnRH antagonist-treated ART cycles is able to support the luteal phase and is compatible with a viable ongoing, pregnancy. This study also suggested that a regimen of three intranasal administrations per day could be at least as effective as 10,000 IU hCG administered subcutaneously, followed by 600 mg/day micronized progesterone administered vaginally in terms of the luteal phase hormonal profile.[105]

RECENT ADVANCES

Zarutskie and Phillips, in 2010,[106] performed a meta-analysis, showed that administration of vaginal progesterone is comparable to administration of intramuscular progesterone for luteal phase support in ART cycles. Their analysis showed a comparable effect between the administration of vaginal progesterone as an oil-in-capsule or as a bioadhesive gel and IM progesterone administration on the endpoints of clinical pregnancy (OR = 0.91, 95% [CI 0.74, 1.13]) and ongoing pregnancy (OR = 0.94, 95% [CI 0.71, 1.26]). A nominally significantly lower rate of miscarriage was observed with vaginal progesterone compared with IM progesterone (OR = 0.54, 95% [CI 0.29, 1.02]).[106]

The recent 2010 meta-analysis by Polyzos et al.,[107] analyzing seven randomized controlled trials, provided solid evidence that no significant difference exists between vaginal gel and all other vaginal progesterone forms in terms of clinical pregnancy rates.

Jee et al.[108] performed a meta-analysis of nine randomized controlled trials to clarify whether the addition of E2 to standard luteal progesterone supplementation is beneficial, both in GnRH agonist and antagonist IVF cycles. The combined data presented suggest that the addition of E2 to progesterone for luteal phase support does not improve IVF outcomes in GnRH agonist and antagonist cycles. Still, there is an obvious need for further large-scale studies regarding GnRH antagonist cycles.

Castillo et al.[109] recently reported very successful luteal support using low-doses of hCG in GnRH antagonist cycles triggered with a GnRH agonist. In their study, a total of 192 patients at risk for OHSS, undergoing a GnRH antagonist protocol (0.25 mg/day Cetrorelix) with recombinant FSH stimulation, were triggered with 1.5 mg subcutaneous Leuprolide administration for ovulation. A total of three hCG boluses were used for luteal support, 1000 IU (Group A, n = 44), 500 IU (Group B, n = 115) or 250 IU (Group C, n = 33) every third day, from the day after oocyte retrieval. The overall pregnancy rate was 51.8 percent and the clinical pregnancy rate was 43.4 percent. Eight cases of moderate (4.2%) and seven cases of severe OHSS (3.6%) were observed in this study. Six out of the seven (85.7%) severe cases were late-onset OHSS related to pregnancy. The authors concluded that a single dose of GnRH agonist for triggering ovulation and low-doses of hCG used as luteal phase support seem to secure a normal pregnancy outcome without increasing the OHSS risk.[109]

CONCLUSION

In conclusion, there is a wide consensus regarding the necessity of luteal support after COH for IVF involving the use of any GnRH analog. Although serial hCG injections offer the most efficient treatment, it is more prudent to administer progesterone to avoid iatrogenic aggravation of possible OHSS. The role of low-dose hCG luteal support, especially with GnRH agonist triggering in GnRH antagonist cycles awaits further evaluation. Intramuscular or vaginal administration of progesterone are both effective but the choice of any specific progesterone preparation should be individualized considering the costs and possible side effects. At present, there is insufficient data in the literature to state that the addition of estradiol to the progesterone for luteal phase support is also mandatory.

REFERENCES

1. Porter RW, Smith J, Craft IL, Abdulwahid WA, Jacobs AS. Induction of ovulation or *in vitro* fertilization using buserelin and gonadotropins. Lancet 2(8414), 1984;1284-5.
2. Wildt T, Diedrich K, Van Der Ven h, Al Hasani S, Hubner H, Klasen R. Ovarian hyperstimulation for *in vitro* fertilization controlled by GNRH agonist administered in combination with human menopausal gonadotropins. Hum Reprod 1986;1:15.
3. Calogero AE, Macchi M, Montanini V, et al. Dynamics of plasma gonadotropin and sex steroid release in polycystic ovarian disease after pituitary-ovarian inhibition with an analog of gonadotropin-releasing hormone. J Clin Endocrinol Metab. 1987;64:980-5.
4. Smitz J, Devroey P, Braeckmans P, Camus M, Khan I, Staessen C, et al. Management of failed cycles in an IVF/GIFT programme with the combination of a GNRH analogue and hMG. Hum Reprod 1987;2:309-14.
5. Smitz J, Devroey P, Camus M, Deschacht J, Khan I, Staessen C, et al. The luteal phase and early pregnancy after combined GNRH-agonist/hMG treatment for superovulation in IVF or GIFT. Hum Reprod 1988;3:585-90.
6. Pellicer A, Miro F. Steroidogenesis *in vitro* of human granulosa lutel cells pretreated *in vivo* with gonadotropin-releasing hormone analogs. Fertil Steril 1990;54:590-6.
7. Van Steirteghem AC, Smitz J, Camus M, Van Weasberghe L, Deschacht J, Khan I, Staessen CV, Wisanto A, Bourgain C, Devroey P. The luteal phase after *in vitro* fertilization and related procedures. Hum Reprod 1988;3:161-4.
8. Macnamee MC, Edwards RG, Howles CM. The influence of stimulation regimens and luteal phase support on the outcome of IVF. Hum Reprod 1988;3:43-52.
9. Bourgain C, Smitz J, Camus M, Erard P, Devroey P, Van Steirteghem AC, Kloppel G. Human endometrial maturation is markedly improved after luteal supplementation of gonadotropin-releasing hormone analogue/human menopausal gonadotropin stimulated cycles. Hum Reprod 1994;9:32-40.
10. Pritts E, Atwood A. Luteal phase support in infertility treatment: A meta-analysis of the randomized trials. Hum Reprod 2002;17:2287-99.
11. Smith EM, Anthony FW, Gadd SC, Masson GM. Trial of support treatment with human chorionic gonadotropin in the luteal phase after treatment with buserelin and human menopausal gonadotropin in women taking part in an *in vitro* fertilization programme. Br Med J 1989;298:1483-6.
12. Belaisch-Allart J, De Mouzon J, Lapouterle C, Mayer M. The effect of hCG supplementation after combined GNRH agonist hMG treatment in an IVF programme. Hum Reprod 1990; 5:163-6.
13. Buvat J, Marcolin G, Guittard C, Herbaut JC, Louvet AL, Dehaene JL. Luteal support after luteinizing hormone releasing hormone agonist for *in vitro* fertilization: Superiority of human gonadotropin over oral progesterone. Fertil Steril 1990;53:490-4.
14. Herman A, Ron El R, Golan A, Raziel A, Soffer Y, Caspi E. Pregnancy rate and ovarian hyperstimulation after luteal human chorionic gonadotropin in *in vitro* fertilization stimulated with gonadotropin-releasing hormone analog and menotropins. Fertil Steril 1990;53:92-6.
15. Albano C, Smitz J, Tournaye H, Riethmuller-Winzen H, Van Steirteghem A, Devroey P. Luteal phase and clinical outcome after human menopausal gonadotrophin/gonadotrophin-releasing hormone antagonist treatment for ovarian stimulation in *in vitro* fertilization/intracytoplasmic sperm injection cycles. Hum Reprod 1999;14:1426-30.
16. Tavaniotou A, Albano C, Smitz J, Devroey P. Effect of clomiphene citrate on follicular and luteal phase luteinizing hormone concentrations in *in vitro* fertilization cycles stimulated with gonadotropins and gonadotropin-releasing hormone antagonist. Fertil Steril 2002;77:733-77.
17. Beckers NG, Macklon NS, Eijkemans MJ, Ludwig M, Felberbaum R, Diedrich K, et al. Nonsupplemented luteal phase characteristics following the administration of r-hCG, r-hLH or GnRH agonist to induce final oocyte maturation in *in vitro* fertilization patients. J Clin Endocrinol Metab 2003;88:4186-92.
18. Kolibianakis EM, Bourgain C, Platteau P, Albano C, Van Steirteghem AC, Devroey P. Abnormal endometrial development occurs during the luteal phase of nonsupplemented donor cycles treated with recombinant follicle-stimulating hormone and gonadotropin-releasing hormone antagonists. Fertil Steril 2003;80:464-6.
19. Daya S. Efficacy of progesterone support in the luteal phase following *in vitro* fertilization and embryo transfer. Meta-analysis of clinical trials. Hum Reprod 1988;3:731-4.
20. Soliman S, Daya S, Collins J, Hughes EG. The role of luteal phase support in infertility treatment: A meta-analysis of randomized trials. Fertil Steril 1994;61:1068-76.
21. Nosarka S, Kruger T, Siebert I, Grové D. Luteal phase support in *in vitro* fertilization: meta-analysis of randomized trials. Gynecol Obstet Invest 2005;60:67-74.

22. Schmidt KLT, Ziebe S, Popovic B, Loft A, Andersen AN. Progesterone supplementation during early gestation after in vitro fertilization has no effect on the delivery rate. Fertil Steril 2001;75:337-41.

23. Nyboe Andersen A, Popovic-Todorovic B, Schmidt KT, Loft A, Lindhard A, Højgaard A, Ziebe S, et al. Progesterone supplementation during early gestations after IVF or ICSI has no effect on the delivery dates: A randomized controlled trial. Hum Reprod 2002;17:357-61.

24. Yoshimi T, Strott CA, Marshall JR, Lipsett MB. Corpus luteum function in early pregnancy. J Clin Endocrinol Metab 1969;29:225-30.

25. Shamma FN, Penzias AS, Thatcher S, DeCherney AH, Lavy G. Corpus luteum function in successful *in vitro* fertilization cycles. Fertil Steril 1992;57:1107-9.

26. Claman P, Domingo M, Leader A. Luteal phase support in in vitro fertilization using gonadotropin–releasing hormone analogue before ovarian stimulation: A prospective randomized study of human chorionic gonadotropin versus intramuscular progesterone. Hum Reprod 1992;7:487-9.

27. McClure N, Leya J, Radwanska E, Rawlins R, Haning RV Jr. Luteal phase support and severe ovarian hyperstimulation syndrome. Hum Reprod 1992;7:758-64.

28. MacDougall MJ, Tan SL, Jacobs HS. *In vitro* fertilization and the ovarian hyperstimulation syndrome. Hum Reprod 1992;7:597-600.

29. Araujo E Jr, Bernardini L, Frederick JL, Asch RH, Balmaceda JP. Prospective randomized comparison of human chorionic gonadotropin versus intramuscular progesterone for luteal phase support in assisted reproduction. J Assist Reprod Genet 1994;11:74-8.

30. Mochtar MH, Hogerzeil HV, Mol BW. Progesterone alone versus progesterone combined with hCG as luteal support in GNRHa/hMG induced IVF cycles: A randomized clinical trial. Hum Reprod 1996;11:1602-5.

31. Penzias AS. Luteal phase support. Fertil Steril 2002;77:318-23.

32. Daya S, Gunby J. Luteal phase support in assisted reproduction cycles (Cochrane Review), in: The Cochrane Library, Issue 3, John Wiley and Sons Ltd., Chichester, 2004.

33. Papanikolaou EG, Pozzobon C, Kolibianakis EM, Camus M, Tournaye H, Fatemi HM, et al. Incidence and prediction of ovarian hyperstimulation syndrome in women undergoing gonadotropin-releasing hormone antagonist *in vitro* fertilization cycles. Fertil Steril 2006;85:112-20.

34. Devroey P, Palermo G, Bourgain C, Waesberghe L, Smitz J, Van Steirteghem AC. Progesterone administration in patients with absent ovaries, Int J Fertil 1989;34:188-93.

35. Bourgain C, Devroey P, Van Waesberghe L, Smitz J, Van Steirteghem AC. Effects of natural progesterone on the morphology of the endometrium in patients with primary ovarian failure. Hum Reprod 1990;5:537-43.

36. Smitz J, Devroey P, Faguer B, Bourgain C, Camus M, Van Steirteghem AC. A prospective randomized comparison of intramuscular or intravaginal natural progesterone as a luteal phase and early pregnancy supplement, Hum Reprod 1992;7:168-75.

37. Tavaniotou A, Smitz J, Bourgain C, Devroey P. Comparison between different routes of progesterone administration as luteal phase support in infertility treatments. Hum Reprod Update 2000;6:139-48.

38. Balasch J, Fabregues F, Ordi J, Creus M, Penarrubia J, Casamitjana R, Manau D, Vanrell JA. Further data favoring the hypothesis of the uterine irst-pass effect of vaginally administered micronized progesterone. Gynecol Endocrinol 1996;10:421-6.

39. Nauhol K, Dehenin L, Jondet M. Profiles of plasma estrogens, progesterone and their metabolites after oral or vaginal administration of estradiol or progesterone. Maturitas 1993;16:185-202.

40. Whitehead MI, Townsend PT, Gill DK, Collins WP, Campbell S. Absorption and metabolism of oral progesterone. Br Med J [Clin Res] 1980;280:825-7.

41. Arafat ES, Hargrove JT, Maxon WS, Desoderio DM, Wentz AC, Anderson RN. Sedative and hypnotic effects of oral administration of micronized progesterone may be mediated through its metabolites. Am J Obstet Gynecol 1988;159:1203-9.

42. Liccardy FL, Kwiatkowski A, Noyes NL, Berkeley AS, Krey LL, Grifo JA. Oral versus intramuscular progesterone for *in vitro* fertilization: A prospective randomized study. Fertil Steril 1999;71:614-8.

43. De Ziegler D, Fanchin R. Progesterone and progestins: Applications in gynecology. Steroids 2000;65:671-9.

44. Levine H. Luteal support in IVF using novel vaginal progesterone gel Crinone 8 percent: Results of an open-label trial in 1,184 women from 16 U.S. centers. Fertil Steril 2000;74:836-7.

45. Penzias AS, Alper MM. Luteal support with vaginal micronized progesterone gel in assisted reproduction. Reprod Biomed Online 2003;6:287-95.

46. Chakravarty BN, Shirazee HH, Dam P, Goswami SK, Chatterjee R, Ghosh S. Oral dydrogesterone versus intravaginal micronized progesterone as luteal phase support in assisted reproductive technology (ART) cycles: Results of a randomized study. Journal of Steroid Biochemistry and Molecular Biology 2005;97:416-20.

47. Balasch J. Dydrogesterone treatment of endometrial luteal phase deficiency after ovulation induced by clomiphene citrate and human chorionic gonadotropin, Fertil Steril 1983;40:469-71.

48. Belaisch-Allart J, Testart J, Fries N. The effect of dydrogesterone supplementation in an IVF program, Hum Reprod 1987;2:183-5.

49. Domitrz J, Wolezynski S, Syrewicz M, Szamatowicz J, Kuezyanski W, Corochowski D, Szamatowicz M. A comparison of the efficiency of supplement in the second phase in the program IVF–ET by dydrogesterone and progesterone, Ginekol. Pol 1999;70:8-12.

50. Chantilis SJ, Zeitoun KM, Patel SI, Johns DA, Madziar VA, McIntire DD. Use of crinone vaginal gel for luteal support in *in vitro* fertilization cycles. Fertil Steril 1999;72:823-9.

51. De Ziegler D, Fanchin R, Massonneau M, et al. Hormonal control of endometrial receptivity. The egg donation model and controlled ovarian hyperstimulaiton. Ann. NY Acad Sci 1994;734:209-20.

52. Miles RA, Paulson RJ, Lobo RJ, Press MF, Dahmoush L, Sauer MV. Pharmacokinetics and endometrial tissue levels of progesterone after administration by intramuscular and vaginal routes: A comparative study. Fertil Steril 1994;62:485-90.

53. De Ziegler D. Hormonal control of endometrial receptivity. Hum Reprod 1995;10:4-7.

54. Fanchin R, De Ziegler D, Bergeron C, Righini C, Torrisi C, Frydman R. Transvaginal administration of progesterone. Obstet Gynecol 1997;90:396-401.

55. Buletti C, De Ziegler D, Flamigni C, Giacomucci E, Polli V, Bolelli GF, et al. Targeted drug delivery in gynaecology: The first uterine pass effect. Hum Reprod 1997;12:1073-9.

56. Ficicioglu C. High local endometrial effect of vaginal progesterone gel. Gynecol Endocrinol 2004;18:240-43.

57. Martinez F, Coroleu B, Parera N, Alvarez M, Traver JM, Boada M, Barri PN. Human chorionic gonadotropin and intravaginal natural progesterone are equally effective for luteal phase support in IVF, Gynecol. Endocrinol 2000;14:316-20.

58. Ludwig M, Diedrich K. Evaluation of an optimal luteal phase support protocol in IVF. Acta Obstet Gynecol Scand 2001;80: 452-66.

59. Ludwig M, Schwartz P, Babahan B, Katalinic A, Weiss JM, Felberbaum R, et al. Luteal phase support using either crinone 8 percent or utrogest: Results of a prospective, randomized study. Eur J Obstet Gynecol Reprod Biol 2002;103:48-52.

60. Salat-Baroux J, Alvarez S, Antoine JM, Tibi C, Cornet D, Mandelbaum J, Plachot M, Junca AM. Pregnancies after replacement of frozen-thawed embryos in a donation program. Fertil Steril 1988;49:817-21.

61. Devroey P, Smitz J, Bourgain C, Camus M, Van Steirteghem A. Micronized progesterone is the method of choice as supplementation therapy in LHRH-agonists superovulated cycles. Contracept Fertil Sex 1991;19:7-8.

62. Friedler S, Raziel A, Shachter M, Strassburger D, Bukovsky I, Ron-El R. Luteal support with micronized progesterone following *in vitro* fertilization using a down regulation protocol with gonadotropin-releasing hormone agonist: A comparative study between vaginal and oral administration. Hum Reprod 1999;14:1944-8.

63. Pouly JL, Bassil S, Frydman R, Hedon B, Nicollet B, Prada Y, Antoine JM, Zambrano R, Donnez J. Luteal support after *in vitro* fertilization: Crinone 8 percent, a sustained release vaginal progesterone gel, versus uterogestan, an oral micronized progesterone. Hum Reprod 1996;11:2085-9.

64. Simunic V, Tomic V, Tomic J, Nizic D. Comparative study of the efficacy and tolerability of two vaginal progesterone formulations, crinone 8 percent gel and utrogestan capsules, used for luteal support. Fertil Steril 2007;87:83-7.

65. Kleinstein J. Efficacy and tolerability of vaginal progesterone capsules (utrogestan) compared with progesterone gel (crinone 8%) for luteal phase support during assisted reproduction. Fertil Steril 2005;83:1641-9.

66. Ng EHY, Chan CCW, Tang OS, Ho PC. A randomized comparison of side effects and patient convenience between cyclogest1 suppositories and Endometrin1 tablets used for luteal phase support in IVF treatment, European Journal of Obstetrics and Gynecology and Reproductive Biology 2006.

67. Posaci C, Smitz J, Camus M, Osmanagaoglu K, Devroey P. Progesterone for the luteal support of assisted reproductive technologies: Clinical options. Hum Reprod 2000;15 (suppl 1):129-48.

68. Nikkanen V, Kresanov I, Makinen J, Vuorento T. The effect of luteal support with human chorionic gonadotropin or progesterone on the daily progesterone profile after different types of ovarian stimulation. Hum Reprod 1992;7:333-6.

69. Friedler S, Zimerman A, Schachter M, Raziel A, Strassburger D, Ron El R. The mid-luteal decline in serum estradiol levels is drastic but not deleterious for implantation after *in vitro* fertilization and embryo transfer in patients with normal or high responses. Fertil Steril 2005;83:54-60.

70. Ghosh D, De P, Sengupta J. Luteal phase ovarian oestrogen is not essential for implantation and maintenance of pregnancy from surrogate embryo transfer in the rhesus monkey. Hum Reprod 1994;9:629-37.

71. Ghosh D, Senupta J. Another look at the issue of peri-implantation oestrogen. Hum Reprod 1995;10:1-2.

72. Edgar DH. Oestrogen and human implantation. Hum Reprod 1995;10:2-4.

73. Kapetanakis E, Pantos KJ. Continuation of a donor oocyte pregnancy in menopause without early pregnancy support. Fertil Steril 1990;54:1171-3.

74. Stassart JP, Corfman RS, Ball GD. Continuation of a donor oocyte pregnancy in a functionally agonadal patient without early oestrogen support. Hum Reprod 1995;10:3061-3.

75. Zegers-Hochschild F, Altieri E. Luteal estrogen is not required for the establishment of pregnancy in the human. J Assist Reprod Genet 1995;12:224-8.

76. De Ziegler D, Bergeron C, Cornel C, Medalie DA, Massai MR, Milgrom E, et al. Effects of luteal oestradiol on the secretory transformation of human endometrium and plasma gonadotropins. J Clin Endocrinol Metab 1992;74:322-31.

77. Younis JS, Ezra Y, Sherman Y, Simon A, Schenker JG, Laufer N. The effect of estradiol depletion during the luteal phase on endometrial development. Fertil Steril 1994;62:103-7.

78. Laufer N, Navot D, Schenker JG. The pattern of luteal phase plasma progesterone and estradiol in fertile cycles. Am J Obstet Gynecol 1982;143:808-13.

79. Muasher SJ, Acosta AA, Garcia J, Jones GS, Jones HW Jr. Luteal phase serum estradiol and progesterone in *in vitro* fertilization. Fertil Steril 1984;41:838-43.

80. Mettler L, Michelmann HW. Estradiol values under gonadotropin stimulation in relation to the outcome of pregnancies in *in vitro* fertilization and embryo transfer. J in vitro Fertil Embryo Transfer 1987;4:303-6.

81. Nylund L, Beskow C, Carlstrom K, Fredricsson B, Gustafson O, Lunell NO, et al. The early luteal phase in successful and unsuccessful implantation after IVF-embryo transfer. Hum Reprod 1990;5:40-2.

82. Sharara FI, McClamrock HD. Ratio of estradiol concentration on the day of human chorionic gonadotropin administration to mid-luteal oestradiol concentration is predictive of *in vitro* fertilization outcome. Hum Reprod 1999;14:2777-82.

83. Ng EHY, Yeung WSB, Lau EYL, So WWK, Ho PC. A rapid decline in serum estradiol concentrations around the mid-luteal phase had no adverse effect on outcome in 763 assisted reproduction cycles. Hum Reprod 2000;15:1903-8.

84. Baird DD, Wilcox AJ, Weinberg CR, Kamel F, McConnaoughey DR, Musey PI, et al. Preimplantation hormonal differences between the conception and nonconception menstrual cycles of 32 normal women. Hum Reprod 1997;12:2607-13.

85. Stewart DR, Overstreet JW, Nakajima ST, Lasley BL. Enhanced ovarian steroid secretion before implantation in early human pregnancy. J Clin Endocrinol Metab 1993;76:1470-6.

86. Lipson SF, Ellison PT. Comparison of salivary steroid profiles in naturally occurring conception and nonconception cycles. Hum Reprod 1996;11:2090-6.

87. Hutchinson-Williams KA, Lunenfeld B, Diamond MP, Lavy G, Boyers SP, DeCherney AH. Human chorionic gonadotropin, estradiol, and progesterone profiles in conception and non-conception cycles in an *in vitro* fertilization program. Fertil Steril 1989;52:441-5.

88. Hutchinson-Williams K, Decherney A, Lavy G, Diamond MP, Naftolin F, Lunenfeld B. Luteal rescue in *in vitro* fertilization-embryo transfer. Fertil Steril 1990;3:495-501.

89. Emperaire JC, Ruffie A, Audebert AJ, Verdauger A. Early prognosis for IVF pregnancies through plasma estrogen. Lancet 1984;2:1151-5.

90. Akman MA, Erden HF, Bener F, Liu JE, Bahceci M. Can luteal phase estradiol levels predict the pregnancy outcome in *in vitro* fertilization cycles of good responders whose excess embryos yield blastocysts? Fertil Steril 2002;77:638-9.

91. Younis JS, Simon A, Laufer N. Endometrial preparation: Lessons from oocyte donation. Fertil Steril 1996;66:873-84.

92. Smitz J, Bourgain C, Van Waesberghe L, Camus M, Devroey P, Van Steirteghem AC. A prospective randomized study on oestradiol valerate supplementation in addition to intravaginal micronized progesterone in buserelin and HMG-induced superovulation. Hum Reprod 1993;8:40-5.

93. Lewin A, Benshusan A, Mezker E, Yanai N, Schenker JG, Goshen R. The role of estrogen support during the luteal phase in *in vitro* fertilization-embryo transplant cycles: A comparative study between progesterone alone and estrogen and progesterone support. Fertil Steril 1994;62:121-5.

94. Farhi J, Weissman A, Steinfeld Z, Shorer M, Nahum H, Levran D. Estradiol supplementation during the luteal phase may improve the pregnancy rate in patients undergoing *in vitro* fertilization-embryo transfer cycles. Fertil Steril 2000;73: 761-6.

95. Unfer V, Casini ML, Gerli S, Costabile L, Mignosa M, Di Renzo GC. Phytoestrogens may improve the pregnancy rate in *in vitro* fertilization-embryo transfer cycles: A prospective, controlled, randomized trial. Fertil Steril 2004;82:1509-13.

96. Gorkemli H, Ak D, Akyurek, Aktan M, Duman S. Comparison of pregnancy outcomes of progesterone or progesterone + estradiol for luteal phase support in ICSI-ET cycles. Gynecol Obstet Invest 2004;58:140-4.

97. Lukaszuk K, Liss J, Lukaszuk M, Maj B. Optimization of estradiol supplementation during the luteal phase improves the pregnancy rate in women undergoing *in vitro* fertilization-embryo transfer cycles. Fertil Steril 2005;83:1372-6.

98. Ata B, Kucuk M, Seyhan A, Urman B. Effect of high-dose estrogen in luteal phase support on live birth rates after assisted reproduction treatment cycles. J Reprod Med 2010;55:485-90.

99. Fatemi HM, MD, Camus M, Kolibianakis EM, Tournaye H, Papanikolaou EG, Donoso P, Devroey P. The luteal phase of recombinant follicle-stimulating hormone/gonadotropin-releasing hormone antagonist *in vitro* fertilization cycles during supplementation with progesterone or progesterone and estradiol. Fertil Steril 2007;87:504-8.

100. Hemminki E, Gissler M, Merilainen J. Reproductive effects of *in utero* exposure to estrogen and progestin drugs. Fertil Steril 1999;71:1092-8.

101. De los Santos MJ, Tarin JJ, Gomez E, Remohi J, Pellicer A. Daily measurement and *in vitro* effects of human chorionic gonadotropin in the early luteal phase. Hum Reprod 1993; 8:2047-51.

102. Grazi RV, Taney FH, Gagliardi CL, Von Hagen S, Weiss G, Schmidt CL. The luteal phase during gonadotropin theraphy: Effects of two human chorionic gonadotropin regiomens. Fertil Steril 1991;55:1088-92.

103. Herman A, Raziel A, Strassburger D, Soffer Y, Bukovsky I, Ron-El R. The benefits of mid-luteal addition of human chorionic gonadotropin in *in vitro* fertilization using a downregulation protocol and luteal support with progesterone. Hum Reprod 1996;11:1552-7.

104. Fujimoto A, Osuga Y, Fujiwara T, Yano T, Tsutsumi O, Momoeda M, et al. Human chorionic gonadotropin combined with progesterone for luteal support improves pregnancy rate in patients with low latemidluteal estradiol levels in IVF cycles. J Assisted Reprod Genetics 2002;19:550-4.

105. Pirard C, Donnez J, Loumaye E. GnRH agonist as luteal phase support in assisted reproduction technique cycles: Results of a pilot study Hum Reprod 2006;21:1894-1900.

106. Zarutskie PW, Phillips JA. A meta-analysis of the route of administration of luteal phase support in assisted reproductive technology: Vaginal versus intramuscular progesterone. Fertil Steril 2009;92:163-9.

107. Polyzos NP, Messini CI, Papanikolaou EG, Mauri D, Tzioras S, Badawy A, Messinis IE. Vaginal progesterone gel for luteal phase support in IVF/ICSI cycles: A meta-analysis. Fertil Steril. 2010;94:2083-7.

108. Jee BC, Suh CS, Kim SH, Kim YB, Moon SY. Effects of estradiol supplementation during the luteal phase of *in vitro* fertilization cycles: A meta-analysis. Fertil Steril 2010;93:428-36.

109. Castillo JC, Dolz M, Bienvenido E, Abad L, Casañ EM, Bonilla-Musoles F. Cycles triggered with GnRH agonist: Exploring low-dose HCG for luteal support. Reprod Biomed Online 2010;20:175-81.

Intracytoplasmic Sperm Injection for All?

Timur Gurgan, Suleyman Guven, Aygul Demirol

OVERVIEW

Since the first assisted human birth in 1978, *in vitro* fertilization (IVF) has been used extensively for the alleviation of infertility by inseminating human oocytes *in vitro* with a 'suspension' of spermatozoa. However, fertilization was often compromised. To overcome such fertilization failure, a new micromanipulation method intracytoplasmic sperm injection (ICSI) was introduced. ICSI refers to a technique in which a single spermatozoon is injected directly into the cytoplasm of a mature oocyte to treat male factor infertility. ICSI was first applied to human gametes in 1988. ICSI is the method of choice in cases of severe oligoasthenoterato-zoospermia (OAT), obstructive and non-obstructive aoospermia. Because of the high fertilization and pregnancy rates achieved with ICSI, the scope of the procedure has been widened to include couples with unexplained infertility, borderline semen, immu-nologic infertility, tubal factor infertility, polycystic ovary syndrome (PCOS), poor responders and previous failure of fertilization in conventional IVF. However, there is not enough data to suggest ICSI for all cases and performing ICSI in the presence of normal sperm parameters is still in debate.

RATIONALE

The main rationale for this chapter is to discuss whether patients with various infertility factors should be treated with conventional IVF or intracytoplasmic sperm injection (ICSI) and also air the main disadvantages of each assisted reproduction technique (ART).

INTRODUCTION

Though IVF is being used extensively for the treatment of infertility for a variety of indications, fertilization rates are often compromised. For severe sperm dysfunctions, more aggressive methods, such as zona drilling, cutting a hole in the zona, partial zona dissection for mechanical insertion of spermatozoa directly into the perivitelline space (subzonal sperm injection (SUZI), were used. However, the high rate of failure of fertilization with these micromanipulation methods obligated researchers to find out a novel micromanipulation technique.[1]

Intracytoplasmic sperm injection (ICSI) refers to a technique in which a single spermatozoon is injected directly into the cytoplasm of a mature oocyte to treat male factor

infertility. ICSI was first applied to human gametes in 1988;[2] the first pregnancies were reported in Belgium in 1992.[3] The ability of ICSI to permit almost any type of spermatozoa to fertilize oocytes has made it the most successful treatment for male factor infertility. The normal fertilization rate following ICSI is approximately 50 to 80 percent.[4] The use of ICSI increased from 39.6 percent of ART cycles in 1997 to 58.9 percent in 2004 (USA 57.5%, Australia/New Zealand 58.6%, Europe 59.3%). The Nordic countries, the Netherlands and the UK used ICSI to a low extent (40.0–44.3%), whereas Austria, Belgium and Germany (68.5–72.9%) and the southern European countries, like Greece, Italy and Spain. used ICSI frequently (66.0–81.2%). The marked increase in the proportion of ICSI cycles seems primarily due to an increased use in couples classified as having mixed causes of infertility, unexplained infertility and advanced age together with a relative decline in tubal factor infertility.[5]

Taking into account the high success rate of ICSI, Orief et al.[6] have recently recommended the consideration of this technique for all cases requiring *in vitro* conception. ICSI is now indicated for male factor infertility when success with standard IVF regimens is considered unlikely, however, in most countries, ICSI is used as a first line treatment to overcome many of the other infertility causes.[7]

ICSI versus IVF for Unexplained Total Fertilization Failure after Conventional IVF

In case of normozoospermia, total fertilization failure and low fertilization (defined as <25% fertilization) occurs in 5 to 15 percent and 20 percent, respectively of the couples undergoing IVF with a recurrence rate of about 30 to 50 percent.[8-10] This failure of oocytes of the female patient to be fertilized by the spermatozoa of the male partner undergoing infertility treatment may be explained by the lack of penetration of the zona pellucida, an oocyte activation failure, or a defect in the oocyte. Intracytoplasmic sperm injection circumvents those obstacles and might therefore, be effective.[11]

In one study, the efficacy of IVF and ICSI after a previous attempt, with total fertilization failure, has been investigated. It was reported that despite the further increased insemination concentration in IVF cycles, no fertilization was observed, whereas with ICSI, excellent fertilization and pregnancy rates were achieved. According to the authors' conclusion, although the technical difficulties, costs and the concerns for safety and long-term effects of ICSI cannot be ignored, currently, ICSI is the most efficacious form of assisted fertilization. Hence, for couples with failed fertilization in a previous IVF attempt with increased insemination concentrations, ICSI should be the treatment of choice. However, most of the couples included in that study suffered from oligoasthenoteratozoospermia.[12]

Based on recent study results, including thirty-eight couples undergoing IVF and ICSI on sibling oocytes after a first IVF attempt with total fertilization failure or with low fertilization, performing ICSI on some oocytes of a cohort may avoid total fertilization failures both, in patients with a history of total fertilization failure and in patients with a history of low fertilization, as the percentage of fertilization is higher after ICSI compared to IVF and the recurrence of total fertilization failure and low fertilization is high after IVF treatment.[11]

Performing ICSI on at least part of the oocytes will avoid unnecessary total fertilization failure both, in patients with a history of total fertilization failure and in patients with a history of low fertilization. Because the contribution of IVF to the total fertilized oocytes is very low, it might be proposed to treat all oocytes with ICSI. Regardless of whether the oocytes have been treated with ICSI or IVF, once fertilized, oocytes seem to be very well-capable of developing into embryos that are competent to establish ongoing pregnancies.[11]

ICSI versus IVF for Unexplained Infertility after Failed Insemination

Unexplained infertility accounts for approximately 15 percent of infertility cases, and is defined as failure to conceive with no known reason when routine fertility examinations show no abnormality in either partner. These patients are first treated with controlled ovarian hyperstimulation (COH) combined with intrauterine (IUI) insemination up to three cycles.[13] Patients who fail to become pregnant are referred for assisted reproduction.

In one recent study, the routine use of IVF and ICSI using sibling oocytes in the first cycle of patients with unexplained infertility was further stressed. The routine use of ICSI is indicated in low responders with unexplained infertility to avoid the high rate of total fertilization failure. Considering patients with less than six oocytes retrieved per cycle, the fertilization rate in IVF cycles was 53.3 percent as compared to 60.7 percent per inseminated oocyte in the ICSI cycles. Complete fertilization failure was higher in conventional IVF (34.3%) than ICSI cycles (10.3%).[14]

Takeuchi, et al.[15] designed a case-control study to determine the prognosis after IVF and subsequent ICSI in couples with unexplained infertility failing to conceive with superovulation and direct intraperitoneal insemination (DIPI). They found that there was a slight but significant difference in the numbers of fertilized oocytes after ICSI between patients with low fertilization rates undergoing IVF after failing to conceive with DIPI (85.8%) and patients with a male factor (90.4%). In patients with unexplained infertility with a failed IVF attempt after failure to conceive with four to six cycles of superovulation and DIPI, ICSI should be the method of choice in a second attempt to avoid failed fertilization or a low fertilization rate, because fertilization failure in couples with unexplained infertility appears to be more likely to recur than in tubal factor patients.[15]

In one prospective, randomized study, investigating the optimal insemination technique in patients undergoing IVF after failed IUI and the role of ICSI, no significant difference in fertilization rates between ICSI (60.4%) and conventional IVF (54.0%) was found. Based on this study result, couples with unexplained infertility and mild endometriosis, failing to conceive with IUI and undergoing IVF, have an 11.4 percent chance of fertilization failure that can be overcome easily by using ICSI in at least some oocytes. ICSI, however, has not been proved superior to IVF as an insemination technique in most cases, as most studies are somewhat limited to the small number of cases.

In another study, two groups of ICSI embryos were compared in unexplained infertility patients: those derived from ICSI when IVF had failed to fertilize (essential), and those derived from ICSI (non-essential group) while their sibling oocytes were fertilized by IVF. Fertilization rates by ICSI were lower in the essential ICSI compared with the non-essential ICSI group, at 65 and 73 percent, respectively. A possible explanation for this observation is that the gamete's quality factor was only partially resolved by micromanipulation. For example, a thickened zona pellucida, which has been overcome by ICSI to allow for fertilization, might still have a deleterious effect on implantation. Thus, a gamete factor may not be limited to fertilization and may affect further events in conception. Accordingly, the better results in the non-essential ICSI group simply represent better quality of the gametes.[16]

ICSI versus IVF for Male Factor Infertility

Decisions concerning the treatment choice for assisted reproduction (IVF or ICSI) are usually made after the evaluation of male fertility factors, or after taking into account the results of previous IVF attempts. There are no widely accepted criteria, hence decisions for couples with male subfertility are often empirical and may lead to complete fertilization failure after IVF, or to the unnecessary use of ICSI.[17]

Most couples with severe male factor infertility can be treated with ICSI. In order to generate normally fertilized oocytes after ICSI, a spermatozoon containing a functional genome and centriole is required. ICSI can also be applied with sperm from the epididymis and testis in case of obstruction of the seminal excretory ducts.

ICSI can be applied in the case of azoospermia caused by impaired spermatogenesis if suffcient sperm can be retrieved from testicular tissue.[7,18] Originally, the indication for ICSI was very poor sperm parameters (severe OAT: less than 500,000 total motile spermatozoa after sperm preparation).[19]

ICSI can be applied with sperm from the epididymis in cases of obstructive azoospermia, congenital bilateral absence of the vas deferens, Young's syndrome, failed vasoepididymostomy, failed vasovasostomy, and a bilateral (iatrogenic) inguinal obstruction of both the ejaculatory ducts.[18] ICSI can also be applied with testicular sperm in all cases where epididymal sperm cannot be used, in the presence of excessive scar tissue preventing retrieval of sperm from the epididymis, in cases of testicular failure due to maturation arrest, partial germ cell aplasia or tubular sclerosis, as well as in the exceptional case of necrozoospermia.[20,21]

For patients with mild male factor infertility ($<15 \times 10^6$ sperm/mL sperm concentration, <32 percent grade A+B motility, <4% normal morphology), the choice of IVF or ICSI is still in debate. In one study, half the oocytes from each patient with mild male infertility were inseminated (conventional IVF) and the other half microinjected (ICSI). The fertilization rate after ICSI only was 32.8 percent, while this Figure was 67.2 percent after IVF and ICSI.[17] Based on this study, results with the use of IVF/ICSI for sibling oocytes for couples with male factor infertility avoided 32.8 percent complete fertilization failures after IVF, but not to decrease significantly the number of ICSI attempts in subsequent cycles. The uncertainties concerning the safety of ICSI suggest that ICSI should still be used cautiously. This study[17] also failed to define a threshold for sperm characteristics for fertilization in conventional IVF.

In patients with mild male factor infertility, the treatment of sibling oocytes with both IVF and ICSI remains the optimal tool to prevent total fertilization failure after conventional IVF.

Preliminary results of a recent study[22] show that the choice for IVF or ICSI is based only marginally on the results obtained in previous cycles. The dominant factors in this decision appear to be sperm parameters, which can vary a lot between treatments within patients. Until more results are available, it is recommended to apply the IVF–ICSI treatment in case of mild male factor infertility when enough oocytes are available and to apply ICSI when the number of oocytes is too small for a fair chance of fertilization through either IVF or ICSI.

The outcome of sibling oocytes, subjected to both conventional IVF and ICSI in the first cycles of severe teratozoospermic patients (with <4 percent normal sperm Kruger's morphology) was also investigated. In this prospective randomized study, it was shown that in couples with severe teratozoospermia as the only male factor, there is a benefit in subjecting sibling oocytes to both IVF and ICSI in the first cycle[24] as 28.2 percent cycles of total fertilization failure were avoided. It also revealed that, despite initially significant higher fertilization rates in ICSI than IVF oocytes, embryo development from ≥6 cells up to blastocyst formation was similar, implying that ICSI should be used with caution because after day 3, ICSI-derived embryo development was compromised.[23] Moreover, in another study, it was shown that high inseminating concentrations in IVF resulted in a higher fertilization rate than ICSI in patients with severe teratozoospermia, however, ICSI produced a significantly higher proportion of morphologically superior embryos with a tendency towards a higher implantation potential.[24]

Conversely, in a recent retrospective study, it was shown that there was no statistical difference in fertilization, fertilization failure, pregnancy, and live birth rates in the first or second IVF cycle when comparing couples with isolated teratozoospermia (<4% normal morphology) to those with a normal semen analysis. Because isolated teratozoospermia generally does not impact on the major IVF indices, these patients need not be subjected to the unnecessary cost and potential risks of ICSI.[25]

ICSI versus IVF for Tubal Factor Infertility

Prospective, randomized[26,27] and retrospective[28] studies in the literature that compared the results of ICSI and IVF in patients with a tuboperitoneal factor as their sole cause of infertility showed that ICSI did not offer any advantage over conventional IVF in such patients. Intracytoplasmic sperm injection is a more expensive and time-consuming technique that requires special equipment and skill. It was suggested that ICSI should not be recommended in patients with strictly tubal factor infertility and that IVF should be the initial treatment of choice.

In another point of view, in IVF patients with non-male factor infertility, subjecting some sibling oocytes to ICSI increased the fertilization rate and formation of good quality embryos per retrieved oocyte. It also avoided the problem of total fertilization failure in almost all cases.[29]

ICSI versus IVF for Poor Responders

Poor responders represent 9 percent of patients undergoing IVF. Some authors have demonstrated an association between the number of retrieved oocytes and low fertilization rates and IVF outcome.[30,31] However, in another study, it was demonstrated that ICSI provides similar fertilization, pregnancy and implantation rates as conventional IVF in poor responders without a male factor. Also, the number and quality of embryos obtained by both the procedures did not differ.[32] ICSI should not be considered as a possible strategy in order to improve the number of embryos available in low responder patients. ICSI should be the method of choice in a second attempt when previous fertilization failure with IVF has occurred in order to determine if the fertilization failure was due to lack of penetration of the zona pellucida or a defect in the oocyte.

In a recent study, the efficiency of IVF and ICSI when few oocytes are available for insemination, was investigated.[33] As pregnancy, implantation and spontaneous abortion rates do not differ significantly between the groups,[33] adopting ICSI in all cases does not seem to be useful and abandoning IVF appears to be a questionable choice.

ICSI versus IVF in Patients with PCOS

In one prospective randomized study, the authors randomly inseminated the sibling oocytes from patients with polycystic ovary syndrome (PCOS), whose husbands had normal semen quality according to the World Health Organization criteria and Kruger's strict criteria, either by conventional IVF or ICSI. They found that (i) the percentage of mature oocytes were not different between patients who had complete fertilization failure or no fertilization failure following IVF; (ii) the oocytes inseminated by ICSI had a significantly higher fertilization rate than those inseminated by conventional IVF; (iii) complete fertilization failure following conventional IVF was as high as 15 percent, whereas there was no fertilization failure in oocytes inseminated by ICSI; (iv) despite the insemination method, the developmental potential in terms of day 2 embryonic morphology and rate of cellular cleavage were similar. However, this study did not randomize patients but instead used sibling oocytes, and such study should be undertaken to compare the pregnancy rate per started cycle and to see whether ICSI should be performed on all, or at least on a portion of oocytes for patients with PCOS undergoing IVF cycles.[34]

Conversely, Stadtmauer et al.[35] performed ICSI in PCOS patients undergoing IVF because they experienced poor fertilization rate following conventional IVF in a number of patients unless ICSI was used.[35]

ICSI versus IVF for Patients with Increased Oocyte Immaturity

During ICSI, only mature oocytes are injected, while immature oocytes are set aside to await the completion of maturation. Because oocyte maturation is unpredictable, most *in vitro* matured oocytes are injected irrespective of the time when they mature. Thus, the timing of ICSI may not always be optimal, especially since research indicates that expulsion of the polar body alone is not enough to determine maturity and that the amount of time between polar body extrusion and time of insemination influences fertilization rates.[36,37] During conventional IVF, oocyte-spermatozoon interaction is not limited or restricted. Thus, fertilization may occur at a more optimal time, after the oocyte has matured.

In an observational study, Taylor et al.[38] compared the ICSI fertilization rates to those achieved with conventional IVF in patients with high rates of oocyte immaturity (patients who had a minimum of 30 percent of their ICSI oocytes in a non-mature stage at the time of microinjection). Their data indicated that conventional IVF resulted in a higher fertilization rate than ICSI. Furthermore, IVF provided more embryos available for transfer or cryopreservation when compared with ICSI, thereby optimizing the patient's cycle. ICSI provides an almost fail-safe method of preventing failed fertilization by assuring the delivery of a single spermatozoon into the oocyte. However, although the technique is newer and more sophisticated, ICSI does not allow for the optimization of an assisted reproductive cycle in patients presenting with high rates of oocyte immaturity.[38]

ICSI for Other Indications

Intracytoplasmic sperm injection, using ejaculated sperm, can be applied in the presence of oligoasthenoteratozoospermia (OAT), in cases of repeated fertilization failure after conventional IVF (<20% fertilization with conventional IVF previously), in the presence of a high concentrations of antisperm antibodies, in cancer patients in remission where sperm were cryopreserved prior to chemo- and radiotherapy, in patients with spinal cord injury, in patients with ejaculatory disturbance, in patients with retrograde ejaculation, and in patients where semen was banked prior to vasectomy. ICSI is also indicated when preimplantation genetic diagnosis (PGD) is applied for monogenetic diseases and polymerase chain reaction (PCR) is used.[7,39]

The Effect ICSI versus IVF on Embryo Quality

In a recent study, the authors compared IVF and ICSI embryos. The results of their study demonstrated no significant differences between the IVF and ICSI groups in the rate of high quality embryos (grade A or grade A1). Thus, after controlling for possible paternal and maternal effects, they demonstrated that embryo quality does not seem to be influenced by the mode of fertilization (IVF or ICSI). It may be concluded that embryo quality depends on intrinsic factors of the gametes involved rather than on the fertilization process per se. Conventional IVF should be the option of choice for every couple requiring ART treatment to avoid the disadvantages of ICSI.[40]

The Effect ICSI versus IVF on the Obstetric Outcome

The perinatal outcome of IVF and ICSI pregnancies is very similar. For singleton pregnancies, a slightly higher incidence of prematurity could be observed in the IVF group. This did not result in a significantly worse outcome in terms of perinatal morbidity and mortality. The obstetric and perinatal outcome of twin pregnancies following IVF and ICSI were also comparable with the only exception of an increased stillbirth rate in the ICSI group. A detailed study of all stillbirths in both groups showed a higher incidence of pregnancy-induced hypertension and/or intrauterine growth retardation in the ICSI group.[41]

In another study, no significant differences were found between pregnancies conceived after either ICSI or IVF, except for the lower birth weights of ICSI children. Thus, infertile couples can be reassured that the ICSI procedure seems to be safe at present, although more long-term follow-up data are needed. With regard to the risk of congenital malformations, it can be concluded that there is no significant difference between ICSI and IVF. However, the increased incidence of congenital malformations found in ICSI and IVF pregnancies compared with the general population is of concern. Thus, genetic counselling and meticulous prenatal care should be offered to all couples treated by ICSI.[42]

CONCLUSION

Intracytoplasmic sperm injection is the method of choice in cases of severe oligoasthenoteratozoospermia, obstructive and non-obstructive azoospermia. Because of the high fertilization and pregnancy rates achieved with ICSI, the scope of the procedure has been widened to include couples with unexplained infertility, borderline semen, immunologic infertility, tubal factor infertility, PCOS, poor responders and previous fertilization failure following conventional IVF. However, there is not enough data to suggest ICSI for all cases and performing ICSI in the presence of normal sperm parameters is still in debate.

REFERENCES

1. Palermo GD, Neri QV, Takeuchi T, Rosenwaks Z. ICSI: Where we have been and where we are going. Semin Reprod Med 2009;27:191-201.
2. Lanzendorf SE, Maloney MK, Veeck LL, Slusser J, Hodgen GD, Rosenwaks Z. A preclinical evaluation of pronuclear formation by microinjection of human spermatozoa into human oocytes. Fertil Steril 1988;49:835-42.
3. Palermo G, Joris H, Devroey P, Van Steirteghem AC. Pregnancies after intracytoplasmic injection of single spermatozoon into an oocyte. Lancet 1992;340:17-8.
4. Van Steirteghem AC, Liu J, Joris H, Nagy Z, Janssenswillen C, Tournaye H, et al. Higher success rate by intracytoplasmic sperm injection than by subzonal insemination. Report of a second series of 300 consecutive treatment cycles. Hum Reprod 1993;8:1055-60.
5. Nyboe Andersen A, Carlsen E, Loft A. Trends in the use of intracytoplasmatic sperm injection marked variability between countries. Hum Reprod Update 2008;14:593-604.
6. Orief Y, Dafopoulos K, Al-Hassani S. Should ICSI be used in nonmale factor infertility? Reprod Biomed Online 2004;9: 348-56.
7. Devroey P, Van Steirteghem A. A review of ten years experience of ICSI. Hum Reprod Update 2004;10:19-28.
8. Barlow P, Englert Y, Puissant F, Lejeune B, Delvigne A, Van Rysselberge M, et al. Fertilization failure in IVF: Why and what next? Hum Reprod 1990;5:451-6.
9. Molloy D, Harrison K, Breen T, Hennessey J. The predictive value of idiopathic failure to fertilize on the first *in vitro* fertilization attempt. Fertil Steril 1991;56:285-9.
10. Roest J, Van Heusden AM, Zeilmaker GH, Verhoeff A. Treatment policy after poor fertilization in the first IVF cycle. J Assist Reprod Genet 1998;15:18-21.
11. van der Westerlaken L, Helmerhorst F, Dieben S, Naaktgeboren N. Intracytoplasmic sperm injection as a treatment for unexplained total fertilization failure or low fertilization after conventional *in vitro* fertilization. Fertil Steril 2005;83:612-7.
12. Kastrop PM, Weima SM, Van Kooij RJ, Te Velde ER. Comparison between intracytoplasmic sperm injection and *in vitro* fertilization (IVF) with high insemination concentration after total fertilization failure in a previous IVF attempt. Hum Reprod 1999;14:65-9.
13. Aboulghar MA, Mansour RT, Serour GI, Amin Y, Ramzy AM, Sattar MA, et al. Management of long-standing unexplained infertility: A prospective study. Am J Obstet Gynecol 1999;181:371-5.
14. Jaroudi K, Al-Hassan S, Al-Sufayan H, Al-Mayman H, Qeba M, Coskun S. Intracytoplasmic sperm injection and conventional *in vitro* fertilization are complementary techniques in management of unexplained infertility. J Assist Reprod Genet 2003;20:377-81.
15. Takeuchi S, Minoura H, Shibahara T, Shen X, Futamura N, Toyoda N. *In vitro* fertilization and intracytoplasmic sperm injection for couples with unexplained infertility after failed direct intraperitoneal insemination. J Assist Reprod Genet 2000;17:515-20.
16. Shveiky D, Simon A, Gino H, Safran A, Lewin A, Reubinoff B, et al. Sibling oocyte submission to IVF and ICSI in unexplained infertility patients: A potential assay for gamete quality. Reprod Biomed Online 2006;12:371-4.
17. Plachot M, Belaisch-Allart J, Mayenga JM, Chouraqui A, Tesquier L, Serkine AM. Outcome of conventional IVF and ICSI on sibling oocytes in mild male factor infertility. Hum Reprod 2002;17:362-9.
18. Tournaye H, Devroey P, Liu J, Nagy Z, Lissens W, Van Steirteghem A. Microsurgical epididymal sperm aspiration and intracytoplasmic sperm injection: A new effective approach to infertility as a result of congenital bilateral absence of the vas deferens. Fertil Steril 1994;61:1045-51.

19. Ubaldi F, Liu J, Nagy Z, Tournaye H, Camus M, Van Steirteghem A, et al. Indications for and results of intracytoplasmic sperm injection (ICSI). Int J Androl 1995;18 (Suppl 2):88-90.

20. Silber SJ, Van Steirteghem AC, Liu J, Nagy Z, Tournaye H, Devroey P. High fertilization and pregnancy rate after intracytoplasmic sperm injection with spermatozoa obtained from testicle biopsy. Hum Reprod 1995;10:148-52.

21. Tournaye H, Liu J, Nagy Z, Verheyen G, Van Steirteghem A, Devroey P. The use of testicular sperm for intracytoplasmic sperm injection in patients with necrozoospermia. Fertil Steril 1996;66:331-4.

22. van der Westerlaken L, Naaktgeboren N, Verburg H, Dieben S, Helmerhorst FM. Conventional *in vitro* fertilization versus intracytoplasmic sperm injection in patients with borderline semen: A randomized study using sibling oocytes. Fertil Steril 2006;85:395-400.

23. Kihaile PE, Misumi J, Hirotsuru K, Kumasako Y, Kisanga RE, Utsunomiya T. Comparison of sibling oocyte outcomes after intracytoplasmic sperm injection and *in vitro* fertilization in severe teratozoospermic patients in the first cycle. Int J Androl 2003;26:57-62.

24. Oehninger S, Kruger TF, Simon T, Jones D, Mayer J, Lanzendorf S, et al. A comparative analysis of embryo implantation potential in patients with severe teratozoospermia undergoing *in vitro* fertilization with a high insemination concentration or intracytoplasmic sperm injection. Hum Reprod 1996;11:1086-9.

25. Keegan BR, Barton S, Sanchez X, Berkeley AS, Krey LC, Grifo J. Isolated teratozoospermia does not affect *in vitro* fertilization outcome and is not an indication for intracytoplasmic sperm injection. Fertil Steril 2007;88:1583-8.

26. Aboulghar MA, Mansour RT, Serour GI, Amin YM, Kamal A. Prospective controlled randomized study of *in vitro* fertilization versus intracytoplasmic sperm injection in the treatment of tubal factor infertility with normal semen parameters. Fertil Steril 1996;66:753-6.

27. Bukulmez O, Yarali H, Yucel A, Sari T, Gurgan T. Intracytoplasmic sperm injection versus *in vitro* fertilization for patients with a tubal factor as their sole cause of infertility: A prospective, randomized trial. Fertil Steril 2000;73:38-42.

28. Staessen C, Camus M, Clasen K, De Vos A, Van Steirteghem A. Conventional *in vitro* fertilization versus intracytoplasmic sperm injection in sibling oocytes from couples with tubal infertility and normozoospermic semen. Hum Reprod 1999;14:2474-9.

29. Khamsi F, Yavas Y, Roberge S, Wong JC, Lacanna IC, Endman M. Intracytoplasmic sperm injection increased fertilization and good-quality embryo formation in patients with nonmale factor indications for *in vitro* fertilization: A prospective randomized study. Fertil Steril 2001;75:342-7.

30. Dor J, Seidman DS, Ben-Shlomo I, Levran D, Karasik A, Mashiach S. The prognostic importance of the number of oocytes retrieved and estradiol levels in poor and normal responders in *in vitro* fertilization (IVF) treatment. J Assist Reprod Genet 1992;9:228-32.

31. Jenkins JM, Davies DW, Devonport H, Anthony FW, Gadd SC, Watson RH, et al. Comparison of 'poor' responders with 'good' responders using a standard buserelin/human menopausal gonadotropin regime for *in vitro* fertilization. Hum Reprod 1991;6:918-21.

32. Moreno C, Ruiz A, Simon C, Pellicer A, Remohi J. Intracytoplasmic sperm injection as a routine indication in low responder patients. Hum Reprod 1998;13:2126-9.

33. Borini A, Gambardella A, Bonu MA, Dal Prato L, Sciajno R, Bianchi L, et al. Comparison of IVF and ICSI when only few oocytes are available for insemination. Reprod Biomed Online 2009;19:270-5.

34. Hwang JL, Seow KM, Lin YH, Hsieh BC, Huang LW, Chen HJ, et al. IVF versus ICSI in sibling oocytes from patients with polycystic ovarian syndrome: A randomized controlled trial. Hum Reprod 2005;20:1261-5.

35. Stadtmauer LA, Toma SK, Riehl RM, Talbert LM. Metformin treatment of patients with polycystic ovary syndrome undergoing *in vitro* fertilization improves outcomes and is associated with modulation of the insulin-like growth factors. Fertil Steril 2001;75:505-9.

36. Balakier H, Sojecki A, Motamedi G, Librach C. Time-dependent capability of human oocytes for activation and pronuclear formation during metaphase II arrest. Hum Reprod 2004;19: 982-7.

37. Hyun CS, Cha JH, Son WY, Yoon SH, Kim KA, Lim JH. Optimal ICSI timing after the first polar body extrusion in *in vitro* matured human oocytes. Hum Reprod 2007;22:1991-5.

38. Taylor TH, Wright G, Jones-Colon S, Mitchell-Leef D, Kort HI, Nagy ZP. Comparison of ICSI and conventional IVF in patients with increased oocyte immaturity. Reprod Biomed Online 2008;17:46-52.

39. Liebaers I, Sermon K, Staessen C, Joris H, Lissens W, Van Assche E, et al. Clinical experience with preimplantation genetic diagnosis and intracytoplasmic sperm injection. Hum Reprod 1998;13(Suppl 1):186-95.

40. Yoeli R, Orvieto R, Ashkenazi J, Shelef M, Ben-Rafael Z, Bar-Hava I. Comparison of embryo quality between intracytoplasmic sperm injection and *in vitro* fertilization in sibling oocytes. J Assist Reprod Genet 2008;25:23-8.

41. Ombelet W, Cadron I, Gerris J, De Sutter P, Bosmans E, Martens G, et al. Obstetric and perinatal outcome of 1655 ICSI and 3974 IVF singleton and 1102 ICSI and 2901 IVF twin births: A comparative analysis. Reprod Biomed Online 2005;11:76-85.

42. Hourvitz A, Pri-Paz S, Dor J, Seidman DS. Neonatal and obstetric outcome of pregnancies conceived by ICSI or IVF. Reprod Biomed Online 2005;11:469-75.

Selection Criteria for Oocyte and Sperm Donors in IVF Programs

Geetha Haripriya

INTRODUCTION

Oocyte Donation

Oocyte donation in humans has been reported as early as 1984 when Lutgen et al.[1] reported the first pregnancy and delivery following *in vitro* fertilization and embryo transfer (IVF-ET) in a patient with primary ovarian failure. Today, the scope of treatment has widened to include a number of conditions. With increasing efficiency and success of IVF, involving the use of donor oocytes, pregnancy rates have remarkably improved to 60 to 65 percent.[2] Impressed with these pregnancy rates, more and more patients are beginning to opt for this form of treatment. Social acceptance of this modality of treatment has also increased both in urban and rural sectors.

Though oocyte donation started off initially to treat patients with premature ovarian failure, more and more indications have now been included.

Although in 1997, the Ethics Committee of the American Society of Reproductive Medicine (ASRM) published guidelines discouraging oocyte donation in women beyond the age of natural menopause,[3] studies have shown that pregnancy outcomes in older recipients are favorable if women are appropriately screened and counseled.[4,5]

Today, women with any of the following indications can opt for the oocyte donation program:[6]

- Primary ovarian failure
- Premature ovarian failure
- Menopause
- Normal ovarian function or functioning ovaries:
  - Genetic abnormalities
  - Chromosomal abnormalities
  - Recurrent IVF failure due to inadequate response to stimulation, poor oocyte quality or recurrent fertilization failure
  - Inaccessible ovaries
  - Advanced age over 40 years to reduce the risk of Down's syndrome and reduce miscarriage rates.

With these expanding indications, the demand for oocyte donors is ever increasing in the USA, with over 10,389 fresh frozen oocyte cycles being reported to the Centre for Disease Control.[2]

CLINICAL DISCUSSION

Sourcing Oocyte Donors

This is a difficult task and several sources have been tried.

1. A sister, relative or a friend willing to be a donor make a great option.
2. Oocyte sharing program among patients was a viable option but very often led to cycle cancellations due to the small number or poor quality of oocytes retrieved. The other problem was the recipient getting pregnant and the donor having a failed cycle. The harvested oocytes may be shared among multiple patients.
3. Voluntary donors, either paid or unpaid, are the best source and anonymity, if strictly maintained, seems the best option.
4. Donor oocyte bank—most IVF programs prefer anonymous donors. Under age 32, pregnancy rates seem to be inversely related to the donor's age.[7,8]
5. With effort, a good donor oocyte bank can be created. The donor details can be computerized with a recall system after 6 months. The maximum number of donations allowed should be no more than 6. Although a few guidelines in the United States exist concerning the number of times an individual donor may participate, the ASRM suggests restricting donors to a maximum of six cycles to limit the circumstative risk. This is done not only to ensure good quality oocytes but also to

prevent the remote chances of ovarian malignancy due to multiple stimulations.[9] If the donor happens to conceive in the interval between stimulations, she should wait for a period of 6 months after completion of lactation. This ensures good quality and number of oocytes. Photographs of donors with a record of age, height, weight, religion, caste, color of skin, hair color and color of the eyes are maintained. Educational qualifications, other interests like music, hobbies and socioeconomic clan are recorded.

Psychological Screening

The donors undergo psychological assessment and go through a counseling session to make sure they understand the procedure involved.

Counseling

Once the donors are selected, they are first counseled regarding the procedure and the service they are rendering to those recipients who need the oocytes. They are assured that the procedure is safe that is done under mild sedation and one with minimal risks. Risks of the donor have been shown to be minimal and are similar to those of women undergoing conventional IVF, which include the risk of anesthesia and ovarian hyperstimulation syndrome (OHSS), postaspiration vaginal or intra-abdominal bleeding.[10] The husbands of the donors also attend this session so that they understand the procedure. The time span of treatment, about 3 to 4 weeks, should be informed and the donor should be willing and able to comply with strict contraceptive measures during any immediately following cycle. An unwilling donor or a donor who does not understand the implications of the whole procedure is unsuitable as this involves wastage of money, time and, most important of all, results in emotional trauma to the recipient.

The donor should understand that reporting to the clinic everyday for injection is mandatory. She should be trained regarding the importance of keeping her appointments for injections and blood tests. A detailed explanation, regarding the timing of oocyte retrieval, the procedure and the post-operative instructions, should be given.

Ideal Oocyte Donors

Oocyte donors must fulfill the following criteria for recruitment to the program:
1. They must be between 20 to 35 years.
2. Donors are encouraged to provide as much non-identifying biological information as possible so that it may be made available to prospective parents and any resulting child.
3. They must not have any family history of any genetically transmitted disease.

4. They must have no personal history of any major medical illness or transmissible infections.
5. They must have normal reproductive systems with adequate response to ovarian stimulation and should have at least one child.
6. They must have normal physical and mental health with a good IQ.
7. They must have a BMI < 25 kg/m^2.

It is ideal to screen the children of donors, their medical history, their IQ and their general health before recruiting the donors.

Screening of Donors

Screening of donors should follow the guidelines recently published by the ASRM.[11] A thorough history and physical examination is mandatory. The donor should be screened thoroughly before entering the program (Table 44.1).

Unlike sperm donation, where a quarantine period for infectious disease is mandatory, limitations in oocyte cryopreservation render the quarantining of oocytes infeasible. Therefore, a careful history of behavioral risk factors, including sexual history, contraception and drug use, body piercing or tattoos and other factors, known to be associated with transmissible disease, such as hepatitis and HIV, is mandatory to minimize the risk of infections to the

Table 44.1: Screening tests for donors to qualify for oocyte donation

- Complete blood count with platelet count
- Blood group and type
- Blood sugar, urea, creatinine
- Hepatitis screen
- VDRL
- HIV screening covering the latent period
- Cervical cultures for Gonorrhea and Chlamydia
- Hormone profile: follicle stimulating hormone (FSH), luteinizing hormone (LH), thyroid function, prolactin and day 2 estradiol
- Pap smear
- Transvaginal ultrasound of the pelvis to assess uterus and ovaries. Transvaginal ultrasound on day 2 is important to assess the uterus and ovaries to rule out polycystic ovaries and to assess the antral follicle count (AFC) and ovarian volume, which indicate the ovarian reserve. An antral follicle count of 12 to 14 would give a good response to ovarian hyperstimulation.
- Appropriate genetic tests for different population groups. The presence of any disorder should exclude her from participation.

recipient. A family history or prior exposure to transmissible spongiform encephalopathy (TSE), such as Cretetzfeldt-Jakob's disease, has also been defined by the recent ASRM guidelines as a risk factor that excludes potential donors. Appropriate genetic tests should therefore be done based on the ethnic background of the egg donors.

Donors should be carefully questioned for any history of Mendelian disorders, whether dominant or recessive, and be tested accordingly. Donors should also be free of any serious malformations of multifunctional origin (e.g. Spina bifida, cleft lip/palate, congenital heart defects) that may recur in future generations. Diseases, such as diabetes, atherosclerosis, and some cancers (e.g. breast, ovarian, colon) may have a familial tendency and may warrant exclusion from the program (Table 44.2).

Consent

Both the donor and the husband should sign a consent form for donation and also compensation for the full procedure and compensation for cancelled procedures.

Compensation to Donors

Monetary benefits may be made to donors in accordance with the policy and the guidelines of the center. If the oocyte donor becomes ill as a direct result of making a donation, the ART center should reimburse any direct expenses that the donor incurs. Appropriate payments should also be made for cancelled cycles.

Donor Anonymity

Maintaining the anonymity of the donor is an important obligation. Most programs warrant that identity disclosure will not occur between recipients and donors.

Selection Criteria for Donor Sperms

The first reported case of human donor insemination was by William Pancoast in 1884 in Philadelphia, USA.[12] Bunge and Sherman[13] first reported the successful use of frozen semen in 1953 but widespread use did not begin until the mid 1970's. The use of cryopreserved semen in donor insemination programs is now mandatory in most countries to minimize the possibility of transmission of human-immunodeficiency virus (HIV) for the recipients.

Like the oocyte donors, semen donors should also be screened thoroughly. A detailed medical history to rule out infections, diabetes, epilepsy and other congenital problems should be taken. A psychological assessment is also made when they are in the list of regular donors. Besides assessing

Table 44.2: Genetic screening for oocyte donors
History of disease
• Family genetic history
• Familial conditions: self, mother, father, siblings
• High blood pressure
• Heart disease
• Deafness
• Blindness
• Severe arthritis
• Juvenile diabetes
• Alcoholism
• Schizophrenia
• Depression or mania
• Epilepsy
• Others
Malformations
• Cleft lip or palate
• Heart defects
• Clubfoot
• Spina bifida
• Others
Mendelian disorders
• Color blindness
• Cystic fibrosis
• Hemophilia
• Muscular dystrophy
• Sickle cell anemia
• Huntington's disease
• Polycystic kidneys
• Glaucoma
• Tay-Sach's disease

general health, they are screened for infection, particularly as leakage of contents into liquid nitrogen following accidental damage to straws or vials remains a possibility.

A list of screening tests is available in Table 44.1.

Details of the donor—color of skin, hair, eyes, height, weight, social status, education qualifications, religion and maintained consent forms should be signed.

Cryopreservation of semen is mandatory and semen is released from semen banks only after a quantative period of 6 months.

CONCLUSION

Oocyte donation is an excellent option for patients whose ovarian reserve is poor and for those who are at a potential risk of transmitting diseases to the offspring. Appropriate selection and screening of donors is important for the success of the donor oocyte program. Proper documentation of consent, investigations, procedures and treatment should be maintained to minimize legal complications and to safeguard the personnel involved in the oocyte donation program.

REFERENCES

1. Lutgen P, Trounson A, Leeton J, et al. The establishment and maintenance of pregnancy using *in vitro* fertilization and embryo donation in patients with primary ovarian failure, Nature 1984;307:174.
2. Centre for diseases control and prevention 2000. Assisted reproductive technology success rates. Department of Health and Human Services, December 2002.
3. Ethical considerations of assisted reproductive technologies. The Ethics Committee of the American Society for Reproductive Medicine. Fertil Steril 1997; 67 (5 Suppl 1):i–iii,1S–9S.
4. Saeur MV, Paulson RJ, Lobo RA. Reversing the natural decline in human fertility, an extended clinical trial of oocyte donation to women of advanced reproductive age. JAMA 1992;268:1275-9.
5. Paulson RJ, Boostanfar R, Saadat P, Mor E, Tourgeman DE, Slater CC, et al. Pregnancy in the sixth decade of life: Obstetric outcome in women of advanced reproductive age. JAMA 2002;288:2320-3.
6. Suja S Sharma, Sucheta Tindal. Oocyte Donation. The ART and science of assisted reproductive techniques 2003;51:352.
7. Faber BM, Mercan R, Hamacher P, Muasher SJ, Toner JP. The impact of an egg donor's age and her prior fertility on recipient pregnancy outcome. Fertil Steril 1997;68:370-2.
8. Cohen MA, Lindherin SR, Sauer MV. Donor age is paramount to success in oocyte donation Human reproduction 1999;14:2755-8.
9. Committee opinion. American Society for Reproductive Medicine: Repetitive oocyte donation 2000;1-4.
10. Saeur MV. Defining the incidence of serious complication experienced by oocyte donors: A review of 1000 cases. Am J Obstetric Gynaecol 2001;184:277-8.
11. The American Society for Reproductive Medicine. Guideliness for oocyte donation. Fertil Steril 2002;77(Suppl 5):S6-S8.
12. Hard AD. Artifical impregnation. Med World 1909;27:253.
13. Bunge RG, Sherman JK. Fertilising capacity of frozen human spermatozoa. Nature (London) 1953;173:767-9.

Did We Really Stop Performing Tubal Procedures?

Kamala Selvaraj, Priya Selvaraj, Deepu Rajkamal Selvaraj

OVERVIEW

An attempt to define and evaluate the emergence of dual-assisted reproductive techniques (ART): (GIFT+IVF-ET or GIFT+ICSI-ET) by a comparative analysis of pregnancy outcomes between dual-ART and the conventional ET (IVF-ET or ICSI-ET) techniques was made. Patients underwent long or short protocol with conventional downregulation and controlled ovarian hyperstimulation (COH) followed by *in vitro* fertilization (IVF) or intracytoplasmic sperm injection (ICSI) and embryo transfer (ET) or dual (GIFT+IVF-ET or GIFT+ICSI-ET). The dual-ART procedures yielded more favorable outcomes in comparison to conventional ART. Dual procedures, when performed on a selected group of patients, proved superior to the conventional ET procedures. This is probably due to immunomodulation favored by the gametes transferred in the lateral-end of the Fallopian tube in the dual procedure.

We have now stopped performing tubal procedure like gamete intrafallopian transfer (GIFT), but we still perform dual procedures in ART like ICSI-ET and blastocyst transfer (BT) for a single patient.

INTRODUCTION

A woman nurtures a child for 9 months in her womb and delivers it in spite of the fact that 50 percent of the child is an allograft, i.e. from the father. How can this be possible? This is possible through a certain understanding between the physiology of the mother's body with that of the developing embryo at the lateral-end of the Fallopian tube, which signals through paracrine secretions, to the rest of the body. Embryo-uterine interaction during implantation is through an internal clock that tunes the harmonic orchestra by generating certain growth factors, which act as a prelude to implantation. The signal from the blastocyst to the mother helps in the immunological adjustments. All this sums up to immunomodulation.

Assisted reproductive techniques (ART) now offers a viable option for the treatment of infertile women. Intrauterine insemination(IUI) was among the first ART procedures to be invented followed subsequently by various others such as *in vitro* fertilization (IVF), gamete intrafallopian transfer (GIFT), zygote intrafallopian transfer (ZIFT) and intracytoplasmic sperm injection (ICSI). These ART procedures can be dual (a combination of tubal and ET procedures). The present chapter discusses about the relative merits and demerits of classical tubal and embryo transfer (ET) procedures, especially GIFT and *in vitro* fertilization (IVF-ET), while comparing them with the dual procedure, recent advances and improvisations in the same with the help of statistical results on a retrospective study.

CLINICAL DISCUSSION

Tubal Procedure

Tubal procedures can be applied to patients with at least on patent healthy tube. GIFT, ZIFT, Pronuclei stage transfer (PROST) and sperm-attached oocytes Fallopian transfer (SOFT) were prominent among the tubal procedures.

Gamete Intrafallopian Transfer[1-3]

Gamete intrafallopian transfer (GIFT) was the first ART procedure that evolved after IUI and follows nature by allowing the oocytes to fertilize and develop in its natural environment of the Fallopian tube and then to make their way into the uterus for implantation. The method was first described by Dr Ricardo H Asch et al.[1] who reported the first pregnancy in 1984. In 1988, Jansen and Anderson reported the first pregnancy both with GIFT and ZIFT.[4]

The principle behind the GIFT procedure is that the gametes (eggs and the sperm) deposited at the lateral-end of the Fallopian tube signal the ovary, endometrium, myometrium and their secretory products provoke the immunological adjustment in the intrauterine environment towards a successful implantation and pregnancy. The embryo signals through its secretion of human chorionic gonadotropin (hCG), which causes luteotrophic action and maintains the secretion of progesterone (P) and 17-beta estradiol (E2). Embryo-uterine interaction occurs during implantation through an internal clock that tunes the harmonic orchestra. Local action at the site of implantation, involving localized vascular response with vasodilatation and increased capillary permeability in the endometrium to form the deciduas, comes via embryo signals. Therefore, the implantation site is markedly improved due to the presence of a gamete or embryo in the lateral end of the Fallopian tube.

Embryo Transfer

The embryo transfer (ET) procedure evolved for patients who have no patent healthy tube, and can also be used in patients with healthy tubes. IVF-ET and ICSI are popular ART procedures that necessitate ET.

In Vitro Fertilization-Embryo Transfer[5]

In *in vitro* fertilization-embryo transfer (IVF-ET), the oocytes and the sperm are collected artificially and made to fertilize outside the body under appropriate laboratory conditions and the resulting embryos are is transferred into the uterine cavity with the hope that a good quality embryo will implant and grow into a healthy baby.

Contrast between Tubal (GIFT) and ET(IVF-ET) Procedures

The advantages of GIFT are that it is done in a single sitting, gametes are fertilized in a natural environment, endometrial trauma is avoided since there is no ET, it can be done during diagnostic laparoscopy[6] when timed with ovulation, involves physiological passage of the embryo into the uterus for implantation, diminished possibility of embryo expulsion and the whole procedure is less expensive than the conventional IVF-ET. The disadvantages are that it is an invasive procedure and fertilization is not proved. Complications related to the procedure, anesthesia and risk of ectopic pregnancy cannot be avoided.

In IVF-ET, the embryo is put back two days ahead of time into the uterus with an unprepared endometrium. There is no proper preparation of the endometrium via an embryo signal. Of course, today we have day 3 transfer and blastocyst (day 5) transfer, which is more in tune with endometrial preparation.

Dual Procedure (Applying Tubal and ET Procedures in Combination)

Dual procedures evolved around the year 1986–87 as, by performing both tubal and ET procedures in combination[7] in that order, the merits of both the procedures could be adopted, yielding higher pregnancy and live birth rates with marginal fetal wastage. Needless to say that dual procedures can be performed only in patients with at least one patent healthy tube.

Patient selection[7] was important not only for the indications but also for the methods of tubal ET and dual procedure.

Results of a Retrospective Study

A retrospective study on 772 ART cycles of tubal (141 cycles), ET (399 cycles) and dual (232 cycles), including own and donor gamete/embryo transfers during 2004–5 at our Fertility Research Centre, GG Hospital, Chennai, reflected the following results.

There was a remarkable increase in the pregnancy rates both, in own gametes/embryo transferred cases (Table 45.1) and the donated gametes/embryos transferred cases (Table 45.2) when the dual procedure was used. Similarly, the pregnancy rates were phenomenally increased (Tables 45.3 and 45.4) with the dual procedure, with marginal fetal wastage, and a lower ectopic and multiple pregnancy rate (Tables 45.5 and 45.6).

Table 45.1: Pregnancy rates-own gametes/embryos

Procedure	Cycles (n)	Positive pregnancies (%)
GIFT	80	10 (12.5)
ET	200	63 (31.5)
Dual	149	55 (36.91)

Table 45.2: Pregnancy rates-donated gametes/embryos

Procedure	Cycles (n)	Positive pregnancies (%)
GIFT	61	18 (29.50)
ET	199	55 (27.63)
Dual	83	41 (49.39)

Table 45.3: Pregnancy outcome-own gametes/embryos

	GIFT	ET	Dual
Singleton	5 (6.3%)	29 (14.5%)	40 (26.8%)
Twins	0 (0%)	14 (7%)	8.0 (5.4%)
Total	5 (6.25%)	43 (21.5%)	48 (32.21%)

Table 45.4: Pregnancy outcome-donated gametes/embryos

	GIFT	ET	Dual
Singleton	12 (19.7%)	27 (13.6%)	20 (24%)
Twins	3 (4.9%)	9 (4.5%)	2 (2.4%)
Total	15 (24.59%)	36 (18.09%)	22 (26.50%)

Table 45.5: Fetal wastage-own gametes/embryos

	GIFT	ET	Dual
Preclinical	2 (2.5%)	6 (3%)	3 (2%)
Missed abortions	3 (3.8%)	8 (4%)	2 (1.3%)
Ectopic	0 (0%)	3 (1.5%)	1 (0.7%)
Inevitable abortions	0 (0%)	3 (1.5%)	1 (0.7%)
Total	5 (6.25%)	20 (10%)	7 (4.69%)

Table 45.6: Fetal wastage-donated gametes/embryos

	GIFT	ET	Dual
Preclinical	1 (1.6%)	8 (4%)	6 (7.2%)
Missed abortions	1 (1.6%)	5 (2.5%)	9 (10.8%)
Ectopic	0 (0%)	4 (2%)	2 (2.4%)
Inevitable abortions	1 (1.6%)	2 (1%)	1 (1.2%)
Total	3 (4.91%)	19 (9.54%)	18 (21.68%)

CONCLUSION

Though GIFT created a sensation when it was first introduced by Asch, it slowly lost its value and IVF and ICSI became more popular, especially in cases of male factor infertility like oligoasthenozoospermia. Hence, we too stopped doing GIFT in between for more than a year. When immunomodulation became evident, we thought of the dual procedure. We found the dual procedure gives better results in terms of pregnancy outcome, less pregnancy wastage and fewer ectopic pregnancies with complete patient satisfaction such that, patients started opting for the dual procedure. The maximum pregnancy rates were achieved in all groups when the endometrial reaction was 0.8 to 1. The implantation site in the uterus, that is the endometrium, which is supposed to be trilaminar at the time of ovulation and implantation should be >0.8 mm. Patients with a male factor and polycystic ovary syndrome (PCOS) seem to benefit from dual procedures. Patients with premature ovarian failure (POF) and those requiring oocyte donation with hormone replacement therapy (HRT) benefitted maximum from this procedure.

REFERENCES

1. Asch RH, Balmeceda JP, Ellsworth LP and Wong PC. Preliminary experiences with gamete intrafallopian transfer (GIFT). Fertil Steril 1987;45:366-71.
2. Borini A, Dal Prato L. Gamete Intrafallopian Transfer. The Art and Science of Assisted Reproductive Techniques. Jaypee, New Delhi 2003;174-9.
3. Carlo Bulletti. Debating tubal transfer in assisted reproductive technologies. Hum Reprod 1996;11:1820-2.
4. Levran D, Farhi J, Nahum H, Royburt M, Glezerman M, Weissman A. Prospective evaluation of blastocyst stage transfer vs zygote intrafallopian tube transfer in patients with repeated implantation failure. Fertil Steril. 2002;77:971-7.
5. Edwards RG, Brody SA. Implantation rates during IVF, GIFT, and other forms of assisted conception. Principles and practice of assisted human reproduction. Saunders, Pennsylvania 1995;475-518.
6. Jansen PPS, Anderson JC. Transvaginal versus Laparoscopic gamete intrafallopian transfer: A case controlled retrospective comparison. Fertil Steril 1992;59:836-40.
7. Taiwan Yi Xue Hui Za Zhi. *In vitro* fertilization, gamete intrafallopian transfer and combined IVF-GIFT results: Three-year experience at Chang Gung Memorial Hospital. Hum Reprod 1989;88:1023-31.

Procreation Options in Human Immunodeficiency Virus-infected Patients

Marialuisa Partisani, Jeanine Ohl, Catherine Rongières

OVERVIEW

Access to potent combination antiretroviral therapy (cART) has improved the health and life expectancy of human immunodeficiency virus (HIV) positive patients and young couples can now consider having children. Medical care is possible for seropositive men and women in assisted reproductive technique (ART) centers, when the HIV infection is well-controlled.

For HIV-positive men, ART is decided after semen virological validation according to legislative recommendations. In case of infected women, the antiretroviral therapy must be reconsidered with regard to a possible pregnancy. In Europe, the results of Centres for Reproductive Assistance Techniques in HIV in Europe (CREAThE) network clustered 9 centers from 6 European countries and data for positive men in ten years (1993–2003). They reported 463 live births and no contamination of the female partner and the offspring.

In Strasbourg, 194 couples underwent an ART procedure. With *in vitro* fertilization (IVF) or intracytoplasmic sperm injection (ICSI), results for women were much lower than for men. Women are more often infertile and ovarian response to stimulation may be impaired as a result of the infection. Nevertheless, these results are acceptable and moreover, no contamination of the partner or child has been found.

Assisted reproductive techniques have represented a real progress in the treatment of infertility by avoiding transmission of the infection to the partner. Nevertheless, ART is expensive and represents a heavy load in everyday life for the couples.

The introduction of cART has offered excellent viral control. Hence, naturally, several teams used these data to avoid ART for fertile couples whose infected partner has a perfectly controlled infection under cART. Recommendations will probably progressively evolve as will the indications of ART for infertile couples or couples not wishing unprotected intercourse.

Nevertheless, is important to keep in mind when following infected women that fertility may be impaired. Pregnancy should probably not be delayed due to a higher risk of failure with age, whether through ART or natural cycle.

INTRODUCTION

Access to potent combination antiretroviral therapy (cART) has improved the health and life expectancy of human immunodeficiency virus (HIV) positive patients[1] and young couples can now consider having children. Adequate care during pregnancy and delivery together with the treatment of the newborn have dramatically decreased the risk of vertical transmission to less than 1 percent.[2] In these subjects, assisted reproductive techniques (ART) permit the avoidance of the risk of virus transmission to the partner and to solve eventual infertility. In France, for 11 years, certain IVF centers have been treating infected couples, in which at least one of the partners was infected with HIV, with encouraging results. New approaches may be discussed and proposed now.

CLINICAL DISCUSSION

That semen contains HIV, is undeniable and explains the worldwide pandemic. Virus can be found in seminal plasma but seldom in sperm cells. The seminal viral load is correlated to the plasmatic viral load.[3] Semen quality seems little affected by the infection.[4] A positive correlation exists between total sperm count, sperm motility and plasmatic CD4 cell count.[5] Antiretroviral toxicity in semen is theoretical, suspected because of its mode of action, but not demonstrated. On the contrary, the effects of cART on semen probably improved the quality. Some results showed better pregnancy rates with treatment (27% vs 9%) and clinical pregnancy rates after intrauterine insemination; p=0.02.[5] For ART, to avoid female contamination, only the final fraction of semen after preparation and virological validation is used.

Additionally, HIV has not been found in oocytes.[6] HIV exists in follicular fluid with an imperfect correlation with plasma.[7] The presence of HIV on granulosa cells is also controversial and not clear. These findings suggest that the infection does not interfere with the ART processes.

The first programs concerned only seropositive men. In Italy, since 1992, more than 2000 IUI, 100 IVF, and some ICSI procedures have been performed for 800 patients and 350 children have been conceived.[8] In Spain, where the experience is more recent,[9] then in Paris (FIV-ICSI),[10] or in Toulouse (IUI),[11] IUI or IVF were performed with semen validated for HIV and no contamination was observed.

The French law has changed in May 2001 and was revised in August 2010: Medical care is possible for seropositive men and women in ART centers, but a specific laboratory must be created, separated in time or in space. Multidisciplinary care must be organized, including a clinical specialist and embryologist for ART, clinical specialist for HIV disease, biology specialist in viruses, pediatrician, obstetrician and psychologist. The clinicians ensure that the HIV infection is well-controlled with CD4 cells count higher than $200/mm^3$ and a stable plasmatic viral load, twice in the six months before inclusion.

Semen is prepared with at least one technique (gradient centrifugation or spontaneous migration). ART is decided after semen virological validation according to the legislative recommendations (Table 46.1).

When the female partner is not infected, she must be controlled as seronegative two weeks before the ART attempt. After the procedure, the serology is controlled after 1, 3 and 6 months and at delivery.

In case of infected women, the antiretroviral therapy must be reconsidered with regard to a possible pregnancy. As the partner is seronegative, he must be controlled as seronegative two weeks before the ART attempt. His semen is prepared in the routine laboratory. When IVF is performed, the follicular fluid is treated in the viral risk lab.

In Europe, the results by CREAThE network clustered 9 centers from 6 European countries and data for positive men over a period of ten years (1993–2003). They reported 463 live births and no contamination of the female partner and the offspring (Table 46.2).[12]

In Strasbourg, 194 couples underwent an ART procedure. IUI is not performed as often as IVF because more than half of the couples include infertile seropositive women. For them, IVF is the procedure of choice. However, even with IVF or ICSI, results when the women are seropositive are much lower than for men. Two main explanations can be taken into account: Women are more often infertile (otherwise self-inseminations would have worked) and ovarian response to stimulation may be impaired as a result of the infection.[13] Nevertheless, these results are acceptable and moreover, no contamination of partner or child has been found (Table 46.3).

ART represented a real progress by avoiding transmission of the infection to the partner and allowing treatment of infertility. Despite many difficulties concerning material and organization, the wish to become a parent can become reality for many seropositive couples. Nevertheless, ART procedures

Table 46.2: CREAThE results for HIV positive men[12]

	IUI	IVF	ICSI	FET	Total
Couples (n)	853	76	262	40	1231
Cycles (n)	2840	107	394	49	3390
Pregnancy rate/cycle (%)	15.1	29.0	30.6	20.4	17.5
Delivery rate/cycle (%)	11.5	20.8	15.8	14.3	12.3
Pregnancy rate/couple (%)	42.7	38.2	43.1	25.0	41.9
Delivery rate/couple (%)	35.1	26.3	21.0	17.5	30.9

Abbreviations: IUI: intrauterine insemination; IVF: *in vitro* fertilization; ICSI: intracytoplasmic sperm injection; FET: frozen-thawed embryo transfer

Table 46.3: ART results in HIV infected couples in Strasbourg 2001–2009 (unpublished)

	Men HIV+	Women HIV +	Both HIV+
Couples	107	72	15
IUI	37	33	6
Pregnancies (n)	11	4	1
IVF/ICSI	200	137	23
Oocyte retrievals (n)	200	122	20
Pregnancies (n)	63	18	4
Pregnancy rate per OR (%)	31.5	13.1	20.0
Babies already born	78	21	2
% couple become parents	49.5	25.0	13.3

Abbreviation: OR: oocyte retrievals

Table 46.1: ART possibilities according to seminal viral load

RNA in seminal plasma (copies/mL)	RNA in final fraction	ART
Undetectable	Useless	Yes
Detected < 100 000	Undetectable	Yes
> 100 000	Useless	No

are expensive and represent a heavy load in everyday life for the couples.

Besides, epidemiologic data have shown that heterosexual transmission is correlated to the plasmatic viral load. The introduction of cART has offered excellent viral control and a drastic decrease in transmission, as observed in several cohorts. Results have been documented in a recent meta-analysis.[14] Naturally, several teams used these data to avoid ART for fertile couples whose infected partner has a perfectly controlled infection with cART. Swiss recommendations are clear: someone with an undetectable plasmatic viral load will not contaminate his or her partner.[15] French recommendations[16] clarify that one cannot speak about zero risk. There is no viral load threshold below which no transmission can occur because of viral sanctuaries in the genital tract. Recommendations from other countries will probably progressively evolve as will the indications for ART for infertile couples or couples not wishing unprotected intercourse.

In this context, it is important to keep in mind when following infected women that fertility may be impaired and the decrease may be noticeable as soon as the age of thirty is reached.[17] Pregnancy should probably not be delayed due to a higher risk of failure with age whether through ART or natural cycle. Soon, a fertility assessment should be made for any couple wishing to conceive, naturally or with the help of ART.

CONCLUSION

Thanks to ART, HIV-infected couples can now have healthy children. Thanks to the improvement in cART and its dissemination, ART will probably, in the future, be reserved only for infertility, as for any other non-infected couple.

REFERENCES

1. Antiretroviral Therapy Cohort Collaboration. Life expectancy of individuals on combination antiretroviral therapy in high-income countries: A collaborative analysis of 14 cohort studies. Lancet 2008;372:293-9.
2. Tubiana R, Le Chenadec J, Rouzioux C, Mandelbrot L, Hamrene K, Dollfus C, et al. Factors associated with mother-to-child transmission of HIV-1 despite a maternal viral load <500 copies/ml at delivery: A case control study nested in the French perinatal cohort (EPF-ANRS C01). J Clin Infect Dis 2010;50:585-96.
3. Kalichman SC, Di Berto G, Eaton L. Human immunodeficiency virus viral load in blood plasma and semen: Review and implications of empirical findings. Sex Transm Dis 2008;35: 55-60.
4. Van Leeuwen E, Prins JM, Jurriaans S, Boer K, Reiss P, Repping S, et al. Reproduction and fertility in human immunodeficiency virus type-1 infection. Hum Reprod Update 2007;13:197-206.
5. Gilling-Smith C, Nicopoullos JD, Semprini AE, Frodsham LC. HIV and reproductive care: A review of current practice. BJOG 2006;113:869-78.
6. Baccetti B, Benedetto A, Collodel G, Crisa N, di Caro A, Garbuglia AR, et al. Failure of HIV-1 to infect human oocytes directly. J Acquir Immune Defic Syndr 1999;21:355-61.
7. Bertrand E, Zissis G, Marissens D, Gerard M, Rozenberg S, Barlow P, Delvigne A. Presence of HIV-1 in follicular fluids, flushes and cumulus oophorus cells of HIV-1-seropositive women during assisted-reproduction technology. AIDS 2004; 18:823-5.
8. Semprini AE, Fiore S, Pardi G. Reproductive counselling for HIVdiscordant couples. Lancet 1997;349:1401-2.
9. Coll O, Vidal R, Martinez de Tejada B, Ballesca JL, Azulay M, Vanrell JA. Management of HIV serodiscordant couples. The clinician point of view. Contracept Fertil Sex 1999;27:399-404.
10. Guibert J, Merlet F, Le Dû A, Mandelbrot L, Leruez-Ville M, Costagliola D, et al. Prise en charge des couples séro-différents pour le VIH. Résultats du protocole NECO (ANRS 092) à Paris. Reprod Humaine Horm 2001;14:363-4.
11. Pasquier C, Daudin M, Righi L, Berges L, Thauvin L, Berrebi A, et al. Sperm washing and virus nucleic acid detection to reduce HIV and hepatitis C virus transmission in serodiscordant couples wishing to have children. AIDS 2000;14:2093-9.
12. Bujan JL, Hollander L, Coudert M, Gilling-Smith C, Vucetich A, Guibert J, et al. Safety and efficacy of sperm washing in HIV-1 serodiscordant couples where the male is infected: Results from the European CREAThE network. AIDS 2007;21:1909-14.
13. Ohl J, Partisani M, Wittemer C, Lang JM, Viville S, Favre R. Encouraging results despite complexity of multidisciplinary care of HIV-infected women using assisted reproduction techniques. Hum Reprod 2005;20:3136-40.
14. Attia S, Egger M, Müller M, Zwahlen M, Low N. Sexual transmission of HIV according to viral load and antiretroviral therapy: Systemic review and meta-analysis. AIDS 2009;23: 1397-404.
15. Vernazza P, Hirschel B, Bernasconi E, Flepp M. Les personnes séropositives ne souffrant d'aucune autre MST et suivant un traitement antirétroviral efficace ne transmettent pas le VIH par voie sexuelle. Bulletin des médecins suisses 2008;89-5:165-9.
16. Yeni P. Prise en charge médicale des personnes infectées par le VIH. Recommandations du groupe d'experts. Rapport 2010. http://www.sante.gouv.fr/IMG/pdf/Rapport_2010_sur_la_prise_en_charge_medicale_des_personnes_infectees_par_le_VIH_sous_la_direction_du_Pr-_Patrick_Yeni.pdf
17. Ohl J, Partisani M, Demangeat C, Binder-Foucard F, Nisand Im Lang JM. Alterations of ovarian reserve tests in Human Immunodeficiency Virus (HIV)-infected women. Gynecol Obstet Fertil 2010;38:313-7.

Management of Poor Ovarian Response in ART: Myths and Facts

Kaberi Banerjee

OVERVIEW

Despite the plethora of predictive tests for low ovarian response, the poor responder is revealed only during ovarian stimulation. The ideal stimulation for poor responders still remains a challenge. The use of very high-doses of gonadotropins to stimulate the ovaries is clearly unavoidable due to the lack of any initial ovarian responsiveness. Nevertheless, the results have been controversial with the prospective randomized trials showing either minimal or no benefit. Additionally, the few available relevant studies have suggested that the use of recombinant follicle stimulating hormone (rFSH) might improve outcome.

Although not derived from authentically prospective trials, optimistic data have been presented, which suggest the beneficial use of flare-up gonadotropin-releasing hormone (GnRH) agonist protocols (standard or microdose) along with high-doses of gonadotropins. The few data available from the use of the GnRH antagonists do not show any benefits at present, though it is possibly too early to comment at this time. Pretreatment with oral contraceptives may help the ovarian response and, therefore, appears to be beneficial. Likewise, adjuvant therapy with growth hormone (GH) or GH-releasing factors causes, in general, either no change or a trend towards non-significant improvement. There appears to be some role of recombinant luteinizing hormone (rLH) in ovarian stimulation protocols for poor responders. Standard intracytoplasmic sperm injection (ICSI) and assisted hatching techniques clearly need to be further assessed in proven poor responders, although the latter approach seems to benefit older *in vitro* fertilization (IVF) patients to a greater extent. Thus, systematic reviews and meta-analyses suggest that insufficient evidence exists to recommend most of the treatments proposed to improve pregnancy rates in poor responders. Currently, there is some evidence to suggest that the addition of GH, as well as performing embryo transfer (ET) on day 2 versus day 3, appear to improve the probability of pregnancy.

INTRODUCTION

Poor ovarian reserve has been a problematic unresolved issue with the reproductive specialists. Unfortunately, there is no universally accepted definition for the 'low', 'poor', 'bad' or 'non-responder', although these patients have much lower pregnancy rates compared with 'normal' responders. Numerous criteria have been used to characterize poor response. The number of developed follicles and/or number of oocytes retrieved after a standard dose ovarian stimulation protocol are two criteria for defining poor ovarian response. This number has varied from 3 to 5 in various studies.[1-3] A peak estradiol level, varying from 300 to 500 pg/mL during stimulation has been suggested by some.[2] An elevated day 3 FSH level, ranging from >7 to >15 mIU/mL has been proposed as an additional criterion to define poor ovarian response.[4,5] There have been other biochemical and radiological markers of poor ovarian response, basal antral follicle count (AFC) being one of the most popular one. So far, poor follicular growth after ovarian stimulation has been considered a common indicator of poor ovarian response.

Many permutations and combinations of treatment have been advised, some proven and some not. In this era of evidence-based medicine, we need to evaluate our practices on the basis scientific data and proof.

This chapter evaluates certain current practices in the field of Reproductive Medicine, which are aimed at improving the ovarian response.

CLINICAL DISCUSSION

Myth: Increasing the dose of gonadotropin to very high-doses (600 IU daily) will improve ovarian response.

Fact: There is a ceiling response to gonadotropins. The only systematic review found in this search for evidence was that of Tarlatzis et al.[6] The authors concluded that studies using high-doses of gonadotropins for ovarian stimulation in poor responders have inconsistent conclusions, and that, the few prospective randomized studies have shown either minimal or no benefit at all. Most studies have concluded no improvement in pregnancy rates when the dose was increased to more than 450 IU daily in women with poor ovarian response. In two recent reviews,[7,8] it was made clear by the authors that increasing the dose of recombinant FSH does not compensate for the decline in retrievable oocytes, and that, higher doses are required only in overweight patients, marginally improving live birth rates. In a review from the Centre for Clinical Effectiveness,[9] searching for evidence for the effectiveness of increasing the total dose of FSH above 3,000 IU for ovulation stimulation of poor responders in assisted reproduction programs, the authors, identifying five studies (included in the present search), concluded that there was no consistent definition of a poor responder and that there was no advantage of the longer, higher dose protocol.

Myth: Increasing the dose, depending on follicular response beyond the early follicular phase, will improve ovarian response.

Fact: Follicular recruitment occurs only in the early follicular phase of the menstrual cycle. Van Hoof et al.[10] reported that a 450 IU daily dose of human menopausal gonadotropin (hMG) given to 46 'low responders' from cycle day 8, had no effect on the number of mature follicles, number of oocytes retrieved and pregnancy rates compared with the 22 controls, being given a 225 IU hMG regime. The authors concluded that such an approach was ineffective in enhancing the ovarian response in low responders, this being in accordance with the hypothesis that follicular recruitment occurs only during the early follicular phases of the menstrual cycle.

Myth: No particular gonadotropin is better than the other in improving pregnancy outcomes in poor responders.

Fact: The use of rFSH versus purified FSH in poor responders was evaluated in a small (15 vs 15 patients), prospective randomized study. The authors found an increased mean number of oocytes collected (7.2 vs 5.6), improved pregnancy rates (33% vs 6%, respectively) and decreased cancellation rates (13% vs 40%, respectively) following stimulation with rFSH compared to purified FSH.[2] Similarly, another prospective study,[11] albeit with historical controls, assessed the efficacy of 300 IU rFSH versus the same dose of purified FSH in the flare-up protocol involving 28 cycles of poor responder patients in each group. These authors suggested that rFSH was associated with a significantly larger number of oocytes retrieved (2.4 vs 1.7, respectively) and significantly increased pregnancy rates (14.3% vs 0%, respectively).[11] It seems therefore, that there is evidence that rFSH produces better results in poor responders, though larger prospective randomized trials are needed to elucidate this issue further.

Myth: Certain gonadotropin regimens have been definitely proven to be superior to others in poor responders.

Fact: Most randomized controlled studies have not documented any significant improvement in pregnancy rates when different protocols were compared. However, certain non-randomized prospective studies have shown better outcomes with specific regimes.

Stop Lupron regimen: This involves stopping the GnRH agonist with the onset of menstruation. This may help in multifollicular recruitment without unnecessary suppression. Two randomized controlled trials compared the effect of the 'stop' versus 'non-stop' long GnRH protocol on pregnancy rates in poor responders undergoing IVF.[12,13] However, pooling the results of the above studies did not suggest that an improvement in pregnancy rates is likely to be present with the stop agonist protocol.

Flare-up regimen: In this protocol, GnRH agonist is started on day 2 and gonadotropins on day 3. The principle is to use the flare response of the agonist and combine it with the gonadotropin to recruit more follicles. This can be further modified by lowering the dose of the agonist (microdose)and stopping the agonist within 3 to 4 days (ultrashort). In another prospective study, 80 poor responders were treated using a classic flare-up GnRH agonist regimen with 450 to 600 IU/day of hMG from cycle day 3 and resulted in a satisfactory number of retrieved oocytes (10 ± 6.6 per cycle), but a low pregnancy rate per transfer of 13.4 percent.[4] In contrast, high pregnancy rates per transfer (29% and 41.7%), but low number of oocytes at retrieval were reported when the same protocol was applied in two other studies of poor responding patients.[3,14] However, based on the results of a single underpowered study,[15] the probability of clinical pregnancy does not seem to be dependent on the type of GnRH agonist protocol used.

GnRH antagonist protocol: The rationale for using GnRH antagonists in patients with poor ovarian response is based on the fact that endogenous gonadotropin secretion is not suppressed during follicular recruitment.[6,16] The use of a GnRH antagonist, Clomiphene citrate and a mean FSH dose of 375 IU/day (reaching doses over 600 IU in some cases) in 24 cycles of poor responders was reported to increase the number of retrieved oocytes per cycle (6.4 vs 4.7, respectively) and the pregnancy rates per transfer (23.5% vs 10%, respectively) when compared with their previous cycles, but not significantly.[16] Based on the results of a single underpowered study,[17] the probability of ongoing pregnancy does not appear to be associated with the type of GnRH analog used for LH surge inhibition. However, because significantly better results were demonstrated with the use of GnRH antagonists with regard to the duration of stimulation and the total dose of gonadotropins required, as well as number of oocyte complexes retrieved, further comparative studies might be necessary. Three eligible randomized trials, which evaluated a GnRH antagonist versus a GnRH agonist protocol in poor responders, were identified. A meta-analysis of these studies suggested that the clinical pregnancy rate is not dependent on the type of analog used, using the above stimulation protocols.

Fact: Addition of recombinant LH to ovarian stimulation protocols in poor responders may improve pregnancy rates.

Although no significant differences in clinical and ongoing pregnancy rates were found, a study conducted by Mochtar et al.[18] in 2007 indicated a beneficial effect of co-treatment with rLH, especially in poor responders.

Myth: A natural cycle IVF definitely improves pregnancy outcomes.

Fact: Some authors have proposed that if a woman does not respond to ovarian stimulation, then the use of her own natural cycle oocyte(s) should be considered. This approach is less invasive and less costly for the patient. Although the results of many studies have been published in the area of natural cycle IVF, very few have involved solely poor responders. In a study, which was prospective in nature and included historical controls,[19] it was suggested that the outcome was improved, with a mean of 0.9 oocytes per cycle versus 1.5 being aspirated. In addition, the cancellation rates were significantly lower (18.8% vs 48%, respectively) and ongoing pregnancy rates per cycle were higher (18.8% vs. 0%, respectively). By contrast, in another prospective study with historical controls,[20] comparable results were reported between the natural and stimulated cycles, in which at least one oocyte was aspirated in 82 percent of the patients while the full-term pregnancy rate was 9 percent. Similar results were found in a prospective study with no controls (44 cycles), in which patients aged over 44 years (i.e. potential but not proven poor responders) were included.[21] Successful oocyte aspiration was achieved in almost half of the cycles (48.5%), and the ongoing pregnancy rate was 2.08 percent per cycle. The study conducted by Morgia et al.[22] in 2004 did not suggest that such a strategy is beneficial, regarding clinical pregnancy rates.

Fact: Oral contraceptive pretreatment helps in improving outcome.

Oral contraceptive pill administration aims to suppress endogenous gonadotropins and, at the same time (through its estrogen component), generates and sensitizes more estrogen receptors. Unfortunately, the administration of combined oral contraceptive (COC) pill acts as a type of pituitary suppression in its own right. A few prospective and randomized studies have shown that COC pretreatment may be beneficial with regard to ovarian response and clinical pregnancy rates.[23,24] This suggestion was not confirmed by pretreatment with progestins alone,[25] although the data were obtained from a patient cohort that excluded poor responders.

Although several investigators have used COC pretreatment in other experimental protocols for poor responders, only one retrospective study has been reported on this topic.[26] These authors showed that COC administration prior to the GnRH-agonist protocol was associated with higher pregnancy rates and lower cancellation rates. In conclusion, although there is a general feeling that COC pretreatment might be of assistance in the ovarian response of poor responders, only a minimal amount of published data exists to further corroborate this.

Fact: Addition of dexamethasone may improve ovarian response in poor responders.

To date, no studies have been reported involving poor responders. In one double-blind, placebo-controlled, prospective, randomized study in 290 cycles of normal responders (aged <41 years), dexamethasone was administered at 1 mg/day in the long luteal protocol until the day prior to oocyte retrieval. The authors found a significantly lower cancellation rate (2.8% vs 12.4%, respectively; P = 0.001).[27] These findings provided great encouragement, as they revealed a very low incidence of poor response with the use of corticosteroids; however, the data are limited and can only be considered as preliminary.

Fact: Addition of other adjuvants may improve ovarian response in poor responders.

Growth hormone: Both, animal and human data have shown that growth hormone (GH) plays an important role in ovarian steroidogenesis and follicular development.[28,29] Treatment with GH enhances the gonadotropin effects on granulosa cells.[30] The results of the quantitative data synthesis, based on limited evidence, suggest that live birth rates are improved when GH is coadministered during ovarian stimulation for IVF in poor responders. GH addition needs to be further evaluated in ovarian stimulation of poor responders undergoing IVF, especially in view of the rate difference observed in live birth following its addition (+16%).

Pyridostigmine: This is an acetylcholinesterase inhibitor which, by enhancing the action of acetylcholine, can inhibit somatostatin release in the brain and thus, increase GH secretion. Based on the results of a small, underpowered study,[31] Pyridostigmine addition does not appear to improve ongoing pregnancy rates in poor responders undergoing IVF.

Oral L-arginine: Nitric oxide (NO), a product of L-arginine is an intra and intercellular modulator in many biologic processes, including ovarian physiology. However, available data from a single, underpowered trial[32] do not seem to confirm the above hypothesis.

Transdermal testosterone: It has been suggested that androgens play a critical role in follicular growth. Androgen receptors have been identified by immunochemistry in the human ovary. The addition of androgen during the early follicular phase might have a beneficial effect on the number of small antral follicles and improve the ovarian sensitivity to FSH. However, regarding the probability of pregnancy, a single, underpowered study[33] did not suggest that live birth/delivery rates are improved with the addition of transdermal testosterone.

Letrozole: The selective inhibition of aromatase prevents the overall production of estrogens, and consequently, their negative feedback effects on the hypothalamus-hypophysis axis. In this way, the pituitary produces more FSH. In addition, the inhibition of aromatase may increase the production of follicular androgens, which might improve follicular sensitivity or stimulate insulin-like growth factor-1 (IGF-1). However, based on the results from a single, underpowered study,[34] no improvement in pregnancy rates was reported with Letrozole addition to FSH.

Myth: ICSI is better than conventional insemination in poor responders.

Because poor responders are usually characterized by the retrieval of a limited number of oocytes, it has been hypothesized that ICSI might improve fertilization rates compared with conventional IVF, and thus, lead to enhancement of the probability of pregnancy in these patients.

Fact: On the basis of a single, underpowered study,[35] it appears that pregnancy rates are not dependent on the method of fertilization.

Fact: Day 2 embryo transfer is better than day 3 transfer in poor responders.

Because of concerns regarding the impact of *in vitro* culture conditions on the limited number of developing embryos in poor responders, it has been proposed that shortening the duration of embryo culture might be associated with an improvement in pregnancy rates by increasing the number of embryos available for transfer. This hypothesis was confirmed in a single study.[36]

Myth: Assisted hatching of zona pellucida improves pregnancy rates in poor responders.

The concept of this intervention is to increase the implantation potential in the few embryos that poor responders produce. The routine use of assisted hatching of the zona pellucida remains controversial, though it has been suggested that women with multiple IVF failures or those aged over 38 years might benefit from the standard application of this technique.[37-39] Nevertheless, the published studies evaluated the use of assisted hatching in patients with poor prognosis for IVF, and not in true poor responders.[40,41] Thus, appropriately powered studies need to be done to evaluate the role of assisted hatching in women producing few oocytes.

CONCLUSION

Despite the plethora of predictive tests for low ovarian response, the poor responder is revealed only during ovarian stimulation. Furthermore, there is no uniformity in the definition of the 'poor' response, thereby rendering many of the clinical trials incomparable. Well-designed, large-scale, randomized, controlled trials are needed to assess the efficacy of the different management strategies. The current results that are available are perhaps, somewhat disappointing, but this should not be too surprising as most poor ovarian response women appear to have occult ovarian failure. Thus, the exhausted ovarian apparatus is unable to react to any stimulation, no matter how powerful this might be.

The ideal stimulation for poor responders still remains a challenge. The use of very high-doses of gonadotropins to stimulate the ovaries is clearly unavoidable due to the lack of any initial ovarian responsiveness. Nevertheless, the results have been controversial with the prospective, randomized trials showing either minimal or no benefit. Additionally, the few available relevant studies have suggested that the use of recombinant FSH might improve outcome.

Although not derived from authentically prospective trials, optimistic data have been presented, which suggest the beneficial use of flare-up GnRH agonist protocols (standard or microdose) along with high doses of gonadotropins. These regimens seem to have better results compared with those of the standard long luteal protocols. A significant improvement was demonstrated with the use of the low-dose, mid-luteal onset, GnRH agonist regimens, that discontinue with the initiation of ovarian stimulation, followed by high-doses of gonadotropins (GnRH agonist 'stop' protocols), according to the prospective studies with historical controls. However, the well-designed, prospective trials failed to confirm this and showed no significant improvement. The few data available from the use of the GnRH antagonists do not show any benefit at present, though it is possibly too early to comment at this time. Certainly, further evaluation in this area is necessary.

Pretreatment with oral contraceptive may help the ovarian response and, therefore, appears to be beneficial. Likewise, adjuvant therapy with GH or GH-releasing factors causes in general, either no change or a trend towards non-significant improvement. There appears to be some role of recombinant LH in ovarian stimulation protocols in poor responders.

Standard ICSI and assisted hatching techniques clearly need to be further assessed in proven poor responders, although the latter approach seems to benefit older IVF patients to a greater extent.

Finally, natural cycle IVF, although a long-standing option, may be an appropriate and also affordable strategy for those poor responders who are capable of producing one or two follicles, with documented results being comparable to those achieved with stimulated cycles.

Thus, systematic reviews and meta-analyses suggest that insufficient evidence exists to recommend most of the treatments proposed to improve pregnancy rates in poor responders. Currently, there is some evidence to suggest that addition of GH, as well as performing embryo transfer on day 2 versus day 3, appears to improve the probability of pregnancy.

REFERENCES

1. Land JA, Yarmolinskaya MI, Dumoulin JC, Evers JLH. High-dose human menopausal gonadotropin stimulation in poor responders does not improve *in vitro* fertilization outcome. Fertil Steril 1996;65:961-5.
2. Raga F, Bonilla-Musoles F, Casan EM, Bonilla F. Recombinant follicle stimulating hormone stimulation in poor responders with normal basal concentrations of follicle stimulating hormone and oestradiol: Improved reproductive outcome. Hum Reprod 1999;14:1431-4.
3. Surrey ES, Bower JA, Hill DM, Ramsey J, Surrey MW. Clinical and endocrine effects of a microdose GnRH agonist flare regimen administered to poor responders who are undergoing *in vitro* fertilization. Fertil Steril 1998;69:419-24.
4. Karande V, Morris R, Rinehart J, Miller C, Rao R, Gleicher N. Limited success using the 'flare' protocol in poor responders in cycles with low basal follicle-stimulating hormone levels during *in vitro* fertilization. Fertil Steril 1997;67:900-3.
5. Faber BM, Mayer J, Cox B, Jones D, Toner JP, Oehninger S. Cessation of gonadotropin-releasing hormone agonist therapy combined with high-dose gonadotropin stimulation yields favorable pregnancy results in low responders. Fertil Steril 1998;69:826-30.
6. Tarlatzis BC, Zepiridis L, Grimbizis G, Bontis J. Clinical management of low ovarian response to stimulation for IVF: a systematic review. Hum Reprod Update 2003;1:61-76.
7. Borini A, Prato L, Dal. Tailoring FSH and LH administration to individual patients. Reprod Biomed Online 2005;11:283-93.
8. Dorn C. FSH: What is the highest dose for ovarian stimulation that makes sense on an evidence-based level. Reprod Biomed Online 2005;11:555-61.
9. Centre for Clinical Effectiveness. In women labelled as poor responders to ovulation stimulation in an assisted reproduction program, is there evidence for the effectiveness of increasing the total dose of FSH above 3000 IU? 2000 Cochrane Database HTA — 20030660.
10. Van Hoof MHA, Alberda AT, Huisman GJ, Zeilmaker GH, Leerentveld K. Doubling the human menopausal gonadotropin dose in the course of an *in vitro* fertilization treatment low responders: A randomized study. Hum Reprod 1993;8:369-73.
11. De Placido G, Alviggi C, Mollo A, Strina I, Varricchio MT, Molis M. Recombinant follicle stimulating hormone is effective in poor responders to highly puried follicle stimulating hormone. Hum. Reprod 2000;15:17-20.
12. Dirnfeld M, Fruchter O, Yshai D, Lissak A, Ahdut A, Abramovici H. Cessation of gonadotropin-releasing hormone analogue (GnRH-a) upon down regulation versus conventional long GnRH-a protocol in poor responders undergoing *in vitro* fertilization. Fertil Steril 1999;72:406-11.
13. Garcia-Velasco JA, Isaza V, Requena A, Martinez-Salazar FJ, Landazabal A, Remohi J. High doses of gonadotropins combined with stop versus nonstop protocol of GnRH analogue administration in low responder IVF patients: a prospective, randomized, controlled trial. Hum Reprod 2000;15:2292-6.
14. Padilla SL, Dugan K, Maruschak V, Shalika S, Smith RD. Use of the flare-up protocol with high-dose human follicle stimulating hormone and human menopausal gonadotropins for *in vitro* fertilization in poor responders. Fertil Steril 1996;65:796-9.
15. Weissman A, Farhi J, Royburt M, Nahum H, Glezerman M, Levran D. Prospective evaluation of two stimulation protocols for low responders who were undergoing *in vitro* fertilization-embryo transfer. Fertil Steril 2003;79:886-92.
16. Craft I, Gorgy A, Hill J, Menon D, Podsiadly B. Will GnRH antagonists provide new hope for patients considered difficult responders to GnRH agonist protocols? Hum Reprod 1999;14:2959-62.
17. Marci R, Caserta D, Dolo V, Tatone C, Pavan A, Moscarini M. GnRH antagonist in IVF poor-responder patients: Results of a randomized trial. Reprod Biomed Online 2005;11:189-93.
18. Mochtar MH, Van der Veen F, Ziech M, van Wely M. Recombinant Luteinizing Hormone (rLH) for controlled ovarian hyperstimulation in assisted reproductive cycles. Cochrane Database Syst Rev 2007;(2):CD005070.
19. Bassil S, Godin PA, Donnez J. Outcome of IVF through natural cycles in poor responders Hum. Reprod 1999;14:1262-5.
20. Feldman B, Seidman DS, Levron J, Bider D, Shulman A, Shine S, Dor J. IVF following natural cycles in poor responders. Gynecol Endocrinol 2001;15:328-34.
21. Bar-Hava I, Ferber A, Ashkenazi J, Dicker D, Ben-Rafael Z, Orvieto R. Natural cycle IVF in women aged over 44 years. Gynecol Endocrinol 2000;14:248-52.
22. Morgia F, Sbracia M, Schimberni M, Giallonardo A, Piscitelli C, Giannini P, et al. A controlled trial of natural cycle versus microdose gonadotropin-releasing hormone analog flare cycles in poor responders undergoing *in vitro* fertilization. Fertil Steril 2004;81:1542-7.
23. Gonen Y, Jacobsen W, Casper R. Gonadotropin suppression with oral contraceptives before *in vitro* fertilization. Fertil Steril 1990;53:282-7.
24. Biljani M, Mahutte N, Dean N, Hemmings R, Bissonnette F, Tan S. Effects of pretreatment with an oral contraceptive on the time required to achieve pituitary suppression with gonadotropin-releasing hormone analogues and on subsequent pregnancy rates. Fertil Steril 1998;70:1063-9.
25. Shaller A, Pittrof R, Zaidi J, Bekir J, Kyei-Mensah A, Tan S. Administration of progestogens to hasten pituitary desensitization after the use of gonadotropin-releasing hormone agonist in *in vitro* fertilization in a prospective randomized study. Fertil Steril 1995;64:791-5.
26. Lindheim S, Barad D, Witt B, Ditkoff E, Sauer M. Short-term gonadotropin suppression with oral contraceptives benefits poor responders prior to controlled ovarian hyperstimulation. J. Assist. Reprod Genet 1996;16:745-7.
27. Keay SD, Lenton EA, Cooke ID, Hull MGR, Jenkins JM. Low-dose dexamethasone augments the ovarian response to exogenous

gonadotropins leading to a reduction in cycle cancellation rate in a standard IVF programme. Hum Reprod 2001;16:1861-5.

28. Jia XC, Kalmijn J, Hsueh AJ. Growth hormone enhances follicle-stimulating hormone-induced differentiation of cultured rat granulosa cells. Endocrinol 1986;118:1401-9.

29. Doldi N, Bassan M, Bonzi V, Ferrari A. Effects of growth hormone and growth hormone-releasing hormone on steroid synthesis in cultured human luteinizing granulosa cells. Gynecol Endocrinol 1996;10:101-8.

30. Lanzone A, Di Simone N, Castellani R, Fulghesu AM, Caruso A, Mancuso S. Human growth hormone Enhances progesterone production by human luteal cells *in vitro*: Evidence of a synergistic effect with human chorionic gonadotropin. Fertil Steril 1992;57:92-6.

31. Kim CH, Chae HD, Chang YS. Pyridostigmine cotreatment for controlled ovarian hyperstimulation in low responders undergoing *in vitro* fertilization-embryo transfer. Fertil Steril 1999;71:652-7.

32. Battaglia C, Regnani G, Marsella T, et al. Adjuvant –L- arginine treatment in controlled ovarian hyperstimulation: A double blind randomized study. Hum Reprod 2002;17:659-65.

33. Massin N, Cedrin-Durnerin I, Coussieu C, Galey-Fontaine J, Wolf JP, Hugues JN. Effects of transdermal testosterone application on the ovarian response to fsh in poor responders undergoing assisted reproduction technique: A prospective, randomized, double-blind study. Hum Reprod 2006;21:1204-11.

34. Goswami SK, Das T, Chattopadhyay R, Sawhney R, Kumar J, Chaudhury K. A randomized single-blind controlled trial of letrozole as a low-cost IVF protocol in women with poor ovarian response: A preliminary report. Hum Reprod 2004;19:2031-35.

35. Moreno C, Ruiz A, Simon C, Pellicer A, Remohi J. Intra-cytoplasmic sperm injection as a routine indication in low responder patients. Hum Reprod 1998;13:2126-9.

36. Bahceci M, Ulug U, Ciray HN, et al. Efficiency of changing the embryo transfer time from day 3 to day 2 among women with poor ovarian response: A prospective randomized trial. Fertil Steril 2006;86:81-5.

37. Cohen J, Alikani M, Trowbridge J, Rosenwaks Z. Implantation enhancement by selective assisted hatching using zona drilling of human embryos with poor prognosis. Hum Reprod 1992;7:685-91.

38. Stein A, Rufas O, Amit S, Avrech O, Pinkas H, Ovadia J, Fisch B. Assisted hatching by partial zona dissection of human pre-embryos in patients with recurrent implantation failure after *in vitro* fertilization. Fertil Steril 1995;63:838-41.

39. Bider D, Liversushits A, Yonish M, Yemini Z, Mashiach S, Dor J. Assisted hatching by zona drilling of human embryos in women of advanced age. Hum Reprod 1997;12:317-20.

40. Schoolcraft W, Schlenker T, Gee M, Stevens J, Wagley L. Improved controlled ovarian hyperstimulation in poor responder *in vitro* fertilization patients with a microdose follicle-stimulating hormone flare, growth hormone protocol. Fertil Steril 1997;67:93-7.

41. Mansour RT, Rhodes CA, Aboulghar MA, Serour GI, Kamal A. Transfer of zona-free embryos improves outcome in poor prognosis patients: A prospective randomized controlled study. Hum Reprod 2000;15:1061-4.

Nuances of Ultrasound-guided Embryo Transfers

Durga Rao

OVERVIEW

Embryo transfer is the final and most crucial step in an assisted reproductive technique (ART) cycle. The procedure being an operator-dependent technique, is what leads to a live birth. The culmination of an *in vitro* fertilization (IVF)/ intracytoplasmic sperm injection (ICSI) cycle, the creation of embryos, and a successful live birth can only result if these embryos are implanted into the uterus in the most competent manner. This chapter details the various aspects that may help in optimizing the technique of embryo transfer.

INTRODUCTION

Since the advent of assisted conception techniques over three decades ago, there has been tremendous development in enhancing and improving the outcome of every facet involved in an assisted reproductive technique (ART).

Advances in pituitary downregulation, ovarian stimulation protocols, media cultures, embryo culture methods, and techniques performed in the laboratory, all have contributed to increasing the success of an assisted reproductive technique (ART) cycle. But disappointingly, embryo implantation, which depends on many factors, broadly and importantly being the quality of embryos, uterine receptivity and the technique of embryo transfer, is still found to be a limiting factor.[1]

Even after the selection of seemingly good quality embryos for transfer, the implantation rates are still only around 15 percent[2] to 20 percent.[3] Despite its apparent simplicity, it seems that the technique of embryo transfer (ET) is of utmost importance in maximizing the chances of pregnancy.[1,4,5] Therefore, over the years, various innovative methods have been tried and tested to improve the procedure of embryo transfer in order to increase the rate of implantation, and thereby, live births. The importance of the embryo transfer technique is also reiterated by the differences seen in pregnancy rates achieved by different practitioners belonging to the same institution who performed the procedure.

The need to increase the efficiency of the procedure is even more imperative now with the move towards introducing single embryo transfers globally to reduce multiple pregnancy.

CLINICAL DISCUSSION

Factors Influencing Embryo Transfer Outcome

The crucial aspect of the technique is to do the procedure 'easily' and be as 'atraumatic' as possible to improve the implantation rate.[6]

The other factors influencing the outcome are:
- The experience of the physician.
- Blood on the tip of the catheter, which may be caused by the endometrial disturbance, which in turn induces myometrial contractions and can, reduce implantations rates. Blood on the tip of the ET catheter was associated with a significant reduction in the clinical pregnancy rate per transfer (14.3% with blood vs 52.4% without blood).[7,8]
- Position chosen for embryo deposition.

The methods that have therefore evolved to improve the procedure include:
- Performing a 'trial or mock' transfer before the actual procedure
- Cleaning the cervix with sterile saline and/or media before embryo transfer
- Removing cervical mucus without trauma before embryo transfer

- Avoiding the use of tenaculum to hold the cervix
- Using soft embryo transfer catheters rather than firm catheters[9]
- Using a fibrin sealant
- Advising a full bladder for the procedure
- Bed rest following embryo transfer
- Performing the procedure under ultrasound guidance.

Different Modes of Embryo Transfer

Traditionally, clinical touch was the method used for ET until ultrasound emerged as a modality to guide embryo transfers. Strickler et al.[10] described the use of ultrasound in ET as far back as 1985. Recent evidence suggests that ultrasound-guided embryo transfer (UGET) makes the procedure easier to perform and helps determine the optimal site for embryo release.[11,12]

Clinical Touch Method

Embryo transfer by clinical touch alone is a procedure where the clinician would rely on tactile perception to place the catheter in position in utero. It is also called the 'blind method', wherein some practitioners would release the embryos at 6 cm of uterocervical length, but the flaw in this technique is that it does not take into consideration the individual variations in sizes of uteri and cervical lengths. Other clinicians introduce the catheter into the upper uterine cavity and release the embryo 1 cm or more from the fundus (assessed just by feel, without touching the fundus). Studies have shown that touching the fundus causes myometrial contractions, causing expulsion of embryos,[13] and could also induce high frequency uterine contractions, lowering the ongoing clinical pregnancy rates.[14] An inadvertent touch of the fundus by this method, therefore, is the main downside to this method.

The other disadvantages with 'clinical touch' alone as a technique is the inability to detect the acute uterocervical angle or cervical stenosis and the possibility of catheter curling in the canal without advancing into the cavity. Woolcott and Stanger et al.[15] demonstrated that during ET, using the clinical touch method, the tip of the catheter was inadvertently placed near the opening of the Fallopian tube (7.4%), abutted the fundal endometrium (17.4%), or below the surface of the endometrium (24.8%), even when perceived to be accurately placed by experienced clinicians.[15]

On the contrary, clinicians using the 'clinical touch' method over the years have acquired the skill of placing embryos just by 'feel', and continue to show good pregnancy rates, questioning the need for UGET.

Ultrasound-guided ET

Strickler et al.[10] were the first to describe the use of ultrasound to negate some of the difficulties with blind procedures.[10]

Advantages of ultrasound-guided ET

The advantages are manifold and include:
- Visualization of the advancement of the catheter through the cervical canal into the uterine cavity.
- Assessment of the uterocervical angle.
- Placement of the tip of the catheter at the desired position in the cavity,[15] or a decrease the chance of improper embryo placement.[15-17,22]
- Observation of the release of fluid containing embryos.
- Relatively atraumatic penetration of the catheter into the uterus.
- Ability to demonstrate to the couple that the catheter is located in the uterus prior to releasing the embryos.
- Detection of early ovarian hyperstimulation syndrome (OHSS).
- Appreciation of the pelvic anatomy as well.

The benefit of UGET seems to be due to the reduction in the incidence of difficult transfers,[18,19] endometrial trauma[15,20] and bleeding[14,19] that can cause strong fundo-uterine contractions.[13] Mirkin's group[21] found that ultrasound made transfers easier and reduced the presence of blood or mucus at the tip of the catheter, and the use of tenaculum, which are factors associated with adverse outcomes.[21]

Disadvantages of ultrasound-guided ET

- Need for a second operator and an abdominal probe,
- Associated cost implications,
- Discomfort of a full bladder, and
- Unknown effects of ultrasound on the embryo.

Additionally, ultrasound may, very rarely, help the clinician negotiate a tight or deviated cervical canal by helping to visualize the course of the catheter. In an obese woman though, visualization of the catheter, even if echogenic, can sometimes be difficult. Lastly, the cost of echogenic catheters that need to be used can be prohibitive.

Evidence Regarding UGET

Current evidence shows improved pregnancy rates following UGET, however, in some studies, no added benefit was demonstrated. A Cochrane database review[11] demonstrated that the live birth/ongoing pregnancies per woman randomized associated with UGET was significantly higher than for clinical touch, with an odds ratio of 1.40 in favor of UGET [95% CI (1.18 to 1.66), P < 0.0001]. This means, for example, that for a population of women with a 25 percent chance of pregnancy using clinical touch alone, the chances of pregnancy would be increased to 32 percent (28% to 46%) by using UGET. The limitations though were the heterogeneity of the studies included in the meta-analysis and lack of data on live birth rates. Another meta-analysis by Abou-Setta[12] showed similar findings, with ultrasound-guided ET significantly increasing the chance of live birth and ongoing clinical pregnancy rates compared with the clinical touch method. Earlier meta-analyses by Buckett[22] and Sallam and Sadek[23] showed similar findings, with no effect on the incidence of ectopic pregnancy, multiple pregnancy, or miscarriage rates. A recent randomized controlled trial (RCT) once again corroborated the above findings.[24]

In comparison to these studies, an RCT by Kosmas et al.[25] showed that an experienced operator was the key to ET, rather than ultrasound guidance. However, their study was done in patients where bladder fullness was left to the patient's choice and was not a prerequisite to performing the procedure. Therefore, it raises the question whether a full bladder could have made some of their transfers easier.[25] The latest and the largest RCT too, did not find that UGET helped improve pregnancy or live birth rates. There was no statistical difference in miscarriage, ectopic pregnancy or multiple pregnancy rates. The ease of the embryo transfer, however, appeared to have a statistically significant effect on the clinical pregnancy outcome, with an easier transfer being more likely to lead to a clinical pregnancy.[26]

In conclusion, it may be said that ultrasound can be more useful in standardizing the procedure of ET in an ART program and shorten the learning curve of specialists in training. Clinical touch alone, as a mode of ET, may be best left to experienced clinicians.

Role of Mock (Trial) Embryo Transfer

Most ART centers perform trial ET prior to the actual embryo transfer. The trial transfer is usually undertaken before mid-cycle. The rationale of this procedure is to identify the group of patients who may have a difficult transfer and for the clinicians to be adequately prepared to initiate any measures to reduce the transfer difficulty and improve pregnancy rates. A suggested use by Shamonki et al.[27] is also to use trial transfer in a practice where ultrasound is not readily available during embryo transfer, either due to a lack of equipment or qualified personnel present to perform the ultrasound.[27] But the same group reported discrepancies in cavity length, even in highly experienced hands (19.4% of their patients had a discrepancy of ≥ 1.5 cm and 29.9% had a discrepancy of ≥ 1 cm) between the length measured at mock transfer and that at ultrasound-guided trial embryo transfer.[28] Tang et al.[29] have also shown that mock transfer performed prior to IVF-stimulated cycles had an inaccuracy of ≥ 1 cm in about 30 percent of patients.[29] These findings are another reason why UGET may, therefore, be preferable to traditional blind transfer because it allows for more accurate placement of embryos in patients where there is a significant discrepancy between actual and blindly perceived uterine cavity length. A recent publication[30] challenged the value of performing a mock embryo transfer and showed that a retroverted uterus at mock transfer might often change position during the actual procedure. The authors suggested that ultrasound guidance during the real transfer is a better method of judging the direction of the uterine axis. Finally, the use of mock transfer may help the physician in choosing the best catheter suitable for the particular uterus and identifying those patients with a stenotic cervix who might benefit from pre-ET treatment with laminaria, cervical dilatation or surgical correction.

Procedure of Ultrasound-guided ET

The whole procedure of UGET can be divided into the following steps:

- *Preparation before ET:* The patient is asked to have a comfortably full bladder before the ET. She is then put in the lithotomy position and a sterile bivalve speculum is inserted into the vagina. The cervix is cleaned with sterile saline or phosphate buffered saline solution. A cotton tip swab dipped in culture media is then used to remove the cervical mucus. Occasionally, a sterile teflon catheter is also used to aspirate the mucus without causing cervical trauma. These measures are taken to decrease the likelihood of introduction of blood, mucus and bacterial contamination from the cervix into the endometrial cavity.

- *Ultrasound visualization:* A second operator is needed to do the abdominal scan during the procedure. The uterus and cervix are visualized in a sagittal plane through the window of a full bladder with a convex probe. The angle of the uterus within the pelvis relative to the midline and also to the axial plane, that is antero, retro or mid position is assessed. Next, the uterocervical angle is measured either by ultrasound or visual estimation. If the angle is acute then the bill of the speculum or a forceps can be used to elevate or displace the cervix to decrease the severity of the angle.[31] In an obese patient, to improve visualization, increasing the depth of the focal zone of the transducer, while decreasing the overall image depth, narrowing the size of the probe sector width, and altering the contrast of the image is advised.

- *Estimation of the position of deposition of the embryo:* Prior to embryo transfer, the endometrial thickness, the distance from the external cervical os to the fundal endometrial surface and the distance from the fundus to the point that the tip of the catheter should reach for proper embryo replacement are measured. Studies have shown that most embryos stay and implant at, or close to where they are extruded from the transfer catheter. A study by Woolcott and Stanger,[32] utilizing transvaginal UGET, assessed the movement of embryo-associated air bubbles by performing a second ultrasound in the standing position immediately after transfer. There was no air bubble movement in 94.1 percent of transfers, a movement of <1 cm in 4.0 percent of transfers, movement of 1 to 5 cm in 2.0 percent transfers and no movement of embryo-associated air out of the uterine cavity, either into the cervix or into the intramural portion of the Fallopian tube.[32] Although embryo-associated air bubble movement may not directly correlate with the actual embryo movement, there may be no better method to assess this variable. A recent study, utilizing 3-dimensional ultrasound, demonstrated that in pregnancies resulting from embryo transfer, 80 percent of embryos implant in areas to which they are initially transferred and 20 percent implant in other areas.[33]

Since current evidence suggests that most embryos implant at or near the place of deposition, it further emphasizes the importance of confirming catheter tip position before release of embryos. Pope et al.[34] in a multivariate logistic regression analysis of 699 embryo transfers, found that for every additional millimeter embryos are deposited away from the fundus, the odds of clinical pregnancy increased by 11 percent.[34] Similar findings were reported by Frankfurter et al.[35,36] The proposed point of deposition of embryos would be mid-uterine cavity or at least 1.5 to 2 cm from the fundus.[37] If the catheter tip is not found to be in position, it is very gently advanced or withdrawn and thus, appropriately relocated, keeping its movement to an absolute minimum.

- *Type of catheter:* A systematic review and meta-analysis, evaluating the firmness of the embryo transfer catheter in relation to a successful transfer, concluded that using soft embryo transfer catheters results in a significantly higher pregnancy rate as compared with firm catheters.[38] There have also been studies showing the benefit of using echogenic catheters, as they can be immediately imaged by transabdominal ultrasonography. Even small movements of the transducer in the transverse plane could track the passage of echogenic catheters through the entire uterine cavity into the fundal region during the first pass. This would reduce the to-and-fro motion necessary to identify the catheter tip which, in turn, would minimize disruption of the endometrium and improve implantation rates.[20] Coroleu's group[39] also showed an increase in implantation rates and a trend towards increased pregnancy rates with the use of echogenic catheters.[39]

- *Introducing the catheter:* The soft inner catheter is introduced under transabdominal ultrasound guidance into the cervix and passed through the internal cervical os without using the outer sheath whenever possible. If resistance is met, the inner sheath is withdrawn and then the outer sheath (with its obturator) is moulded according to the uterocervical angle measured while still in its sterile sleeve. The outer sheath of the catheter is then passed through the endocervix and placed up to or just through the internal os, and not advanced into the uterine cavity. In difficult cases, grasping the cervix with a tenaculum can be performed to facilitate this maneuver. The inner catheter is now threaded through the outer sheath and advanced under real-time ultrasound guidance to the preselected position.

- *Loading the catheter:* The catheter is first loaded with medium, taking care to avoid air bubbles. The embryos are then loaded into the catheter. The catheter is held with the tip slightly down to avoid the embryos traveling through the liquid column to the syringe-end and brought to the clinician. A longer 'interval loading-discharging embryos' would favor the influence of some environmental factors, such as exposure to light, temperature, inappropriate O_2 and CO_2 concentrations, potentially having detrimental effects on oocytes and embryos, and would decrease the implantation rates.[40] Another study showed that the duration of the embryo transfer procedure from the moment when the loaded catheter was handed to the physician and up to embryo discharge was significantly shorter in the echogenic catheter group (having a higher implantation rate) than in the standard catheter group.[39] The shorter duration of the embryo transfer procedure with the use of the echogenic catheter could be explained by better catheter identification under ultrasound.

Finally, the catheter is withdrawn very slowly after keeping it still for a few seconds and examined for blood, mucus and retained embryos under the microscope.

Vaginal Ultrasound and ET

Vaginal ultrasound can also be used as a modality to visualize the introduction of the catheter into the uterine cavity. The proximity of the transducer helps in providing better visualization. An empty bladder is patient friendly too, but simultaneous placement of transducer and catheter in the vagina may require the speculum to be opened slightly more, causing discomfort to the patient and it may also be cumbersome for the clinician to use both hands together.

Three-dimensional Ultrasound and ET

Three-dimensional (3D) ultrasound provides volume data and means of assessing three planes simultaneously. A study done with 3D ultrasound observed migration of embryos in unintended directions, in spite of reassuring images on two-dimensional (2D) ultrasound, suggesting a role in enhancing the precision of placement of embryos.[41] Porter[31] suggests that in cases of Müllerian anomalies, where the uterine cavity shape may be altered, 3D ultrasound may show better clarity of the fundal endometrial contours and be of benefit in obtaining a measurement of the mid-cavity.[31] A study suggests that uterine cavity and catheter placement may be better achieved with 3D sonography than 2D sonography, and improve the embryo transfer technique.[42] However, the use of 3D ultrasound has not shown to increase sensitivity.

Gergly et al.[43] evaluated the use of maximal implantation potential (MIP) point in conjunction with a 3D/4D ultrasound and stated that embryos placed at this point improved implantation and pregnancy rates.[43] More studies are needed to fully evaluate the advantage, taking higher cost of the machine into view and assessing the added benefit over two-dimensional ultrasound before it can be recommended for routine use.

CONCLUSION

To get the best outcome from an embryo transfer, the use of soft catheters, ultrasound guidance, deposition of embryos in the mid-cavity, and most importantly, an atraumatic technique has proven to be beneficial.

Trial transfers, removal of cervical mucus, use of fibrin sealants, are supported with only limited evidence. Ultimately, all these modalities depend on the experience and skill of the clinician performing the transfer.

REFERENCES

1. Sallam HN. Embryo transfer: Factors involved in optimizing the success. Curr Opin Obstet Gynecol 2005;17:289-98.
2. Edwards RG. Clinical approaches to increasing uterine receptivity during human implantation. Hum Reprod 1995;10 (Suppl 2):60-6.
3. Eytan O, Elad D, Zaretsky U, Jaffa AJ. A glance into the uterus during *in vitro* simulation of embryo transfer. Hum Reprod 2004;19:562-9.
4. Mansour RT, Aboulghar MA. Optimizing the embryo transfer technique. Hum Reprod 2002;17:1149-53.
5. Pasqualini RS, Quintans S. Clinical practice of embryo transfer. Reprod Biomed Online 2002;4:83-92.
6. Matorras R, Urquijo E, Mendoza R, Corcostegui B, Exposito A, Rodriguez-Escudero F. Ultrasound-guided embryo transfer improves pregnancy rates and increases the frequency of easy transfers. Hum Reprod 2002;17:1762-6.
7. Goudas VT, Hammitt DG, Damario MA, Session DR, Singh AP, Dumesic DA. Blood on the embryo transfer catheter is associated with decreased rates of embryo implantation and clinical pregnancy with the use of *in vitro* fertilization embryo transfer. Fertil Steril 1998;70:878-82.
8. Alvero R, Hearns-Stokes RM, Catherino WH, Leondires MP, Segars JH. The presence of blood in the transfer catheter negatively influences outcome at embryo transfer. Hum Reprod 2003;18:1848-52.
9. Abou-Setta AM, Al-Inany HG, Mansour R, Serour GI, Aboulghar MA. Soft versus firm embryo transfer catheters for assisted reproduction: A systematic review and meta-analysis. Hum Reprod 2005;20:3114-21.
10. Strickler RC, Christianson C, Crane JP, Curato A, Knight AB, Yang V. Ultrasound guidance for human embryo transfer. Fertil Steril 1985;43:54-61.
11. Brown JA, Buckingham K, Abou-Setta A, Buckett W. Ultrasound versus 'clinical touch' for catheter guidance during embryo transfer in women. Cochrane Database Syst Rev 2007; CD006107. Review
12. Abou-Setta AM, Mansour RT, Al-Inany HG, Aboulgar MM, Aboulgar MA, Serour GI. Among women undergoing embryo transfer, is the probability of pregnancy and live birth improved with ultrasound-guided over clinical touch alone? A systematic review and meta-analysis of prospective randomized trials. Fertil Steril 2007;88:333-41.
13. Lesny P, Killick SR, Tetlow RL, Robinson J, Maguiness SD. Embryo transfer- can we lean anything new from the observation of junctional zone contractions. Hum Reprod 1998;13:1540-46.
14. Fanchin R, Righini C, Olivennes F, Taylor S, de Ziegler D, Frydman R. Uterine contractions at the time of embryo transfer alter pregnancy rates after *in vitro* fertilization. Hum Reprod 1998;13:1968-74.
15. Woolcott R, Stanger J. Potentially important variables identified by transvaginal ultrasound-guided embryo transfer. Hum Reprod 1997;12:963-6.
16. Coroleu B, Barri PN, Carreras O, Martinez F, Parriego M, Hereter L, Parera N, Veiga A, Balasch J. The influence of the depth of embryo replacement into the uterine cavity on implantation rates after IVF: A controlled, ultrasound-guided study. Hum Reprod 2002;17:341-6.
17. Pope CS, Cook EK, Arny M, Novak A, Grow DR. Influence of embryo transfer depth on *in vitro* fertilization and embryo transfer outcomes. Fertil Steril 2004;81:51-8.
18. Hearns-Stokes RM, Miller BT, Scott L, Creuss D, Chakraborty PK, Segars JH. Pregnancy rates after embryo transfer depend on the provider at embryo transfer. Fertil Steril 2000;74:80-6.
19. Sallam HN, Agameya AF, Rahman AF, Ezzeldin F, Sallam AN. Ultrasound measurement of the uterocervical angle before embryo transfer: A prospective controlled study. Hum Reprod 2002;17:1767-72.
20. Letterie GS, Marshall L, Angle M. A new coaxial catheter system with an echodense tip for ultrasonographically guided-embryo transfer. Fertil Steril 1999;72:266-8.
21. Mirkin S, Jones EL, Mayer JF, Stadtmauer L, Gibbons WE, Oehninger S. Impact of transabdominal ultrasound guidance on performance and outcome of transcervical uterine embryo transfer. J Assist Reprod Genet 2003;20:318-22.
22. Buckett WM. A meta-analysis of ultrasound-guided versus clinical touch embryo transfer. Fertil Steril 2003;80:1037-41.
23. Sallam HN, Sadek SS. Ultrasound-guided embryo transfer: A meta-analysis of randomised controlled trials. Fertil Steril 2003; 80:1042-6.
24. Eskandar M, Abou-Setta AM, Almushait MA, El-Amin M, Mohmad SE. Ultrasound guidance during embryo transfer: A prospective, single-operator, randomized, controlled trial. Fertil Steril 2008;90:1187-90.
25. Kosmas IP, Janssens R, DeMunck L, Al Turki HF, Tournaye H, Van Steirteghem AC, Devroey P. Ultrasound guidance during embryo transfer does not offer any benefit in clinical outcome: A randomized controlled trial. Hum Reprod 2006;21:i101.
26. Drakeley AJ, Jorgensen A, Sklavounos J, Aust T, Gazvani R, Williamson P, Kingsland CR. A randomized controlled clinical trial of 2295 ultrasound-guided embryo transfers. Hum Reprod 2008;23:1101-6.
27. Shamonki MI, Schattman GL, Spandorfer SD, Chung PH, Rosenwaks Z. Ultrasound-guided trial transfer may be beneficial in preparation for an IVF cycle. Hum Reprod 2005;20:2844-9.

28. Shamonki MI, Spandorfer SD, Rosenwaks Z. Ultrasound-guided embryo transfer and the accuracy of trial embryo transfer. Hum Reprod 2005;20:709-16.

29. Tang OS, Ng EHY, So WWK, Ho PC. Ultrasound-guided embryo transfer: A prospective randomized controlled trial. Hum Reprod 2001;16:2310-5.

30. Yang WJ, Lee RK, Su JT, Lin MH, Hwu YM. Uterine position change between mock and real embryo transfers. Taiwan J Obstet Gynecol 2007;46:162-5.

31. Porter MB. Ultrasound in assisted reproductive technology. Semin Reprod Med 2008;26:266-76.

32. Woolcott R, Stanger J. Ultrasound tracking of the movement of embryo-associated air bubbles on standing after transfer. Hum Reprod 1998;13:2107-9.

33. Baba K, Ishihara O, Hayashi N, Saitoh M, Taya J, Kinoshita K. Three-dimensional ultrasound in embryo transfer. Ultrasound Obstet Gynecol 2000;16:372-3.

34. Pope CS, Cook EK, Arny M, Novak A, Grow DR. Influence of embryo transfer depth on *in vitro* fertilization and embryo transfer outcomes. Fertil Steril 2004;81:51-8.

35. Frankfurter D, Silva CP, Mota F, et al. The transfer point is a novel measure of embryo placement. Fertil Steril 2003; 79:1416-21.

36. Frankfurter D, Trimarchi JB, Silva CP, Keefe DL. Middle to lower uterine segment embryo transfer improves implantation and pregnancy rates compared with fundal embryo transfer. Fertil Steril 2004;81:1273-7.

37. Coroleu B, Barri PN, Carreras O, Martinez F, Parriego M, Hereter L, Parera N, Veiga A, Balasch J. The influence of the depth of embryo replacement into the uterine cavity on implantation rates after IVF: A controlled, ultrasound-guided study. Hum Reprod 2002;17:341-6.

38. Abou-Setta AM, Al-Inany HG, Mansour RT, Serour GI, Aboulghar MA. Analysis. Hum Reprod 2005;20:3114-21.

39. Coroleu B, Barri PN, Carreras O, Belil I, Buxaderas R, Veiga A, Balasch J. Effect of using an echogenic catheter for ultrasound-guided embryo transfer in an IVF programme: A prospective, randomized, controlled study. Hum Reprod 2006;21:1809-15.

40. Matorras R, Mendoza R, Expósito A, Rodriguez-Escudero FJ. Influence of the time interval between embryo catheter loading and discharging on the success of IVF. Hum Reprod 2004; 19:2027-30.

41. Letterie GS. Three-dimensional ultrasound-guided embryo transfer: a preliminary study. Am J Obstet Gynecol 2005; 192:1983-7.

42. Fang L, Sun Y, Su Y, Guo Y. Advantages of 3-dimensional sonography in embryo transfer. J Ultrasound Med 2009;28: 573-8.

43. Gergely RZ, DeUgarte CM, Danzer H, Surrey M, Hill D, DeCherney AH. Three-dimensional/four-dimensional ultrasound-guided embryo transfers using the maximal implantation potential point. Fertil Steril 2005;84:500-3.

Follicular Fluid Environment and ART Outcome

Ernesto Bosch

OVERVIEW

The follicular fluid environment has a strong influence on the maturation of the oocyte. Its variations have a significant impact on the quality of the oocyte, and therefore, on embryo viability and cycle outcome. During follicular development in the natural cycle, there is a precise sequence of hormonal changes in the follicular microenvironment that are related to those observed in the plasma. In ovarian stimulation cycles, the presence of a mature oocyte is generally related to a higher concentration of estradiol and progesterone. On the other hand, while fertilization is usually related to high estradiol levels, abnormal fertilization and cleavage is related to high progesterone, and no fertilization to high androstenedione. Pregnancy has shown to be associated with a high estradiol/androgens ratio in the follicular fluid. The hormonal composition of the follicular fluid varies depending on the stimulation protocol used. Either total concentrations or the relationships between them are different depending on pituitary suppression and the combination of gonadotropins used. It is up to the clinicians to individualize the stimulation protocols for each patient in order to provide the most favorable follicular milieu for optimizing the oocyte quality.

INTRODUCTION

Follicular fluid is usually not considered for clinical practice, as in most Reproduction Units, it is discarded once the oocytes are isolated after follicular aspiration. However, follicular fluid has a prognostic value, because its environment has a strong influence on the maturation of the oocyte. Follicular fluid can be considered as a mirror of oocyte quality, and therefore, of embryo quality. Consequently, follicular fluid composition is directly related to cycle outcome.

In this chapter, a review of the variations in follicular fluid composition under different ovarian stimulation protocols and its relationship to laboratory and clinical parameters is presented.

CLINICAL DISCUSSION

Synthesis of Follicular Fluid

In its preantral stage, the ovarian follicle is not dependent on gonadotropic stimulation. Nevertheless, its granulosa cells are able to synthesize ovarian steroids, although in very limited amounts. At the end of the preantral stage, the theca interna layer is developed, and follicle stimulating hormone (FSH) receptors will appear on the granulosa cells. Thus, theca cells will start producing androgens, while granulosa cells are able to aromatize them into estrogens, through the action of the cytochrome P450 complex.

When receptors for luteinizing hormone (LH) are expressed on the theca cells, androgen substrate production for aromatization is increased, and the follicle grows much faster due to cellular multiplication and the accumulation of follicular fluid.

Besides receptors for FSH, LH and steroids, gap junctions develop among granulosa cells and also between the oocyte and granulosa cells. They allow the exchange of hormones and molecules in a way that they form a functional unity (Fig. 49.1).

Composition of Follicular Fluid

Non-hormonal Components

Follicular fluid is partially composed of follicular secretions, partially from plasma exudates. Thus, its composition reflects both changes in granulosa and theca cells secretions,

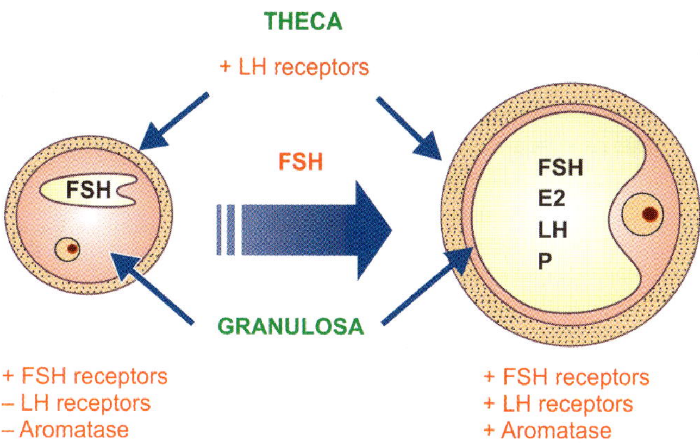

Fig. 49.1: Receptor expression in the antral and the preovulatory follicle

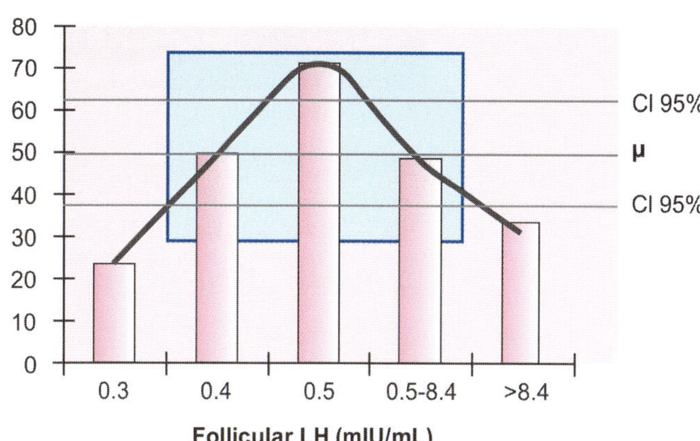

Fig. 49.2: Follicular fluid LH concentrations and its relationship with the fertilization rate

and alterations in plasma due to physiologic or pathologic processes.

The concentration of inorganic compounds is very similar to those observed in plasma. While pO_2 is very variable among follicles of the same patient, pCO_2 is quite constant, and similar to plasma values.[1] Na^+ and K^+ concentrations in plasma mainly determine follicular fluid osmotic pressure.[2]

Additionally, different carbohydrates, mucopolysaccharides, lipids and proteins have been described in the follicular fluid.[2]

Hormonal Components

Steroid hormones were identified in the follicular fluid of rabbits for the first time in 1929,[3] and several studies by Short in the 60's classified different estrogens and androgens in the follicular fluid of cows and mares.[4] Lately, steroid hormones have been quantified in the human follicular fluid with a variation in their concentrations in healthy women and in patients with some kind of disorder. Elevated concentrations of androgens have been identified in the follicular fluid of Stein-Leventhal syndrome patients,[5] and high levels of progesterone (P) have been observed during the follicular phase of patients with dysfunctional uterine bleeding.[6]

Pituitary hormones were lately evaluated by McNatty and colleagues[7] in the 70's,[7] and penetration of gonadotropin-releasing hormone (GnRH) agonists in the follicle,[8] as well as the presence of systemic hormones, such as insulin and cortisol, was also described.

Paracrine Factors

In the last decade, research has focussed on the description and role of paracrine factors, such as cyclic AMP, insulin-like growth factors (IGF), IGF binding proteins (IGF-BP), fibroblast growth factor (FGF), growth and differentiation factors, bone morphogenic protein (BMP), vascular endothelial growth factor (VEGF), and diverse cytokines, such as interleukins, tumor necrosis factor (TNF)-α, or leukotriene B-4, some of which are shown to play a crucial role in the communication between the follicular fluid and the cumulus-oocyte complex (COC).

Follicular Fluid in the Natural Cycle

In the mid 70's, McNatty and colleagues[7] analyzed steroids and gonadotropin concentrations in the follicular fluid along the menstrual cycle, and their relationship to their plasma levels. They observed that estradiol (E2) was higher in the mid-follicular phase while LH increased significantly in the late follicular phase. Preovulatory follicles contained elevated concentrations of estradiol and progesterone (P), low levels of prolactin (PRL), and LH and FSH concentrations corresponding to 30 to 60 percent of those found in blood.

On the other hand, progesterone was obviously higher in the mid-luteal phase. The authors concluded that during follicular development, there is a precise sequence of hormonal changes in the follicular microenvironment that is related to that observed in plasma.

These same authors cited the relationship between hormonal follicular fluid concentrations and the mitotic activity of granulosa cells,[9] and observed that those follicles with higher FSH levels in the early follicular phase had a higher mitotic index, and grew faster. As the mitotic activity of granulosa cells increased, receptors for LH appeared on them. Once LH entered in the follicle, the mitotic activity stopped and progesterone secretion started (Fig. 49.2). Oocytes with the capacity to resume meiosis originated from follicles with lower androgens/estrogens ratio compared to those oocytes that degenerated.[10]

Other authors also demonstrated that oocytes in metaphase I and II stages originated from follicles with higher levels of LH, while oocytes that were degenerating corresponded to follicles with elevated levels of androgens and high androgens/estrogens ratio.[11]

Table 49.1: Follicular fluid findings related to cycle outcome parameters in ovarian stimulation cycles	
Lobo et al. (1984)	Mature oocytes: ↑ P, ↑ P/E2
Tarlatzis et al. (1985)	Fertilization and pregnancy: ↑ E2, ↓ P/E2
Ben Rafael et al. (1987)	Abnormal fertilization and cleavage: ↑ P
Lindner et al. (1988)	Fertilization: ↑ PRL
Brzyski et al. (1990)	Mature oocytes and fertilization: ↑ E2 and ↑ P
Tonetta et al. (1990)	Fertilization and cleavage: ↑ E2 and ↑ PRL Abnormal cleavage: ↑ P
Kobayashi et al. (1991)	Mature oocytes and fertilization: ↑ E2 and ↑ P Mature oocytes but not fertilized: ↑ A
Andersen et al. (1993)	Pregnancy: ↑ E2/A, ↑ E2/T, = E2/P

Follicular Fluid in Ovarian Stimulation Cycles

In the late 80's and early 90's, a number of studies related cycle outcome parameters with follicular fluid hormonal concentrations. In Table 49.1, some of the most relevant of these studies, in which the data observed were quite consistent, are shown. The presence of a mature oocyte is generally related to a higher concentration of E2 and progesterone. On the other hand, while fertilization is usually related to high E2, abnormal fertilization and cleavage is related to high progesterone, and no fertilization to high androstenedione (Δ4). Andersen and colleagues[12] demonstrated that pregnancy was associated with a high estradiol/androgens ratio in the follicular fluid, with no relationship with the E2/progesterone the ratio.

In the previous years, we and others have analyzed the impact of different ovarian stimulation protocols on follicular fluid composition, and the relationship of these variations with the cycle outcome.

GnRH Agonists vs No GnRH Agonists

This first study was performed in order to analyze the difference between downregulated and non-downregulated cycles.[13] We included 20 young patients, with exclusively tubal infertility undergoing IVF. Ten of them followed a classic GnRH agonist long protocol, while the other 10 did not receive any GnRH agonist. Patients both the groups were stimulated with equal doses of highly purified-FSH.

The first relevant finding of this study was that all the analyzed hormones except progesterone and FSH showed significantly higher follicular fluid concentrations in non-downregulated patients, providing a consequently higher E2/progesterone ratio in these cycles (Table 49.2). When follicular LH levels were correlated with the other determined hormones, positive correlations with estrogens and androgens (A) were observed. However, the most relevant finding of this study was the description of an intrafollicular LH window, determining that very low and very high levels of follicular LH could be detrimental for oocyte functionality, in terms of fertilization capability (Fig. 49.2).

GnRH Agonist Long vs Short Protocol

Hormone levels in follicular fluid were compared in patients undergoing IVF with a flare protocol versus a control group of patients undergoing the long protocol.[14] They observed that all the steroid concentrations were higher in the short protocol group, but Δ4 was especially, significantly higher in this group. This group of patients also showed higher levels of serum LH on the day of human chorionic gonadotropin (hCG) administration. They concluded that the flare up regimen provides a poorer outcome than the long protocol due to a less favorable serum and follicular fluid endocrine milieu. In other words, surpassing the LH ceiling could lead to excessive follicular androgenization that leads to deleterious follicular maturation with unfertilized oocytes, and poor oocyte maturation.

GnRH Agonists vs GnRH Antagonists

Garcia Velasco and co-workers[15] analyzed the different steroid follicular concentrations according to the use of a GnRH agonist versus a GnRH antagonist. Thirty-six patients, aged 32.2 years undergoing IVF due to tubal factor, male or unexplained infertility were enrolled. Stimulation was performed in both the cases with recombinant FSH (rFSH) alone, and in the case of the GnRH antagonists group, a single dose of 3 mg of Cetrorelix was administered on the 7th day of stimulation, while the GnRH agonist group followed the classical long protocol.

The main finding of the present study was that follicular E2 was significantly lower among patients who were treated with a GnRH antagonist as was the E2/testosterone (T) ratio. These findings suggest that there is a direct effect of GnRH antagonists on ovarian cells, inducing lower granulosa cells aromatase activity. However, the number of metaphase II

Table 49.2: Follicular fluid hormonal concentrations in downregulated and non-downregulated cycles

Hormones in follicular fluid	Downregulated	Non-downregulated	Student's p value
E2 (pg/mL)	1108 ± 876	2071 ± 1751	p < 0.05
P (µg/mL)	29.9 ± 27.5	25.4 ± 35.7	NS
A (ng/mL)	3.8 ± 3.6	12.8 ± 13.9	p < 0.05
T (ng/mL)	7.1 ± 5.7	10.0 ± 7.3	p < 0.05
DHEAS (mIU/mL)	1669 ± 845	2232 ± 1252.2	p < 0.05
FSH (mIU/mL)	6.8 ± 2.4	7.9 ± 4.4	NS
LH (mIU/mL)	0.7 ± 0.7	3.6 ± 3.0	p < 0.05
hCG (mIU/mL)	137.7 ± 85.1	283 ± 149.7	p < 0.05

Abbreviations: E2: estradiol; P: progesterone; A: androgens; T: testosterone; DHEAS: dehydroepiandrosterone sulfate; FSH: follicle stimulating hormone; LH: luteinizing hormone; hCG: human chorionic gonadotropin

oocytes, and the fertilization, implantation and pregnancy rates were comparable between both the groups, which suggests that follicular development and functionality was not affected.

Recombinant FSH vs hp-hMG in GnRH Long Protocol Cycles

One of the largest studies analyzing follicular fluid hormone levels and cycle outcome with controlled ovarian hyperstimulation (COH) protocols was developed by Westergaard and co-workers.[16] They included 280 patients following a GnRH agonist long protocol, administered either subcutaneously (SC) or intranasal (IN) Buserelin, and undergoing stimulation with highly purified human menopausal gonadotropin (hp-hMG) or with recombinant FSH (r-FSH).

When serum hormone determinations, drawn on the day of oocyte retrieval were compared, FSH, LH and progesterone were shown to be significantly higher in the hp-hMG group, while hCG was higher in the r-FSH group. On the other hand, no differences were observed between groups for E2 and Δ4 determinations. Regarding follicular fluid concentrations, FSH, LH, E2 and Δ4 were higher in the hp-hMG group while hCG and progesterone were lower compared to the r-FSH group. The E2/Δ4 ratio was similar between the groups.

Authors suggest that these differences could be due on one hand to the longer half-life of the FSH isoforms contained in the urinary preparations compared to recombinant compounds, while differences in LH are obvious as the FSH group had only the endogenous residual levels. These higher concentrations of gonadotropins resulted in higher concentrations of E2 and Δ4 in the hMG group, maintaining similar E2/Δ4 ratios. Patients who followed ovarian stimulation with hMG showed higher pregnancy and delivery rates compared to stimulated with FSH alone, although differences were not statistically significant. Results according to the route of GnRH agonist administration were comparable.

When follicular fluid hormonal concentrations were related to cycle outcome, it was observed that FSH and LH levels were higher in the conception cycles, while there was a trend to statistically significance with E2 levels. No differences were seen regarding hCG, P, Δ4 and the different hormonal ratios. The authors concluded that a stimulation protocol that creates a preovulatory follicular environment rich in FSH and LH, and probably, also E2, might be especially favorable for an oocyte to mature, fertilize and develop into an embryo with a high chance to implant after embryo transfer.

Follicular Fluid Hormonal Variations: Impact on Oocyte Quality

Impact of LH Administration

In order to analyze the impact of LH administration on the follicular environment and its subsequent effect on oocyte quality, and therefore, the cycle outcome, we performed a prospective trial in which 30 oocyte donors following a GnRH agonist (IN Nafarelin) long protocol were randomized for stimulation with r-FSH alone (300 IU/day) or a combination of r-FSH and r-LH, (225/75 IU per day, or 150/150 IU per day). All donors were normovulatory and younger than 35 years. During stimulation, only variations in the r-FSH dosage were permitted. On the day of hCG administration, serum E2, P, FSH, LH, hCG, T, Δ4 and dehydroepiandrosterone (DHEAS) were measured. Two follicles were aspirated from each ovary of an individual donor and its correspondent oocyte was labelled and followed for morphological classification. In follicular fluid, E2, P, LH, T, Δ4 and DHEAS were determined and their values correlated with oocyte morphology, maturation, and fertilization. Embryo quality and recipients' cycle outcomes in terms of implantation and pregnancy rates were also evaluated.

When serum hormone determinations on the day of hCG were compared, interestingly, there were no significant differences among the groups for E2, progesterone or androgens. Moreover, serum LH levels were comparable among groups, reflecting a poor impact of LH addition on the serum LH profile. Only serum FSH was significantly higher in the group that did not receive LH. It is also interesting to mention that in this group, the serum progesterone was higher than in the other groups, although differences were not significant (Table 49.3). But, if serum hormone values are analyzed per obtained oocyte, it can be observed that there is a trend towards higher E2 levels per oocyte, and also to higher androgen levels per oocyte, reaching statistically significance in the case of T (Table 49.4).

These findings clearly correlated with those observed in follicular fluid. E2 follicular levels increased with the increase in LH stimulation doses. Additionally, ovarian androgens and T were also significantly higher in the group that received 150 IU/day of LH (Fig. 49.3).

When follicular fluid hormone values were correlated with the nuclear stage of the obtained oocyte, it was observed that metaphase I oocytes originated from follicles where the estradiol levels were significantly lower and T and Δ4 were higher when compared to the follicles that provided either metaphase II or germinal vesicle (GV) oocytes (Table 49.5).

When they were correlated with oocyte morphology, no differences were observed regarding E2 and progesterone levels. However, the LH concentration was significantly higher in the follicles in which the oocytes showed multiple alterations, while androgens were higher in follicles in which the oocytes showed anomalies in their perivitelline space. (Table 49.6).

None of the hormones determined in the follicular fluid showed any relationship with the likelihood of fertilization of the contained oocyte. Similarly, there was no correlation with embryo quality. The proportion of good quality embryos among the groups was comparable and there were no significant differences regarding implantation and pregnancy rates. The conclusion of this study was that an intrafollicular E2 defect is related with metaphase I oocytes, while excess a LH and androgens are related to oocyte anomalies. However, no relationship between follicular hormonal levels and embryo quality was observed.

Markers of Oocyte Developmental Potential

Mendoza and co-workers[17] attempted to identify hormonal and growth factor intrafollicular markers of oocyte developmental quality. They analyzed the follicular fluid composition of 54 young patients undergoing a GnRH

Table 49.3: Serum hormone levels on the day of hCG administration according to the dose of FSH and LH received

	FSH 300 IU	FSH/LH 225/75 IU	FSH/LH 150/150 IU	p value
E2 (pg/mL)	2662 ± 1239	2208 ± 852	2700 ± 1339	NS
P4 (ng/mL)	1.1 ± 0.7	0.6 ± 0.3	0.6 ± 0.5	NS
FSH (mIU/mL)	13.4 ± 4.5a	8.6 ± 4.1b	7.5 ± 1.3b	0.009 (a > b)
LH (mIU/mL)	2.0 ± 1.9	1.6 ± 1.5	2.2 ± 1.8	NS
T (ng/mL)	0.6 ± 0.2	0.5 ± 0.2	0.8 ± 0.3	NS
A (ng/mL)	2.7 ± 0.7	2.4 ± 0.4	2.9 ± 1.1	NS
DHEAS (μg/dL)	206 ± 57	190 ± 142	192 ± 78	NS

Table 49.4: Serum hormone levels on the day of hCG administration per obtained oocyte according to the dose of FSH and LH received

	FSH 300 IU	FSH/LH 225/75 IU	FSH/LH 150/150 IU	p value
E2 (pg/mL)	149 ± 52	166 ± 69	199 ± 58	NS
P4 (ng/mL)	0.065 ± 0.039	0.046 ± 0.025	0.037 ± 0.023	NS
FSH (mIU/mL)	0.96 ± 0.81	0.64 ± 0.29	0.63 ± 0.21	NS
LH (mIU/mL)	0.15 ± 0.06	0.14 ± 0.05	0.17 ± 0.04	NS
T (ng/mL)	0.03 ± 0.01a	0.04 ± 0.02	0.07 ± 0.02b	0.003 (a < b)
A (ng/mL)	0.16 ± 0.05	0.19 ± 0.10	0.22 ± 0.05	NS
DHEAS (μg/dL)	12.8 ± 7.1	15.1 ± 5.0	16.3 ± 3.6	NS

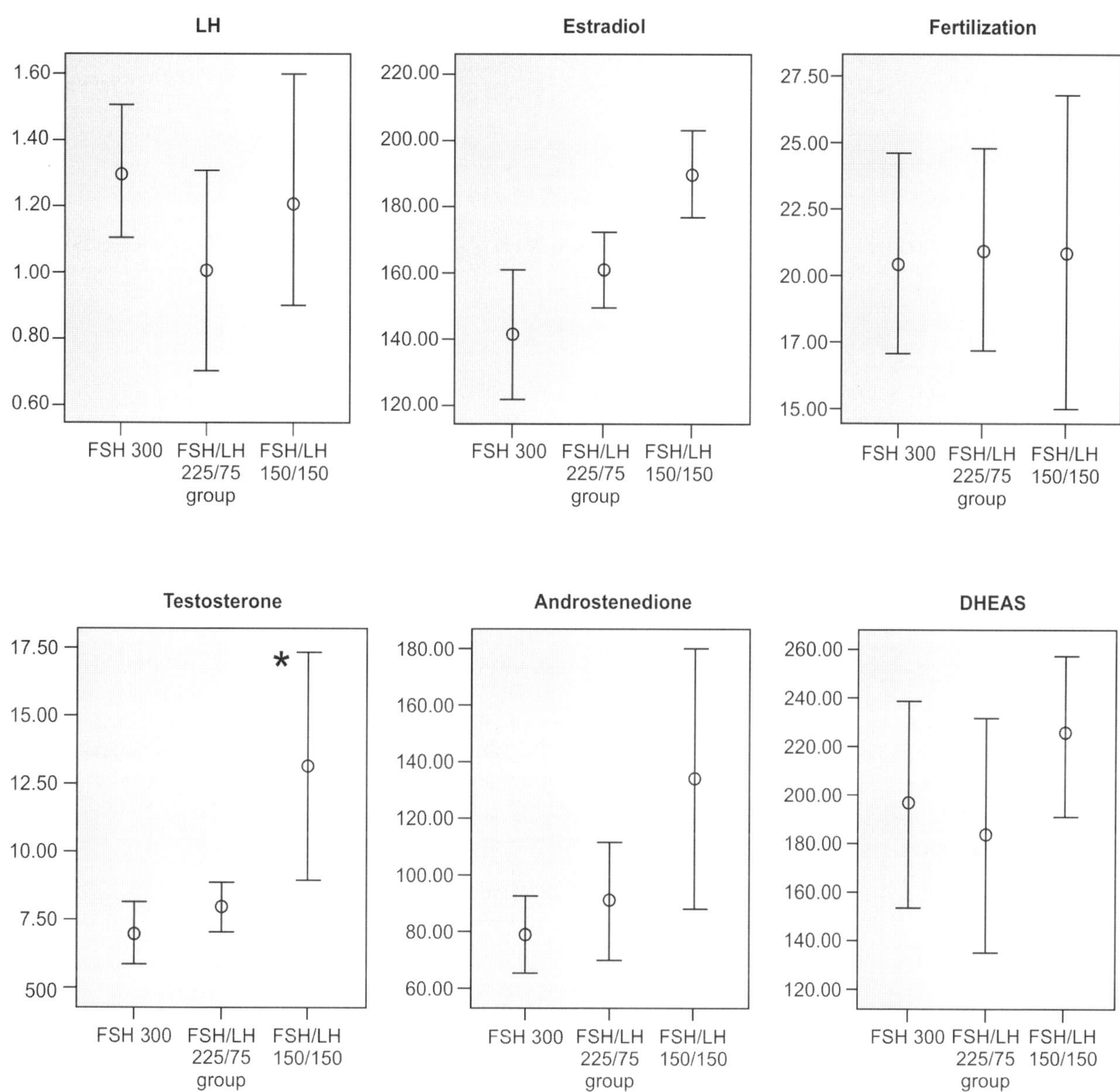

Fig. 49.3: Follicular fluid hormone determinations according to FSH and LH doses received

Table 49.5: Follicular fluid hormone determinations according to oocyte nuclear stage			
	Metaphase II	*Metaphase I*	*Germinal vesicle*	*p value*
E2 (pg/mL)	165 ± 60a	91 ± 79b	175 ± 19a	0.04 (a > b)
P4 (ng/mL)	17.5 ± 6.3	15.0 ± 13.0	23.7 ± 15.1	NS
LH (mIU/mL)	$1.4 + 0.7$	1.1 ± 0.8	1.3 ± 0.7	NS
T (ng/mL)	7.8 ± 6.2b	21.6 ± 30.7a	12.4 ± 0.6	0.007 (a > b)
A (ng/mL)	94.1 ± 54.1b	302 ± 281a	161 ± 5.7	< 0.001 (a > b)
DHEAS (µg/dL)	219 ± 94	270 ± 212	228 ± 10.6	NS

Table 49.6: Follicular fluid hormone determinations according to oocyte morphology				
	Normal	*Perivitelline space anomalies*	*Polar body and cytoplasm anomalies*	*Multiple anomalies*	*p value*
E2 (pg/mL)	167 ± 44	266 ± 85	164 ± 58	193 ± 62	NS
P4 (ng/mL)	19.2 ± 5.3	13.4 ± 6.4	17.2 ± 5.6	17.9 ± 9.7	NS
LH (mIU/mL)	1.6 ± 0.7b	1.5 ± 0.2b	1.3 ± 0.6b	3.0 ± 1.8a	<0.001 (a > b)
T (ng/mL)	7.8 ± 6.0b	19.0 ± 0.5a	7.2 ± 5.9b	14.0 ± 0.3	0.011 (a > b)
A (ng/mL)	87.0 ± 36.2b	280 ± 49a	86.7 ± 48.4b	125 ± 31b	<0.001 (a > b)
DHEAS (µg/dL)	207 ± 101b	453 ± 281a	214 ± 80b	230 ± 21	0.003 (a > b)

agonist long protocol and stimulation with a combination of hp-FSH and hMG for *in vitro* fertilization. They observed that E2, LH, growth hormone (GH), prolactin (PRL) and insulin-like growth factor 1(IGF-I) were higher in the follicles of the patients who got pregnant when compared to those who did not. Moreover, follicles that provided an oocyte that resulted in an embryo that finally implanted, contained higher concentrations of these hormones compared to those determined in follicles from which the resulting embryo failed to implant. On the other hand, interleukin (IL)-1 was higher in follicles related to a negative outcome.

The authors suggested that GH plays an important role in enhancing intrafollicular metabolic events required for oocyte maturation, promoting FSH and LH action. IGF-1 may also play a role as a mediator of GH action, at least partially. IL-1 would not be related to postfertilization oocyte viability.

Impact of Letrozole Administration

In a pilot study recently published by our colleagues from Madrid, to evaluate the impact of aromatase inhibitors as an adjuvant treatment in IVF cycles, intraovarian androgens were determined and related to cycle outcome.[18] It was performed in 147 low responder patients with a previous cancelled IVF cycle; 71 patients were treated with Letrozole, 2.5 mg plus a high-dose FSH/hMG-antagonist regimen; 76 patients were similarly treated but Letrozole was not employed. Letrozole was administered during the first 5 days of stimulation and hormones were evaluated in both the serum and follicular fluid. The number of oocytes retrieved, fertilization, implantation and pregnancy rates were compared; Δ4, T, E2, and pro-gesterone values were determined in serum and follicular fluid.[18]

Results showed that Letrozole-treated patients showed significantly higher levels of follicular fluid T and Δ4 (80.3 pg/mL vs 43.8 pg/mL and 57.9 vs 37.4 mg/mL, respectively). Similarly, these patients had a higher number of oocytes retrieved (6.1 vs 4.3) and a higher implantation rate (25% vs 9.4%) despite similar doses of FSH/hMG (3,627 IU vs 3,804 IU). These data suggest that in poor responders, providing a higher intrafollicular androgen milieu, can improve their cycle outcome.[18]

Intrafollicular Paracrine Factors

Most recent research has been focussed on determining the role of different intrafollicular paracrine factors and analyzing the relationship between their intrafollicular concentration and cycle outcome. Thus, it has been demonstrated that there is no correlation between intrafollicular tumor necrosis factors (TNF) and cycle outcome, while high levels of vascular endothelial growth factor (VEGF) or leptin have been associated with poor outcomes.[19]

Antiphospholipid molecules have also been analyzed in the follicle and related to lower, although non-significant implantation rate, and comparable live birth rates.[20] On the other hand, Fanchin and colleagues[21] have determined intrafollicular anti-Müllerian hormone (AMH) levels, and have shown that there is a positive correlation between its values and antral follicular count (AFC) and the number of oocytes retrieved. They also demonstrated that peripheral AMH levels reflect its follicular production.

CONCLUSION

It is well-known that the follicular fluid composition varies along the natural menstrual cycle, following a perfect sequence that determines oocyte maturation and functionality. This physiologic composition is altered under conditions of ovarian stimulation, the different ovarian stimulation protocols causing different intrafollicular hormonal con-centrations affecting oocyte maturation and therefore, the cycle outcome. In this sense, an extensive number of studies have determined steroid and gonadotropin levels in the follicular fluid after different ovarian stimulation protocols, and have compared their values and correlated them to the cycle outcome parameters.

There is a large amount of data and conclusions that can be drawn from these studies, but only a few of them remain consistent across the variety of studies. Thus, there is wide consensus suggesting that a rich FSH and LH intrafollicular milieu provides higher E2 and androgen concentrations, which are related to a better cycle outcome. An important role of GH and IGF-1 has also been described.

It is also commonly accepted that excess intrafollicular androgens, as related to the flare up protocol or to excess LH levels a during ovarian stimulation are related to a poor outcome due to poor oocyte quality. However, patients with a background of low response with high concentrations of intrafollicular androgens benefit from the use of the aromatase inhibitor, Letrozole.

On the other hand, a defect in intrafollicular LH, which can occur when stimulation is performed with FSH alone and/or GnRH antagonists, can affect oocyte functionality in terms of fertilization, as can as an excess of it, defining an intrafollicular LH window, similarly to what has been described regarding serum LH levels during the follicular phase.

Summarizing, the composition of follicular fluid can be crucial for an IVF cycle, as its variations due to the use of different protocols and different gonadotropin compounds have a direct impact on the biological quality of the oocyte, and therefore, on the overall outcome of the procedure. It is up to the clinician to individualize the stimulation protocol for each patient in order to provide the most favorable follicular milieu for optimizing the quality of the oocyte.

REFERENCES

1. Shalgi R, Kraicer PF, Soferman N. Gases and electrolytes of human follicular fluid. J Reprod Fert 1972;28:335-41.
2. Edwards RG. Follicular fluid. J Reprod Fert 1974;37:189-219.
3. Parkes AS. Internal secretions of the ovary. Longmans Green. London 1929.
4. Short RV. Steroids present in the follicular fluid of the mare. J Endocr 1960;20:147-64.
5. Gorgi EP. The determination of steroids in the cyst fluid from polycystic ovaries. J Endocr 1963;27:225-40.
6. Gorgi EP. Steroids in cyst fluid from ovaries of normally menstruating women and of women with functional uterine bleeding. J Reprod Fert 1965;10:309-18.
7. McNatty KP, Hunter WM, McNely AS, Sawers RS. Changes in the concentrations of pituitary and steroids and hormones in the follicular fluid of human Graafian follicles throughout the menstrual cycles. J Endocrinol 1975;64:555-71.
8. Pellicer A, Tarín JJ, Miró F, Sampaio BA, De los Santos MJ, Remohí J. The use of gonadotropin-releasing hormone analogues (GnRHa) in *in vitro* fertilization: Some clinical and experimental investigations of a direct effect on the human ovary. Hum Reprod 1992;7 (Suppl 1):39-47.
9. McNatty KP, Sawers RS. Relationship between the endocrine environment within the Graafian follicle and the subsequent rate of progesterone secretion by human granulosa cells in vitro. J Endocr 1975;66:391-40.
10. McNatty KP, Smith DM, Makris A, Osathannondth R, Ryan KJ. The microenvironment of the human antral follicle: Inter-relationships among the steroid levels in antral fluid, the population of granulosa cells, and the status of the oocyte in vivo and in vitro. J Clin Endocrinol Metab 1979;49:851-60.
11. Seibel MM, Smith D, Dlugi M, Levesque L. Preovulatory follicular fluid hormone levels in spontaneous human cycles. J Clin Endocrinol Metab 1989;68:1073-7.
12. Andersen YC. Characteristics of human follicular fluid associated with successful conception after *in vitro* fertilization. J Clin Endocrinol Metab 1993;1227-34.
13. Bosch E. Influence of follicular LH levels on oocyte quality in *In Vitro* Fertilization. Doctoral Thesis. Valencia School of Medicine. Valencia University, 1999.
14. Bo-Abbas YY, Martin KA, Liberman RF, Cramer DW, Barbieri RL. Serum and follicular fluid hormone levels during in vitro fertilization after short or long-course treatment with a gonadotropin-releasing hormone agonist. Fertil Steril 2001; 75:694-9.
15. Garcia-Velasco JA, Isaza V, Vidal C, Landazabal A, Remohi J, Simon C, Pellicer A. Human ovarian steroid secretion *in vivo*: effects of GnRH agonist versus antagonist (cetrorelix). Hum Reprod 2001;16:2533-9.
16. Westergaard LG, Erb K, Laursen SB, Rasmussen PE, Rex S, Westergaard CG, Andersen CY. Concentrations of gonadotropins and steroids in preovulatory follicular fluid and serum in relation to stimulation protocol and outcome of assisted reproduction treatment. Reprod Biomed Online 2004; 8:516-23.
17. Bosch E, Pau E, Albert C, Zuzuarregui J, Remohí J, Pellicer A. Impact of different amounts of LH in controlled ovarian hyperstimulation oocyte donation cycles. Fertil Steril 2006; 86;S425.
18. Garcia-Velasco JA, Moreno L, Pacheco A, Guillen A, Duque L, Requena A, Pellicer A. The aromatase inhibitor letrozole increases the concentration of intraovarian androgens and improves *in vitro* fertilization outcome in low responder patients: A pilot study. Fertil Steril 2005;84:82-7.
19. Asimakopoulos B, Nikolettos N, Papachristou DN, Simopoulou M, Al-Hasani S, Diedrich K. Follicular fluid levels of vascular endothelial growth factor and leptin are associated with pregnancy outcome of normal women participating in intra-cytoplasmic sperm injection cycles. Physiol Res 2005;54:263-70.
20. Buckingham KL, Stone PR, Smith JF, Chamley LW. Anti-phospholipid antibodies in serum and follicular fluid—is there a correlation with IVF implantation failure? Hum Reprod 2006; 21:728-34.
21. Fanchin R, Louafi N, Mendez Lozano DH, Frydman N, Frydman R, Taieb J. Per-follicle measurements indicate that anti-Müllerian hormone secretion is modulated by the extent of follicular development and luteinization and may reflect qualitatively the ovarian follicular status. Fertil Steril 2005;84:167-73.

The ART Laboratory

Improving Implantation: Choosing the Right Embryo

Padma Rekha Jirge

OVERVIEW

The field of assisted reproductive techniques (ART) has seen changes in all the concerned aspects, i.e. clinical, endocrinological and laboratory. This has led to an improvement in the outcome of *in vitro* fertlization (IVF) cycles. However, in view of the health and economic burden created by multiple pregnancy resulting from IVF, there is an ever-increasing need to minimize the number of embryos transferred and indeed, limit them to single embryo transfer electively in majority of the women undergoing IVF. This necessitates the use of effective means to select euploid embryos with the highest implantation potential. This chapter will look into the current practice of embryo assessment and the future possibilities.

INTRODUCTION

The past decade has witnessed improvements in laboratory culture techniques and the development of stage-specific sequential media. This has led to a better and stable environment for the preimplantation embryos. Increasing experience in *in vitro* fertilization (IVF)/intracytoplasmic sperm injection (ICSI) has helped in appreciating the complexities of oocyte and embryo physiology. Cumulatively, these factors have resulted in an improvement in the implantation and pregnancy rates. This is also reflected in multiple pregnancy, which constitutes up to 30 percent of all IVF/ICSI pregnancies. However, such an occurrence is increasingly being considered as an unacceptable complication of ART cycles.[1] There is a trend towards the elective transfer of a single embryo in many countries. In addition, there are restrictions in certain countries, such as Germany and Italy, as to the number of oocytes to be fertilized and the number of embryos to be cultured. Hence, it becomes imperative to select embryos with the best implantation potential for optimal results.

Apart from a good stimulation protocol, additional pharmacological interventions in the form of low-dose Aspirin and glucocorticoids do not improve the implantation rate in an unselected population of women undergoing IVF/ICSI.[2,3] The prime factor influencing implantation is the embryo itself. Traditionally, we have based the selection of embryos with good implantation potential on the cleavage stage embryo morphology. However, it is now understood that a proportion of cleavage stage embryos with 'normal morphology' do have an abnormal chromosomal component. Additional information obtained from early stages, such as oocyte quality, zygote morphology, and in selected cases, extended culture is considered to be important towards the selection of the right embryos for transfer. There is also work done to identify metabolites, which may prove to be biochemical markers. In certain situations, resorting to invasive modalities, such as preimplantation genetic diagnosis (PGD), may be the only way of confirming the genetic normalcy of embryos.

We will look into the various methods used for assessing embryo quality in the current practice, followed by a discussion on role of each of these in predicting the embryo quality.

CLINICAL DISCUSSION

Assessment of Embryo Quality: Non-invasive Methods

Morphology

Oocytes

The size of the oocyte cohort and the number of mature oocytes (metaphase II), present at oocyte retrieval, influence all the *in vitro* events. The intra- and extracytoplasmic compartments of oocytes have been examined to identify markers of good fertilization and implantation. Cytoplasmic inclusions, vacuoles, extensive granulation, particularly centrally located, may all indicate impaired cytoplasmic maturity and constitute oocyte dysmorphism. Increased cytoplasmic viscosity, as evidenced by delayed return of the oolemma to its original position following injection of the spermatozoon in ICSI, may indicate increased cytoplasmic turbulence.

First polar body (PB1) morphology has been studied as well, as it reflects the genetic make of the oocyte itself. Morphological variants are graded as follows: round with a smooth surface (Grade 1), oval with a rough surface (Grade 2), fragmented (Grade 3) and huge PB1 (Grade 4).[4] The size of the perivitelline space has been considered in the evaluation of oocyte morphology as well.[5] A few studies have used spindle view to identify the presence of the spindle and its alignment with the PB1.

Zygote Scoring

The oocyte is routinely examined 16 to 20 hours after insemination or injection for the presence of two pronuclei, which confirms fertilization. The pronuclear size, alignment, location and the number, distribution and appearance of nucleoli within them have all been studied to identify zygotes with high implantation potentials.[6-9] Another scoring method incorporates the position of polar bodies as well, in an effort to improve the predictive value of zygote scoring.[10] A simple system of assessing pronuclei and nucleoli, as described by Tesarik and Greco,[8] is described here (Table 50.1 and Fig. 50.1). Pattern 0 is considered to be normal whilst all other patterns are considered to exhibit abnormal morphology.

In the progressive embryo assessment, the next stage of examination is at 25 to 27 hours or early cleavage stage. The presence of embryos, which have entered syngamy and cleaved with two equal sized and mononuclear blastomeres, is considered as an additional predictor of implantation potential.

The most conventional and widely used method to choose good embryos is morphological assessment on day 2 at 41 to 44 hours and on day 3 at 66 to 71 hours. Table 50.2 shows the parameters used for assessing cleavage stage embryos.

According to a strict criteria, 'top quality' embryos constitute those with four or five blastomeres on day 2, and seven or more on day 3, 20 percent fragmentation or less on day 3 and no multinucleated blastomeres.[12]

Majority of the units perform embryo transfer on day 2 or 3. However, some routinely allow extended culture, whilst others may selectively do this for certain indications. Various groups use criteria such as the presence of 8 good oocytes or zygotes or 4 good cleavage stage embryos to allow for extended culture. Blastocyst evaluation is performed at 120 hours on day 5 of *in vitro* culture.[13,14] The blastocyst scoring system

Table 50.1: Definition of patterns of pronuclear stage morphology (Adopted from Tesarik and Greco[8])

Pattern	Description
0	Similar number of NPB in both pronuclei; NPB always polarized if <7 and never polarized if >7; polarized or non-polarized in both pronuclei.
1	Big difference (>3) in the number of NPB in both pronuclei.
2	Small number (<7) of NPB without polarization in at least one pronucleus.
3	Large number (>7) of NPB with polarization in at least one pronucleus.
4	Very small number (<3) of NPB in at least one pronucleus.
5	Polarized distribution of NPB in one pronucleus and non-polarized in the other.

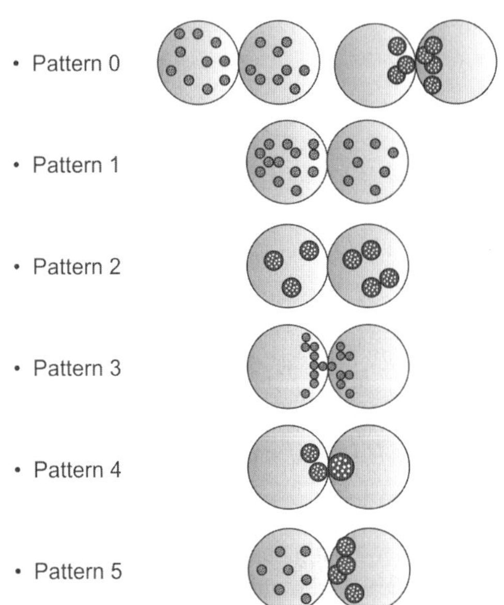

Fig. 50.1: Zygote scoring based on pronuclear morphology *(Adopted from Tesarik and Greco[8])*

Table 50.2: Pre-embryo grading (Adapted from Veeck, 1990)[11]

Grade	Blastomeres	Fragments
1	Equal size	No
2	Equal size	Minor or blebs
3	Unequal size	No
4	Equal or unequal size	Moderate to heavy
5	Any size	Major or complete fragmentation

is based on three parameters: (i) blastocoele formation and degree of expansion, (ii) development of the inner cell mass (ICM) and (iii) development of the trophectoderm (TE).

Grade 1 : Fully expanded blastocyst (distinct ICM, TE and blastocoele, thin zona pellucida, fully expanded diameter);

Grade 2 : Expanding blastocyst (distinct ICM, TE, and blastocoele, thin zona pellucida, substantial increase in embryo diameter, but not fully expanded);

Grade 3 : Early blastocyst (distinct ICM, TE and blastocoele);

Grade 4 : Late cavitating embryo with >50 percent blastocoele (distinct blastocoele, ICM and TE not laid down);

Grade 5 : Early cavitating embryo with <50 percent blastocoele (first signs of blastocoele);

Grade 6 : Compacted embryo;

Grade 7 : Compacting embryo;

Grade 8 : Arrested embryo.

It is useful to combine the findings of the evaluation from different stages and adopt a Graduated Embryo Score (GES), which has a high predictive value for blastocyst formation and pregnancy (Figs 50.2A to D).[15]

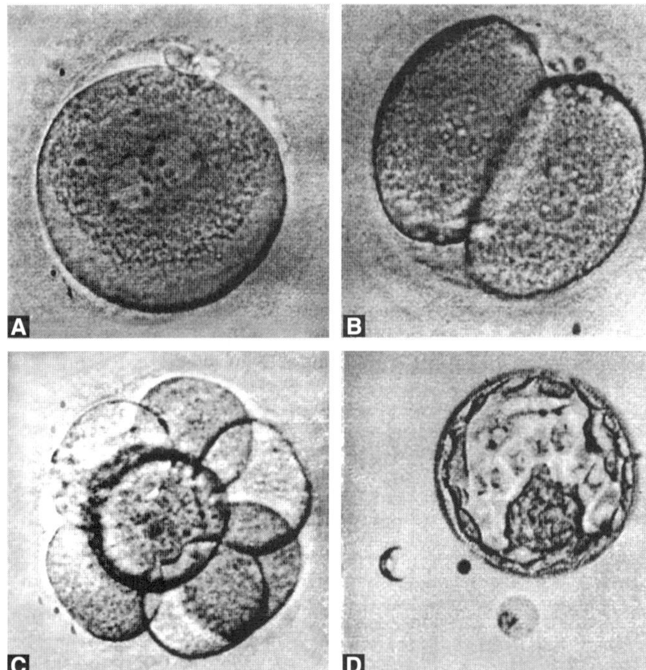

Figs 50.2A to D: (A) Embryo evaluated after at 16–18 hours postinsemination demonstrating nucleolar alignment along the pronuclear axis; (B) Embryo evaluated at 25–27 hours post-insemination demonstrating symmetrical blastomere cleavage and no fragmentation; (C) Embryo evaluated at 64–67 hours post-insemination demonstrating symmetrical cleavage, eight cells and no fragmentation; (D) Fully expanded blastocyst at 120 hours post- insemination. (*Adopted from Fisch et al.*[15])

Omics

In an effort to improve the ability to select embryos with a high implantation potential, non-invasive methods of assessment of the embryo metabolism have been investigated in the recent years. Amino acid consumption at different stages of development, secretion of embryonic proteins and assessment of embryo respiration are some of the technologies being studied. Looking at the secretome, differential secretion of various embryonic proteins into the surrounding culture media, may assist in identifying embryos with the highest implantation potential.[16] Raman and near-infrared technologies are capable of detecting specific changes in the 'secretome' and the findings correlate well with morphological assessment.[17] However, the clinical implications of these novel technologies need to be proven with adequately powered prospective studies.[18]

Time-lapse Imaging of Embryos (EmbryoScope)

Another innovative technology is monitoring the embryo development with time-lapse imaging built within the incubator. Initial evidence suggests that time-lapse imaging provides a morphological, temporal and spatial assessment of embryo development without impairing the embryo quality.[19] Ongoing work on this novel technology should define its role in clinical practice.

Doppler Studies

Color Doppler indices of ovarian perifollicular blood flow have been compared with various outcome measures in IVF/ICSI cycles. More recently, power Doppler has been used as it is more sensitive at detecting low velocity flow and hence, improves visualization of small vessels. Oocytes from follicles with good blood flow are considered to yield embryos with good implantation potential.

Invasive Methods

It is now known that none of the morphological features in an embryo can ascertain a normal chromosomal complement. Preimplantation genetic diagnosis (PGD), following embryo biopsy, overcomes this problem. If subjected to aneuploidy screening, normal embryos can be transferred at the blastocyst stage in the same cycle. However, for more complex situations, the embryos need to be cryopreserved, to be transferred in a subsequent cycle. At present, its application is restricted for use in women with specific indications.

Predicting the Embryo Quality

The availability of stage-specific culture media and extended culture have contributed to a better understanding of pre-implantation embryo physiology. However, this has not always led to a dramatic improvement in the implantation rate. On the other hand, we have seen an increase in multiple pregnancy along with the associated burden of maternal and fetal morbidities. In addition, there are laws limiting the number of oocytes and embryos that can be cultured and subsequently transferred in some countries. All these factors necessitate limiting the number of embryos transferred. Recent data shows that the application of single embryo transfer with appropriate selection criteria does not result in a significant reduction in the overall pregnancy rate compared to the transfer of two embryos.[20] Hence, the selection of the 'best' embryo, which has the highest chance of successful implantation amongst a cohort of embryos and, at the same time, minimizes the risk of multiple pregnancy, has become an urgent need.

The most widely used method for assessing embryo quality is cleavage stage embryo morphology. However, this method alone is increasingly recognized to be inadequate to predict blastocyst formation[21] and implantation potential.[22] One of the reasons is the presence of undiagnosed aneuploidy and altered gene expression in some embryos.[23,24] Hence, attempts have been made to use more rigorous criteria for better selection of embryos. Strict grading, as described above, and transferring one or two 'top quality' embryos, is associated with an increased implantation rate of 42 to 47 percent, compared to an implantation rate of 8 to 18 percent in those with an abnormal day 2 cleavage rate.[1,25] Further, embryos conforming to the above criteria on day 2, and exhibiting fast cleavage on day 3 and subsequent early compaction may indicate a genuinely good growth potential. Expanded blastocysts, resulting from embryos with >10 percent fragmentation on day 3, implant less well than those with <10 percent fragmentation (30% vs 49%, respectively).[18] Embryos with multinucleate balstomeres (MNB) can grow to blastocysts and implant as well though they are more likely to be associated with early developmental arrest. MNB embryos are known to lack normal RNA synthesis, suggesting a defective transcription of genes that eventually leads to developmental arrest.[26] Thus, simple observations of cleavage rate, fragmentation and the presence of MNB improve the predictive value of implantation potential at this stage itself.

There is growing evidence that assessment of embryos and selection of good quality embryos should start much earlier as certain morphological features at different stages are strong markers of a healthy embryo.

The size of the cohort and the number of mature oocytes at retrieval have a direct impact on the implantation potential of resultant embryos. Adequate number is also a prerequisite, if a graded embryo score is to be successfully implemented. Though approximately 20 percent of the oocytes are immature at the time of oocyte retrieval, a proportion of them do mature *in vitro* prior to ICSI. They have similar fertilization rates as *in vivo* matured oocytes. However, the available data suggests that their further development

potential is hampered. Asynchrony between nuclear and cytoplasmic maturity appears to have an adverse impact on the developmental competence of such oocytes.[27,28] It is known that oocytes with normal cytoplasm, intact polar body and normal perivitelline space have a better fertilization rate and yield better quality embryos (67%) when compared to oocytes with cytoplasmic inclusions (45%)[5] or a large perivitelline space (53%).[29] Conversely, oocyte dysmorphism, such as granular cytoplasm, when extensive, is associated with impaired embryo development and implantation without any apparent adverse effect on the fertilization rate.[30,31] Increased viscosity of ooplasm as evidenced by slow return of the oolemma to its original shape after ICSI,[32] may interfere with the dynamic activities occurring during fertilization, including alignment of pronuclei and hence, further embryo development. This is reflected in zygote and blastocyst quality and clinical pregnancy rate at a later stage though no apparent effect may be seen during the cleavage stage.[32] The presence of vacuoles in the cytoplasm can have an adverse impact on fertilization. The later they arise, the more likelihood of a developmental arrest.[33]

The significance, if any, of varying morphology of PB1 is not understood. Though there is concern about the functional competence of oocytes with large and fragmented PB1,[4] no correlation has been established between any particular morphology and fertilization rate, embryo quality, blastocyst development and implantation rate. PB1 morphology, so far, has not proved to be a reliable predictor of developmental potential of the oocytes, as evidenced by PGD.[34]

Recently, a computer assisted polarization microscopy system (Polscope) is used to view the birefringent meiotic spindle to avoid any damage during oocyte manipulation. The meiotic spindle is always aligned with the first polar body and any misalignment noted in *in vivo* matured oocytes is due to the displacement of first polar body during manipulation for denuding the cumulus and corona. Very limited evidence shows that such oocytes may exhibit abnormal fertilization.[35] As damage to the oocytes during manipulation occurs in as less as 4 to 5 percent of the oocyte cohort, the role of the polscope in routine practice is unclear. However, the availability of very few oocytes for ICSI and manipulation of frozen and thawed oocytes may constitute some of the indications for its use in future.

As opposed to the abundance of work on oocyte quality, very little is understood about the impact of sperm quality on early embryo development. However, it is accepted that abnormal sperm can affect fertilization and embryo development at all stages. Conversely, even sperm with abnormal sperm DNA can fertilize oocytes and lead to live births.[36,37] At present, apart from simple morphological criteria, there is no better way of selecting sperm for intracytoplasmic injection.

However, the use of intracytoplasmic morphologically selected sperm injection (IMSI) may prove to be beneficial in couples undergoing ICSI for poor semen parameters and repeated ICSI failures.[38]

Most ethical concerns can be solved and work load on the laboratory personnel reduced if embryos endowed with the potential to implant can be identified as early as possible during the period of embryonic development. Selection of embryos at an early stage has the advantage of allowing for blastocyst transfer and reducing the number of embryos transferred, provided a good cryopreservation system is in place. Pronuclear stage zygotes provide the very first sign of fertilization and give valuable information about polarity of the cell, which is associated with normal protein synthesis and genetic component. The failure of alignment of the pronuclei is indicative of incomplete progression of events during fertilization and any inequality in the sizes of male and female pronuclei is a strong indicator of chromosomal abnormality. Pronuclei with 3 to 7 large, even-sized nucleoli indicate synchrony between the male and female pronuclei. The nucleoli are the areas where rRNA synthesis occurs. Unequal numbers, sizes or very unequal distribution of nucleoli might be markers of chromosomal abnormalities or aberrant meiotic events, leading to breakdown of normal development and resulting in embryos with lack of implantation potential. Zygotes with pattern 0 have the highest implantation potential with an implantation rate of 30 percent and pregnancy rate of 45 percent as compared to 11 percent and 22 percent, respectively with non-pattern 0 embryos, when embryo transfer is performed on day 2.[7,9,39] In addition, a higher incidence of multiple pregnancy is noted when more than one pattern 0 zygote is transferred, suggesting an association between normal embryos and pattern 0. Patterns 1 and 3 are more likely to show arrest at cleavage stage (30%) and patterns 1 and 5 are more likely to exhibit multinucleated blastomeres (30%).[8] Further, Grade 1 and 2 blastocysts showed a significantly high implantation rate of 27.2 to 58 percent when they were derived from pattern 0 zygotes compared to 11.1 to 39 percent with abnormal PN patterns and a high multiple pregnancy rate of 50 percent.[7,40] Further support to this morphological assessment comes from studies incorporating fluorescent *in situ* hybridization (FISH) analysis of oocytes or cleavage stage embryos. The highest proportion of euploid embryos (59%) were derived from zygotes with aligned equal-sized pronuclei, either at the center of the cell with large aligned or scattered nucleoli in both pronuclei and polar bodies along the longitudinal axis of the pronuclei. This was followed by those with aligned but peripherally placed pronuclei with nucleoli and polar body distribution as above (25%). Complex chromosomal abnormalities were very high in all other patterns. This again supports that polarity is a strong indicator of the association between energy availability and correct alignment of chromatin onto the mitotic plate and disturbance could represent errors occurring at meiosis and mitosis with gene-

ration of chromosomal abnormalities.[41] The pronuclear morphology corresponds with cleavage morphology in 84 percent of the embryos.[42] It is now important to evaluate the relative importance of any particular scoring system over others with randomized controlled trials.

Recent data shows that further evidence of good implantation potential comes from the occurrence of early cleavage at 25 to 27 hours.[43-45] In embryo transfers including at least one embryo derived from a polarized zygote, which cleaved early, a 51 percent pregnancy rate has been reported compared to 38 percent when no such embryos were available for transfer. In a cohort of morphologically good embryos, assessment of alignment or polarization of nucleoli and occurrence of early cleavage can serve as a simple non-invasive method for selection of embryos with high implantation potential.[46]

The availability of sequential culture media capable of supporting *in vitro* development of the human embryo to the blastocyst stage, and higher implantation rates (50%) reported after blastocyst transfer,[47] have encouraged many centers to move towards blastocyst transfer. In addition, this is considered as an important step towards reducing the number of embryos transferred in an individual and hence, in reducing the risk of multiple pregnancy. Blastocyst culture has the potential advantage that it allows the identification of embryos with good developmental potential, better synchronization between the embryo developmental stage and uterine environment and decreased uterine contractility. However, it is known that majority of the embryos do not reach blastocyst stage and a proportion of them would have good implantation potential at the cleavage stage.[48] It also implicates increased cost and workload. Hence, controversy still exists in the literature regarding the merits of blastocyst transfer.[18]

In a selective group of good responders, when combined evaluation of pronuclear and cleavage stage morphology is used for selection criteria, the rates of implantation (35% and 38%) and pregnancy (58% and 62%) were similar with day 3 and day 5 transfers, respectively. When the data from cryopreserved embryo transfer is included, day 3 transfer may be superior to day 5 transfer.[42] As more than 50 percent of the embryos derived from IVF patients with a poor prognosis are genetically abnormal,[49] and 40 percent of blastocysts exhibit some chromosomal mosaicism of the ICM,[50] development up to the blastocyst stage in itself does not indicate a normal chromosomal complement as well. Hence, the GES and the use of embryos, which have conformed to a predefined growth pattern for embryo transfer and cryopreservation, may provide the only non-invasive opportunity to choose genetically normal embryos.

Periovarian blood flow characteristics and their association, if any, to the outcome of IVF cycles is yet controversial.[51,52] If proven to be of any value, it can be incorporated into the assessment system without much difficulty.

Analysis of follicular fluid and culture media for certain specific classes of metabolites, such as glycolytic products and amino acids, which are end products of known cellular processes, may be a useful predictor of embryo implantation potential. At present, only a few metabolites can be evaluated and the full potential of this methodology is yet to be explored.[53] Although far from understanding it completely, such knowledge may lead to the development of non-invasive assays to assess the quality of oocytes and introduce any necessary changes in the culture media.

In women with advanced maternal age, recurrent implantation failure and recurrent miscarriage, preimplantation genetic screening (PGS) and aneuploidy screening has been done to enhance embryo selection. However, its role in an unselected population is still controversial.[54]

CONCLUSION

The changing social and clinical scenario demands replacement of minimal number of embryos without compromising the implantation or pregnancy rates. Hence, choosing the 'best' embryo becomes imperative. Despite their limitations, morphometric parameters remain the most practical way of assessing embryo potency. Rather than a single static observation during the cleavage stage, regular assessment at every stage of preimplantaion development leads to selection of embryos with good implantation potential. To be most effective, the assessment should start as early as oocyte retrieval and follow every stage of development until embryo transfer. It is of utmost importance to avoid any impairment of the embryo environment. Once such criteria are implemented into our routine practice, in an unselected population, day 3 and day 5 transfers are expected to provide similar results. Randomized trials incorporating GES for embryo evaluation should help in this endeavor. The presence of a successful embryo cryopreservation program is an important part of such a system. The impact of ovarian blood flow assessment on the outcome of treatment is still to be understood. In future, it may become possible to use metabolic assays to assess the quality of embryos in routine clinical practice. Additionally, the EmbryoScope may provide a useful insight into the selection of embryos with high implantation potentials. Until such a time, we continue to rely on specific time-dependent morphologic features of the embryos for choosing the right embryo. Preimplantation genetic screening and diagnosis offer the only way to success in a small group of women with specific indications.

REFERENCES

1. Gerris J, De Neubourg D, Mangelschots K, Van Royen E, Van de Meerssche, Valkenburg M. Prevention of twin pregnancy after *in vitro* fertilization or intracytoplasmic sperm injection based on strict embryo criteria: A prospective randomized clinical trial. Hum Reprod 1999;14:2581-7.

2. Pakkila M, Rasanen J, Heinonen S, Tinkanen H, Toumivaara L, Makikallio K, et al. Low-dose aspirin does not improve ovarian responsiveness or pregnancy rate in IVF and ICSI patients: A randomized, placebo-controlled double-blind study. Hum Reprod 2005;20:2211-4.

3. Ubaldi F, Rienzi L, Ferrero S, Anniballo R, Iacobelli M, Cobellis L, Greco E. Low-dose prednisolone administration in routine ICSI patients does not improve pregnancy and implantation rates. Hum Reprod 2002;17:1544-7.

4. Ebner T, Yaman C, Moser M, Sommergruber M, Feichtinger O, Tews G. Prognostic value of first polar body morphology on fertilization rate and embryo quality in intracytoplasmic sperm injection. Hum Reprod 2000;15:427-30.

5. Xia P. Intracytoplasmic sperm injection: Correlation of oocyte grade based on polar body, periviteline space and cytoplasmic inclusions with fertilization rate and embryo quality. Hum Reprod 1997;12:1750-5.

6. Scott L, Smith S. The successful use of pronuclear embryo transfers the day following oocyte retrieval. Hum Reprod 1998;13:1003-13.

7. Scott L, Alvero R, Leondires M, Miller B. The morphology of human pronuclear embryo is positively related to blastocyst development and implantation. Hum Reprod 2000;5:2394-403.

8. Tesarik J, Greco E. The probability of abnormal preimplantation development can be predicted by a single static observation on pronuclear stage morphology. Hum Reprod 1999;14:1318-23.

9. Zollner U, Zollner KP, Hartl G, Dietl J, Steck T. The use of a detailed zygote score after IVF/ICSI to obtain good quality blastocysts: The German experience. Hum Reprod 2002;17:1327-33.

10. Gianaroli L, Magli MC, Ferraretti AP, Fortini D, Grieco N. Pronuclear morphology and chromosomal abnormalities as scoring criteria for embryo selection. Fertil Steril 2003;80:341-9.

11. Veeck LL. The morphological assessment of human oocytes and early concepti. In: Keel BA and Webster BW (Eds), Handbook of the Laboratory diagnosis and Treatment of Infertility. CRC Press, Raton, FL; 1990. p. 353.

12. Van Royen E, Mangelschots K, De Neubourg D, et al. Characterisation of a top quality embryo, a step towards single-embryo transfer. Hum Reprod 1999;14:2345-9.

13. Gardner DK, Schoolcraft WB. *In vitro* culture of human blastocysts. In: Jansen R, Mortimer D, (Eds). Towards reproductive certainty: infertility and genetics beyond. Carnforth, Parthenon Press, 1999. pp. 378-88.

14. Bongso A. Handbook on Blastocyst culture. Sydney Press Induspint (S) Pte Ltd. Singapore 1999.

15. Fisch JD, Rodriguez H, Ross R, Overby G, Sher G. The Graduated Embryo Score (GES) predicts blastocyst formation and pregnancy rate from cleavage-stage embryos. Hum Reprod 2001;16:1970-5.

16. Katz-Jaffe MG, McReynolds S, Gardner DK, Schoolcraft WB. The role of proteomics in defining the human embryonic secretome. Mol Hum Reprod 2009;15:271-5.

17. Nagy ZP, Sakkas D, Behr B. Symposium: Innnovative techniques in human embryo viability assessment. Noninvasive assessment of embryo viability by metabolomic profiling of culture media ('metabolomics'). Reprod Biomed Online 2008;17:502-7.

18. Nel-Tehmaat L, Nagy ZP. A review of the promises and pitfalls of oocyte and embryo metabolomics. Palcenta 2011;32 (Suppl 3): S257-63.

19. Cruz M, Gadea B, Garrido N, Pedersen KS, Martinez M, Perez-Cano I, et al. Embryo quality, blastocyst, and ongoing pregnancy rates in oocyte donation patients whose embryos were monitored by time-lapse imaging. J Assist Reprod Genet 2011;28:569-73.

20. De Sutter P, Van der Elst J, Coetsier T, Dhont M. Single embryo transfer and multiple pregnancy rate reduction in IVF/ICSI: A 5-year appraisal. Reprod Biomed Online 2003;6:464-9.

21. Graham J, Han T, Prter R, Levy M, Stillman R, Tucker MJ. Day 3 morphology is a poor predictor of blastocyst quality in extended culture. Fertil Steril 2000;74:495-7.

22. Ragione T, Verheyen G, Papanikolaou EV, Van Landuyt L, Devroey P, Van Steirteghem. Developmental stage on day-5 and fragmentation rate on day-3 can influence the implantation potential of top-quality blastocysts in IVF cycles with single embryo transfer. Reprod Biol Endocrinol 2007;5:2.

23. Munne S, Cohen J. Chromosome abnormalities in human embryos. Hum Reprod Update 1998;4:842-55.

24. Wells D, Bermudez MG, Steurwald N, Malter HE, Thornhill AR, Cohen J. Association of abnormal morphology and altered gene expression in human preimplantation embryos. Fertil Steril 2005;84:343-55.

25. Van Royen E, Mangelschots K, De Neubourg D, Laureys I, Ryckaert G, Gerris J. Calculating the implantation potential of day 3 embryos in women younger than 38 years of age: A new model. Hum Reprod 2001;16:326-32.

26. Tesarik J, Kopecny V, Plachot M, Mandelbaum J. Ultrastructural and autoradiographic observations on multinucleated blastomeres of human cleaving embryos obtained by *in vitro* fertilisation. Hum Reprod 1987;2:127-36.

27. Shu Y, Gebhardt J, Watt J, Lyon J, Dasig D, Behr B. Fertilization, embryo development, and clinical outcome of immature oocytes from stimulated intracytoplasmic sperm injection cycles. Fertil Steril 2007;87:1022-7.

28. Trounson A, Anderiesz C, Jones G. Maturation of human oocytes *in vitro* and their developmental competence. Reproduction 2001;121:51-75.

29. Plachot M, Selva J, Wolf JP, Bastit P, de Mouzon J. Consequences of oocyte dysmorphy on the fertilization rate and embryo development after intracytoplasmic sperm injection. A prospective multicenter study. Gynecol Obstet Fertil 2002; 30:772-9.

30. Serhal PF, Ranieri DM, Kinis M, Machant S, Davies M, Khadum IM. Oocyte morphology predicts outcome of intracytoplasmic sperm injection. Hum Reprod 1997;12:1267-70.

31. Kahraman S, Yakin K, Donmez E, Samli H, Bahce M, Cengiz C, Sertyel A, et al. Relationship between granular cytoplasm of oocytes and pregnancy outcome following intracytoplasmic sperm injection. Hum Reprod 2000;15:2390-93.

32. Ebner T, Moser M, Sommergruber M, Puchner M, Wiesinger R, Tews G. Developmental competence of oocytes showing increased cytoplasmic viscosity. Hum Reprod 2003;18:1294-8.

33. Ebner T, Moser M, Sommergruber M, Gaiswinkler U, Shebl O, Jesacher K, Tews G. Occurrence and developmental consequences of vacuoles throughout preimplantation development. Fertil Steril 2005;83:1635-40.

34. Verlinsky Y, Lerner S, Illkevitch N, Kuznetsov V, Kuznetsov I, Cieslak J, Kuliev A. Is there any predictive value of first polar body morphology for embryo genotype or developmental potential? Reprod Biomed Online 2003;7:336-41.

35. Rienzi L, Ubaldi F, Martinez F, Iacobelli M, Minasi MG, Ferrero S, et al. Relationship between meiotic spindle location with regard to the polar body position and oocyte developmental potential after ICSI. Hum Reprod 2003;18:1289-93.

36. Menezo YJ. Paternal and maternal factors in preimplantation embryogenesis: Interaction with the biochemical environment. Reprod Biomed Online 2006;12:616-21.

37. Agarwal A, Allamaneni SS. The effect of sperm DNA damage on assisted reproduction outcomes. A review. Minerva Ginecol 2004;56:235-45.

38. Knez K, Zorn B, Tomazevic T, Vrtacnik-Bokal E, Virant-Klun I. The IMSI procedure improves poor embryo development in the same infertile couples with poor semen quality: A comparative prospective randomized study. Reprod Biol Endocrinol 2011; 29:123.

39. Wittemer C, Bettahar-Lebugle K, Ohl J, Rongieres C, Nisand I, Gerlinger P. Zygote evaluation: An efficient tool for embryo selection. Hum Reprod 2000;15:2591-7.

40. Balaban B, Urman B, Isiklar A, Alatas C, Aksoy S, Mercan R, et al. The effect of pronuclear morphology on embryo quality parameters and blastocyst transfer outcome. 2001;6:2357-61.

41. Gianorali L, Magli MC, Ferraretti AP, Lappi, Borghi E, Ermini B. Oocyte euploidy, pronuclear zygote morphology and embryo chromosomal complement. Hum Reprod 2007;22:241-9.

42. Rienzi L, Ubaldi F, Iacobelli A, Ferrero S, Minasi MG, Martinez F, Tesarik J, Greco E. Day 3 embryo transfer with combined evaluation at the pronuclear and cleavage stages compares favourably with day 5 blastocyst transfer. Hum Reprod 2002;17: 1852-5.

43. Lawler C, Baker HW, Edgar DH. Relationships between timing of syngamy, female age and implantation potential in human *in vitro* fertilized oocytes. Reprod Fertil Dev 2007;19:482-7.

44. Terriou P, Giorgetti C, Hans E, Salzmann J, Charles O, Cignetti L, Avon C, Roulier R. Relatioship between even early cleavage and day 2 embryo score and assessment of their predictive value for pregnancy. Reproductive Biomed Online 2007;14:294-9.

45. Giorgetti C, Hans E, Terriou P, Salzmann J, Barry B, Charbert-Orsini V, et al. Early cleavage: an additional predictor of high implantation rate following elective single embryo transfer. Reprod Biomed Online 2007;14:85-91.

46. Lundqvist M, Johansson U, Lundkvist O, Milton K, westin C, Simberg N. Does pronuclear morphology and/or early cleavage rate predict embryo implantation potential? Reprod Biomed Online 2001;2:12-6.

47. Gardner DK, Lane M, Stevens J, Schlenker T, Schoolcraft WB. Blastocyst score affects implantation and pregnancy outcome: towards a single blastocyst transfer. Fertil Steril 2000;73:1155-8.

48. Alper MM, Brinsden P, Fischer R, Wikland M. To blastocyst or not to blastocyst? That is the question. Hum Reprod 2001; 16:617-9.

49. Gianaroli L, Magli MC, Ferraretti AP, Fiorentino A, Garrisi J, Munné S. Preimplantation genetic diagnosis increases the implantation rate in human *in vitro* fertilization by avoiding the transfer of chromosomally abnormal embryos. Fertil Steril 1997;68:1128-31.

50. Magli MC, Jones GM, Gras L, Gianaroli L, Korman I, Trounson AO. Chromosome mosaicism in day 3 aneuploid embryos that develop to morphologically normal blastocysts *in vitro*. Hum Reprod 2000;15:1781-6.

51. Van Blerkom J, Antezac M, Schrader R. The developmental potential of human oocyte is related to the dissolved oxygen content of follicular fluid: Association with vascular endothelial growth factor levels and perifollicular blood flow characteristics. Hum Reprod 12:1047-55.

52. Palomba S, Russo T, Falbo A, Orio F, Manguso F, Nelaj E, et al. Clinical use of perifollicular vascularity assessment in IVF cycles: a pilot study. Hum Reprod 2006;21:1055-61.

53. Singh R, Sinclair KD. Metabolomics: Approaches to assessing oocyte and embryo quality. Theriogenology 2007;68 (Suppl 1): S56-62.

54. Donoso P, Staessen C, Fauser BC, Devroey P. Current value of preimplantation genetic aneuploidy screening in IVF. Hum Reprod Update 2007;13:15-25.

Oocyte Cryopreservation

Andrea Borini, C Lagalla, V Bianchis

OVERVIEW

Oocyte cryopreservation is a relatively old technique, since the first pregnancy was obtained in the late 80s. Nevertheless, due to the few clinical studies and the scarcity of the results, it has not been applied routinely for a long period. One of the main factors driving the research in this field has been the law restrictions in Italy, where just three eggs can be inseminated. Freezing the remaining oocytes has represented the best way to optimize the stimulation cycles.

Once cryopreservation started being used consistently in several clinics, another important issue was raised about which technique to use. Mainly, the two main alternatives are slow freezing and vitrification. Both the procedures have been applied with success in the animal field, but slow freezing was first used to cryopreserve human oocytes. Since then, different protocols have been developed and different results obtained worldwide.

RATIONALE

The rationale of oocyte cryopreservation is mainly to preserve the supernumerary oocytes in *in vitro* fertilization (IVF) cycles to avoid freezing an excess of extra embryos and to optimize ovarian stimulation in countries with restrictive laws. Moreover, oocyte cryopreservation represents an important chance for women at risk for fertility loss due to malignant disease or premature ovarian failure in addition to women who choose to postpone motherhood for personal or professional reasons. The possibility to cryopreserve oocytes as a routine IVF procedure is an important option to maximize oocyte donation, avoiding donor/recipient synchronization and making the quarantine of specimens possible. Last but not least, oocyte cryopreservation allows potential conflicts associated with legal ownership of cryopreserved embryos in the event of divorce to be bypassed.

INTRODUCTION

Nowadays, oocyte cryopreservation is considered as a reliable option to maximize the clinical efficiency of each cycle, while avoiding repeated pharmacological stimulations. For several years, the unique nature of the human oocyte together with the lack of cryobiological data and the empirical approach of early studies resulted in a general lack of interest in the technique. For many years, the most widespread method to cryopreserve oocytes has been the slow cooling propane-1,2-diol (PrOH)-based protocol, originally set-up to freeze cleaving embryos.[1] Nevertheless, ever since the first pregnancy was achieved,[2] oocyte cryopreservation has been considered for a long period as an experimental procedure with episodic clinical studies.

After the introduction of intracytoplasmic sperm injection (ICSI) as an elective technique for the insemination of thawed oocytes, fertilization problems were mostly overcome. In fact, one of the main consequences of freezing is the premature release of cortical granules and the phenomenon known as zona hardening[3] that may limit fertilization with standard IVF.

In 2001, Fabbri et al.[4] proposed a modified slow-cooling protocol to improve survival after thawing but, despite the good biological outcome, its clinical efficiency was unsatisfactory.[5-7]

In 2007, our group[8] modified the freezing and thawing solutions with a differential sucrose concentration in an attempt to minimize the stress during the cooling phase. This mixture has been used in the past for human biopsied cleavage-stage embryos[9] with appreciable results. The survival, fertilization and cleavage rates were still comparable to those obtained by Fabbri et al.[4] but pregnancy and implantation rates were significantly improved.

Besides the slow freezing technique, the vitrification technique has been reintroduced lately in several clinics. Although it has been applied for the long-term preservation of human MII oocytes since 1989,[10] with the first delivery being achieved in 1999,[11] clinical results need more confirmation. At the beginning, several studies on oocyte vitrification[12-16] with few oocytes showed that this method may represent a valid alternative to slow freezing but, even though it has been said that vitrification will be the future of oocyte cryopreservation,[17] many questions are still open and further studies are necessary.

CLINICAL DISCUSSION

Freezing Procedures

An aim of slow freezing protocols is to reduce the damage caused by intracellular ice formation; this is achieved by dehydrating the cells prior to freezing (Figs 51.1A and B).

As human oocytes contain a large amount of water in their cytoplasm, the formation of intracellular ice may interfere with the cell viability. It is important to point out that the ultrastructure of the human oocyte is very complex and delicate. The meiotic spindle and the cortical granules as the calcium signalling can be compromised during the freeze-thaw procedures.

To partially overcome these aspects, cryoprotectants are normally used in the cryopreservation mixtures despite their potential toxic effect on the cells. In fact, they protect the cells from ice crystal damage and reduce the concentration of the solute. There are two categories of cryoprotectants, depending on their ability to penetrate the cells: Intracellular (penetrating) and extracellular (nonpenetrating) agents.

Slow Cooling

This is the most widely used protocol and the one that for many years has yielded the best clinical results. Relatively low concentrations (typically 1.5 M) of penetrating cryoprotectants, such as Pr-OH or dimethyl sulfoxide (DMSO), and very slow cooling rates are applied in the attempt to ensure a finely tuned control over the various factors that may contribute to cell damage. Sucrose is used in the vast majority of protocols, although more recently, choline has been taken into consideration as a substitute for Na^+ in the freezing solutions.[18]

Rapid Thawing

It is a rapid thawing procedure that removes the cryoprotectant by stepwise dilutions (usually 1.5 M; 1.0 M; 0.2 M Pr-OH) to reduce the osmotic shock that might cause swelling or bursting of the oocyte. High sucrose concentrations in the thawing solutions compensate for the high intracellular concentration of cryoprotectants and control the water inflow inside the cell.

Vitrification

Vitrification causes a glass-like solidification of living cells while preventing ice crystallization during cooling and warming. However, a negative consequence of this strategy is the increased probability of nearly all forms of injury except those caused by ice crystal formation. To achieve vitrification, a radical increase in both, the cooling rate and cryoprotectant concentrations is required. The solutions to vitrify contain an increased amount of cryoprotectants, up to 7 M, much higher than in the slow-cooling procedure. During vitrification, the samples are plunged directly into liquid nitrogen. Under these conditions, cells are rapidly dehydrated and the high viscosity of the freezing solution causes their glass-like solidification (hence the term vitrification) without ice crystal formation. However, although cryoprotective agents are fundamental for cell cryopreservation, their toxicity is a key-limiting factor. The higher the cooling rate, the lower is the required cryoprotectant concentration, and vice versa.

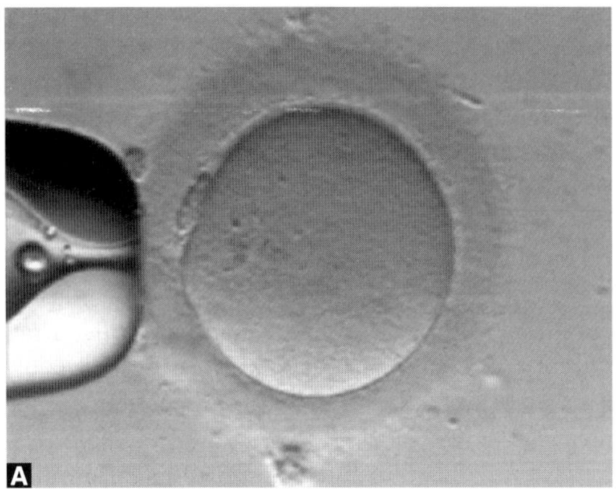

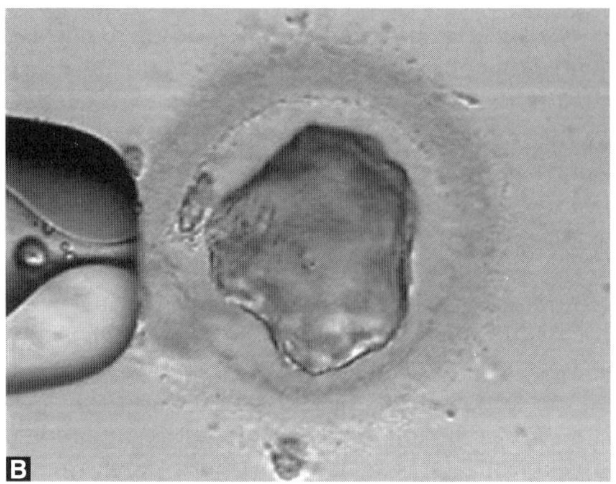

Figs 51.1A and B: Osmotic response generated by exposure to 1.5 M ethylene glycol at 25°C

The most commonly accepted cryoprotectant for vitrification is ethylene glycol (EG). Another successful approach is the combination of two or, more frequently, three cryoprotectants to decrease the specific toxicity of each one. Among the non-permeable cryoprotectants, sucrose has recently become a standard component of vitrification mixtures.

Warming: Vitrified oocytes are warmed with a multi-step dilution, using decreasing concentrations of osmotic buffers (usually sucrose). This has to counteract the swelling caused by the permeable cryoprotectants that leave the cells.[17]

Possible Damage to the Oocyte due to Cryopreservation

Influence of Cryoprotectants on Oocyte Function

The main function of cryoprotectants is to preserve cells from damage due to ice crystal formation but, at the same time, they may induce negative effects such as osmotic stress. A side effect that seems to be caused by cryoprotectants is the premature cortical granules (CG) release. Fluorescence and electronic microscopy studies[19] found that mere exposure to Pr-OH leads to a significant reduction in CG staining in human oocytes. Ultrastructural analyses confirmed that freezing and thawing procedures induce extensive loss of CG from the cortex of mature oocytes. In particular, our group published that subcortical CG decrease in oocytes frozen with Pr-OH (Fig. 51.2A) correlated with the applied protocol:

A low concentration of sucrose (0.1M) was associated with a slightly more significant loss of CG than a higher sucrose concentration (0.3 M) (Figs 51.2A to C).[20] Experimental data in mice showed that zona hardening may occur after thawing as a consequence of CG release. However, an immunostaining study on frozen-thawed oocytes, conducted by Li et al.[21] on a small number of oocytes, did not show any difference in CG loss after thawing.

An alternative and interesting hypothesis concerning CG release is related to $[Ca^{2+}]_I$ regulation that may be disrupted by cryopreservation. This not only would affect the conversion of oocytes into zygotes but also the expression of the normal pattern of fetal development. Jones et al.[22] and Larman et al.[23] found evidence that the oocyte Ca^{2+} release mechanism may be affected by cryopreservation.

On the other hand, in 1993, Carroll et al.[24] cryopreserved mouse oocytes that were then successfully fertilized by standard IVF. The important implication is that ICSI may be avoided if the appropriate cooling conditions are applied. The same matter is described in another publication from our group.[25]

Cytoskeletal Damage after Cryopreservation

Another main aspect to analyze is the possible damage caused by freezing on the meiotic spindle. The debate concerning this relation has been going on for a number of years, with several authors having different opinions and results.

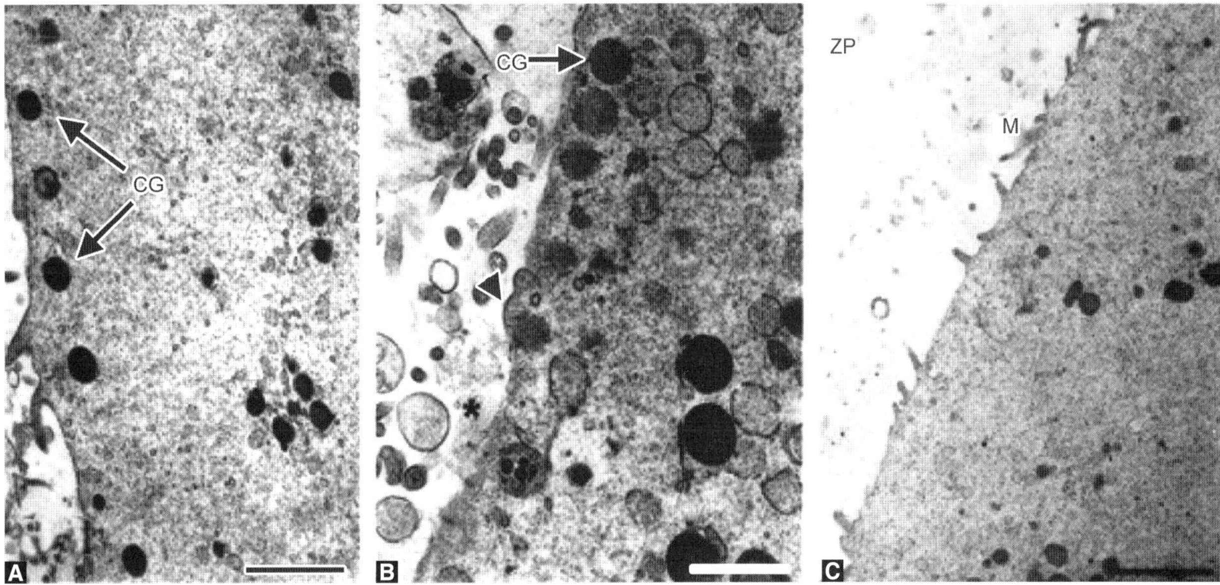

Figs 51.2A to C: Human mature oocytes. Presence, amount and density of cortical granules are shown. A single, regular row of electron dense cortical granules (CG plus arrows) is seen just beneath the oolemma in (A) (control group). Cortical granules (CG plus arrow) appear instead reduced in density in (B) (sucrose 0.1 mol/L group) and frankly absent in (C) (sucrose 0.3 mol/L group). (*Nottola et al. Ultrastructure of human mature oocytes after slow cooling cryopreservation using different sucrose concentrations. Hum Reprod 2007;22:1123-33*).

A confocal microscopy study, conducted by our group,[26] showed a correlation between the freezing procedure and the loss of normal spindle organization. This confirmed our previous analyses using electron microscopy[27] on oocytes frozen with high sucrose concentrations, where we observed that the structure of the MII spindle does not change when the cryopreservation conditions are appropriate. Consequently, this finding can be correlated with our clinical experience, where the abortion rate in fresh and frozen-thawed cycles is the same.[5,8]

Another important feature of the oocyte cytoskeletal apparatus is the cortical meshwork of actin filaments, whose integrity is fundamental for cytokinesis, including PBII extrusion and first cleavage after fertilization. The predictable consequence due to damage in this region would be the retention of PBII and the inhibition of cleavage after fertilization. By using fluorescence microscopy and phalloidin staining in an unpublished study, still in progress, Albertini found no changes in the subcortical actin meshwork of oocytes cryopreserved with high sucrose concentrations. Our observations, conducted on the pronuclear stage in two separate series of treatment using frozen oocytes, confirmed these findings, where a low incidence of one or three-pronuclear fertilization and a high cleavage rate were observed.[5,8]

Solution Effect during Slow Cooling

During slow cooling, dehydration is caused at first by cryoprotectants, which create an osmotic gradient, and then, by the progressive solidification of water into ice. This determines the concentration of the solutes, mainly sodium, in the unfrozen fraction of the system and possible biochemical toxicity in the intracellular membranes and plasmalemma. Hence, the adoption of sodium-depleted freezing media, where sodium is replaced by equimolar amounts of the cation choline.[27] However, studies on human oocytes[28,29] suggest that the usefulness of these new media is uncertain: in the study of Stachecki et al.[29] only 20 to 30 oocytes were analyzed and no control group (frozen with sodium-rich media) was included; moreover, although high survival rates were reported (90%), the cleavage rate was low (78%).

Results with Slow Cooling

From 1986, when the first pregnancy with frozen-thawed oocytes was reported,[2] only few other live births were obtained for several years. After the introduction of ICSI on thawed oocytes,[3] a number of reports were published. The first protocol employed was the same used for embryos, i.e. 1.5M Pr OH and 0.1M sucrose, but the oocyte survival rate and clinical outcome did not yield appreciable results.[7,30,31]

After a long period, during which oocyte cryopreservation was virtually dismissed by the scientific community, Porcu et al.[32] published a paper on oocyte freezing using a slow cooling method with 1.5M PrOH plus 0.2M sucrose. A high survival rate was obtained (54.1%) but the fertilization rate was still low (57.7%). Even though 16 pregnancies were obtained, the implantation rate was only 1.2 percent when calculated on the number of thawed oocytes. This value is four times smaller compared to the implantation rate with embryo cryopreservation.[33]

In 2001, Fabbri et al.[4] published a modified slow cooling protocol using a higher sucrose concentration (0.3M) on the assumption that it might increase oocyte dehydration.[4] The oocyte survival rate improved dramatically (>80%), but unfortunately, no clinical results were described. Using the same protocol, Porcu et al.[32] obtained a 90 percent survival rate and a 50 percent pregnancy rate; the study, however, involved only 88 oocytes harvested from seven donor women. The group directed by Chen et al.[6] reported a higher implantation rate per oocyte (5%) from 21 freeze-thaw cycles. The rate obtained was comparable to embryo freezing. Later on, using the same protocol in a much larger number of oocytes, our group obtained very different results that confirmed high survival, fertilization and cleavage rates, but also low pregnancy and higher miscarriage rates.[5] Only a small fraction of embryos that progressed beyond the first cleavage stage was observed. These data have been confirmed by De Santis et al.[7] and La Sala et al.[34] in large groups of patients recruited in their studies. In another study,[35] a reduced early cleavage rate at 25h was noticed in frozen-thawed oocytes using the 0.3M sucrose protocol compared with embryos from fresh sibling oocytes (7.1% vs 59.5%).

A study published by Bianchi et al.[8] on 1083 frozen and 403 thawed oocytes was conducted using a modified sucrose protocol, which involved a lower sucrose concentration in the freezing solution (0.2M) and a higher amount of sucrose in the thawing mixture. This lower concentration allows the oocyte to dehydrate more gradually and thus, less traumatically.[36] Also, as previously suggested by the original work of Lassalle et al.[1] the thawing solution should maintain a higher sucrose concentration to allow a progressive and controlled rehydration. Results were encouraging, with a survival rate of 75.9 percent, pregnancy rate per transfer and per patient of 21.3 percent and 21.8 percent, respectively and implantation and miscarriage rates of 13.5 percent and of 11.8 percent, respectively.

A different approach has been applied used for mouse oocytes by Stachechi et al.[27] who replaced sodium with the less toxic organic ion choline in the freezing solutions, a measure believed to reduce the solution effect. This protocol was adopted by Quintans et al.[37] and by Boldt et al.[18] with very good clinical results: The former reported pregnancy and implantation rates of 50 percent and 25 percent respectively, but the miscarriage rate was 50 percent; the latter achieved a pregnancy rate of 36.4 percent. The two studies, however, involved only a small group of patients (12 and 15, respectively).

More recently, a multicenter study in Italy was reported by Borini et al.[38] after the application of the Italian law permitting the insemination of only three oocytes. The protocol consisted of a 2- step PROH — sucrose-based solution with the same sucrose concentration previously described by Bianchi et al.[8] Despite the good results, the implantation per oocyte was lower (10.1%) than before.

Results with Vitrification

Since its first application to embryo cryostorage by Rall and Fahy in 1985,[39] vitrification has suffered from two drawbacks related to the difficulties of the technique and the possible cross-contamination risk due to the direct contact with liquid nitrogen. This has raised strong arguments against the method and limited its application for sometime.[17]

The early clinical results of oocyte vitrification were rather discouraging. In 1999, Kuleshova et al.[11] reported the birth of a healthy baby born using a relatively low number of oocytes and an open pulled straw device. No other reports have since been published under identical parameters. Later on, other vitrification approaches failed to produce considerable improvements in the outcome.[17] Only in 2003 did Yoon et al.[40] report a survival rate of 68.6 percent following thawing of 474 vitrified oocytes. However, only 41 percent of them were suitable for microinjection, and although pregnancy and implantation rates were 21.4 percent and 6.4 percent, respectively, the implantation rate per thawed oocyte was only 1.6 percent.

The major breakthrough was obtained by Kuwayama et al.[41] in 2005 with the introduction of a new open device called the Cryotop. The author in fact reported a high blastocyst formation rate (50%) after ICSI on vitrified-thawed oocytes and achieved 12 pregnancies from 29 embryo transfers, resulting in the birth of 10 healthy babies.[41]

Using the same approach, Lucena et al.[42] vitrified 707 mature oocytes obtained from 33 donor women and 40 patients undergoing infertility treatment. Oocyte thawing resulted in high fertilization, cleavage, and pregnancy rates. The best results, however, have been obtained in donor replacement cycles. In a clinical study, Antinori et al.[12] vitrified 463 supernumerary oocytes using the Cryotop device; 328 out of 330 (99.4%) of them survived the warming procedure. Fertilization, pregnancy and implantation rates per embryo were 92.9 percent, 32.5 percent and 13.2 percent respectively. The birth of healthy babies was reported.[42]

Other developed devices also seem to be successful in oocyte vitrification. Using the Cryoloop open system, a total of 235 oocytes were vitrified and thawed in a study conducted by Chen et al.[13] The survival and fertilization rates were 71.9 percent and 72.5 percent, respectively. Forty-one embryos were transferred to 11 patients and 2 had a positive pregnancy outcome. One patient delivered two healthy females while the other patient still had an ongoing pregnancy at 16 weeks of gestation at the time of publication.

A prospective clinical research was conducted by Yoon et al.[43] utilizing slush nitrogen [SN (2)]. Twenty-eight infertile women underwent 30 cycles of IVF-ET using previously vitrified oocytes. Three hundred-sixty-four surplus oocytes from 28 patients were vitrified. Three hundred and two (85.1% ± 2.9%) of the oocytes survived warming. Fertilization and cleavage rates were 77.4 percent ± 3.5 percent (168/218) and 94.3 percent ± 2.1 percent (158/168), respectively. Thirteen pregnancies (43.3%) resulted from 30 uterine transfers of 120 embryos, with an implantation rate of 14.2 percent (17/120).[43]

More recently, Cobo et al.[44] compared the outcomes using fresh and cryopreserved donor oocytes vitrified with an open device (Cryotop). The vitrified group included 231 MII oocytes while the fresh group had 219 oocytes. The survival rate after thawing was very high at 96.9 percent. The fertilization rates (82.2% vs 76.3%, respectively) and cleavage rates on day 3 (84.6% vs 77.6%, respectively) were higher in the fresh group compared to the vitrified group, but the differences were not significant. The blastocyst formation rate was 47.5 percent in the fresh group and 48.7 percent in the frozen/thawed specimens. The pregnancy and implantation rates for the frozen/thawed group were very high when compared to other clinics (65.2% and 40.8%, respectively).[44]

Ubaldi et al.[45] reported the cumulative pregnancy rate obtained using the Cryotop vitrification device. The author considered 182 ICSI cycles with an overall pregnancy rate of 53.3 percent. This result is comparable to the data published by our group in 2006.[46]

One of the main issues still under debate concerns the likelihood of disease transmission using an open device to vitrify samples. This can happen because there is a direct contact between the samples and the liquid nitrogen. The closed system (Cryotip) instead, is sealed at both ends and can overcome this problem.

RECENT ADVANCES

In 2006, Oktay et al.[47] published a meta analysis in which he showed that a higher mean number of embryos were transferred following vitrification rather than slow freezing.[47] More recently, Smith et al.[48] compared slow cooling and vitrification and it has been evidenced that the survival rate (81% vs 67%, respectively) and the clinical pregnancy rates (38% vs 13%, respectively) were significantly higher following vitrification compared with slow cooling. Even though, up to now, vitrification seems to work better, the protocol used for slow freezing was not the most successful.

Another report published by Grifo et al.[49] showed that survival rates were not different between the two techniques (88% for slow cooling and 95% for vitrification) as were the fertilization and blastocyst formation rates.

Noyes et al.[50] published a paper analyzing a total of 58 publications (43 using slow freezing, 12 vitrification and three using both the methods) from 1986 to 2008. Three hundred eight babies were born from slow freezing and 289 from vitrification while 12 came from either protocol. The rate of single pregnancies was 81 percent compared to 19 percent for multiples. It is very important to point out that the overall rate of birth anomalies was not different from standard IVF. Eight anomalies were reported: Three ventricular septal cardiac defects, one choanal atresia, one biliary atresia, one Rubinstein-Taybi syndrome, one clubfoot and one skin hemangioma. Three of these anomalies resulted from slow freezing while five from vitrification, showing no difference between the techniques.

Chian et al.[51] reported the obstetric and perinatal outcomes in 165 pregnancies and 200 infants conceived following oocyte vitrification. The author showed that the mean birth weight and the incidence of congenital anomalies were the same as in IVF or in natural conception.

CONCLUSION

Oocyte cryopreservation is a relatively complex technique to apply due to the unique nature of the human oocyte. Even though this option in IVF has been considered experimental for several years,[25] it is now becoming a reliable tool in the IVF routine.

New approaches to the study of oocyte cryobiology have clarified many of the critical points that play a role in oocyte cooling efficiency: (i) critical changes in the plasmalemma regulate the passage of water and small molecules, including cryoprotectants, between intra- and extracellular compartments, thus influencing oocyte survival; (ii) Pr-OH causes activation in the mouse, but not in human oocytes; (iii) cortical granules are not always released, suggesting that insemination via microinjection may be avoided; (iv) under appropriate storage conditions, the risk of chromosome and meiotic spindle disorganization is limited; (v) increased solute concentrations during freezing have been thought to cause cryodamage, even though the experience in humans so far has failed to show that the solution effect is the main factor responsible for oocyte survival and viability.

Recently, on the other hand, vitrification has raised considerable enthusiasm. For a long period, it was not considered as an alternative to slow freezing because of the few pregnancies and live births obtained. In the last few years, several studies have reported appreciable numbers of frozen oocytes and good clinical results. These works almost unanimously support the application of vitrification and emphasize its advantages: It causes less harm to the oocyte and is a simple and rapid procedure, leading to higher survival and development rates than alternative methods.[17]

Nevertheless, comparative studies conducted so far, have not shown a big difference between slow freezing and vitrification even though further randomized studies with the best protocols available are needed to draw a line.

REFERENCES

1. Lassalle B, Testart J, Renard JP. Human embryo features that influence the success of cryopreservation with the use of 1,2 propanediol. Fertil Steril 1985;44:645-51.
2. Chen C. Pregnancy after human oocyte cryopreservation. Lancet 1986;1:884-6.
3. Gook DA, Schiewe MC, Osborn SM, Asch RH, Jansen RP, Johnston WI. Intracytoplasmic sperm injection and embryo development of human oocytes cryopreserved using 1,2-propanediol. Hum Reprod 1995;10:2637-41.
4. Fabbri R, Porcu E, Marsella T, Rocchetta G, Venturoli S, Flamigni C. Human oocyte cryopreservation: new perspectives regarding oocyte survival. Hum Reprod 2001;16:411-6.
5. Borini A, Sciajno R, Bianchi V, Sereni E, Flamigni C, Coticchio G. Clinical outcome of oocyte cryopreservation after slow cooling with a protocol utilizing a high sucrose concentration. Hum Reprod 2006;21:512-7.
6. Chen SU, Lien YR, Chen HF, Chang LJ, Tsai YY, Yang YS. Observational clinical follow-up of oocyte cryopreservation using a slow-freezing method with 1,2-propanediol plus sucrose followed by ICSI. Hum Reprod 2005;20:1975-80.
7. De Santis L, Cino I, Rabellotti E, Papaleo E, Calzi F, Fusi FM, et al. Oocyte cryopreservation: Clinical outcome of slow-cooling protocols differing in sucrose concentration. Reprod Biomed Online 2007;14:57-63.
8. Bianchi V, Coticchio G, Distratis V, Di Giusto N, Flamigni C, Borini A. Differential sucrose concentration during dehydration (0.2 mol/l) and rehydration (0.3 mol/l) increases the implantation rate of frozen human oocytes. Reprod Biomed Online 2007;14:64-71.
9. Jericho H, Wilton L, Gook DA, Edgar DH. A modified cryopreservation method increases the survival of human biopsied cleavage stage embryos. Hum Reprod 2003;18:568-71.
10. Pensis M, Loumaye E, Psalti I. Screening of conditions for rapid freezing of human oocytes: Preliminary study toward their cryopreservation. Fertil Steril 1989;52:787-94.
11. Kuleshova L, Gianaroli L, Magli C, Ferraretti A, Trounson A. Birth following vitrification of a small number of human oocytes: case report. Hum Reprod 1999;14:3077-9.
12. Antinori M, Licata E, Dani G, Cerusico F, Versaci C, Antinori S. Cryotop vitrification of human oocytes results in high survival rate and healthy deliveries. Reprod Biomed Online 2007;14: 72-9.
13. Chen ZJ, Li Y, Hu JM, Li M. Successful clinical pregnancy of cryopreserved human oocytes after vitrification. Zhonghua Yi Xue Za Zhi 2006;86:2037-40.
14. Kuleshova LL, Lopata A. Vitrification can be more favourable than slow cooling. Fertil Steril 2002;78:449-54.
15. Kuwayama M, Vajta G, Kato O, Leibo SP. Highly efficient vitrification method for cryopreservation of human oocytes. Reprod Biomed Online 2005;11:300-8.
16. Selman H, Angelini A, Barnocchi N, Brusco GF, Pacchiarotti A, Aragona C. Ongoing pregnancies after vitrification of human

oocytes using a combined solution of ethylene glycol and dimethyl sulfoxide. Fertil Steril 2006;86:997-1000.

17. Vajta G, Nagy ZP. Are programmable freezers still needed in the embryo laboratory? Review on vitrification. Reprod Biomed Online 2006;12:779-96.

18. Boldt J, Cline D, McLaughlin D. Human oocyte cryopreservation as an adjunct to IVF-embryo transfer cycles. Hum Reprod 2003;18:1250-5.

19. Ghetler Y, Skutelsky E, Ben Nun I, Ben Dor L, Amihai D, Shalgi R. Human oocyte cryopreservation and the fate of cortical granules. Fertil Steril 2006;86:210-6.

20. Nottola SA, Macchiarelli G, Coticchio G, Bianchi S, Cecconi S, De Santis L, et al. Ultrastructure of human mature oocytes after slow cooling cryopreservation using different sucrose concentrations. Hum Reprod 2007;22:1123-33.

21. Li XH, Chen SU, Zhang X, Tang M., Kui YR, Wu X et al. Cryopreserved oocytes of infertile couples undergoing assisted reproductive technology could be an important source of oocyte donation: a clinical report of successful pregnancies. Hum Reprod 2005;20:3390-94.

22. Jones A, Van Blerkom J, Davis P, Toledo AA. Cryopreservation of metaphase II human oocytes effects mitochondrial membrane potential: implications for developmental competence. Hum Reprod 2004;19:1861-6.

23. Larman MG, Sheehan CB, Gardner DK. Calcium-free vitrification reduces cryoprotectant-induced zona pellucida hardening and increases fertilization rates in mouse oocytes. Reproduction 2006;131:53-61.

24. Carroll J, Wood MJ, Whittingham DG. Normal fertilization and development of frozen-thawed mouse oocytes: Protective action of certain macromolecules. Biol Reprod 1993;48:606-12.

25. Coticchio G, Bonu MA, Sciano R, Sereni E, Bianchi V, Borini A. Truths and myths of oocyte sensitivity to cryopreservation. Reprod Biomed Online 2007;15:24-30.

26. Bromfield JJ, Coticchio G, Hutt K, Sciajno R, Borini A, Albertini DF. Meiotic spindle dynamics in human oocytes following slow-cooling cryopreservation. Hum Reprod 2009;24:2114-23.

27. Stachecki JJ, Cohen J, Willadsen S. Detrimental effects of sodium during mouse oocyte cryopreservation. Biol Reprod 1998;59:395-400.

28. Boldt J, Tidswell N, Sayers A, Kilani R, Cline D. Human oocyte cryopreservation: 5-year experience with a sodium-depleted slow freezing method. Reprod Biomed Online 2006;13:96-100.

29. Stachecki JJ, Cohen J, Garrisi J, Munne S, Burgess C, Willadsen SM. Cryopreservation of unfertilized human oocytes. Reprod Biomed Online 2006;13:222-7.

30. Porcu E, Fabbri R, Seracchioli R, Ciotti PM, Magrini O, Flamigni C. Birth of a healthy female after intracytoplasmic sperm injection of cryopreserved human oocytes. Fertil Steril 1997;68:724-6.

31. Borini A, Bonu MA, Coticchio G, Bianchi V, Cattoli M, Flamigni C. Pregnancies and births after oocyte cryopreservation. Fertil Steril 2004;82:601-5.

32. Porcu E, Fabbri R, Damiano G, Giunchi S, Fratto R, Ciotti PM, et al. Clinical experience and applications of oocyte cryopreservation. Mol Cell Endocrinol 2000;169:33 7.

33. Gook DA, Edgar DH. Cryopreservation of the human female gamete: Current and future issues. Hum Reprod 1999;14:2938-40.

34. La Sala GB, Nicoli A, Villani MT, Pescarini M, Gallinelli A, Blickstein I. Outcome of 518 salvage oocyte-cryopreservation cycles performed as a routine procedure in an *in vitro* fertilization program. Fertil Steril 2006;86:1423-7.

35. Bianchi V, Coticchio G, Distratis V, Di Giusto N, Borini A. Early cleavage delay in cryopreserved human oocytes. Hum Reprod 2005a;(Suppl 1):i54.

36. Paynter SJ. A rational approach to oocyte cryopreservation. Reprod Biomed Online 2005;10:578-86.

37. Quintans CJ, Donaldson MJ, Bertolino MV, Pasqualini RS. Birth of two babies using oocytes that were cryopreserved in a choline-based freezing medium. Hum Reprod 2002;17:3149-52.

38. Borini A, Levi Setti PE, Anserini P, De Luca R, De Sants L, Porcu E, et al. Multicenter observational study on slow-cooling oocyte cryopreservation: Clinical outcome. Fertil Steril 2010; 94:1662-8.

39. Rall WF, Fahy GM. Ice-free cryopreservation of mouse embryos at -196 degrees C by vitrification. Nature. 1985;313:573-5.

40. Yoon TK, Kim TJ, Park SE, Hong SW, Ko JJ, Chung HM, Cha KY. Live births after vitrification of oocytes in a stimulated *in vitro* fertilization-embryo transfer program. Fertil Steril. 2003;79:1323-6.

41. Kuwayama M, Vajta G, Kato O, Leibo SP. Highly efficient vitrification method for cryopreservation of human oocytes. Reprod Bio Med Online 2005;11:300-8.

42. Lucena E, Bernal DP, Lucena C, Rojas A, Moran A, Lucena A. Successful ongoing pregnancies after vitrification of oocytes. Fertil Steril 2006;85:108-11.

43. Yoon TK, Lee DR, Cha SK, Chung HM, Lee WS, Cha KY. Survival rate of human oocytes and pregnancy outcome after vitrification using slush nitrogen in assisted reproductive technologies. Fertil Steril 2007;952-6.

44. Cobo A, Kuwayama M, Perez S, Ruiz A, Pellicier A, Remohi J. Comparison of concomitant outcome achieved with fresh and cryopreserved donor oocytes vitrified by the Cryotop method. Fertil Steril 2008;89:1657-64.

45. Ubaldi F, Anniballo R, Romano S, Baroni E, Albricci L, Colamaria S, et al. Cumulative ongoing pregnancy rate achieved with oocyte vitrification and cleavage stage transfer without embryo selection in a standard infertility program. Hum Reprod 2010;25:1199-205.

46. Borini A, Lagalla C, Bonu MA, Bianchi V, Flamigni C, Coticchio G. Cumulative pregnancy rates resulting from the use of fresh and frozen oocytes: 7 years' experience. Reprod Biomed online 2006;12:481-6.

47. Oktay K, Cil AP, Bang H. Efficiency of oocyte cryopreservation: A meta-analysis. Fertil Steril 2006;86:70-80.

48. Smith GD, Serafini PC, Fioravanti J, Yadid I, Coslovsky M, Hassun P, et al. Prospective randomized comparison of human oocyte cryopreservation with slow-rate freezing or vitrification Fertil Steril 2010;94:2088-95.

49. Grifo J, Noyes N. Delivery rate using cryopreserved oocytes is comparable to conventional *in vitro* fertilization using fresh oocytes: Potential fertility preservation for female cancer patients. Fert and Steril 2010;93:391-6.

50. Noyes N, Porcu E, Borini A. Over 900 oocyte cryopreservation babies born with no apparent increase in congenital anomalies. Reprod Biomed Online 2009;18:769-76.

51. Chian RC, Huang JY, Tan SL, Lucena E, Saa A, Rojas A, et al. Obstetric and perinatal outcome in 200 infants conceived from vitrified oocytes. Reprod BioMed Online 2008;16:608-10.

Comparison of Two Freezing Techniques for Human Embryos: Slow Freezing and Vitrification

Ramadevi Papolu, Charulata Chatterjee, A Rajyalakshmi, J Vijayalakshmi

OVERVIEW

The need for human cryopreservation arose as a direct consequence of improvements in *in vitro* fertilization (IVF) techniques that have led to a greater number of viable embryos being available for transfer. Traditional slow cooling methods of cryopreservation have certain disadvantages. They are time-consuming, require expensive freezing equipment and result in ice crystal formation. These disadvantages can be avoided by the use of the vitrification technique.

In a retrospective comparative study on 54 patients undergoing assisted reproductive techniques (ART) at our Institute, we aimed to assess the outcome of thawing cryopreserved human blastocysts by either vitrification or the conventional slow cooling technique. We observed that vitrification is a reliable method with high efficacy, convenience, and high rates of blastocyst survival (80.4%) and pregnancy (42.55%), making it a superior alternative to the conventional slow cooling method (65% survival rate; 16.6% pregnancy rate). We also aimed to examine the effect of artificial shrinkage (induced collapse of the blastocyst) before vitirification on blastocyst survival and the subsequent pregnancy rate. We observed that artificial shrinkage before vitrification is a useful technique for attaining better survival (82.7%) and pregnancy rates (50%).

INTRODUCTION

The need for human embryo cryopreservation arose as a direct consequence of the rapid development and success of human IVF. An increase in the number of oocytes recovered after improved methods of superovulation and higher fertilization and cleavage rates have resulted in a greater number of viable embryos available for transfer. Since replacement of more than 3 embryos increases the risks associated with multiple gestation, human embryo cryopreservation has become an ethical necessity in order to provide an acceptable method for the preservation of extra embryos.[1-4]

The traditional slow-cooling methods of cryopreservation are referred to as equilibrium cooling and vitrification as non-equilibrium cooling.[5] The time taken in the slow-cooling method ranges from 90 min to 5 hours. Freezing includes the precipitation of water as ice, with the resulting separation of the water from the dissolved substances. Both, intracellular ice crystal formation and the high concentration of dissolved substances pose problems. Therefore, a slow rate of cooling attempts to maintain a very delicate balance between those factors that may result in damage, mostly by ice crystallization but also by osmotic and chilling injury, zona and blastomere fracture, and alteration of the cytoskeleton.

Disadvantages of slow-cooling like time, expensive freezing equipment and ice crystallization can be avoided through the use of vitrification protocols.

Vitrification is the solidification of a solution (water is rapidly cooled and formed into a glassy, vitrified state from the liquid phase) at low temperature, not by ice crystallization but by an extreme elevation in viscosity during cooling.[6] Vitrification of water inside the cells is achieved either by increasing the speed of temperature conduction or by increasing the concentration of cryoprotectant.

The chief difference between vitrification and traditional cryopreservation methods is that it is an 'open system', defined by (i) direct contact between the solution containing the embryos and liquid nitrogen (liqN$_2$) and (ii) storage of embryos in only partially sealed containers. To promote extremely rapid cooling, this system lacks any significant thermoinsulating layer around the specimen. In the scientific literature, the terms 'cryopreservation' and 'thawing' are commonly used for conventional cryopreservation and the terms 'vitrification' and 'warming' for vitrification. Accordingly, this terminological separation will be utilized hereafter.

From the outcome of both techniques, certain benefits of the vitrification protocol are that, it is a simple, faster and inexpensive procedure. Further, the need for controlled rate freezing equipment, which requires routine calibration and maintenance is eliminated. The cells are placed into very small volumes of cryoprotectant. Furthermore, to reduce the volume of cryoprotectant, special carriers are used. These include open pulled straws,[7] flexipet denuding pipettes,[8] microdrops,[9] electron microscopic copper grids,[10] hemi straw system,[8,11] nylon mesh,[12] and the cryo loop.[13]

Reasons for our personal preference for blastocyst freezing include:

- Blastocyst transfer in routine IVF programs reduce the number of embryos for uterine transfer, thereby reducing multiple pregnancy.
- Better post-thaw survival and implantation rate as compared to early stage embryos.[14]
- Consistent blastocyst cryopreservation is a necessary adjunct to maximize cumulative pregnancy rates from each oocyte retrieval.[15]

The vitrification method is dependent on blastocyst development and has been negatively correlated with the size of the blastocele. Large blastoceles might decrease the cryoprotective potential due to ice crystal formation during the cooling steps. Artificial shrinkage of the blastocelic cavity is an effective approach to reduce the volume and also to obtain a statistical increase in the survival of expanded and larger blastocysts.

Cryopreservation induces hardening of the zona pellucida (ZP), which may impair spontaneous hatching after warming. Hatching before embryo transfer improves pregnancy rates. Hatching should be performed within 10 minutes after warming because the blastocele has not fully expanded yet and perivitelline space is present.

CLINICAL DISCUSSION

In our first study (Study I), we attempted to compare cryopreservation of human blastocysts using either a traditional slow freezing procedure or a vitrification procedure. We therefore analyzed retrospectively, the reproductive outcome of both the techniques and the relative pregnancy rates following transfer of cryopreserved-thawed blastocysts.

The pilot study II was carried out to confirm the effectiveness of the Cryoloop technique with artificial shrinkage of the blastocelic cavity and assisted hatching of blastocysts.

Materials and Methods

Patients and IVF

- The standard long protocol, using gonadotropin-releasing hormone (GnRH) analogs and gonadotropins for controlled ovarian hyperstimulation (COH) was used for all the women. They were administered human chorionic gonadotropin (hCG) when the dominant follicles reached a diameter of ~17 mm. Oocytes were collected 36 hrs after hCG administration using a vaginal ultrasound-guided procedure. The oocytes were inseminated using either conventional IVF or intracytoplasmic sperm injection (ICSI) and incubated in universal IVF media (Medicult) in a CO_2 incubator at 37°C in an atmosphere of 5 percent CO_2.
- Fertilization was assessed at 15 to 18 hours after insemination by the presence of two pronuclei. Embryos were cultured in Blast Assist Medium 1 (Medicult) and then placed into Blast Assist Medium 2 (Medicult) for 48 to 72 hours. In some cases, 4 to 8 cell stage embryos were transferred into the patient after 48 to 56 hours of culture in the first medium; only supernumerary embryos were cultured in the second medium.

Blastocyst Grading

- All the patients agreed to use their supernumerary embryos for freezing. The mean age of the women was 34.2 ± 5 years.
- Supernumerary blastocysts were scored depending on the developmental stage and were graded according to the system of Gardner and Lane,[16,17] with slight modification.

Blastocysts were given a numerical score, based on the rate of development and expansion.

Grade 1: Early blastocysts with a blastocele < 50 percent of the embryo volume.

Grade 2: Early blastocysts with a blastocele ≥ 50 percent of the embryo volume.

Grade 3: Full blastocysts with a blastocele completely filling the embryo but not expanded.

Grade 4: Expanded blastocysts with a blastocele volume larger than that of the early embryo, with a thinning zona.

We add to this numeric score two alphabetic scores to grade first the inner cell mass (ICM) and second the trophectoderm.

Blastocysts were graded A (high cell number with good cell-cell adhesion), B (lower cell number with poorer cell-cell attachment), or C (no ICM apparent, sparse granular cells in the IE).

Supernumerary blastocysts graded C were not cryopreserved. Patients not achieving a clinical pregnancy returned for a frozen blastocyst transfer cycle. In some cases, with the patients consent, the blastocysts were transferred to the recipients.

Transfer of Blastocysts and Assessment of Pregnancy

All women received transdermal estradiol (German Remedies) with GnRH agonists for the preparation of the endometrium. Administration of progesterone (50 mg in oil, daily) was initiated when the endometrial thickness was >10 mm. Five days after the initiation of progesterone treatment, blastocysts were thawed/warmed and surviving blastocysts were transferred into the recipient's uterus. Most recipients received one to three blastocysts. Chemical pregnancy was assessed based on serum hCG levels at 9 to 10 days after blastocyst transfer, after which a clinical pregnancy was confirmed by the presence of fetal heart activity or a gestational sac at ~30 days after blastocyst transfer.

Between February 2005 to March 2006, we performed cycles of vitrified/warmed and slow-frozen/thawed blastocyst transfers.

Vitrification of Blastocysts

The protocol for the vitrification of blastocysts was adopted from previous reports described by Mukaida et al.[18]

Blastocysts were placed in equilibration solution, which is the base medium [Hepes-buffered human tubal fluid (HTF) with 20% human serum albumin (HSA)] containing 7.5 percent (v/v) ethylene glycol (EG) and 7.5 percent (v/v) dimethyl sulfoxide (DMSO). After 2 mins, the blastocysts were suspended in the base medium containing 15 percent (v/v) EG, 10 mg/mL Ficoll 70 and 0.65 mol/L sucrose. Both the cryoprotectant solutions had been warmed briefly in incubator at 37°C, and blastocysts were handled on the stage warmer of a dissecting microscope at 37°C. After loading the blastocysts into the straws, they was plunged into liquid Nitrogen.

For Study II, we had used the Cryoloop. The Cryoloop consisted of a nylon loop (20 μm wide, 0.5–0.7 mm diameter) mounted on a stainless steel pipe that was inserted into the lid of a cryovial. While the blastocysts were suspended in cryoprotectant solution I, a cryoloop was dipped into cryoprotectant solution II in order to create a thin, filmy layer of solution by surface tension on the nylon loop. The blastocysts were then washed quickly in solution II and transferred on the filmy layer of the nylon loop using a micropipette or a flexipet. Immediately after the loading of blastocysts, the cryoloop was plunged into liquid nitrogen. The duration for which the blastocysts were exposed to the vitrification solution II before cooling was ≤ 30 seconds. Using a stainless steel rod, the cryoloop with blastocysts were sealed in a cryovial, which was previously submerged in liquid Nitrogen. The vials were stored in a cryocan.

Blastocyst Warming and Assessment of Survival

To remove the cryoprotectant, blastocysts were warmed and diluted in a two-step process. Blastocysts were removed from liquid Nitrogen and placed directly into a prewarmed culture dish containing 1 mL of 0.33 mol/L sucrose solution. After 2 minutes, the blastocysts were transferred to the 0.2 mol/L sucrose solution. After 3 mins, blastocysts were washed and kept in the base medium for 5 mins and then returned to the culture medium (Medicult) until transfer.

For Study II: Volume of the blastocele cavity was reduced either by puncturing it with a glass microneedle or by laser system. Blastocysts were held by placing the ICM at 12 or 6 o'clock position and a needle or laser puncture was made through the trophectoderm cells into the blastocele cavity until it shrunk. Contraction of the blastocyst was observed for 30 seconds. After complete shrinkage of the blastocysts, they were vitrified as described above.

Assisted hatching with laser (1,480-nm diode laser, RI instruments) was performed within 10 mins after warming, as, at this stage, the blastocele had not fully expanded and the perivitelline space was present.[19,20]

Slow-frozen blastocysts were originally frozen in modified protocols containing glycerol and sucrose, based on Menezo's two-step method previously described.[21,22] Briefly, blastocysts were exposed for 10 minutes into 5 percent glycerol, then moved into 9 percent glycerol + 0.2 mol/L sucrose.

Blastocysts were transferred into straws, sealed and loaded in a rate controlled freezer (cryologic-CL-2200). The initial blastocyst cooling was achieved at a rate of –2°C / min to –6°C. The temperature was held for 10 minutes. Cooling from –6°C to –40°C was done in steps of 0.3°C/min and from –40°C to –150°C in steps of 35°C/min, after which, the blastocysts were plunged directly into liquid Nitrogen (–196°C) for cryostorage. Blastocysts were thawed by removing the straws from the liquid Nitrogen and disappearance of all intracellular ice crystals occurred during initial blastocyst thawing, carried out for 30 seconds at room temperature. The straw was cut open onto a Petridish and the contents expelled into the dish. Blastocysts were placed in a serial dilution of cryoprotectant at room temperature through two concentrations of glycerol (9%, 5%, 10 min/dilution) in 0.2 mol/L sucrose. Blastocysts were washed in the base medium (Hepes-buffered HTF with 10% HSA) and returned to culture medium (Medicult) until transfer.

Survival of blastocysts was assessed based on the morphological integrity of the blastomeres, ICM, trophectoderm and re-expansion of the blastocele. The surviving blastocysts were scored according to the developmental stage and graded for quality as described before.

Results

Study I

Table 52.1 shows the clinical outcome of patients who completed the conventional slow-freezing or vitrification program. The mean age of the women for both the groups was 34.2 ± 5.0 years. Out of a total of 117 vitrified blastocysts, 94 (80.4%) survived. An average of 2.0 vitrified blastocysts were replaced per embryo transfer, resulting in a pregnancy rate of 42.55

Table 52.1: Retrospective data of conventional slow-freezing vitrification method for blastocysts

Parameters	Slow freezing	Vitrification
Patient's age (years)	34.2 ± 5.0	34.2 ± 5.0
No. of blastocysts warmed/thawed	117	117
No. of blastocysts survived (%)	76 (65)	94 (80.4)
No. of blastocysts transferred	76	94
Mean no. of blastocysts transferred	2.5	2.0
No. of transfers	30	47
No. of clinical pregnancies (%)	5 (16.6)	20 (42.55)

Note: p > 0.05 for every comparison

Table 52.2: The survival and development of blastocysts following cryoloop vitrification with artificial shrinkage

Parameters	Results
Patient's age (years)	34.2 ± 5.0
No. of blastocysts warmed	29
No. of blastocysts survived (%)	24 (82.7)
No. of blastocyst hatched (%)	12 (50)
Mean number of blastocysts transferred	3
No. of transfers	8
No. of clinical pregnancies (%)	4 (50)

percent (20/47), concurrently 117 slow-frozen blastocysts were thawed and 76 (65%) survived the thaw process. An average of 2.5 slow-frozen blastocysts were replaced per embryo transfer, resulting in a pregnancy rate of 16.6 percent (5/30). The blastocyst survival rate was higher in the vitrified group than in the slow-frozen group.

When the vitrified-warmed blastocysts were divided into day-5 or day-6 group, there was no significant difference in the survival and pregnancy rates, so it was not taken into consideration [p < 0.1].

Study II

The survival and development of blastocysts vitrified by the Cryoloop method are summarized in Table 52.2.

The blastocyst survival rate using Cryoloop was 82.7 percent. In 50 percent of the surviving blastocysts, hatching was performed post warming.[8] Embryo transfer resulted four clinical pregnancies, accounting for 50 percent. However, further studies should be conducted for statistical significance.

CONCLUSION

Both the studies demonstrated encouraging results with vitrification, which proved to be an attractive alternative to the conventional slow-freezing protocol with no ice crystal formation and ease of operation. Several articles report that survival rates in cryopreserved expanded blastocele can be improved by artificial reduction of the blastocele cavity.[23-26] Furthermore, the high percentage of pregnancies might be due to laser assisted hatching.

Our pilot study shows encouraging results, but further studies may be required to achieve statistical significance.

In general, vitrification shows promise as a successful alternative to conventional freezing technology. The advantages of vitrification include greater cryosurvival, lesser time, simplicity of method, surety of embryo transfer and thus, ease in patient management, with the ability to cryopreserve individual blastocysts at their optimal stage of development and expansion.

REFERENCES

1. Staessen C, Janssenswillen C, Van Den Abbeel E, Devroey P, Van Steirteghem AC. Avoidance of Triplet pregnancies by elective transfer of two good embryos. Hum Reprod 1993;8:1650-3.
2. Staessen C, Nagy ZP, Liu J, Janssenswillen C, Camus M, Devroey P, Steirteghem AC. One year's experience with elective transfer of two good quality embryos in the human *in vitro* fertilization and intracytoplasmic sperm injection programmes. Hum Reprod 1995;10:3305-12.
3. Fujii S, Fukai A, Yamaguchi E, Sakamoto T, Sato S, Saits Y. Reducing multiple pregnancies by restricting the number of embryos transferred to two at the first embryo transfer attempt. Hum Reprod 1998;13:3550-4.
4. Ludwig M, Schopper B, Katalinic A, Sturm R, Al-Hasani S, Diedrich K. Experience with the elective transfer of two embryos under the conditions of the German embryo protection law: Results of a retrospective data analysis of 2573 transfer cycles. Hum Reprod 2000;15:319-24.
5. Fahy GM, MacFarlane DR, Angell CA, Meryman HT. Cryobiology 1984;21:407-26.
6. Fahy GM. Vitrification, a new approach to organ cryopreservation. In: Mery Man HT (Ed). Transplantation approaches to graft rejection. New York: Alan R Liss; 1986;305-35.
7. Vajta G, Booth PJ, Holm P, Greve T, Callesen H. Successful vitrification of early stage bovine invitro produced embryos with the open pulled straw (OPS) method. Cryo LeH 1997;18:191-5.
8. Libermann J, Tuker MJ. Effect of carrier system on the yield of human oocytes and embryos as assessed by survival and developmental potential after vitrification. Reproduction 2002;124:483-9.
9. Papisk, Shimizu M, Izaike Y. Factors affecting the survivability of bovine oocytes vitrified in droplets. Theriogenology 2000;54:651-8.
10. Park SP, Kim EY, KimDZ, Park NH, Won YS, Yoon SH, Chung KS, Lim JH. Simple, efficient and successful vitrification of bovine blastocysts using electron microscopic grids. Hum Reprod 1999;14:2838-43.
11. Kuwayama M, Kato O. Successful vitrification of human oocytes. Fertil Steril 2000;74:Suppl 349 (Abstract 127).

12. Matsumoto H, Jiang JY, Tanaka T, Sasada H, Sats E. Vitrification of large quantities of immune bovine oocytes using nylon mesh. Cryobiology 2001;42:139-44.

13. Mukaida T, Nakamora S, Tomiyama T, Ishikawa Y, Makita M, Ased T, Araki Y. Successful birth after transfer of vitrified human blastocysts with use of a cryoloop containerless technique. Fertil Steril 2001;76:618-23.

14. Longley MT, Marek DM, Gardner DK, Doody KM, Doody KJ. Extended Embryo culture in human assisted reproduction treatments. Hum Reprod 2001;6:902-8.

15. Mandelbeum J, Belaisch-Allart J, Junca AM, Antine JM, Plachot M, Alvarez S, et al. Cryopreservation in human assisted reproduction is now routine for embryos but remains a research procedure for oocytes. Hum Reprod 1998;13(Suppl 3):161-77.

16. Gardner DK, Lane M. Embyo culture systems. In: Trousan AO, Gardner DK (Eds). Handbook of *in vitro* Fertilization 2nd edn, Boca Raton (FL) (RC press : 2000 P205-64).

17. Tucker MJ, Liebermann J. Morphological scoring of human embryos and its relevance of Blastocyst transfer: In: Patrizio P, Tucker MJ. Guelman V (Eds). Color atlas of human assisted reproduction: Laboratory and clinical insight. Philadelphia; Lippincott, Williams and Wilkins: 2003. pp. 99-108.

18. Mukaida T, Nakamura S, Tomiyama T, Wada S, Oka C, Kasai M, Takahashi K. Vitrification of human blastocysts using cryoloops: clinical outcome of 223 cycles. Hum Reprod 2003;18:384-91.

19. Tucker MJ, Cohen J, Massey JB, Mayer MP, Wiker SR, Wright G. Partial dissection of the zona pellucida of frozen-thawed human embryos may enhance blastocyst hatching, implantation, and pregnancy rates. Am J Obstet Gynecol 1991;165:341-4.

20. Tucker M. Relevance of assisted hatching with blastocysts stage transfer, Proceedings of the 1st World Congress on controversies in Obstetrics, Gynaecology and Infertility; 1999, Oct 28-31 Prague, Bologna, Italy: Monduzzi, Editore: 1999;49-52.

21. Menezo Y, Veigh A. Cryopreservation of blastocysts proceedings of the 10th world congress on IVF and Assisted Reproduction: 1997 May 24-28: Vancouver, British Columbia. Bologna, Italy: Monduzzi Editore 1997. pp. 41-5.

22. Sills ES, Sweitzer CL, Morton PC, Perloe M, Kaplan CR, Tueker MJ. Dizygotic twin delivery following *in vitro* fertilization and transfer of thawed blastocysts cryopreserved at day 6 and 7. Fertil Steril 2003;79: 4234-7.

23. Vanderzwalmen P, Bertain G, Debauche Ch, Standaert V, Van Roosendaal E, Vandervorst M, et al. Births after vitrification at morula and blastocysts stages: Effect of artificial reduction of the blastocelic cavity before vitrification. Hum Reprod 2002;17:744-51.

24. Son WY, Yoon SH, Yoon HJ, Lee SM, Lim JH. Pregnancy outcome following transfer of human blastocysts vitrified on electron microscopy guides after induced collapse of the blastocoele. Hum Reprod 2003;18:137-9.

25. Zench NH, Lejeune B, Zech H, Vanderzwalmen P. Vitrification of hatching and hatched human blastocysts: effect of an opening in the zona pellucida before vitrification. Reprod Biomed Online 2005;11:355-61.

26. Hiraoka K, Hiraoke K, Kinutani M, Kinutani IC. Blastocoele Collapse by micropipetting prior to vitrification gives excellent survival and pregnancy outcomes for human day 5 and 6 expanded blastocysts. Hum Reprod 2004;19:2884-8.

The Role of Co-culture in Implantation

Natachandra Chimote, Meena Chimote, Nirmalendu Nath, Amiya Mukherjee

OVERVIEW

Co-cultures have been advocated in assisted reproduction owing to the shortcomings of simple media to support embryo development beyond the cleavage stage. Various types of human and non-human cells and cell lines have been used for co-cultures. High rates of blastocyst formation have been reported with the use of co-cultures, and they have been proposed as a rescue treatment option in couples with repeated implantation failures. Since the advent of complex sequential media, which yield very high blastocyst formation and blastocyst implantation rates, the need for co-cultures has been obviously questioned. Upon review of the literature, it is evident that well-designed randomized studies that compare co-cultures with simple or sequential media do not exist. The progression of cleavage stage embryos to the blastocyst stage, for embryos that are cultured in modern sequential media, appears to be similar, if not better, rendering the use of co-cultures obsolete. Furthermore, there is no consensus regarding the inevitability of sequential media, as similar results have been obtained with a single medium formulation that supports all stages of the preimplantation period. Whether co-cultures are advantageous in patients with repeated implantation failures, however, should be investigated in randomized trials. Co-cultures still serve as powerful tools for understanding embryo metabolism. Furthermore, co-cultures may be instrumental in studying expression of implantation-related genes and embryo-endometrium interaction.

INTRODUCTION

Despite the rapid development of assisted reproduction techniques (ART) in recent years, implantation rates after replacement of embryos into the uterine cavity remains low, whereas the abortion rate is relatively high (15% to 45%). Reproductive wastage in ART may be attributed to:

- Chromosomal anomalies in stimulated oocytes.[1]
- Poor egg and/or sperm quality.[2]
- Asynchronization between the embryo stage and endometrial development at the time of embryo replacement.

Several techniques have been adopted in recent years to improve embryo viability *in vitro* and implantation rates. The optimal embryo culture medium for *in vitro* fertilization (IVF) and embryo transfer (ET) has not been established. Attempts to improve *in vitro* culture conditions by changes in media formulations and supplements have met with little success despite stringent quality control on embryo culture media components and instruments. The quality of the *in vitro* culture conditions for human embryos is one of the most critical aspects of a successful IVF-ET. Attempts to improve culture conditions based on formulations of human tubal fluid (HTF) has yielded certain improvement in embryo quality.[3] Allowing fertilization and early embryonic development to take place *in vivo* by ART techniques, such as gamete intrafallopian transfer (GIFT), zygote intrafallopian transfer (ZIFT), and tubal ET, has been suggested to overcome embryonic-endometrial asynchronization.[4] The pregnancy rate (PR) and take home baby rates for GIFT have been reported to be slightly higher in most centers.[5]

Another physiological approach to simulate the endometrial environment has been the use of co-culture systems to allow embryonic development *in vitro* up to the blastocyst stage. Cells from different reproductive and non-reproductive sources, such as uterus, cumulus, ovary, kidney and spleen,[6] showed positive co-culture effects and improved embryonic viability *in vitro*. However, these intricate techniques although effective, are reserved for clinical use only in few specialized laboratories.

Recent evidence suggests that co-culture of human embryos with various cellular monolayers results in increased rates of embryo development, decreased fragmentation and improvement in implantation and pregnancy rates following IVF-ET.[7-13] This beneficial impact on IVF outcome is supported by substantial evidence from animal studies.[4-18] Although this evidence suggests a positive effect of co-culture cells on IVF, the rate of development has been lower when the embryos have been cultured *in vitro* as compared with *in vivo* development. Further improvements are therefore needed if the *in vitro* maturation and fertilization of oocytes and the *in vitro* culture of the resulting embryos are to be used more reliably for research and clinical purposes.

CLINICAL DISCUSSION

Types of Co-culture

The variability in success rates associated with co-culture systems can be attributed to differences in types of cell lines, maintenance of the cells, and various environmental factors within each laboratory.

The most commonly used cell lines in human IVF-ET include:

- Bovine reproductive tract cells[19]
- African green monkey kidney cells (Vero)[8]
- Human oviduct and granulosa cells lines.[20,21]

The inherent fear of using xenologous and heterologous cell lines is the risk of disease transmission to the exposed embryos. A number of studies have evaluated the effect of various somatic cell lines on human embryo development. Only recently have autologous endometrial cells been used in human IVF.[22,23] When surplus human embryos were co-cultured on Fallopian tube epithelium, significantly higher rates of blastocyst formation with more nuclei per blastocyst were demonstrated compared with conventionally cultured pre-embryos.[20]

Endometrial Co-culture

An autologous endometrial co-culture system, using first passaged cryopreserved stroma and glandular epithelial cells has been reported.[24] In this study, a cohort of embryos was cultured alternatively on conventional medium and co-culture. The embryos placed on the patient's own endometrial cells had fewer cytoplasmic fragments and a greater number of blastomeres at the time of transfer. Therefore, it appears that autologous endometrial co-culture cells may provide a more suitable environment for embryo growth than the conventional medium.

Efforts to formulate a medium based on the composition of human tubal fluid have suggested that the ratio of Na^{+1} to K^{+1} ions in the culture medium are important for determining the quality of the embryos and subsequent pregnancy rates. Others have demonstrated that the addition of glutamine, absence of glucose in the initial stages of cleavage, and addition of ethylenediaminetetraacetic acid (EDTA) may be beneficial in improving embryo development.[25] Unfortunately, these media are devoid of growth factors secreted by reproductive tract cells and potential paracrine signals, which could enhance embryo growth and development.

It is becoming increasingly apparent that the embryo is a dynamic organism that is able to respond to both autocrine as well as paracrine signals from the surrounding environment. When human embryos are cultured in groups, morphological characteristics appear to improve, suggesting that factors released by the embryos may enhance their quality.[26] Embryonic signals also have been shown to stimulate endometrial stromal cell synthesis and secretion of insulin-like growth factor-binding protein (IGFBP) that, in turn, may modify insulin growth factor action on mouse embryo development.[16] A recent study[27] demonstrated enhanced gene expression of activin receptors from deselected human preimplantation embryos when co-cultured on human endometrial stromal cells. Because the activin ligand was expressed only in the co-cultured cells while the activin receptor was detected only in the developing embryo, a paracrine mechanism for activin in early preimplantation development was postulated. Therefore, the autocrine and paracrine interactions between the embryo and its culture environment may play a role in enhancing embryo quality and possibly, improving pregnancy rates in IVF-ET.

It was also found that co-cultured embryos grown on bovine oviductal cells had significantly more blastomeres and fewer cytoplasmic fragments than conventionally grown embryos in randomly allocated patients.[19] A few researchers, with the aid of videocinematography, noted that a number of morphological features were improved significantly for co-cultured compared to non-cocultured embryos on bovine oviductal cells.[28] In addition, a recent prospective randomized trial found a significantly higher percentage of fertilized oocytes developed to the eight-cell stage on three different co-culture systems compared with serum-supplemented media.[29]

This study suggests that *in vitro* culture conditions may be enhanced with the use of autologous endometrial co-culture, as reflected by improved embryo quality. There is evidence of a correlation between embryo morphology and clinical pregnancy rates, which would suggest that this co-culture system ultimately, might have a beneficial effect on IVF-ET success.[30,31] In addition, by using the patient's own reproductive tract cells, the potential infectious risks of heterologous and xenologous co-culture systems will be avoided.

Blastocyst Transfer after Co-culture with Human Endometrial Epithelial Cells

Blastocyst transfer is currently an attractive option for IVF teams in the treatment of infertile couples, as it may improve implantation rates while decreasing the rate of multiple pregnancy.[32] Blastocyst transfer is suitable when an appropriate number of oocytes are obtained. Considering an average 80 percent fertilization rate, 90 percent cleavage rate, and 50 percent blastocyst formation rate, the patient must produce at least seven metaphase II oocytes in order to transfer two blastocysts. Blastocyst transfer has also been presented as an appealing option for patients with recurrent implantation failure, those in whom multiple pregnancy should be avoided,[33] and those undergoing preimplantation genetic diagnosis (PGD).

A crucial issue in blastocyst transfer is the development of culture techniques that produce acceptable blastocyst rates. Currently, commercially available culture media cannot sufficiently support embryo development. Approximately 60 percent of embryos are blocked during *in vitro* development, probably owing to external conditions in the embryology laboratories.[34] Extended culture of embryos can be performed with sequential media alone or over a monolayer of different cell types.[35] The co-culture system is designed to improve embryo development, as cells may provide trace elements or growth factors not present in defined media and may perform scavenging functions. Several studies provide evidence of a molecular dialog between the developing embryo and the maternal endometrial epithelium.[36-41] This embryonic–endometrial cross talk may be beneficial in not only improving blastocyst rates, but also for the activation of specific paracrine molecules, which improves the prospects for the implantation of the embryo.

Using a physiologic approach, Mercader et al.[42] developed a co-culture program in which human embryos are developed to the blastocyst stage on a monolayer of primary human endometrial epithelial cells. Endometrial tissue is simple to obtain (endometrial biopsy), safe (no risk of viral disease transmission among species), physiologic (endometrial epithelial cells are the first cells with which the embryo comes into contact when it reaches the uterine cavity), and easy to grow.[36] The co-culture system yielded excellent blastocyst formation rates in patients undergoing IVF (50.8%) or oocyte donation (58.2%). Therefore, a patient with four good quality embryos on day 2 had two blastocysts for transfer, decreasing the possibility of multiple pregnancy without compromising the pregnancy rates.

Improvements in culture techniques,[39] a more delicate ET technique,[40] and more refined patient selection may contribute to these results. Optimal laboratory conditions, with a larger incubator and delicate embryo handling, are required to prolong embryo culture beyond 3 days. In addition, the use of endometrial epithelial cells to co-culture human embryos increases the number of blastomeres while decreasing the fragmentation rate per embryo compared with non-cocultured embryos from the same patient.[41]

Blastocyst Culture after Intracytoplasmic Sperm Injection

It is suspected that blastocyst development rather reflects the competence of the oocyte itself and is relatively independent of a paternal genomic effect.[43] In this regard, a theoretical impact of cumulus cells (CCs) may be raised. These somatic cells are mediators[44] of oocyte maturation, development and fertilization[45] and are, in turn, regulated by oocyte factors.[46-48] Therefore, in intracytoplasmic sperm injection (ICSI), where oocytes are denuded before injection, any potential positive effect of surplus CCs on further development cannot exert further influence. This might result in lower numbers of blastocysts as compared to conventional IVF, in which CCs are not removed until the day of fertilization. Thus, the attached cumulus tissue on ICSI oocytes could somehow mimic the suggested effect of co-culture with homologous granulosa[49,50] or CCs[51-53] on further outcome.

Ebner et al.[54] in their study, prospectively split sibling oocytes into two groups; in the first cohort, gametes were denuded completely, and in the second, numerous CCs were left attached to the zona pellucida (ZP) before ICSI. Thus, any impact of those CCs on preimplantation development and pregnancy outcome could be evaluated. It was found that the surplus cumulus cells on the oocyte impaired fertilization and the ability to cleave compared with the control oocytes having no cumulus cells. By contrast, quality of the embryos on days 2 and 3 turned out to be improved in the presence of abundant CCs. Prolonged culture to day 5 led to an overall blastocyst formation rate of 53.9 percent; however, 36.5 percent were of optimal quality, as assessed by the morphology of the inner cell mass (ICM) and trophoectoderm (TE). While the rate of blastocyst formation was significantly increased in the study group, the rate of top quality blastocysts was not affected.

A recent review[44] emphasized that intercellular communication between oocytes and granulosa cells (CCs and mural granulosa cells) is essential for normal follicular differentiation and oocyte developmental competence. In detail, two separate ways of signalling between gametes and somatic cells occur, either paracrine or via gap junctions, with both forms being essential for normal oogenesis.[46,55] Several key molecules produced by the oocyte (e.g. growth differentiation factor 9 or bone morphogenic protein 15) play an important role in granulosa cell function and differentiation.[56,57] In addition, gametes promote their own development via metabolic co-operation with CCs, e.g. inducing amino acid uptake[58] or glycolysis.[59]

By contrast, CCs play an important role during early maturational steps and after resumption of meiosis, although at this time, transzonal cytoplasmic processes are mostly withdrawn, because paracrine communication compensates for the loss of gap junctional connection. This is supported by the finding that IVF results are compromised if the CCs are removed prior to IVF compared to post-IVF.[60,61] In order not to loose any beneficial effect of the CC mass on *in vitro* development of early embryos, several authors introduced co-culture with either mural granulosa cells or CCs.[49-53] The mechanisms, which contribute to better embryonic development following co-culture with homologous granulosa cells, are still unclear; however, it can be hypothesized that that is the result of detoxifying and/or embryotrophic factors.

Of course, the more physiological approach would be to leave the majority of the cumulus oophorus intact 24 hours past IVF, which has successfully been used in order to increase embryo quality and pregnancy rate.[53,62,63] In ICSI, however, evidence of any effect of attached CCs on further competence of the oocyte is scarce. Actually, as of the date of this article, only one ICSI study that deals with partly denuded rabbit oocytes exists.[64] These authors did not find any benefit in terms of fertilization, cleavage or blastocyst formation. However, they removed all remaining CCs as early as 8 hours after injection in order to guarantee adequate pronuclear evaluation. Thus, any possible long-term effect of the additional presence of CC on further developmental competence of the conceptus is reduced. To realize any impact of *in situ* co-culture of CCs on the rates of implantation and pregnancy, prospective transfer of incompletely denuded oocytes has to be favored.

Cumulus Co-culture

It is believed that the feeder or helper cells stimulate development of morphologically sound embryos by removing toxins from the culture medium and by the addition of growth factors such as insulin-like growth factor (IGF)-I and IGF-II, vascular endothelial growth factor (VEGF), transforming growth factor—TGF α and TGF β, platelet activating factor (PAF), and epidermal growth factor (EGF).[65] It has been postulated that the feeder cells metabolize the glucose present in the medium, thus allowing the embryos to be exposed to tolerable levels of glucose.[66] Several studies have demonstrated faster cleavage rates, less fragmentation, and better implantation rates using a co-culture system. Co-culture systems reportedly increase blastulation rates to as high as 55 to 70 percent.[3,8,9,67]

Three main growth factors and cytokines—IGF-I and IGF-II,[68-70] interleukin (IL)-1 and IL-6,[71,72] and VEGF,[73,74] are expressed by cumulus cells and are known to improve embryo morphology and play a putative role in the implantation process.

In an effort to improve implantation rates, the search has been ongoing for a "glue" that will allow more intimate contact between the embryo and the uterus.[75] Parekh et al.[76] demonstrated a significant increase in implantation rates and a significant increase in the pregnancy rates (PRs), using the combination of co-culture and cumulus-aided embryo transfer with autologous cumulus cells. These cells may not only aid in embryonic development, but also provide a natural mechanism to improve embryo-uterine adhesion. This study also suggested that sequential media could be modified to contain those embryotrophic factors that are present in cumulus cells to enhance PRs. The continued secretion of growth factors by the cumulus cells in utero appears to be plausible because the study demonstrated the secretion of three growth factors (IL-6, IGF-I, and VEGF) in an *in vitro* culture system. Besides their cytokine action, the fact that these expanded cumulus cells may continue to contribute to the increase in adhesiveness between the embryo and the uterus in utero was demonstrated in an *in vitro* system.

Experience at Our Center

Patient Selection

Forty patients were enrolled into the study. All patients underwent their IVF treatment following the ovulation induction protocol. Indications for IVF in this group of patients were mechanical factor (n = 15), polycystic ovaries (n = 14), and unexplained infertility (n = 11). Patients with a male factor were not included.

Ovarian Stimulation Protocol

The ovarian stimulation protocol used a gonadotropin-releasing hormone (GnRH) analog (Lupride), which was given as an injection, starting from day 21 of the previous cycle. When the laboratory test indicated pituitary suppression [17-estradiol (E2) ~ < 20 pg/mL], the dose of Lupride was decreased to 6 × 100 g/day, and stimulation with pure follicle stimulating hormone (FSH) (Ovufol, 225 IU/day; VHB Pharma, India) was initiated. Lupride treatment was continued until the evening of human chorionic gonadotropin (hCG) administration. When at least 3 to 4 leading follicles reached a diameter of 18 to 20 mm and serum E2 levels were >500 pg/mL, 5,000 IU of hCG (Ovutrig, VHB Pharma, India) was administered intramuscularly (IM) to trigger the final stage of follicular maturation. Oocyte pick-up was performed transvaginally under ultrasound guidance 34 to 36 hours after hCG administration.

Establishment of Co-culture System

In Vitro Culture

In the study group, at 17 to 19 hours after insemination, the cumulus mass was removed from the oocytes partially by a mechanical method, using fine needle assisted micro-dissection to observe fertilization (Fig. 53.1). Fertilized oocytes were placed individually for co-culture with the attached partial cumulus mass, in pre-equilibrated single droplets (each 10–15 µL) containing mechanically separated cumulus cells in cleavage media in another pre-equilibrated culture oil dish. The system was cultured at 37°C in 5 percent CO_2 and 100 percent humidity. This resulted in an actively growing monolayer covering approximately 50 percent of the culture area. The proliferating monolayer of cells from the original oocytes during maturation culture was left undisturbed until after 48 hours, The percentage of cleavage and the morphological appearance criteria of embryos were recorded daily for 72 hours in the system using an inverted phase-contrast microscope. The embryos that reached the compaction stage were transferred individually into a single droplet of blastocyst media along with the naturally formed monolayer of cumulus cells from the cleavage media. After 48 hours, blastocyst formation was observed (Fig. 53.2).

On the other hand, in the control group completely denuded fertilized oocytes were kept in cleavage and blastocyst culture—single droplets just like in the study group but without any cumulus mass cells, which was removed at the time of observing fertilization. A comparative study was carried out in terms of fertilization, cleavage (gradation), blastocyst formation and pregnancy rate. The results are given in Table 53.1. It was observed that though the fertilization rates in both the groups did not differ, the cleavage (gradation), blastocyst formation and pregnancy rate per blastocyst transfer was higher in the study group.

Though the biological basis of this phenomenon is not fully understood from these results, possible functions of co-culture cells include:

i. Detoxifying the culture medium, for example by chelation of heavy metal ions,

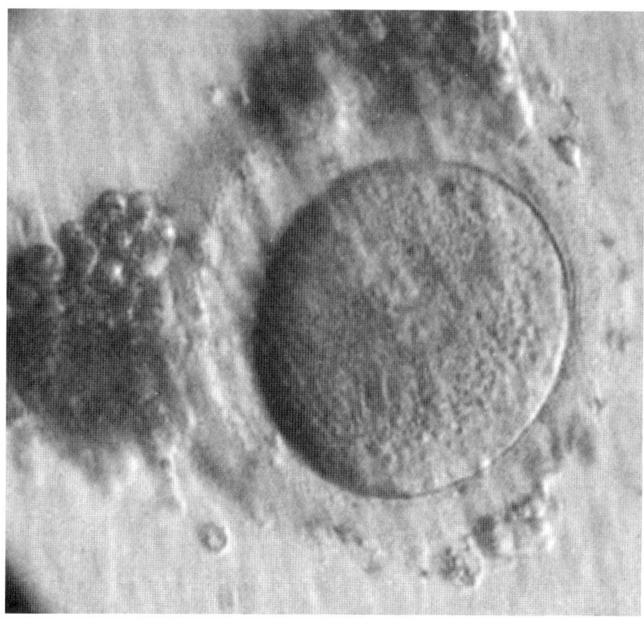

Fig. 53.1 Partially denuded fertilized oocyte

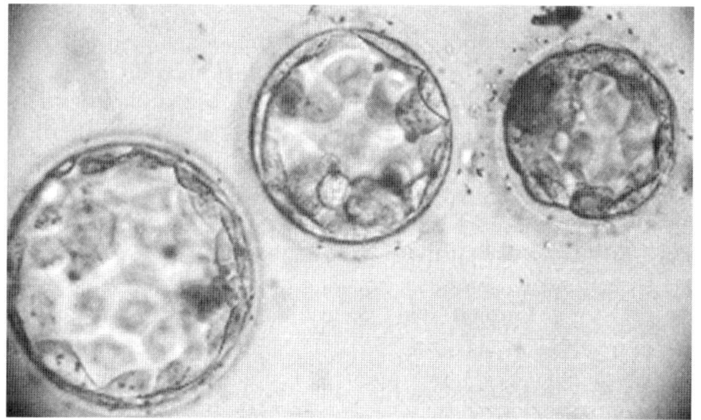

Fig. 53.2 Early and expanded blastocysts after co-culture

Table 53.1 Comparison of the pregnancy outcome in IVF-ET patients following transfer of embryos with and without co-culture

Parameters	Control Group (without co-culture)	Study Group (with co-culture)	P value
No. of oocytes inseminated	175	145	–
2 PN (fertilization)	161 (92%)	139 (96%)	NS
Cleavage D2	133 (83%)	136 (98%)	0.014
No. of Gr. A embryos on D2	61 (46%)	101 (74%)	0.0027
No. of Gr. A embryos on D3	58 (44%)	96 (71%)	0.002
No. of 2 PN for BC	89	80	NS
No. of blastocysts	27 (30%)	43 (54%)	0.001
No. of blastocyst transfers	15	25	0.001
No. of pregnancies	5 (33%)	12 (48%)	0.001

Abbreviations: PN: pronuclei; BC: blastocyst culture

ii. Reducing the concentration of normal constituents in the medium, such as glucose, that inhibit embryo development,

iii. Secretion of factors into the medium that stimulate embryos or enhance the maternal embryonic genome shift and improve cell organelle structure, such as (a) nutrients and substrates, including amino acids or pyruvate, or (b) proteins or 'growth factor'.

iv. Stabilization of the physiochemical conditions, such as pH, O_2/CO_2 concentrations, or the culture medium, or

v. A combination of several of these possible mechanisms.

It is therefore concluded that either embryos, not exposed to the co-culture environment during early cleavage may be unable to overcome the damage that was incurred earlier, or that co-cultured embryos obtain certain beneficial factors for normal development *in vitro*.

Results

The results of this study are summarized in Table 53.1.

CONCLUSION

In conclusion, human embryos may require additional embryotrophic factor(s) not present in simple culture media for continued development of an increased proportion of embryos beyond the second to third day after fertilization. Co-culture of embryos with monolayers of granulosa cells can enhance the development of early human embryos and possibly overcome a block to development. This method may also be used to culture embryos for an extra day to reduce asynchrony between the embryo and uterus, as well as to enhance the possibility of embryo selection and preimplantation genetic diagnosis. Collectively, these findings may provide useful information, enabling a human assisted reproduction program to develop the optimum culture system to increase the quality of human embryos available for replacement.

REFERENCES

1. Bongso A, Ng SC, Ratnam SS. Co-cultures: Their relevance to assisted reproduction. Hum Reprod 1990;5:893-900.
2. Bongso A, Ng SC, Mok H, Lira MN, Teo HL, Wong PC, et al. Effect of sperm motility on human *in vitro* fertilization. Arch Androl 1989;22:185-92.
3. Quinn P, Kerin JF, Warnes GM. Improved pregnancy rate in human *in vivo* fertilization with the use of a medium based on the composition of human tubal fluid. Fertil Steril 1985;44:493-8.
4. Wong PC, Bongso TA, Ng SC, Chan CLK, Hagglund L, Anandakumar C, et al. Pregnancies after human tubal embryo transfer: A new method of infertility treatment. Singapore J Obstet Gynaecol 1988;19:41-8.
5. Yovich JL, Yovich JM, Edirsinghe WR. The relative chance of pregnancy following tubal uterine transfer procedures. Fertil Steril 1988;49:858-64.
6. Bongso A, Ng S-C, Fong C-Y, Ratnam S. Co-cultures: A new lead in embryo quality improvement for assisted reproduction. Fertil Steril 1991;56:179-91.
7. Wiemer KE, Cohen J, Amborski GF, et al. *In vitro* development and implantation of human embryos following culture on fetal bovine uterine fibroblast cells. Hum Reprod 1989;4:595-600.
8. Menezo Y, Guerin JF, Czyba JC. Improvement of human early embryo development *in vitro* by co-culture on monolayers of Vero cells. Biol Reprod 1990;42:301-6.
9. Menezo Y, Hazout A, Dumont M, Herbaut N, Nicollet B. Co-culture of embryos on Vero cells and transfer of blastocysts in humans. Hum Reprod 1992;7:101-6.
10. Gregory L, Booth AD, Wells C, Walker SM. A study of the cumulus-corona cell complex *in vitro* fertilization and embryo transfer, a prognostic indicator of the failure of implantation. Hum Reprod 1994;9:1308-17.
11. Mansour RT, Aboulghar MA, Serour IG, Abbass AM. Co-culture of human pronucleate oocytes with their cumulus cells. Hum Reprod 1994;9:1727-9.
12. Tucker MJ, Ingargiola PE, Massey JB, Morton PC, Wiemer KE, Wiker SR, Wright G. Assisted hatching with or without bovine oviductal epithelial cell co-culture for poor prognosis *in vitro* fertilization patients. Hum Reprod 1994;9:1528-31.
13. Freeman MR, Whitworth CM, Hill GA. Granulosa cell co-culture enhances human embryo development and pregnancy rate following *in vitro* fertilization. Hum Reprod 1995;10:408-14.
14. Thibodeaux JK, Godke RA. *In vitro* enhancement of early-stage embryos with co-culture. Arch Pathol Lab Med 1992;116:364-72.
15. Bongso A, Fong CY, Ng SC, Ratnam S. The search for improved *in vitro* systems should not be ignored, embryo co-culture may be one of them. Hum Reprod 1993;8:1155-60.
16. Cart JW. Bovine embryo co-culture. Cell Biol Int 1994;18:1155-62.
17. Feng HI, Yang QZ, Sun QY, Qin PC, Liu JM. Development of early bovine embryos in different culture systems. Vet Rec 1994;135:304-6.
18. Leppens G, Saklcas D. Differential effect of epithelial cell conditional medium fractions on preimplantation mouse embryo development. Hum Reprod 1995;10:1178-83.
19. Weimer KE, Hoffman DI, Maxson WS, Eager S, Muhlenberg B, Fiore I, et al. Embryonic morphology and rate of implantation of human embryos following co-culture on bovine oviductal epithelial cells. Hum Reprod 1993;8:97-101.
20. Vald M, Walker D, Kennedy RC. Nuclei number in human embryos co-cultured with human ampullary cells. Hum Reprod 1996;11:1678-86.
21. Quinn P, Margalit R. Beneficial effects of co-culture with cumulus cells on blastocyst formation in a prospective trial with supernumerary human embryos. J Assist Reprod Genet 1996;13:9-14.
22. Nieto FS, Watkins WB, Lopata A, Gordon Baker HW, Edgar DH. The effects of co-culture with autologous cryopreserved endometrial cells on human *in vitro* fertilization and early embryo morphology: A randomized study. J Assist Reprod Genet 1996;13:386-9.

23. Jayot S, Parneix I, Verdaguer S, Discamps G, Audebert A, Emperaire JC. Co-culture of embryos on homologous endometrial cells in patients with repeated failures of implantation. Fertil Steril 1995;63:109-14.

24. Barmat LI, Hung-Ching Liu, Spandorfer SD, Xu K, Veeck L, Damario MA, Rosenwaks Z. Human pre-embryo development on autologous endometrial co-culture versus conventional medium. Fertil Steril 1998,70:6,1109-13.

25. FitzGerald L, DiMattina M. Improved medium for long-term culture of human embryos overcomes the *in vitro* developmental block and increases blastocyst formation. Fertil Steril 1992;57:641-7.

26. Moessner J, Dodson WC. The quality of human embryo growth is improved when embryos are cultured in groups rather than separately. Fertil Steril 1995;64:1034-5.

27. Liu H-C, Mele C, Catz D, Noles N, Rosenwaks Z. Production of insulin-like growth factor binding proteins (IGFBPs) by human endometrial stromal cells is stimulated by the presence of embryos. J Assist Reprod Genet 1995;12:78-87.

28. Morgan K, Wiemer K, Steuerwald N, Hoffman D, Maxson W, Godke R. Use of videocinematography to assess morphological qualities of conventionally cultured and co-cultured embryos. Hum Reprod 1995;10:2371-6.

29. Feng HL, Wen XH, Amet T, Pesser SC. Effect of different co-culture systems in early human embryo development. Hum Reprod 1996;11:1525-8.

30. Veeck L. Oocyte assessment and biologic performance. Ann NY Acad Sci 1989;541:259-74.

31. Roseboom TJ, Vermeiden JPW, Schoute E, Lens JW, Schats R. The probability of pregnancy after embryo transfer is affected by the age of the patient, cause of infertility, number of embryos transferred and the mean morphology score as revealed by multiple logistic regression analysis. Hum Reprod 1995;10:3035-41.

32. Gardner DK, Schoolcraft WB, Wagley L, Schlenker T, Stevens J, Hesla J. A prospective randomized trial of blastocyst culture and transfer in *in vitro* fertilization. Hum Reprod 1998;13: 3434-40.

33. Patton PE, Sadler-Fredd K, Burry KA, Gorrill MJ, Johnson A, Larson JM, et al. Development and integration of an extended embryo culture program. Fertil Steril 1999;72:418-22.

34. Van Langendonckt A, Demylle D, Wyns C, Nisolle M, Donnez J. Comparison of G1.2/G2.2 and Sydney IVF cleavage/blastocyst sequential media for the culture of human embryos: a prospective, randomized, comparative study. Fertil Steril 2001;76:1023-31.

35. Garcia-Velasco JA, Simon C. Blastocyst transfer: Does it improve clinical outcome? Curr Opin Obstet Gyn 2001;13:299-304.

36. De los Santos MJ, Mercader A, Frances A, Portoles E, Remohi J, Pellicer A, et al. Role of endometrial factors in regulating secretion of components of the immunoreactive human embryonic interleukin-1 system during embryonic development. Biol Reprod 1996;54:563-74.

37. Simon C, Gimeno MJ, Mercader A, O'Connor JE, Remohi J, Polan ML, et al. Embryonic regulation of integrins b3, a4 and a1 in human endometrial epithelial cells *in vitro*. J Clin Endocrinol Metab 1997;82:2607-16.

38. Meseguer M, Aplin D, Caballero-Campo P, O'Connor JE, Martin JC, Remohi J, et al. Human endometrial mucin MUC1 is upregulated by progesterone and downregulated *in vitro* by the human blastocyst. Biol Reprod 2001;64:181-92.

39. González RR, Caballero-Campo P, Jasper M, Mercader A, Devoto L, Pellicer A, et al. Leptin and leptin receptor are expressed in the human endometrium and endometrial leptin secretion is regulated by the human blastocyst. J Clin Endocrinol Metab 2000;85:4883-8.

40. Galan A, O'Connor E, Valbuena D, Herrer R, Remohi J, Pampfer S, et al. The human blastocyst regulates endometrial epithelial apoptosis in embryonic adhesion. Biol Reprod 2000;63:430-9.

41. Caballero-Campo P, Dominguez F, Coloma J, Meseguer M, Remohi J, Pellicer A, et al. Hormonal and embryonic regulation of chemokines IL-8, MCP-1 and RANTES in the human endometrium during the window of implantation. Mol Hum Reprod 2002;8:375-84.

42. Mercader A, Garcia-Velasco JA, Escudero E, Remohi J, Pellicer A, Simon C. Clinical experience and perinatal outcome of blastocyst transfer after co-culture of human embryos with human endometrialepithelial cells: A 5-year follow-up study. Fertil Steril 30:3,1162-8.

43. Banerjee S, Lamond S, McMahon A, Campbell S, Nargund G. Does blastocyst culture eliminate paternal chromosomal defects and select good embryos? Hum Reprod 2000;15:2455-9.

44. Sutton ML, Gilchrist RB, Thompson JG. Effects of *in-vivo* and *in vitro* environments on the metabolism of the cumulus-oocyte complex and its influence on oocyte developmental capacity. Hum Reprod Update 2003;9:35-48.

45. McKenzie LJ, Pangas SA, Carson SA, Kovanci E, Cisneros P, Buster JE, Amato P, Matzuk MM. Human cumulus granulosa cell gene expression: A predictor of fertilization and embryo selection in women undergoing IVF. Hum Reprod 2004;19:2869-74.

46. Albertini DF, Combelles CM, Benecchi E, Carabatsos MJ. Cellular basis for paracrine regulation of ovarian follicle development. Reproduction 2001;121:647-53.

47. Eppig JJ. Oocyte control of ovarian follicular development and function in mammals. Reproduction 2001;122:829-38.

48. Matzuk MM, Burns KH, Viveiros MM, Eppig JJ. Intercellular communication in the mammalian ovary: Oocytes carry the conversation. Science 2002;21:2178-80.

49. Dirnfeld M, Goldman S, Gonen Y, Koifman M, Calderon I, Abramovici H. A simplified co-culture system with luteinized granulosa cells improves embryo quality and implantation rates: A controlled study. Fertil Steril 1997;67:120-2.

50. Fabbri R, Porcu E, Marsella T, Primavera MR, Cecconi S, Nottola SA, Motta PM, Venturoli S, Flamigni C. Human embryo development and pregnancies in a homologous granulosa cell culture system. J Assist Reprod Genet 2000;17:1-12.

51. Quinn P, Margalit R. Beneficial effects of co-culture with cumulus cells on blastocyst formation in a prospective trial with supernumary human embryos. J Assist Reprod Genet 1995;13:9-14.

52. Saito H, Hirayama T, Koike K, Saito T, Nohara M, Hiroi M. Cumulus mass maintains embryo quality. Fertil Steril 1995; 62:937-8.

53. Carrell DT, Peterson CM, Jones KP, Hatasaka HH, Udoff LC, Cornwell CE, Thorp C, Kuneck P, Erickson L, Campbell B. A

simplified co-culture system using homologous, attached cumulus tissue results in improved human embryo morphology and pregnancy rates during *in vitro* fertilization. J Assist Reprod Genet 1999;16:344-8.

54. T Ebner1, M Moser, M Sommergruber, O Shebl, G Tews. Incomplete denudation of oocytes prior to ICSI enhances embryo quality and blastocyst development. Hum Reprod 2006;21:11, 2972-7.

55. Dong J, Albertini DF, Nishimori K, Kumar TR, Lu N, Matzuk MM. Growth differentiation factor-9 is required during early ovarian folliculogenesis. Nature 1996;383:531-5.

56. Galloway SM, McNatty KP, Cambridge LM, Laitinen MP, Juengel JL, Jokiranta TS, McLaren RJ, Luiro K, Dodds KG, et al. Mutations in an oocyte-derived growth factor gene (BMP 15) cause increased ovulation rate and infertility in a dosage-sensitive manner. Nat Genet 2000;25:279-83.

57. Li R, Norman RJ, Armstrong DT, Gilchrist RB. Oocyte-secreted factor(s) determine functional difference between bovine mural granulosa cells and cumulus cells. Biol Reprod 2000;63:839-45.

58. Eppig JJ, Pendola FL, Wiggleswoth K, Pendola JK. Mouse oocytes regulate metabolic co-operativity between granulosa cells and oocytes: Amino acid transport. Biol Reprod 2005;73,351-7.

59. Sugiura K, Pendola FL, Eppig JJ. Oocyte control of metabolic cooperativity between oocytes and companion granulosa cells: Energy metabolism. Dev Biol 2005;279:20-30.

60. Fatehi AN, Zeinstra EC, Kooij RV, Colenbrander B, Bevers MM. Effects of cumulus cell removal of *in vitro* matured bovine oocytes prior to *in vitro* fertilization on subsequent cleavage rate. Theriogenology 2002;57:1347-55.

61. Wongsrikeao P, Kaneshige Y, Ooki R, Taniguchi M, Agung B, Nii M, Otoi T. Effect of the removal of cumulus cells on the nuclear maturation, fertilization and development of porcine oocytes. Reprod Domest Anim 2005;40:166-70.

62. Mansour RT, Aboulghar MA, Serour GI, Abbass AM. Co-culture of human pronucleate oocytes with their cumulus cells. Hum Reprod 1994;9:1727-9.

63. Khamsi F, Roberge S, Lacanna IC, Wong J, Yavas Y. Effects of granulosa cells, cumulus cells, and oocyte density on *in vitro* fertilization in woman. Endocrine 1999;10:161-6.

64. Zheng YL, Jiang MX, Zhang YL, Sun QY, Chen DY. Effects of oocyte age, cumulus cells and injection methods on *in vitro* development of intracytoplasmic sperm injection rabbit embryos. Zygote 2004;12:75-80.

65. Desai N, Lawson J, Goldfarb J. Assessment of growth factor effects on post-thaw development of cryopreserved mouse morulae to the blastocyst stage. Hum Reprod 2000;15:2, 410-8.

66. Bavister BD. Culture of preimplantation embryos: facts and artifacts. Hum Reprod Update 1995;1:91-148.

67. Ben-Chetrit A, Jurisicova A, Casper RF. Co-culture with ovarian cancer cell enhances human blastocyst formation *in vitro*. Fertil Steril 1996;65:664-6.

68. Echternkamp SE, Spicer LJ, Gregory KE, Canning SF, Hammond JM. Concentrations of insulin-like growth factor-I in blood and ovarian follicular fluid of cattle selected for twins. Biol Reprod 1990;43:8-14.

69. Rabinovici J, Dandekar P, Angle MJ, Rosenthal S, Martin MC. Insulinlike growth factor I (IGF-I) levels in follicular fluid from human preovulatory follicles: Correlation with serum IGF-I levels, Fertil. Steril 1990;54:428-33.

70. Mason HD, Willis DS, Holly JM, Franks S. Insulin preincubation enhances insulin-like growth factor-II (IGF-II) action on steroidogenesis in human granulosa cells. J Clin Endocrinol Metab 1994;78:1265-7.

71. Zolti M, Ben-Rafael Z, Meirom R, Shemesh M, Bider D, Mashiach S, et al. Cytokine involvement in oocytes and early embryos. Fertil Steril 1991;56:265-72.

72. Austgulen R, Arntzen KJ, Vatten LJ, Kahn J, Sunde A. Detection of cytokines (interleukin-1, interleukin-6, transforming growth factorbeta) and soluble tumour necrosis factor receptors in embryo culture fluids during *in vitro* fertilization. Hum Reprod 1995;10:171-6.

73. Kamat BR, Brown LF, Manseau EJ, Senger DR, Dvorak HF. Expression of vascular permeability factor/vascular endothelial growth factor by human granulosa and theca lutein cells. Role in corpus luteum development. Am J Pathol 1995;146:157– 65.

74. Abbas MM, Evans JJ, Sin IL, Gooneratne A, Hill A, Benny PS. Vascular endothelial growth factor and leptin: regulation in human cumulus cells and in follicles. Acta Obstet Gynecol Scand 2003;82:997-1003.

75. Schoolcraft W, Lane M, Stevens J, Gardner DK. Increased hyaluronan concentration in the embryo transfer medium results in a significant increase in human embryo implantation rate. Fertil Steril 2002;78: Abstract Book O-11.

76. Parikh F, Nadkarni SG, Naik NJ, Naik DJ, Uttamchandani SA. Cumulus co-culture and cumulus-aided embryo transfer increases pregnancy rates in patients undergoing *in vitro* fertilization. Fertil Steril 2006;86:4, 839-47.

Oocyte and Embryo Wastage in ART: It is in the Seed, not the Soil

Sujata Kar

OVERVIEW

Natural human reproduction is very inefficient in achieving live births. A number of studies have shown that the maximum chances of conceiving a clinically recognized pregnancy in one natural menstrual cycle is about 30 percent under optimal conditions for conception. This implies that, in nature, almost 70 percent of human embryos are lost at various stages from the preimplantation embryo to full term pregnancies. Clinical pregnancy loss is only the tip of the iceberg. The vast majority of conceptions are lost even before the woman realizes she might be pregnant. The reproductive loss that occurs even before a first missed period is substantial. Following fertilization about 30 percent embryos fail to implant, another 30 percent are lost after the embryo has started implanting but before the pregnancy is clinically recognized.

This massive biological loss can be traced to the time of formalities of the primary germ cell in the fetal ovaries. As we know, 80 percent of the oocytes undergo apoptosis even before the human female is born. This huge loss of oocytes in such a short time has been described as mass cellular suicide. Similarly, we encounter high rates of embryo and oocyte wastage with the use of assisted reproductive techniques (ART) from the time of oocyte retrieval to the formation of cleavage stage embryos, low implantation rates and high rates of pregnancy loss. This raises the obvious question of how far we can take the success of *in vitro* fertilization (IVF)? Have we reached the limits of improving pregnancy rates in IVF? Is it possible that majority of oocytes and embryos are intrinsically abnormal and not capable of implantation or developing further?

Thus, it has become clear that right from the time of fetal germ cell production to live births, human reproduction is an extremely wasteful exercise both in nature and also in assisted reproduction. A process of continuous reduction or selection against aneuploid embryos starts right from the time of fertilization.

The availability of sensitive assays for determining human chorionic gonadotropin (hCG) levels and assisted reproductive techniques like IVF have made it possible to observe the events from ovulation to the ongoing pregnancy. Intense research is on in the field of implantation with focus on biomarkers of early embryos, cytogenetics, and genetic regulation of implantation. Current methods used in the laboratory for embryo selection do help to choose better embryos but are still inaccurate. Preimplantation genetic screening (PGS) and metabolomic profiling are techniques that may help to select chromosomally normal embryos, however, they are not practical and cost-effective yet.

The future probably lies in identifying genes in the oocytes, which control embryo development and implantation, and genes that regulate programmed cell death.

INTRODUCTION

Natural Human Reproduction

Although planet earth is facing a population explosion, it is a known fact that the fecundity of the human race is very low. Human reproduction is very inefficient in achieving live births right from the time of the formation of the primary germ cell line in the fetal ovaries. This was first highlighted in a publication by Roberts and Lowe in 1975, where the number of births registered in England in 1970 was compared with the number of births that might have been expected, given the estimated number of fertile ovulatory cycles exposed to coitus in the same year and population.[1] The authors put forth the question "Where have all the conceptions gone?" since only 22 percent of the cycles at risk of pregnancy resulted in live birth.

A number of studies have since reported[2,3] that the maximal chance of conceiving a clinically recognized pregnancy in one cycle is about 30 percent when the circumstances for conception are optimal. Pregnancies may be lost at any time between fertilization and implantation or up to term. Clinical pregnancy loss is only the tip of the iceberg. The vast majority of conceptions are lost even before the woman realizes she might be pregnant.

The reproductive loss that occurs even before a missed period is substantial. Following fertilization, about 30 percent embryos fail to implant, another 30 percent are lost after the embryo has started implanting but before the pregnancy is clinically recognized.[4]

Availability of sensitive assays for determination of serum levels of human chorionic gonadotropin (hCG) and *in vitro* fertilization (IVF) technologies have made it possible to observe the events from ovulation to ongoing pregnancy. Intense research is on in the field of implantation, biomarkers of early embryos, cytogenetics, genetic regulation of implantation and so on.

This has literally opened up the previously elusive black box of early pregnancy.[5] Our understanding of the natural limits of human fecundity has thus improved. In nature, human pregnancy wastage occurs on a scale that only about 25 to 30 percent of conceptions will progress to live births.

This raises the obvious question of how far we can take the success of IVF? Have we reached the limits of improving pregnancy rates in IVF?

Present Success of ART

The practice of ART has come a long way since 1978—birth of the first test-tube baby. In clinical practice, the availability of purified and recombinant products have made ovulation induction very comfortable for the patients and clinician. Many softer ovulation induction protocols are being tried without compromising on the success rates. Highly researched and scientifically prepared culture media are now easily available and along with improved culture conditions in the laboratory, have ensured the production optimal embryos in the laboratory. The success of frozen embryo transfer has made IVF cycles more cost-effective in many patients. Assisted laser hatching and preimplantation genetic diagnosis are likely to further improve pregnancy rates in assisted reproduction.

Over the last decade, clinicians are striving to reduce multiple pregnancy. Embryologists have concentrated on choosing top quality embryos using various morphological criteria. Elective single embryo and double embryo transfer policies are being adopted by many centers. Emphasis is on choosing high quality embryos, and the process starts right from grading the oocytes.

The 2003 assisted reproductive technology (ART) surveillance data from the USA[6] reported that the overall, 42 percent of embryo transfer procedures following ART resulted in a pregnancy and 35 percent resulted in a live birth delivery (delivery of one or more live born infants). The highest live birth rates were observed among ART

procedures utilizing freshly fertilized embryos from donor eggs (51%) while the multiple pregnancy rate ranged from 35 to 40 percent. Current data available from IVF practices in the USA indicate that there is a 27 percent live birth rate from all initiated cycles, which does show some improvement over previous years.[7] Despite improvements in laboratory and clinical practice, ongoing pregnancy rates from IVF remain 20 to 25 percent per started cycle.[5]

The role of early pregnancy loss in determining clinical outcomes of IVF is uncertain as there are very few studies reporting the true rate of pregnancy loss following IVF. In one of the early studies Liu et al.[8] reported a 4 percent occult pregnancy loss rate, which was much lower than that following natural conception. Later studies have shown the IVF premenstrual pregnancy loss to be more prevalent.

Data from oocyte donation studies suggest that impaired implantation may explain the early pregnancy loss observed in IVF. Oocyte donation is associated with higher implantation rates than routine ART (SART/ASRM 2002). A possible explanation for this observation is the more physiological endometrial milieu into which embryos are transferred in oocyte donation cases. Unlike routine IVF, the endometrium of the recipient is neither exposed to supraphysiological levels of hormones in the follicular phase nor the high luteal progesterone levels that may alter the endometrial receptivity.[9-12]

Thus, IVF cycles are marred with low implantation rates and high early pregnancy loss rates.

Enormous Biological Loss: Both in Nature and Assisted Reproduction

In nature, almost 70 percent of human embryos are lost at various stages from the preimplantation embryo to full term pregnancies. Similarly, there are high rates of embryo wastage with the use of ART. This biological wastage of gametes and embryos becomes even more pronounced if comparison is made between the number of oocytes retrieved with the live birth rate. This section will discuss two different issues of embryo and oocyte wastage.

CLINICAL DISCUSSION

Embryo and Oocyte Wastage

In a recent study reported in Fertility Sterility by Kovalevsky et al.[13] statistics for ART cycles using fresh, non-donor eggs and embryos were derived and the percentage of embryos wasted each year was calculated. Trends over time were evaluated for percentage of embryos wasted, the average number of embryos transferred, and the delivery per transfer rate. The percentage of embryos transferred that did not produce a live birth was 90.8 percent in 1995 and decreased to 84.9 percent in 2001. It was also noted that this trend correlated with a reduction in the number of embryos transferred (3.9–3.1) and an improvement in delivery rate per transfer (25–33.4%). The authors concluded that possibly, only a small fraction of embryos has the capacity to become a live birth. Clinicians should strive to reduce embryonic wastage without an adverse effect on the delivery rates by perfecting methods of ovarian stimulation, embryo screening and reducing the number of embryos transferred.

Patrizio et al.[14] in a very interesting study, reported the overall biological wastage from oocytes inseminated to ongoing pregnancy. The study group consisted of patients undergoing preimplantation genetic screening (PGS) for advanced maternal age, recurrent pregnancy loss and multiple failed IVF cycles. Of 333 oocytes inseminated, 183 (55%) provided embryos for biopsy, of which only 33 (18% per embryo and 9.9% per oocyte) were normal. 26 embryos were finally found suitable for transfer (14% per embryo and 7.8% per oocyte), of which five (1.5%) implanted and three (1%) resulted in live birth. Thus, 333 oocytes resulted in 3 live births.[14]

Cytogenetic studies of oocytes and preimplantation embryos support the concept that majority of the embryos and oocytes obtained during IVF are intrinsically chromosomally abnormal and therefore, lack the capacity to develop into good quality embryos and implant. Under current *in vitro* culture conditions, high rates of oocyte and embryo wastage are observed. The underlying causes for embryo demise could be DNA damage, poor embryo metabolism, suboptimal culture conditions, or intrinsic chromosomal imbalance. Abnormalities in zygotes and preimplantation embryos are observed during IVF/intracytoplasmic sperm injection (ICSI) right from fertilization.

Rates of abnormal fertilization vary from 2 to 9 percent.[5] The two main categories are haploid (one pronucleus) or triploid (three pronuclei). One pronucleus may be due to non-decondensation of the sperm nuclear material or by pathogenetic activation of the oocyte. Embryos originating from a single pronuclear zygote may be considered for transfer only if normally fertilized two pronuclear zygotes are not available for transfer.[15] Tripronuclear zygotes may be a result of dispermy or nonextrusion of the 2nd polar body. They cleave fast and may develop into blastocysts, but should not be considered for transfer.

Chromosomal Abnormalities in Preimplantation Embryos

Analysis of Cleavage Stage Embryos

Embryos cultured *in vitro* show various morphological features, which are very commonly used as embryo selection criteria.

a. Morphologically normal embryos
b. Multinucleation in blastomeres
c. Cytoplasmic fragmentation
d. Dominant blastomere
e. Abnormal or delayed cell division
f. Embryo arrest.

1. *Karyotype analysis of morphologically normal embryos*: Reports have been published giving a 20 to 40 percent rate of chromosomal abnormalities in normal appearing preimplantation embryos. Munne et al.[16] report a 29 percent abnormality rate. Similar rates were reported for human blastocysts, although there have also been reports of almost 100 percent chromosomal mosaicism at the blastocyst stage.[17]

   The observations reported from these studies is complicated and there is disparity in the results. From the recent data, it is becoming apparent that many factors could determine the chromosomal aneuploidy rates. Additionally, the timing and technique used for analysis could give variable results. There is a need to find improved techniques for chromosomal analysis of cleavage stage embryos.

2. *Chromosomal abnormalities in fragmented and multinucleated embryos*: The percentage of fragmentation has been associated with chromosomal abnormalities, mostly mosaicism.[18] Detected by fluorescent *in situ* hybridization (FISH), embryos with 45 to 100 percent fragmentation showed 89 percent mosaics and 11 percent aneuploidy, i.e. an almost 100 percent abnormality rate, whereas 0 to 15 percent fragmentation showed 29 percent and 11 percent mosaics and aneuploids, respectively.[19] Embryos with multinucleated blastomeres are normally associated with abnormal embryo development and/ or dysmorphism. A recent study has reported that the presence of multinucleated cells in viable embryos could indicate up to 74 percent chromosomal abnormality (extensive mosaicism and/or polyploidy).

3. *Chromosomal abnormalities and embryo development*: Majority (71%) of arrested embryos are chromosomally abnormal, the dominant disorder being polyploidy followed by mosaicism and aneuploidy. Around 57 percent of slow developing embryos are abnormal, showing aneuploidy (23%) in the majority, followed by mosaicism (22%) and polyploidy (13%).[16]

   Few external factors have been implicated in high rates of chromosome abnormalities in cleaving embryos. The type of hormonal stimulation, temperature, water and air quality may influence chromosomal abnormalities (19%).

Programmed Cell Death and Embryo Wastage

Programmed cell death is a finely co-ordinated set of events involving at least 100 gene products that can either suppress or activate cellular self destruction.[20] The fate of a cell i.e. whether it lives, differentiates or dies is determined by the balance between cell death suppressor versus cell death inducers. Increasing evidence now indicates that cell fate is determined by the outcome of specific intracellular interactions between pro- and anti-apoptotic proteins, many of which are expressed during oocyte and preimplantation embryo development.

Recent data shows that the onset of apoptosis seems to be developmentally regulated in a stage-specific manner, however, the underlying molecular mechanisms are yet to be determined. Of course, chromosomal abnormalities are one cause of developmental arrest, fragmentation of oocytes and embryos. Activation of programmed cell death pathways play an important role in preimplantation embryo survival. Cell death triggers could be DNA damage, poor embryo metabolism, suboptimal culture conditions and so on.

Current concepts and advances in the understanding of the regulation of cell death gene expression in the preimplantation embryo is beyond the scope of this chapter.

Programmed Cell Death and Massive Oocyte Loss in the Human Ovarian Germ Cell Line

Primordial germ cells are the direct precursors of oocytes. They start proliferating by the sixth gestational week, reaching 6 to 7 million oogonia by 16 to 20 weeks. Loss of germ cells starts from this time onwards. A massive loss of oocytes (close to 4.5 million) occurs over the next 20 weeks. The new born female is born with 1 to 2 million oocytes per ovary, having lost 80 percent of her oocytes much much before even attaining reproductive potential. This huge loss of oocytes in such a short time has been described as mass cellular suicide.[21] The functional lifespan of the female gonads is determined by the size and rate of depletion of the oocyte stock in the ovaries at birth. This is also described as the female biological clock, which is driven by a genetic program of cell death. This programmed cell death (apoptosis) claims up to 99.9 percent of the mammalian germ cell line, which is ultimately responsible for menopause, ovarian failure and infertility.[22] The study of germ cell death is still at its infancy. However, many interesting questions arise:

How and why does the female body create so many germ cells only to deplete them?

Is it possible to prolong the lifespan of a female by manipulating oocyte depletion?

Can this information be used therapeutically to treat infertility and the aging process?

Implications for ART

Despite the advances today, IVF has low implantation and high embryo wastage rates. Current studies put forth the hypothesis that a large number of human oocytes and embryos are chromosomally abnormal (aneuploides) and possibly, not capable of producing a healthy pregnancy. Additionally, genes regulating programmed cell death claim a large number of gametes and zygotes, which may be morphologically and chromosomally normal. Thus, it is fair to presume that success rates greater than the maximal rates reported in spontaneous cycles will not be achieved unless the aneuploid embryo is eliminated from the selection process.

In both IVF and ICSI, the most challenging and difficult step is to select the most competent embryo for transfer.

What is a Good Embryo (The Seed)?

Selection of the most competent embryo is generally based on morphological criteria. Morphological characteristics are, however, notoriously hard to describe, are often unambiguous and findings often do not correlate between early and late stages of development. Moreover, considerable interobserver variability is not unusual. Many scoring systems, currently being used, are crude, using only a few characteristics like fragmentation, cell number, and general appearance of the blastomeres and that too, only on the day of embryo transfer. Such traditional practices do not tap the full potential of morphological scoring. Careful observation and documentations should be a part of every IVF laboratory. The embryologist should consider information from all stages of development starting from the oocyte, zygote and embryo by which, a much better prediction can be achieved rather than by only using day 2 morphology.

Oocyte morphology and embryonic development have been well correlated.[23,24] Many transcription factors (indicating upregulation of certain genes) have a polarized distribution in the oocyte. Oocytes with dark, coarse or pitted cytoplasm are much more likely to be aneuploid. Abnormal cytoplasm in the oocyte is associated with poor development and this factor should be considered while selecting embryos for transfer or freezing.[25]

Polar body morphology has been well-correlated with subsequent blastocyst development and implantation. Polar body shape (round or ovoid), fragmentation, orientation and size of the perivitelline space has been used by researchers to grade oocytes. Round or ovoid, unfragmented polar bodies with a small perivitelline space has been associated with better development potential.[25]

Scoring the pronuclear (PN) and nucleolus morphology for predicting the developmental potential of zygotes has been in use. Normally, the two PNs appear within a short interval and rapidly migrate to the center of the cytoplasm, nucleoli form and become polarized at adjacent poles of the apposed PNs. Asynchrony of nucleolar dynamics are associated with lower developmental potential. PN and nucleolar morphology seem to have a strong correlation with blastocyst development and should be considered for embryo selection.[25]

Blastomere size, shape and number are a regular part of all embryo scoring systems. It is generally agreed that uneven, irregular, cleared and unequal blastomeres have poor developmental potential. Multinucleated blastomeres should be assessed with multiple charts. They are highly likely to be chromosomally abnormal, especially if all the blastomeres are multinucleated. If normal embryos are not available, only then those with minimal and late multinucleation may be considered for embryo transfer.

The appearance of the zona pellucida, as an indicator of embryo quality, has been described.[26,27] Embryos with uneven zona may make it easier to hatch and thus, implant.

Embryo cytoplasmic fragmentation is commonly used for embryo scoring. The pattern and degree of fragmentation are both used according to the definition of Alikari et al.[28] Pattern comprises of (a) minimal volume in one blastomere, (b) localized fragments in the perivitelline space (PVS) (c) small fragments all over the embryo and (d) large fragments resembling a whole blastomere. The degree of fragmentation is expressed in percentage and defined as the volume of the PVS and/or the cleavage cavity occupied by the enucleated cytoplasmic fragments.

Cleavage rate has now emerged as a major determinant of development.[25] Embryos that start cleaving early and are at the four-cell stage 42 hours postinsemination have a better developmental potential. Thus, it would appear that systematic observation, recording and analysis of morphological characteristics starting from the oocyte, significantly increase the ability to select good embryos.

Yet, to improve the current pregnancy rates, we need newer techniques to identify the aneuploid embryos. Many of the morphologically normal embryos are aneuploid or chromosomally abnormal.

Role of Preimplantation Genetic Screening in Embryo Selection

Preimplantation genetic diagnosis (PGD) was first introduced in 1990. Today, PGD has become a clinically established procedure in ART. Initially, PGD was being performed for monogenic disorders like—X-linked disorders, cystic fibrosis, Tay Sach's disease, etc. With the development of FISH, PGD is now being used for aneuploidy detection for a number of clinically significant chromosomes.

The genetic material for PGD is derived from three possible sources:
a. Polar bodies
b. Blastomeres from early cleaving embryos (D3, 6 to 10 cell stage)
c. Trophectoderm cells from blastocysts.

Preimplantation genetic screening (PGS) is being using generally for the following indications:
- Advanced maternal age
- Repeated IVF failure
- Repeated miscarriage
- Testicular sperm extraction (TESE)-ICSI.

Currently, PGD can be used for about 50 monogenic disorders and chromosomal aneuploidy screening for chromosome number X,Y,13,14,15,16,18,21,22.

Although PGS for aneuploidy is being used more and more often for selecting embryos for transfer, its effectiveness is still unclear.

A Cochrane Database Review[29] reported the latest analysis results in 2006. The authors concluded that there is insufficient data to determine whether PGS is an effective intervention in IVF/ICSI to improve birth rates.

Available data on PGS for advanced maternal age showed no difference in live birth and ongoing pregnancy rates. More properly conducted randomized controlled trials are needed.

Role of Metabolic Profiling of the Embryo

Today, there are no biological criteria or objective analytical methods to assist in the process of embryo selection. Morphological criteria is the primary determinant of embryo viability, unfortunately, morphological analysis does not equate to biological functionality. Embryologists have to depend on this grading in the absence of alternative methods. New technology that is capable of selecting only functionally competent oocytes and embryos can lead to markedly improved success rates in an IVF program. PGS and genomic testing have limitations. They are labor intensive procedures, lack sensitivity and specificity, and are considered controversial, since they require a single cell biopsy at the early embryo stage. Prenatal genetic diagnosis (PGD) is still regarded as an experimental procedure by the Food and Drug Administration (FDA) and American Society of Reproductive Medicine (ASRM).

Metabolomic profiling is new technology used in the laboratory. Semen, follicular fluid, culture media of the embryo during culture and prior to transfer are specimens that are usually discarded and can be analyzed for multiple biomarkers of oxidative stress. This is a non-invasive test, performed on normally discarded culture media. An embryo, which is healthy and likely to result in pregnancy, has a different metabolism than a non-healthy embryo and these differences can be picked up from the fluid in which the embryo is cultured. The embryo literally eats and breaths into it.

Quantification may be possible using spectroscopic analysis and advanced bioinformatics. The technology of metabolomic profiling of the embryo is now commercially available in the USA from a company called Molecular Biometrics. If proven to be accurate and reliable, this breakthrough technology could provide IVF practitioners a new tool for accurate selection of the embryo for transfer.

CONCLUSION

The embryo or the endometrium (seed or the soil): The role of the endometrium in establishing a pregnancy is now becoming very clear. The implantation window is the self-limiting period of endometrial receptivity during which the endometrium opens up to receive the embryo. Various morphological and biochemical markers are being proposed to define the implantation window. Recently, genes regulating the implantation window have been recognized. It is obvious that extreme fine tuning or perfect co-ordination of ovulation induction, luteal support and timing of embryo transfer is of prime importance for successful nidation.

However, within the implantation window, it will have to be the biological competence of the embryo which will determine pregnancy.

It has become clear that right from the time of fetal germ cell production to live births, human reproduction is an extremely wasteful exercise, both in nature and also in assisted reproduction. A process of continuous reduction or selection against aneuploid embryos starts right from the time of fertilization.

REFERENCES

1. Roberts J, Lowe R. Where have all the conceptions gone? Lancet 1975;1:636-7.
2. Zinaman MJ, Clegg ED, Brown CC, O'Connor J, Selevan SG. Estimates of human fertility and pregnancy loss. Fertil Steril 1996;65:503-9.
3. Slama R, Eustache F, Ducot B, Jensen TK, Jørgensen N, Horte A, et al. Time to pregnancy and semen parameters: A cross sectional study among fertile couples from four European cities. Hum Reprod 2002;17:503-15.
4. Leon Speroff, Marc A. Fritz, Clinical Gynecological endocrinology and infertility 7th edition, 2005, Lippincott Williams and Wilkins, Fertilization and implantation: 245-6.
5. Macklon NS, Geraedts JP, Fauser BC. Conception to ongoing pregnancy: The 'black box' of early pregnancy loss. Hum Reprod Update 2002;8:333-43.
6. Wright VC, Chang J, Jeng G, Macaluso M. Assisted reproductive technology surveillance: United States, 2003. MMWR Surveill Summ. 2006;55:1-22.
7. Jain T, Missmer SA, Hornstein MD. Trends in embryo-transfer practice and in outcomes of the use of assisted reproductive technology in the United States. N Engl J Med 2004;350:1639-45.
8. Liu HC, Jones GS, Jones HW Jr, Rosenwaks Z. Mechanisms and factors of early pregnancy wastage in *in vitro* fertilization: Embryo transfer patients. Fertil Steril 1988;50:95-101.
9. Horcajadas JA, Riesewijk A, Polman J, van Os R, Pellicer A, Mosselman S, Simón C. Effect of controlled ovarian hyperstimulation in IVF on endometrial gene expression profiles. Mol Hum Reprod 2005;11:195-201.
10. Devroey P, Bourgain C, Macklon NS, Fauser BC. Reproductive biology and IVF: Ovarian stimulation and endometrial receptivity. Trends Endocrinol Metab 2004;15:84-90.
11. Bourgain C, Devroey P. The endometrium in stimulated cycles for IVF. Hum Reprod Update 2003;9:515-22.
12. Fauser BC, Devroey P. Reproductive biology and IVF. Ovarian stimulation and luteal phase consequences. Trends Endocrinol Metab 2003;14:236-42.
13. Kovalevsky G, Patrizio P. High rates of embryo wastage with the use of assisted reproductive technology: A look at the trends between 1995 and 2001 in the united states. Fertil Steril 2005;84:325–30.
14. Patrizio P, Bianchi V, Lolioti MD, Garasimova T, Sakkas D. High rate of biological loss in assisted reproduction: It is in the seed, not in the soil. Reprod Biomed ONLINE. 2007;14:92-5.
15. A Color Atlas for Human Assisted Reproduction. Pasquale Patrizio, Michael J Tucker, Vanessa Guelman, Lippincott Wiliams and Wilkins – 2003.
16. Munné S, Alikani M, Tomkin G, Grifo J, Cohen J. Embryo morpohology, development rates and maternal age are correlated with chromosome abnormalities. Fertil Steril 1995;64:382-91.
17. Ruangvutilert P, Delhanty JD, Serhal P, Simopoulou M, Rodeck CH, Harper JC. FISH analysis on day 5 postinsemination of human arrested and blastocyst stage embryos. Prenat Diagn 2000;20:552-60.
18. Pellestor F, Sèle B. Assessment of aneuploidy in the human female by using cytogenetics of IVF failure. Am J Hum Genet 1988;42:274-83.
19. Munné S, Cohen J. Chromosome abnormalities in human embryos. Hum Reprod Update. 1998;4:842-55.
20. Jurisicova A, Acton BM. Deadly decisions: The role of genes regulating programmed cell death in human preimplantation embryo development. Reproduction 2004;128:281-91.
21. Morita Y, Tilly JL. Oocyte apoptosis: like sand through an hourglass. Dev Biol 1999;213:1-17.
22. Tilly JL. Commuting the death sentence: how oocytes strive to survive. Nat Rev Mol Cell Biol 2001;2:838-48.
23. Van Blerkom J, Henry G. Oocyte dysmorphism and aneuploidy in meiotically mature human oocytes after ovarian stimulation. Hum Reprod 1992;7:379-90.
24. Antczak M, Van Blerkom J. Oocyte influences on early development: The regulatory proteins leptin and STAT3 are polarized in mouse and human oocyte and differentially distributed within the cells of the preimplantation stage embryo.Mol Hum Reprod 1997;3:1067-86.
25. Sjöblom P, Menezes J, Cummins L, Mathiyalagan B, Costello MF. Prediction of embryo developmental potential and pregnancy based on early stage morphological characteristics. Fertil Steril 2006;86:848-61.
26. Cohen J, Inge KL, Suzman M, Wiker SR, Wright G. Video cinematography of fresh and cryopreserved embryos, a retrospective analysis of embryonic morphology and implantation. Fertil Steril 1989;51:820-7.
27. Palmstierna M, Murkes D, Csemiczky G, Andersson O, Wramsby H. Zona pellucida thickness variation and occurrence of visible mononucleated blastomeres in pre-embryos are associated with a high pregnancy rates in IVF treatment. J Assist Reprod Genet 1998,15:70-5.
28. Alikani M, Cohen J, Tomkin G, Garrisi GJ, Mack C, Scott RT. Human embryo fragmentation *in vitro* and its implications for pregnancy and implantation. Fertil Steril 1999;71:836-42.
29. Twisk M, Mastenbroek S, van Wely M, Heineman MJ, Van der Veen F, Repping S. Preimplantation genetic screening for abnormal number of chromosomes (aneuploidies) in *in vitro* fertilisation or intracytoplasmic sperm injection. Cochrane Database Syst Rev 2006;(1):CD005291.

Preimplantation Genetic Diagnosis

Preimplantation Genetic Diagnosis: Expansion of Indications and Technical Advances

Sanjeev Khot, Manisha Joshi

OVERVIEW

The use of preimplantation genetic diagnosis (PGD) to assist the identification and preferential transfer of healthy euploid embryos should improve implantation rates, reduce miscarriages and trisomic offspring, and ultimately lead to an increase in live birth rates. Preimplantation genetic diagnosis is a technique by which early human embryos are genetically screened for genetic diseases and then discarded or transferred into the womb using assisted reproductive techniques (ART). PGD is proved to be a boon to couples with a high risk of transmitting an inherited condition like—monogenic disorder, autosomal recessive, autosomal dominant or X-linked disorder, or a chromosomal structural aberration such as a balanced translocation. It is an alternative to prenatal diagnosis. The main advantage of PGD is that it avoids selective pregnancy termination as the method ensures a pregnancy free of the disease under consideration, thus avoiding the difficult choice of abortion. PGD is helpful for mitochondrial DNA (mtDNA) mutations, which are usually serious pleiotropic disorders with maternal inheritance like Neurogenic ataxia retinitis pigmentosa (NARP). The topic also throws light on PGD for Alzheimer's disease, cancer disposition syndromes, as is discussed with case studies, breast cancer antigen (BRCA) 1 and BRCA 2 gene testing and non-medical traits like inherited deafness. In this chapter, we have discussed about pregenetic screening (PGS), which is offered to patients with a history of recurrent miscarriages, non-obstructive azoospermia and advanced maternal age. The technical aspects of PGD cover the topics of denudation of oocytes, intracytoplasmic sperm injection (ICSI), and evaluation of the embryo. The various biopsy procedures involved, like blastocyst biopsy, polar body biopsy, laser assisted biopsy, cleavage stage biopsy, and the merits and demerits of each biopsy technique has also been discussed in this chapter. Fluorescent *in situ* hybridization (FISH) and polymerase chain reaction (PCR) are the two most commonly used techniques in PGD, and the demerits of using these techniques is also a topic in this article. Preimplantation genetic haplotyping (PGH) is a new clinical method of PGD. The topic covers the ethical aspects of PGD and the regulatory authority in the world and the Indian scenario.

INTRODUCTION

Preimplantation genetic diagnosis (PGD) is an option for couples who are at risk of transmitting serious genetic diseases that enables them to have unaffected progeny without facing the risk of pregnancy termination after prenatal diagnosis, as currently practised. It is also one of the practical tools used in assisted reproduction techniques to improve the chance of conception for infertility cases with a poor prognosis. Because PGD is performed using a single biopsied cell, technological advances are important to improving PGD accuracy.[1]

Before PGD, couples at a high risk for conceiving a children with particular disorders would have to initiate the pregnancy and then undergo chorionic villus sampling (CVS) in the first trimester or amniocentesis in the second trimester to test the fetus for the presence of disease. If the fetus tested positive for the disorder, the couple would be faced with the dilemma of whether or not to terminate the pregnancy. With PGD, couples are much more likely to have healthy babies.

In 1967, Robert Edwards and David Gardner reported the successful sexing of rabbit blastocysts, setting the first steps towards PGD.[2] It was not until the 1980s that human IVF was fully developed, which coincided with the breakthrough of the highly sensitive polymerase chain reaction (PCR) technology. Handyside and collaborators' first successful attempts at testing were in October 1989, with the first births in 1990 though the preliminary experiments had been published some years earlier.[3]

In these first cases, PCR was used for sex determination for patients carrying X-linked diseases. With the development of interphase single cell fluorescent *in situ* hybridization (FISH) in the early 1990s, the indications for PGD are expanding to include a plethora of chromosomal disorders, as discussed further. More than 3000 PGD cycles have been performed until now with a pregnancy rate of around 24 percent. The procedure is safe and the incidence of abnormalities is equivalent to that in the general population.[4] This has contributed to the avoidance of misdiagnosis in PGD for single gene disorders, and extensive experience in PGD for chromosomal disorders suggests strategies for more reliable evaluation of the chromosomal status of the preimplantation embryo.[1]

CLINICAL DISCUSSION

Indications and Conditions for PGD

Couples are at Risk of Transmitting a known Genetic Abnormality to their Children

Only healthy and normal embryos are transferred into the mother's uterus, thus diminishing the risk of inheriting a genetic abnormality and late pregnancy termination (after positive prenatal diagnosis).

Couples who are at a risk are those with the following disorders:

- Monogenic disorders
- Autosomal recessive disorders (cystic fibrosis, beta-thalassemia, sickle cell disease, spinal muscular atrophy type 1, Tay-Sachs disease).
- Autosomal dominant or X-linked disorders (myotonic dystrophy, Huntington's disease, Charcot-Marie-Tooth disease).
- X-linked diseases (Fragile X syndrome, Hemophilia A, Duchenne's muscular dystrophy).

Preimplantation Genetic Screening

Early pregnancy losses can be attributed to aneuploidy. In preimplantation genetic screening (PGS), only chromosomally normal embryos are transferred into the uterus, thus reducing the risk of first and second trimester losses.

Preimplantation genetic diagnosis (PGD) is helpful for patients with unexplained infertility, recurrent miscarriages, unsuccessful *in vitro* fertilization (IVF) cycles, advanced maternal age, or male factor infertility. In these cases, the most likely cause is a chromosome abnormality.

Chromosome abnormalities include aneuploidy and structural abnormalities. Aneuploidy is the most common chromosomal abnormality. Aneuploidy can occur in both oocytes and sperm. Structural abnormalities include translocations, inversions, and deletions. Structural chromosome abnormalities can also be present in oocytes and sperm. The transmission of a chromosome abnormality to an embryo can result in a low implantation rate, miscarriage or the birth of

a baby with a genetic disorder. Using FISH, the scientists in our PGD laboratory can identify the absence of these specific genetic disorders in each normally developing embryo. As a result, only those embryos free of genetic disease will be transferred to the patient's uterus so as to increase the chance of conception and ultimately, a healthy baby.

The term preimplantation genetic screening (PGS) is used to denote procedures that do not look for a specific disease but use PGD techniques to identify embryos at risk. PGD is a poorly chosen phrase because, in Medicine, to diagnose means to identify an illness or determine its cause. An oocyte or early-stage embryo has no symptoms of disease. They are not ill. Rather, they may have a genetic condition that could lead to disease. To screen means to test for anatomical, physiological, or genetic conditions in the absence of symptoms of disease. Hence, both PGD and PGS should be referred to as types of embryo screening.

Advanced Maternal Age

Women of advanced maternal age (≥ 37 years) are at a higher risk of producing aneuploid embryos, resulting in implantation failure, a higher risk of miscarriage or the birth of a child with a chromosome abnormality (e.g. Down's syndrome). This is due to the fact that all of the woman's oocytes are present at birth. Over time, the chromosomes within the oocytes are less likely to divide properly, resulting in cells with too many or too few chromosomes.

Aneuploidy is also believed to be a major reason for the decrease of fertility with age. Several studies have determined that approximately 70 percent of embryos from women of advanced maternal age may be aneuploid. Table 55.1 represents the incidence of chromosmal abnormalities with advanced age.[5]

For women aged 37 years and older undergoing IVF, PGD for aneuploidy significantly improves pregnancy rates, reduces miscarriage rates, and decreases the chance of a chromosomally abnormal pregnancy if six or more embryos of good quality are available for analysis.

Recurrent Pregnancy Loss

Fertile couples with repeated miscarriages should be evaluated for the presence of a chromosomal abnormality. The female

Table 55.1: Chromosomal abnormalities in advanced age[5]			
Age (years)	*Normal embryos (%)*	*Aneuploid embryos (%)*	*Other abnormality (%)*
25–35	61	8	31
36–37	60	10	30
38–39	47	18	35
40–41	43	26	31
42–44	39	30	31

or male partner may be a carrier of a balanced translocations or be an aneuploid mosaic. Approximately 5 to 8 percent of couples with a history of recurrent pregnancy loss have an abnormal karyotype, usually a balanced translocation. PGD can be performed for couples with a balanced translocation, allowing them to implant only chromosomally balanced embryos, thus reducing their risk of miscarriage. The use of PGD for translocations is technically more complicated than for aneuploidy.

Unsuccessful IVF Cycles and Unexplained Infertility

Preimplantation genetic diagnosis dramatically improves the chances of a successful IVF pregnancy in couples where prior IVF failures have remained unexplained. It has been estimated that over half of all IVF failures cannot be explained by an apparent problem with embryo quality. For many couples, however, this statistic is quite misleading. In most IVF centers, a close look at the appearance of embryos under the microscope is essential as they most often attempt to determine a good or high quality embryo from those of lesser quality. Generally, embryos are given good marks when they demonstrate an appropriate number of cell divisions at a given time in their growth cycle, when the individual cells of the embryo appear to have a uniform size and when there is an absence of cellular fragments that may or may not represent problems in the growth progress of the embryo.

Recent advances, however, have shown that even embryos receiving the highest ratings from scientists based on their normal or excellent appearance under the microscope may, in fact, be highly abnormal and totally incapable of ever producing a pregnancy. This discovery was brought about by the addition of PGD to the tools available to scientists in the IVF laboratory. PGD has offered physicians and scientists, for the first time ever, the ability to examine far beyond the superficial appearance of an embryo. We are now able to examine the most important internal genetic code of the embryo as well. And with these new genetic tools, we have come to learn that some embryos that appear on the surface to be of the highest quality may carry a genetic code that makes them poor choices for attempting to establish a healthy pregnancy.

Male Factor Infertility

In couples with severe male factor infertility, PGS/PGD may not only increase pregnancy rates but also limit the prevalence of chromosome abnormalities. Various genetic defects have been found to be associated with male factor infertility. This includes aneuploidy, most commonly Klinefelter's syndrome, Robertsonian translocations, Y chromosome microdeletions, androgen receptor mutations, and other autosomal gene mutations (e.g. cystic fibrosis transmembrane conductance regulator gene and sex hormone-binding globulin gene

mutations). Therefore, a high risk of transmission of genetic mutations to the patient's offspring is associated with IVF and particularly involving ICSI. This risk can be reduced by PGD.

Mitochondrial Disorders

Diseases arising from mitochondrial DNA (mtDNA) mutations are usually serious pleiotropic disorders with maternal inheritance. Owing to the high recurrence risk in the progeny of carrier females, 'at-risk' couples often ask for prenatal diagnosis. However, the reliability of such practices remains under debate. Preimplantation diagnosis, a theoretical alternative to conventional prenatal diagnosis, requires that the mutant load, measured in a single cell from an eight cell embryo, accurately reflect the overall heteroplasmy of the whole embryo, but this is not known to be the case.[6]

PGD for Neurogenic Ataxia Retinitis Pigmentosa

Mitochondrial DNA-associated (mtDNA-associated) Leigh syndrome and Neurogenic ataxia retinitis pigmentosa (NARP) (neurogenic muscle weakness, ataxia, and retinitis pigmentosa) are part of a continuum of progressive neurodegenerative disorders caused by abnormalities of mitochondrial energy generation. Leigh syndrome or subacute necrotizing encephalomyelopathy is characterized by the onset of symptoms typically between 3 and 12 months of age, often following a viral infection. Decompensation [often with elevated lactate levels in blood and/or cerebrospinal fluid (CSF)] during an intercurrent illness is typically associated with psychomotor retardation or regression. Neurologic features include hypotonia, spasticity, movement disorders (including chorea), cerebellar ataxia, and peripheral neuropathy. Extraneurologic manifestations may include hypertrophic cardiomyopathy. About 50 percent of affected individuals die by age three years, most often as a result of respiratory or cardiac failure. NARP is characterized by proximal neurogenic muscle weakness with sensory neuropathy, ataxia, and pigmentary retinopathy. Mutations in the mitochondrial genes MT-ATP6, MT-TL1, MT-TK, MT-TW, MT-TV, MT-ND1, MT-ND3, MT-ND4, MT-ND5, MT-ND6 and MT-CO3 are associated with mtDNA-associated Leigh's syndrome. MT-ATP6 is the only gene associated with NARP. Approximately 10 to 20 percent of individuals with Leigh's syndrome have either the m.8993T>G or m.8993T>C MT-ATP6 mutations; approximately 10 to 20 percent have mutations in other mitochondrial genes. Mitochondrial DNA-associated Leigh's syndrome and NARP are transmitted by maternal inheritance. The father of a proband is not at risk of having the disease-causing mtDNA mutation. The mother of a proband usually has the mtDNA mutation and may or may not have symptoms. In most cases, the mother has a much lower mutant load than the proband and usually remains asymptomatic or develops only mild symptoms. Occasionally, the mother has a substantial mutant load and develops severe symptoms in adulthood. The offspring of males with a mtDNA mutation are not at risk; all offspring of females with a mtDNA mutation are at risk of inheriting the mutation. The risk to the offspring of a female proband of developing symptoms depends on the tissue distribution and mutant load of the disease-causing mtDNA mutation. Prenatal diagnosis and PGD for couples at increased risk of having children with mitochondrial DNA-associated Leigh's syndrome and NARP may be possible by analysis of mtDNA extracted from non-cultured fetal cells or from single blastomeres, respectively; however, the use of molecular genetic test results to predict long-term outcome is difficult.[7]

Human Leukocyte Antigen Matching

Among the new indications of PGD is preimplantation human leukocyte antigen (HLA) matching. This technique cannot only be applied to exclude the presence of a genetic disorder, but also to provide a potential donor for stem cell or bone marrow transplantation to an affected child with recessive diseases, including thalassemias or acquired malignancies such as leukemia. This has been previously used to avoid the birth of a child with Fanconi anemia, an autosomal recessive disorder, whose HLA-matched cord blood stem cells were successfully transplanted to cure the affected sibling.[8]

RECENT ADVANCES IN PGD

Late Onset Diseases

PGD for Alzheimer's Disease

Verlinsky et al.[9] have reported the use of PGD by a woman who carried a gene for early onset Alzheimer's disease (AD), and who wished to have a child that would be free of that condition. PGD was carried out, and she gave birth to a child free of that condition.[9]

Cancer Predisposition Syndromes

Preimplantation genetic diagnosis can be used to avoid the birth of children who are healthy at birth but face a higher than average risk of having cancer or some other serious disease. Recently, Rechitsky et al.[13] have used PGD for a group of couples at risk for producing children with cancer predisposition. The procedure was performed for patients with predisposition to familial adenomatous polyposis coli (FAP), Von Hippel-Lindau syndrome (VHL), retinoblastoma, Li-Fraumeni syndrome, determined by p53 tumor suppressor gene mutations, neurofibromatosis types I and II and familial posterior fossa brain tumor (hSNF5). Overall, 20 PGD cycles were performed for 10 couples, resulting in preselection and transfer of 40 mutation-free embryos, which resulted in five

unaffected clinical pregnancies and four healthy children were born.[10,11]

PGD can also be used to identify genetic mutations like BRCA-1, BRCA-2, which do not cause a specific disease but increases the risk of a set of diseases if present in the family. In May 2006, the UK Human Fertilisation and Embryology Authority (HFEA) approved the use of PGD for lower penetrance, late onset cancer susceptibility syndromes such as hereditary breast and ovarian cancer.[10-12]

PGD for Sex Selection

Sex Selection

Many couples request PGS for sex selection, which can be motivated by cultural, social, ethnic, psychological, and other reasons, such as the desire for family balancing, which is possible because of PGD.

The use of PGS for sex selection unrelated to disease is controversial and has elicited moral outrage about not implanting normal embryos when they are found to be of the undesired sex. Frequent objections include the danger of sex discrimination, the perpetuation of oppression against females, the ethics of expanding control over non-essential characteristics (those not required for life) of offspring, and the relative importance of sex selection when weighed against medical and financial burdens to parents. Personal, religious, ethical, and moral norms vary among different populations, and proper respect must be given to these views when discussing the performance of PGS for sex selection. Much discussion is still necessary to achieve a reasonable consensus and acceptance of PGD for sex selection.[13]

PGD for Non-medical Traits

Inherited Deafness

Tests for GJB2 mutations—the largest known contributor to inherited deafness, if available, will lead people with a family history of deafness to possibly request PGD to screen out embryos with the mutation, in order to increase their chances of having a child without a hearing disability. Because hearing is clearly beneficial to a child, a major ethical concern with this practice would be the prejudice to the deaf community that it might cause.[12]

Technical Aspects of PGD

Before requesting PGD, candidates should consult a geneticist or a genetic counselor to evaluate the risk of transferring their genetic abnormality to their offspring. Tests should be performed to confirm the diagnosis of the affected parent, to pinpoint the genetic change leading to the condition in question, and to ensure that the currently available technology can identify that genetic change in a polar body, cleavage state, or blastocyst embryo biopsy. In order to have embryos to biopsy for PGD/PGS, patients must undergo *in vitro* fertilization (IVF).

Intracytoplasmic Sperm Injection

In the majority of the reported cycles, intracytoplasmic sperm injection (ICSI) is used instead of IVF. The main reasons are to prevent contamination with residual sperm adhered to the zona pellucida and to avoid unexpected fertilization failure.

Evaluation of Embryos

Non-affected or normal embryos transferred into the uterus, are found to be free of any inherited disease by FISH or PCR for subsequent implantation/pregnancy.

Biopsy Procedures

Preimplantation genetic diagnosis can be performed on cells from different developmental stages; the biopsy procedures vary accordingly. After fertilization of the oocyte with sperm, embryos are allowed to develop into cleavage-stage embryos. On day 3 after egg retrieval (equivalent to 2 days after fertilization), a single blastomere is removed from the developing embryo for performance of FISH or PCR for genetic evaluation of the embryo. A biopsy may be performed

- On unfertilized and fertilized oocytes [for polar bodies (PBs)].
- On day three, cleavage-stage embryos (for blastomeres).
- On blastocysts (for trophectoderm cells).

Polar Body Biopsy

Polar body biopsy works only for female chromosomal disorders. The mature metaphase II oocyte extrudes a single polar body. This polar body can be removed and tested, providing information on only the chromosomal content of the oocyte.

Disadvantages of polar body biopsy: The disadvantages of PB biopsy is that, it only provides information about the maternal contribution to the embryo, which is why cases of autosomal dominant and X-linked disorders, that are maternally transmitted, can be diagnosed, and autosomal recessive disorders can only partially be diagnosed. Another drawback is the increased risk of diagnostic error, for instance, due to the degradation of the genetic material or events of recombination that lead to heterozygous first PBs. It is generally agreed that it is best to analyze both PBs in order to minimize the risk of misdiagnosis. This can be achieved by sequential biopsy, necessary if monogenic diseases are diagnosed, to be able to differentiate the first from the second PB, or simultaneous biopsy if FISH is to be performed. In Germany, where the legislation bans the selection of preimplantation embryos, PB analysis is the only possible method to perform PGD.

The biopsy and analysis of the first and second PBs can be completed before syngamy, which is the moment from which the zygote is considered an embryo and becomes protected by the law. Because only information about the mother can be obtained by analyzing polar bodies, chromosomal abnormalities occurring after fertilization (when the sperm meets the egg) are not detected.

This technique is infrequently used given the limitations listed above.

Cleavage-stage Biopsy (Blastomere Biopsy)

One of the most common approaches for PGD/PGS is to biopsy a single blastomere from day 3 embryos; this allows the extraction of a single blastomere from a developing embryo. The biopsy is usually performed on embryos with less than 50 percent anucleated fragments at the 8-cell or later stage of development. A hole is made in the zona pellucida and one or two blastomeres containing a nucleus are gently aspirated or extruded through the opening.

Advantages and disadvantages of cleavage-stage biopsy over PB biopsy: The main reasons are that it allows for a safer and more complete diagnosis than PB biopsy and still leaves enough time to finish the diagnosis before the embryo transfer, unlike blastocyst biopsy. Of all cleavage-stages, it is generally agreed that the optimal moment for biopsy is at the eight-cell stage. It is diagnostically safer than the PB biopsy and, unlike blastocyst biopsy, it allows for the diagnosis of embryos before day 5. In this stage, the cells are still totipotent and the embryos are not yet compacting. Although it has been shown that upto a quarter of a human embryos can be removed without disrupting its development, it still remains to be studied whether the biopsy of one or two cells correlates with the ability of the embryo to further develop, implant and grow into a full-term pregnancy.

The main advantage of cleavage-stage biopsy over PB analysis is that the genetic input of both partners can be studied. On the other hand, cleavage-stage embryos are found to have a high rate of chromosomal mosaicism, putting into question whether the results obtained on one or two blastomeres will be representative for the rest of the embryo. Therefore a combination of PBs and cleavage biopsy are used many a times. Cleavage-stage biopsy yields a very limited amount of tissue for diagnosis, necessitating the development of single-cell PCR and FISH techniques. Although theoretically, PB biopsy and blastocyst biopsy are less harmful than cleavage-stage biopsy, this is still the prevalent method.[14]

Blastocyst Biopsy

Blastocyst formation begins on day 5 post-egg retrieval and is defined by the presence of an inner cell mass (ICM) and the outer cell mass or trophectoderm. At this stage of development, the embryo is formed of more than 100 cells. A hole is breached in the zona pellucida and further, the procedure as outlined above is followed. Genetic analysis is further performed using PCR or FISH techniques.

Disadvantages of blastocyst biopsy: A limitation of this procedure is the potential acquisition of cells from the trophectoderm that are not representative of the developing embryo (inner cell mass) due to mosaicism (having multiple different types of cell lines). In addition, genetic/aneuploidy testing is completed approximately 24 to 48 hours of the embryo biopsy; due to the limited viability of embryos in the laboratory ($\leq$ 6 days after egg retrieval), many embryos do not survive until the time of embryo transfer. Therefore, biopsied blastocysts must be cryofrozen.[13]

Genetic Analysis Testing

In most instances, the genetic testing can be completed within 24 hours of the embryo biopsy, allowing for a day 4 or day 5 embryo transfer. Due to limited viability of the embryos in the laboratory, fewer than half of the chromosomes can be evaluated for aneuploidy by FISH or PCR.

Fluorescent *in situ* Hybridization

Fluorescent *in situ* hybridization (FISH) is used for the determination of sex for X-linked diseases, chromosomal abnormalities and aneuploidy screening. FISH is used more commonly in PGS, secondarily due to its utility as an aneuploidy screen. Probes (i.e. small pieces of DNA that are a match for the chromosomes being analyzed) bind to a particular chromosome. Each probe is labeled with a different fluorescent dye. These fluorescent probes are applied to the cell biopsy sample and are expected to attach to the specific chromosomes. They can be visualized under a fluorescent microscope.[13] Currently, a large panel of probes are available for different segments of all chromosomes, but the limited number of different fluorochromes confines the number of signals that can be analyzed simultaneously. Thus, in order to be able to analyze more chromosomes on the same sample, consecutive rounds of FISH need to be carried out with a maximum of three rounds. The FISH technique is considered to have an error rate between 5 and 10 percent.[4]

Polymerase Chain Reaction

Polymerase chain reaction (PCR) is used for the diagnosis of single gene defects, including dominant and recessive disorders. PCR, sometimes called DNA amplification, is a technique in which a particular DNA sequence is copied many times in order to facilitate its analysis. PCR rapidly multiplies a single DNA molecule into billions of molecules. As a result of this, PCR provides the possibility to obtain a large quantity of copies of a particular stretch of the genome, making further analysis possible. It is a highly sensitive and specific technology, which makes it suitable for all kinds of genetic diagnosis, including PGD.

Diagnosis and Misdiagnosis of PGD Applications Categorized by FISH and PCR

Polymerase chain reaction is a relatively fast and convenient way to test DNA. The method has been used in a variety of preimplantation genetic testing protocols. However, it requires sufficient amounts of a pure, high-quality sample of DNA, which is sometimes difficult to obtain from a single cell such as a polar body or blastomere. In addition, laboratory contamination and allele dropouts are possible complications.

Only one cell should be amplified; however, if another cell or piece of DNA enters the tube, it is also amplified. ICSI must be used to minimize this problem and to ensure that no excess sperm are present (paternal contamination) and that all the cumulus cells have been removed (maternal contamination).

Errors in PCR can result in misdiagnoses leading to an affected embryo being transferred or the discarding of a normal embryo. One error is caused by a phenomenon known as allele dropout. This refers to the preferential amplification of one allele over another during the PCR process and is mainly a problem for PGD of dominant disorders or when two different mutations are carried for a recessive disorder and only one mutation is being analyzed. In autosomal dominant diseases, the risk of transferring an affected embryo is 11 percent, while it is 2 percent for recessive disorders.[13]

Preimplantation Genetic Haplotyping

Preimplantation genetic haplotyping (PGH) is a new clinical method of preimplantation genetic diagnosis (PGD). PGH was first developed in 2006 at London's Guy's Hospital that greatly advances PGD by using DNA fingerprinting rather than identifying the actual genetic signature (such as point mutations).[15]

PGH versus Previous PGD Techniques

- PGH has the ability to screen male embryos, especially for X-linked disorders like Duchenne's muscular dystrophy and Becker's muscular dystrophy.
- Higher success rates.
- Increased reliability.

Embryo Transfer and Cryopreservation of Surplus Embryos

Embryo transfer is usually performed on day three or day five post-fertilization, the timing depending on the techniques used for PGD and the standard procedures of the IVF center where it is performed.

With the introduction of the single-embryo transfer policy in Europe, which aims at the reduction of the incidence of multiple pregnancy after ART, usually, one embryo or an early blastocyst is replaced in the uterus. Serum hCG is determined on day 12. If a pregnancy is established, an ultrasound examination at 7 weeks is performed to confirm the presence of the fetal heartbeat. Couples are generally advised to undergo prenatal diagnosis (PND) because of the, albeit low, risk of misdiagnosis.

It is not unusual that after the PGD, there are more embryos suitable for transferring back to the woman than necessary. For couples undergoing PGD, those embryos are very valuable, as their current cycle may not lead to an ongoing pregnancy. The cryopreservation and later thawing and replacement of these embryos would give them a second chance to pregnancy without undergoing the cumbersome and expensive ART and PGD procedures another time.

Ethical Issues

Preimplantation genetic diagnosis has raised ethical issues. The technique can be used to determine the gender of the embryo, and thus, can be used to select embryos of one gender in preference to the other in the context of family balancing. It may be possible to make other social selection choices in the future. While controversial, this approach is less destructive than fetal deselection during the pregnancy. Costs are substantial and insurance coverage may not be available. Thus, PGD widens the gap between people who can afford the procedure versus a majority of patients who may benefit but cannot afford the service.

PGD has the potential to screen for genetic issues unrelated to medical necessity. The prospect of a designer baby is closely related to the PGD technique.

Regulatory Authority

World Scenario

In the UK, the Human Fertilisation and Embryology Authority-(HFEA) has legal authority over whether a clinic is licensed to do PGD at all and for what indications. While some physicians have challenged the scope of the HFEA's regulatory authority, the HFEA has provided a regulatory model that other nations should emulate.[16]

The situation in the United States is quite different. No agency exists at the state or federal level that plays a role comparable with that of the HFEA. The Congress exercises some control by refusing to fund research or the use of PGD, but this often means that the activity escapes meaningful external review in the private sector. A few States have laws restricting embryo research, but several of them have been struck down as unconstitutionally vague or intrusive on reproductive rights, and the others are vulnerable to the same charges. State malpractice and tort law will apply, but those restrictions provide little oversight of the ethical acceptability of new procedures. How PGD is used and for what indications is thus left largely to the discretion of providers offering those services and the patients who seek it.[12]

The Indian Council of Medical Research (ICMR) has issued guidelines for the use of PGD in 2005, which are available on www.icmr.nic.in and can be downloaded from the internet. However, these need to be updated as the scope for PGD is increasing and more and more centers in India have started offering PGD. As of now, there are only guidelines which need to be followed. However, there is no law pertaining to PGD except the prenatal diagnostic testing (PNDT) act, as sex determination is banned in India.[17]

CONCLUSION

Preimplantation genetic diagnosis is increasingly available for the detection of aneuploidy in low prognosis IVF patients and for single gene mutations that cause genetic disease, susceptibility to cancer, and late onset disorders. If PGD is acceptable to prevent offspring with serious genetic disease, then these additional uses should be acceptable as well. There is also ethical support for using PGD to assure that a child is a HLA match with an existing child. More controversial is the use of PGD for gender selection, particularly, for the first child. Equally controversial would be its use to screen embryos for hearing, sexual orientation, and other non-medical traits, uses that are now highly speculative. Careful ethical analysis and open public debate is essential if new uses of PGD are to become acceptable methods for having children.[12]

REFERENCES

1. Kuliev A, Verlinsky Y. Preimplantation genetic diagnosis: technological advances to improve accuracy and range of applications. Reprod Biomed Online 2008;16:532-8.
2. Edwards RG, Gardner RL. Choosing Sex Before Birth. New Scientist 1968;38:218-20.
3. Handyside AH, Kontogianni EH, Hardy K, Winston RM. Pregnancies from biopsied human preimplantation embryos sexed by Y-specific DNA amplification. Nature 1990;344:768-70.
4. International Working Group on Preimplantation Genetics, International Congress of Human Genetics: Preimplantation genetic diagnosis: Experience of three thousand cycles. Report of the 11th Annual Meeting of International Working Group on Preimplantation Genetics, in association with 10th International Congress of Human Genetics. Vienna, Austria; May, 2001.
5. Molina B Dayal. Ioanna Athanasiadis Medical Director of Egg Donation Program, Department of Obstetrics and Gynecology, Division of Reproductive Endocrinology and Infertility, Medical Faculty Associates, George Washington University School of Medicine 14 Dec 2010.
6. Dean NL, Battersby BJ, Ao A, Gosden RG, Tan SL, Shoubridge EA, Molnar MJ. Prospect of preimplantation genetic diagnosis

for heritable mitochondrial DNA diseases. Mol Hum Reprod 2003;9:631-8.

7. Thorburn DR, Rahman S. Mitochondrial DNA-Associated Leigh Syndrome and NARP. In: Pagon RA, Bird TD, Dolan CR, Stephens K, Adam MP, (Eds). SourceGeneReviews™ [Internet]. Seattle (WA): University of Washington, Seattle; 1993-2003 Oct 30 [updated 2011 May 03].

8. Verlinsky Y, Rechitsky S, Schoolcraft W, Strom C, Kuliev A. Preimplantation diagnosis for Fanconi anemia combined with HLA matching. JAMA 2001;285:3130-3.

9. Verlinsky Y, Rechitsky S, Verlinsky O, Masciangelo C, Lederer K, Kuliev A. Preimplantation diagnosis for early-onset Alzheimer disease caused by V717L mutation. JAMA 2002;287:1018-21.

10. Menon U, Harper J, Sharma A, Fraser L, Burnell M, ElMasry K, Rodeck C, Jacobs I. Views of BRCA gene mutation carriers on preimplantation genetic diagnosis as a reproductive option for hereditary breast and ovarian cancer. Hum Reprod 2007;22:1573-7.

11. Rechitsky S, Verlinsky Y, Chistokhina A, Sharapova T, Ozen S, Masciangelo C, Kuliev A, Verlinsky Y. Preimplantation genetic diagnosis for cancer predisposition. Reprod Biomed Online 2002;5:148-55.

12. Robertson JA. Extending preimplantation genetic diagnosis: the ethical debate. Ethical issues in new uses of preimplantation genetic diagnosis. Hum Reprod 2003;18:465-71.

13. www. Preimplantationgeneticdiagnosis.eu

14. Amit Patki, Shashikant Umbardand. An introduction to genetic and fetal medicine; FOGSI books 2009-195.

15. Renwick PI, Pamela J, Trussler J, Jane, et al. Proof of principle and first cases using preimplantation genetic haplotyping: A paradigm shift for embryo diagnosis. Reproductive BioMedicine Online, 2006;13(1):110-9.

16. ESHRE PGD Consortium Steering Committee. ESHRE Preimplantation Genetic Diagnosis Consortium: data collection III (May 2001). Hum Reprod 2002;17:233-46.

17. www.icmr.nic.in (2007).

Preimplantation Genetic Diagnosis for Single Gene Disorders

KK Gopinath

INTRODUCTION

Preimplantation genetic diagnosis (PGD) offers couples at high risk of transmitting serious genetic diseases the possibility of avoiding repeated elective terminations or invasive prenatal diagnostic procedures. The detection of genetic disease in the human embryo before implantation gives parents the chance of starting a pregnancy knowing that the baby will be free of the inherited disorder that is prevalent in their family.

Single gene disorders can be transmitted in a number of different ways and to decide upon which technique to be used for PGD of single gene disorder, we must understand the inheritance of these genetic diseases. Autosomal recessive inheritance requires two copies of a defective or mutated gene, so that a carrier has one normal and one mutated gene. If both partners are carriers or there is consanguinity, there is a one in four chance that they will have an affected child, e.g. cystic fibrosis, β-thalassemia. Autosomal dominant inheritance requires a single copy of the mutant gene to manifest the disease and if one parent is affected, there is a 50 percent risk that their offspring will be affected. If none of the parents is affected but if they have a previous child affected by an autosomal dominant disorder, then it indicates a *de novo* mutation with a 1 percent recurrence risk. Achondroplasia and Huntington's disease are examples of dominant disorders. X-linked recessive conditions are almost exclusively seen in males as the mutant gene is present on the X-chromosome, and males have only one copy of the X-chromosome, therefore manifesting the disease, however, females have two X-chromosomes, so they are not affected but are carriers. She is at 50 percent risk of passing on the abnormal X-chromosome to her sons, e.g. hemophilia.

A PGD program requires the involvement of a Clinical Genetics unit, an IVF unit and diagnostic testing laboratories.

Timely, clear and comprehensive communications between these different units is imperative as a single embryonic cell is generally available for diagnosis, which should be accurate.

CLINICAL DISCUSSION

Genetic Counseling

Genetic counseling is the sharing of information and advice about inherited conditions. Counseling depends on an accurate diagnosis and is mandatory for PGD. It provides appropriate and sufficient information to allow patients to give informed consent to PGD treatment.

It includes the following issues:[1]

- Explanation of the nature and severity of the inherited genetic disorder
- Mode of inheritance of the disorder and recurrence risk
- Number of embryos expected to be affected according to Mendelian ratios
- Testing only for genetic disorders previously characterized for that couple and for which testing is available
- Information on specific laboratory tests to be used and their limitations
- Reliability of PGD, chances of misdiagnosis or adverse outcomes, and possibility of allele dropout
- Decision-making about transfer of carrier embryos and disposition of affected embryos or undiagnosed embryos.

Treatment-Related Counseling

- Description of and details regarding IVF/ICSI procedures
- Number of embryos to be transferred and the possibility that all embryos are affected
- Risk of multiple pregnancy and miscarriage
- Cost of treatment and the risk of medical complications during ovarian stimulation or oocyte retrieval.

Patient Selection

For appropriate patient selection for PGD, a team approach involving the geneticist and gynecologist is required. In appropriate cases, a DNA study has to be carried out on the parent or family members before starting the treatment. A complete explanation of IVF and PGD is required and relevant documentation to be maintained.

This includes the following:
- Written informed consent.
- Genetic counseling report including detailed pedigree and family history data.
- Documents of DNA tests or other specific tests of affected child and appropriate family members. For example, the markers to be used for Fragile 'X' need to be checked for each couple to see if they are informative. If the precycle work-up is informative, then it is recommended to go ahead with PGD.
- Other preliminary tests in conjunction with IVF/ICSI with respect to both male and female reproductive history also have to be carried out.

Intracytoplasmic Sperm Injection

Intracytoplasmic sperm injection (ICSI) (Fig. 56.1) is the recommended method of choice for insemination in all PGD cases. This is because of two important reasons, i.e. to eliminate sperm contamination, which is important when polymerase chain reaction (PCR) is used, and for efficient fertilization, which reduces the possibility of fertilization failure after regular IVF.

Embryo Biopsy

Embryo biopsy can be performed at three stages, polar body, cleavage stage and blastocyst, although in a recent survey of practices among 50 centers performing PGD, the majority performed only cleavage stage biopsy.[1]

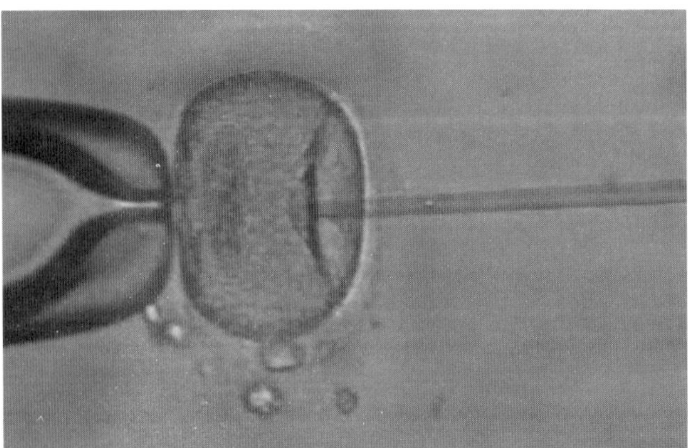

Fig. 56.1: Intracytoplasmic sperm injection. Right side holding pipette. Left side injecting pipette

First and Second Polar Body Biopsy

The rationale behind this type of biopsy is that the polar bodies, the first as well as second, contain the complementary genotype to the oocyte.[2] Thus, if the first polar body is shown to contain the affected gene, it can be concluded that the oocyte contains the normal gene and can therefore, be fertilized and transferred safely to the mother. Technically, polar body biopsy is quite straightforward, where the first polar body is removed on the day of the oocyte collection and the second polar body removed from the zygote between 18 and 22 hours post insemination.[3] With a thin pipette, the polar bodies are removed from under the zona and transferred to a PCR tube or a glass slide. Sequential removal of the polar bodies has been proposed and has been applied to PGD for the detection of cystic fibrosis,[4] β-thalassemia[5] and maternal chromosome translocation.[6]

There are a number of disadvantages, which severely limit the potential use of this technique, as for instance, the approach can only be applied to maternally inherited diseases, only a single cell is available for analysis and polar body biopsy cannot be used for gender determination.

Cleavage Stage Biopsy

Cleavage stage biopsy is the most widely used technique, and has an advantage over polar body biopsy, as the genetic constitution of the embryo is completely formed and thus, comparable to genetic material obtained at prenatal diagnosis. There are different methods for the removal of blastomeres from cleavage stage embryos, but the most accepted is zona drilling, using acid tyrode solution and aspiration of blastomere(s). Laser zona drilling has also come up, which is more precise and obviates the need for disposable or reusable tools.[7]

Blastocyst Biopsy

Blastocyst biopsy is performed on day 5 to 8 after fertilization and the advantage is that more amount of tissue can be obtained than at the cleavage stage, making diagnosis more reliable (Figs 56.2A to F).

Diagnostic Methods

Gender Determination and Diagnosis of Chromosome Aneuploidies

Sex selection was done in the early days of PGD to avoid the transfer of embryos affected with X-linked disease such as hemophilia.[8] PGD for sex selection, in order to prevent the birth of healthy female carriers of X-linked recessive disorders, thereby avoiding reproductive dilemmas for future children related to serious heath risks for the grandchildren, has also come up.

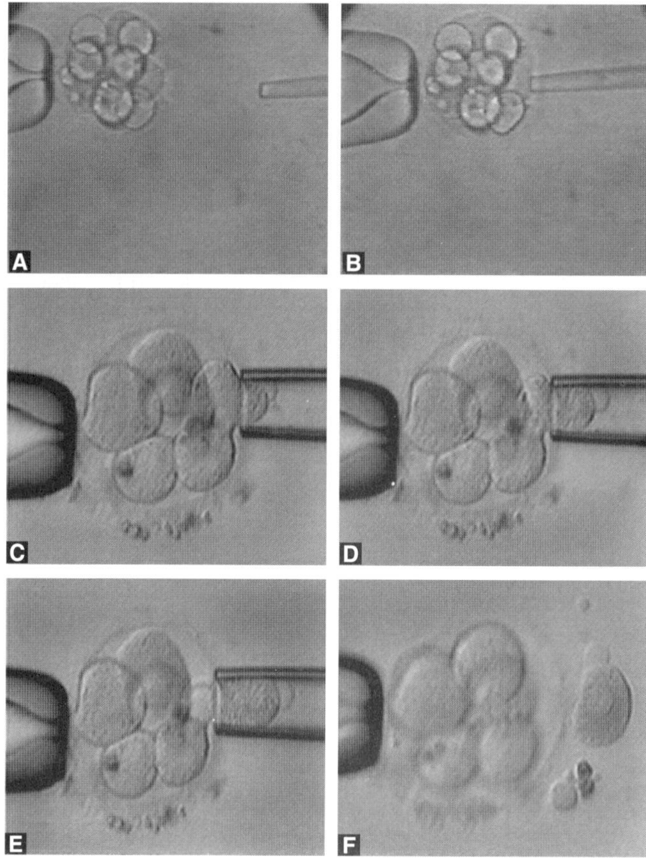

Figs 56.2A to F: Blastomere biopsy: (A) Laser zona drilling (B to E) Steps in blastomere aspiration using a blastomere aspiration pipette (right) (F) Blastomere separated from the embryo

At present, fluorescent *in situ* hybridization (FISH) is used for sexing of the embryos and to detect the most common chromosomal aneuploidies associated with birth defects and early pregnancy loss. FISH has also been used for PGD for chromosomal abnormalities such as translocations.

Fluorescence in situ Hybridization

Fluorescence *in situ* hybridization is a molecular cytogenetic technique for enumerating chromosomes. FISH uses DNA probes that are fluorescently tagged and bind to complementary sequences on specific chromosomes. After hybridization, nuclei can be examined under a fluorescent microscope and the number of fluorescent signals will indicate the number of chromosomes present.[9] Several probes can be hybridized simultaneously if each is labeled with a different colored fluorochrome. This enables enumeration of more than one chromosome in a single cell, thereby making it possible to do sexing of the embryo and screening for aneuploidy.[10,11]

X-linked recessive disease accounts for 6 to 7 percent of single gene defects and includes conditions like Duchenne's muscular dystrophy (DMD), hemophilia and various mental retardation syndromes. PGD for sexing included one of the largest group of patients treated in the data collected by the ESHRE-PGD consortium, and the majority of these used FISH for the diagnosis.[12]

PCR-based Diagnosis

Polymerase chain reaction (PCR) allows the amplification of well-defined DNA sequences enzymatically in an exponential way. Two short oligonucleotide primers, based on the known sequences of the region of interest are added in great molar excess. Genomic DNA acts as a template. Taq polymerase, with the help of four deoxynucleotide triphosphates (dNTPs) and with differential temperature gradient is able to synthesize the DNA strands from the 3' end of the annealed primer. The amount of DNA synthesized doubles at every cycle and thus, there is an exponential increase in the amount of DNA between the two primers.

Rapid amplification of the specific gene fragments from a single cell using PCR has been successfully applied to pre-implantation genetic diagnosis.

Before attempting to do PCR from a single cell and ensuring that the test yields the expected results, assay validation should be performed on appropriate DNA samples of the affected individuals (autosomal dominant), carrier (autosomal recessive, X-linked recessive) and unaffected samples for the mutation to be tested.[1] It is recommended that for single gene defect cases, each clinical cycle should include the appropriate positive control samples. These should include for recessive diseases, one heterozygous and one homozygous normal; and for linked markers, the two parents and if possible, the genotype of an affected child. For each blastomere analyzed, there should be an appropriate negative control and reagent control (no DNA).[1]

Nested PCR

Holding and Monk[13] showed that the specificity and efficiency of the PCR technique could be greatly enhanced by using nested PCR. Here, the first PCR reaction of typically 20 to 30 cycles is followed by a second PCR round, with a few microliters of the first PCR product used as a template. The primers in the second PCR amplify a sequence smaller than in the first PCR, i.e. with primers that have boundaries inside the first PCR product (Fig. 56.3). Most authors describing single cell PCR for PGD to date have used this strategy.

Fluorescent PCR

The use of the more sensitive fluorescent PCR was introduced by Findlay and co-workers.[14] The principle is quite

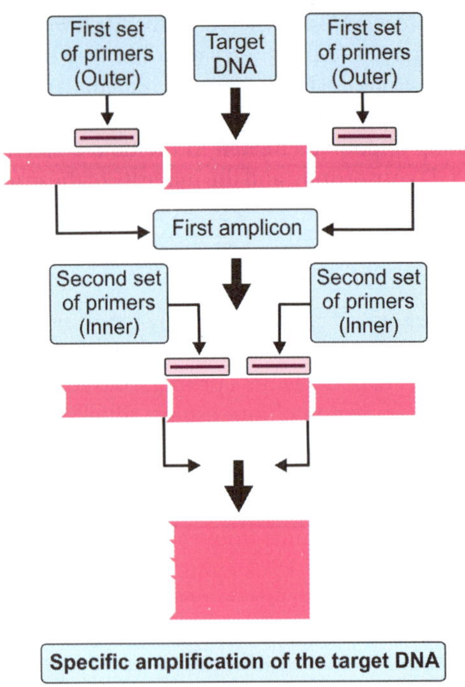

Fig. 56.3: Nested PCR

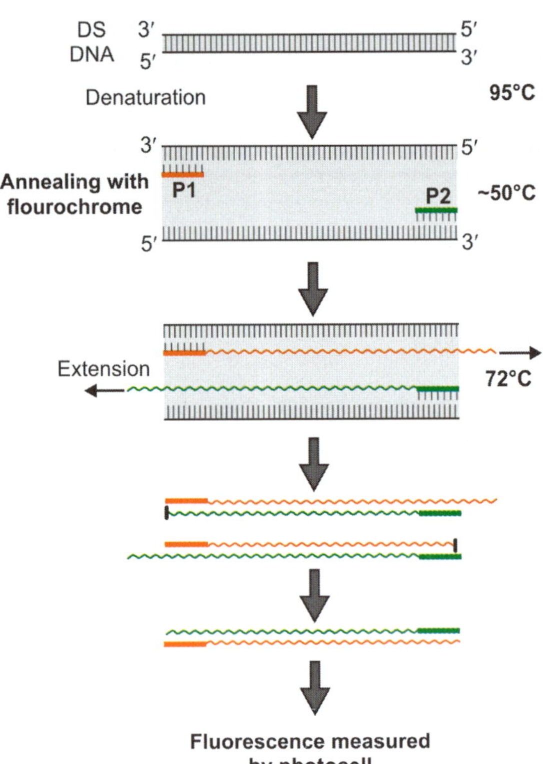

Fig. 56.4: Fluorescent PCR

straightforward. A fluorescent oligonucleotide, labeled at the 5′ end with a fluorochrome, can be substituted for one of the primers used for the gene amplification by PCR. This will produce fluorescent DNA fragments that can be separated by electrophoresis on a polyacrylamide gel. A laser beam is sent through the gel perpendicular to the direction of current. Whenever a fluorescently labeled fragment passes through the laser beam, the resulting fluorescence is measured by a photocell behind the gel, which facilitates the sizing of an amplicon to single nucleotide accuracy (Fig. 56.4).

Fluorescent PCR is so sensitive and accurate that even a 3bp cystic fibrosis deletion ΔF508 can be clearly differentiated from the normal allele and therefore, can be successfully applied to PGD.[15] The sensitivity of the fluorescent PCR product detection is over thousand times greater than the conventional PCR product analysis, and moreover, the time required is also lesser. As time is a crucial factor in PGD, this allows speedy diagnosis and transfer of unaffected embryos. With the analysis of PCR products from a single cell, possible after a single round of amplification, this also eliminated the need for post-PCR processing.[15]

Multiplex PCR

With multiplex genomic analysis (multiplex PCR) it is possible to amplify and screen multiple segments of a gene for mutation analysis. This rapid and simple technique permits the detection of many single gene disorders from one cell within 6 to 8 hours, allowing embryo transfer the same working day, which is a great advantage for patients undergoing preimplantation genetic diagnosis.

Several sets of PCR primers, specific for independent loci, can be included within the same PCR cocktail. Successful multiplex reactions enable the simultaneous assessment of numerous loci. Strategies for the multiplex PCR amplification of mutations and linked polymorphisms have been reported for cystic fibrosis[16] and β-thalassemia,[5] and have been performed for medium chain acyl coA dehydrogenase deficiency (MCAD) and myotonic dystrophy.[15]

Multiplex PCR can also be employed to circumvent problems caused by allele dropout.[5]

Single cell PCR usually consists of the following steps:

- The cell to be analyzed (e.g. polar body or blastomere) is washed in phosphate buffer saline twice using a sterile transfer pipette before transfer into the PCR tube with or without the aid of a microscope. The PCR tube usually contains the solution in which the cells will be lysed.
- Several lysis procedures have been described, of which, the most used is freeze-thawing, boiling in water, incubation at 37°C with proteinase K and sodium dodecyl sulfate (SDS) and incubation at 65°C in alkaline lysis buffer.[17]
- The PCR reaction is set up with the addition of PCR components, such as primers dNTPs, MgCl$_2$, KCl, Tris HCL and buffer, to the genomic DNA isolated in the previous step.

- During the first round of PCR, 25 to 30 cycles are typically carried out. A few microliters of the first PCR product are added to the reaction mix of the second PCR consisting of the same components as the first PCR.[17] In case of nested PCR, the primers of the second PCR are different from the first PCR. The use of appropriate positive, negative and reagent control is always recommended for accuracy and efficacy of the procedure. When fluorescent PCR is used, only 35 to 40 cycles of PCR are usually required.
- For conventional PCR, the products after PCR amplification are analyzed by agarose gel or polyacrylamide gel. Fluorescent PCR products have to be analyzed on automated sequencing systems. Sometimes, additional techniques, such as restriction enzyme digestion and heteroduplex formation are needed for mutation identification.

Allele Specific Drop-out: A Problem

Ray and co-workers[18] were the first to describe allele specific drop-out (ADO) in blastomeres obtained after PGD for the Δ F508 mutation in cystic fibrosis: 25 percent of the heterozygous blastomeres revealed ADO. ADO is recognized in nearly every PCR tested. Allele drop-out is a phenomenon, whereby only one of the two alleles present is successfully amplified.[18] Allele drop-out is equally likely to affect either of the alleles in a heterozygous cell and although its frequency can be estimated, it is not possible to predict which allele will be affected in a given reaction. Allele drop-out may lead to misdiagnosis of heterozygous embryos, and is the most significant obstacle to the reliable diagnosis of dominant disorders in a single cell (Fig. 56.5).

A number of explanations for ADO have been put forward. The presence of haploid cells in an otherwise diploid embryos could partly explain ADO in blastomeres. The other hypothesis is of imperfect PCR conditions or incomplete cell lysis and degradation of the DNA strand.

A series of experiments on blastomeres demonstrated that the denaturation temperature at the start of the first PCR is critical, and an increase in the denaturing temperature from 90° to 96°C causes a four-fold reduction in ADO at the cystic fibrosis locus and an eleven-fold reduction at the β globin locus.[19] Strategies other than raising the denaturation temperature can be used for reducing or at least, detecting ADO. Findlay and associates[14] showed that, because of its higher sensitivity, much lower rates of ADO could be achieved with fluorescent PCR. Using this strategy, ADO in an affected embryo would always be detected and the embryo would not be transferred. This strategy has been proposed for Tay-Sach's disease and for β-thalassemia.[20,21]

Once DNA from a single cell has been amplified to a detectable level, any of the manifold mutation detection techniques currently available for standard PCR analysis can be employed for its examination.

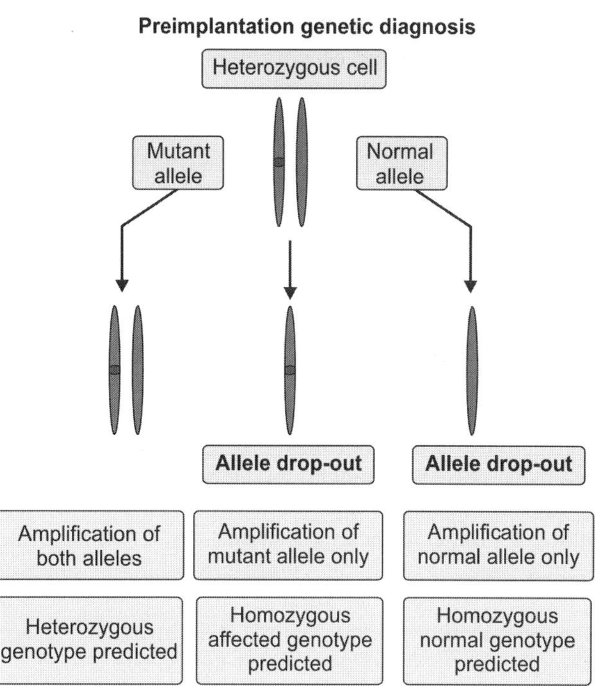

Fig. 56.5: Allele specific drop-out

Primed *in situ* Labeling

The primed *in situ* labeling (PRINS) technique represents a relatively new approach to the detection of specific DNA or RNA sequences *in situ*, and therefore, can be used for single blastomeres spread on microscopic slides. This method consists of annealing of chromosome-specific primers, followed by Taq polymerase driven extension and thus, resembles PCR. However, in this case, replication occurs on the glass slide rather than in a tube and in the presence of labeled nucleotides. This leads to the generation of a fluorescent signal on chromosomal nuclei. Pellestor and co-workers[22] developed this method at the single cell level and showed its potential for preimplantation diagnosis. Using primers for satellite sequences on chromosomes 9, 16, 18, 21, X and Y in a two-step protocol, they were able to clearly show these chromosomes in six morphologically abnormal pre-embryos.

Restriction endonuclease digestion: Restriction endonucleases are bacterial enzymes that recognize specific DNA sequences and cleave the DNA strand at or near the recognition site. Differences in DNA sequences, such as those caused by mutation, can often be revealed by digestion of the normal and mutant DNA with restriction enzymes. A restriction enzyme selected will be such that it will cleave a normal DNA strand while a mutant strand remains undigested. The digestion products can be distinguished from the undigested PCR product following electrophoresis. An enzyme that does the reverse (digests the mutant allele but not the wild type) can also be used, however, in this case, incomplete or failed digestion could lead to the embryo being wrongly diagnosed as normal. Amplification of DNA followed by restriction enzyme digestion has allowed single cell diagnosis of Marfan's syndrome, Lesch-Nyhan syndrome, sickle cell anemia, β-thalassemia, cystic fibrosis and spinal muscular atrophy.[15]

Linkage analysis using polymorphic markers: Even when the exact mutation causing a disorder is unknown, the particular disease may still be avoided by preimplantation detection of a linked marker. Any informative marker (polymorphic site), which is in close proximity to the disease locus, can be used as a tool to indicate the presence/absence of the mutation without its direct detection. Markers that are intragenic or situated close to the gene are preferred for this approach, as they are unlikely to be separated from the mutation by recombination during meiosis. For linkage analysis to be employed, the pedigree of the family concerned must be obtained and the DNA of these family members must be tested in advance to determine which polymorphic variant is inherited along with the disease phenotype. The most commonly used polymorphic markers are short tandem repeats (STR), also known as microsatellites. These are highly polymorphic and widely spread through the human genome and subsequently, have the greatest probability of being informative for a given family. Linkage analysis was employed for the diagnosis of Marfan's syndrome, where the affected embryos were identified by tracing the inheritance of a dinucleotide repeat polymorphism linked to the causative fibrillin gene.[23] Recently, PGD has been successfully achieved based on linked marker analysis for polycystic kidney disease (PKD).[24] Autosomal dominant polycystic kidney disease is caused by the genes PKD1 or PKD2, with their loci on chromosome 16p and 4q, respectively for which no direct testing is yet available, making linkage analysis a method of choice. Verlineky and associates[24] used three closely linked markers to PKD1 and four closely linked markers to PKD2 for PGD of autosomal dominant polycystic kidney disease, which resulted in a twin pregnancy and the birth of two unaffected children.

Heteroduplex analysis: Heteroduplex analysis can identify a wide variety of mutations, but is particularly likely to detect small deletions or insertions, which can be used for the identification of single gene disorders in PGD. The heating and cooling that occurs during PCR causes the amplified DNA first to become single stranded and then to reanneal, becoming double stranded DNA again. Usually, this results in the original homoduplexes being formed again, but in heterozygous samples heteroduplexes may also be formed.

These consist of complementary DNA strands from different alleles, which anneal together. The only region that does not anneal is the mutation site (where the normal and mutant alleles differ in sequence). This area of mismatch retards the migration of heteroduplexes during polyacrylamide gel electrophoresis and thus, they can be resolved from homoduplexes. The presence of a heteroduplex indicates that the DNA sample is heterozygous (Fig. 56.6).

In the case of the ΔF 508 mutation that causes cystic fibrosis, homozygous affected samples are revealed by the formation of heteroduplexes after the equivalent wild type PCR product has been added.[25] Homozygous normal genotypes are revealed by heteroduplex formation following addition of ΔF 508/ΔF 508 PCR product. Heteroduplex analysis has been used in PGD of cystic fibrosis, Tay-Sachs disease and familial adenomatous polyposis.[15]

Single strand conformation polymorphism: Single strand conformation polymorphism (SSCP) is a mutation scanning

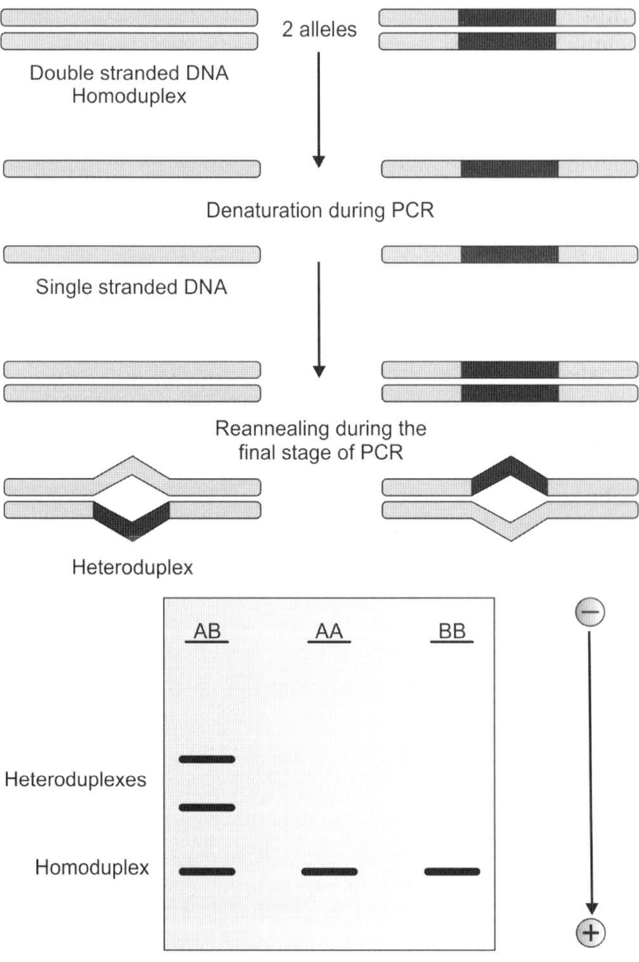

Fig. 56.6: Heteroduplex analysis

technique to detect point mutations, small deletions and insertions. In this technique, PCR amplification is the first step followed by denaturation, which leads to a single strand of DNA that takes on sequence-specific conformations, which are then subjected to electrophoresis. DNA strands of differing base sequences (e.g. strands derived from different alleles) will usually adopt distinct conformations; indeed, a single base alteration can result in a radical change of conformation. Different conformations migrate at distinct rates if they are subjected to non-denaturing using polyacrylamide gel electrophoresis and thus, different alleles can be distinguished. SSCP was employed for PGD of the dominant cancer syndrome familial adenomatous polyposis coli.[15]

Whole Genome Amplification (WGA)

Non-specific amplification of the entire genome (whole genome amplification) has also been applied to single cell analysis. Using these techniques, a single genome can be amplified numerous times, thus providing sufficient DNA templates for many independent PCR amplifications. This technique has great future promise, and will be applied for more applications in PGD. This technique has been clinically applied to the PGD of the dominant cancer syndrome familial adenomatous polyposis coli.[15]

Embryo Transfer

Embryo transfer is done on a day appropriate to the diagnostic test turn around time. It is recommended that selection criteria for embryo transfer are based primarily on unaffected diagnosis and secondarily favorable embryo morphology. Transfer of carrier embryos (autosomal recessive or X-linked disorder) is acceptable since adverse health consequences to the resulting child are unlikely. Each situation needs careful evaluation and fully informed discussion with the couple. Embryo transfer on either day 3, 4, 5 or 6 can be carried out as in routine IVF practice. Following PGD, sometimes, no unaffected embryos may be available for transfer. In such cases, transfer of affected embryos is not recommended[1] and couples should be counseled accordingly.

Another important aspect with PGD is the confirmation of the diagnosis by follow-up of pregnancies (including multiple pregnancy rate and outcome), prenatal testing, deliveries, the health of children at birth and beyond, which should be carried out along with appropriate data.

CONCLUSION

Preimplantation genetic diagnosis is a very early form of prenatal diagnosis; embryos from couples at risk for a genetic disease are obtained *in vitro* through classic IVF techniques and are analyzed for the presence of the genetic disease under consideration before the transfer of healthy embryos. To diagnose disease in the embryos, polar bodies are taken from fertilized oocytes, or blastomeres are biopsied from cleavage stage embryos. The cell can be analyzed by various methods like FISH and PCR. Worldwide, more than 100 children have been born after PGD and it is expected that PGD will show an exponential growth, confirming its clinical importance.

REFERENCES

1. Thornhill AR, deDie- Smulders CE, Geradts JP, et al. ESHRE PGD consortium Best Practice guidelines for clinical pre-implantation genetic diagnosis (PGD) and preimplantation genetic screening (PGS). Hum Reprod 2004;20:35-48.
2. Verlinsky Y, Kuliev A, Dyban A. Preconception diagnosis of single gene and chromosomal disorders. Hum Reprod 1994;9: 182-3.
3. Verlinsky Y, Ginsberg N, Lifchez A, Valle J, Moise J, Strom CM. Analysis of polar body: preconception genetic diagnosis. Hum Reprod 1990;5:826-9.
4. Strom CM, Ginsberg N, Rechitsky S, Cieslak J, Ivakhenko V, Wolf G, et al. Three births after preimplantation genetic diagnosis for cystic fibrosis with sequential first and second polar body analysis. Am J Obstet Gynecol 1998;178:1298-306.
5. Kuliev A, Rechitsky S, Verlinsky O, Ivakhnenko V, Evsikov S, Wolf G, Angastiniotis M, Georghiou D. Preimplantation genetic diagnosis of thalassemias. J Assist Reprod Gene 1998;15:219-25.
6. Munne S, Scott R, Sable D, Cohen J. First pregnancies after preconception diagnosis of translocations of maternal origin. Fertil Steril 1998;69:675-81.
7. Harper J, Thornhill A. Embryo biopsy. In: Preimplantation Genetic Diagnosis. Wiley, Chichester 2001;141-63.
8. Klipstein S. Preimplantation genetic diagnosis; Technological promise and ethical perils. Fertil Steril 2005;83:1347-53.
9. Harper J, Wilton L. FISH and embryo sexing to avoid X-linked disease. In: Preimplantation Genetic Diagnosis Wiley, Chichester 2001;191-201.
10. Munne S, Magli C, Bache M, Fung J, Legator M, Morrison L, et al. Preimplantation diagnosis of the aneuploidies most commonly found in spontaneous abortions and live births, X, Y, 13,14,15,16,18,21,22. Prenat Diagn 1998;18:1459-66.
11. Wilton L. Preimplantation genetic diagnosis for aneuploidy screening in early human embryos: A review. Prenat Diagn 2002; 22:1-7.
12. ESHRE PGD consortium. Preliminary assessment of data from January 1997 to September 1998. Hum Reprod 1999;14:3138-48.
13. Holding C, Monk M. Diagnosis of beta-thalassemia by DNA amplification in single blastomeres from mouse preimplantation embryos. Lancet 1989;2:532-5.
14. Findlay I, Urquhart A, Quirke P, Sullivan K, Rutherford AJ, Lilford RJ. Simultaneous DNA fingerprinting diagnosis of sex and single gene defect status from single cells. Hum Reprod 1995;10:1005-13.
15. Wells D, Sherlock J. Diagnosis of single gene disorders. In: Pre-implant Genetic Diagnosis. Wiley, Chichester; 2001.pp.165-90.
16. Rechitsky S, Strom C, Verlinsky O, et al. Allele drop out polar bodies and blastomeres. J Assist Reprod Genet 1998;15:253-7.

17. Serman K, Liebaeras I. Preimplantation genetic diagnosis.In: Molecular biology in reproductive medicine. Parathenon, New York 1999;409-31.

18. Ray P, Winston RML, Handyside AH. Single cell analysis for diagnosis of cystic fibrosis and Lesch-Nyhan syndrome in human embryos before implantation. Miami Bio/Technology short reports: Proceedings of the 1994 Miami Bio/Technology European symposium, Advances in Gene Technology: Molecular Biology and Human Genetic Disease 1994;5:46.

19. Ray PF, Handyside AH. Increasing the denaturiation temperature during the first cycles of amplification reduces allele dropout from single cells for preimplantation genetic diagnosis. Mol Hum Reprod 1996;2:213-8.

20. Sermon K, Lissens W, Nagy ZP, Van Steirteghem A, Liebaers I. Simultaneous amplification of the two most frequent mutations of infantile Tay-Sachs disease in single blastomeres. Hum Reprod 1995;10:2214-7.

21. Ray PF, Kaeda JS, Bingham J, Roberts I, Handyside AH. Preimplantation diagnosis of β-thalassaemia major. Lancet 1996;347:1696.

22. Pellestor F, Girard et A, Andreo B, Letfort G, Charlieu JP. The PRINS technique: Potential use for rapid preimplantation embryo chromosome screening. Mol Hum Reprod 1996;2:135-8.

23. Harton GL, Tsipouras P, Sisson ME, Starr KM, Mahoney BS, Fugger EF, et al. Preimplantation genetic testing for Marfan syndrome. Mol Hum Reprod 1996;2:713-5.

24. Verlinsky Y, Rechitsky S, Verlinsky O, Ozen S, Beck R, Kuliev A. Preimplantation genetic diagnosis for polycystic kidney disease. Fertil Steril 2004;82:926-9.

25. Handyside AH, Lesko JG, Tarin JJ, Winston RM, Hughes MR. Birth of a normal girl after in vitro fertilization and Preimplantation diagnostic testing for cystic fibrosis N. Engl J Med 1992;327:905-9.

Preimplantation Genetic Diagnosis for Selecting HLA Compatible Embryos

Semra Kahraman, Cagri Beyazyurek

OVERVIEW

Preimplantation Genetic Diagnosis (PGD) in combination with human leukocyte antigen (HLA) matching is being used to detect a particular gene mutation in an unaffected child who can be a HLA donor for its sibling. Stem cells from the resulting baby's umbilical cord blood therefore, of a great therapeutic value for hematopoietic and other life threatening diseases, as these stem cells can be used for transplantation without graft rejection, thus saving an affected child's life.

It has been ten years since the first PGD technique with are HLA matching for Fanconi anemia was reported, allowing successful hemopoietic reconstitution in the affected sibling by transplantation of stem cells obtained from an HLA-matched offspring.[1,2]

The selection of embryos for HLA typing necessitates the application of assisted reproductive technique (ART) even though the vast majority of the couples are fertile. The successful outcome of ART cycles is highly dependent on female age and ovarian reserve. This technique is made crucially important by the fact that the theoretical probability of finding a HLA identical embryo in cases of acquired diseases is 25 percent (1/4) and the probability of finding both a HLA identical and mutation free embryo in cases of single gene disorders is not more than 18 percent (3/16). Using a standard *in vitro* fertilization (IVF) procedure, oocytes or embryos are tested for causative gene mutations simultaneously with HLA alleles, selecting and transferring only those unaffected embryos, which are HLA matched to the affected sibling.

INTRODUCTION

More than 2000 healthy children have already been born after PGD and the expanding indications include chromosomal abnormalities, single gene disorders, HLA tissue typing of the embryos, predisposition of adult onset disorders, translocations and cancer predispositions.[3-10] In fact, PGD can be carried out for any disorder in which molecular testing can be performed. A partial list of disorders for which PGD be applied is shown in Table 57.1.

Although the majority of these disorders are due to rare genetic defects, the incidence of some, such as β-thalassemia, sickle cell anemia and cystic fibrosis are very common in certain parts of the world, such as the Mediterranean region, which include Turkey, Italy, Greece and Cyprus. In Turkey, β-thalassemia carrier frequency is around 4 percent, however, this rate is found to be as high as 14 percent in some areas where consanguineous marriages are common.[11]

In particular, for blood-borne disorders, hematopoietic stem cells (HSC) from HLA-identical siblings provide the highest success rate according to the Pesaro low-risk score,[12] and the current results indicate that about 90 percent of the cases can be cured successfully after HSC transplantation.[13] The use of cord blood as a stem cell source also results in reduced incidence of graft rejection and other serious complications associated with bone marrow transplantation. However, in most cases, a suitable donor cannot be found in the family, and due to a small number of children per family, only one-third of patients are able to find a HLA-identical sibling.[14] The probability of having an unaffected child, who may also be a HLA match for an affected sibling, is only one in five; these families often go through multiple cycles of pregnancy before conceiving an unaffected HLA match. In the remaining patients, the only resort is the identification of a matched unrelated donor. However, the probability of finding HLA-matched unrelated donor cord blood from the cord blood units is extremely low. Therefore, PGD is a much more attractive option with this technique, enabling sufficient number of embryos to be tested at one time, thus increasing the chances of identifying an appropriate match.

Table 57.1: Some of the current indications for PGD

Achondroplasia (FGFR3)	Hypophosphatasia (ALPL)
ADA (Adenosine Deaminase) deficiency	Incontinentia pigmenti (KBKG-NEMO)
Adrenal hyperplasia	Kennedy disease (AR)
Adrenoleukodystrophy (ABCD1)	Krabbe (GALC)
Agammaglobulinemia-Bruton (TyrsKnse)	LCHAD
Alpha thalassemia (HBA1)	Lesch-Nyhan (HPRT1)
Alpha-antitrypsin (AAT)	Leukemia, acute lymphocytic (for HLA)
Alport syndrome (COL4A5)	Leukemia, acute myelogenous (for HLA)
Alzheimer (very early onset-PSEN1)	Leukemia, chronic myelogenous (for HLA)
Beta thalassemia (HBB)	Leukocyte adhesion deficiency (ITGB2)
Bloom syndrome (Blm)	Li-Fraumeni syndrome (TP53)
Canavan disease (ASPA)	Lymphoproliferative disorder (X-linked)
Charcot-Marie-Tooth, type IA-IB	Marfan syndrome (FBN1)
Charcot-Marie-Tooth neuropathy-2E	Menkes (ATP7A)
Charcot-Marie-Tooth neuropathy-XL	Metachromatic leukodystrophy (ARSA)
Choroideremia (CHM)	Mucolipidosis 2 (I-Cell)
Chronic granulomatous Dz (CYBB)	Multiple epiphyseal dysplasia
Citrullinemia (ASS)	Myotonic dystrophy
Cleidocranial dysplasia (RUNX2)	Myotubular myopathy
Congenital adrenal hyperplasia (CYP31A2)	Neurofibromatosis (NF1 & NF2)
Congenital erythropoietic porphyria (UROS)	Niemann-pick type C (NPC1)
Crigler Najjar (UGT1A1)	Ornithine transcarbamylase deficiency (OTC)
Cystic fibrosis (CFTR)	Osteogenis imperfecta (COL1A1)
Darier disease (ATP2A2)	Pachyonychia congenita (KRT16 & KRT6A)
Diamond Blackfan (DBA-RSP19)	Periventricular heteropia (PH)
Duchenne muscular dystrophy (DMD)	Phenylketonuria (PKU)
Dystrophy myotonica (DMPK)	Polycystic kidney disease (AR-PKD1) polycystic
Emery-Dreifuss muscular dystrophy	Kidney disease (PKD1) retinoblastoma 1 (RB1)
Epidermolysis bullosa	Retinitis pigmentosa
Epidermolytic hyperkeratosis (KRT10) Factor	Rhesus blood group D (RHD)
F13 deficiency (F13A1)	Rhizomelic chondrodysplasia puncta RCDP1
Familial adenomatous polyposis (APC)	Sacral agenesis (HLXB9)
Familial dysautonomia (IKBKAP)	Sanfilippo A (MPSIIIA)
Fanconi anemia A (FANCA)	Sandhoff disease
Fanconi anemia C (FANCC)	SCID-X1 (SevereCmbndImmuneDefic (IL2RG)
Fanconi anemia F (FANC F)	Shwachman-Diamond syndrome (SBDS)
Fanconi anemia G (FANCG)	Sickle cell (HBB)
Fragile X (FMR1)	Smith-Lemli-Opitz (SLOS)
Friedreich ataxia I (FRDA)	Spinal muscular atrophy (SMN1)
Gaucher disease (GBA)	Spinocerebellar ataxia-3 (SCA3)
Glycogen storage disease, type 1A	Spinocerebellar ataxia-2 (SCA2)
Glutaric acidemia-2A	Tay-Sachs (HEXA)
Hemophilia A (F8)	Treacher Collins (TOCF1)
Hemophilia B (F9)	Tuberous sclerosis 1 (TSC1)
Hunter syndrome (IDS)	Von-Hippel Lindau
Huntington disease (HD)	Wiskott-Aldrich syndrome (WAS)
Hurler syndrome (MPSI-IDUA)	X-linked hydrocephalus
Hyper IgM (CD40-ligand; TNFSF5)	

The HLA complex is located on chromosome 6 and represents one of the most polymorphic regions of the human genome. Comparative DNA sequence analysis of the HLA complex has shown the presence of a high number of alleles in this region. Of these regions, we are studying HLA-A, HLA-B, HLA-C (Class I) and HLA-DR (Class II) as these regions are the most polymorphic regions. Linked short tandem repeat (STR) markers scattered through the HLA complex have also been studied to increase the accuracy of the analysis and to detect potential contaminations and crossing over occurrence between the HLA genes.

The single cell polymerase chain reaction (PCR) technique has several pitfalls, such as contamination by extraneous DNA, amplification failure, preferential amplification, and allele dropout (ADO), which is the failure of PCR to amplify one of the two alleles. If ADO occurs, only a single allele is amplified and detected after PCR, giving a heterozygous cell the appearance of homozygosity. This may lead to harmful consequences, such as failure to amplify the mutant allele and the consequent transfer of affected embryos in the case of a dominant disease. The ADO rate and the efficiency of amplification of targeted regions depend on efficient lysis methods[15] and also the type of cell analyzed. With the simultaneous usage of linked STR markers with multiplex single cell PCR techniques, the accuracy of single cell PCR is approximately 98 percent.[16] ADO rates in single cells can be decreased by analyzing more than one cell, which is possible with blastocyst-stage biopsy. Trophectoderm biopsy

is a good alternative to cleavage stage biopsy as it enables the evaluation of approximately 2 to 5 cells, thus decreasing both the rate of amplification failures and ADO associated with single cell PCR.[17,18] There are many advantages of blastocyst stage biopsy such that since the trophectoderm cells are extra-embryonic tissue, the removal of these cells avoids the risk of affecting the development of the fetus. Additionally, the proportion of cells that are removed is much lower compared to cleavage stage biopsy. Furthermore, blastoscyst stage embryos have a higher implantation potential compared to day 3 or day 4 embryos, so a higher rate of implantation could be achieved by trophectoderm analysis.[10,17]

Figure 57.1 shows the polymorphic STR markers scattered through the HLA region, which were used to detect any possible ADO in relation to HLA typing.

CLINICAL DISCUSSION

Patients and Methods

The study group consisted of a total of 157 couples who underwent a total of 303 cycles. Between 2003 and mid of 2010 at Istanbul Memorial Hospital, ART and Reproductive Genetics Center, 127 couples were referred for both mutation analysis for a specific genetic disorder and HLA typing, while 30 couples were referred for the sole purpose of HLA typing for acquired disorders. The detailed list of diseases can be found in Table 57.2.

Table 57.2: Cycle participations of patients and indications for HLA typing		
HLA typing combined with mutation analysis	*Patients*	*Cycles*
Beta-thalassemia	112	224
Wiskott-Aldrich syndrome	3	4
X-Adrenoleukodystrophy	3	3
Fanconi anemia	2	3
Hurler syndrome	2	3
Alpha mannosidosis	1	4
Gaucher disease	1	4
Hyperimmunoglobulinemia D syndrome	1	1
Sickle cell anemia	1	1
Glanzmann's disease	1	2
HLA typing for aquired diseases	*Patients*	*Cycles*
Acute lymphoblastic leukemia	12	16
Acute myelogenous leukemia	8	14
Diamond blackfan anemia	3	11
Hystiocytosis	1	3
Chronic myelogenous leukemia	1	2
Burkitt's lymphoma	1	2
Aplastic lymphoma	2	2
Anaplastic lymphoma	1	2
Myelodysplastic syndrome	1	2
Total	**157**	**303**

Preclinical Work-up

First, a haplotype analysis of mother, father and child, and when available, of the other family members, was performed for each family prior to preimplantation HLA typing. A panel of 50 different STR markers (Fig. 57.1) were tested on genomic DNAs to ensure the presence of sufficient informative markers (Fig. 57.2) to aid the identification of monosomy, trisomy, recombination, ADO and uniparental disomy (UPD) of the analyzed chromosomes and regions. For each family, at least 12 heterozygous markers spanning the HLA-A, HLA-B, HLA-C, HLA-DR,HLA-DQ regions (HLA Classes I, II, and III) were selected for PGD analysis.

The study period was divided into two according to the methods used, which included lysis of single cells, mutation testing, PCR conditions and primers used in the PGD study. Oocyte retrievals, inseminations, culture, biopsies and embryo transfers were performed in the Istanbul Memorial Hospital ART unit and all the PGD studies and evaluations were performed in the Istanbul Memorial Hospital Reproductive Genetics Unit.

PGD Study

The methods can be found elsewhere.[19] In the first period, the alkaline lysis method was used as described.[20] Cells were lysed by incubation at 65°C for 10 minutes in a sterile PCR tube containing 5 µL of lysis buffer (200 nmol/L KOH, 50 nmol/L DDT). The lysis buffer was then neutralized prior to adding the first round PCR mix which contained all external primers for co-amplification of all selected HLA markers and mutation linked markers. The second-round PCR reaction for each locus was then performed using 2 µL of the first round product.

In the second period, the proteinase K method was used for lysis of the cells as described previously.[2] The biopsied single cells were placed into a lysis solution containing 0.5 µL of 10 × PCR buffer, 0.5 µL of 1 percent tween-20, 0.5 µL of 1 percent triton X-100, 3.5 µL of water, and 0.05 µL of proteinase K. The lysis reaction was as follows: 45°C for 15 minutes for the lysis of the cells and 96°C for 20 minutes for inactivation of proteinase K. Although the reaction conditions were different in the two periods, both can be briefly summarized as follows; DNA testing was performed by two rounds of PCR reactions: in the first round, using multiplex PCR which allows simultaneous amplification of HLA regions and mutation-linked markers and in the second round, using singleplex PCR, which is a fluorescent PCR with semi or hemi-nested primers. Primer sequences and PCR conditions used in this study have been reported previously.[2,5,20-22]

Between 2003 and 2008, mutation analysis was performed using the mini sequencing technique as described elsewhere.[23] After mid-2008, restriction enzyme digestion reactions and subsequently, polyacrylamide gel electrophoresis analysis[21]

were used. Since mid-2009, both the methods are being used according to preference.

IVF and Embryo Biopsy Procedure

The stimulation protocols used were as outlined previously.[24] Oocyte retrievals were performed by transvaginal ultrasound guidance 36 h after recombinant human chorionic gonado-tropin (rhCG-Ovitrel) injection. Approximately 2 to 3 hours after oocyte retrieval, cumulus cells were enzymatically removed. Intracytoplasmic sperm injection (ICSI) was performed on metaphase II oocytes. One blastomere was removed from cleavage stage embryos (Fig. 57.3A) from an opening made using laser (IodoLaser, Research Instruments). Subsequently, after diagnosis, embryo transfer was performed, usually on day 4 but rarely on day 5. Recently, since 2009, trophectoderm tissue biopsies have also been performed. Blastocyst-stage biopsy was performed by making a hole in the zona pellucida on day 3 of embryonic development, which allowed the developing trophectoderm cells to protrude after blastulation, facilitating the biopsy. On day 5 postfertilization, approximately 4 to 5 cells were excised using laser energy without the loss of the inner cell mass (Fig. 57.3B). After diagnosis, the embryos were replaced during the same cycle, on day 5 or 6. Pregnancy was first evaluated by evaluation of serum beta-hCG, 12 days after embryo transfer and a clinical pregnancy was diagnosed by ultrasonographic visualization of one or more gestational sacs.

Results

In the HLA + mutation testing group (Group I), out of 262 initiated cycles, 166 cycles (63.35%) reached the embryo transfer stage. In the HLA-only group (Group II), 70.8 percent of the initiated cycles reached the embryo transfer stage. The detailed distribution of indications and overall results for each group are shown in Tables 57.2 and 57.3.

In total, 2989 blastomeres were biopsied and in 2751 (92.0%), a full diagnosis was achieved. In Group I, 17.9 percent of the analyzed embryos were found to be HLA compatible. Out of these compatible embryos, 4.6 percent were found to be free of mutations, 8 percent were found to be carriers of the analyzed disease and 4.9 percent were found to be affected. In group II, 16 percent of embryos were found to be HLA matched and 70.4 percent HLA non-matched.[19]

A total of 74 clinical pregnancies (34.9%) were achieved from 212 embryo transfer cycles with 6 ongoing pregnancies. To date, with 52 deliveries, 59 healthy and HLA compatible children have been born. 21 sick children have already been cured with cord blood cell and/or bone marrow transplantation. 23 children are waiting for their newborn siblings to gain sufficient weight and maturity for the donation of stem cells (Table 57.3). The 21 successful transplantations have been performed for the following

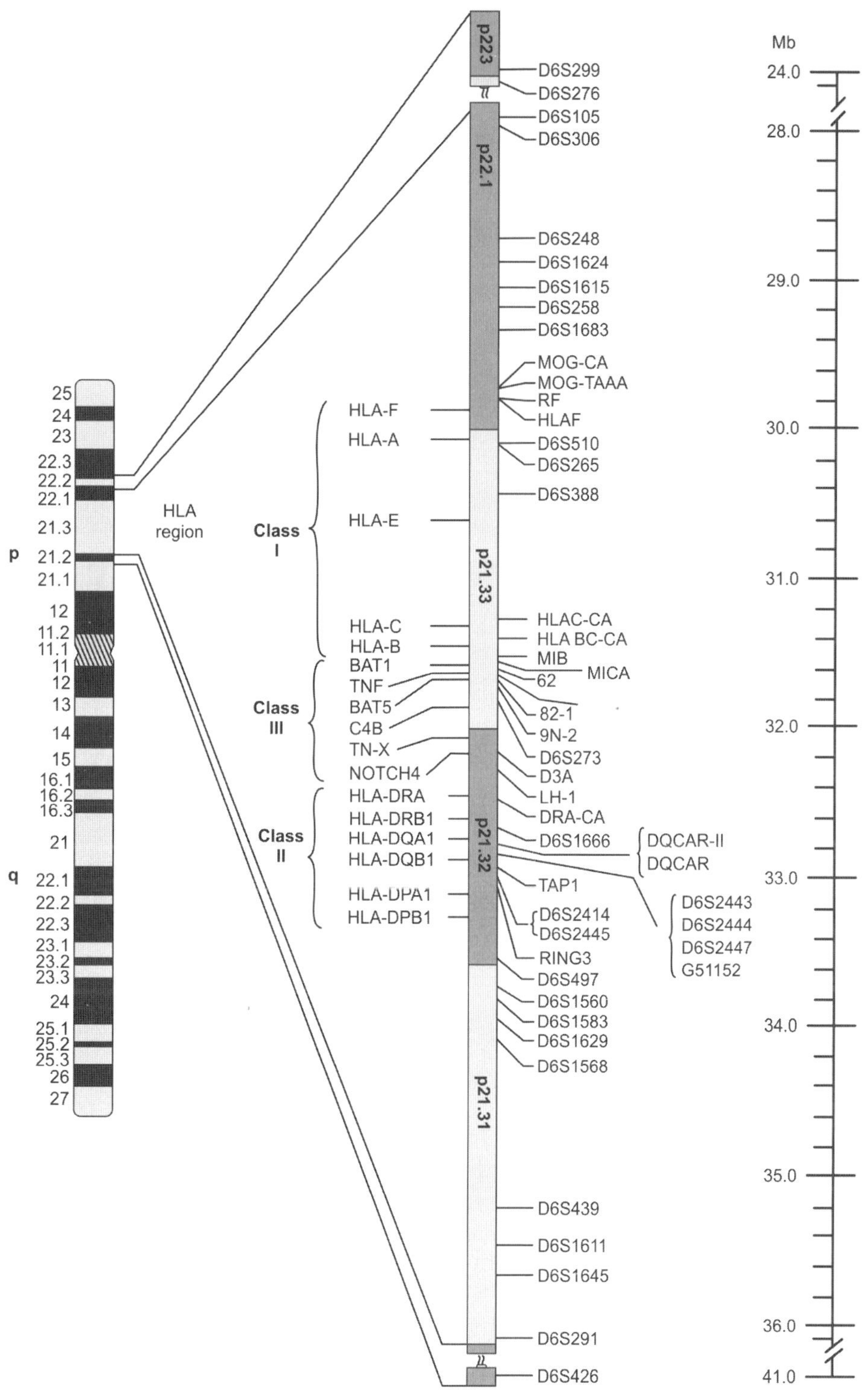

Fig. 57.1: Polymorphic STR markers used in HLA typing of the embryos

indications: β-thalassemia (n = 16), Wiskott Aldrich syndrome (n = 1), thrombasthenia (n = 1), X-ALD (n = 1), acute myeloid leukemia (n = 1) and Diamond Blackfan anemia (n = 1).

The majority of our HLA typing combined with PGD cases were β-thalassemia carriers (88.2%). The detailed outcomes of these cycles are shown in Table 57.4.

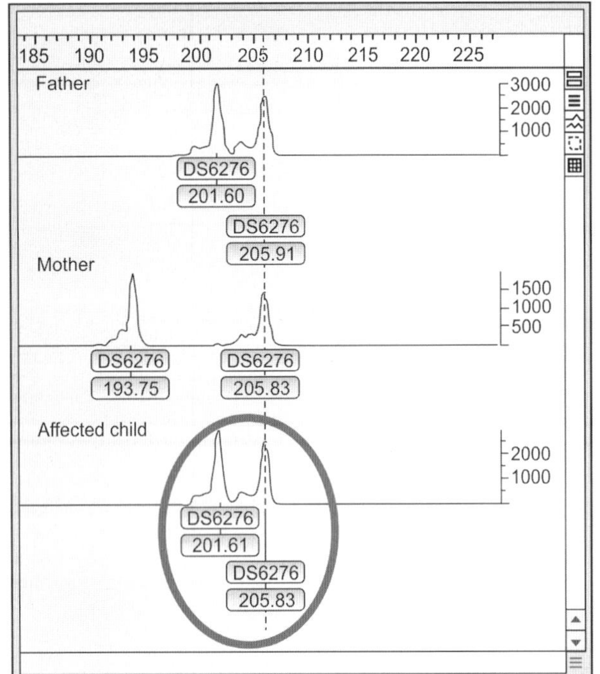

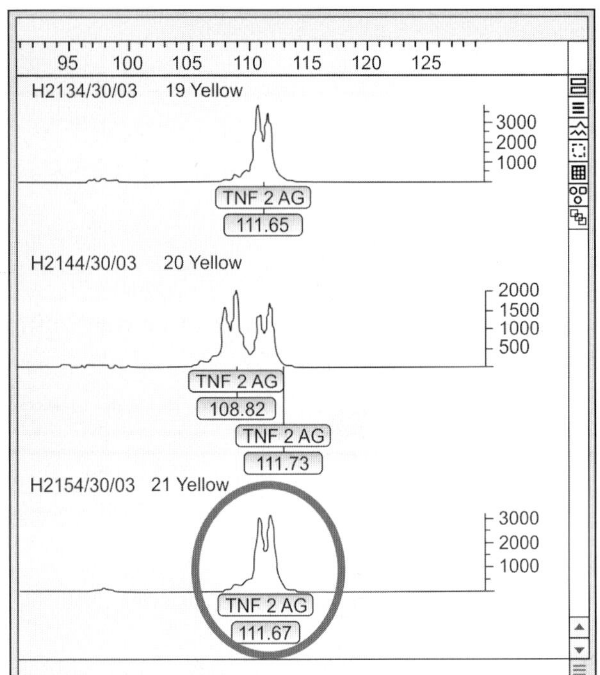

Fig. 57.2: Identification of informative markers during the HLA set-up study

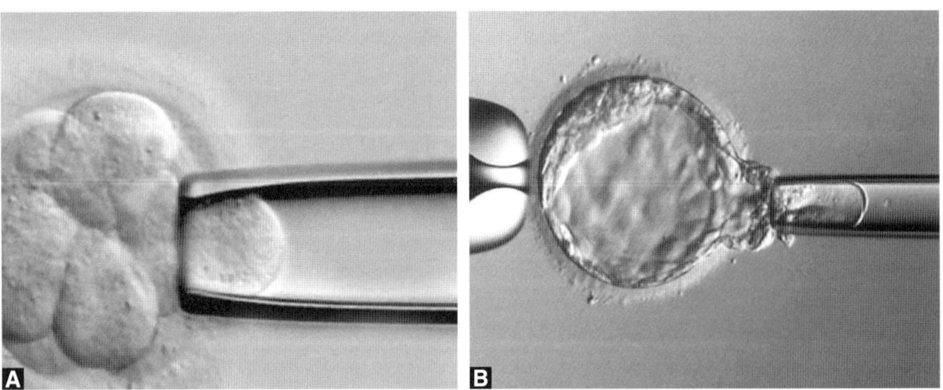

Figs 57.3A and B: Biopsy techniques: (A) Cleavage stage biopsy; (B) Blastocyst stage biopsy

The effect of maternal age and ovarian reserve on the success rate was compared between β-thalassemia carriers, since this group provided sufficient homogenous data. According to Table 57.5A, maternal age has little impact on the conception rate if at least one transferable embryo was found. However, miscarriage rates were different in these two groups (p < 0.05). When the groups were compared according to the clinical pregnancy rate (CPR) per cycle initiated, the difference became more pronounced (e.g. 23.4% vs 14.3%), however, it still did not reach statistical significance (Table 57.5A). However, the number of patients was not homogenous in both groups (201 patients below and only 35 patients ≥ 38 years), which may have reduced the statistical power of the comparison. Similarly, when the numbers of retrieved oocytes were classified as ≤5, 5< to ≤10, 10< to ≤20 and >20, a threshold number for retrieved oocytes-cumulus complexes was not identified (Table 57.5B). The probable reason for that may be the fertility status of the couples. The fact that all of these couples were fertile increased their chances of achieving pregnancy. On the other hand, the lack of use of morphological and developmental criteria for embryo transfer decreased the success of the outcome.

Table 57.3: Overall clinical results of HLA typing			
	HLA + mutation testing	*HLA only*	*Total*
No. of patients/cycles	136/262	35/65	171/327
Maternal age, mean (min-max)	32.0 ± 4.83 (21–43)	34.2 ± 5.65 (23–45)	32.44 (21–45)
BMI	25.77 ± 3.96	24.56 ± 5.2	25.52 ± 4.26
Total dosage of gonadotropins (mean)	3359.1 ± 1340	2715 ± 1337	3234.11 ± 1361
Ooctytes retreived (mean)	15.87 ± 8.81	16.86 ± 7.86	16.02
Mature oocytes injected (mean)	12.18 ± 6.73	12.86 ± 6.11	12.31
Oocytes fertilized (%)	87.90 ± 12.34	83.96 ± 13.65	87.33
Cycles with transfer (%)	63.4	70.8	64.8
β-hCG+ (%)	41.6	37	40.56
Clinical pregnancy rate per transfer (%)	36.1	30.4	34.9
Clinical miscarriages (n)	14	3	17
Implantation rate (%)	26.7	23.3	26
No. of embryos transfered (mean)	1.58 ± 0.71	1.59 ± 0.72	1.58
No. of pregnancies reaching to term (n)	43	8	52
No. of pregnancies ongoing (n)	3	3	5
No. of babies born (n)	51	10	62
No. of succsessful transplantations (n)	19	2	21[a]

[a]23 children are awaiting an appropriate time for HSC transplantation, Kahraman, et al.[19]

Table 57.4: Clinical and molecular analysis results of HLA typing and mutation analysis for β-thalassemia carriers	
Patient/cycle	120/236
Mean maternal age (min-max)	31.85 (21–43)
Oocytes retreived (mean)	16.03
Matured oocytes injected (mean)	12.21
Oocytes fertilized (%)	88.41
Embryos biopsied (n)	2132
Embryos diagnosed for HLA (%)	93.6
• Compatible (%)	17.9
• Not compatible (%)	71.1
• Other (polyploidy, aneuploidy, recombination and UPD) (%)	11.0
Diagnosed for mutation (%)	85.2
• Normal (%)	25.4
• Carrier (%)	45.0
• Affected (%)	25.2
• Other (polyploidy, aneuploidy, recombination and UPD) (%)	4.4
Compatible normal (%)	4.3
Compatible carrier (%)	8.4
Compatible affected (%)	4.8
Compatible other (%)	0.4
Transferable (%)	12.7
Cycles with embryo transfer (%)	62.7
Clinical pregnancies per transfer cycle (%)	35.1
No of transfered embryos (mean)	1.6
Implantation rate (%)	26.8
Ongoing pregnancies (n)	2
Birth (n)	37/44
aHSC transplantations (n)	16*

*19 children are awaiting an appropriate time for transplantation

Table 57.5: Clinical results of β-thalassemia carriers

(A) Clinical results of β-thalassemia carriers according to maternal age.

	Maternal age		
	<38	*≥ 38*	*p-value*
Cycles initiated (n)	201	35	
Maternal age (mean)	30.4 ± 3.72	40.14 ± 1.74	
Oocytes collected (mean)	17.30 ± 8.82	8.63 ± 4.16	<0.001
Body mass index (BMI)	25.39 ± 3.93	26.15 ± 5.5	NS
Total dosage of gonadotropins (IU)	3043.96 ± 1254.97	4152.59 ± 1488.80	<0.001
Matured oocytes injected (mean)	13.15 ± 6.77	6.80 ± 3.30	<0.001
Oocytes fertilized (%)	88.33 ± 11.63	85.90 ± 15.99	NS
Embryos biopsied (mean)	10.06 ± 5.40	5.03 ± 3.07	<0.001
Cycles with ET (n)	133 (66.2)	15 (42.9)	<0.01
Transferred embryos (mean)	1.60 ± 0.72	1.47 ± 0.74	NS
Positive β-hCG per ET cycle (%)	40.6	40.0	NS
CPR per ET cycle (%)	35.3	33.3	NS
CPR per cycle initiated (%)	23.4	14.3	NS
Clinical miscarriages (n)	7	3	<0.05
Implantation rate (%)	27	23	NS

Abbreviations: NS: not significant; ET: embryo transfer; CPR: clinical pregnancy rate

(B) Clinical results of β-thalassemia carriers according to the ovarian reserve.

	Cumulus oocyte complexes				
	≤ 5	*5 < to ≤ 10*	*10 < to ≤ 20*	*> 20*	*p-value*
Cycles initiated (n)	20	55	93	68	
Maternal age (mean)	35.1 ± 4.73	33.8 ± 5.09	31.3 ± 4.78	29.8 ± 3.47	<0.001
Oocytes collected (mean)	3.80 ± 0.95	8.15 ± 1.42	15.20 ± 2.97	27.07 ± 6.32	<0.001
Body mass index (BMI)	27.12 ± 3.9	25.46 ± 4.23	25.29 ± 4.05	25.47 ± 4.61	NS
Total dosage of gonadotropins (mean)	4490 ± 1539	4216.51 ± 1462	2861.79 ± 1115.23	2657.55 ± 841.9	<0.001
Matured oocytes injected (mean)	3.45 ± 1.00	6.22 ± 1.41	11.72 ± 2.91	20.29 ± 5.28	<0.001
Oocytes fertilized (%)	89.42 ± 15.82	85.83 ± 15.33	88.61 ± 11.05	88.41 ± 10.13	NS
Embryos biopsied (mean)	2.5 ± 1.67	4.6 ± 1.70	9.2 ± 3.17	15.1 ± 4.80	<0.001
Cycles with ET (n)	7 (35.0)	22 (40.0)	64 (68.8)	53 (77.9)	<0.001
Transfered embryos (mean)	1 ± 0.00	1.2 ± 0.54	1.6 ± 0.68	1.8±0.79	<0.005
+β-hCG per ET cycle (%)	57.2	36.4	39	41.5	NS
CPR per ET cycle (%)	57.2	31.8	32.8	35.8	NS
CPR per cycles initiated (%)	22.2	13	22.6	28	NS
Clinical miscarriages (n)	0	2	3	4	NS
Implantation rate (%)	57.2	27	24.5	27	NS

Abbreviations: NS: not significant; ET: embryo transfer; CPR: clinical pregnancy rate

CONCLUSION

This data presents one of the world's largest experiences on preimplantation HLA typing, and the results with stem cell transplantation are by far the best from one center. The data demonstrates that once a mutation-free and HLA-compatible embryo is found, acceptable pregnancy rates can be obtained with this approach, even in the presence of some cycle-related limitations such as advanced maternal age and/or diminished ovarian reserve. Our results indicate that HLA typing with or without mutation analysis is a promising and effective therapeutic tool for curing an affected sibling.

REFERENCES

1. Verlinsky Y, Rechitsky S, Schoolcraft W, Strom C, Kuliev A. Designer babies – are they a reality yet? Case report: Simultaneous preimplantation genetic diagnosis for Fanconi anaemia and HLA typing for cord blood transplantation. Reprod Biomed Online 2000;1:31.
2. Verlinsky Y, Rechitsky S, Schoolcraft W, Strom C, Kuliev A. Preimplantation diagnosis for Fanconi anemia combined with HLA matching. JAMA 2001;285:3130-3.
3. Simpson JL. Changing indications for preimplantation genetic diagnosis (PGD) Mol Cell Endocrinol 2001;183 (suppl. 1); S69-S75.
4. Kuliev A, Verlinsky Y. Preimplantation HLA typing and stem cell transplantation: Report of International meeting, Cyprus 2004.
5. Fiorentino F, Biricik A, Karadayi H, Berkil H, Karlikaya G, Sertyel S, et al. Development and clinical application of a strategy for preimplantation genetic diagnosis of single gene disorders combined with HLA matching. Mol Hum Reprod 2004;10:445-60.
6. Fiorentino F, Biricik A, Nuccitelli A, De Palma R, Kahraman S, Iacobelli M, et al. Strategies and clinical outcome of 250 cycles of Preimplantation Genetic Diagnosis for single gene disorders. Hum Reprod 2006;21:670-84.
7. Kahraman S, Findikli N. Effect of Italian referendum on global IVF: a comment from Turkey. Reprod Biomed Online 2005;11:662-3.
8. Kahraman S, Findikli N, Karlikaya G, Sertyel S, Karadayi H, Saglam Y, Fiorentino F. Medical and social perspectives of preimplantation genetic diagnosis for single gene disorders and/or HLA typing. Reprod Biomed Online 2007;14(Suppl 1):104-8.
9. Van de Velde H, Georgiou I, De Rycke M Schots R, Sermon K, Lissens W, Devroey P, Van Steirteghem A, Liebaers I. Novel universal approach for preimplantation genetic diagnosis of β-thalassemia in combination with HLA matching of embryos. Hum Reprod 2004;19:700-8.
10. Kokkali G, Traeger-Synodinos J, Vrettou C, Stavrou D, Jones GM, Cram DS, et al. Blastocyst biopsy versus cleavage stage biopsy and blastocyst transfer for preimplantation genetic diagnosis of beta-thalassaemia: A pilot study. Hum Reprod 2007;22:1443-9.
11. Arcasoy A. Thalasemia. Science and Technology 1999;374:54-6.
12. Lucarelli G, Galimberti M, Giardini C, Polchi P, Angelucci E, Baronciani D, Erer B, Gaziev D. Bone marrow transplantation in thalassemia: The experience of Pesaro. Ann NY Acad Sci 1998;850:270-5.
13. Gaziev J, Lucarelli G. Stem cell transplantation for thalassemia. Reprod Biomed Online 2005;10:111-5.
14. Costeas PA. Bone marrow donor registry and availability of HLA matched donors. Abstracts of International Seminar on Preimplantation HLA Typing and Stem Cell Transplantation, Limassol, Cyprus, 2004. p. 9. (http//:www.pgdis.org).
15. Shirazi A, Ahadi AM, Farzaneh DF, Sadeghizade M. Effect of lysis strategy in accuracy and repeatability of sex determination by single cell polymerase chain reaction method. Journal of Biological Sciences 2009;9:78-82.
16. Rechitsky S, Verlinsky O, Amet T, Rechitsky M, Kouliev T, Strom C, Verlinsky Y. Reliability of preimplantation diagnosis for single gene disorders. Mol Cell Endocrinol 2001;183:65-8.
17. McArthur SJ, Leigh D, Marshall JT, Gee AJ, De Boer KA, Jansen RP. Blastocyst trophectoderm biopsy and preimplantation genetic diagnosis for familial monogenic disorders and chromosomal translocations. Prenat Diagn 2008;5:434-42.
18. Pangalos CG, Hagnefelt B, Kokkali G, Pantos K, Konialis CP. Birth of a healthy histocompatible sibling following preimplantation genetic diagnosis for chronic granulomatous disease at the blastocyst stage coupled to HLA typing. Fetal Diagn Ther 2008;24:334-9.
19. Kahraman S, Beyazyurek C, Ekmekci GC. Seven years of experience on preimplantation HLA typing: a clinical overview of 327 cycles. Reprod Biomed Online 2011;23:363-71.
20. Fiorentino F, Kahraman S, Karadayi H, Biricik A, Sertyel S, Karlikaya G, et al. Short tandem repeats haplotyping of the HLA region in preimplantation HLA matching. Eur J Hum Genet 2005;8:953-8.
21. Rechitsky S, Tur-Kaspa, Kuliev A, Verlinsky Y. Preimplantation genetic diagnosis with HLA matching. Reprod Biomed Online 2004;9:210-21.
22. Verlinsky Y, Rechitsky S, Sharapova T, Morris R, Taranissi M, Kuliev A. Preimplantation HLA typing. JAMA 2004;291:2079-85.
23. Fiorentino F, Magli MC, Podini D, Ferraretti AP, Nuccitelli A, Vitale N, et al. The minisequencing method: an alternative strategy for preimplantation genetic diagnosis of single gene disorders. Mol Hum Reprod 2003;7:399-410.
24. Kahraman S, Karlikaya G, Sertyel S, Karadayi H, Findikli N. Clinical aspects of preimplantation genetic diagnosis for single gene disorders combined with HLA typing. Reprod Biomed Online 2004;5:529-32.

Preimplantation Genetic Diagnosis: Clinical Applications

Mirudhubashini Govindarajan

OVERVIEW

The successful clinical application of preimplantation genetic diagnosis (PGD) was first reported in 1990 from Hammersmith Hospital in London. This had been performed for a patient at risk of an X-linked genetic disorder. The procedure seemed to be the ideal alternative to the prenatal diagnostic procedure in early pregnancy and termination thereafter. Now, more than 2 decades later, more than 100 single gene disorders and a large number of chromosomal defects are detectable by PGD. However, the technique has also introduced many controversial questions for the medical community to address. Clinicians have to be aware of what this technology can and cannot deliver, especially real success in terms of live birth per cycle started as a denominator—not often discussed or published in the literature.

Preimplantation genetic screening (PGS) has evolved out of PGD—to try and select the most suitable embryos for transfer. The use of PGD has dramatically increased in the past few years, particularly in the US. The indications for this procedure arise from infertility clinics and not genetic clinics. The procedure, in fact, has been advocated to improve *in vitro* fertilization (IVF) outcome in selected situations. However, the clinical value of PGS is still being debated, while in theory, the argument for PGS looks persuasive. As more clinicians and patients look for PGS to improve their IVF outcome, it has become more critical to understand whether PGS actually improves the IVF success rate or not. The recommendations of the PGD consortium of European Society for Human Reproduction and Embryology (ESHRE) have recently been published. Some of these recommendations are discussed.

INTRODUCTION

The first ever baby conceived using the IVF technique was delivered in 1978 (Steptoe and Edwards). Since then, more than a million babies, conceived as a result of assisted reproductive techniques, have been born worldwide. The last two decades have seen numerous technological advances in this field. It is now possible to diagnose genetic abnormalities in the early embryo. Preimplantation genetic studies have become established diagnostic procedures. Several of the existing and possible applications of PGD are at an interface between Reproductive Medicine and Clinical Genetics. ART is now being used for genetic reasons as well as infertility treatments, and an entirely new dimension has been added. The UNESCO report in 2003 aptly states, "IVF aims at having a child, PGD aims at having a healthy child, and PGD/HLA typing aims at having a healthy and helpful child". However, these procedures are still not very widely practised owing to high technological demands, costs, relatively low pregnancy rates and strict licensing procedures in many countries. Very

few studies have so far been performed or published, offering an integrated analysis of technological, patient-related, ethical and economic aspects of PGD and PGS.[1]

Preimplantation genetic studies have become clinically useful in two major areas—PGS for identifying abnormal aneuploid embryos and PGD for diagnosing specific inherited genetic abnormalities in the embryo. These studies utilize methodologies such as fluorescent *in situ* hybridization (FISH) and polymerase chain reaction (PCR). Polymerase chain reaction amplifies specific fragments of DNA from a single cell and has contributed tremendously for diagnosing inherited genetic abnormalities at a single cell level. FISH and the newer array based technologies facilitate the diagnosis of aneuploidies in a single cell. This allows PGS of all the available embryos and explores the possibility of improving success with IVF procedures.

Preimplantation genetic diagnosis was developed in 1989[2] in an effort to avoid transferring affected embryos to couple who carried serious genetic disorders such as hemophilia, cystic fibrosis (CF) and the like. Only unaffected embryos can be selected for transfer. Diagnosis can be made before pregnancy starts, avoiding the need for invasive prenatal diagnostic procedures and selective abortion later.[3] There is consensus among professionals that PGD is acceptable for medical indications if there is a high risk of transmitting serious genetic disorders. In addition, PGD has also been used for other reasons such as matching tissue type of the embryo to an existing sibling for therapeutic donor purposes. However, the demand for using PGD for non-medical purposes, such as sex selection for social or cultural reasons, also exists.[4] This extended use of PGD is controversial.

Preimplantation genetic screening (PGS) previously called PGD–AS, or aneuploidy screening is performed for different indications. PGS is usually carried out for infertile couples undergoing *in vitro* fertilization (IVF) procedures in an effort to improve poor pregnancy outcomes. This is sought to be achieved by transferring embryos, which have numerically normal chromosomes. Although the use of PGS is steadily increasing,[5] the importance and place of this technique is still being debated.[6,7] This discussion is particularly relevant where this methodology is applied at IVF clinics without the necessary genetic expertise.

Preimplantation Studies: The Techniques

The two main steps of the preimplantation genetic studies are:
1. Obtaining nuclear material for genetic analysis.
2. Analyzing methodologies.

Obtaining Nuclear Material

The human oocyte and embryo upto the stage of expanded blastocyst are enclosed within the zona pellucida. Sampling techniques require micromanipulation, techniques to penetrate the protective glycoprotein layer. Target cells are then removed by micromanipulation, causing minimal damage to the embryo. There are three different methods for obtaining nuclear material for genetic studies from the oocytes/embryo.

Polar body biopsy: Verlinsky et al.[8] in Chicago, pioneered polar body biopsy and PGD both, for aneuploidy screening and single gene defects involving maternal mutations. Both first and second polar bodies are biopsied from zygotes following IVF/ICSI procedures for either chromosomal or single gene defect analysis.

The first polar body is extruded as a byproduct of the first meiotic division. This occurs inside the follicle before ovulation. The polar body contains counterparts of the chromosomes in the developing oocyte. It is trapped in the space between the oocyte and the zona pellucida.

Following fertilization and activation of sperm chromatin, the oocyte enters second meiosis. Duplicated chromatids of the haploid oocyte separate. One set of chromatid remains in the oocyte. The other set is expelled in the second polar body.

The polar bodies are distinguished on the basis of morphology. The first polar body tends to have crinkled bodies and tend to fragment. The second polar body is generally smoother and may have a visible interface.

The polar bodies do not contribute structurally to the developing embryo. The embryo integrity is maintained in polar body biopsy and therefore, it is a safe technique. However, the main drawback is that the polar body analysis can detect only maternally transmitted genetic or chromosomal abnormalities. Paternally derived defects and those originating after fertilization postzygotic cannot be diagnosed by this technique.[9] Low quality of polar body chromosomal spreading can limit the accuracy and reliability of FISH analysis.

Cleavage stage biopsy: Cleavage stage biopsy or blastomere biopsy is the most commonly used biopsy technique. Non-contact infrared lasers are now used for zona drilling and embryo biopsy. One or two blastomeres are biopsied for analysis on the third day when the embryos reach the eight-cell stage. Cleavage stage biopsy is performed before compaction, the process of intercellular adhesion and junction formation. Embryo transfer is performed on day 4/5, allowing time for analysis. Disorders of both maternal and paternal origin, as well as those originating after fertilization, can be checked from the blastomeres obtained on the 3rd day.

The implantation rates for the biopsied embryo is lower.[9,10] There is evidence for significant chromosomal mosaicism in cleavage stage embryos. Therefore, biopsied cells may not be representative of the whole embryo.[11]

Blastocyst biopsy: On day 5/6, the embryo becomes a blastocyst containing approximately 150 cells. Cells are differentiated into an inner cell mass and trophectoderm cells. The trophectoderm cells may be biopsied safely. More number of cells can be obtained for examination at this stage without compromising the embryo. However, the time left for diagnosis is very small, as the embryos should be transferred before day 5 or 6. The clinical application of this technology is recent and only limited data has been reported. Its application on a large scale needs validation (PGDIS 2004).

Analyzing Methodologies

Polymerase Chain Reaction (PCR)

The PCR technique was introduced in the mid-1980s. This technique enriches DNA for a specific oligonucleotide fragment (amplicon). After 30 to 40 cycles, an initial minute quantity of DNA is amplified several times. This then, is subjected to analytical techniques to determine the presence of point mutations deletions, insertions and other genetic markers. Direct sequencing of DNA can also be performed. Studies on DNA are performed using ethidium bromide staining of separated DNA fragments on agarose gels. Currently, fluorescent PCR has been used where fragments are separated and identified using color flurochromes. This method is more sensitive and accurate. This technique is primarily used for analysis of genes in monogenic diseases.[5] Amplification of a specific region of DNA by PCR allows for the analysis of disease causing changes in DNA or markers linked to a disease, e.g. microsatellitis and single nucleotide proteins (SNPs).[12]

Whole Genome Amplification

The PCR technique amplifies only the genetic area of interest, where as the whole genome amplification (WGA) technology amplifies the whole genome, producing many times more DNA for analysis. This can then be applied for diagnosing a huge range of genetic disorders.

Fluorescent in situ Hybridization (FISH)

The FISH technique is most commonly used for the analysis of chromosomes. FISH applies chromosome specific probes for upto 9 chromosomes on a single blastomere. FISH probes are labeled with different colored fluorochromes that bind to specific gene sequences on specific chromosomes. Although it allows the evaluation of only a limited number of chromosomes (between 5–9), FISH can still detect over 80 percent of all chromosomal abnormalities. The common probes used are those most likely to be aneuploid in spontaneous abortions such as 13, 16, 18, 21, 22, X and Y. Because probes hybridize to a specific locus, FISH provides information only about a very small segment of the chromosome. This allows for selecting out abnormal embryos and choosing normal embryos for transfer

In polar body biopsy procedures, the first polar body is a byproduct of the first meiotic division. Normally, there is a double signal for each chromosome. Each signal represents a single chromatid. In meiotic errors the number of signals may vary from 1 to 4. The genotype of the oocytes is usually the opposite of the polar body I genotype—(i.e. missing signals in the polar body suggests extra chromosome material in the oocyte and vice versa). In contrast, the normal FISH pattern in polar body II is represented by a single signal for each chromosome (single chromatid). Any deviation from this suggests a meiotic error.

The primary use of FISH is to determine sex chromosomal content for couples at risk of various sex-linked disorders such as hemophilia and for chromosomal abnormalities.

The FISH technique is limited because only a few chromosomes can be identified at a time. A complete karyotype that will provide maximum information cannot be obtained by the FISH technique.

Comparative Genomic Hybridization

Comparative genomic hybridization (CGH) is a relatively new and still experimental technique. It is a molecular cytogentic technique based on the analysis of genomic DNA and does not require metaphase chromosomes. CGH analyzes the entire chromosomal complement. However, polyploidy and balanced translocations cannot be detected by CGH. The disadvantage is that the whole procedure takes about 72 hours, which limits its use.[13] Technology is being improved to decrease the time taken for the procedure as well as to improve the resolution using microarrays.

CLINICAL DISCUSSION

Preimplantation Genetic Diagnosis (PGD)

Preimplantation genetic diagnosis is an effective technique for diagnosing recurrent genetic conditions. It is performed for ruling out a specific inherited genetic disorder in the offspring of a carrier couple at risk. The referrals for these procedures usually originate in the genetics clinic. It can be considered as an alternative to prenatal diagnostic procedures (PND). First, such diagnostic PGD techniques were reported from Hammersmith Hospital, London in 1990, and were used to diagnose an X-linked genetic disorder. Now, well over 100 single gene disorders are detectable using this technology. More than 5000 couples have been treated in the last decade with this technology.

Main Indications for PGD

Monogenic Disorders

Carriers of monogenic disorders fall into the following categories:

1. *Autosomal recessive disorders with a 1:4 risk:* The most common indications for PGD in this category have been cystic fibrosis, β-thalassemia, spinal muscular atrophy, Tay-Sach's disease and the like.
2. *Autosomal dominant disorders with a 1:2 risk:* These may be disorders such as mytonic dystrophy, amyloid polyneuropathy, Charcot-Marie tooth disease, achrondroplasia and the like.
3. *X-linked recessive disorders with 1:2 risk in males:* Common disorders are Fragile-X syndrome, Duchenne's muscular dystrophy, hemophilia A and B and the like.

These disorders are carried on the X-chromosome, the female being the carrier. Genetic disease, however, is usually expressed in males. The FISH technique can be used to identify X and Y-chromosomes and the sex of the embryo. Only female embryos are transferred. However, one-half of these are carriers. All male embryos are discarded although only one-half of these are affected by the condition. This may be unacceptable for some. The options for using PCR to diagnose these genetic disorders are becoming available now.

Chromosomal Rearrangements

The application of PGD for Robertsonian and reciprocal translocations is on the rise. Reproductive risks in these situations are dependent on the chromosomes involved and the sex of the carrier.[14]

Late Onset Disorders

In autosomal dominant disorders with full penetrance, PGD may be justifiable if the disease is severe, debilitating or lethal, e.g. Huntington's disease.

The PGD technique is justified if the child will have several decades of unimpaired living and the disease is treatable. Screening for common late onset diseases, such as BRCA 1 and BRCA 2 genes for breast cancer and familial adenomatous polyposis, is not considered ethically acceptable by majority of the workers.

Mitochondrial Disorders

For any given condition, PGD should be evaluated against offspring prenatal diagnostic procedures (PND). It should also be evaluated against allowing nature to take its own course. PGD offers the advantage of earlier diagnosis prior to implantation. It also avoids the need for termination of a pregnancy and the emotional trauma associated with it.

PGD has certain drawbacks also. Assisted reproductive techniques (ART) need to be done in an otherwise fertile couple. This becomes technically demanding, expensive and has attendant maternal and fetal risks. There is a need for ART specialists, clinicians, geneticists and molecular biologists to work together. The real success rate in terms of live birth rate per cycle started is not often reported in the results table, and is probably low in the order of 10 to 15 percent. Many couples do not have embryos left for transfer. According to one estimate, upto 40 percent of the patients may not get to an embryo transfer.[15] According to the PGD consortium 2006,[16] there is a misdiagnosis rate of 2 to 3 percent, and most centers advise a chorionic villus sampling (CVS) or amniocentesis after conceiving to safeguard against errors.

Directional counseling should be avoided when PGD is suggested to patients. They should be given complete information on all the available procedures and be allowed to decide between PGD and PND without interference. At present, PGD can be offered as an alternative to PND but cannot replace it entirely.

Preimplantation Genetic Screening (PGS)

Preimplantation genetic screening is at present, used for couples undergoing ART in order to improve the procedure outcome. Aneuploid embryos can result in failed cleavage, failed implantation or miscarriage, compromising the reproductive outcome. PGS selects out aneuploid embryos. Chromosomally normal embryos are selected by this procedure for transfer in an IVF/ICSI cycle.

Indications for PGS

The use of PGS has increased tremendously all over the world in the last few years for improving IVF results in the following situations:
- Advanced maternal age
- Recurrent implantation failure
- Recurrent early pregnancy losses
- Poor morphology embryos
- Severe male factor problems
- Improving success rates.

Various studies on spontaneous abortion have shown that more than half the abortions are associated with chromosomal abnormalities. IVF with PGS and selected transfer of euploid embryos is now considered as an established treatment for couples with recurrent pregnancy loss when one parent carries a balanced chromosomal translocation.

Aneuploidy, resulting from non-dysjunction of chromosomes, increases with maternal age. Maternal age may also increase the incidence of chromosomal mosaicism.[17] Poor embryo morphology is also associated with polyploidy and mosaicism.[13] IVF with PGS for reasons of advanced maternal age or unexplained pregnancy loss can increase the implantation rates and decrease the miscarriage rates. Nevertheless, a modest improvement in live birth rates achieved thus far, cannot justify the associated costs and risks in couple without other specific indications for IVF.

The experience of the efficacy, reliability and safety of PGS is growing, but is still limited.[5,18,19] Some consider this procedure still as experimental.[20] PGS raises concern because of the risk of misdiagnosis due to the high rate of mosaicism in cleavage stage embryos.[7] The only randomized large-scale trial so far has been from the Dutch-speaking Free University of Brussels that consisted of over 400 cycles. This study failed to demonstrate an improved pregnancy rate in screened cycles.

Technical Problems and Limitations

Methods involved in preimplantation genetics can be technically challenging and have distinct limitations.

- An older woman produces less number of embryos, making it inappropriate to apply the technique in this situation.
- PGD/PGS does not detect mosaicism.
- Increasing embryonic mosaicism with increasing maternal age makes PGD less accurate in older women.
- The FISH probe binds to a very small area of the chromosome and does not provide information on the rest of the chromosome.
- FISH does not detect chromosomal structural abnormalities.
- Other technical problems that may be encountered are:
  - Contamination of the PCR sample
  - Failure of DNA amplification
  - Loss of nuclear material during fixation
  - Overlapping of signals
  - Background staining
  - Split spots
  - Non-diagnosis due to allele drop-out
  - Misdiagnosis.

CONCLUSION

At present, the advantage of applying preimplantation genetic studies on a larger scale has not been demonstrated conclusively and harder data are needed. The ESHRE reproductive group statement (2006) states that benefits are not clearly proven yet, and that, there are not enough published studies to promote PGS as a routine tool. To sum up, even though it is widely used, PGS should be still considered experimental and offered in a trial setting. As yet, it cannot be offered as a panacea for every form of reproductive failure.

REFERENCES

1. Ingerslav HJ, Poulsen PB, Hojgaard A, Anderson A, Kolvraa S, Hindkjaer J, Larsen RJ, Dinesen J, Jespergaard C. Preimplantation diagnostic –En medicinsk teknologivundering http://www.sat.dk/applikationer/cemtv/publikationer/docs/Preimplantation/html/sum.htm) 2002.
2. Handyside AH, Kontogianni, EG Hardy K, Winston RM. Pregnancies from biopsied human preimplantation embryos sexed by Y-specific DNA amplification. Nature 1990;344:768-70.
3. Boyle KE, Vlahos N, Jarow JP. Assisted Reproductive Technology in the new millennium II. Urology 2004;63:217-24.
4. Knoppers BM, Isasi RM. Regulatory approaches to reproductive genetic testing. Hum Reprod 2004;17:1391-8.
5. Sermon K, Moutou C, Harper J, Geraedts, Scriven P, Wilton lMagli MC, Michiels A, Viville S, De Die C. ESHRE PGD data collection IV: May–December 2001. Hum Reprod 2005;20:19-34.
6. Wilson L. Preimplantaion genetic diagnosis for aneuploidy screening in early embryos: A review. Prenat. Diagn 2002;22:312-8.
7. Staesson C, Platteau P, Van Assche E, An Michielss H, Tournaye MC, Devroye P, Liebaers I, Van steirteghem A. Comparison of blastocyst transfer with or without preimplantation genetic diagnosis for aneuploidy screening in couples with advanced maternal age: A prospective randomized controlled trial. Hum Reprod 2004;19:2849-58.
8. Verlinsky Y, Cohen J, Munne S, Giananoli L, Simpson JL, Ferraretti AP, Kuliev A. Over a decade of experience with preimplantation genetic diagnosis: a multicenter report. Fertil Steril 2004;82:292-4.
9. Gianaroli L, Magli MC, Ferreretti AP. Preimplantation genetic diagnosis. In Current Practices and Controversies in Assisted Reproduction. Report of a WHO meeting 2001. WHO Geneva 2002.
10. Sermon K, Moutou C, Harper J, Geraedts, Scriven P, Wilton lMagli MC, Michiels A, Viville S, De Die C. ESHRE PGD data collection IV: May–December 2001. Human Reproduction 2005;20:19-34.
11. Staesson C, Platteau P, Van Assche E, An Michielss H, Tournaye MC, Devroye P, Liebaers I, Van steirteghem A. Comparision of blastocyst transfer with or without preimplantation genetic diagnosis for aneuploidy screening in couples with advanced maternal age: A prospective randomized controlled trial. Human Reproduction 2004;19:2849-58.
12. Boyle KE, Vlahos N, Jarow JP. Assisted reproductive technology in the new millennium II. Urology 2004;63:217-24.
13. Sermon K, Van Steiteghem A, Liebaers I. Preimplantation genetic diagnosis: Lancet 2004;363:1633-41.
14. Seriven PN, Flinter FA Braude PR, Ogilvie CM. Robertsoinian translocations–reproductive risks and indications for preimplantation genetic diagnosis. Hum Reprod 2001; 16:2267-73.
15. Brande PR, de Wert GMWR, Evers-Kiebooms G, Pettigrew RA, Geraedts JP. Non disclosure preimplantation genetic diagnosis for Huntigton's disease: Practical and ethical dilemma. Prenatal Diagnosis 1998;18:1422-6.
16. PGD consortium 2006—ESHRE Monographs Oct 2006.
17. Munne S. Preimplantation genetic diagnosis of numerical and structural chromosome abnormalities. Reprod Biomed Online 2002;4:183-96.
18. Briggs DA, Power NJ, Lamb V, Rutherford JA, Gsden RG. Amplification of DNA sequences in polar bodierm human oocs for diagnosis of mitrochodrialease. Ancet 2000;355:1520-1.
19. Wilton L. Preimplantation genetic diagnosis for aneuploidy screening early human embryos: A review Prenatal Diagnosis 2002;22:312-8.
20. IFFS. IFFS surveillance 04, Fertil Steril 2004;81 (Suppl 4) S9-54.

Preimplantation Genetic Diagnosis: The Current State of the Art

Sulochana Gunasheela

INTRODUCTION

There are couples with family members affected with genetically carried diseases. Some women happen to have recurrent miscarriages due to chromosomal abnormalities and there are some patients who have repeated attempts at *in vitro* fertilization (IVF) wherein, morphologically normal looking embryos fail to implant. All these are couples, who are eager to find out what the cause of reproductive failure is due to, and they wish to circumvent their malady by having a choice of conception by embryos, which are free from such diseases.

Only some genetic diseases are inherited and many are *de novo* mutations caused by factors unknown (e.g. viral, chemical and environmental factors). While *de novo* mutations are most unlikely to repeat in the same couple, inherited genetic diseases have a good chance of recurrence, the incidence being 25 percent with X-linked or autosomal recessive diseases and 50 percent with autosomal dominant diseases.

The first attempt at choosing the right pregnancy was made by prenatal diagnosis (PND). PND consists of diagnosing the chromosomal abnormality of a pregnancy that has already occurred by methods like chorionic villi sampling (CVS), culture of amniocytes from amniotic fluid and aspirated blood from the umbilical cord of the fetus. Some genetic diseases can be diagnosed by ultrasound only. Several thousand cases of PND have been performed with a high level of accuracy and low risk to fetal life, unlike preimplantation genetic diagnosis (PGD), which is still in an experimental stage.[1]

Commonly, there are two types of embryos or embryonic material taken up for biopsy. These are blastomeres aspirated from a day 2 to day 3 embryo (cleavage stage biopsy) and trophectoderm taken from a 5-day embryo (blastocyst biopsy); a biopsy may also be taken from oocytes in metaphase II even before fertilization-polar body biopsy.

CLINICAL DISCUSSION

Preimplantation Genetic Diagnosis (PGD)

Blastomere Biopsy

The embryos are usually obtained after intracytoplasmic sperm injection (ICSI) to avoid contamination from cumulus cells around the zona or supernumeric spermatozoa lying in the subzonal space. Two blastomeres are removed from a day 2 to 3 embryo which has at least 7 to 8 blastomeres. An opening is made in the zona pellucida either by use of laser or by application of acid tyrode solution. The embryos are held at the opposite pole by a suction pipette; the blastomeres are gently aspirated through the hole made. The embryos are incubated in media free from Ca^{2+} and Mg^{2+} for a while before the biopsy, if they have already compacted. The blastomeres are taken up immediately either for fluorescent *in situ* hybridization (FISH) for the detection of aneuploidy or for polymerase chain reaction (PCR), if it is being tested for monogenic disorders.

Preimplantation genetic diagnosis makes it mandatory for the couple to undergo IVF and most preferably, ICSI even though they have established their ability to achieve pregnancy by the natural method several times. This makes the PGD program cost prohibitive as compared to PND. The technique of PGD, being highly precise and labor-intensive, makes it inaccessible for most centers to develop. A single blastomere, or even a double blastomere biopsy may not give a consistent result due to genetic mosaicism noted between individual blastomeres of a single embryo, using both, cytogenic methods and the FISH technique, suggesting that the genetic diagnosis made on small number of cells cannot be totally relied upon.[2] Further, biopsy of every available embryo has to be done in order to select the right embryos for transfer. Excess embryos with a normal genetic karyotype may be frozen, but so far, there are very few reports of babies born out of frozen biopsied embryos. The procedure of aspirating

25 to 30 percent of blastomeres from a day 3 embryo itself can occasionally cause death of the embryo even if it were normal, thus causing unnecessary loss of embryos.

Blastocyst Biopsy

Blastocyst biopsy (BB) produces a large number of cells for scrutiny, and it is ethically more acceptable and less injurious to the embryo than removal of blastomeres, each one of which is capable of becoming a total embryo. The genetic structure of the cells of the trophectoderm will be representative of the embryo itself. Another argument in favor of BB is that, there is a good chance of only robust and healthy embryos to become blastocysts, thus making PGD less labor-intensive.

Blastocyst biopsy is ethically more acceptable because the tissue sample taken consists of trophectoderm, which is the outermost portion of the embryo, which does not participate in the formation of the true embryo.

The downside of BB is that in many laboratories, embryos are lost steadily at each stage of growth in culture, and the number of blastocysts available at the end stage of the culture procedure would be much reduced. This, added to the occasional death of an embryo, caused by the technique of PGD itself, may result in some couples not having any embryo left for transfer. Since the program of PGD is in an experimental stage, with a misdiagnosis of upto 4 percent, many workers believe that even after transferring 'disease-free embryos', it may be worthwhile doing a PND to confirm the normality of the pregnancy.[3]

Polar Body Biopsy (Oocyte Biopsy)

Polar body biopsy (PBB) is one form of study of pre-implantation genetics. While blastomere analysis from a 2 to 3-day old embryo and blastocyst biopsy from a 5 day old embryo gives the genomic details of the embryo as a whole, PBB genetic analysis focuses only on maternally derived chromosomal anomalies.

There are two polar bodies—polar body 1 (PB1) and polar body 2 (PB2). The PB1 is removed from a preovulatory mature oocyte, which is not yet fertilized. The PB2 is extruded from the oocyte at the time of fertilization. Removal of polar bodies for biopsy is less traumatic to the oocyte because these are lying in the subzonal region and outside the oolemma. In view of this, the blastomeres inside the oolemma are left undisturbed. Although the objection to the PBB is that it relates entirely to maternal genomic anomalies, it is still valuable because 90 percent of the embryo aneuploidies occur during maternal meiosis I, and meiosis II, particularly when they are age-related. The PB1 and PB2 can be subjected to analysis by using FISH probes. Upto 5 chromosomes can be detected by FISH at the single cell level, allowing screening for the most common aneuploidies for chromosomes 13,18, 21 and sex chromosomes.

Clinical experimental evidence shows that by analysis of PB1 and PB2 for aneuploidies in women aged 38 years and above, 50 percent of the embryos are found to carry chromosomal aberrations and these can occur in both meiosis I and meiosis II. One of the disadvantages of PBB is that the first polar body can sometimes disappear before the second polar body is extruded. So, one may have to do the duplication procedure of zona drilling and aspiration as each polar body arrives, making it labor-intensive.

Polar body biopsy can be performed by a mechanical or laser technique. It does not interfere with the embryo structure and cell allocation. It also satisfies some of the controversial ethical problems of removing a potential totipotent blastomere. The hole required in the zona is the same as that required for assisted hatching (AH). However, it will not detect other abnormalities, such as polyploidy, haploidy and mosaicism, that can occur inside the cells after fertilization is completed.[4] Such a situation occurs in at least 19 percent of embryonic chromosome abnormalities.

There are two groups among couples who are referred for PGD.

PGD for Group 1 Diseases (Aneuploidy)

Group one consists of diseases caused by chromosomal abnormalities, either numerical or structural. These can be detected by FISH analysis, which is based on detection of chromosome-specific signals in the nuclei of the blastomeres as the color of each signal is chromosome-specific. Currently, a mixture of FISH probes are available for the detection of 13, 16, 18, 21, X and Y chromosomes.[4]

The following conditions can be diagnosed by the FISH technique:
- Structural chromosomal abnormalities:
  - Reciprocal translocations
  - Robertsonian translocations
  - Inversions
  - Deletions.
- Couples at high risk for aneuploidy:
  - Klinefelter's syndrome
  - Sex chromosomal mosaicism
  - Male meiotic abnormalities.

Use of PGD in IVF Treatment

Women, who have undergone repeated IVF failures or recurrent abortions, and all women above the age of 38 to 39 undergoing IVF.

Preimplantation genetic diagnosis for aneuploidy (PGD-A) amounts to the detection of multiple chromosomal abnormalities simultaneously in order to increase the ongoing pregnancy rate in every assisted reproductive technique (ART) cycle, thus improving the implantation rate and decreasing the abortion rate. The present criteria for selection of the 'best' embryos for transfer appears to be tragically inadequate, since the implantation rate is anywhere between 10 to 20 percent. PGD-A may be done for all women over 37 years of age, those with repeated implantation failure after the transfer of morphologically normal embryos, and in women with unexplained recurrent abortions.[5]

Gianaroli et al.[6] have reported on effect of the FISH technique for PGD-A for women older than 38 years of age and including those with more than 3 IVF failures.[6] The probe mixture used contained chromosomes X, Y, 13, 18 and 21. The 11 patients underwent PGD-A, while 17 controls did not. 55 percent were chromosomally abnormal out of 61 embryos analyzed. In 10 cycles, at least one normal embryo was transferred. 4 clinical pregnancies ensued with an implantation rate of 28 percent. In 17 women, who were kept as controls, 4 pregnancies occurred with an implantation rate of 11.9 percent.

The FISH technique has been applied on polar bodies biopsied from the oocytes of 425 patients more than 35 years of age.[7] Chromosomes 13, 18 and 21 were tested in 659 IVF cycles. There were 3943 oocytes available for biopsy. Aneuploidy was present in 43.1 percent oocytes (1388). Embryo transfer was done in 614 cycles resulting in 131 clinical pregnancies and the birth of 88 healthy children.[7]

Preimplantation genetic diagnosis for aneuploidy, using probes for 4 to 8 chromosome pairs was performed in couples of advanced maternal age, showing a marginal increase in the implantation rate from 14 percent in the test group to 18 percent in the PGD group.[8] However, spontaneous abortions decreased 2.5 times from 23 percent in controls to 9 percent in the PGD group. With the slight increase in implantation rate in PGD, added to the decrease in abortion rates, there was a significant increase in deliveries from 11 percent in controls to 16 percent in the PGD group. The low percentage of increase in the implantation rate with PGD-tested embryos in women of advanced age is attributed to a few other factors. It is possible that embryos of advanced maternal age may be having other non-chromosomal causes for reduced implantation. Another factor for affecting implantation might be the procedure of embryo biopsy itself. Embryos can be damaged due to opening of the zona for embryo biopsy. The diameter of the hole is between 40 to 50 μm, whereas the puncture made for assisted hatching is between 20 to 30 μm diameter. While the latter is recommended for increasing the implantation rate, the former can actually subject the embryo to attacks from cytotoxic cells in the uterine fluid. Another effect of embryo biopsy could be interference with compaction by the use of media free from Ca^{+2} and Mg^{+2} ions.

The FISH technique can be used for the diagnosis of X-linked recessive disorders, Klinefelter's males, XXX syndrome and patients with Turner's syndrome (45 XO). Embryo sexing may be done for the transfer of female embryos, for Yq microdeletions, and for reciprocal translocations such as t(11 ; 22) and t(3 ; 8).[9]

PGD for Group 2 Diseases

These diseases are inherited monogenic disorders, known to be running in the families. They do not belong to structural or numerical anomaly or abnormality of chromosomes. These have to be diagnosed by the application of the PCR technique.

The Technique of PCR in PGD

The technique of PCR was first introduced in the mid-1980s. The principle of PCR is to enrich a DNA sample for one oligonucleotide fragment called the PCR product or amplicon. The technique consists of stretching of genomic DNA at a locus of interest. The quantity of amplified DNA may be insufficient in a single cell analysis for completing the diagnosis.

The precise diagnosis of PCR relies on several key elements, which include reagents such as primers and DNA templates; there should be no possibility of DNA contamination from any source. PCR has 3 pitfalls: amplification failures, allele drop-out (ADO) and contamination.

Amplification Failure

Amplification failure (AF) occurs in about 10 percent of isolated blastomeres, the main causes being the biopsy technique, premature cell lysis and PCR conditions. Cells that appear to be anucleate, and those derived from arrested or fragmented embryos, have a low amplification efficiency.[10,11] In such cells, the DNA may be degraded or may be entirely absent. This is of great importance where diagnosis is based on the detection of deletions such as Duchenne's muscular dystrophy (DMD). In such cases, if an allele is not amplified, one has to be very sure that it is not secondary to amplification failure, as this would cause a gross mistake in the diagnosis.

Allele Drop-out

Allele drop-out (ADO) occurs when only one of the two alleles present in a cell is amplified to a detectable level. ADO may affect either of the alleles in a heterozygous cell. The absence of a mutated allele may be due to drop-out, and this may result in misdiagnosis of an affected fetus as a normal one. The causes of ADO are not fully understood. Many hypotheses are made—denaturing temperature, incomplete cell lysis and DNA degradation prior to PCR. The significant frequency of ADO has been the reason for many centers insisting on obtaining at least 2 cells from each embryo for genetic diagnosis.

Contamination

One of the greatest obstacles to the genetic analysis of a single cell is contamination. Three main sources are known for possible contamination. First, paternal genome contamination may arise from the fact that many spermatozoa are still lying in the subzonal space after IVF. This may be mistakenly sampled with the blastomere, second polar body or even the trophectoderm cells during embryo biopsy. This is the reason why geneticists insist on embryos obtained by ICSI and not by traditional IVF.

Traditional IVF also results in embryos having several layers of cumulus cells adherent to them and one may mistakenly aspirate cumulus cells along with the blastomeres. Thirdly, external contamination may occur from the buccal cells of laboratory technicians or from PCR products generated during the previous experiment.

Laboratory technicians should take special care while using template preparations. PCR assembly, product analysis equipment, and reagents used for a single cell PCR should never be allowed to come into contact with the previously used samples. Laboratory technicians should wear disposable outer clothing, caps, and gloves kept in the room to avoid external contamination. Many centers use rooms under constant positive pressure. All reagents and solutions should be DNA-free, sterilized by autoclaving and filtered through a 0.22 micron filter or by ultraviolet irradiation. PCR reagents should be tested against contamination prior to any clinical use. To detect contamination in the analyzed sample, a negative control should be used.

Common Diseases Referred for PCR (Group 2)

Autosomal Recessive Disorders (PCR)

- Cystic fibrosis
- Thalassemia
- Spinal muscular atrophy
- Tay-Sach's disease
- Miscellaneous

Autosomal Dominant Disorders (PCR)

- Myotonic dystrophy
- Huntington's disease
- Charcot-Marie-Tooth disease
- Miscellaneous

X-linked Disorders (FISH)

- Duchenne's muscular dystrophy
- Fragile X syndrome
- Hemophilia
- Wiskott-Aldrich syndrome
- Miscellaneous

Results of PGD Conducted by ESHRE Consortium Steering Committee[12]

The European Society for Human Reproduction and Embryology (ESHRE) PGD consortium collected data on 1318 PGD cycles over a period of 7 years, from January 1994 to May 2000.

Group I (Aneuploidy for FISH Technique)

In Group 1, 465 ART cycles were taken up. IVF was done on 123 cycles and ICSI on 342 cycles. Polar body biopsy was done on 25 cycles and cleavage embryo biopsy on 440 cycles. There were 6025 oocytes in all and only 2994 oocytes turned into embryos, which could be biopsied. Diagnosis was made on 1859 embryos and 676 embryos were declared as transferable, but in some centers, they transferred even those embryos, which were thought to show aneuploidy, since this was only a trial program; thus, 908 embryos were transferred. This resulted in 133 embryos with heartbeats (28%). The clinical pregnancy rate was 29 percent per oocyte retrieval and 36 percent per embryo transfer procedure.

Group II (Inherited Monogenic Recessive and Dominant Disorders) (ESHRE PGD 2000)

There were 853 cycles taken up for PGD for inherited disorders. 771 cycles had reached the stage of oocyte retrieval; 619 cycles had ICSI only, while 2 had IVF and ICSI combined and for the remaining 50 cycles, traditional IVF was conducted.

PCR was performed on 377 cycles, FISH in 381 cycles, while 9 cycles had both FISH and PCR. A small discrepancy in the number is explained in some cycles as the procedures were slightly deviated from protocol.

On oocyte retrieval, 10,267 oocytes were collected with a fertilization rate of 63 percent (6465). 81 percent of the embryos were suitable for biopsy, and successful biopsy was done on 5041 embryos and a diagnosis was made in 4323 embryos. The number of transferable embryos were 1838 in 639 cycles of oocyte retrieval. A positive heartbeat was seen in 141 cycles, with a clinical pregnancy rate of 16.5 percent per cycle started, 18 percent per oocyte retrieval and 22 percent per embryo transfer procedure. Out of 141 clinical pregnancies, 138 reached more than 12 weeks (192 fetuses) and there were 123 deliveries. 162 babies were born with a mean birth weight of 3167 g for singleton and 2344 g for twins. 116 gestational sacs were again taken up for PND; 109 were reported to be normal, 4 were reported as abnormal and 3 results were not announced.

The consortium expressed distress that there were 4 cases misdiagnosed for monogenic diseases, which were tested by PCR. This was thought to be due to contamination, thus calling for stricter guidelines to be issued by the PGD consortium. The application of recent technical developments, such as multiplex PCR, may decrease the misdiagnosis rate (3.4 %).[12]

The ESHRE PGD 2000 reported a pregnancy loss of 20 percent, which included biochemical pregnancies, blighted oocytes, clinical abortions and extrauterine pregnancies. PGD has shown that the list of a variety of diseases, which can be diagnosed is continuously increasing, giving a great challenge to molecular biologists.[12]

FURTHER ADVANCES IN PGD

Multiplex PCR

Multiplex PCR refers to the simultaneous amplification of more than one fragment in the same cell taken up for the

PCR reaction, using more than one pair of unrelated primers. The amplification of more than four different loci have been reported in single cells. This requires more careful primer design and optimization of reaction to ensure that all primer sets amplify sufficiently under the same condition. The product of each PCR primer pair is of a different size so that it may be distinguished by gel electrophoresis.[13]

Fluorescent PCR

The PCR products are commonly separated by gel electrophoresis and their migration depends chiefly on their size. The identification of these products is by either radio-active labeling, ethidium bromide or silver staining. Such techniques are rather insensitive and they cannot distinguish between products of a relatively similar size. This problem is solved by the fluorescent PCR technique, which consists of tagging the primers with different fluorescent markers so that the products may be distinguished according to their specific wavelengths and the relative fluorescence intensities.[14]

PCR for Embryo Selection in IVF

The goal of PGD is to weed out unhealthy embryos and make a choice of embryos compatible with life and free from disease for transfer ultimately into the uterus. This is also done with a view to enhance the implantation rate and reduce the abortion rate. Unfortunately, as the state of the art goes today, the incidence of multiple pregnancy in IVF-ET settings has gone up from a rate of 16.5 to 33 percent. This is because of the anxiety still lurking in the minds of both the PCR scientists and the clinicians. PGD technology involves the loss of embryos at each step of growth to diagnosis and later on, selection for embryo transfer.

The loss of blastomeres due to punching of holes in the zona pellucida can allow premature hatching or leakage of retained blastomeres endangering the life of the whole embryo. In view of this, one is afraid to reduce the number of healthy embryos fit for transfer. This situation is still responsible for high incidence in multiple pregnancy.

CONCLUSION

Preimplantation genetic diagnosis still remains a complicated matter, involving Clinical, Reproductive Medicine and Molecular Genetics. There is a place for every type of biopsy. Several questions are yet to be answered like at what stage should we do a biopsy? Should we conduct a polar body biopsy or a blastomere biopsy at the 4 to 8 cell stage? Is it practical to restrict biopsy only to blastocysts? How much can the FISH technique help us and how does one reduce the problems related to PCR technology, since there are so many pitfalls of mosaicism, allele drop-outs, and contamination in every type of biopsy? As the current state of the art stands, one may still have to supplement the test with a PND. The ultimate goal is to improve the implantation rate in IVF, reduce the incidence of chromosomally or genetically transferred diseases and give solace to women who are victims of recurrent abortions or IVF failure.

REFERENCES

1. Elejalde BR, de Elejalde MM, Acuña JM, Thelen D, Trujillo C, Karrmann M. Prospective Study of amniocentesis performed between weeks 9 and 16 of gestation: Its feasibility, risks, complications and use in early genetic prenatal diagnosis: Am J Med Genet 1990;35:188-96.
2. Angell RR, Sumner AT, West JD, Thatcher SS, Glasier AF, Baird DT. Postfertilization polyploidy in human preimplantation embryos fertilized *in vitro*. Hum Reprod 1987;2:721-7.
3. Liu J, Lissens W, Silber S, Devroey P, Liebaers I, Van Steirteghem A. Birth after preimplantation diagnosis of the cystic fibrosis ΔF 508 mutation by polymerase chain reaction in human embryos resulting from Intracytoplasmic Sperm Injection with epididymal sperm. J Am Med Assoc 1994;272:1858-60.
4. Munne S, Daily T, Sultan KM, Grifo J, Cohen J. The use of First polar bodies for preimplantation diagnosis of aneuploidy. Mol Hum Reprod 1, Hum Reprod 1995a;10:1014-20.
5. Gianaroli L, Magli C, Ferraretti AP, et al. Preimplantation diagnosis for aneuploidies in patients undergoing *in vitro* fertilization with a poor prognosis: Identification of the categories for which it should be proposed. Fertil Steril 1999;72: 837-44.
6. Gianoroli L, Magli C, Ferraretti AP, Munné S. Preimplantation genetic diagnosis increases the implantation rate in human *in vitro* fertilization by avoiding the transfer of chromosomally abnormal embryos. Fertil Steril 1997;68:1128-31.
7. Verlinsky Y, Cieslak J, Ivakhnenko V, Lifchez A, Strom C, Kuliev A. Birth of healthy children after preimplantation diagnosis of common aneuploidies by polar body fluorescent *in situ* hybridization analysis. Fertil Steril 1996;66:126-9.
8. Munne S, Magli C, Cohen J, Morton P, Sadowy S, Gianaroli L. Positive outcome after preimplantation diagnosis of aneuploidy in human embryos. Hum Reprod 1999;14:2191-9.
9. Van Assche E, Staessen C, Vegeti W, Bonduelle M, Vandervorst M, Van Steirteghem A, Liebaers I. Preimplantation genetic diagnosis and sperm analysis by fluorescence in-situ hybridization for the most common reciprocal translocation t(11 ; 22). Mol Hum Reprod 1999;5:682-90.
10. Cui KH, Matthews CD. Nuclear structural conditions and PCR amplification in human preimplantation diagnosis. Mol Hum Reprod 1996;2:63-71.
11. Ray PF, Ao A, Taylor DM, Winston RM, Handyside AH. Assessment of the reliability of single blastomere analysis for preimplantation diagnosis of the ΔF508 deletion causing cystic fibrosis in clinical practice. Prenat Diagn 1998;18:1402-12.
12. ESHRE PGD Consortium Steering Committee: Data collection II (May 2000). Hum Reprod 2000;15:2673-83.
13. Dreesen JCFM, Jacobs LJAM, Bras M, Herbergs J, Dumoulin JC, Geraedts JP. Multiplex PCR of polymorphic markers flanking the CFTR gene; A general approach for preimplantation genetic diagnosis of cystic fibrosis. Mol Hum Reprod 2000;6:391-6.
14. Sherlock J, Cirigliano V, Petrou M, Tutschek B, Adinolfi M. Assessment of diagnostic quantitative fluorescent multiplex PCR assay performed on single cell. Ann Hum Genet 1998;62: 9-23.

ART Outcome and Beyond

Can We Improve the IVF Outcome?

Mohinder Kochhar

INTRODUCTION

Louise Brown, the first *in vitro* fertilization (IVF) baby was born on 25th July 1978. Edwards and Steptoe used oocytes recovered during a normal cycle. Since then, controlled ovarian stimulation (COH) has been widely used. New products have revolutionized the management of infertility. Patient treatment with the use of gonadotropin-releasing hormone agonists (GnRHa) or antagonists prevents a premature luteinizing hormone (LH) surge. The introduction of recombinant gonadotropins has led to more uniform and stable formulations and better results. The use of drugs, designated to treat type II diabetes, such as Metformin, has begun as an adjunct to the treatment of patients with polycystic ovaries (PCO) with improved results.

CLINICAL DISCUSSION

Factors Responsible for Success

Cause of infertility: Age of the patient, the quality of embryos, endometrial receptivity, number of embryos transferred and the embryo transfer technique, laboratory environment and culture media will influence success.

The cause of infertility is important. Patients with a history of tuberculosis, endometriosis, fibroid uterus, and polycystic ovaries are likely to have a poor result. Treating these conditions prior to the IVF cycle improves the result. Pelvic inflammatory disease (PID) and hydrosalpinges are known to reduce the pregnancy rate. Sharara et al.[1] have demonstrated that in cases with hydrosalpinges, the window of implantation, which is expressed by the appearance of avB_3, endometrial integrin is impaired and might be corrected by salpingectomies.[1]

Age of patient: Older patients and patients with premature ovarian failure with high follicle stimulating hormone (FSH) levels and previous repeated failed fertilization should be advised adoption or donor oocytes. Cohen et al.[2] demonstrated that by removing cytoplasm from younger women's ovaries and injecting into the oocytes of older women will increase the chance of implantation.[2] This new technology is a significant scientific advance, however, it raises new ethical and legal implications of a child inheriting genes from two mothers.

In applied clinical research, our aim should be to improve embryo viability, implantation and reduce ovarian hyper-stimulation syndrome (OHSS) and multiple pregnancy rate.

The success rate for *in vitro* fertilization (IVF) and embryo transfer (ET) depends on embryonic viability and uterine receptivity.

New procedures have improved success. Intracytoplasmic sperm injection (ICSI) has revolutionized the treatment for male infertility and for previous failed fertilization.

Improving Embryo Quality

In the process of human embryonic development, a cleavage arrest generally occurs at the four to eight cell stage as first reported by Brande et al.[3] Sequential serum-free media is used for the development of the pronuclei and 8-cell embryo, respectively. Selection of the embryos, which develop into blastocysts would increase the pregnancy rates and on the other hand, decrease the multiple pregnancy by replacing only one or two blastocysts. Gardner and Lane[4] demonstrated that it was possible to obtain a 50 percent blastocyst development and a 70 percent pregnancy rate, and the rest can be cryopreserved.[4] The only risk is that none of the embryos may reach the blastocyst stage, thus resulting in a failure to transfer embryos, and no embryos being available for embryo transfer. Chen et al.[5,6] demonstrated that to improve cryopreservation techniques, some biophysical research is needed.[2] This would be useful in better freezing of embryos, oocytes, ovarian tissue, testicular tissue and individual spermatozoa or spermatids. It will permit preservation of healthy oocytes prior to irradiation or chemotherapy or even to delay conception for personal reasons.[5,6]

Preimplantation genetic diagnosis is a technique that permits the diagnosis of the genotype of an embryo before implantation and the diagnosis of aneuploidy, especially in older women with a history of recurrent miscarriages and avoids the transmission of genetic abnormalities.

Assisted Hatching

It is believed that a thin zona pellucida has a better implantation rate. In older women, assisted hatching improves implantation.

The Role of the Endometrium

It is seen that for implantation to occur, a co-ordinate molecular dialog must be established between the prime and receptors on the apical surface of the luminal epithelium and trophoblast of the hatched blastocyst. If the dialog is not established, implantation is interrupted. Uterine blood flow may be increased by using low-dose Aspirin, nitroglycerine and Viagra. Practitioners of traditional Chinese medicine believe that acupuncture improves blood supply to the uterus and ovaries, relaxes the uterus and increases endometrial receptivity.

The embryo transfer technique, whether a single or a double transfer, with a soft catheter under ultrasound guidance gives better results, especially in previous difficult transfers.[7]

In vitro maturation (IVM) offers a cheaper alternative to conventional stimulation cycles and avoids the associated risk of hyperstimulation. IVM is likely to gradually become more widely used and knowledge gained from follicles studied *in vitro* will surely bring the benefit of new knowledge of Reproductive Medicine. The conquest of infertility is an incredible achievement. It is the victory of human will, endurance and technology. In the near future, we expect significant advances in basic reproduction, applied research, diagnostic tools, stem cell research, drug development and clinical management of infertility and an improvement in IVF success.[8]

CONCLUSION

The path to success lies in patient selection, quality of ovulation induction, which produces healthy oocytes, appropriate culture media and a proper environment, good endometrium and atraumatic embryo transfer under ultrasound guidance. In spite of good quality embryos, the implantation rate is still low. Future research is required to improve endometrial receptivity.

How do we define success? Is it by the pregnancy rate, chemical or biochemical, positive beta human chorionic gonadotropin (hCG) levels, clinical evidence of gestational sac or detection of a heartbeat? From the patient's point of view, it is birth of a child and the 'take home baby rate.'

REFERENCES

1. Sharara FI. Effects of hydrosalpinx on IVF outcome: The search goes on. Hum Reprod 1997;12:2853-4.
2. Cohen J, Scott R, Schimmel T, Levron J, Willadsen S. Birth of infant after transfer of anucleate donor oocyte cytoplasm into recipient eggs. Lancet 1997;350:186-7.
3. Braude P, Bolton V, Moore S. Human gene expression first occurs between the four and eight-cell stages of preimplantation development. Nature 1988;332:459-61.
4. Gardner DK, Lane M. Culture and selection of viable blastocysts: A feasible proposition for human IVF? Hum Reprod Update 1997;3:367-82.
5. Chen C. Pregnancies after human oocyte cryopreservation. Ann NY Acad Sci 1988;541:541-9.
6. Chen C. Pregnancy after human oocyte cryopreservation. Lancet 1986;1:884-6.
7. Malpani A, Malpani A. How to improve success rates in IVF? The Art and Science of Assisted Reproductive Techniques (ART); In: Allahbadia GN, Basuray R (Eds). Jaypee Brothers Medical Publishers (P) Ltd, New Delhi 2003.pp.289-92.
8. Lunenfeld B. Present and future of infertility therapy. The Art and Science of Assisted Reproductive Techniques (ART); In: Allahbadia GN, Basuray R (Eds). Jaypee Brothers Medical Publishers (P) Ltd, New Delhi 2003.pp.537-44.

Does Seasonal Variability Affect ART Outcome?

Lata Kamble, Anil Gudi, Amit Shah

OVERVIEW

Epidemiologists throughout the world have consistently demonstrated a seasonal distribution in human natural conception and birth rates. The reasons for this phenomenon are not very well-understood; possible explanations might be the variations in semen quality, showing a significantly lower sperm count in the summer compared to the winter. The direct and indirect effects of the light/dark cycle, associated with season and location on the female reproductive process have also been demonstrated. Both, ovulation rates and endometrial receptivity have been shown to be reduced during long, dark winters in northern countries, where a summer peak in conception and multiple pregnancy rates are observed. In northern countries, which have strong seasonal contrasts, the activity of the anterior pituitary-ovarian axis, and accordingly, the conception rate, decreases during the dark winter. For areas without such a seasonal contrast, data are conflicting. Melatonin, a hormone secreted during darkness, plays a role in the regulation of reproduction. These seasonal variations may be mediated through hypothalamic-pituitary or pineal output and possibly, through brain neurotransmitters such as serotonin, dopamine, and endogenous opioids. Modern life provides conditions that approach constancy and non-seasonality. This has probably diminished the impact of seasonal changes on the human reproductive process.

However, the influence of seasonal variation on the results of assisted reproduction in humans still remains debated. Some studies have suggested possible seasonal variations during assisted reproductive treatment of humans, although variations of the ovulation rate due to varying endogenous gonadotropin secretion are suppressed by the hormonal therapy given during assisted conception treatment and lower sperm counts in non-treated ejaculates (observed during the summer months) are compensated in assisted conception treatment cycles by utilizing a concentrated and constant amount of motile sperm to inseminate or inject the oocytes. Several other studies could not confirm the presence of seasonal variations. Data from these studies are inconsistent.

INTRODUCTION

Our bodies evolved to be 'in tune' with their environment. This connection is vital for reproduction, as birth of the young ones has to coincide with optimal weather conditions and availability of food, thus giving them a high chance of survival.[1] Most mammals are therefore, 'seasonal breeders' and switch their sexual behavior and fertility on and off, guided by the amount of daylight (photoperiod), but influenced also by other factors, such as energy intake/output balance (that is, availability of food).[1,2] This biological programming of births, or synchronization of reproductive response to appropriate environmental conditions, clearly leads to distinct advantages for the offspring being born at the time of optimum weather conditions and maximal food availability during the early part of the offspring's life.[3,4] Although humans are not 'seasonal breeders', they show sexual behaviour and reproduce all year round, their fertility being influenced by the environment, including season and food intake.

The effects of seasonal changes on the reproductive life of animals, in particular daylight length, are well-known across the world. This effect of seasonal variation and daylight length on mammalian reproduction, leading to spring births, has been well-established, and is known as photoperiodism.[5] However, the influence of seasonal variation and its mechanism on human reproduction is less well-understood than in animals.

Seasonality in Human Reproduction

Epidemiological studies have shown distinct geographical differences on the impact of seasonality on natural conceptions and births in humans.[6] These studies observed a decline in natural conception and birth rates during the spring in warm climates in nonequatorial regions.[7-10] The causes for this decline are not very well-understood; possible explanations might be the variations in semen quality, showing a significantly lower sperm count in the summer compared to the winter,[11-17] variations in the ovulation rate[18-20] and variations in endometrial receptivity[18,21] throughout the seasons; these variations might be linked to the light-dark effect of the female reproductive axis and may be mediated through fluctuations in the hypothalamo-pituitary, pineal or adrenal function and also possibly, through brain neurotransmitters such as serotonin, dopamine and endogenous opioid peptides.[6] Soltriol (Vitamin D_3), a steroid mediator of sunlight, has also been implicated in various reproductive events.[22] Both ovulation rates and endometrial receptivity were shown to be reduced during long, dark winters in northern countries, where a summer peak in conception and multiple pregnancy rates are observed. Thus, it is suggested that while male fertility potential seems to be in influenced by temperature, the female reproductive axis is probably influenced by light. Data regarding varying frequencies of intercourse as a function of season remains inconsistent.

Other studies with regard to seasonal variation in tropical latitudes amongst populations, which face seasonal variation in food availability, have suggested that the availability of food, both in human and animal populations may influence fertility. It is suggested that poor calorific intake or high energy expenditure to gather food would delay menarche, suppress the frequency of ovulation in non-lactating adults and prolong lactational amenorrhea in these populations.[23] In more temperate latitudes, a clear difference is noted, with most studies showing the major peak in birth rate in spring, consistent with a peak in conception during the summer months and a smaller secondary peak in births in September.[6,24-26] These differences are seen both, throughout Europe and in the northern latitudes of the United States,[27] and seem to clearly demonstrate the possible effect of light variation on conception with an increase in fertility related to an increase in exposure to light.[6]

In Western societies, however, even though factors such as seasonal availability of food are of little relevance, seasonal variations in birth rate are still seen. However, confounding factors, such as contraceptive use, family planning, diet and stress-related variables associated with modern lifestyle, make evaluation of seasonal effects in developed countries more difficult.

Mediators of the Seasonal Effect on Reproduction

Melatonin

Melatonin is secreted by the pineal gland and is thought to play a major role in controlling the process of reproduction. In humans, studies on the pituitary-ovarian axis and the pineal gland during light and dark seasons have demonstrated an increase in melatonin concentrations during the dark season, with a corresponding decrease in estrogen levels at the time of ovulation and during the luteal phase, leading to an increase in the level of luteal phase gonadotropins, increased sex hormone binding globulin (SHBG) and decreased testosterone.[28] This suggested, but could not prove, that melatonin secretion in response to decreased light availability is associated with an inhibition of ovarian function.

During the daylight hours, the secretion of melatonin is minimal in humans and in all other mammals studied so far.[29] However, with the onset of darkness, the sympathetic nerves become active, releasing norepinephrine onto the pineal's parenchymal cells and thereby initiating synthesis and release of melatonin. As the pineal melatonin level rises, the lipid soluble hormone enters the blood stream via passive diffusion down a concentration gradient. The resulting daily rhythm in circulating melatonin levels gives rise to the normal day-night light-dark cycle.[30,31] Most studies support the idea that melatonin exerts its main reproductive effects at the level of the pituitary or central nervous system by suppressing the pituitary responses to gonadotropin-releasing hormone (GnRH)[32] or by directly inhibiting hypothalamic GnRH pulses.[33] However, melatonin could also exert direct effects on the gonads and ovarian steroidogenesis. The ovary takes up circulating melatonin in cats and rats more effectively than most other tissues.[34] This has also been demonstrated in hamster and human ovaries.[35]

A positive correlation has been demonstrated between plasma melatonin and prolactin levels[36] as shown in Figure 61.1. Melatonin levels were reported to be high in several cases of hyperprolactinemia.[37] The mechanism by which melatonin might exert its effect on serum prolactin levels remains unclear. The theories postulated are that it could inhibit the release of hypothalamic dopamine or it might act centrally by enhancing serotonin-mediated neurotransmission.[38] Melatonin, through these putative mechanisms, may mediate seasonal effects on reproductive processes.

Soltriol (Vitamin D_3)

Vitamin D_3 or Soltriol—$[1,25(OH)_2$—vitamin $D_3]$ has recently been proposed as a regulator and modulator of reproductive processes in both sexes. This steroid hormone has been suggested as a transducer and hormonal messenger of sunlight, mediating the seasonal adaptation of growth, development and procreation. Evidence from the literature suggests its involvement in the onset of puberty, fertility, pregnancy, lactation and probably, sexual behavior. Nuclear receptors for Soltriol have been discovered in the rat uterus, oviduct and ovary, as well as in the testis, epididymis, prostate, pituitary and hypothalamus.[39]

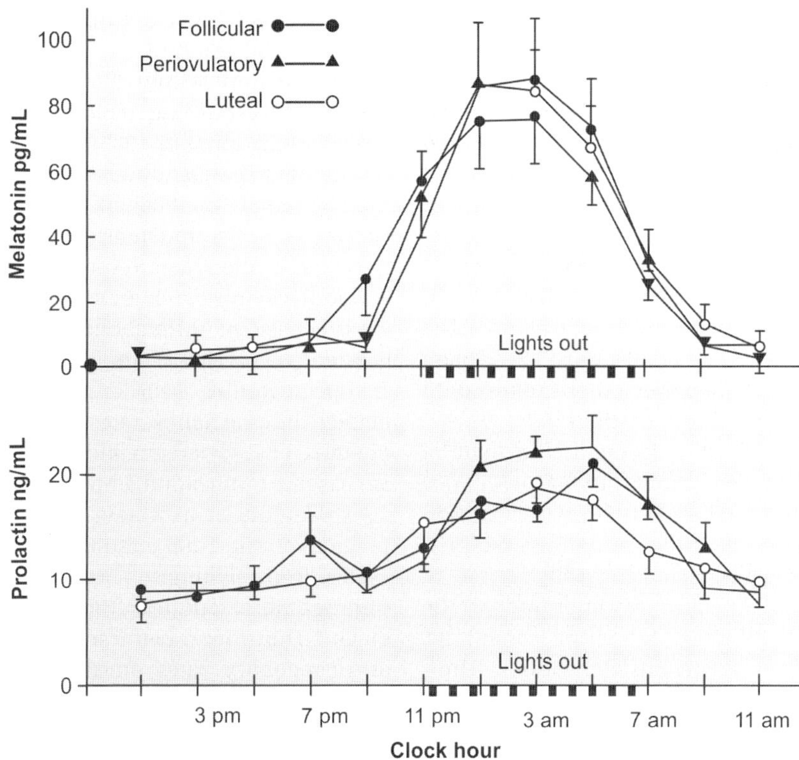

Fig. 61.1: Mean (±SE) plasma melatonin and prolactin levels sampled at 2-hour intervals over 24-hour periods during the early follicular, periovulatory and mid-luteal phases of the menstrual cycle in 14 regularly ovulating women (*Brzezinski, et al. 1988*)

Soltriol may be involved in facilitating ovulation. Because of the presence of Soltriol receptors in the germinal epithelium, it has been suggested that Soltriol has a complimentary action with estradiol in producing and labilizing lysosomes, which weakens the tunica albuginea and enhances ovum release. It is likely that Soltriol promotes certain cellular activities to facilitate egg transport and fertilization in the oviduct. Its presence in the uterus, especially in the glands of the endometrium and corpus luteum, may also point to a possible role in endometrial development and receptivity.[39,40] Studies of antibodies to LH suggest that Soltriol acts directly on a sub-population of gonadotrophs in the pituitary gland,[41] or it may operate indirectly through hypothalamic structures associated with the control of gonadotropin secretion, such as the arcuate and the ventromedial nuclei, by altering the negative feedback of ovarian hormones on gonadotropin release.[42]

It has been proposed that the actions of Soltriol and estradiol complement each other, since these two steroids show corresponding changes in blood levels and have related sites of nuclear receptors in various tissues. Thus, Soltriol, through elevated blood levels after exposure to sunlight, may participate in the regulation and seasonal modulation of reproductive functions.[39]

Complementary relationships between the actions of Soltriol, the hormone of sunlight, and melatonin, the hormone of darkness, are postulated. Such an agonist-antagonist relationship of Soltriol and melatonin on reproductive processes in many mammalian species has been reported in the literature. Retraction of melanin in the skin, through melatonin, to facilitate exposure to sunlight is just one example of this interrelationship.[40]

Thus, season seems to be a significant predictor of sperm quality and may substantially influence the ovulation rate. Although more studies are needed in order to elucidate its mechanism and impact, the specific time of the year seems to have implications for the treatment of infertility.

Seasonality in Assisted Reproduction

The impact of seasonality on human assisted conception has not yet been completely clarified as conflicting reports have been published, and therefore, the influence of seasonal variation on the results of assisted reproduction in humans still remains debated. Assisted reproductive techniques (ART) exert an extensive control over reproductive mechanisms, and a huge effort has been made to standardize pharmacological and laboratory protocols to minimize every external influence on assisted conception results. The whole hormonal milieu during the treatment cycle is manipulated to control the process of ovarian stimulation and ovulation. Furthermore, lower sperm counts in non-treated ejaculates (observed during the summer months) are compensated in assisted conception treatment cycles by selecting a concentrated and constant amount of best quality motile sperm to inseminate/inject the oocytes. Therefore, it is very tempting, to speculate that any influence the seasonal variation might have on the assisted conception cycle might be negligible. Nevertheless, while significant season-related changes that impact the effectiveness of human assisted conception have been reported by some authors,[6,43-47] however, other studies could not confirm the presence of seasonal variations.[48,49]

Every clinician and biologist working in the field of Reproductive Medicine wonders about varying pregnancy rates because success rates fluctuate without a clear reason from excellent to very poor. This often cannot be explained by the group a patient belongs to (e.g. advanced age of the woman, poor responders, primary infertility of the female, multiple infertility factors), by culture conditions, technical failures or other comprehensible reasons. Thus, we do wonder whether the different seasons of the year can have good or bad influences on the characteristics of the oocytes and on the fertilization and pregnancy rates during assisted conception in humans. Seasonal rhythms have been suspected to influence both natural and assisted human reproduction.

There is lack of good quality evidence in the literature, regarding the influence of seasonal variation on the outcome of assisted conception. The few studies done so far have been small, low power and mostly retrospective studies. A careful evaluation of the literature on the influence of seasonal variations on the outcome of IVF shows that the extent of discrepancies among the studies is remarkable. One point is the difference in the stimulation protocols used. In some studies, cycles with down regulation were included, but absent in others. In addition, there was no consistency between the studies about the criterion for the inclusion of a patient to the corresponding season: in some studies it was the day of the beginning of stimulation, in others it was the day of oocyte retrieval, resulting in a difference upto 17 days. Also, the published studies have been conducted in different climates. Because of the widely diverse environments with different temperatures and light changes, the different studies are not comparable. Regarding the heterogeneous study results, it is also remarkable that the seasonal effects observed are very complex. The results between the different studies were highly inconsistent, with some showing the best pregnancy rates in the months of November, December, January and February,[44] while others showing the worst pregnancy rates in the months of January, February and March in IVF cycles with a spontaneous luteinizing hormone (LH) surge, whereas no differences in IVF cycles with human chorionic gonadotropin (hCG) administration.[50]

Several studies from different parts of the world that have examined seasonal fluctuations in IVF programs have yielded conflicting results. In 1985, Wood, et al.[43] were the first to report lower pregnancy rates in summer (December through March) in their Australian (Melbourne) IVF clinic population. Casper, et al.[50] from Ontario, Canada, reported significantly lower conception rates in spontaneous LH-surge IVF cycles in winter (December to March), but found that pregnancy rates were consistent throughout the year in human chorionic gonadotropin (hCG)-stimulated cycles. In contrast, in European studies, Daya, et al.[51] failed to show any seasonal change in pregnancy rates in 2674 IVF cycles. Similarly, Fleming, et al.[48] were unable to demonstrate any fluctuations in seasonal fertilization, implantation and conception rates.

Chamoun, et al.[45] have reported seasonal variation in pregnancy and implantation rates in 230 consecutive IVF cycles from Baltimore, Maryland (eastern USA). Similar findings were reported from the Netherlands by Stolwijk, et al.[44] They found better fertilization rates, embryo quality and pregnancy rates during the period of November to February in a study of 1154 first-time IVF cycles. These authors concluded, however, that some of the variation could be explained by the women's ages, type of infertility and indications for IVF. These confounders, together with a possible effect of intraclass correlation between observations, the technique of ART used, and the impact of different geographical areas, may explain the disparity in the results of the studies on IVF seasonality.

In a study done in Jerusalem, Rojansky, et al.[52] looked into 1072 cycles retrospectively and found significant seasonal variability in fertilization and embryo quality rates in the human IVF process, the highest fertilization and grade A embryo rates in spring and the lowest in autumn. The conception rates, which showed a trough in the spring and rose gradually to an autumn acme, did not reach statistical significance. These seasonal fluctuations in fertilization and embryo quality were positively correlated with the annual light changes but not with temperature, humidity or any other seasonal factor studied. Since the hypothalamic-pituitary function is suppressed and ovulation is exogenously manipulated in women undergoing IVF, the authors suggested that the observed seasonal effect in fertilization and embryo quality rates, and possibly, on conception rate, might be related to a direct melatonin or neurotransmitter effect on the end organ, namely the ovary (oocyte), or endometrium (receptivity). The authors also concluded that the lower conception rates during spring, the time period when both fertilization and embryo quality rates are at their highest, could only be explained by reduced endometrial receptivity during the spring season. If this seasonal decrease in receptivity occurs in spite of the exogenous endometrial stimulation regimens used in IVF programs, it might be deduced that factors other than gonadotropins and gonadal hormones may play a role in mediating this effect on the endometrium.

A study by Weigert, et al.[53] from Austria, included 8185 *in vitro* fertilization-embryo transfer (IVF-ET) cycles, the highest number published so far. They found that the best pregnancy rates were obtained in December. They postulated that the better quality of sperm during winter months could have influenced fertilization as well as pregnancy rates, particularly during the years when intracytoplasmic sperm injection (ICSI) had not yet come into practice. However, they concluded that parameters, like age and number of embryos transferred, have a stronger influence on a positive outcome than any temporal aspects.

Gindes, et al.[49] from Israel, evaluated 3522 consecutive assisted reproduction cycles conducted over a 4-year period in a single assisted reproduction technology unit. Their findings demonstrated fluctuations (with no seasonal pattern) in pregnancy rates which, although impressive, could only be explained by chance alone. Furthermore, other variables, such as estrogen level on day of hCG administration and fertilization rate, also fluctuated at random, with no correlation with each other. The authors were unable to identify any reason for these observed fluctuations and believe that they might be explained by chance alone.

Revelli, et al.[54] from Italy, retrospectively studied 2067 patients undergoing their first IVF attempt. They observed that the highest pregnancy rate was found in spring and the lowest in summer, but this did not reach statistical significance. They concluded that their findings reinforce the notion that seasonality has no significant effect on the results of human assisted reproductive techniques (ART) and that, it appears likely that in human ART, the pharmacological control of ovarian function as well as the standardization of laboratory equipment and procedures prevail over seasonal rhythms and lower the impact of any seasonal influence.

Wunder, et al.[55] from Switzerland, retrospectively analyzed 7368 IVF cycles and showed no significant seasonal differences in the fertilization rate, the pregnancy or implantation rates. Their results, which show no significant seasonal differences in the implantation rate, pointed to an absence of a seasonal change in endometrial receptivity. The best pregnancy and implantation rates were found in December, despite a significantly lower number of embryos transferred. However, these differences did not reach statistical significance. Their results also showed and confirmed that the statistically significant variables influencing the outcome of an IVF cycle are—age, etiology of infertility, day of transfer and center. However, the suspected seasonal variability of the outcome of IVF cycles could not been confirmed. They concluded that following IVF there is no statistically significant variability in fertilization, implantation or pregnancy rates between the seasons.

More recently, a study from UK by Wood et al.[5] retrospectively analyzed 2709 standardized cycles of IVF/ICSI. Their results suggest an optimal outcome in summer months compared to winter months, in contrast to the above studies from other parts of Europe. The results showed that there was significant improvement in assisted conception outcomes in cycles performed in summer (lighter) months with more efficient ovarian stimulation. There was similarly a significantly improved implantation rate per embryo transferred and greater clinical pregnancy rate during summer cycles. This study appears to demonstrate a significant benefit of increased daylight length on the outcomes of IVF/ICSI cycles. Whilst the exact mechanism of this is unclear, it would seem probable that melatonin may have actions at multiple sites and on multiple levels of the reproductive tract, and may exert a more profound effect on outcomes of assisted conception cycles than has been previously considered. When data was analyzed in patients, who had undergone at least two cycles of treatment, one during restricted daylight and another during months with increased daylight, again clear benefits were seen in these matched cycles performed during extended daylight hours.

Thus, it can be seen from the above studies that the results of these studies are highly inconsistent, conflicting and not comparable due to the wide variation and diverse environments with different temperatures and light changes. Therefore, from these studies it is difficult to either confirm or refute the influence of seasonality on the outcome of ART and to draw a meaningful conclusion. However, majority of the studies suggest that seasonal variations may not have a significant effect on the results of ART and that, other factors, such as age, etiology of infertility, and day of transfer, play a major role on the outcome of ART. But on the other hand, few studies suggest a significant seasonal effect on the outcome of ART and although the exact mechanism by which the seasonal variations exert their effect on the outcome of ART is not clear, it is postulated that melatonin may have a role in modulating the process of reproduction even in assisted reproduction.

CONCLUSION

While there is some evidence on the influence of seasonality on human reproduction, there is a paucity of good quality evidence on the influence of seasonality on assisted reproduction. Some studies have shown a significant effect of seasonality on the outcome of assisted reproduction. Whilst the exact mechanism of this is unclear, it has been postulated that melatonin may have actions at multiple sites and on multiple levels of the reproductive tract, and may exert a more profound effect on outcomes of assisted conception cycles than has been previously considered. It has also been suggested that melatonin may be involved in steroidogenesis in human ovaries, and so, it seems to be possible that melatonin is an additional seasonally influenced and influencing factor for IVF-ET. However, the role of melatonin in assisted reproductive techniques remains to be investigated.

There are other studies that could not find any such effect. These studies suggested that in human assisted conception, the pharmacological control of ovarian function as well as the standardization of laboratory equipment and procedures prevail over seasonal rhythms and lower the impact of any seasonal influence.

The current available evidence is conflicting and therefore, it is not completely clear as to whether seasonality has any effects on the outcome of ART. It seems that, in spite of great advances in reproductive technique, primitive endogenous factors within the human, modulated by melatonin secretion either directly or via complex hormonal and neurological interactions in response to light, exert greater influence on the reproductive outcome than had been previously thought. More studies need to be undertaken in humans undergoing assisted conception to establish the exact mechanism for these variations and then find ways to manipulate these factors to improve success rates in assisted conception cycles.

REFERENCES

1. Lincoln GA, Short RV. Seasonal breeding: Nature's contraceptive. Rec Progr Horm Res 1980;36:1-52.
2. Lincoln GA, Rhind SM, Pompolo S, Clarke IJ. Hypothalamic control of photoepriod-induced cycles in food intake, body weight and metabolic hormones in rams. Am J Physiol Regul Integr Comp Physiol 2001;281,R76-R90.
3. Immelmann K. Role of environment in reproduction as source of predictive information. In: DS Farner (Ed.). Breeding biology of birds. Washington, DC: National Academy of Sciences 1973. pp. 121-47.
4. Pang SF, Ayre EA, Pang CS, Lee PP, Xu RK, Chow PH, et al. Neuroendocrinology of melatonin in reproduction: Recent developments. J Chem Neuroanat 1998;14:157-66.
5. Simon Wood, Alison Quinn, Stephen Troupe, Charles Kingsland, Iwan Lewis-Jones. Seasonal variation in assisted conception cycles and the influence of photoperiodism on outcome in *in vitro* fertilization cycles. Hum Fertil (Camb) 2006;9:223-9.
6. Rojansky N, Brzezinski A, Schenker JG. Seasonality in human reproduction: An update. Hum Reprod 1992;7:734-45.
7. Huntington E. Season of birth: Its relation to human abilities. John Wiley, New York 1938.
8. Lamar JK, Rodgers R. Season and human fertility in Galveston, Texas. Anat Rec 1943;87:453-4.
9. Rosenberg HM. National Center of Health Statistics. Seasonal variation of births: United States 1933-63. Vital and Health Statistics. Series 21, No. 9 (PHS publication no. 1000). US Government Printing Office, Washington, DC 1966.
10. Becker S. Seasonality of fertility in Matlab, Bangladesh. J Biosoc Sci 1981;13:97-105.
11. Tjoa WS, Smolensky MH, Hsi BP, Steinberger E, Smith KD. Circannual rhythm in human sperm count revealed by serially independent sampling. Fertil Steril 1982;38:454-9.
12. Levine RJ, Bordson BL, Mathew RM, Brown MH, Stanley JM, Starr TB. Deteriorations of semen quality during summer in New Orleans. Fertil Steril 1988;49:900-7.
13. Reinberg A, Smolensky MH, Halleck M, Smith KD, Steinberger E. Annual variation in semen charcteristics and plasma hormone levels in men undergoing vasectomy. Fertil Steril 1988;49:309-15.
14. Politoff L, Birkhaeuser M, Almendral A, Zorn A. New data confirming a circannual rhythm in spermatogenesis. Fertil Steril 1989;52:486-9.
15. Saint Pol P, Beuscart R, Leroy-Martin B, Hermand E, Jablonski W. Circannual rhythms of sperm parameters of fertile men. Fertil Steril 1989;51:1030-3.
16. Levine RJ, Mathew RM, Chenault CB, Brown MH, Hurtt ME, Bentley KS, Mohr KL, Working TK. Differences in the quality of semen in outdoor workers during summer and winter. New Engl J Med 1990;323:12-6.
17. Levine RJ. Seasonal variation in human semen quality. In Zorginotti AW (ed) Temperature and Environmental Effects on the Testis. Plenum Press, New York 1991.pp.89-96.
18. Timonen S, Franzas B, Wichmann K. Photosensitivity of the human pituitary. Ann Chir Gynecol Fenn 1964;53:165-70.
19. Kivela A, Kauppila A, Ylostalo P, Vakkuri O. Seasonal, menstrual and circadian secretions of melatonin, gonadotropins and prolactin in women. Acta Physiol Scand 1988;132:321-7.
20. Rameshkumar K, Thomas JA, Mohammed A. Atmospheric temperature and anovulation in south Indian women with primary infertility. Ind J Med Res 1992;96:27-8.
21. Kottler ML, Coussieu C, Valensi P, Levy F, Dergrelle H. Ultradian, circadian and seasonal variation of plasma progesterone and LH concentrations during the luteal phase. Chronobiol Int 1989;6:267-77.
22. Stumpf WE, Denny EM. Vitamin D (Solitrol), light and reproduction. Am Obstet Gynecol 1989;161:1375-84.
23. Bronson FH. Seasonal variation in human reproduction: Environmental factors. Q Rev Biol 1995;70:141-64.
24. James WH. Seasonal variation in human births. J Biosoc Sci 1990;22:113-9.
25. Lerchl A, Simoni M, Nieschlag E. Changes in seasonality of birth rates in Germany from 1951 to 1990. Naturwissenschaften 1993;80:516-8.
26. Eriksson AW, Fellman J. Seasonal variation of livebirths, stillbirths, extramarital births and twin maternities in Switzerland. Twin Res 2000;3:189-201.
27. Lam DA, Miron JA. Global patterns of seasonal variation in human fertility. Ann N Y Acad Sci 1994;709:9-28.
28. Kauppila A, Kivela A, Pakarinen A, Vakkuri O. Inverse seasonal relationship between melatonin and ovarian activity in humans in a region with strong seasonal contrast in luminosity. J Clin Endocrinol Metab 1987;65:823-8.
29. Wurtman RJ, Waldhauser F. Melatonin in humans. J Neural Transm Springer-Verlag, Vienna 1986.

30. Pelham RW, Vaughan GM, Sandock KL, Vaughan MK. 24-hour cycle of a melatonin-like substance in the plasma of human males. J Clin Endocrinol Metab 1973;37:341-4.

31. Lynch HJ, Wurtman RJ, Moskowitz MA. Daily rhythm in human urinary melatonin. Science 1975;187:169-71.

32. Martin JE, Engel J, Klein DC. Inhibition of the *in vitro* pituitary response to luteinizing hormone-releasing hormone by melatonin, serotonin, and 5-methoxytryptamine. Endocrinology 1977;100:675-81.

33. Bittman EL, Kaynard AH, Olster DH, Robinson JE, Yellon SM, Karsch FJ. Pineal melatonin mediates photoperiod control of pulsatile luteinizing hormone in the ewe. Neuroendocrinology 1985;40:409-18.

34. Wurtman R J, Axelrod J, Potter LT. The uptake of H3-melatonin in endocrine and nervous tissues and the effects of constant light exposure. J Pharmacol Exp Ther 1964;143:314-9.

35. Cohen M, Rosella D, Chabner B. Evidence for a cytoplasmic melatonin receptor. Nature 1978;274:894-6.

36. Brzezinski A, Wurtman RJ. The pineal gland: Its possible roles in human reproduction. Obstet Gynecol Surv 1988;43:197-207.

37. Wetteberg L. Clinical importance of melatonin. Progr Brain Res 1979;52:539-47.

38. Anton-Tay F, Chou C, Anton S, Wurtman RJ. Brain serotonin concentrations: Elevation following intraperitoneal administration of melatonin. Science 1968;162:277-81.

39. Stumpf WE, Denny EM. Vitamin D (soltriol), light and reproduction. Am J Obstet Gynecol 1989;161:1375-84.

40. Stumpf WE. The endocrinology of sunlight and darkness: Complementary roles of vitamin D and pineal hormones. Naturwissenschaften 1988;75:247-51.

41. Stumpf WE, Sar M, O'Brien LP. Vitamin D sites of action in the pituitary studied by combined autoradiography-immuno-histochemistry. Histochemistry 1988;8:11-6.

42. Stumpf WE, O'Brien LP. 1,25(OH)2 Vitamin D3 sites of action in the brain: An autoradiographic study, Histochemistry 1987; 87:393-6.

43. Wood C, McMaster R, Rennie G, Trounson A, Leeton J. Factors influencing pregnancy rate following an embryo transfer. Fertil Steril 1985;43:245-50.

44. Stolwijk AM, Reuvers MJCM, Hamilton CJCM, Jongbloet PH, Hollanders JMG, Zeilhuis GA. Seasonality in the results of *in vitro* fertilization. Hum Reprod 1994;2300-5.

45. Chamoun D, Udoff L, Scott L, Madger L, Adashi EY, McClamrock HD. A seasonal effect on pregnancy rates in an *in vitro* fertilization program. J Assist Reprod Genet 1995;12:585-9.

46. Weigert M, Feichtinger W, Kulin S, Kaali SG, Dorau P, Bauer P. Seasonal influences on *in vitro* fertilization and embryo transfer. J Assist Reprod Genet 2001;18:598-602.

47. Ossenbühn S. Exogenous influences on human fertility: Fluctuations in sperm parameters and results of *in vitro* fertilization coincide with conceptions in the normal population. Hum Reprod 1998;13:2165-71.

48. Fleming C, Nice L, Hughes AO, Hull MGR. Apparent lack of seasonal variation in implantation rates after *in vitro* fertilization. Hum Reprod 1994;9:2164-6.

49. Gindes L, Yoeli R, Orvieto R, Shelef M, Ben-Rafael Z, Bar-Hava I. Pregnancy rate fluctuations during routine work in an assisted reproduction technology unit. Hum Reprod 2003;18: 2485-8.

50. Casper RF, Erskine HJ, Armstrong DT, Brown SE, Daniel SA, Graves GR, Yuzpe AA. *In vitro* fertilization: Diurnal and seasonal variation in luteinizing hormone surge onset and pregnancy rates. Fertil Steril 1988;49:644-8.

51. Daya I, Garcia JE, Smith RD, Padilla SL. Seasonal variation in *in vitro* fertilization pregnancy rate: An analysis of 2,674 oocyte retrievals. Infertility 1993;15:21-6.

52. Rojansky N, Benshushan A, Meirsdorf S, Lewin A, Laufer N, Safran A. Seasonal variability in fertilization and embryo quality rates in women undergoing IVF. Fertil Steril 2000; 74:476-81.

53. Weigert M, Feichtinger W, Kulin S, Kaali SG, Dorau P, Bauer P. Seasonal influences on *in vitro* fertilization and embryo transfer. J Assist Reprod Genet 2001;18:598-602.

54. Revelli A, La Sala GB, Gennarelli G, Scatigna L, Racca C, Massobrio M. Seasonality and human *in vitro* fertilisation outcome. Gynecol Endocrinol 2005;21:12-7.

55. Wunder DM, Limoni C, Birkhäuser MH and the Swiss FIVNAT Group. Lack of seasonal variations in fertilization, pregnancy and implantation rates in women undergoing IVF. Hum Reprod 2005;20:3122-9.

Natural Killer Cells as Predictors of Successful Implantation

Stefan Kostadinov, Surendra Sharma

OVERVIEW

A balanced maternal immune system seems to be necessary for a normal pregnancy outcome. Antifetal, antiplacental, and antipaternal antibodies are detectable in sera of women with successful pregnancies. It appears that the immune responses during pregnancy differ from the rules of the classic transplantation immunity. It is well-recognized now, that the maternal immune system not only recognizes pregnancy but reacts in a differential way resulting in either success or failure. The two-way immunological relationship between the mother and the fetus is determined by both, fetal antigen presentation and recognition of and reaction to these antigens by the maternal immune system. It appears that the early immune tolerance, allowing survival of the embryo, relies mainly on maternal factors. As with other mucosal sites, the cycling endometrium is seeded with T and B lymphocytes, as well as with macrophages, dendritic cells, and natural killer (NK) cells, of which, the latter are the predominant cell type.

Phenotypically, decidual NK cells differ from NK cells in peripheral blood. It has been suggested that decidual NK cells represent a distinct subpopulation of circulating NK cells or that, they have undergone some tissue-specific differentiation. It has been shown that decidual NK cells in early pregnancy mediate angiogenesis and control trophoblast invasion at the implantation site.

The process of implantation, currently thought to be the most critical step in achieving successful early pregnancy, remains one of the key events to be elucidated in Reproductive Medicine. What happens with the NK cells in the decidua when implantation is unsuccessful? Do dNK cells play a role in an unsuccessful *in vitro* fertilization (IVF)? A complete understanding of the migration and role of the decidual NK cells is expected to have a considerable clinical impact in women's reproductive health areas such as infertility and gestational complications.

INTRODUCTION

The circumstances that permit the human fetus to escape rejection by the mother's immune system have been a subject of profound interest for decades. It appears plausible that the paternally-derived fetal antigens should be recognized by the maternal immune system as foreign, resulting in deleterious consequences. It appears that non-recognition of fetal antigens should be favorable for a normal pregnancy outcome. However, this is not exactly the case. What is fascinating is that the immune responses during pregnancy differ from the rules of the classic transplantation immunity. There is ample evidence now that pregnancy is indeed recognized by the maternal immune system. Antifetal, antiplacental, and antipaternal antibodies are detectable in sera of women with successful pregnancies,[1] clearly showing that maternal recognition of fetus-derived antigens does not compromise pregnancy.

It is well-discussed now that the maternal immune system not only recognizes pregnancy but reacts in a differential way resulting in either success or failure. In fact, inadequate recognition of fetal antigens might result in failed pregnancy. A balanced maternal immune system seems to be necessary for a normal pregnancy outcome. It has been shown that non-specific immunostimulation of the pregnant female reduces the originally high resorption rates in an abortion-prone murine strain combination. It has been shown that human lymphocyte antigen (HLA) matching between the parents is associated with spontaneous abortion.[2]

CLINICAL DISCUSSION

Peri-implantation Events and Placentation

The bidirectional immunological relationship between the mother and the fetus is determined on one hand by fetal antigen presentation and on the other hand, by the recognition of and reaction to these antigens by the maternal immune system. The fetus itself does not come into direct contact with maternal tissue. Following fertilization of the ovum in the Fallopian tube, the developing embryo moves towards the uterus in a process of remodeling for implantation. The endometrium undergoes hormonally-programmed decidualization. Until approximately week 10 of human gestation, the embryo develops in a hypoxic environment while the uterine spiral arteries are constricted. The decidua contains not only cells that provide nourishment to the embryo, but also a carefully selected set of maternal leukocytes that are ultimately encountered by migrating, invasive fetal cells (trophoblast).[3]

On the fetal side of the maternal-fetal interface, trophoblast cells derived from the outermost trophectoderm layer of the blastocyst form the external cell layers of the placenta and comprise the chorion membrane. These cells surround and enclose the fetus throughout pregnancy and interact directly with elements of the maternal immune system. Trophoblast cells are subdivided by anatomic location, type of differentiation, and role in inducing tolerance in the pregnant uterus. The placental villi are encircled by two subpopulations: villus cytotrophoblast and syncytial trophoblast, which are responsible for bidirectional transport of nutrients from the mother to the fetus and removal of fetal waste, as well as producing critical pregnancy hormones, such as progesterone. Within the villi, mesenchymal cells that include early macrophages, called Hofbauer cells, fibroblasts, and undifferentiated cells, that ultimately become sources of endothelial cells for the developing placental vasculature, are generated from the inner cell mass of the embryo.

A third subpopulation of trophoblast cells, termed the extravillous cytotrophoblast cells, invades the decidua. These cells are generated from villus cytotrophoblast cells that proliferate, form columns, and head toward the decidualizing endometrium. These cells permeate with apparent ease through the interstitium to locate and invade the maternal spiral arteries, where they replace the endothelial cells.[4,5] During this process, the smooth muscle cells surrounding the spiral arteries are lost. Thus, controls on vasodilatation and vasoconstriction are removed, permitting maternal blood to flow over the placenta. As pregnancy progresses, the extravillus cytotrophoblast regresses to form the chorion membrane, which remains in immediate proximity to the maternal decidua.

This type of placentation, where neither endothelial cells nor basement membrane intervenes between maternal blood or tissue containing leukocytes and fetal trophoblast cells, is called hemochorial. The functional result is that placental and extraplacental trophoblast cells play a major role in achieving an immunologically compatible relationship between the mother and the fetus. Many of the same maternal-fetal physical arrangements of placentation are found in mice, which are popular models for studying human pregnancy.[6]

Immune Cells of Decidua

One fact of immune privilege in human pregnancy is clear; the embryo/fetus survives as a consequence of conjunctive interactions between the fetus and the mother.[7] It appears that the early immune tolerance relies mainly on maternal factors. Progesterone, an immunosuppressive hormone, is produced in the ovary in the secretory phase of the cycle and in the early stages of pregnancy. Implantation is accompanied by a flush of inflammatory cytokines from a pool of white blood cells, with neutrophils and macrophages predominating, as documented in the mouse,[8] alerting the mother to the implant. Subsequently, dramatic accommodations are made in the cellular composition of the decidualizing human endometrium. As with other mucosal sites, the cycling uterus is seeded with T and B lymphocytes and with macrophages, dendritic cells, and natural killer (NK) cells. Following implantation, the pregnant uterus is redesigned as a site of innate immunity rather than acquired immunity. Macrophages are consistently present throughout gestation, constituting 10 to 20 percent of the leukocytes. There are also small number of T cells and dendritic cells detected.

Natural Killer Cells

Analysis of the leukocytes in the uterus has shown that natural killer (NK) cells are the predominant population.[8] They are also referred to as large granular lymphocytes (LGL) because of the prominent granules in their cytoplasm. The total number of these cells in the uterine mucosa varies throughout human menstrual cycle. They are sparse during the proliferative phase, increase significantly throughout the secretory phase, and remain in high numbers in the decidua during the early stages of gestation.[9] Their numbers are particularly high in decidua basalis at the site where trophoblast cells invade into the uterus. This temporal association with the menstrual cycle implies a potential role of estrogen and progesterone in the recruitment and/or proliferation of uterine NK cells.

Phenotypically, decidual NK cells (CD56^{bright} CD16$^-$) differ from NK cells in peripheral blood (CD56^{dim} CD16$^+$). This fact suggests that either decidual NK cells represent a distinct subpopulation of circulating NK cells or that they have undergone some tissue-specific differentiation. It is still not entirely clear which of these possibilities is the correct one. Interestingly, it has been reported that uterine NK cells share many phenotypic features with NK cells isolated from the fetal liver. This indicates that NK cells with the uterine phenotype are already present very early in ontogeny, even before the appearance of T cells. Macrophages are also abundant at the implantation site, but have not been studied extensively. However, the observation that NK cells and macrophages, but not T and B cells, comprise the major population of leukocytes in the uterus suggests that implantation is likely to involve an innate immune system that is distinct from that seen in organ transplantation, where rejection is mediated by cells of the specific immune system, T and B cells.

The main effector functions of NK cells *in vivo* are cytotoxicity and cytokine production. Both of these activities are regulated by receptors for major histocompatibility complex (MHC) class I antigens. MHC genes are organized into three regions encoding the class I and class II human leukocyte antigens (HLA) while class III products are complement proteins. The NK cell receptors, which bind HLA class I molecules in humans, belong to three structurally distinct families: CD94/NKG2 heterodimers, killer cell Ig-like receptors (KIR) and Ig-like transcripts (ILT).[10]

NK cells are almost absent during the preovulatory phase of the endometrium of non-pregnant women, are highly proliferative after ovulation, and constitute around 70 percent of the lymphocytes in the decidua.[11] Decidual NK (dNK) cells differ in many ways from their peripheral blood counterparts in terms of gene expression, phenotype and functions.[12] The two subsets identified in peripheral blood NK cells are also present in the decidua, but in an almost inverse proportion: the cytolytic subset (CD56[dim] CD16[+]) accounts for only 5 percent of this population, and the cytokine-secreting subset-95 percent. Although the decidual NK cells possess the essential machinery required for target lysis, their cytolytic function is substantially reduced.[13] In addition, the decidual NK cells produce several cytokines, including some angiogenic factors, which are not normally secreted by NK cells in the peripheral blood.

NK Cell Localization and Trafficking

The variation in the number of decidual NK cells with the menstrual cycle is well-established but the mechanism for the marked increase in dNK cells seen in the mid and late secretory phase of the menstrual cycle continuing into early pregnancy is uncertain. It has been shown that upto 40 percent of CD56[+] dNK cells isolated from the late secretory phase endometrium express Ki67, a proliferation marker.[14] It could be stipulated that local proliferation of dNK cells accounts for their dramatic increase in number. Another explanation of the dramatic increase in dNK cell population could be the influx of peripheral blood NK cells from the circulation with subsequent modification to the specialized dNK cell phenotype within the uterine microenvironment. Expression of various adhesion molecules by dNK cells and by endometrial endothelium could explain homing of dNK cell to the endometrium and may account for their distribution in a perivascular position. Recruitment of CD56[bright] CD16[-]

cells from the peripheral circulation has also been suggested and an increase in circulating CD56[bright] NK cells has been reported in the peripheral blood of women of reproductive age compared with males.

Fate of dNK Cells

The reduction of dNK cells in later pregnancy and also at the end of the menstrual cycle is still incompletely understood. Death by both apoptosis and necrosis has been proposed for the loss of uterine NK cells in the late stages of mouse pregnancy,[15] but information regarding the fate of the cells in human pregnancy is lacking. It is possible that dNK cells degranulate in late pregnancy[16] or interact with the invading trophoblast in a non-compatible hormonal milieu leading to their demise.[9]

dNK Cells Control Trophoblast Invasion and Vascular Remodeling in the Decidua

In a set of milestone studies using NK-deficient mice, Croy and colleagues[17] began to understand the function of these unique NK cell subpopulations in the pregnant uterus of mice. They showed that mouse uterine NK cells, through interferon-γ secretion, control uterine vascular remodeling[17]—a vital characteristic of pregnancy. It is also possible that dNK cells direct the trophoblast invasion.[18] Since then, much attention has been directed at understanding whether these cells have the same role in humans. The observation that decidual NK cells in early human pregnancy are often in close contact with the invading trophoblast has led to the hypothesis that they could have a role in the control of this crucial invasion.

Hanna et al.[19] found that decidual NK cells in early pregnancy mediate angiogenesis and trophoblast chemo-attraction, two key functions of early pregnancy. First, they showed that decidual NK cells, but not NK cells derived from the peripheral blood, control trophoblast invasion; this control occurs through the release of interleukin-8 (IL-8) and interferon-inducible protein-10 (IP-10), chemokines that bind to receptors expressed on invasive trophoblast cells. Second, they provided evidence that decidual NK cells also produce proangiogenic factors, including vascular endothelial growth factor (VEGF) and placental growth factor (PLGF); both these factors favor vascular growth in the decidua. Finally, the researchers uncovered the NK receptor ligand interactions that seem to trigger release of these crucial factors. They identified two decidual NK-cell activating receptors (NKp30 and NKp44) and found that their specific ligands may be provided by two types of cells in the decidua, namely trophoblast cells and maternal stromal cells. Much of this evidence was obtained using human tissue, with animal models providing further proof of functionality.

NK Cells — Killers or Builders, or Both

Ample evidence substantiates the fact that maternal NK cells in the uterus of pregnant healthy women do not use their cytotoxic functions. Most studies to date have shown a pregnancy-compatible role for dNK cells in reproduction, mainly through their regulation of decidualization, production of pregnancy-compatible cytokines, and cross-talk with the trophoblast. During pregnancy, NK cell-deficient mice display abnormalities in decidual artery remodeling and trophoblast invasion, possibly due to the lack of dNK cell-derived IFN-γ.[20] In humans, it has been suggested that defective trophoblast invasion and placental development are associated with altered dNK cell function and pre-eclampsia.[21,22] Curiously, although dNK cells display an activated phenotype to date, no *in vivo* role for dNK cell cytotoxicity has been identified. It is tempting to speculate that although dNK cells normally contribute to the success of pregnancy, they may exert a negative role given aberrant intrauterine conditions. Our own experiments implicate dNK cells as critical mediators in inflammation-induced fetal demise.[23] Moreover, IL-10, an anti-inflammatory cytokine, with pivotal intrauterine immunomodulating properties, appears to play a crucial role in the protection of the fetus from inflammation-associated dNK cell aggression. Most likely, both inflammation and IL-10 deficiency are required for initiation of an antifetal immune responses. During normal pregnancy, mild inflammation, either systemically or locally at the maternal-fetal interface, may not lead to fetal demise due to the protective anti-inflammatory effects of the physiological presence of IL-10 or other modulators.[24,25] However, with insufficient IL-10 production, inflammatory processes may proceed unchecked, leading to increased dNK cell cytotoxic activation, invasiveness, and eventual fetal demise. This could explain why NK cell activity is increased in some women experiencing recurrent spontaneous abortion compared with that during normal pregnancy.

NK Cells and IVF Success

The process of implantation, currently thought to be the most critical step in achieving successful early pregnancy, remains one of the key events to be elucidated for reproductive medicine. The presently available techniques to predict implantation success are limited and mostly controversial.[26] The psychological and financial burden associated with the unpredictability of *in vitro* fertilization (IVF) treatment outcome can be significant to the patients. One of the key determinants of implantation success is the mechanism underlying uterine receptivity.[27]

As it was mentioned previously, uterine immune cell populations undergo remarkable changes during the course of each ovulatory cycle. In decidualized tissue, CD56^{bright}, CD16^{null} NK cells predominate and remain there until the onset of menses. In response to successful implantation and as pregnancy advances through the first trimester, this population of NK cells increases significantly.

What happens with the NK cells in the decidua when implantation is unsuccessful? Do dNK cells play a role in unsuccessful IVF? Recent elegant experiments by Heuvel, et al.[28,29] suggest that a subpopulation of NK cells shows propensity for adherence to uteroplacental tissue.[28,29] It appears that this may be an integral step during implantation of the embryo and points to the angiogenic properties of a special type of NK cells. Based on what we know regarding the similarities between mouse and human placentation, it is temping to speculate, that NK cells from women prone to implantation failure will not/minimally attach to the mouse decidua from wild type and IL-10 knockout strains, whereas NK cells from women who are going to have a successful implantation will attach to a greater degree. We have set up an experimental design to evaluate and confirm the degree of attachment of NK cells isolated from the peripheral blood of women undergoing IVF treatment, to the mouse gestational tissue subjected to a variety of *in vivo* treatments at four different stages of the IVF cycle through the first hCG-positive reading as shown in Figure 62.1.

We are performing these studies on women experiencing recurrent implantation failure and women undergoing IVF for the first time. We also analyzed peripheral blood mononuclear cells from the study subjects for phenotypic and functional properties, particularly for NK cell content and cytotoxic activity. Interestingly enough, in our preliminary experiments using blood from normal first trimester pregnant women and non-pregnant women and male subjects, we demonstrated that peripheral blood NK cells from pregnant women attached in large numbers to wild type (WT) pregnant mouse decidua. Attachment of labeled NK cells from non-pregnant women and male subjects was not observed (Figs 62.2A and B).

CONCLUSION

It is clear that the maternal-fetal immune interactions differ from those between an organ allograft and recipient. Implantation appears to be influenced by an NK cell interaction with the fetal trophoblast and maternal decidua. It seems that NK cell adherence to gestational tissue provides a unique conducive microenvironment for implantation and early pregnancy. A complete understanding of the migration and role of the decidual CD 56 ^{bright} NK cells is expected to have a considerable clinical impact in women's reproductive health areas such as infertility and gestational complications (i.e. recurrent spontaneous abortion and pre-eclampsia).

ACKNOWLEDGMENT

This work was supported by a grant from NIH (P20RR018728).

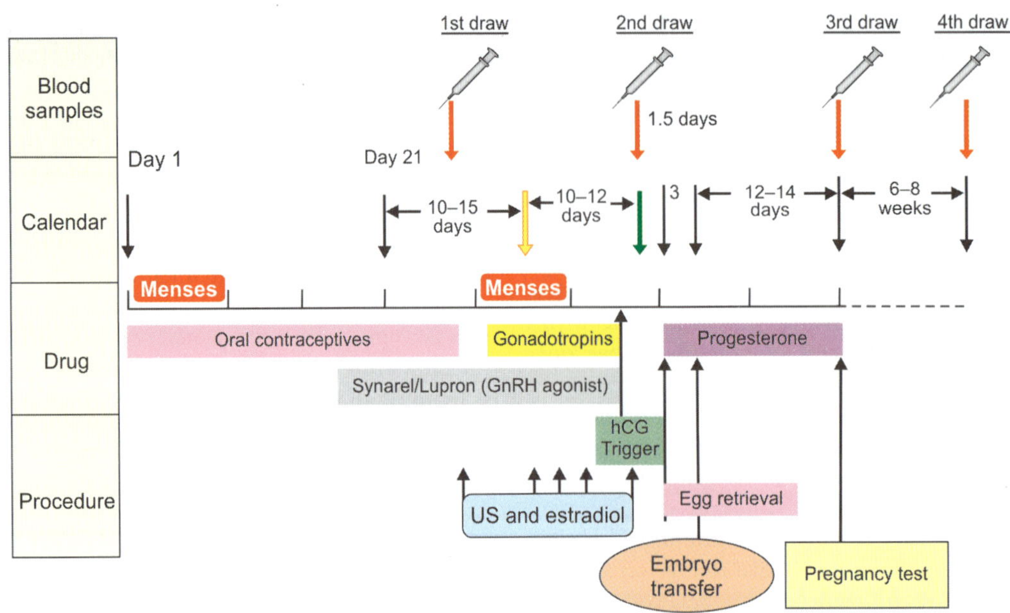

Fig. 62.1: IVF cycle diagram with blood draw points. Red arrows under syringes indicating the time of blood samples: 1st — baseline, prior to gonadotropin treatment; 2nd — at hCG triggering; 3rd — at first pregnancy test; 4th — at 8 weeks of pregnancy

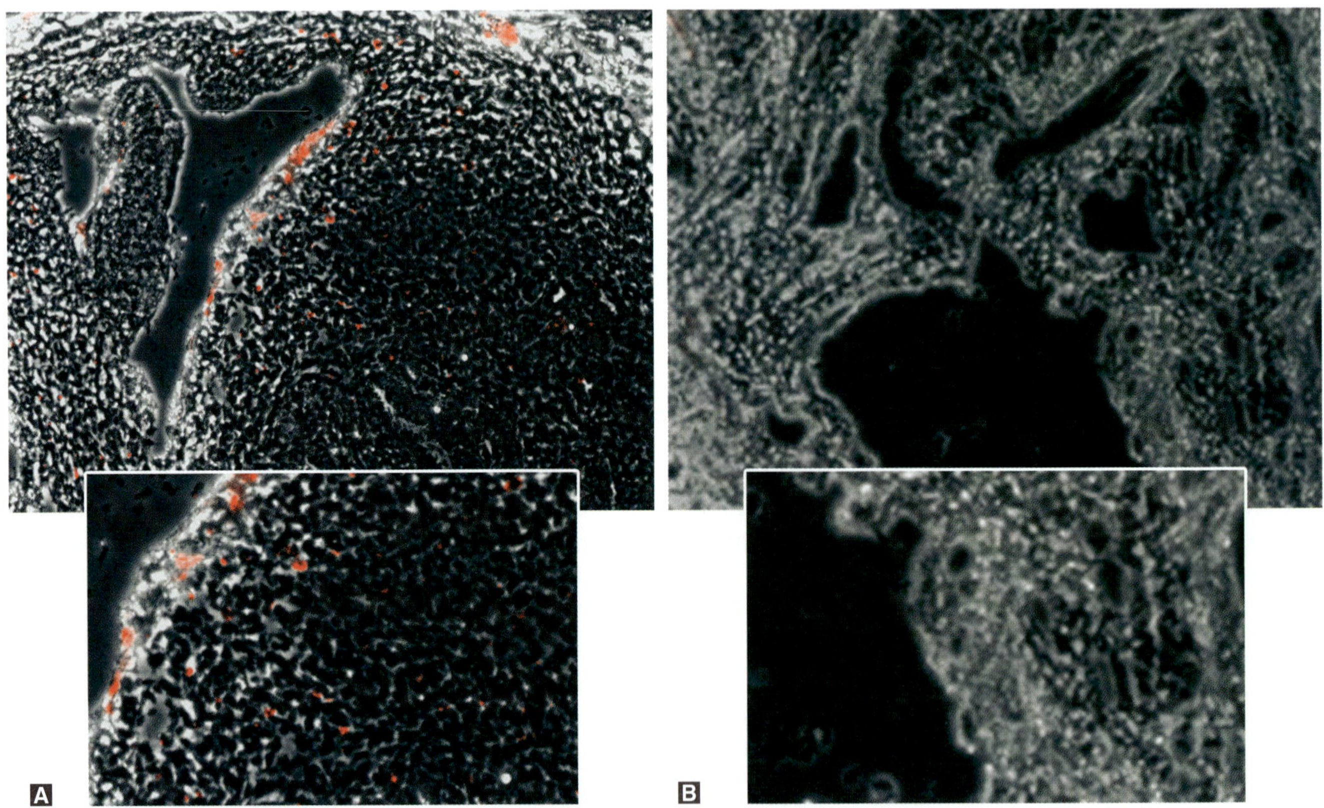

Figs 62.2A and B: Adhesion assay of PB CD56+ cells to pregnant d7 wild type mouse decidua: (A) CD 56+ cells from a first trimester pregnant woman attach in large numbers to frozen sections of the mouse uterus, exhibiting red fluorescence (200X); (B) No visible red fluorescence was observed when CD 56-labeled cells from a non-pregnant woman were applied to frozen sections from the same mouse uterus (200X). (inserts showing higher power magnification, 400X)

REFERENCES

1. Billington WD. Transfer of antigens and antibodies between mother and fetus. In: Coulam CB, Faulk WP, McIntyre J (Eds). Immunological Obstetrics, New York: WW. Norton and Co 1992.pp.290-304.
2. Ober C, Hyslop T, Elias S, Weikamp LR, Hauck WW. Human elucocyte antigen matching and fetal loss: Results of a 10 years prospective study. Hum Reprod 1998;13:33-8.
3. Bulmer JN, Pace D, Ritson A. Immunoregulatory cells in human decidua: Morphology, immunohistochemistry and function. Reprod Nutr Dev 1988;28:1599-613.
4. Moffett A, Loke C. Immunology of placentation in eutherian mammals. Nat Rev Immunol 2006;6:584-94.
5. Norwitz ER, Schust DJ, Fisher SJ. Implantation and the survival of early pregnancy. N Engl J Med 2001;345:1400-8.
6. Rossant J, Cross JC. Placental development: Lessons from mouse mutants. Nat Rev Genet 2001;2:538-48.
7. Hunt JS, Petroff MG, McIntire RH, Ober C. HLA-G and immune tolerance in pregnancy. FASEB J 2005;9:681-93.
8. McMaster MT, Newton RC, Dey SK, Andrews GK. Activation and distribution of inflammatory cells in the mouse uterus during the preimplantation period. J Immunol 1992;148:1699-1705.
9. Bulmer JN, Lash GE. Human uterine natural killer cells: A reappraisal. Mol Immunol 2005;42:511-21.
10. Lanier LL. NK cell receptors. Annual Review of Immunology 1998;16:359-93.
11. Moffett-King A. Natural killer cells and pregnancy. Nat Rev Immunol 2002;2:656-63.
12. Koopman LA, Kopcow HD, Rybalov B, Boyson JE, Orange JS, Schatz F, et al. Human decidual natural killer cells are a unique NK cell subset with immunomodulatory potential. J Exp Med 2003;198:1201-12.
13. Kopcow HD, Allan DS, Chen X, Rybalov B, Andzelm MM, Ge B, Strominger JL. Human decidual NK cells form immature activating synapses and are not cytotoxic. Proc Natl Acad Sci USA 2005;102:15563-8.
14. Jones RK, Searle RF, Stewart JA, Turner S, Bulmer JN. Apoptosis, bcl-2 expression, and proliferative activity in human endometrial stroma and endometrial granulated lymphocytes. Biol Reprod 1998;58:995-1002.
15. Kusakabe K, Okada T, Sasaki F, Kiso Y. Cell death of uterine natural killer cells in murine placenta during placentation and preterm periods. J Vet Med Sci 1999;61:1093-1100.
16. Spornitz UM. The functional morphology of the human endometrium and decidua. Adv Anat Embryol 1992;124:1-99.
17. Croy BA, Xie X. *In vivo* models for studying homing and function of murine uterine natural killer cells. Methods Mol Med 2006;122:77-92.
18. Ain R, Canham LN, Soares MJ. Gestation stage-dependent intrauterine trophoblast cell invasion in the rat and mouse: novel endocrine phenotype and regulation. Dev Biol 2003;260:176-90.
19. Hanna J, Goldman-Wohl D, Hamani Y, Avraham I, Greenfield C, Natanson-Yaron S, et al. Decidual NK cells regulate key developmental processes at the human fetal-maternal interface. Nat Med 2006;12:1065-74.
20. Ashkar AA, Croy BA. Functions of uterine natural killer cells are mediated by interferon-γ production during murine pregnancy. Semin Immunol 2001;13:235-41.
21. Hiby SE, Walker JJ, O'shaughnessy KM, Redman CW, Carrington M, Trowsdale J, Moffett A. Combinations of maternal KIR and fetal HLA-C genes influence the risk of pre-eclampsia and reproductive success. J Exp Med 2004;200:957-65.
22. Parham P. NK cells and trophoblasts: Partners in pregnancy. J Exp Med 2004;200:951-5.
23. Murphy SP, Fast LD, Hanna NN, Sharma S. Uterine NK cells mediate inflammation-induced fetal demise in IL-10-null mice. J Immunol 2005;175:4084-90.
24. Hanna N, Hanna I, Hleb M, Wagner E, Dougherty J, Balkundi D, Padbury J, Sharma S. Gestational age-dependent expression of IL-10 and its receptor in human placental tissues and isolated cytotrophoblasts. J Immunol 2000;164:5721-8.
25. Sargent IL, Borzychowski AM, Redman CW. NK cells and human pregnancy. An inflammatory view. Trends Immunol 2006;27:399-404.
26. Yuval Y, Lipitz S, Dor J, Achiron R. The relationships between endometrial thickness, and blood flow and pregnancy rates in *in vitro* fertilization. Hum Reprod 1999;14:1067-71.
27. Red-Horse K, Zhou Y, Genbacev O, Prakobphol A, Foulk R, McMaster M, Fisher SJ. Trophoblast differentiation during embryo implantation and formation of the maternal-fetal interface. J Clin Invest 2004;114:744-54.
28. van den Heuvel MJ, Horrocks J, Bashar S, Hatta K, Burke S, Evans SS, Croy BA, Tekpetey FR. Periovulatory increases in tissue homing potential of circulating CD56 (bright) cells are associated with fertile menstrual cycles. J Clin Endocrinol Metab 2005;90:3606-13.
29. van den Heuvel MJ, Horrocks J, Bashar S, Taylor S, Burke S, Hatta K, Lewis JE, Croy BA. Menstrual cycle hormones induce changes in functional interactions between lymphocytes and decidual vascular endothelial cells. J Clin Endocrinol Metab 2005;90:2835-42.

Medical Treatment with Misoprostol for Early Failure of Pregnancies Conceived Following ART

Daniel S Seidman, Micha Baum, David Stockheim, Ronit Machtinger

OVERVIEW

Medical treatment with Misoprostol for early pregnancy failure offers a safe and cost-effective management option with a low rate of side effects. Significant complications, including infection and excessive bleeding, are rare. The role of pretreatment with Mifepristone has not been proven. Patients with early pregnancy failure, who had conceived through controlled ovarian hyperstimulation (COH) or *in vitro* fertilization (IVF) were found to have a significantly higher response rate to medical treatment with Misoprostol. Long-term follow-up data shows that intrauterine adhesions are rare after medical compared with surgical management of spontaneous abortions and that, reproductive outcome is good. Infertility patients, always concerned about their next pregnancy, often prefer medical treatment over surgical evacuation, despite more discomfort and lower success rates associated with the more conservative approach.

INTRODUCTION

Early pregnancy failure is one of the most common complications of first trimester pregnancy. Its incidence is reported to be as high as 50 percent of conceptions, 12 to 15 percent of clinically diagnosed pregnancies and 2 to 6 percent of pregnancies where a fetal heart pulse was demonstrated.[1,2] Surgical evacuation is still commonly recommended as early as possible following the diagnosis of pregnancy failure. The reason for this, dating back to the first half of the previous century, was prompt treatment designed to prevent blood loss and infection.[3] In practice, these complications are hardly ever seen or reported in the literature in association with conservative follow-up of early pregnancy failure. However, prompt surgical evacuation carries a small risk of surgical complications, including anesthesia-related problems, uterine perforation, intrauterine adhesions, cervical trauma and infection.

CHANGING TRENDS

Two relatively new developments in the last decade have led to a revival in the use and more intensive investigation of medical management of early pregnancy loss (spontaneous abortion or blighted ovum). This first innovation was the introduction of transvaginal sonography (TVS), and the second advancement was the growing experience with induced medical termination of ongoing pregnancies, using a protocol that includes Mifepristone and Misoprostol.

The wide availability of TVS currently allows close and simple monitoring of the intrauterine cavity. Thus, pregnancy failure can be reliably diagnosed at an earlier stage. Furthermore, TVS facilitates accurate monitoring of the response to medical management of early pregnancy failure, the emerging alternative to surgical termination.

Over the past decade, elective medical termination of pregnancy, using a protocol that includes Mifepristone and Misoprostol, was widely accepted into practice. This drug regimen was consistently shown to be associated with high success rates of 90 to 95 percent.[4,5]

CLINICAL DISCUSSION

Medical Treatment

Medical treatment of pregnancy failure is slowly gaining wider acceptance in many countries. Various drug protocols, mainly using prostaglandin (PG) analogs, have been studied.[6]

Table 63.1: Advantages of the PGE1 analog Misoprostol (Cytotec)

- Inexpensive
- Easily stored
- Readily available
- Multiple administration modes

The PGE1 analog, Misoprostol, has the advantage of being inexpensive, easily stored and readily available (Table 63.1). Reported success rates following the administration of PG range from 62 percent to 88 percent.[2,7-17] This wide range of results could be attributed to differences in patient selection, varying dosing regimens, routes of administration, follow-up periods and definitions of success.

Mifepristone Pretreatment

Mifepristone pretreatment was expected to increase the success of treatment with PG as it is known to increase uterine smooth muscle contractility.[5] The first progesterone antagonist to be accepted into clinical practice was Mifepristone, also known as RU-486. It binds to the progesterone receptor with an affinity greater than that of progesterone, inhibits transcription, and causes decidual necrosis and detachment of the products of gestation. This drug also promotes uterine contractions by increasing myometrial excitability and causes cervical dilatation.[18]

Protocols composed of the combination of Mifepristone and PG analogs have been used with a success rate ranging from 52 to 84 percent.[2,7,19,20] However, to date the only randomized study reported, found no improvement in the success rate of Misoprostol for the termination of early pregnancy failure following Mifepristone pretreatment.[19]

We recently undertook a prospective randomized trial to compare the effectiveness and safety of Mifepristone pretreatment prior to Misoprostol treatment compared to only Misoprostol treatment of early pregnancy failure.[8] In a non-blinded controlled trial, a total of 115 consecutive women, diagnosed with a blighted ovum or a missed abortion of less than 9 weeks gestation were prospectively enrolled.

After providing an informed consent, the participants were randomized into two groups. Group I received 600 mg Mifepristone (Mifegyne, Exelgyn, SA Paris, France) and were discharged after two hours of observation. Group II received an oral administration of 800 µg Misoprostol (Cytotec, Searle, High Wycombe, England) divided in two equal doses three hours apart. Patients were observed for six hours following the first Misoprostol dose. All the patients, from both the groups were requested to return 48 hours later to receive Misoprostol, 800 µg orally, again divided into two equal doses. Women, who experienced significant vaginal bleeding, underwent a TVS examination. Misoprostol was not given to women who had an empty uterine cavity diagnosed by TVS. Women were discharged within six hours following the first Misoprostol dose, depending on the severity of bleeding and pain.

The success rate was defined as the nonrequirement for surgical intervention. Follow-up included a clinical interview and all the patients underwent a TVS assessment of the uterine cavity. When a woman from either group did not bleed within 48 hours after completing the drug protocol, she was requested to return for a TVS scan. If a gestational sac was still found on TVS examination, surgical evacuation was performed.

Ten to fourteen days following the treatment, patients were invited for a clinical interview to assess their bleeding pattern and conduct a TVS examination. The TVS follow-up included an evaluation of the uterine cavity contents. A well-defined endometrial line, with a maximum thickness of less than 15 mm combined with the absence of vaginal bleeding, was defined as complete abortion according to the Royal College of Obstetricians and Gynaecologists (RCOG) guidelines[9] for spontaneous abortions. In the absence of any clinical complaint, these patients were not invited for further follow-up.

Women with suspected retained products of conception (antero-posterior diameter >15 mm or presence of blood vessels in the suspicious tissue) were invited for a follow-up clinical and TVS examination after the first menstruation. According to our protocol, women with suspected TVS retained products of conception following menstruation, underwent diagnostic, and if necessary, operative hysteroscopy.[10] Retained intrauterine products of conception were suspected postmenstruation based on the results of TVS imaging or patients' complaints of prolonged bleeding. In such cases, hysteroscopy was performed in order to confirm the diagnosis and evacuate the gestational remnants.

Our success rate was similar in Groups I and II; 38 of 58 (65.5%) patients vs 42 of 57 (73.6%) patients respectively [odds ratio 0.68 (95% confidence interval 0.28-1.63)]. Pretreatment with Mifepristone resulted in a non statistically significant lower rate of retained intrauterine gestational sac requiring curettage; 10.3 percent and 17.5 percent of the cases in Groups I and II, respectively [odds ratio 0.54 (95% confidence interval 0.15-1.79)]. No cases of severe infection or bleeding, necessitating blood transfusion, occurred.

Complete evacuation of the uterus, in our study, was achieved in approximately two-thirds of the women who received Misoprostol for early pregnancy failure, with similar success rates following Mifepristone pretreatment. Patient's age, parity, past pregnancy failures or the amount of gestational products did not significantly influence the success rate. Similar success rates (74 percent in women treated with a combination of Mifepristone and Misoprostol versus a 71 percent success rate after treatment with Misoprostol alone) were previously reported by Gronlund, et al.[19] However, in contrast to our study, the latter authors used a crossover design with alternating regimens every 4 months, which is not considered an adequate randomization technique. Furthermore, the percentages of surgical evacuation according to the cause (i.e. retained gestational sac, suspected residua) were not provided.[19]

Among the 58 patients in Group I, who received both Mifepristone and Misoprostol, the success rate was 65.5 percent. This success rate is within the range of 52 to 95 percent reported in previous studies.[2,7,19,20] The main differences between the studies were in the dosing protocols, routes of administration and follow-up regimens.

Of the 57 women in Group II, who received Misoprostol only, the success rate was 73.6 percent. Our results fall well within that range of 25 to 95 percent reported in the literature.[1,6,11,12] In the largest study reported to date, Zhang, et al.[13] found that of the 491 women with early pregnancy failure, assigned to receive 800 µg of Misoprostol vaginally, 71 percent had complete expulsion by day 3 and 84 percent by day 8.

Comparison of the results of the present study with those of previous studies is difficult due to differences in patient selection criteria, medication dosing protocols, routes of administration, follow-up regimens and definition of outcome end-points. Our study is also unique with regard to the relative long follow-up of all cases, extending at least until after the first menstrual cycle. Furthermore, it is worth noting that in our follow-up, we applied extensively diagnostic and operative hysteroscopy in cases of suspected residua. The major methodological limitation of the present study is the non-blinded randomization method used. However, it is reasonable to assume that this did not significantly bias our results since the primary end-point was the need for surgical evacuation, and this was determined by the physician who performed the TVS and was blinded to the random treatment assignment.

There is a lack of consensus at present regarding the indication for surgical intervention following medical treatment of missed abortion. El-Refaey, et al.[19] and Creinin, et al.[14] postulated that surgical interventions should be done only in cases of retained gestational sacs. Reynolds, et al.[15] stated that absence of a gestational sac on transvaginal ultrasound should be the criterion used to document success after medical management of first-trimester missed abortion, as it is associated with the highest short and long-term success rates, as well as mild and self-limited symptoms in the days following treatment. Other authors, including Nielsen, et al.[2], Gronlund et al.[19] and Leung et al.[16] performed surgical evacuation in all cases with suspected retained products of gestation by TVS (antero-postero diameter of more than 15 or 20 mm/ homogenous intrauterine dimension of more than 11 cm[2] in combined transverse and sagittal planes). We chose the latter definition for the present study. The definition used

may strongly influence the interpretation of the findings, since we found that women who were treated with the protocol containing Mifepristone had lower curettage rates, due to retained intrauterine gestational sac, compared with women treated with Misoprostol only.

The complete expulsion of the products of gestation from the uterus, using the uterotonic agent Misoprostol, may be dose-dependent. This assumption is based on our results and the fact that in our study, patients who were given a combination of Mifepristone and Misoprostol received half the dose of Misoprostol in comparison to the patients treated with Misoprostol alone. This difference in the Misoprostol dose between the groups was also noted in one previous study that compared a similar treatment protocol.[19] The results of the combined regimen reported by Wagaarachchi, et al.[7] where a higher dose of Misoprostol was given according to response, but not in a randomized manner, may further support this assumption.

Medical Treatment in Infertility Patients

As medical management of early pregnancy failure is currently gaining wider recognition, it seems that this non-invasive treatment option should be especially useful and psychologically acceptable to women undergoing infertility treatment.

Women who conceive following infertility treatment seem to have greater and more immediate concern regarding future pregnancies. They are also often more worried about the potential harm to the endometrium inflicted by curettage. Furthermore, early pregnancy loss may have unique characteristics among infertility patients. For instance, in patients who conceived by COH or IVF, pregnancy loss is often detected earlier, multiple corpus lutea may be present in the ovaries, and progesterone supplementation for luteal phase support is a common practice.

We therefore tried to compare the success rate of medical treatment with Misoprostol for early pregnancy failure among pregnancies achieved following assisted reproductive techniques (ART) versus spontaneous pregnancies. We prospectively recruited all women who underwent medical treatment for early pregnancy failure with a CRL up to 25 mm in our medical center between 9/2001 and 8/2005. The treatment protocol included vaginal administration of 800 mcg Misoprostol. A second dose of Misoprostol was given 1 to 3 days later if the TVS evaluation showed an endometrial thickness ≥15 mm and TVS was performed again after the next menstrual bleeding. Those with a persistent gestational sac underwent curettage. When residual tissue was suspected, diagnostic follow-up, if required, was performed by operative hysteroscopy.

We found that of the 201 women enrolled, 48 women conceived following COH or IVF and 153 women had a spontaneous pregnancy. Success rates, defined as non-requirement for surgical intervention, were achieved in 91.7 percent (44/48) of the infertility patients and in 73.2 percent (112/153) of the patients who conceived spontaneously (p = 0.009). The success rates were 87.5 percent in 17 patients who conceived through COH and 93.3 percent in the 31 patients who underwent IVF. No major complications were reported. One patient experienced severe pain, necessitating administration of nonoral analgesia.

A stepwise unconditional logistic regression analysis was performed. The following variables were considered: manner of conception (spontaneous vs ART), gestational age of the fetal demise, gestational age at diagnosis, and the time interval between those dates. According to the logistic regression results, the success rate was influenced only by the manner of conception. The chance of success with medical abortion was increased by 3.7 folds for ART pregnancies compared with spontaneous pregnancies (OR 3.7, 95% CI 1.22–11.1, P < 0.009).[8]

We concluded that medical treatment seems to be an especially valuable treatment option for early fetal loss in pregnancies achieved by ovulation induction or IVF. Infertility patients, who experience early fetal loss, seem to prefer the less invasive nature of medical management. However, only future research will determine if medical management offers long-term advantages in terms of time to new conception.[8]

CONCLUSION

Medical treatment of early pregnancy failure offers a safe management option with a low rate of side effects (Table 63.2). From our experience, complications are rare. Only few patients experience fever after receiving Mifepristone pretreatment and/or Misoprostol, but they usually do not require antibiotic treatment. In our series, none of the patients needed blood transfusion due to excessive bleeding. Pretreatment with Mifepristone was not found to clearly enhance the treatment outcome with Misoprostol in our study.[8]

Patients with early pregnancy failure, who had conceived through COH or IVF, were found to have a significantly higher response rate to medical treatment with Misoprostol.

Table 63.2: The benefits of medical management of early pregnancy loss with the PGE1 analog, Misoprostol (Cytotec)

1. Reduction in the need for curettage in most women with early pregnancy failure; effective in 70–80 percent of cases.

2. Low level of associated major complications (<1%).

3. Avoidance of laminaria in failed cases.

4. Elimination of the potential risks of surgical evacuation, including anesthesia-related complications, uterine perforation, intrauterine adhesions and cervical trauma, in successful cases.

5. Highly cost-effective in most settings.

This may be due to a tendency to detect miscarriages earlier in patients undergoing infertility, a greater propensity to follow these patients conservatively before referring them for intervention and perhaps, due to other yet undetermined confounding factors. Recently, long-term follow-up data has become available showing that intrauterine adhesions are rare after medical compared with surgical management of spontaneous abortions,[17] and that, the reproductive outcome is good.[21,22] Infertility patients, always concerned about their next pregnancy, seem to prefer medical treatment over surgical evacuation.[23] When treatment with Misoprostol fails, it can still dilatate and soften the cervix, and can therefore, negate the need for inserting a laminaria before vacuum aspiration of the uterine contents.[24-26] Misoprostol treatment of early pregnancy failure may also offer a very cost-effective advantage compared to curettage.[27,28]

REFERENCES

1. Chung TKH, Cheung LP, Leung TY, Heines CJ, Chang AMZ. Misoprostol in the management of spontaneous abortion. BJOG 1995;102:832-5.

2. Nielsen S, Hahlin M, Platz-Christensen J. Unsuccessful treatment of missed abortion with a combination of an anti-progesterone and a prostaglandin E1 analogue. BJOG 1997; 104:1094-6.

3. Ankum WM, Waard MW, Bindels PJE. Management of spontaneous miscarriage in the first trimester: An example of putting informed shared decision making into practice. BMJ 2001;322:1343-6.

4. Comparison of two doses of mifepristone in combination with misoprostol for early medical abortion: A randomized trial. World Health Organization task force on postovulatory methods of fertility regulation. BJOG 2000;107:524-30.

5. Peyron R, Aubeny E, Targosz V, Silvestre L, Renault M, Elkik F, et al. Early termination of pregnancy with Mifepristone (RU 486) and the orally active prostaglandin Misoprostol. NEJM 1993;328:1509-13.

6. Herabutya Y, Prasertsawat PO. Misoprostol in the management of missed abortions. Int J Gynecol Obstet 1997;56:263-6.

7. Wagaarachchi PT, Ashok PW, Narvekar N, Smith NC, Tempelton A. Medical management of early fetal demise using a combination of Mifepristone and Misoprostol. Hum Reprod 2001;16:1849-53.

8. Stockheim D, Machtinger R, Wiser A, Dulitzky M, Soriano D, Goldenberg M, et al. A randomized prospective study of Misoprostol or Mifepristone followed by Misoprostol when needed for the treatment of women with early pregnancy failure. Fertil Steril 2006;86:956-60.

9. Luise C, Jermy K, May C, Costello G, Collins WP, Bourne T. Outcome of expectant management of spontaneous first trimester miscarriage: Observational study. BMJ 2002;324:873-5.

10. Goldenberg M, Schiff E, Achiron R, Lipitz S, Mashiach S. Managing residual trophoblastic tissue: Hysteroscopy for directing curettage. J Reprod Med 1997;42:26-8.

11. Chung TKH, Lee DTS, Cheung LP, Heines CJ, Chang AMZ. Spontaneous abortion: A randomized controlled trial

comparing surgical evacuation with conservative management using misoprostol. Fertil Steril 1999;71:1054-9.

12. Demetroulis C, Saridogan E, Kunde D, Naftalin AA. A prospective randomized control trial comparing medical and surgical treatment for early pregnancy failure. Hum Reprod 2001;16:356-9.

13. Zhang J, Gilles JM, Barnhart K, Creinin MD, Westhoff C, Frederick MM. National Institute of Child Health Human Development (NICHD) Management of Early Pregnancy Failure Trial. A comparison of medical management with misoprostol and surgical management for early pregnancy failure. NEJM. 2005;353:761-9.

14. Creinin MD, Harwood B, Guido RS, Fox MC, Zhang J. NICHD Management of Early Pregnancy Failure Trial. Endometrial thickness after Misoprostol use for early pregnancy failure. Int J Gynaecol Obstet 2004;86:22-6.

15. Reynolds A, Ayres-de-Campos D, Costa MA, Montenegro N. How should success be defined when attempting medical resolution of first-trimester missed abortion? Eur J Obstet Gynecol Reprod Biol 2005;118:71-6.

16. Leung SW, Pang MW, Chung TK. Retained products of gestation in miscarriage: An evaluation of transvaginal ultrasound criteria for diagnosing an 'empty uterus'. Am J Obstet Gynecol 2004;191:1133-7.

17. Tam WH, Lau WC, Cheung LP, Yuen PM, Chung TK. Intra-uterine adhesions after conservative and surgical management of spontaneous abortion. J Am Assoc Gynecol Laparosc 2002; 9:182-5.

18. Christin-Maitre S, Bouchard P, Spitz IM. Medical termination of pregnancy. NEJM 2000;342:946-56.

19. Gronlund A, Gronlund L, Clevin L, Andersen B, Palmgren N, Lidegaard O. Management of missed abortion: Comparison of medical treatment with Mifepristone + Misoprostol or Misoprostol alone with surgical evacuation. A multi-center trial in Copenhagen County, Denmark. Acta Obstet Gynecol Scand 2002;81:1060-5.

20. El-Refaey H, Hinshaw K, Henshaw R, Smith N, Tempelton A. Medical management of missed abortion and an embryonic pregnancy. BMJ 1992;305:99.

21. Graziosi GC, Bruinse HW, Reuwer PJ, Teteringen O, Mol BW. Fertility outcome after a randomized trial comparing curettage with Misoprostol for treatment of early pregnancy failure. Hum Reprod 2005;20:1749-50.

22. Tam WH, Tsui MH, Lok IH, Yip SK, Yuen PM, Chung TK. Long-term reproductive outcome subsequent to medical versus surgical treatment for miscarriage. Hum Reprod 2005;20:3355-9.

23. Graziosi GC, Bruinse HW, Reuwer PJ, van Kessel PH, Westerweel PE, Mol BW. Misoprostol versus curettage in women with early pregnancy failure: Impact on women's health-related quality of life. A randomized controlled trial. Hum Reprod 2005;20:2340-7.

24. MacIsaac L, Grossman D, Balistreri E, Darney P. A randomized controlled trial of laminaria, oral Misoprostol, and vaginal Misoprostol before abortion. Obstet Gynecol 1999;93:766-70.

25. Burnett MA, Corbett CA, Gertenstein RJ. A randomized trial of laminaria tents versus vaginal Misoprostol for cervical ripening in first trimester surgical abortion. J Obstet Gynaecol Can 2005; 27:38-42.

26. Goldberg AB, Drey EA, Whitaker AK, Kang MS, Meckstroth KR, Darney PD. Misoprostol compared with laminaria before early second-trimester surgical abortion: A randomized trial. Obstet Gynecol 2005;106:234-41.

27. Graziosi GC, van der Steeg JW, Reuwer PH, Drogtrop AP, Bruinse HW, Mol BW. Economic evaluation of Misoprostol in the treatment of early pregnancy failure compared to curettage after an expectant management. Hum Reprod 2005;20:1067-71.

28. Stockheim D, Carp H. Misoprostol for early pregnancy failure. Isr Med Assoc J 2010;12:375-6.

Management of Recurrent Miscarriages

Yadava Bapurao Jeve

OVERVIEW

Recurrent miscarriage is disheartening to the couple and to the treating clinician. Recurrent miscarriage is defined as three or more consecutive miscarriages. It affects 1 percent of women. The etiological factors involved in recurrent early pregnancy loss include genetic factors, endocrine disorders, anatomical defects, immunological factors, infectious factors, environmental factors[1] and unexplained factors (Table 64.1). We may succeed to assign the cause in 60 percent of women.

This topic is aimed to discuss the management of recurrent miscarriage in clinical practice. Recurrent miscarriages are post-implantation failures in natural conception, whereas repeated reproductive failures in assisted reproductive techniques (ART) are majorly implantation failures. The investigations and management are similar for the recurrent miscarriages of clinically diagnosed pregnancy in assisted conception as they are postimplantation failures. These patients should be referred to the recurrent miscarriage clinic before the next treatment cycle or attempt of pregnancy. There is strong association between subfertility and spontaneous miscarriages. The evidence suggests higher frequency of spontaneous miscarriages amongst subfertile couples and a higher prevalence of subfertility in women with recurrent spontaneous miscarriages when compared with the general population.[2] Many known and unknown etiological factors in both clinical conditions significantly overlap to cause reproductive failure.

Recently, assisted reproductive techniques have been used to prevent further miscarriages in women with recurrent miscarriage with known genetic causes.[3] There is tremendous psychological impact of recurrent miscarriage. Women with unexplained recurrent pregnancy loss still have a 60 to 70 percent chance of delivering a viable infant[4] without any treatment. The key treatment is psychological support for unexplained recurrent miscarriages. Women with recurrent miscarriage are at high risk for adverse obstetric outcomes, including fetal abnormalities, stillbirths and neonatal deaths, even when the pregnancies are ongoing.[5] Hence, it is relevant to discuss the management of this challenging clinical condition when we study assisted conception.

INTRODUCTION

Spontaneous miscarriage is a major loss for pregnant women, especially for those who achieve pregnancy through expensive and stressful ART treatments. Most of the pregnancies are lost even before implantation. The incidence of spontaneous miscarriage may be much greater than is clinically recognized. Spontaneous abortion occurs in 12 to 15 percent of all pregnancies. Thirty percent of the pregnancies are lost between implantation and the 6th week. Studies have shown that the risk of recurrent spontaneous miscarriage is much higher in patients with previous losses. A review of 10 retrospective, cohort and prospective studies showed that the risk of miscarriage after two consecutive losses is 17 to 25 percent and the risk of miscarrying a fourth pregnancy after three consecutive losses is between 25 and 46 percent.[6]

The risk of miscarriage increases with age.[7] Study shows spontaneous miscarriage in 29 percent of women 40 years and older, undergoing *in vitro* fertilization (IVF), after the demonstration of fetal heartbeat by ultrasonography.[8]

Etiology

Genetic Causes

The most common cause of sporadic spontaneous miscarriage is a chromosomal abnormality of the embryo. Approximately 50 to 60 percent of early spontaneous miscarriage are associated with a chromosomal anomaly of the conceptus.[9] The most common abnormality is aneuploidy, with auto-somal trisomy accounting for more than 50 percent of chromosomally abnormal abortuses. Other common types of aneuploidy include XO, XXX, XXY and XYY. Polyploidy

Table 64.1: Etiological factors

Genetic disorders	• Aneuploidy • Polyploidy • Translocation • Euploid Miscarriages	Infectious	• Toxoplasma • Ureaplasma • Chlamydia • Cytomegalovirus • Listeria • Herpes virus
Anatomical defects	• Müllerian fusion defect • Uterine synechiae • Leiomyomas • Cervical incompetence	Immunological factors	• Autoimmunity-Antinuclear antibody, Lupus anticoagulant, Anticardiolipin antibody • Alloimmunity-HLA homozygosity
Thrombophilia	• Antithrombin III deficiency • Protein C deficiency • Protein S deficiency • Factor V Leiden mutation • Prothrombin gene mutation	Endocrine disorders	• Endocrine abnormalities during the follicular phase • Luteal phase defect • Insulin resistance • PCOS • Hyperprolactinemia, hypoprolactinemia • Hyperthyroidism, hypothyroidism • Diabetes mellitus
Environmental	• Occupational/chemical exposure • Stress, alcohol • Radiation	Aging gametes, Endothelial dysfunction, Inferility	
Unexplained factors			

accounts for approximately 22 percent of chromosomally abnormal abortuses. The euploid miscarriages peak at 13 weeks of gestation and incidence increases with maternal age. A genetic abnormality as a single or polygenic mutation, and various maternal and some paternal factors are responsible for euploid miscarriage.[9] Parental genetic abnormalities are a much less common cause of recurrent miscarriage.

Endocrine Causes

Endocrine abnormalities during the follicular phase

Both phases of the menstrual cycle have to be considered together, as luteal defects are frequently associated with inadequate follicular growth, premature luteinization or basal hormone imbalances during the follicular phase, and an increased rate of prolactin and androgen abnormalities in women with recurrent spontaneous miscarriage. Increased frequencies of hyperprolactinemia and of hypersecretion of luteinizing hormone (LH) have been reported in women with miscarriage.[10]

Luteal phase defect

Most previous studies have focused on the association between recurrent spontaneous miscarriage and luteal phase defects, based on retarded endometrium, or decreased progesterone concentrations or short duration of the second phase of the cycle. Insufficient progesterone production by the corpus luteum or placenta was blamed for miscarriages. Most recent studies have found that 20 to 25 percent of women with recurrent miscarriages have an inadequate luteal phase. There is strong evidence that progestational treatment makes no difference.[7]

Unfortunately, reduced levels of these hormones are the consequence rather than the cause.[9] Immunomodulator action of progesterone may have some value in this management, and is explained in the management section.

PCOS and insulin resistance

Recent insights into polycystic ovary syndrome (PCOS) have transformed it from a fertility or cosmetic problem into a more surreptitiously menacing systemic malady, at whose heart lies insulin resistance. When women with polycystic ovary syndrome finally achieve pregnancy (often after a long, arduous, and expensive course of fertility treatments), they are faced with the distressing prospect of a substantially increased risk of miscarriage during the first trimester.[11-13] Rates of early pregnancy loss, defined as miscarriage during the first trimester, are reported to be 30 to 50 percent in women with polycystic ovaries or the polycystic ovary syndrome[11,12] Insulin resistance (IR) is a key factor behind the link between PCOS/obesity and the risk of spontaneous miscarriage.

Mechanism by which insulin resistance causes miscarriages

- Hyperinsulinemia increases androgen production.[14] Hyperandrogenimia is a known risk factor for recurrent miscarriages.
- Hyperinsulinemia adversely affects the preimplantation environment by decreasing the expression of glycodelin and insulin-like growth factor (IGF)-binding protein-1. Glycodelin may play a role in inhibiting the endometrial immune response of the embryo, and IGF-binding protein-1 seems to facilitate adhesion processes at the feto-maternal interface. It is suggested that higher levels of plasminogen activator inhibitor 1 are related to an increased risk of spontaneous miscarriage, presumably because it induces a hypofibrinolytic state.[15]

Obesity

Other reported risk factors for early pregnancy loss in the polycystic ovary syndrome include obesity.[16] Overweight women have an increased risk of miscarriage independent of maternal age, and a weight loss of 10 kg has been shown to reduce the chance of miscarriage from 75 percent to 18 percent.[17]

Elevated LH

It has been reported that hypersecretion of basal LH with or without polycystic ovaries is a risk factor for miscarriage.[7] High basal LH concentrations leading to premature luteinization may be found in up to 33 percent women with recurrent spontaneous miscarriages. Previous studies have suggested that women who hypersecrete LH, a frequent feature of the polycystic ovary syndrome, are at increased risk for miscarriage after either spontaneous or assisted conception.[11,12] However, it was recently reported that suppression of endogenous LH release before conception, in women with elevated circulating LH concentrations and a history of recurrent miscarriage, did not improve the live birth rate.[13] Tonic hypersecretion of LH appears to induce premature oocyte maturation, causing problems with fertilization and miscarriage.

Thyroid dysfunction

There is a relatively low prevalence of abnormal thyroid function (~2%) in women with recurrent spontaneous miscarriage, but thyroid screening is important because both hypothyroidism and hyperthyroidism are easy to correct medically. There is controversy in the findings of antithyroid antibodies in women with recurrent miscarriages.[9] Thyroid peroxidase antibody (TPO)-positive women have an increased risk of miscarriage.

Diabetes mellitus

Spontaneous abortions are increased in women with insulin dependent diabetes. Lack of glycemic control results in an increase in the miscarriage rate.[9]

Other endocrinological anomalies

Recently, amenorrhea, immunoendocrinological disorders and hyperandrogenism, have been identified in a substantial proportion of women with recurrent spontaneous miscarriages.[10]

Anatomical Causes

Structural anomalies in the uterus can result in impaired vascularisation of a pregnancy and distorted space for the fetus. Congenital or acquired defects like Müllerian fusion defect, uterine synechiae, leiomyomas, and cervical incompetence can be diagnosed and treated.

Infections

There is currently no hard evidence that bacterial or viral infections cause recurrent pregnancy losses.[7] In various studies, no association has been detected between *antichlamydia* antibodies and recurrent miscarriages.[18] The infective agent to be implicated as the cause of repeated pregnancy loss, must be capable of persisting in the genital tract without any significant symptoms Toxoplasmosis, Rubella, Cytomegalovirus, Herpes and Listeria infections do not fulfill these criteria and hence, routine TORCH screening should be abandoned. The presence of bacterial vaginosis in the first trimester of pregnancy has been reported as a risk factor for second trimester miscarriage. Hence, a vaginal swab culture and treatment with antibiotics, if positive for bacterial vaginosis, reduces the risk of second trimester miscarriage.

Immunological Factors

Autoimmunity (self antigens): The studies show that 15 percent of the recurrent miscarriages are attributed to autoimmune factors.[9]

Antiphospholipid antibodies: The lupus anticoagulant and anticardiolipin antibodies are antiphospholipid antibodies. They cause placental thrombosis, infarction, and also block prostacyclin formation. They facilitate a thrombogenic and vasoconstrictive milieu. Whilst this is certainly important, *in vitro* evidence suggests an alternative mechanism. It has recently been reported that thrombin, in its role as a cell signalling agent, increases trophoblast apoptosis and impairs trophoblast invasion.[19] At later gestational ages, this hypercoaguability is amplified, leading to uteroplacental vascular insufficiency and subsequent fetal loss.

Alloimmunity (foreign antigens): The defective recognition of fetal alloantigens by the maternal immune system is associated with recurrent pregnancy failure and may be prevented by boosting the maternal immune response with paternal or third party leucocyte immunization.[20] In terms of immunology the success of pregnancy means, that the fetus as a semi-allogeneic graft is not rejected by the mother's/recipient's immune system. Besides a variety of specific and nonspecific mainly locally acting substances, a process of active tolerance induction is responsible for fetal survival. In response to paternally inherited fetal antigens, the maternal immune system produces so-called blocking factors. In most women with unexplained recurrent spontaneous miscarriage, these blocking factors cannot be detected.[21] Antibodies against fetal histocompatibility antigens are found in healthy pregnant women, whereas they are not demonstrable in the serum of patients with recurrent spontaneous miscarriages.[22] In most women the alloimmune cause of recurrent spontaneous miscarriages includes increased sharing of human leukocyte antigens (HLA) that may prohibit the mother from making antipaternal cytotoxic antibodies (APCA), anti-idiotypic antibodies (Ab2) and mixed lymphocyte reaction blocking antibodies (MLR-Bf). Over activity of T helper-1 (Th-1) cytokines and natural killer (NK) cells have been also reported to be the major alloimmune cause of recurrent spontaneous miscarriage.[23]

Thrombophilia

The major cause of thrombosis in pregnancy is an inherited predisposition for clotting. Antithrobin III deficiency, Protein S deficiency, and Protein C deficiency are inherited in autosomal dominant patterns. Factor V Leiden mutation and prothrombin gene mutation are the most common inherited causes of venous thromboembolism.[7] Women with recurrent miscarriages, who have no obvious identified cause should consider hematological screening. Thrombosis of the utero-placental vasculature, trophoblast apoptosis and impaired trophoblast invasion[19] are suggested mechanisms for fetal loss.

Aging Gametes

The aging of gametes in the female genital tract before fertilization increases the chances of miscarriage. Also, infertility patients over the age 35 had a higher incidence of small amniotic sac syndrome and euploidic miscarriages. Maternal age and the number of previous miscarriages are two independent risk factors for a further miscarriage. The risk of miscarriage is highest among couples where the woman is ≥35 years of age and the man ≥40 years of age.

Endothelial Dysfunction

It has been reported that women with recurrent pregnancy loss also demonstrated a significantly lower endothelium-independent vasodilatation. Endothelial dysfunction may represent a link between pre-eclampsia and increased cardiovascular disease later in life and predisposes women with unexplained recurrent miscarriages to an increased cardiovascular risk.[24]

Environmental Factors

Occupational and chemical exposure, stress, alcohol, and radiation have been reported to be associated with an increased risk of recurrent miscarriages.[7]

Recurrent Miscarriages and Infertility

Women with unexplained secondary infertility have 44 percent spontaneous miscarriage.[2] Women with unexplained secondary infertility experienced a three-fold increase in the frequency of spontaneous miscarriages and half the number of live births compared with the general population. The association between infertility and spontaneous miscarriage includes a higher frequency of spontaneous miscarriage among infertile couples, as well as a higher prevalence of infertility among patients with recurrent spontaneous miscarriages compared with the general population.

Investigations

Developing a comprehensive and efficient plan for evaluating and managing the patient with recurrent spontaneous miscarriage is always a challenging task, given the multifactorial nature of the problem. The evaluation should start after two consecutive fetal losses rather than waiting till three losses.

History is a very useful tool to rule out any endocrine, medical, or familial disorder. A strong family history of habitual miscarriage or genetic anomaly suggests a parental karyotypic abnormality, and a chromosomal analysis of the affected partner is appropriate in the primary evaluation. Any history suggestive of recurrent mid-trimester losses with painless cervical dilatation, or cervical incompetence should be suspected. Physical findings suggest Müllerian fusion defects, leiomyomas or other structural defects. Cervical and endometrial cultures and viral titers should be pursued in the evaluation only after other possible causes have been investigated.

Enocrinological causes are suspected on history and examination. It is diffucult to establish the diagnosis of luteal phase defect. Repetitive endometrial biopsies to detect a histological lag of more than two days may be required to establish the diagnosis.[7] A short luteal phase is considered as one that lasts less than 11 days; when this situation is coupled with a mid-cycle progesterone level of less than 10 ng/mL (32 nmol/L), luteal phase defect is diagnosed. It has been suggested that greater sensitivity and specificity may be achieved by measuring progesterone levels on day 25 or day 26 of the menstrual cycle. The significance of this diagnosis is still questionable. Insulin resistance can be determined by homeostasis model assessment (HOMA-IR). It is calculated as fasting insulin in microunits/mL multiplied by fasting glucose in mmol/L divided by 22.5. When this value is more than 4.5, it is labeled as insulin resistance. Occult diabetes mellitus can be screened by a glucose challenge test or by directly opting for glucose tolerence test in high-risk women.

Immunological Abnormalities

An immunological abnormality has a history of immunological disorder (e.g. Raynaud's phenomenon, lupus erythematosus, rheumatoid arthritis) or of idiopathic deep venous thrombosis suggesting the presence of abnormal antibodies. These antibodies often exist without historical or physical evidence of disease. The screening and evaluation for these abnormalities includes measurement of activated partial thromboplastin time (APTT), antinuclear antibody and anticardiolipin antibody titers. A prolonged APTT suggests the possible presence of lupus anticoagulant. Thrombophilia coagulation studies and screening for inherited predisposition for thrombosis is diagnostic. Antiphospholipid syndrome (APS) is diagnosed if the woman has two positive tests at least 12 weeks apart for either lupus anticoagulant or anticardiolipin antibodies of immunoglobulin G (IgG) and/ or immunoglobulin M (IgM) class present in a medium or high titers over 40 g/L or above the 99th percentile. The dilute Russell's viper venom time test with a platelet neutralization procedure is more sensitive and specific than either the APTT test or the kaolin clotting time test. There is a significant variation among different laboratory values and hence, they should be interpreted carefully.

Thromboelastography

It has been demonstrated that whole-blood hemostasis testing, using thromboelastography, identifies that a proportion of women with recurrent early miscarriages are in a pro-thrombotic state outside of pregnancy, and that, women in such a state are at increased risk of future miscarriage compared with those with a lower thromboelastograph index of coagulability.[19]

Natural Killer Cells and Cytokines

Peripheral blood natural killer (NK) cells are phenotypically and functionally different from uterine NK (uNK) cells, hence, there is no justification to use blood NK cells as markers for uterine NK cells. Alloimmune disorders are difficult to diagnose as no routine laboratory tests can detect them. The suggested evaluation is maternal and paternal HLA comparison, cytotoxic antibodies to paternal leukocytes, and blocking factors for mixed lymphocyte reactions.[9] Monoclonal antibodies have also been produced that identify many of these mediators and leukocyte markers associated with immune function. It is now possible, using biochemical mediators of immunological responses as new immunological reagents, to probe the immune mechanisms and immunoregulatory events responsible for the success and failure of reproduction.[25] Cytokines are immune molecules that control both immune and other cells. Cytokine responses are of two types, either as T-helper-1 (Th-1) type, which produce the proinflammatory cytokines, interleukin 2, interferon and tumor necrosis factor (TNF) alpha, or as T-helper-2 (Th-2) type, which produce the anti-inflammatory cytokines, interleukins 4, 6 and 10. Normal pregnancy is the result of a predominantly Th-2 cytokine response, but women with recurrent miscarriage have a higher Th-1 cytokine response. Further research is required before recommending the use of cytokines and NK cells to diagnose recurrent miscarriage.

Karyotype

Routine karyotyping of couples with recurrent miscarriage is not advisable. Cytogenetic analysis should be performed on products of conception with recurrent miscarriage and if it shows an unbalanced structural chromosomal abnormality, parental peripheral blood karyotyping may be performed.

Thrombophilia

Second trimester miscarriage is strongly associated with inherited thrombophilia due to Factor V Leiden deficiency, Factor II (prothrombin) gene mutation and Protein S deficiency. Hence, thrombophilia factors should be screened.

Special Investigations for Assisted Reproductive Techniques (ART)

Pregnancies obtained after *in vitro* fertilization and embryo transfer (IVF-ET) are at increased risk for an adverse outcome compared with natural pregnancies. Therefore, there is a need for markers that accurately detect the establishment of pregnancy and predict its outcome as early as possible, allowing for modification of monitoring and treatment if required. Ultrasound examination is part of the routine follow-up after in vitro fertilization, but a gestational sac is not reliably visible until 33 to 37 days after ovulation induction. As a result, there is an ongoing effort to find endocrine markers that can earlier detect the establishment of pregnancy and forecast its outcome.[26] (1) Day 11 total beta-hCG can be used to compare human chorionic gonadotropin (hCG) levels in samples from different sampling days and to predict early pregnancy losses and multiple ongoing pregnancies with high sensitivity and specificity. (2) Inhibin-A concentrations are more accurate than day 11 hCG levels for predicting preclinical miscarriage after IVF, but they have no advantage in forecasting ongoing or multiple ongoing pregnancies. (3) Prognostic accuracy of CA-125 measurements for the prediction of pregnancy as well as its outcome is inferior to that achieved with inhibin-A.[27] Table 64.2 presents specific investigations for ART.

Table 64.2: Specific investigations for ART	
Genetic factors: Karyotyping of both parents	*Infectious causes:* As it has limited role, cultures only if clinically indicated (high vaginal swab)
Anatomical defects: Transvaginal sonography, HSG, if needed MRI in selective cases	*Endocrine disorders:* TSH, prolactin, fasting and postprandial sugar, fasting insulin, GTT Serum LH, Progesterone
Thrombophilia: Thrombin time, APTT, Fibrinogen, Anticardiolipin antibody titer, Homocysteine level, Antithrombin III, Thromboelastography, Screening for inherited thrombophilia	*Immunological factors:* Autoimmunity—APTT, PT, kaolin clotting time, antinuclear antibody titer, lupus anticoagulant, anticardiolipin antibody titer Alloimmunity—Maternal and paternal HLA comparison, cytotoxic antibodies to paternal leukocytes, blocking factors for mixed lymphocyte reactions (many are under research)
Environmental: No specific investigation	*Special investigations in ART:* Inhibin-A, Day 11 total beta-hCG, CA-125, preimplantation genetic screening (PGS)/preimplantation genetic diagnosis (PGD) aneuploidy testing

Abbreviations: HSG: hysterosalpingography; MRI: magnetic resonance imaging; APTT: activated partial thromboplastin time; TSH: thyroid stimulating hormone; LH: luteinizing hormone; GTT: glucose tolerance test

Preimplantation Genetic Diagnosis (PGD)

Aneuploidy testing in couples with poor prognosis undergoing ART cycles is a useful tool to increase the chance of ART success. Furthermore, abnormal gamete cell morphology should be considered as one of the major indications.[28] Various trials provide no arguments in favor of PGD for aneuploidy screening (PGD-AS) for improving the clinical outcome per initiated cycle in patients with advanced maternal age.[29] Preimplantation genetic screening (PGS)/ preimplantation genetic diagnosis, and aneuploidy testing are thus, the vital investigations. Table 64.3 presents a list of routinely recommended investigations in clinical settings.

CLINICAL DISCUSSION

Management

A recurrent miscarriage clinic and expert advice help to improve the reproductive outcome. If all of above investigations are not available with given clinical settings, it is worth considering management based on the clinical picture or managing as unexplained recurrent miscarriage.

Tender Loving Care

A cause for recurrent miscarriage can be identified approximately 50 to 60 percent of the time.[4,30] There is tremendous psychological impact of recurrent miscarriage. Psychologic support in the form of frequent discussions and sympathetic counseling are crucial to the successful evaluation and treatment of the anxious couple. When no etiologic factor is

Table 64.3: List of routinely recommended investigations in clinical settings
• *Structural:* Pelvic ultrasound, further investigations and imaging if anomaly is suspected.
• *Hematological:* Anti-cardiolipin IgG, Anti-cardiolipin IgM, Lupus Anticoagulant, Anti-protein C resistance, Prothrombin time, Antinuclear antibody
• *Thrombophilia screen:* Antithrombin activity, Protein C activity, Protein S levels
• *Genetic thrombophilia screen:* Factor V Leiden mutation, PTG20210A (Prothombin gene) mutation
• *Endocrine disorders:* Thyroid function, thyroid antibodies (TPO), glucose tolerance tests, prolactin
• *Genetic disorders:* Karyotype in selective couples
• High vaginal swab if clinically indicated (history of pre-term labor and or mid trimester loss)

identified, and no treatment started a 60 to 80 percent fetal salvage rate still may be expected.[30]

Tender loving care with regular antenatal check-ups goes a great way in achieving live term pregnancy. Hence, couples with unexplained recurrent miscarriage should be offered appropriate emotional support and reassurance that they have a good prognosis for future pregnancies.[1]

Once a patient conceives, serial ultrasonography, beta-hCG determination, and estradiol determination may be useful in detecting the stage of the embryonic death if subsequent miscarriage occurs. A karyotype analysis of the products of conception should be performed if fetal loss occurs.

Lifestyle modification and stress reduction should be emphasized by pointing out that a healthier lifestyle, free from tobacco, alcohol, illicit drugs and undue stress, cannot hurt and may significantly improve the couple's chances for a successful pregnancy.

Management of Specific Disorders

Genetic Disorders

According to McDonough,[31] the treatment of endocrine disorders yields a 90 percent rate of having a normal child correction of anatomical factors yields a 60 to 70 percent rate, but known genetic factors are associated with only a 32 percent chance for a normal child.[31] Karyotyping is vital when the couple has a malformed fetus in addition to habitual recurrent miscarriages. Karyotyping detects only a small perce centage of pregnancy loss. In most cases, couple is chromosomally normal but fetal chromosomal anomaly is a random event. These may occur at gametogenesis or at fertilization. Even if the karyotyping is abnormal, nothing can be done to prevent future miscarriages. They may have a chance of a normal pregnancy. To decrease the risk of having an abnormal child, amniocentesis or chorionic villus sampling (CVS) is advisable. A couple with serious high risk chromosomal abnormalities should be offered donor sperm or in vitro fertilization with donor oocytes. Preimplantation genetic screening (PGS) with IVF treatment in women with unexplained recurrent miscarriage does not improve live birth rates.

Anatomic Defects

Anatomical defects are treated with surgical measures. Minimally invasive surgeries are a better option for the treatment of structural defects. Cervical incompetence is treated with prophylactic cervical cerclage. Transvaginal ultrasound examination in a subsequent pregnancy is indicated with a history of mid-term loss due to cervical incompetence. Cervical length <25 mm before 24 weeks is an indication for a cervical stitch.

Infections

The treatment of bacterial vaginosis reduces the risk of second trimester miscarriages. The TORCH test and treatment is not useful to improve the outcome.

Endocrine Disorders

Though elevated LH is associated with an increased risk of miscarriage, suppression of LH secretion with a GnRH agonist prior to ovulation induction yielded no difference in the outcome.[7] Hyperprolactinemia can be treated with dopamine agonist or Cabergoline. Thyroid disorders can be treated medically to achieve a euthyroid status. Thyroid

antibodies and the Levothyroxine (TABLET) study is a randomized controlled trial of the efficacy and mechanism of Levothyroxine treatment on the pregnancy and neonatal outcomes in women with thyroid antibodies. This study will help to find the role of thyroxin treatment in women with normal thyroid function tests but raised thyroid peroxidase (TPO) antibodies.

Luteal Phase Defect (LPD) and the Role of Progesterone

The treatment of luteal phase defect is even more controversial than its diagnosis. Common treatments include progesterone vaginal suppositories. Yet, it is by no means certain that progestational treatment makes a difference. A meta-analysis failed to find any evidence of positive effect of progestational treatment on the maintenance of pregnancy.[32] Only when repetitive endometrial biopsies suggest LPD, it is reasonable to treat with progesterone or Clomiphene. Progesterone acts as an immunomodulator and it shifts from the proinflammatory Th-1 cytokine responses to anti-inflammatory Th-2 cytokine response, which is more favorable and pregnancy-protective.

Dihydrogesterone is a potential immunomodulator that produces progesterone-induced blocking factors (PIBF), which is protein produced by pregnancy lymphocytes following exposure to progestorone. PIBF inhibits cell mediated cytotoxicity and natural killer cell activity. Thus, it is immunoprotective for pregnancy.[33] A large multicenter study[34] is currently under way to assess the benefit of progesterone supplementation in women with unexplained recurrent miscarriage.[34]

Polycystic Ovary Syndrome (PCOS) and Metformin Use during Pregnancy

Insulin resistance is an independent risk factor for spontaneous miscarriage in spontaneous pregnancy as well as women conceiving after ART treatment. Patients with IR should be advised to improve their insulin sensitivity through lifestyle changes or medical intervention before infertility treatment to reduce their risk of spontaneous miscarriage. Metformin administration decreases the rate of early pregnancy loss by several potential mechanisms.[15,35,36]

1. *Androgen reduction*: Elevated serum androgen concentrations have been reported to be a risk factor for early pregnancy loss in the polycystic ovary syndrome. In women who receive Metformin at 6 to 10 weeks of pregnancy, serum-free testosterone levels decrease by 57 percent compared those who do not receive Metformin.[15,35] Its testosterone-lowering effect, which, like prevention of weight gain, is probably mediated through its insulin-sensitizing action.

2. *Reduction of circulating plasminogen activator inhibitor-1*: Metformin administration has been reported to decrease circulating plasminogen activator inhibitor-1 in women with polycystic ovary syndrome. Metformin

counteracts the adverse effect of hyperinsulinemia on the preimplantation environment.

3. *Prevention of gestational diabetes (GD) and Type 2 diabetes mellitus (DM)*: One major benefit of continuing a Metformin–diet through pregnancy is avoidance of major weight gain in women with PCOS. Metformin during pregnancy causes modulation of the 'natural' augmentation of IR changes during gestation. To the extent that metformin reduces insulin, IR and insulin secretion during pregnancy, while blocking weight gain, and reducing GD, it should play a role in the primary prevention of type 2 DM.

Safety of Metformin use in pregnancy: Metformin is classified as a category B drug, which means that no teratogenic effects have been demonstrated in animal studies. To date, Metformin use during pregnancy has not been associated with any adverse effects on the mother or the fetus.[36]

Thus, it improves endometrial function, implantation and pregnancy outcome. Data on the use of metformin to decrease the chance of miscarriage are contradictory as no adequately powered trials have been published. Yet, the use of Metformin is not lincensed in UK for this indication.[37]

Thrombophilia

When inherited deficiencies are the cause of recurrent miscarriages, women should be treated with anticoagulant regimens. Low molecular weight heparin is a preferred choice when pregnancy is diagnosed.

Immunological Factors

Autoimmunity: When significant titers of antiphospholipid antibodies are present, various studies suggest simultaneous application of low-doses of acetylsalicylic acid and low molecular weight heparin seems to be the best solution in women suffering from recurrent spontaneous miscarriage. This treatment combination of low-dose aspirin and low molecular weight heparin reduces the miscarriage rate by 54 percent. The occurrence of anticardiolipin antibodies in the blood serum of patient's suffering from antiphospholipid syndrome is a better foretelling factor for the future pregnancy outcome than the occurrence of lupus anticoagulant antibodies.[38-40] Glucocorticoids should not be given in antiphospholipid antibodies syndrome without connective tissue disorder. Low-dose Prednisone is given when lupus is present. Immunoglobulin therapy is reserved for women with overt disease or heparin-induced thrombocytopenia.

Alloimmunity: Immunotherapy in the form of infusion of the partner's lymphocytes is given to stimulate antibody formation and a favorable maternal immune response to protect the fetus. Immunotherapy is to produce blocking factors and therefore, to protect a conceptus from rejection.[21]

It is proposed that antibodies can be induced by leucocyte injections, a high percentage (60 to 85%) of patients have a next pregnancy without complications. In previous studies, the passive transfer of antibodies by infusion of intravenous gammaglobulins has shown similar results.[22] Some studies had reported successful outcomes upto 68 percent. It was revealed from extensive updated analysis of this subject that paternal lymphocytes immunotherapy may play a significant role in the prevention of alloimmune causes of fetal loss in women with recurrent miscarriages. These alloimmune parameters are suppressed in successful immunotherapy, which is comparable to normal pregnancy.[23] Paternal lymphocyte (PL) immunotherapy results in the development of mixed lymphocyte reaction blocking antibodies (MLR-Bf).[41] However all these studies have significant limitations in their design and analysis, hence the evidence does not support use of any immunotherapy to improve the reproductive outcome.

There is no specific immunologic test or clinical method, which will predict the need for treatment: There is risk of possible complications such as undesirable immune responses and the possibility of transmitting infectious diseases like Cytomegalovirus. The possible complications should be carefully weighed against the anticipated effects, since no vital indication exists in the case of recurrent miscarriage, unlike most situations, where the transfusion of blood products is contemplated.[42]

Role of active immunotherapy in idiopathic recurrent miscarriage: Studies indicate a general trend favoring paternal over maternal lymphocyte immunization, but reinforces the need for larger multicentric controlled trials, as well as more detailed biological study in humans to understand the nature of the maternal-fetal interface and its breakdown.[43]

Unexplained recurrent miscarriage: Most of the times, it is not possible to find a cause for recurrent pregnancy loss. Psychological support and more frequent attendance at a dedicated early pregnancy clinic improves the outcome. There is room to investigate the woman for thyroid antibodies and rechecking antiphospholipid antibodies. Empirical treatment approaches, using Aspirin, low molecular weight heparin (LMWH), progesterone supplementation, Metformin and Thyroxin are not supported by strong evidence yet. There are ongoing trials to answer these questions. Meanwhile, the clinical decision would be the appropriate approach. Table 64.4 presents a summary of treatment for recurrent miscarriages.

CONCLUSION

ART as a Treatment for Recurrent Miscarriages

Recently, assisted reproductive techniques have been used to prevent further miscarriages in women with recurrent miscarriage. One approach uses either screening or diagnosis of embryonic chromosomes prior to embryo replacement

Table 64.4: Summary of treatment for recurrent miscarriages			
Cause	*Evidence of benefit with treatment*	*No evidence of any benefit with treatment but treatment may cause risk to woman/baby*	*Evidence awaited (research ongoing)*
Uterine septum			Surgical correction
Cervical weakness	Cervical cerclage		
Antiphospholipid syndrome	Aspirin 75 mg daily plus LMWH throughout pregnancy	Corticosteroids or intravenous immunoglobulin	
Inherited thrombophilia	LMWH throughout pregnancy		
Elevated LH		Pre-pregnancy pituitary suppression	
PCOS			Metformin supplementation
Hyperprolactinemia	Cabergoline		
Thyroid dysfunction	Medical management		
TPO antibodies			Thyroxin supplementation (Tablet study)
Infection	Treatment of bacterial vaginosis if present	TORCH test or treatment	
Unexplained	Psychological support		Progesterone supplementation (promise trial)
Unexplained			Human chorionic gonadotrophin supplementation
Unexplained			Aspirin/LMWH
Unexplained		Paternal cell immunization, third-party donor leukocytes, trophoblast membranes and immunoglobulin	
Unexplained		PGD /IVF	

Abbreviations: LH: luteinizing hormone; LMWH: low molecular weight heparin; PCOS: polycystic ovary syndrome; TPO: thyroid peroxidase antibodies; TORCH: Toxoplasma, other infections, Rubella, Cytomegalovirus, Herpes simplex virus-2; PGD: preimplantation genetic diagnosis; IVF: *in vitro* fertilization

[preimplantation genetic screening (PGS)/preimplantation genetic diagnosis (PGD)]. The second approach involves surrogacy. However, PGS/PGD assumes that the embryo is chromosomally abnormal, and that the mother should receive a chromosomally normal embryo. Surrogacy assumes that the embryo is normal and that the maternal environment needs to be substituted. In repeated fetal aneuploidy or in the older patient, PGS or PGD is preferable. However, with high numbers of miscarriages, or in autoimmune pregnancy loss, surrogacy is preferable. In the light of recent work, it is uncertain which treatment mode is indicated in balanced parental chromosome aberrations. In conclusion, both techniques have a place, but probably only in those patients with a poor prognosis in whom assisted reproductive techniques will be shown to improve the subsequent live birth rate above the spontaneous rate.[3]

REFERENCES

1. Horne AW, Alexander CI. Recurrent miscarriage. J Fam Plann Reprod Health Care 2005;31:103-9.
2. Coulam CB. Association between infertility and spontaneous abortion. Am J Reprod Immunol 1992;27:128.
3. Carp HJ, Dirnfeld M, Dor J, Grudzinskas JG. ART in recurrent miscarriage: Preimplantation genetic diagnosis/screening or surrogacy? Hum Reprod 2004;19:1502-5.
4. Katz VL, Kuller JA. Recurrent miscarriage. Am J Perinatol 1994;11:386-97.
5. Yang CJ, Stone P, Stewart AW. The epidemiology of recurrent miscarriage: A descriptive study of 1214 prepregnant women with recurrent miscarriage. Aust N Z J Obstet Gynaecol 2006; 46:316-22.
6. Rand SE. Recurrent spontaneous abortion: Evaluation and management. Am Fam Physician 1993;1-5
7. Leon Speroff, Robert Glass, Nathan Kase. clinical gynecologic endocrinology and infertility: Sixth edition: Lipincott Williams; Baltimore. P 1044-52.

8. Deaton JL, Honore GM, Huffman CS, Bauguess P. Early transvaginal ultrasonography following an accurately dated pregnancy: the importance of finding a yolk sac or fetal heart motion.Hum Reprod 1997;12:2820.

9. Williams Obstetrics; 21st edition, McGraw-Hill Publication New York P 856-877.

10. Bussen S, Sütterlin M, Steck T. Endocrine abnormalities during the follicular phase in women with recurrent spontaneous abortion The Journal of Clinical Endocrinology and Metabolism 87:524-2529.

11. Omburg R, Armar NA, Eshel A, Adams J, Jacobs HS. Influence of serum luteinising hormone concentrations on ovulation, conception and early pregnancy loss in polycystic ovary syndrome. BMJ 1988;297:1024-6.

12. Egan L, Owen EJ, Jacobs HS. Hypersecretion of luteinising hormone, infertility, and miscarriage. Lancet 1990;336:1141-4.

13. Atson H, Kiddy DS, Hamilton-Fairley D, Scanlon MJ, Barnard C, Collins WP, Bonney RC, Franks S. Hypersecretion of luteinizing hormone and ovarian steroids in women with recurrent early miscarriage. Hum Reprod 1993;8:829-33.

14. Tian L, Shen H, Lu Q, Norman RJ, Wang J. Insulin resistance increases the risk of spontaneous abortion after assisted reproduction technology treatment. J Clin Endocrinol Metab. 2007;92:1430-3.

15. Jakubowicz DJ, Iuorno MJ, Jakubowicz S, Roberts KA, Nestler JE. Effects of metformin on early pregnancy loss in the polycystic ovary syndrome. J Clin Endocrinol Metab 2002;87:524-9.

16. Edorcsak P, Storeng R, Dale PO, Tanbo T, Abyholm T. Obesity is a risk factor for early pregnancy loss after IVF or ICSI. Acta Obstet Gynecol Scand 2000;79:43-8.

17. Knee J, Ong, Efstathios T, William L. Long-term consequence of polycystic ovarian syndrome. COG 2006;16:333-6.

18. Osser S, Persson K. Chlamydial antibodies in women who suffer miscarriage. Br J Obstet Gynecol 1996:103:137.

19. Rai R, Tuddenham E, Backos M, Jivraj S, El'Gaddal S, Choy S, Cork B, Regan L. Thromboelastography, whole-blood hemostasis and recurrent miscarriage. Hum Reprod 2003;18:2540-3.

20. Agrawal S, Kishore R. Paternal leucocyte immunotherapy for recurrent pregnancy loss. Natl Med J India 1995;8:121-3.

21. von Ditfurth M, Kuhn U, Kuntz BM, Distler W. The immuno-logically-caused early abortion. Z Geburtshilfe Perinatal 1989; 193:247-50.

22. Schwartz D, Jungl E. Neumeister A. Immunologic diagnosis and therapy in habitual abortion. Wien Med Wochenschr 1990;140(22):547-50.

23. Pandey MK, Thakur S, Agrawal S. Lymphocyte immunotherapy and its probable mechanism in the maintenance of pregnancy in women with recurrent spontaneous abortion. Arch Gynecol Obstet 2004;269:161-72.

24. Germain AM, Romanik MC, Guerra I, Solari S, Reyes MS, Johnson RJ, et al. Endothelial dysfunction: A link among preeclampsia, recurrent pregnancy loss, and future cardiovascular events? Hypertension 2007;49:15-6.

25. Hill JA, Anderson DJ. Immunological mechanisms in recurrent spontaneous abortion. Arch Immunol Ther Exp (Warsz) 1990; 38:111-9.

26. Hauzman E, Murber A, Fancsovits P, Papp Z, Urbancsek J. Use of biochemical markers to predict the outcome of pregnancies conceived by *in vitro* fertilization. Orv Hetil 2006;147:1409-20.

27. Schmidt T, Rein DT, Foth D, et al. Prognostic value of repeated serum CA 125 measurements in first trimester pregnancy. Eur J Obstet Gynecol Reprod Biol 2001;97:168-73.

28. Kahraman S, Benkhalifa M, Donmez E, Biricik A, Sertyel S, Findikli N, Berkil H. The results of aneuploidy screening in 276 couples undergoing assisted reproductive techniques. Prenat Diag 2004;24:307-11.

29. Staessen C, Platteau P, Van Assche E, Michiels A, Tournaye H, et al. Comparison of blastocyst transfer with or without preimplantation genetic diagnosis for aneuploidy screening in couples with advanced maternal age: a prospective randomized controlled trial. Hum Reprod 2004;19:2849-58.

30. Rock JA, Zacur HA. The clinical management of repeated early pregnancy wastage. Fertil Steril 1983;39:123-40.

31. Mc donough PG. Reapeated first trimester loss; Evaluation and management. Am J Obstet Gynecol 1985;153:1.

32. Goldstein P, Berrier J, Rosen S, Sacks HS, Chamers TC, A meta-analysis of randomized control trial of progestational agents in pregnancy. BJOG 1989;96:265-74.

33. Raj Raghupathy, Esraa Al M, Ma'asoumah M, et al. Modulation of cytokine production by dydrogesterone in lymphocytes from women with recurrent miscarriage. BJOG 2005;112:1096-101.

34. PROMISE, http://www.medscinet.net/promise

35. Glueck CJ, Goldenberg N, Wang P, Loftspring M, Sherman A. Metformin during pregnancy reduces insulin, insulin resistance, insulin secretion, weight, testosterone and development of gestational diabetes: Prospective longitudinal assessment of women with polycystic ovary syndrome from preconception throughout pregnancy. Hum Reprod 2004;19:510-21.

36. Nestler JE. Should patients with polycystic ovarian syndrome be treated with metformin? An enthusiastic endorsement. Hum Reprod 2002;17:1950-3.

37. Knee J, Ong, Efstathios T, William L. Long term consequence of polycystic ovarian syndrome. COG 2006;16:333-6.

38. Malinowski A, Dynski MA, Maciolek-Blewniewska G, Glowacka E. Treatment outcome in women suffering from recurrent miscarriages and antiphospholipid syndrome. Ginekol Pol 2003;74:1213-22.

39. Triolo G, Ferrante A, Ciccia F, Accardo-Palumbo A, Perino A, Castelli A, et al. Randomized study of subcutaneous low molecular weight heparin plus aspirin versus intravenous immunoglobulin in the treatment of recurrent fetal loss associated with antiphospholipid antibodies. Arthritis Rheum 2004;50:1017-8.

40. Rai R, Cohen H, Dave M, Regan L. Randomized control trial of aspirin and aspirin plus heparin in pregnant women with recurrent miscarriage associated with phospholipid antibodies. Br Med J 1997;314:253.

41. Pandey MK, Agrawal S. Induction of MLR-Bf and protection of fetal loss: A current double blind randomized trial of paternal lymphocyte immunization for women with recurrent spontaneous abortion. Int Immunopharmacol 2004;4:289-98.

42. Marzusch K, Mayer G, Dietl J. Active immunotherapy of habitual abortion: Is the danger greater than the therapeutic gain? Geburtshilfe Frauenheilkd 1991;51:1009-13.

43. Sterzik K, Strehler E, De Santo M Oblinger E, Rosenbusch B. Idiopathic habitual abortion: Experiences with active immunotherapy. Geburtshilfe Frauenheilkd 1995;55:493-9.

Current Concepts in Multifetal Pregnancy Reduction and Selective Termination

Alon Shrim, Rivka Peltz, Shlomo Lipitz

OVERVIEW

The incidence of higher-order multiple gestations have dramatically increased in the last two decades, mainly due to rise in assisted reproductive techniques (ART) procedures being performed. Higher-order multiple gestations carry both maternal risks as well as high rates of perinatal and neonatal morbidity and mortality, mainly due to pregnancy loss prior to 24 weeks and premature deliveries.

The goal of first trimester multifetal pregnancy reduction (MFPR) is to reduce the number of fetuses in a higher-order multiple gestation. This will decrease the chance of premature delivery and improve the outcome for the remaining fetuses.

Selective termination (ST) refers to fetal reduction due to a fetal anomaly diagnosed in one fetus of a multiple pregnancy. It usually takes place in the second trimester of pregnancy.

INTRODUCTION

The incidence of higher-order multiple gestations have dramatically increased in the last two decades, mainly due to a rise in assisted reproductive techniques (ART) procedures being performed. In *in vitro* fertilization (IVF) cycles, the chances to achieve higher-order multiple gestations correlate with the number of embryos transferred. In the last decade, the number of transferred embryos has been better controlled, thus, some decrease in the incidence of higher-order multiple gestations has been observed.

Since higher-order multiple gestations carry maternal risks as well as high rates of perinatal and neonatal morbidity and mortality, mainly due to pregnancy loss prior to 24 weeks and premature deliveries, the goal of first-trimester multifetal pregnancy reduction is to reduce the number of fetuses in a higher-order multiple gestation. This will decrease the chance of premature delivery and improve the outcome for the remaining fetuses.

Although some groups are in disagreement regarding the risk of pregnancy loss due to multifetal pregnancy reduction, all are in agreement that multifetal pregnancy reduction significantly reduces the rates of delivery before 32 weeks gestation and thus, increases the chances of delivering healthy baby/babies.

CLINICAL DISCUSSION

Technique

Verifying chorionicity is of paramount importance and is mandatory prior to multifetal pregnancy reduction.

The described technique is relevant only to cases where all fetuses have their own chorion and amnion (trichorionic-triamniotic, etc.). Special cases where fetuses share the chorion/amnion are described separately.

The first multifetal pregnancy reductions were reported in 1986 and involved 15 cases. The fetal number in the beginning was 3 to 6 and pregnancy was reduced to singleton or twins. The procedure was carried out by dilatation of the cervix and ultrasound-guided, transvaginal aspiration of the selected gestational sac.

Later, a transabdominal approach was described that involved ultrasound-guided injection of potassium chloride (KCl 15%) into the fetal chest at 11 to 13 weeks of gestation. This is the most common method used today and is straightforward. The patient is given a single oral antibiotic dose (e.g. Amoxicillin, 500 mg) immediately before the procedure. Ultrasonography is used to map the location of all gestations precisely within the uterus, and measurements of crown-rump length and nuchal translucency thickness (see timing of reduction) are taken. If an abnormality is found or these measurements are abnormal in a particular fetus, that fetus is selected for reduction. Otherwise, the fetus or fetuses that are technically easiest to access are chosen, with the exception of the fetus overlying the internal os, which is rarely selected. A 21-gauge needle is used and 2 to 5 mL of 15 percent KCl solution is injected under ultrasound guidance into the fetal chest of each selected fetus. If considered necessary, the procedure is repeated for every additional fetus. Post procedure asystole should be observed for 3 minutes. We are adamant on verifying asystole immediately following the procedure as well as 1 hour later. After the procedure, patients should be observed for the usual complications of multiple gestations as well as for psychological aspects of agreeing to actively terminate one pregnancy.

Transvaginal multifetal pregnancy reduction (MFPR) is another option, less commonly practiced nowadays. It involves ultrasound-guided aspiration of the selected fetus(es) between 6 to 8 weeks gestational age. A significant advantage of this method is the relatively lower psychological burden on the woman and her partner, as it is done in a very preliminary stage of pregnancy. On the other hand, it might (not often) necessitate general anesthesia, it does not allow for preMFPR prenatal testing at 11 to 13 weeks, and in addition, some triplet pregnancies might be spontaneously reduced between 6 to 13 weeks.

Thus, and since it is associated with relatively higher loss rates when compared with the transabdominal approach (12% versus 5% in one study),[1] it is less commonly performed, however, it might be considered for quadruplets and higher order pregnancies.

Timing

Multifetal pregnancy reduction is typically performed between 10 and 13 weeks' gestation. As some of the higher-order multiple gestations will have one or more gestational sac spontaneously arrested, it is our interest not to intervene ahead of time. Performing nuchal translucency measurement and selectively reducing an abnormal fetus is another rationale. Most studies[1] did not find different rates of pregnancy loss when the procedure was done between 8 and 13 weeks gestational age. In our series as well,[2] the rate of pregnancy loss was not significantly different when multifetal pregnancy reduction was performed as early as 11 to 12 weeks vs reductions that were performed at 13 to 14 weeks' gestation (pregnancy loss rates of 4.3% vs 4%). Several groups offer chorionic villi sampling (CVS) (11–12 weeks) with fluorescent *in situ* hybridization (FISH) analysis prior to MFPR.

Results

Evans et al.[1] have summarized more than eight years of 3513 multifetal pregnancy reductions from 11 centers. During the study period, increasing rates of multifetal pregnancy reductions were noted. With increasing experience of the operators, results are continuously improved, measured by both parameters of pregnancy loss rates prior to 24 weeks (13.2% prior to 1990 vs 6.4% between 1995-1998) as well as prematurity rates.

Overall loss rates in the last period of the study (1995-1998) were correlated strongly with starting and finishing number of fetuses (starting number ≥6, 15.4%; starting number 5, 11.4%; starting number 4, 7.3%; starting number 3, 4.5%; starting number 2, 6.2%: finishing number 3, 18.4%; finishing number 2, 6.0%; finishing number 1, 6.7%).

The proportion of cases with a starting number ≥5 diminished from 23.4 to 15.9 to 12.2 percent.

Triplet pregnancies are currently, by far, the most common type of higher-order multiple gestations and finishing number of 1 or 2 fetuses does not seem to significantly alter the pregnancy outcome.

A 2006 study[3] reported as low as 4.4 percent pregnancy loss rate (prior to 24 weeks) for triplets that were followed expectantly versus 8 percent for triplet pregnancies that were reduced to twins. However, rates of preterm delivery (24–31 weeks) were almost 3 times higher in the triplets that were followed expectantly; 27 percent versus 10 percent for triplet pregnancies that were reduced to twins.

On the other hand, and in concordance with other studies,[4] in our prospective series,[5] loss of the entire pregnancy before 25 gestational weeks occurred in 20.7 percent of the triplet pregnancies managed expectantly as compared with 8.7 percent in the group with reduction to twins. Fetal reduction from triplet pregnancy to twins was associated with a significantly lower incidence of prematurity, low-birth-weight and very-low-birth-weight infants.

We believe that for a patient with higher-order multiple gestations the following factors should be discussed:
- Procedure- related pregnancy loss rates are estimated as 4.5 percent in triplet pregnancy, 8 percent for quadruplet pregnancy and 11 to 15 percent for higher order multiple gestations.
- Several groups are in disagreement regarding the risk of pregnancy loss due to multifetal pregnancy reduction. However, all are in agreement that in the long run, and in any higher-order multiple gestations, multifetal pregnancy reduction significantly reduces the rates of delivery before 32 weeks' gestation and thus, increases the chances of delivering healthy baby/babies.

This decision should be individualized in all cases.

Special Cases

A triplet pregnancy that contains monochorionic twins (trichorionic diamniotic) deserves special consideration. Several options for MFPR are present:
- Reducing the single fetus and keeping the monochorionic-diamniotic twins. This option exposes the pregnancy to the complications of monochorionic-diamniotic twin pregnancies, including Twin to Twin Transfusion Syndrome (TTS).

- Reducing the monochorionic-diamniotic twins, leaving one fetus and decreasing the risks of monochorionic-diamniotic twin pregnancies.

The risk in either of the options is not significantly higher and currently, if a monochorionic pair of fetuses exists within a higher-order multiple gestation, that pair is usually selected for reduction.

A third option exists, which is much more difficult; to reduce one of the monochorionic twins. This procedure cannot be done by KCl injection due to risk of mortality or brain damage to the co-twin. It is done later in pregnancy and carries higher rates of pregnancy loss.

Selective Termination

Selective termination (ST) refers to fetal reduction due to fetal anomaly diagnosed in one fetus of a multiple pregnancy. It usually takes place in the second trimester of pregnancy.

The incidence of malformations is considered higher in multiple pregnancy. In monozygotic pregnancies typically, the risk for an anomaly is more than twice the risk in a singleton pregnancy. Micromanipulation as part of IVF is also considered as risk for higher rate of anomalies.

Newer techniques, such as CVS, amniocentesis, fetal blood sampling, fetoscopy, advanced ultrasound, etc. as well as new lab techniques, such as advanced Molecular Genetics, all enable early detection of fetal anomalies nowadays. When such an anomaly is diagnosed in one of two (or more) fetuses, the pregnant woman and her partner will usually have to decide from several treatment options:

- Continuation of the pregnancy as is—so that the healthy fetus is not endangered
- Selective termination of the affected fetus
- To terminate the pregnancy in an early stage, which is an option in minority of the patients.

Prior to any decision, chorionicity must be clearly defined. It is best diagnosed in the first or early second trimester ultrasound (number and location of placentas, gender, width of the intertwin membrane and/or lambda/twin peak sign). When chorionicity is unclear and ST is suggested, amniocentesis should be considered for DNA fingerprinting in order to diagnose the correct fetus for termination.

Selective Termination in Dichorionic Diamniotic Twins

Selective termination in dichorionic-diamniotic twin pregnancies is performed using transabdominal, ultrasound-guided injection of 5 to 10 cc of potassium chloride (KCl 15%) to the fetal heart. The patient is given a single oral antibiotic dose (e.g. Amoxicillin, 500 mg) immediately before the procedure.

Identification of the embryo with the anomaly prior to the ST is mandatory. When anatomical anomaly is the case, or when the fetuses are discordant for gender, identification is usually straightforward. However, in cases of chromosomal abnormality in one of concordant gender twins, amniocentesis might be needed for fast detection and relocalization of the affected fetus (e.g FISH technique) prior to performing the termination. Inadvertent termination of a healthy fetus has been reported. It emphasizes the importance of accurate identification of the affected fetus. The risk of a false report regarding the location of the affected twin is especially manifested if 2 to 3 weeks have passed since the initial procedure for diagnosis was done. In cases of chromosomal anomalies, some centers suggest that fetal blood be collected during the procedure in order to confirm that the sick fetus was indeed the one to be terminated.

In our institution, one hour after termination, ultrasound should be done to reconfirm asystole.

RECENT ADVANCES

Selective Termination in Monochorionic Diamniotic Twins

Blood circulatory anastomosis between the placentas of monochorionic twins does not allow KCl injection to the affected fetus's heart due to the increased risk to the healthy twin. The injected KCl might pass to the healthy twin or alternatively, blood flow changes between the dead and surviving fetus might injure the healthy twin.

Numerous methods have been tried and reported for the termination of monochorionic twins, including hysterotomy, embolization of the umbilical vessels using hystoacril, endoscopic-guided ligation of the umbilical cord or ablation by bipolar cautery, radio frequency (RFA) or laser. The later three are currently the most frequent.[6]

Laser coagulation is usually done using a 400 to 600 micrometer fiber YAG laser, and the absence of blood flow, detected using color Doppler methods, is expected. This method carries relatively higher failure rates when performed later than 20 weeks gestational age, thus, for termination beyond 20 to 21 weeks bipolar cautery is usually used.[7]

Either bipolar cautery or RFA is usually used. In bipolar cautery of the umbilical cord, a 2 to 3 mm trocar is inserted to the gestational sac of the selected fetus, guided by ultrasound, and the cautery device is inserted through the trocar. Ultrasound-guided grasp of the umbilical cord follows with the bipolar device and coagulation is performed for 30 second periods. The Doppler study is repeated until the absence of flow is detected. The procedure is usually repeated in two locations along the umbilical cord.

In RFA, under continuous ultrasound guidance, a 17-gauge radiofrequency needle is inserted into the fetal abdomen just cephalad to the umbilical cord insertion. After confirmation of the location, the prongs of the device are deployed and 40W of energy delivered until the average temperature of the three prongs reach a target temperature of 100°C. This is usually achieved within 2 to 3 minutes. The radiofrequency energy is then continued for an additional 3 minutes.

Follow-up after ST includes assessment every 2 weeks for fetal monitoring by a non-stress test (NST) and/or bio-physical profile. In monochorionic twins, Doppler studies of the middle cerebral artery (MCA) might be considered as well to rule out anemia of the surviving twin. Magnetic resonance imaging (MRI) is recommended at 30 to 32 weeks of gestation for the surviving fetus.

Disseminated intravascular coagulation (DIC) is a concern following singleton intrauterine fetal death (IUFD). It is extremely rare in twin pregnancies following IUFD of one fetus and in our department, coagulation tests are not part of the follow-up after ST. Assessment of the risk for preterm delivery is performed by NST, fetal fibronectin (FFN) testing and/or by measurement of cervical length by transvaginal ultrasound. Tocolysis is not routinely given and Betamethasone should be considered after 24 weeks gestational age.

Timing

Theoretically, when fetal anomaly/malformation is detected, and if the couple is interested and ST is allowed by law, the ST may take place at either of the following timings:

- As the anomaly is detected
- Following Betamethasone, at 30 to 32 weeks gestational age
- After 36 weeks or when delivery begins, in order to minimize as much as possible the risks of prematurity. This option carries difficult ethical issues and is forbidden in many Western countries.

As ST carries a relatively low-risk of losing the entire pregnancy or of preterm delivery, we recommend performing the termination once it is diagnosed, prior to viability of the fetus.

Results

Dichorionic-diamniotic twins: The first reports on ST appeared in the early 80s. In 1999, Evans and colleagues[8] reported 402 cases of ST using KCl injection into the fetal heart, with 100 percent technical success.[8] Thirty women (7.5%) lost the entire pregnancy prior to 24 weeks gestational age. Pregnancy loss rates were not significantly correlated to gestational age at the time of procedure (8.7% loss rate when ST was done between 13 to 18 weeks, 6% loss rate when ST was done between 19 to 24 weeks and 9.1% loss rate after 25 weeks). 78 percent live births occurred later than 33 weeks gestational age and only 6 percent between 25 to 28 weeks.

Monochorionic-diamniotic twins: Ultrasound-guided bipolar coagulation and RFA has become more popular in recent years. Data regarding both bipolar coagulation as well as laser ablation is relatively limited. Lewi et al.[6] reported eighty cases of cord coagulation (73 twins, 7 triplets), where ST was performed by either bipolar or laser coagulation at a median gestational age of 21 weeks. The survival rate was 83 percent (72/87). There were 9 intrauterine fetal deaths (10%); 5 within 24 hours and 4 between 4 and 10 weeks after the procedure. There was 1 termination of pregnancy because of chorioamnionitis. Median gestational age at delivery was 35.4 weeks, with 79 percent of patients delivering after 32 weeks. Preterm prelabor rupture of the membranes occurred in 38 percent of the cases and accounted for all the perinatal deaths prior to 25 weeks (n = 5).

It seems that in spite of the relatively high neonatal mortality rates following ST in monochorionic-diamniotic twin pregnancies, umbilical cord occlusion is a relatively accepted option, especially as opposed to the other option, which is termination of the pregnancy.

CONCLUSION

First-trimester multifetal pregnancy reduction is a relatively safe treatment option to reduce the number of fetuses in a higher-order multiple gestation. As such, it decreases the complications of premature delivery and improves the outcome for the remaining fetuses.

REFERENCES

1. Evans MI, Berkowitz RL, Wapner RJ, Carpenter RJ, Goldberg JD, Ayoub MA, et al. Improvement in outcomes of multifetal pregnancy reduction with increased experience. Am J Obstet Gynecol 2001;184:97-103.
2. Lipitz S, Shulman A, Achiron R, Zalel Y, Seidman DS. A comparative study of multifetal pregnancy reduction from triplets to twins in the first versus early second trimesters after detailed fetal screening. Ultrasound Obstet Gynecol 2001;18:35-8.
3. Papageorghiou AT, Avgidou K, Bakoulas V, Sebire NJ, Nicolaides KH. Risks of miscarriage and early preterm birth in trichorionic triplet pregnancies with embryo reduction versus expectant management: New data and systematic review. Hum. Reprod 2006;21:1912-7.
4. Evans MI CDBDFC. Multifetal Pregnancy Reduction. In: Blickstein IKL, (Ed). Multiple Pregnancy. Taylor and Francis 2009. pp. 535-43.
5. Lipitz S, Reichman B, Uval J, Shalev J, Achiron R, Barkai G, et al. A prospective comparison of the outcome of triplet pregnancies managed expectantly or by multifetal reduction to twins. Am J Obstet Gynecol 1994;170:874-9.
6. Lewi L, Gratacos E, Ortibus E, Van SD, Carreras E, Higueras T, et al. Pregnancy and infant outcome of 80 consecutive cord coagulations in complicated monochorionic multiple pregnancies. Am J Obstet Gynecol 2006;194:782-9.
7. Challis D, Gratacos E, Deprest JA. Cord occlusion techniques for selective termination in monochorionic twins. J Perinat. Med 1999;27:327-38.
8. Evans MI, Goldberg JD, Horenstein J, Wapner RJ, Ayoub MA, Stone J, et al. Selective termination for structural, chromosomal, and mendelian anomalies: international experience. Am J Obstet Gynecol 1999;181:893-7.

The Association Between Congenital Malformations and Infertility, Infertility Treatment and ART

Jacob Farhi, Benjamin Fisch

OVERVIEW

The data reported in the literature to date indicate that *in vitro* fertilization (IVF) is probably related to an excess occurrence of major malformations, even in singleton infants. The congenital malformation rate in the general population ranges from 1 to 3 percent. The 30 percent increase associated with IVF increases this rate to 1.3 to 3.9 percent. There is apparently no association of major congenital malformations with specific laboratory maneuvers of oocyte, sperm or embryos, or to the medication used for ovarian stimulation or luteal support. Moreover, children born to infertile couples following infertility treatments other than IVF also have an increased risk for specific congenital malformations as do infants of couples with infertility who conceived spontaneously. All this suggests that there may be an inherent risk of a congenital abnormality in the infertile population.

Within the infertile population, those who were diagnosed with male factor infertility have the highest risk, as indicated by outcome analysis of singleton pregnancies resulting from IVF versus artificial insemination, with or without ovarian stimulation agents and with or without sperm donation.

Basic research is also required to elucidate the biological mechanisms underlying the genetic and epigenetic effects of infertility per se or the different modalities of infertility treatment. Large-scale prospective epidemiological studies would establish the magnitude of risk and the cause of congenital malformations in the infertile population and its relation to the infertility treatments.

INTRODUCTION

The exposure of human gametes to *in vitro* handling and *in vitro* culture conditions at the early stages of embryonic development has been of major concern to scientists, physicians, and patients with regard to enhanced development of congenital malformations since the introduction of assisted reproductive techniques (ART).[1] Theoretically, there are several putative factors in infertility treatments, which may affect embryo development. The high doses of gonadotropins used to stimulate folliculogenesis, which lead to a high estradiol environment, can alter the maturation process of oocytes, the physiological environment of implantation and the first stages of embryo development.[2] Animal studies demonstrated that exposure of embryos to different culture conditions can alter the expression and imprinting of various genes.[3] In intracytoplasmic sperm injection (ICSI), the artificial selection of sperm for fertilization and the injection process may bypass the natural barriers that prevent abnormal sperm cells from penetrating the zona pellucida. Furthermore, the process of embryo cryopreservation may have deleterious effects on DNA and embryonic gene expression.[4,5] Prolonged exposure of embryos grown to the blastocyst stage under *in vitro* culture conditions may lead to abnormal adhesion properties and abnormal splitting of the inner cell mass, resulting in an increased rate of monochorionic twins and conjoined twins.[6]

CLINICAL DISCUSSION

The Association Between Congenital Malformations and IVF Treatment

Early studies from Australia, France, England and Israel did not find an increased risk of congenital malformations in IVF babies. These studies reported a similar incidence of congenital malformations in infants born to couples who underwent ART to the observed rate in the general fertile population.[7-15] New evidence gathered recently has reached the opposite conclusion. This data from several large cohort studies, multicenter studies, and meta-analyses suggests a potential elevated risk. The first reports were by Bergh, et al.[16] and Hansen, et al.[17] Bergh, et al.[16] in a study on 5856 Swedish babies, found that 5.4 percent of those born following *in vitro* fertilization (IVF) had a major malformation, especially neural tube defects (anencephaly, hydrocephaly and spina bifida) and esophageal atresia. Hansen, et al.[17] from Western Australia, reported major congenital malformation rates of 9 percent for infants born after IVF and 8.6 percent for infants born after intracytoplasmic sperm injection (ICSI), compared to 4.5 percent for naturally conceived babies.

This new data prompted a worldwide reassessment of the issue, which yielded similarly high rates of congenital malformations in IVF babies.[2,18-22] Hansen, et al.[23] published a comprehensive meta-analysis of the pooled epidemiological data (7 studies) on birth defects following ART. The odds ratio for all congenital malformations was 1.40 (95% CI 1.28–1.53), indicating a significantly increased risk in the order of 30 to 40 percent compared to the general fertile population. When the analysis was restricted to major birth defects, the odds ratio was 2.0. These findings agreed with the 4.3 percent rate of major congenital malformations reported by Klemetti, et al. [24] compared to 2.9 percent in naturally conceived children. The adjusted odds ratio for congenital malformations in the IVF group in this study was 1.3 (95% confidence interval, 1.1–1.6). The risk was higher in boys of both singleton and multiple pregnancies and lower for girls of multiple pregnancies (OR = 0.5, 95% CI 0.2–0.9). Statistically, singleton infants born by IVF had more major congenital malformations than control singletons. Three-way analysis of sex, multiplicity, and affected organ yielded an increased risk for urogenital and musculoskeletal congenital malformations in singleton boys of IVF pregnancies. A recent study from our center, comparing newborns conceived by IVF before (1986–1994) and after (1995–2002) the introduction of ICSI also found that major malformation rates were two to three-fold higher than those in the general population in the first period (9.35% vs 4.05%) and 1.75-fold higher in the second period (9.0% vs 5.18%, respectively).[25]

There are two meta-analyses that limited their data to singleton IVF pregnancies in order to eliminate the effect of multiple pregnancies, which by themselves are a risk factor for congenital malformations. Lambert, et al.[26] failed to establish an association between congenital malformation and singleton IVF pregnancies or between congenital malformations and the presence of infertility alone or exposure to infertility treatments. However, McDonald, et al.[27] who included both case-control and cohort studies, found an increased risk in the IVF/IVF-ICSI group (OR 1.41; CI 1.06–1.88) compared with spontaneously conceived singletons matched for maternal age.

The Association Between Various Elements of IVF Treatment and the Risk of Congenital Malformations

Olson, et al.[28] evaluated different aspects of the IVF procedure in relation to congenital malformations. Overall, he found an incidence of 6.2 percent for major birth defects in children born after IVF compared with 4.4 percent in naturally conceived children. The adjusted odds ratio of a major birth defect in all IVF-conceived children was 1.30 (95% confidence interval, 1.00–1.67). The birth defect rate increased in the IVF group when the analysis was limited to term singletons. There was also no effect of duration of incubation in the laboratory from egg collection to embryo transfer [short exposure, zygote intra fallopian tube transfer (ZIFT), or longer exposure and transfer on day 2 or 3] (OR 1.10, 95 percent CI 0.65–1.86 for ZIFT), and no correlation of birth defects with type of medication for ovulation induction. Regarding exposure to fertility drugs after embryo transfer, although estrogen supplementation was prescribed more often for mothers of the malformed than the non-malformed children in the IVF group, most of the mothers of malformed children did not use them.[24] Cryopreservation did not seem to affect singleton pregnancies, but it was associated with a higher incidence of major birth defects in twin IVF pregnancies compared to twin conception after 'fresh' embryo transfer (OR 2.11, 95% CI 1.03–4.33, P = .041).[28]

Intracytoplasmic Sperm Injection (ICSI) and Congenital Malformations

Intracytoplasmic sperm injection (ICSI) involves the selection of a single sperm cell and its manual injection into the oocyte. The lack of relevant experimental studies, the non-natural selection of the fertilizing sperm, and the potentially oocyte-damaging injection procedure have raised concerns that ICSI may increase the risk of birth defects. A comparison between IVF and IVF + ICSI in relation to congenital malformations may reveal the related risk for ICSI in this regard. A survey of the Swedish Medical Birth Register for all children born by IVF from 1982 to 2001 showed a higher rate of congenital malformations among IVF children, but no difference between ICSI and non-ICSI cycles, other than an excess of cases of hypospadias after ICSI.[29] Lie, et al.[30] in an analysis of the pooled data on 5,395 children conceived by ICSI, calculated that the risk of major congenital malformations was increased by 1.12-fold over children conceived by standard IVF (95% confidence interval 0.97–1.28, P = 0.12). Bonduelle, et al.[31] in a multicenter cohort study, noted similar results, and attributed the higher rate of congenital malformations in the ICSI group to the excess of malformations in the urogenital system of the male infants. Olson, et al.[28] found that after controlling for age, plurality, and parity, there was no difference in the birth defect rate between IVF and ICSI pregnancies, for all children

(OR 0.86, 95% CI 0.54–1.38 for ICSI) and for singletons only (OR 1.06, 95% CI 0.53–2.08 for ICSI). Unlike the other studies, there was no difference in the particular organ systems affected. Klemetti, et al.[24] also noted a similar rate of major malformations between the ICSI and IVF groups (4.6%). The above data seems to indicate that the use of ICSI does not increase the risk of congenital malformations compared to the risk observed in standard IVF with *in vitro* insemination of oocytes.

Imprinting Disorders and IVF

Experimental studies have noted a relationship of manipulative procedures such as sperm cryopreservation, embryo culture, and somatic cell cloning with abnormal methylation of genes that control imprinting at early embryonic stages of development.[32-34] These data were supported by more recent cumulative evidence of a possible link between IVF and epigenetic abnormalities,[35] specifically Beckwith-Wiedemann syndrome, caused by hypomethylation of the control center of 5q,[36-38] and Angelman syndrome, which involves imprinted gene clusters.[39,40] However, a recent seven-year Danish cohort study of 442,349 singleton non-IVF and 6052 IVF children found 54 cases of imprinting in the non-IVF group compared to zero in the IVF group.[41] These findings agree with the suggestion of Ludwig, et al.[42] that imprinting disorders are associated with infertility per se rather than to ICSI or IVF methodology.

The Association Between Diagnosis of Infertility and the Risk of Congenital Malformations in Non-IVF Conceptions

It is possible that the culprit is not the infertility treatment/IVF procedure per se but a factor or factors inherent to infertile patients, and specifically those who require ART, who may differ demographically or genetically from the general population of the same age group.

Spontaneous Conceptions

Data on spontaneous pregnancies and their outcome are sparse because couples with infertility who conceive spontaneously are often difficult to identify. The most striking data relating the infertility state to major malformations in offspring were presented recently by Zhu, et al.[43] in a study of the time needed to conceive in spontaneous pregnancies. In this study, they used the standard definition for infertility of more than one year to achieve conception. Their cohort included 50,897 singletons and 1,366 twins born to fertile couples, 5,764 singletons and 100 twins born to infertile couples who conceived naturally, and 4588 singletons and 1690 twins born after infertility treatment. Overall, the prevalence of congenital malformations increased with an increase in time to conception. Singletons of infertile couples,

whether conceived naturally or after infertility treatment, had a higher prevalence of congenital malformations than singletons born to fertile couples; hazard ratios were 1.20 and 1.39, respectively. No such findings were noted for twins. Additionally, babies born after infertility treatment had more genital organ malformations than babies conceived naturally. These findings were in line with the study of Ludwig, et al.[42] relating imprinting disorders to spontaneous conception in infertile patients, regardless of the use of IVF or ovarian stimulation. Others found that infertile couples that conceive spontaneously have generally poorer perinatal outcomes than the general population.[44]

Studies comparing natural cycles and semen donor insemination (DI) cycles can provide important information on the possible effect of *in vitro* sperm manipulation or sperm cryopreservation on the occurrence of congenital malformations. As most women treated with DI are fertile, and all sperm donors are considered fertile, their pregnancy outcome would be expected to be similar to that of the general population, taking into account the relatively advanced age of women who require DI. However, if laboratory sperm manipulation harbors a risk for congenital malformations, there should be an increased rate of congenital malformation following this exposure even in theoretically otherwise fertile population. Two prospective and large population-based studies included data on congenital malformations associated with DI. The first, from France, reported malformations in 1.9 percent in 1298 deliveries,[45] and the second, from Australia, reported malformations in 2.4 percent of 242 term pregnancies or midtrimester abortions.[46] Both these values were similar to the rates in the general population of the respective countries, corrected for maternal age. Regarding the effect of sperm cryopreservation and thawing process, the use of frozen thawed spermatozoa for AID was not found to affect the health of children following this procedure.[47] By contrast, the use of sperm samples from males diagnosed with male factor infertility and exposed to similar *in vitro* manipulations were found to be associated with a high incidence of genetic abnormalities.[48] Buckett, et al.[49] reported that chromosomal abnormalities are more frequent in men with oligo-, terato-asthenozoospermia who are referred for ICSI.

Ovulation Induction and the Risk of Congenital Malformations

Most studies on the association of congenital malformations with ovulation induction also included children born after IVF. In this section, the focus is only on the data related to ovulation induction. In the largest and most detailed study on this subject, Klemetti, et al.[24] detected at least one major congenital malformation in 3.7 percent of 4467 children born after ovulation induction compared with 2.9 percent of a random sample of 27,078 naturally conceived children. In the study group, boys were affected more than girls in both singleton and multiple gestations. Stratification by organ showed that girls in singleton pregnancies had a slightly higher risk of major heart anomalies, and boys, of urogenital malformations. The occurrence of malformations was not related to the drug used for ovarian stimulation or to the medications used for luteal support, either natural or synthetic progestin. Olson, et al.[28] found no significant difference in the rate of major malformations between children conceived by ovulation induction or IUI (5.0%) and a matched cohort of naturally conceived children (4.4%). The adjusted odds ratio of a major birth defect after ovulation induction/IUI was 1.11. Although this difference was not statistically significant, when stratified according to organ affected, the children born after ovulation induction/IUI had a significantly higher incidence of major congenital malformations in the musculoskeletal system. Kallen, et al.[50] reported from the Swedish Medical Birth Register on 4029 women who delivered following ovulation induction treatment. The OR for major congenital malformations was 1.21 following treatment with ovulation induction. This risk was corrected when adjustment for subfertility was made indicating that the risk for congenital malformation was related to subfertility and not to the treatment effect. Lai, et al.[51] reported that the rate for positive findings on first trimester screen for Down syndrome's was significantly higher in IUI pregnancies than in spontaneous conceptions (14.3% vs 7.1%).

The above studies show that although the overall risk for congenital malformations in infertile patients seems similar or slightly increased in relation to that observed in the general fertile population, infertile patients who conceive with ovulation induction treatments have a higher incidence of major congenital malformations in specific organs-heart, urogenital or musculoskeletal.

CONCLUSION

Although the absolute risk of having a child with birth defects is low for the individual couple, people contemplating infertility treatment and specifically IVF, and their counselors need to take the current data into consideration. Their decisions should be tempered by the awareness that the current classification of malformations into major and minor does not take into account later functional impairments, their potential treatability, or their long-term consequences, and further studies of these issues are still needed.

REFERENCES

1. Edwards RG, Sharpe DJ. Social values and research in human embryology. Nature 1971;14;231:87-91.
2. Winston RM, Hardy K. Are we ignoring potential dangers of *in vitro* fertilization and related treatments? Nat Med 2002; (Suppl.):S14-8.
3. Lonergan P, Rizos D, Gutierrez-Adan A, Fair T, Boland MP. Effect of culture environment on embryo quality and gene expression—experience from animal studies. Reprod Biomed 2003;7:657-63.
4. Bouquet M, Selva J, Auroux M. Cryopreservation of mouse oocytes: Mutagenic effects in the embryo? Biol Reprod 1993; 49:764-9.
5. Emiliani S, Van den Bergh M, Vannin AS, Biramane J, Englert Y. Comparison of ethylene glycol, 1,2-propanediol and glycerol for cryopreservation of slow-cooled mouse zygotes, 4-cell embryos and blastocysts. Hum Reprod 2000;15:905-10.
6. Shimizu Y, Fukuda J, Sato W, Kumagai J, Hirano H, Tanaka T. First trimester diagnosis of conjoined twins after *in vitro* fertilization-embryo transfer (IVF-ET) at blastocyst stage. Ultrasound Obstet Gynecol 2004;24:208-9.
7. Saunders DM, Lancaster P. The wider perinatal significance of the Australian *in vitro* fertilization data collection program. Am J Perinatol 1989;6:252-7.
8. French National Registry, Analysis of data 1986 to 1990. FIV-NAT (French *in vitro* national). Fertil Steril 1995;64:746-56.
9. Friedler S, Mashiach S, Laufer N. Births in Israel resulting from *in vitro* fertilization/embryo transfer, 1982-1989: National Registry of the Israeli Association for Fertility Research. Hum Reprod 1992;7:1159-63.
10. MRC Working Party on Children Conceived by *in Vitro* Fertilisation, Births in Great Britain resulting from assisted conception, 1978-87. Br Med J 1990;300:1229-33.
11. Morin NC, Wirth FH, Johnson DH, Frank LM, Presburg HJ, Van De Water VL, Chee EM, Mills JL. Congenital malformations and psychosocial development in children conceived by *in vitro* fertilization. J Pediatr 1989;115:222-7.
12. Sutcliffe AG, D'Souza SW, Cadman J, Richards B, McKinlay IA, Lieberman B. Minor congenital anomalies, major congenital malformations and development in children conceived from cryopreserved embryos. Hum Reprod 1995;10:3332-7.
13. Verlaenen H, Cammu H, Derde MP, Amy JJ. Singleton pregnancy after *in vitro* fertilization: Expectations and outcome. Obstet Gynecol 1995;86:906-10.
14. Isaksson R, Gissler M, Tiitinen A. Obstetric outcome among women with unexplained infertility after IVF: a matched case-control study. Hum Reprod 2002;17:1755-61.
15. Zadori ZJ, Kozinszky Z, Orvos H, Katona M, Kaali SG, Pal A. The incidence of major birth defects following *in vitro* fertilization. J Assist Reprod Genet 1995;20:131-2.
16. Bergh T, Ericson A, Hillensjo T, Nygren KG, Wennerholm UB. Deliveries and children born after *in vitro* fertilisation in Sweden 1982-95: A retrospective cohort study. Lancet 1999; 354:1579-85.
17. Hansen M, Kurinczuk JJ, Bower C, Webb S. The risk of major birth defects after intracytoplasmic sperm injection and *in vitro* fertilization. N Engl J Med 2002;346:725-30.
18. Barlow DH. The children of assisted reproduction. The need for an ongoing debate. Hum Reprod 2002;17:1133-4.
19. Lambert RD. Safety issues in assisted reproduction technology: The children of assisted reproduction confront the responsible conduct of assisted reproductive technologies. Hum Reprod 2002:17:3011-5.

20. Schultz RM, Williams CJ. The science of ART. Science 2002;21; 296:2188-90.

21. Kovalevsky G, Rinaudo P, Coutifaris C. Do assisted reproductive technologies cause adverse fetal outcomes? Fertil Steril 2003; 79:1270-2.

22. Powell K. Fertility treatments: seeds of doubt. Nature 2003; 422:656-8.

23. Hansen M, Bower C, Milne E, de Klerk N, Kurinczuk J. Assisted reproductive technologies and the risk of birth defects—a systematic review. Hum Reprod 2005;20:328-38.

24. Klemetti R, Gissler M, Sevona T, Koivurova S, Ritvanen A, Hemminki E. Children born after assisted fertilization have an increased rate of major congenital anomalies, Fertil Steril 2005; 84:1300-7.

25. Merlob P, Sapir O, Sulkes J, Fisch B. The prevalence of major congenital malformations during two periods of time, 1986-1994 and 1995-2002 in newborns conceived by assisted reproduction technology. Eur J Med Genet 2005;48:5-11.

26. Lambert RD. Safety issues in assisted reproductive technology: aetiology of health problems in singleton ART babies. Hum Reprod 2003;18:1987-91.

27. McDonald SD, Murphy K, Beyene J, Ohlsson A. Perinatal outcomes of singleton pregnancies achieved by *in vitro* fertilization: A systematic review and meta-analysis. J Obstet Gynaecol Can 2005;27:449-59.

28. Olson CK, Keppler-Noreuil KM, Romirtti PA, Budelierc WT, Ryan G, Sparks AET, Van Voorhis BJ. *In vitro* fertilization is associated with an increase in major birth defects. Fertil Steril 2005;84:1308-15.

29. Kallen B, Finnstrom O, Nygren KG, Olausson PO. *In vitro* fertilization (IVF) in Sweden: Risk for congenital malformations after different IVF methods. Birth Defects Res A Clin Mol Teratol 2005;73:162-9.

30. Lie RT, Lyngstadaas A, Orstavik KH, Bakketeig LS, Jacobsen G, Tanbo T. Birth defects in children conceived by ICSI compared with children conceived by other IVF methods; a meta-analysis. Int J Epidemiol 2005;34:696-701.

31. Bonduelle M, Wennerholm UB, Loft A, Tarlatzis BC. A multi-centre cohort study of the physical health of 5-year-old children conceived after intracytoplasmic sperm injection, *in vitro* fertilization and natural conception. Hum Reprod 2005;20: 413-9.

32. Young LE, Fernandes K, McEvoy TG, Butterworth SC, Gutierrez CG, Carolan C, Broadbent PJ, Robinson JJ, Wilmut J, Sinclair KD. Epigenetic change in IGF2R is associated with fetal overgrowth after sheep embryo culture. Nat Genet 2001;27:153-4.

33. Khosla S, Dean W, Brown D, Reik W, Feil R. Culture of preimplantation mouse embryos affects fetal development and the expression of imprinted genes. Biol Reprod 2001;64:918-26.

34. Doherty AS, Mann MR, Tremblay KD, Bartolomei MS, Schultz RM. Differential effects of culture on imprinted H19 expression in the preimplantation mouse embryo. Biol Reprod 2000;62:1526-35.

35. Gosden R, Trasler J, Lucifero D, Faddy M. Rare congenital disorders, imprinted genes, and assisted reproductive technology. Lancet 2003;361:1975-7.

36. Maher ER, Brueton LA, Bowdin SC, Luharia A, Cooper H, Cole TR, Macdonald F, Sampson JR, Barrett CR, Reik N, Hawkins MM. Beckwith-Wiedemann syndrome and assisted reproduction technology (ART). J Med Genet 2003;40:62-4.

37. Gicquel C, Gaston V, Mandelbaum J, Siffroi JP, Flahault A, Le Bouc Y. *In vitro* fertilization may increase the risk of Beckwith-Wiedemann syndrome related to the abnormal imprinting of the KCN1OT gene. Am J Hum Genet 2003;72:1338-41.

38. DeBaun MR, Niemitz EL, Feinberg AP. Association of *in vitro* fertilization with Beckwith-Wiedemann syndrome and epigenetic alterations of LIT1 and H19. Am J Hum Genet 2003; 72:156-60.

39. Cox GF, Burger J, Lip V, Mau UA, Sperling K, Wu BC, Horsthemke B. Intracytoplasmic sperm injection may increase the risk of imprinting defects. Am J Hum Genet 2002;71:162-4.

40. Orstavik KH, Eiklid K, van der Hagen CB, Spetalen S, Kierulf K, Skjedal O, Buiting K. Another case of imprinting defect in a girl with Angelman syndrome who was conceived by intracytoplasmic semen injection. Am J Hum Genet 2003;72: 218-9.

41. Lideaard O, Pinborg A, Andersen AN. Imprinting diseases and IVF: Danish National IVF cohort study. Hum Reprod 2005; 20:950-4.

42. Ludwig M, Katalinic A, Gross S, Sutcliffe A, Varon R, Horsthemke B. Increased prevalence of imprinting defects in patients with Angelman syndrome born to subfertile couples. J Med Genet 2005;42:289-91.

43. Zhu JL, Basso O, Obel C, Bille C, Olsen J. Infertility, infertility treatment, and congenital malformations: Danish national birth cohort. BMJ 2006;30;333:665-6.

44. Draper ES, Kurinczuk JJ, Abrams KR, Clarke M. Assessment of separate contributions to perinatal mortality of infertility history and treatment (a case control analysis). Lancet 1999;353: 1746-9.

45. Thepot F. 1997 results of medical assisted procreation with third-party donation and autopreservation: CECOS French Federation. Contracept Fertil Sex 1998;26:476-80.

46. Virro MR, Shewchuk AB. Pregnancy outcome in 242 conceptions after artificial insemination with donor sperm and effects of maternal age on the prognosis for successful pregnancy. Am J Obstet Gynecol 1984;1;148:518-24.

47. Lansac J, Royere D. Follow-up studies of children born after frozen sperm donation. Hum Reprod Update 2001;7:33-7.

48. Gekas J, Thepot F, Turleau C, Siffroi JP, Dadoune JP, Briault S, et al. Chromosomal factors of infertility in candidate couples for ICSI (an equal risk of constitutional aberrations in women and men). Hum Reprod 2001;16:82-90.

49. Buckett W, Aird L, Luckas M, Kingsland C, Lewis-Jones I, Howard P. Intracytoplasmic sperm injection. Karyotyping should be done before treatment. Br Med J 1996;313:1334.

50. Kallen B, Olausson PO, Nygren KG. Neonatal outcome in pregnancies from ovarian stimulation. Obstet Gynecol 2002; 100:414-9.

51. Lai TH, Chen SC, Tsai MS, Lee FK, Wei CF. First-trimester screening for Down syndrome in singleton pregnancies achieved by intrauterine insemination. J Assist Reprod Genet 2003;20:327-31.

Preservation of Ovarian Tissue: Pioneers Close to a New Border?

René Frydman, Antoine Torre

OVERVIEW

Progress in the anticancer treatments of young adults was done to the detriment of their fertility. For girls, these treatments induce a premature ovarian failure that nothing can stop. Traditional assisted reproduction techniques (ART) reach their limits. However, infertility remains a major concern for these young women; does one have to choose between life and the possibility of having children?

Although cryopreservation of ovarian strips is still at the stage of research, three births, recently obtained by this technique, give birth to the hope. These descriptions follow several years of constant progress in the field, as well in animals (litters obtained for goats and macaques) as in women (ten attempts of autograft biologically successful, reappearance of folliculogenesis and even obtained embryo).

In 2004, Donnez described the first birth after autograft of ovarian strips, cryopreserved before sterilizing treatment for Hodgkin's lymphoma. Since, then, two other attempts of ovarian grafting concluded with the birth of healthy children, and an ongoing pregnancy in Belgium, while two other attempts led to biochemical or clinical pregnancies that unfortunately ended in miscarriages. Obviously, progress in this promising technique seems to be quicker and quicker.

With each new technique, a few details must be improved. For example, the ischemia of the freshly reintroduced fragments must be controlled. Nevertheless, this technique must at least be exposed, or taught to any person interested in infertility.

INTRODUCTION

Iatrogenic Female Infertility and the Failure of Conventional Treatments

There are many circumstances, irrespective of malignancy, for which a woman of childbearing age could receive gonadotoxic chemotherapy. Indeed, some kind of cancers impose treatments likely to deteriorate fertility. These diseases often touch young adults or children and do not allow the use of traditional embryonic preservation, for which, a partner is necessary. The problem is less serious with the boy since assisted reproduction techniques (ART), employed in the event of male infertility [intracytoplasmic injection (ICSI), testicular biopsy)] are efficient, and gamete banking (sperm cryopreservation) is well mastered. On the other hand, for girls or young women, when premature ovarian failure occurs, no effective solution is available. Oocyte cryopreservation, at the stage of research and is insufficiently powerful to save fertility, mature oocytes being poorly resistant to thawing. Thus, alternative strategies were developed and have started to bear their fruits.

Young Women and Anticancer Treatment: Surviving but Sterile

The incidence of childhood cancers seem to be on the rise. Treatments, whose immediate toxicity is better controlled, allow a much higher survival but with long-term side effects as the deterioration of fertility. In 2010, in the United Kingdom, one person out of 750 survived a childhood cancer.[1] For these future adults, sterility will undoubtedly be a major cause of deterioration of the quality of life.

For girls, it is clearly established that the anticancer treatments deteriorate the ovarian reserve. The ovary is twice more sensitive to radiotherapy than the testicle. The sterilizing dose of radiation decreases with age. Moreover, the effects of radiotherapy are unlikely to be limited to the ovary

Table 67.1: Chemotherapy and fertility risk[1]

Pediatrics cancers			*Cancers of the young adult*
High risk (>80%)	**Medium risk**	**Low risk (<20%)**	
Whole-body irradiation	Acute myeloblastic leukemia (difficult to quantify)	Acute lymphoblastic leukemia	Genital rhabdomyosarcoma
Localized radiotherapy—pelvic or testicular	Hepatoblastoma	Wilms' tumor	Retroperitoneal sarcoma
Chemotherapy conditioning for bone-marrow transplantation	Osteosarcoma	Soft-tissue sarcoma—stage I	Bone tumors
Hodgkin's disease—treatment with alkylating-drugs	Ewing's sarcoma—non-metastatic	Germ-cell tumors (with gonadal preservation and no radiotherapy)	Ovarian cancer
Soft-tissue sarcoma—stage IV (metastatic)	Soft-tissue sarcoma—stage II or III	Retinoblastoma	Breast cancer
Ewing's sarcoma—metastatic	Neuroblastoma	Brain tumor—surgery only, cranial irradiation <24 Gy	Cancer of the cervix
	Non-Hodgkin lymphoma		Rectum and colon cancer
	Hodgkin's disease—alternating treatment		
	Brain tumor—craniospinal radiotherapy, cranial irradiation >24 Gy		

since the fetuses of patients irradiated in the pelvis are found to have a higher incidence of fetal hypotrophy, suggesting a uterine effect.

Chemotherapy is also likely to decrease the ovarian reserve, especially when it contains alkylating drugs. Unfortunately, to our knowledge, no fundamental work contributing to the molecular explanation of this gonadic toxicity has been published yet. Hence, gonadic protection measures, intuitive but simplistic, seem ineffective. Nevertheless, infertility induced by anticancer treatment is a real clinical problem. For a teenager treated with chemotherapy, the risk of premature ovarian failure increases by a factor of 4 while it increases by a factor of 27 among women from 21 to 25 years old.[2] Several studies showed that among women younger than 20 years old, the rate of amenorrhea after chemotherapy ranges from 20 to 50 percent, and these women show a higher statistical risk for premature menopause. Among all the women treated for a cancer (all ages inclusive), 17 percent will suffer from a premature ovarian failure (in average at 26 years old)[3] and 42 percent will have it in the third decade.[4] The overall rate of premature ovarian failure is about 60 percent. Spontaneous pregnancies could occur in 28 percent of young women treated for cancer, in spite of a documented deterioration in their ovarian function.[3,5] Among women older than 25 years treated for cancer, the rate of amenorrhea can reach 80 to 90 percent; all these patients will potentially undergo premature ovarian failure and only 5 percent will spontaneously

Table 67.2: Chemotherapeutic agents and fertility risk[1]

High risk	*Medium risk*	*Low risk*
Cyclophosphamide	Cisplatin	Vincristine
Ifosfamide	Carboplatin	Methotrexate
Chlormethine	Doxorubicin	Dactinomycin
Busulfan		Bleomycin
Melphalan		Mercaptopurine
Procarbazine		Vinblastine
Chlorambucil		

get pregnant.[6] The bone marrow transplantation, with its associated treatments, undoubtedly bear the darkest prognosis as regards the fertility[7,10] even when it involves a child. Indeed, only 19 percent of the treated girls will have a normal ovarian function.[8] In the older patients, menopause is quasi-systematic.[9] As you can see, the fertility among women who require chemotherapy is a major public health problem, unfortunately too often ignored. Table 67.1 summarizes cancers and their relation to infertility. The disease can also deteriorate fertility, by it own presence. Table 67.2 summarizes chemotherapeutic agents and their correlation with infertility.

Other Situations and their Fertility Risk

Few systemic diseases (Systemic lupus erythematosus, Behçet's disease, Scleroderma) may benefit from immunosuppressive but gonadotoxic treatments. It is the same for certain steroid resistant inflammatory diseases (Glomerulonephritis, Inflammatory bowel disease).

The problem is also acute for patients carrying BRCA1 or BRCA2 mutations, for which a prophylactic ovariectomy is recommended because of increased risk of ovarian and tubal cancers in these patients. The risk of degeneration must lead to prudence owing to the reintroduction of these ovarian fragments.

Lastly, some pathologies, like the Turner's syndrome or repeated endometriomas, induce accelerated ovarian atresia. For example, at the age of 12 years, 80 percent of the girls with Turner's syndrome still have follicles. Safeguarding the fertility would probably be possible at this age (without any future risk of gonadoblastoma, this one reaching only the rare forms of Turner's with mosaicism Y).[10]

Conventional Solutions for Safeguarding Female Fertility

When a disease imposes an irradiation located on the pelvis (i.e. seldom), it is of good sense to remove the ovaries away from the site of irradiation.

Initial studies on animal models suggested that blocking the gonadotropic axis by gonadotropin-releasing hormone (GnRH) agonists could preserve the germinal cells when a gonadotoxic drug must be used. In humans two non-randomized studies and two uncontrolled studies on a small number of patients (120, 21, 125 and 5 patients) have suggested that this practice could protect fertility.[4,11-13] In the absence of evidence-based data we must not recommend this practice.

Cryopreservation of embryos is the most well-tried technical solution when the patient has a partner, when she can postpone her anticancer treatment to perform an ovarian stimulation and if the couple accepts, the idea of an *in vitro* fertilization (IVF).

Newer Methods

Less than 10 percent of the mature oocytes cryopreserved after ovarian stimulation survive thawing. However, a hundred pregnancies have been obtained thanks to this technique.[14]

In vitro maturation of primordial follicles starting from cryopreserved ovarian strips exposed to GDF9 has been carried out in the mouse.[15,16] The human oocyte growth seems more complex.

The xenografting of human ovarian strips on SCID mice is still explored in research.[17,18]

Lastly, some consider the removal of embryonic stem cells from aborted fetuses in order to graft them into patients with premature ovarian failure. This sensitive subject, still very theoretical, is the object of an ethical controversy.[19]

Finally, apart from the cryopreservation of the mature oocytes, the only innovative technique that permits conception is the autograft of ovarian strips.

CLINICAL DISCUSSION

Cryopreservation of Ovarian Tissues

To date, the autografting ovarian strips is the only technique that has allowed the preservation of fertility. Transplantation of the whole ovary gave good results only with the fresh ovary (hormonal persistence in the goat and the monkey,[20] litters obtained in the rat,[21] persistence and folliculogenesis in humans[20,22]). The cryopreservation of the isolated primordial follicles is under study. The fundamental fact is that only primordial follicles correctly resist freeze-thaw.

The Autograft of Ovarian Strips

The idea is to take small fragments of ovarian cortex (in which the primordial follicles are present) and to place them in a cryoprotecting solution at low temperature. In this state, preservation in liquid nitrogen. When thawed at ambient temperature, they can be reintroduced.

There has been tremendous success with the technique (i.e. with litters) in rodents (guineapigs, rats, mouse, rabbits). Recently, it was also successful in larger animals:

- The goat in which regrafting of ovarian strips, after cryopreservation resulted in the birth of a young one.[23]
- The macaque, littered a young after ovariectomy and immediate grafting of fresh ovarian fragments.[24]

In women, seven attempts of reintroduction of fresh ovarian cortex fragments were reported with varying outcomes of the five heterotopic grafts reported (i.e. apart from the abdominal cavity), two of them resulted in hormonal success, while folliculogenesis resumed in three. Two orthotropic grafts with fresh fragments were recently attempted on two patients suffering from recurring endometriomas (indicating the ovariectomy). To date, only the follicular survival report has been published,[25] but, is the graft still in progress?

The autograft after cryopreservation gave better results. Folliculogenesis resumed in a certain number of patients[26] in whom a heterotopic graft had been carried out (such as, for example, in this 37-year-old patient treated for cervix cancer).[27]

In 2004, a heterotopic graft of ovarian cortex strips under the abdominal skin made it possible to obtain an embryo following *in vitro* fertilization (IVF) in a 30-year-old woman, six years after a sterilizing treatment for breast cancer.[28]

A few months later, Donnez, et al.[29] described the first pregnancy obtained after orthotopic regrafting of cryopreserved ovarian strips in the subperitoneum. This 31-year-old patient had been treated six years before by sterilizing chemotherapy for Hodgkin's lymphoma. Nine months after the reintroduction of these fragments, a pregnancy was diagnosed.[29] Two spontaneous ovulations in the remaining ovaries during a nineteen-month period preceding this pregnancy while the hormonal substitution was stopped, led some to cast doubt on the implication of the graft on this pregnancy.[30,31] Nevertheless, many consider that it is certainly the first pregnancy obtained by this way.[1,32]

In 2005, the American team Silber, et al.[33] also obtained a pregnancy after an orthotopic graft, but this time, with fresh ovarian cortex. Two 26-year-old homozygote twin women were unmatched for their ovarian function. One had been amenorrheic for 10 years with histological ovarian atrophy, whereas the other had three children and a normal genital life. After an unfruitful attempt at oocyte donation, the twin whose ovaries were functional, gave one of her ovaries to her sister. After dissection, the whole ovarian cortex was grafted on the ovarian stroma of the twin suffered from menopause. Five months later, the recipient conceived naturally, perhaps due to the grafted fragments.[33]

Almost simultaneously, the Israeli team comprising of Meirow, et al.[34] also reported the birth of a child obtained after orthotopic grafting of cryopreserved ovarian strips. This 28-year-old patient had taken advantage of cryopreservation while she had chemotherapy for non-Hodgkin's lymphoma. The following months were marked by all the signs of premature ovarian failure. After having cured this lymphoma, the ovarian strips were reintroduced into her ovarian subcortex, which was followed by, a hormonal standardization and two spontaneous menstrual cycles. A four-celled embryo obtained by *in vitro* fertilization in a semi-natural cycle, gave rise to the birth of a healthy child.[34] As before, nothing proves that this pregnancy really comes from the reintroduced fragments.[35]

In France, Poireau and Lefebvre recently reported the result of their first replacement of ovarian strips. The removed tissue, a whole ovary, had been replaced in 2000 in a 20-year-old patient, who suffered from Hodgkin's lymphoma. Once cured, two-thirds of the ovarian cortex was introduced under the skin of the abdomen (i.e. heterotopic grafting). Five months were necessary for the graft to be functional. Then, 11 cycles of ovarian stimulation yielded 22 oocytes and 4 transferred embryos, but unfortunately, without a pregnancy. The harmful effect of the pelvic irradiation could be responsible for the lack of pregnancy. Indeed, the endometrial thickness of the patient had never exceeded 6 mm, which is a known pejorative factor in the success of IVF. The graft functioned for one year and the team considers the grafting of the remaining ovarian strips.

Since then, in Belgium, Demeestere et al.[36] announced encouraging results following a mixed graft (ortho and heterotopic) in a 29-year-old patient after marrow transplantation for aggressive Hodgkin's lymphoma. They obtained a spontaneous pregnancy that unfortunately ended in a miscarriage after 7 weeks of amenorrhea. The cytogenetic analysis showed karyotypic abnormality (70 XXY, +10).[36] However, a new pregnancy could be in progress by his team. Lastly, the Danish team of Andersen, et al.[37] reported a possible biochemical pregnancy after a mixed graft in a 31-year-old patient with Hodgkin's lymphoma. Three semi-natural cycles of IVF were performed on this patient. Two oocytes were retrieved from the heterotopic graft both of which fertilized and the transfer of these two embryos was followed by an increase in serum human chorionic gonadotropin (hCG) levels up to 22 IU/mL.[37] In our opinion, this rate seems too low to assert the reality of this biochemical pregnancy.

Recent successes should not make us forget that it is a new and thus, a technique that requires perfection. Several parameters have been studied:

- The cryopreservation is overall well controlled. The majority use dimethyl sulfoxide (DMSO) as a cryoprotectant. The use of an automat allows reproducibility and freezing-thawing seems responsible only for about 9 percent of the primordial follicle loss.[38]
- The site of transplantation (orthotopic or heterotopic) seems to play an important part in favoring intra-abdominal grafting. Thus, in the mouse, replacement under the renal capsule is more effective than in sub-cutaneous region.[39] According to their experiment, Oktay and Buyuk[40] are of the opinion that heterotopic grafting could deteriorate oocyte maturation and would modify the maturity criteria (obtained at 10 mm in diameter and not at 17 mm, as is traditional when maturation takes place in the abdominal cavity).[40]
- The small size of the grafts could also be important as it was shown in the sow.[38]

In fact, during the first 48 hours following grafting, follicles suffer from ischemia and this could be responsible for the loss of 50 to 75 percent of follicles that determines for how long the graft will be in progress. It is in this area that progress must be made.

Autograft of Whole Ovary

This technique consists in dissecting the lumbo-ovarian pedicle while ensuring that the ligature of the utero-ovarian pedicle does not cause ovarian ischemia. Once the arteries and veins are identified, they are cut. Then, in case of cryopreservation, the ovary must be catheterized and infused with a cryoprotectant solution, placed in a limp of slow freezing and cooled to 80°C. After 12 hours, the ovary can be transferred into liquid nitrogen. After thawing, the pedicle is supposed to be reconnected to blood vessels.

The experiment was reported only on fresh ovaries with various good results. In the goat and the monkey, the hormonal secretion of the ovary persisted.[20] In the rat, a litter was obtained.[21] In the woman, the description of such a technique exists since 1987 (autotransplantation in the arm with an ongoing hormonal secretion).[22] It even allowed the persistence of folliculogenesis in a 29-year-old woman with cervix cancer, who thus needed pelvic radiotherapy, for which ovarian grafting was performed in her arm.[20]

As you see, this technique is not fully controlled. One of the limits is the skill of the vascular surgeon. Freezing does not seem to deteriorate the vitality of the follicles.[41] However, as to date, cryopreservation of a whole organ has always showed failures, it is astonishing that the ovary makes an exception.

The Cryopreservation of Primordial Follicles

This technique allowed the pioneer in ovarian physiology to understand follicular growth.[42] The concept consists in purifying the primordial follicles contained in the ovarian cortex before cryopreservation. Once the disease is cured, these thawed primordial follicles would be included in an inert matrix and grafted. Indeed, it is known that the primordial follicles resist freezing-thawing. Moreover, it seems that follicle density has an impact on the ovarian physiology. Paracrine interaction between follicles seems necessary for correct ovarian functioning. By controlling the follicular density (which would be possible here), perhaps the graft would work longer. The use of an inert matrix is judicious to decrease the period of ischemia following grafting. Lastly, purifying the primordial follicles would have the great advantage of eliminating any risk of metastases (possibly contained in the ovarian stroma) from the autograft, which will not be a luxury for young patients cured of cancer.

This technique is not even validated in the animal. The principal problem remains the purification of a great number of primordial follicles, a problem not yet solved. Enzymatic digestion gropes even if it seems that, in *in vitro* studies, the liberase enzyme is preferable to the collagenases.[43] A purification method, using a gradient of Ficoll showed that it has no detrimetal effect on follicular survival, unfortunately without clearly purifying them (thus without concentrating them).[44] For the moment, primordial follicle recovery is achieved by vacuuming with the mouth with the help of a microscopic catheter under the objective of a binocular magnifying glass.

Control of the Metastasis Risk

Reintroduction of cancer in a cured patient is a major risk of the technique. That is why grafting is considered only in the event of a weak probability of ovarian metastasis. Table 67.3 recapitulates cancers that risk ovarian metastasis.

Table 67.3: Cancers that risk for ovarian metastasis[47]

Low risk of ovarian involvement	Moderate risk of ovarian involvement	Cancers with high risk of ovarian involvement
Breast cancer, stage I–III, infiltrative ductal	Breast cancer, stage IV, infiltrative lobular	Genital rhabdomyosarcoma
Squamous cell carcinoma of the cervix	Adeno/ adenosquamous carcinoma of the cervix	Leukemia
Hodgkin's and non-Hodgkin's lymphomas	Colon cancer (including tumors of rectum and appendix)	Burkitt's lymphoma
Wilm's tumor	Upper gastrointestinal system malignancies	Neuroblastoma
Osteogenic sarcoma		
Non-genital rhabdomyosarcoma		
Ewing's sarcoma		

When the disease is at high risk, as in the case of BRCA1 and BRCA2 mutations, in which 2 to 18.5 percent of the patients carry an occult ovarian cancer,[45] advances in knowledge (xenotransplantation) will perhaps bring solutions in the future and it remains elicit to cryopreserve fertility cells.[14] For low risk diseases, immunodeficient mice grafted with ovarian strips from women suffering from lymphoma, did not develop the disease,[46] which is reassuring.

FUTURE PROSPECTS

The molecular and cellular processes induced early by the graft of cortical fragments must be understood. Indeed, the knowledge of these mechanisms appears as an essential step in improving the ovarian strips grafting techniques. Differential analysis of this genetic expression between the follicular cells, the stromal cells of the graft and the host should also be carried out.

The understanding of why the heterotopic graft gives worse results may pass through a comparison of the genetic expression profiles within the various cellular types on the ungrafted fragments, the subperitoneal graft (a quite vascularized site) and the subcutaneous graft (which offers a worse vascularization and obviously involves an important follicular loss). This approach could make possible the identification of the mechanism of angiogenic induction and highlight the comparison with the usual pathway induced by hypoxia. This could help to fight against the follicular loss.

Strategies to fight against ischemia should also be particularly studied by protecting the transplant from oxidative stress or by stimulating the growth of vessels.

CONCLUSION

Since pregnancies can be obtained after grafting the ovarian strips, safeguarding of fertility should absolutely be considered before the use of any gonadotoxic treatment on young women. Many developments have yet to be made, but the idea will remain the same-to preserve the cells able to give to a woman, once cured, the possibility of having children. The cryopreservation of ovarian strips allows that and must thus be studied, taught and improved.

The molecular comprehension of the mechanisms involved will probably help to find treatments likely to improve the results that have so far not been so good.

Nevertheless, this promising technique excites almost all of fertility specialists, who dream of reproducing by themselves this nice story.

REFERENCES

1. Wallace WH, Anderson RA, Irvine DS. Fertility preservation for young patients with cancer: Who is at risk and what can be offered? Lancet Oncol 2005;6:209-18.
2. Larsen EC, Müller J, Schmiegelow K, Rechnitzer C, Andersen AN. Reduced ovarian function in long-term survivors of radiation- and chemotherapy-treated childhood cancer. J Clin Endocrinol Metab 2003;88:5307-14.
3. Larsen EC, Müller J, Rechnitzer C, Schmiegelow K, Andersen AN. Diminished ovarian reserve in female childhood cancer survivors with regular menstrual cycles and basal FSH <10 IU/l. Hum Reprod 2003;18:417-22.
4. Franke HR, WM Smit, I Vermes. Gonadal protection by a gonadotropin-releasing hormone agonist depot in young women with Hodgkin's disease undergoing chemotherapy. Gynecol Endocrinol 2005;20:274-8.
5. Mackie EJ, Radford M, Shalet SM. Gonadal function following chemotherapy for childhood Hodgkin's disease. Med Pediatr Oncol 1996;27:74-8.
6. Schilsky RL, Sherins RJ, Hubbard SM, Wesley MN, Young RC, DeVita VT. Long-term follow-up of ovarian function in women treated with MOPP chemotherapy for Hodgkin's disease. Am J Med 1981;71:552-6.
7. Clark ST, Radford JA, Crowther D, Swindell R, Shalet SM. Gonadal function following chemotherapy for Hodgkin's disease: A comparative study of MVPP and a seven-drug hybrid regimen. J Clin Oncol 1995;13:134-9.
8. Thibaud E, Rodriguez-Macias K, Trivin C, Espérou H, Michon J, Brauner R. Ovarian function after bone marrow transplantation during childhood. Bone Marrow Transplant 1998; 21:287-90.
9. Meirow D. Reproduction post-chemotherapy in young cancer patients. Mol Cell Endocrinol 2000;169:123-31.
10. Hovatta O. Cryobiology of ovarian and testicular tissue. Best Pract Res Clin Obstet Gynaecol 2003;17:331-42.
11. Blumenfeld Z, Dann E, Avivi I, Epelbaum R, Rowe JM. Fertility after treatment for Hodgkin's disease. Ann Oncol 2002;13:138-47.
12. Pereyra Pacheco B, Méndez Ribas JM, Milone G, Fernández I, Kvicala R, Mila T, et al. Use of GnRH analogs for functional protection of the ovary and preservation of fertility during cancer treatment in adolescents: a preliminary report. Gynecol Oncol 2001;81:391-7.
13. Recchia F, Saggio G, Amiconi G, Di Blasio A, Cesta A, Candeloro G, Rea S. Gonadotropin-releasing hormone analogues added to adjuvant chemotherapy protect ovarian function and improve clinical outcomes in young women with early breast carcinoma. Cancer 2006;106:514-23.
14. Sonmezer M, Oktay K. Fertility preservation in female patients. Hum Reprod Update 2004;10:251-66.
15. Liu J, Van der Elst J, Van den Broecke R, Dhont M. Live offspring by *in vitro* fertilization of oocytes from cryopreserved primordial mouse follicles after sequential in vivo transplantation and *in vitro* maturation. Biol Reprod 2001; 64:171-8.
16. Hreinsson JG, Scott JE, Rasmussen C, Swahn ML, Hsueh AJ, Hovatta O. Growth differentiation factor-9 promotes the growth, development, and survival of human ovarian follicles in organ culture. J Clin Endocrinol Metab 2002;87:316-21.
17. Gook DA, Edgar DH, Borg J, Archer J, Lutjen PJ, McBain JC. Oocyte maturation, follicle rupture and luteinization in human cryopreserved ovarian tissue following xenografting. Hum Reprod 2003;18:1772-81.
18. Paris MC, Snow M, Cox SL, Shaw JM. Xenotransplantation: a tool for reproductive biology and animal conservation? Theriogenology 2004;61:277-91.
19. Mavroforou A, Michalodimitrakis E. Moral arguments on the use of ovarian tissue from aborted foetuses in infertility treatment. Hum Reprod Genet Ethics 2005;11:6-11.
20. Hilders CG, Baranski AG, Peters L, Ramkhelawan A, Trimbos JB. Successful human ovarian autotransplantation to the upper arm. Cancer 2004;101:2771-8.
21. Wang X, Chen H, Yin H, Kim SS, Lin Tan S, Gosden RG. Fertility after intact ovary transplantation. Nature 2002;415:385.
22. Leporrier M, von Theobald P, Roffe JL, Muller G. A new technique to protect ovarian function before pelvic irradiation. Heterotopic ovarian autotransplantation. Cancer 1987;60: 2201-4.
23. Gosden RG, Baird DT, Wade JC, Webb R. Restoration of fertility to oophorectomized sheep by ovarian autografts stored at -196 degrees C. Hum Reprod 1994;9:597-603.
24. Lee DM, Yeoman RR, Battaglia DE, Stouffer RL, Zelinski-Wooten MB, Fanton JW, Wolf DP. Live birth after ovarian tissue transplant. Nature, 2004;428:137-8.
25. Donnez J, Squifflet J, Dolmans MM, Martinez-Madrid B, Jadoul P, Van Langendonckt A. Orthotopic transplantation of fresh ovarian cortex: A report of two cases. Fertil Steril 2005;84:1018.
26. Oktay K, Buyuk E, Rosenwaks Z, Rucinski J. A technique for transplantation of ovarian cortical strips to the forearm. Fertil Steril 2003;80:193-8.

27. Kim SS, Hwang IT, Lee HC. Heterotopic autotransplantation of cryobanked human ovarian tissue as a strategy to restore ovarian function. Fertil Steril 2004;82:930-2.

28. Oktay K, Buyuk E, Veeck L, Zaninovic N, Xu K, Takeuchi T, Opsahl M, Rosenwaks Z. Embryo development after heterotopic transplantation of cryopreserved ovarian tissue. Lancet 2004;363:837-40.

29. Donnez J, Dolmans MM, Demylle D, Jadoul P, Pirard C, Squifflet J, Martinez-Madrid B, van Langendonckt A. Livebirth after orthotopic transplantation of cryopreserved ovarian tissue. Lancet 2004;364:1405-10.

30. Oktay K, Tilly J. Live birth after cryopreserved ovarian tissue autotransplantation. Lancet 2004;364:2091-2.

31. Hubinont C, Debieve F, Biard JM, Debauche C, Bernard P. Livebirth after cryopreserved ovarian tissue autotransplantation. Lancet 2004;364:2093.

32. Smitz J, Cortvrindt R. First childbirth from transplanted cryopreserved ovarian tissue brings hope for cancer survivors. Lancet 2004;364:1379-80.

33. Silber SJ, Lenahan KM, Levine DJ, Pineda JA, Gorman KS, Friez MJ, Crawford EC, Gosden RG. Ovarian transplantation between monozygotic twins discordant for premature ovarian failure. N Engl J Med, 2005;353:58-63.

34. Meirow D, Levron J, Eldar-Geva T, Hardan I, Fridman E, Zalel Y, Schiff E, Dor J. Pregnancy after transplantation of cryopreserved ovarian tissue in a patient with ovarian failure after chemotherapy. N Engl J Med 2005;353:318-21.

35. Siegel-Itzkovich J. Woman gives birth after receiving transplant of her own ovarian tissue. BMJ 2005;331:70.

36. Demeestere I, Simon P, Buxant F, Robin V, Fernandez SA, Centner J, et al. Ovarian function and spontaneous pregnancy after combined heterotopic and orthotopic cryopreserved ovarian tissue transplantation in a patient previously treated with bone marrow transplantation: case report. Hum Reprod 2006;21:2010-4.

37. Rosendahl M, Loft A, Byskov AG, Ziebe S, Schmidt KT, Andersen AN, et al. Biochemical pregnancy after fertilization of an oocyte aspirated from a heterotopic autotransplant of cryopreserved ovarian tissue: case report. Hum Reprod 2006;21:2006-9.

38. Jeremias E, Bedaiwy MA, Nelson D, Biscotti CV, Falcone T. Assessment of tissue injury in cryopreserved ovarian tissue. Fertil Steril 2003;79:651-3.

39. Hernandez-Fonseca H, Bosch P, Sirisathien S, Wininger JD, Massey JB, Brackett BG. Effect of site of transplantation on follicular development of human ovarian tissue transplanted into intact or castrated immunodeficient mice. Fertil Steril 2004;81:888-92.

40. Oktay K, Buyuk E. Fertility preservation in women undergoing cancer treatment. Lancet 2004;363:1830.

41. Martinez-Madrid B, Dolmans MM, Van Langendonckt A, Defrère S, Donnez J. Freeze-thawing intact human ovary with its vascular pedicle with a passive cooling device. Fertil Steril 2004;82:1390-4.

42. Gougeon A, Ecochard R, Thalabard JC. Age-related changes of the population of human ovarian follicles: increase in the disappearance rate of non-growing and early-growing follicles in aging women. Biol Reprod 1994;50:653-63.

43. Dolmans MM, Michaux N, Camboni A, Martinez-Madrid B, Van Langendonckt A, Nottola SA, Donnez J. Evaluation of Liberase, a purified enzyme blend, for the isolation of human primordial and primary ovarian follicles. Hum Reprod 2006;21:413-20.

44. Martinez-Madrid B, Dolmans MM, Langendonckt AV, Defrère S, Van Eyck AS, Donnez J. Ficoll density gradient method for recovery of isolated human ovarian primordial follicles. Fertil Steril 2004;82:1648-53.

45. Kauff ND, Satagopan JM, Robson ME, Scheuer L, Hensley M, Hudis CA. Risk-reducing salpingo-oophorectomy in women with a BRCA1 or BRCA2 mutation. N Engl J Med 2002;346:1609-15.

46. Kim SS, Battaglia DE, Soules MR. The future of human ovarian cryopreservation and transplantation: fertility and beyond. Fertil Steril 2001;75:1049-56.

47. Sonmezer M, Shamonki MI, Oktay K. Ovarian tissue cryopreservation: benefits and risks. Cell Tissue Res 2005;322:125-32.

Is Aspirin Useful in ART Protocols?

Kaberi Banerjee

INTRODUCTION

Aspirin (acetyl-salicylic acid) was discovered in the late nineteenth century and was marketed by Bayer as an effective cure for headache and rheumatic pain. It is widely used for its analgesic, anti-inflammatory and antipyretic action but over the past few decades, its use as an antithrombotic, when used in low doses, has been increasing. Its use in patients with coronary artery disease has been firmly established[1,2] and in Obstetrics, a number of randomized control trials (RCT) and meta-analyses have been conducted to establish its benefit in preventing pre-eclampsia and associated intrauterine growth retardation (IUGR).[3-5]

Antithrombotic Effect

Aspirin inhibits cyclooxygenase production by platelets at a low dose (60–150 mg/day). This inhibits thromboxane production and leads to the inhibition of platelet aggregation. At higher doses, it inhibits cyclooxygenase production by the endothelial vessel wall and this leads to inhibition of prostacyclin production. Since prostacyclin is a vasodilator, higher doses of Aspirin leads to vasoconstriction.

CLINICAL DISCUSSION

Aspirin and IVF

The proposed mechanism for the beneficial effect of Aspirin *in vitro* fertilization (IVF) is thought to be through its anti-thrombotic effect, which in turn, could improve tissue perfusion. A good blood supply to the ovaries might optimize delivery of exogenous gonadotropins to the gland and hence, could improve ovarian response in patients undergoing IVF. This might be useful for patients who have reduced ovarian response. Low-dose Aspirin (LDA) might also improve uterine blood flow and improve the endometrial receptivity and therefore, improve implantation. This could be beneficial in patients with failed implantation and in those with a thin endometrium.

A large RCT (n = 298) was conducted in patients undergoing IVF for tubal infertility, using 100 mg of aspirin versus placebo from day 21 of the cycle up to 12 weeks of pregnancy.[6] The study showed improved ovarian responsiveness, measured by the number of follicles more than 15 mm, number of oocytes retrieved, mean pulsatility index of uterine and ovarian arterties, implantation and clinical pregnancy rates in the group that took Aspirin as compared to the group who took placebo. The clinical pregnancy rates in the Aspirin group were 45 percent as compared to 28 percent in the placebo group, which was significantly different (p < 0.05).

Another large RCT (n = 1380) concluded that Aspirin improves success rates in IVF cycles. In Group 1, 75 mg of Aspirin was started from the day of embryo transfer and continued till the determination of a pregnancy test.[7] In Group 2, no medication was given. Administering Aspirin improved live birth rates from 23.2 percent to 27.2 percent (odds ratio:1.2, confidence interval:1-1.6).

The role of Aspirin in women with a thin endometrium (< 8 mm) in a previous evaluation cycle of oocyte donation has also been studied.[8] The study of population was randomized into those who received 81 mg of Aspirin (n = 15) and those who did not receive any medication (n = 13) from 1 week before estrogen therapy to 9 weeks after embryo transfer, if the pregnancy test was positive. Though there was no increase in the endometrium thickness, the implantation rate was significantly higher in the Aspirin group (24% vs 9%).

Another study attempted to evaluate the role of Aspirin in improving the uterine blood flow in patients with reduced uterine perfusion documented on Doppler flowmetry.[9] Ninety-nine women undergoing frozen embryo replacement cycle were recruited. The study population was divided into two groups, Group 1 with reduced uterine perfusion and Group 2 with normal uterine perfusion. In their first attempt, Group 1 received LDA (150–300 mg) starting from day 13 of hormone replacement. Those in Group 2 did not receive any Aspirin. In subsequent attempts, Group 1 was arbitrarily allocated to start Aspirin on day 1 or day 13 of estrogen supplementation and 10 women from Group 2 were arbitrarily selected to receive Aspirin from day 1. In Group 2 addition of Aspirin did not improve the pregnancy rates. In Group 1 improved blood flow and pregnancy rates (47% vs 17%, respectively) were achieved in those taking Aspirin from day 1. It thus appears that Aspirin improves uterine perfusion and pregnancy rates in those with already reduced blood flow.

There have been other studies which concluded that Aspirin does not make any significant difference to the implantation or clinical pregnancy rate. Two hundred and seventy-nine unselected patients undergoing intracytoplasmic sperm injection (ICSI) were randomized into two groups, one receiving 80 mg of Aspirin from day 1 of ovarian hyperstimulation and group 2, which did not receive any treatment.[10] The study concluded that low-dose Aspirin did not improve implantation and pregnancy rates in this study population. Lok, et al.[11] conducted a double blind randomized control trial (n = 60) and concluded that addition of Aspirin in poor responders (raised FSH, previous cancelled cycles, age <40 years) did not improve ovarian and uterine blood flow or ovarian responsiveness.[11] They used 80 mg Aspirin from the day of gonadotropin-releasing hormone (GnRH) downregulation to the day of oocyte collection or transfer. Another small study (n = 36) concluded that in women with previous failed cycles, who are undergoing a frozen embryo replacement cycle, the addition of Aspirin from day 2 of cycle till pregnancy continued, if pregnancy test was positive, made no difference to the clinical pregnancy rate or the implantation rate.[12]

What is the role of Aspirin in antiphospholipid antibody (APA) positive patients undergoing IVF? Though a few studies have claimed that Aspirin in combination with Heparin or Prednisolone improves pregnancy rates, there has recently been strong evidence to doubt the role of APA positivity in patients undergoing IVF.[13,14] Chilcott, et al.[15] found that though the prevalence of the APA in an IVF population was higher than expected in a normal population, there was no difference in pregnancy and live birth outcomes, regardless of APA status.[15] In a recent meta-analysis, the clinical pregnancy rate and live birth rate (LBR) of APA positive and APA negative was comparable.[16] Thus, it appears that medical intervention just for the sake of APA positivity is not required in patients undergoing IVF.

Thus, one study has concluded that administration of 100 mg of the Aspirin from day 21 of the cycle up to 12 weeks of pregnancy improved pregnancy rates.[6] Four studies have been conducted to see if Aspirin is beneficial when given after embryo replacement.[7-9,12] Two studies were conducted on frozen cycles,[9,12] one was in a fresh cycle,[7] and one study was conducted to see if it was beneficial in patients undergoing oocyte donation and where a previous evaluation cycle has shown that the endometrium does not grow beyond 8 mm.[8] Most of these studies have concluded that using Aspirin improves the chances of success. One study conducted in poor responders failed to show its benefit.[11]

The drawback of the above studies lies in their inconsistencies in the dose of Aspirin used, the use of placebo, time of starting or time of stopping Aspirin. Regardless of the above flaws, the above studies indicate that the use of Aspirin in IVF is promising. There are however, many issues to be resolved. What is the right dose? When should it be started? Until when should it be continued? Which group of patients will benefit most from it?

Meta-analysis of the Role of Aspirin in Patients Undergoing IVF-ICSI[17]

A decision was made to conduct a meta-analysis to find out if Aspirin should be routinely given to patients undergoing IVF-ICSI treatment at Guys and St Thomas Hospital, London. Searches were conducted in MEDLINE, EMBASE, Cochrane Library, National Research Register, and SCISEARCH, and all randomized controlled trials that evaluated the effectiveness of Aspirin compared to placebo or no treatment in women undergoing IVF-ICSI treatment were included. Seven relevant trials, including a total of 1241 women, were identified.[6,8,10-12,18,19] The largest study to date reporting on the use of LDA in IVF was a quasi-randomized study.[7] This study reported a trend of beneficial effect of LDA on both clinical pregnancy and live birth rates [OR 1.3, 95% CI (1.0–1.6)] and 1.2, 95% CI (1.0–1.6), respectively. This study however, was excluded as it reported on 1022 patients in 1380 cycles, which means that some patients must have contributed to more than one cycle of treatment. As observations from this study are not independent, pooling of results using data from it would invalidate the meta-analysis. Despite the persistence of the trend of beneficial effect of LDA in a subgroup analysis for outcomes using the first cycles of treatment only, the lack of proper randomization (by alternate days to Aspirin or 'no treatment' in this study) and more importantly, lack of allocation concealment might have introduced bias with a tendency of overestimating the treatment effect by upto 40 percent.[20] This would negate drawing valid conclusions by pooling results of first cycles of treatment of this study together with other studies in the meta-analyses. A meta-analysis of the other randomized controled trials did not show a significant benefit of Aspirin therapy in improving the clinical pregnancy rate (RR 1.11, 95% CI 0.95, 1.31) or live birth rate (RR 0.94, 95%

CI 0.64, 1.39) in patients undergoing IVF or ICSI treatment. There was no significant difference in the miscarriage rate (RR 1.06, 95% CI 0.53, 2.11) or ectopic pregnancy rate (RR 2.24, 95% CI 0.70, 7.24) between the treatment and control groups. There was a significant improvement in uterine artery pulsatility index in patients taking low dose Aspirin [(weighted mean difference (WMD) –0.78, 95% CI –0.87, –0.69)] and in the number of oocytes retrieved (WMD 2.46, 95% CI 1.65, 3.27). The evidence regarding other surrogate outcomes was either not significant or contradictory.

CONCLUSION

Based on the findings of our review, Aspirin therapy cannot currently be recommended for routine clinical use, outside the context of a clinical trial. However, given the paucity of the existing evidence, the lack of power in the available trials to detect minimally important treatment effects in clinically meaningful outcomes and the trend of benefit demonstrable in the point estimate of clinical pregnancy in this review, a double-blinded, placebo controlled randomized trial with an adequate sample size is needed to reach a definitive conclusion on the effect of low dose Aspirin on the important clinical outcomes as pregnancy and/or live birth rates in an IVF setting.

REFERENCES

1. Elwood PC, Stillings MR. Use of aspirin in cardiovascular prophylaxis. Cardiovasc J S Afr 2000;11:155-60.
2. European Action on Secondary Prevention by Intervention to reduce Events. EUROASPIRE 1 and 2 Group. Clinical reality of coronary prevention guidelines: a comparison of EUROASPIRE 1 and 2 in nine countries. EUROASPIRE 1 and 2 Group. Lancet 2001;31:995-1001.
3. Dekker G, Sibai B. Primary, secondary and tertiary prevention of pre-eclampsia. Lancet 2001;357:209-15.
4. Duley L, Henderson-Smart DJ, Knight M, King JF. Antiplatelet agents for preventing pre-eclampsia and its complication. Cochrane Database Syst Rev. 2004(1):CD004659.
5. Coomarasamy A, Honest H, Papaioannou S, Gee H, Khan KS. Aspirin for prevention of pre-eclampsia in women with historical risk factors: a systematic review. Obstet Gynecol 2003;101:1319-32
6. Rubinstein M, Marazzi A, Polak de Fried E. Low dose aspirin treatment improves ovarian responsiveness, uterine and ovarian blood flow velocity, implantation and pregnancy rates in patients undergoing *in vitro* fertilization: a prospective, randomized, double-blind placebo-controlled assay. Fertil Steril 1999;71:825-9.
7. Waldenstom U, Hellberg D, Nilsson S. Low dose aspirin in a short regimen as standard treatment in *in vitro* fertilization: a randomized, prospective study. Fertil Steril 2004;81:1560-4.
8. Weckstein LN, Jacobson A, Galen D, Hampton K, Hanmel J. Low dose aspirin for oocyte donation recipients with a thin endometrium: prospective, randomized study. Fertil Steril 1997;68:927-30.
9. Wada I, Hsu CC, William G, Macnamee MC, Brinsden PR. The benefits of low dose aspirin therapy in women with impaired uterine perfusion during assisted conception. Hum Reprod 1994;10:1954-7.
10. Urman B, Mercan R, Alatas C, Balaban B, Isiklar A, Nuhoglu A. Low dose aspirin does not increase implantation rates inpatients undergoing ICSI: a prospective randomized study. J Assist Reprod Genet 2000;17:586-90.
11. Lok IH, Yip SK, Cheung LP, Yin Leung PH, Haines CJ. Adjuvant low dose aspirin therapy in poor responders undergoing *in vitro* fertilization: a prospective, randomized, double-blind, placebo-controlled trial. Fertil Steril 2004;81:556-61.
12. Check JH, Dietterich C, Lurie D, Nazari A, Chuong J. A matched study to determine whether low dose aspirin therapy in women with impaired uterine perfusion during assisted conception. Hum Reprod 1994;10:1954-7.
13. Geva E, Amit A, Lerner-Geve L, Yaron Y, Daniel Y, Schwartz, et al. Prednisolone and aspirin improve pregnancy rates in patients with reproductive failure and autoimmune antibodies: a prospective study. Am J Reprod Immunol 2000;43:36-40.
14. Sher G, Zouves C, Feinman M, Massarani G, Matzer W, Chong P, et al. A rational basis for use of combined heparin/aspirin and IVIG immunotherapy in the treatment of recurrent IVF failure associated with antiphospholipid antibodies. Am J Reprod Immunol 1998;39:391-4.
15. Chilcott IT, Raul M, Cohen H, Rai R, Skull J, Pickering W, et al. Pregnancy outcome is not affected by antiphospholipid antibody status in women referred for *in vitro* fertilization. Fertil Steril 2000;73:526-30.
16. Hornstein M, Davis OK, Massey JB, Paulson R, Collins JA. Antiphospholipid antibodies and *in vitro* fertilization success: a meta-analysis. Fertil Steril 2000;73:526-30.
17. Khairy M, Banerjee K, El-Toukhy T, Coomarasamy A, Khalaf Y. Aspirin in women undergoing IVF treatment: a systematic review and meta-analysis. Fertil Steril (in press).
18. Van Doreen IM, Schoot BC, Dargel E, Maas P. Low dose aspirin demonstrates no positive effect on clinical results in the first *in vitro* fertilization (IVF) cycle. Fertil Steril 2004;82:O-46 S18.
19. Pakkila M, Rasanen J, Heinonen S, Tinkanen H, Tuomivaara L, Mäkikallio K, et al. Low dose aspirin does not improve ovarian responsiveness or pregnancy rate in IVF and ICSI patients: a randomized, placebo-controlled double-blind study. Human Reproduction 2005;20:2211-4.
20. Schulz KF, Chalmers I, Hayes RJ, Altman DG, et al. Empirical evidence of bias: dimensions of methodological quality associated with estimates of treatment effects in controlled trials. JAMA 1995;273:408-12.

Cytokines and Embryo Implantation

Gérard Chaouat, Fabrice Petit, Mona Rahmati, Marie Petitbarat, Sylvie Dubanchet, Nathalie Ledée

OVERVIEW

In this review, we discuss some of the aspects of the role of cytokines in implantation and immediate postimplantation, which might govern the onset of recurrent spontaneous miscarriages as well as pre-eclampsia. We briefly describe the implantation in steps, and then summarize the status of embryo signals research. This allows us to describe the possibility of embryo selection for an optimized single embryo transfer policy. This is followed by the role of inflammation in early implantation, focusing on leukemia inhibitory factor (LIF) and colony stimulating factor (CSF) as well as of seminal fluid cytokines. This step is followed by the establishment of the Th2 predominance, briefly described before turning on to the control of angiogenesis by the uterine natural killer (NK) cells, which of course, leads to summarize the status of vascular endothelial growth factor (VEGF) as well as angiopoietins. We then turn to the regulation of these by the IL-15/IL-18 tripod, and the role of Tregs, and finish with the role of the complement pathway. We conclude by highlighting the complexity revealed by transcriptomics.

INTRODUCTION

Normal embryo implantation occurs in the uterus, which is the only place where an embryo normally cannot implant except in a precisely timed period, where uterine and embryo programs coincide, which defines the 'implantation window'.

This does not mean that the embryo cannot implant elsewhere, and extrauterine and tubal pregnancies are here to testify for that, as are the very few cases reported each year of term cesarean deliveries of abdominal pregnancies.

These pregnancies are a surgical emergency due to massive intraperitoneal hemorrhages, except when peritoneal adherence prevents intra-abdominal bleeding, and creates a pseudodecidua.

Such a problem is due to the lack of dilatable arteries at the ectopic implantation site, a function exerted at normal implantation one by the spiral arteries, the first key determinant of implantation. The second one is of course, adhesion and proper control of invasion. The third one is the establishment of a materno-fetal immune dialog, which is key to postimplantation pregnancy maintenance, since it precludes the lack of a maternal anti-fetal immune rejection process, what is often termed 'maternal tolerance to the fetal allograft'*.[1]

But first, it has indeed been an important discovery of the last years made by Reproductive Immunologists that the development of such arteries is controlled by cytokines, that are either secreted or regulated by uterine natural killer cells (uNK).[2,3] It is not a hazard that such cells are absent from the 'implantation' site of tubal pregnancies as well as in the case of abdominal pregnancies.[4]

For the second aspect, cytokines not only control the angiogenic process, but they are also involved in the induction of adhesion molecules, as well as in the establishment of a proper balance between matrix metalloproteases (MMP) versus tissue inhibitors of metalloproteases (TIMP).[5]

Finally, we will see that immune 'tolerance' is linked to the role of Th2 cytokines.

---

* As discussed in (1), it is NOT a real immunological tolerance to paternal alloantigens but a transient local one, which is at best associated with systemic anti-paternal hyporesponsiveness in the first pregnancy.

Implantation Steps

Cytokine networks are themselves at least partly hormone dependent, as is the preparation of the uterus to the very process of implantation. This preparation in the cycle involves cytokines. The most classical example is the uterine secretion of LIF, which is the first cytokine, if not the first molecule, which was demonstrated to be absolutely required for successful implantation in mice,[6] and appears important for implantation in humans (see below).

The proper uterine secretion of LIF is clearly dependent upon a progesterone signal,[7] up to the point that in the mink, where there is a delayed implantation, the awakening of the previously 'dormant' embryo in spring is provoked by such a signal.[8]

Let us recall here that the implantation process itself is divided into four stages; orientation, apposition, adhesion, and invasion (Fig. 69.1).

Grossly, LIF, as well as several inflammatory cytokines, control adhesion, while other cytokines control invasion, and the immediate post implantation steps involve 'tolerance mechanisms', and this is where Th2 cytokines intervene. However, it may be observed that this is slightly more complex than it seems.

Embryo Signals

The first stages, which occur immediately after fecundation are characterized by an intense blastocyst metabolic activity, amongst which is the secretion of soluble mediators.

The question of whether some of these are 'embryonic signals' required for successful implantation is an important one. It could either directly be a cytokine or a factor acting on cytokine production. Amongst the latter is soluble HLA-G (sHLA-G), which is now well-known to inhibit killer cell activity and regulate local angiogenesis.[9]

Great hopes have followed the initial report by Fuzzi, et al.[10] which concluded that sHLA-G was a reliable marker of embryo implantation, since only those embryos which produced it in embryo culture supernatants would have the capacity to implant. However, many other workers do not report such a 'black and white correlation' and there are even scientists who do not detect any sHLA-G in such supernatants, and even suspect that such a detection could be an artefact.[11]

The reasons for such discrepancies are various, and discussed in detail,[12] where a study of our own network is also described.

At present, we believe that the commercial kits available do not permit a reproducible and reliable dosage, nor that sHLA-G measurement would permit an absolute selection of the embryos, which will implant versus those which will not. At present, the aim must be to establish robust reproducible systems that function identically in all laboratories.[12]

Embryo signals nevertheless, do exist: two excellent examples are trophoblast interferons in ovine species, and Wnt/beta catenin pathways in rodents.

In ruminant species, there is no chorionic gonadotropin. The search for an equivalent material lead to the discovery of 'trophoblastin'- ovine trophoblast protein (oTP), which was found to define a new class of interferons (tau) that is highly conserved across species.[13]

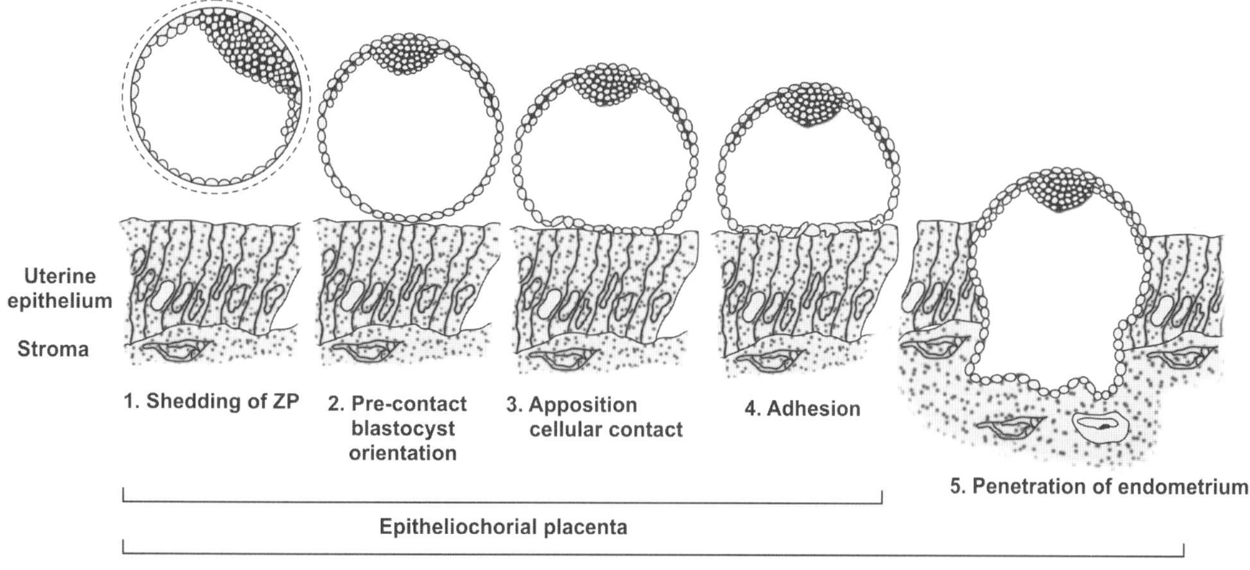

Fig. 69.1: Stages of implantation

In contrast to gamma interferons, which are abortifacient at high doses, tau interferons are neither cytostatic nor cytotoxic for the trophoblasts, which secrete them at the trophoblast/trophectoderm 'elongation' stage. It has a series of immunoregulatory and antiviral activities, while also maintaining the corpus luteum.[13,14]

Trophoblast interferons have been demonstrated in mice,[15] where they were previously thought not to exist. However, despite the initial results from Imakawa's group, presented in the 90s,[16] the search for tau interferon equivalents in humans has been negative.

The second example is the Wnt beta catenin pathway in mice: Dufort, et al.[17] have shown that activation of this pathway is mandatory for implantation, and this depends on yet uncharacterized soluble embryonic factors plus estrogens.[17]

The action is dependent upon two steps. First, there is a transient activation of the circular smooth muscle on early day 4. Subsequently, embryonic factors activate the luminal epithelium at the future implantation site, and involve regulation of LIF production, an inflammatory cytokine (see below).[17] More interesting is the fact that using Luminex based assays, or in the future, adapted enzyme-linked immunosorbent assay (ELISA)-based assays, one might be able to select the embryos which have a good potential for implantation before even IVF itself, based on the determination of the cytokine content of the follicular fluid (FF).

Indeed, the EMBIC groups have shown on sHLA-G and we have cited EMBIC conclusions elsewhere. But most important in our opinion, it seems possible to predict the embryo implantation potential as early as oocyte retrieval for *in vitro* fertilization (IVF)/intracytoplasmic sperm injection (ICSI), with a key role for follicular fluid (FF), granulocyte colony-stimulating factor (G-CSF) and IL-15.[18-20]

In a first pilot study under the co-direction of Ledée and Piccinni, Florence, we measured by Luminex the cytokine content (28 cytokines and chemokines) of each individual FF after oocyte collection and traced the fate of the subsequent embryos. The most important result was that the level of G-CSF in individual FF samples was correlated with the implantation potential of the corresponding embryo.[18]

A second study involved modified natural IVF/ICSI cycles, and reproducibility of follicular composition was evaluated over two cycles for 15 patients, which is important if one wants to be sure that there is no variation between each cycle. A multiple analysis confirmed the value of G-CSF, but in addition, we found that a combination of both FF G-CSF and IL-15 was the optimal model to predict birth.[19,20]

Inflammation and Implantation

As far as the uterus is concerned, a series of studies indeed point out to the role of inflammatory cytokines in implantation, some of them being triggered by the mating itself.[21,22] Amongst these, an important one may be IL-1. The initial studies of Simon, et al.[23] showing that blocking the IL-1 receptor by IL-1Ra totally prevented implantation[23] have never been reproduced, and IL-1 KO or IL-1 receptor KO mice breed normally.[24]

Yet, there is a lot of evidence for IL-1 presence in murine and, more important, human reproductive tract,[25] and it has been shown, for example, that IL-1 can regulate the production of LIF in explants culture of human endometrial biopsy fragments.[26]

LIF, as stated, was the first cytokine shown to be absolutely necessary for murine implantation: LIF KO results in total implantation failure, and even LIF+/LIF+ embryos do not implant in a LIF–/LIF– mother. This is corrected by osmotic pump delivery of recombinant LIF.[6]

In humans, a proportion of sterile women have no or few LIF when LIF production is assessed by ELISA in the supernatants of endometrial explants or in flushing liquids,[26,27] and some sterile women have LIF mutations, which render it ineffective in the uterus.[28,29]

A trial of recombinant LIF (r-LIF) was conducted by an important pharmaceutical firm, but was negative. It should be stated, however, that r-LIF was given to an unselected group of patients, e.g. without assessing beforehand their status as LIF non-producers. Since only a small proportion of sterile patients are (positive for uterine) LIF or harbor LIF mutations, this negative result was highly predictable and we indeed, did forecast a negative outcome of the trial.

CSF-1 or, in line with Simon's observations, IL-1 are LIF inducers in a progesterone prepared environment.[30]

Recently, in mice, LIF has been linked to the Wnt beta catenin pathways.[17] Another important cytokine is IL-11, and mice KO for the IL-11 R alpha receptor have abnormal decidualization, leading to implantation failure.[31]

In addition, the trophoblast differentiates and expresses placental lactogen-I in such mice, but they do not expand and the decidual vasculature, as well as the number of uterine natural killer cells, is abnormal at the implantation sites of IL-11R alpha mutant mice. Very low levels of endometrial IL-11 have been reported in women suffering implantation defects or infertile with endometriosis.[32,33]

Keeping with the data of Ledée, et al.[34] suggesting that natural cycles may be better alternatives in some cases,[34] a report exists showing reduced expression of interleukin-11 and interleukin-6 in the peri-implantation endometrium of excessive ovarian responders.[33]

Colony-stimulating factors are known to be important. CSF-1 is a major growth factor for trophoblasts, and increases in a programmed fashion in the uterus.[35]

However, the sterility observed in CSF-1 negative mice involves both female and male defects, rendering the final interpretation of the data confusing.

As for granulocyte macrophage colony-stimulating factor (GM-CSF) (as well as GM-CSF+ CSF KO) mice have small litter size due to fetal loss by resorbtion post-implantation,[36] in agreement with the 'immunotrophic' hypothesis of Wegmann, et al.[37] and our own data of prevention by rGM-CSF of abortion in a murine model.[38]

The data on CSF prompted studies by the Robertson's group[39] on the effects of mating itself. It lead them to discover that mating prepares the uterus for implantation, as well as future 'tolerance' to the embryonic 'allograft,' and obviously also pre-eclampsia, with a cardinal role for GM-CSF and TGF beta.[39] The effects could be linked to the local recruitment of local regulatory T cells.[40,41]

Besides, conflicting results have been found in mice (mice are fertile for some, reduced litter size for others, and one group correlates high IL-6 levels with abortion in the CBA × DBA/2 murine model.[42] One should rather state here that in humans, the Robertson group reports a low IL-6 (and IL-1alpha) mRNAs in secretory endometrium in case of recurrent miscarriage.[43]

The Th1/Th2 Cytokine Balance

The classical view is the Th1/Th2 paradigm.[44,45] Investigations in a murine model of early pregnancy loss have revealed very high levels of tumor necrosis factor (TNF) and gamma interferon, and almost absence of the classical Th2 cytokines (IL-3, IL-4, IL 10) in aborting mice, and more precisely, in those uterine chambers where early resorption occurs.[46]

Additionally, it was well-known that the humoral immune responses and associated pathologies, such as lupus, flare during pregnancy, while cell-mediated ones, such as rheumatoid polyarthritis, often remit. In parallel, peripheral blood NK cell lytic units as measured by a ^{51}Cr CRT test, are lowered in pregnant women. Therefore, in an Immunology Today 1993 citation classic, Tom Wegmann enunciated that 'successful pregnancy is a Th2 phenomenon.'[44]

Indeed, the classical Th1 cytokines synergized in inducing abortion, and incidentally their neutralization rescue the mice from abortion.[46] Their action is on maternal vessel coagulation,[47,48] explaining the role of Aspirin and heparin in miscarriage treatment, which was claimed by Alan Beer himself to be rather effective.[49]

In this context, it is important to quote that progesterone receptors are expressed by activated T cells. This allows them, in such a progesterone rich environment, to secrete progesterone induced blocking factor (PIBF), which blocks NK activity, and further promotes the Th2 bias.[50] It has now been tested in human implantation defects upon induction with dihydrogesterone.[51]

In humans, excess gamma interferon and TNF was earlier termed by Joe Hill as 'immunodystrophism' in case of IVF failures.[52]

As for recurrent spontaneous pregnancy loss, a great number of studies reported that Th1 cytokines were incompatible with successful pregnancy, and for example, Raghupathy's group showed that lymphocytes from spontaneous aborters display a clear Th1 bias in an *in vitro* model of anti-placental immune responses, as was confirmed later by several cohort studies, such as those of Jenkins, who also extended the Th1 bias to IL-12.[53,54]

In the same vein, Piccini, et al.[55] used cloned decidual T cell but also associated the Th2 bias with a parallel involvement of non Th1/Th2 cytokines, the M-CSF, -immunotrophic and LIF (see above).[55]

It is in this context that the neutralization of TNF by anti-TNF drugs for implantation failure or recurrent spontaneous abortions was proposed.

The results by Winger and Reed were extremely interesting in that context,[56,57] but we expressed concerns about their use during pregnancy itself,[58] and indeed, such concerns were the prime reason why we did not start lymphokine or anti-TNF therapy ourselves despite our murine data,[38,46] especially neutralization of TNF and gamma interferon.[46] Recent data, however, levitates these concerns, since the treatment seems efficient even if given before IVF itself.[59]

Closer to our earlier murine data about the effects of CSF,[38] Scarpellini and Sbrascia[60] have reported the use of recombinant G-CSF in treatment of early pregnancy loss.[60] This might be linked to GM-CSF control of Th1/Th2 balance as well as the immunotrophic properties of this cytokine, or both. It should be stated, however, that these results need confirmation and, because of a possible epigenetic action on the embryo, a follow-up register is highly necessary.

A Cardinal Role for Uterine Natural Killer (NK) Cells

A significant development has been the emergence of a new role for uterine NK cells (uNKs). Until recently, these cells were seen as 'bad guys' by the classical Th1/Th2 paradigm, whose activation would cause abortion.[44] However, at the time of implantation, the uterine stroma is replete with NK cells (60 to 80% of the stroma in mice and human), which are indeed activated to massively secrete IL-18, viewed otherwise as abortogenic in an established pregnancy.

Even more confusing for the classical Th1/Th2 bias, there is more IL-18, in a murine non abortion-prone mating than in control ones.[61] The explanation comes from the studies of Croy's group and those of Guimond, et al. initially showing that uNK deficient mice harbor massive reproductive defects, such as reduced placental size and very thick uterine arteries, leading to fetal deaths.[2,62-64] Such thick vascular walls are also seen in IL-15 KO mice, but in this case, it does not cause fetal death,[65] a lack of lethality also observed in the Il-2 receptor common gamma chain KO mice.[66] Also, it must be stated that implantation per se, is not affected in any of those NK-deficient mice.

Subsequent experiments have shown that interferon gamma is required at the implantation site to 'properly activate' uNK, which control the uterine vascular bed remodelling and indeed, interferon gamma receptor KOs display implantation defects as well vascular anomalies.

The common explanation for these phenomena is that uterine NK cells secrete angiogenic factors, including angiopoietin 2 and VEGF.[64]

Angiogenic Cytokines

As far as VEGF is concerned, it also is expressed in the pre- and peri-implantation uterine stroma and not solely by uNK cells in the human,[67,68] and animals, including in species with delayed implantation such as the mink. Its expression is also regulated by hormones during the cycle as well as chorionic gonadotropin at implantation,[67-69] as well as the level of soluble VEGF receptor. It is outside the scope of this study to detail that, but it must be mentioned that sVEGF-R excess is likely an important determinant of pre-eclampsia since the work of Karumanchi (see below for the role of complement in that respect). These observations have prompted implantation blockade assays in rhesus monkeys by injecting neutralizing antibody to VEGF,[70] an eventual prelude to anti-angiogenic drug-mediated abortion/contraception in humans.

Angiopoietin-2 is secreted essentially by uNK cells by mice and humans, rather than uterine stroma during estrogen-dominated cycling phase and the progesterone-dominated mated phase, whereas another cytokine with angiogenic effects, Ang-1 is seen only in the 2nd phase in the uterus, angiopoietin 1 is also expressed by preimplantation mouse embryos and may synergize and complement the uterine one at implantation.[71-75]

Local gamma interferons + IL-15 properly activate pre/peri-implantation uNK, which also seems to depend upon a proper interaction of uterine NK receptors with major histocompatibility complex (MHC) antigens of the invading trophoblasts, mostly HLA-G and HLA-C in humans, which might link implantation defects and pre-eclampsia.[76] Indeed, angiopoietin and VEGF deregulations have been observed in miscarriages[77] and defective interactions with HLA-G/HLA-C are also suspected in recurrent miscarriages.[78]

HLA-G also interacts directly with the vascular endothelium,[3,9,79] and studies in mice confirm the role of maternal cells/paternal antigen recognition in regulating optimal utero-placental vascularization.[80]

Other Regulations of Importance

In addition, there is intervention of IL-12, IL-18 and EBI3 (Epstein Barr virus–induced protein) chain of IL-27, or IL-18 binding protein (IL-18 BP).

In humans, abnormal levels of these correlate with pathologic sub-endometrial vascular flow index (VFI), and IL-15 levels decline with IL-18 in sterile patients, but not really with excess NK counts. Therefore, effects are likely NK cytotoxic versus angiogenic activation rather than NK replication, which depends more on the ratio IL-18/IL-18BP.[81-83] Further, developments imply Tweak as well.[84,85] Tailored therapies and schemes are being tested by N Ledée.

Stress-related implantation failure or early pregnancy loss also involves cytokines, notably TNF,[86] which is also important in 'occult' loss, whose animal models exist, such as in C57 Bl/6 mice.[87]

In line with the last data and other linking excess of some Th1 cytokines and early pregnancy losses abortion, high levels of IL-23 or IL-27 are abortifacient,[88] as are paradoxically excess levels of the Th2-like cytokines, IL-13, which appears to be involved in some abortions.[89]

Regulatory T cells (Tregs) secrete the immunosuppressive molecule IL-35[90] in mice and the optimal presence of Tregs (Fox P3 T cells) seems important in the prevention of early post-implantation pregnancy loss/abortion in allogeneic murine pregnancy as well as, as quoted, in humans.[91-93] In a study,[40] Fox P3 mRNA was reduced 2-fold in the infertile uterus, but even if Treg cell differentiation is controlled by TGF beta, the relative abundance in endometrial tissue of TGF beta1, TGF beta2, TGF beta3 mRNAs was not changed. Cytokines influencing Th1 and Th2 cell differentiation, including interferon (IFN) gamma, IL-2, IL-4, IL-5, IL-10 and IL-12p40, as well as dendritic cell-regulating cytokines IL-1alpha, IL-1beta, IL-6, LIF, GM-CSF and TNF alpha were also expressed similarly, regardless of the fertility status.[40] Arruvito, et al.[94] have shown that Treg cells are in fact, not only quantitatively, but qualitatively decreased in women with recurrent spontaneous abortions (RSA).[94]

Finally, cytokines are also involved in the induction/regulation of MMP/TIMPs, which are crucial for implantation and invasion as well as regulating integrins and integrin receptors. A very good review of this topic (very well studied in India), is evident in the work of Das and Basak.[95]

Complement

The discovery that complement neutralization at a very early stage prevents abortion in a murine abortion model,[96] is important because it shows another pathway by which innate immunity can be regulated in a murine embryo system. In this system, showing the role of very early embryo quality signals, Tartakowsky's group[97] obtained almost complete prevention of abortion in a CBA × DBA/2 embryo transfer system into CBA/J mice, a variation of the classical model, by pre-culturing embryos in CSF-1 before transfer.[97] In the classical system, Girardi, et al.[96] have shown that the embryo resorption process is initiated very early, much earlier than initially thought,[98] is complement activation-dependent, and implies complement-dependent local dysregulation of VEGF production, since both, embryo loss and abnormal vessel formation/low VEGF levels are corrected by neutralizing the complement very early,[96] as is also seen in a murine model of Antiphospholipid syndrome,[99] thus linking several immune pathways of early pregnancy loss.

Quite important in that respect is the fact that prevastatin prevents miscarriages in both antiphospholipid and immune abortion in mice,[100,101] as well as eclampsia-like syndromes in such animals.[101] This set of data was confirmed at the ISIR meeting of the Japanese Society for Immunology of Reproduction in Osaka (August 28–29, 2010), where Dr Keiichi Kumasawa from Osaka University presented 'placenta-specific gene manipulation and its application for the study of pre-eclampsia'. He showed that placenta-specific SFlt transgenic mouse also display hypertension and albuminuria in pregnancy, with abnormal placental development and that, prevastatin treatment corrects these symptoms.[102]

This set of data link angiogenic cytokines and immune ones, as well as bridges malimplantation and pre-eclampsia. It is on that basis that clinical multicenter trials are started.

The reasons for such a deregulation of complement remains to be established, albeit we believe it is due to environmental factors[103] affecting the MBL-controlled pathway. Indeed, we have traced such a deregulation in mice and human.[104,105]

Microarrays

The interactions, however, are complex, as reveal a variety of microarrays conducted in cyclic and pregnant endometrium in mice and animals. The data show, as was already predicted long ago when we revised the Th1/Th2 paradigm, spatial and temporal variations in the distribution of cytokines, and the variations are different in sterile versus fertile patients and in miscarriages versus fertile individuals. A detailed comparative analysis is outside the scope of this manuscript, so we would refer the reader to selected reviews.[106-110] For our own studies, the reader may refer to Chaouat, et al.[110] We have illustrated here a Venn diagram pointing out that before pregnancy, the uteri of fertile and sterile or RPL women do differ, and that, RPL and sterility have different profiles (Fig. 69.2).

CONCLUSION

The last 10 years have seen a real explosion in the field of Reproductive Immunology, which has indeed, confirmed two predictions of pioneers in the field: one, by Tom Wegmann, that 'the embryo is bathing in a sea of cytokines'. The second, by Charlie Loke in 1991, that 'uterine NK cells may have a role in the control of implantation and the transformation of the uterine vasculature by trophoblast on which the blood supply to the fetoplacental unit depends'. The data now bridge innate and adaptive immunity, but appear very complex.

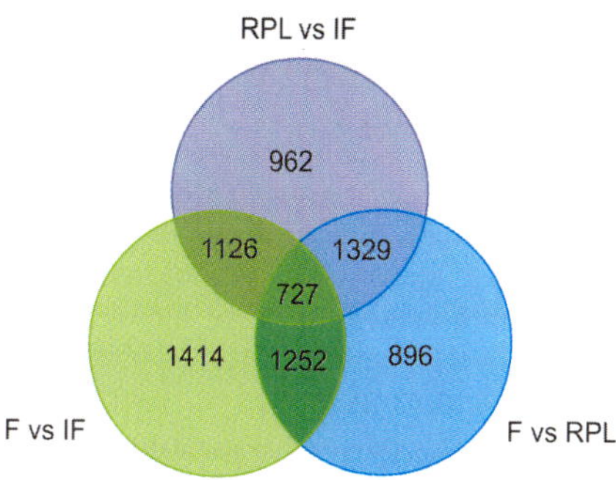

Fig. 69.2: Venn diagram fertile (F), implantation failure (IF) and recurrent pregnancy loss (RPL)

We are likely to be able very soon, to select the embryos with good implantation potential on a precise, defined molecular basis without the burden of complex instrumentation (whose costs are, anyhow, decreasing every year).

We already have treatments for a certain number of etiologies of implantation failure, recurrent spontaneous pregnancy losses, and possibly, for the diagnosis and treatment of pre-eclampsia, which is a major leap forward. It is likely that more will be developed very soon, filling several of the existing gaps in our knowledge. But as suggested by Chris Redman and Ian Sargent in their recent review on pre-eclampsia, 'For the first time, the pathogenesis of pre-eclampsia, can be related to defined immune mechanisms that are appropriate to the feto-maternal frontier. Now, the challenge is to prove the detail'. It may be a bit premature to issue such a statement for embryo implantation, but we are not so far from such a goal.

Notwithstanding, in many cases, larger scale double-blind clinical trials are needed before we can translate such advances in routine. And, on the other hand, as testified by the microarrays data, much still remains to be deciphered. Yet, already, a gain for the clinician is obviously emerging.

REFERENCES

1. Chaouat G, Petitbarat M, Dubanchet S, Rahmati M, Ledée N. Tolerance to the foetal allograft? Am J Reprod Immunol 2010;63:624-3.
2. Zhang J, Chen Z, Smith GN, Croy BA. Natural killer cell-triggered vascular transformation: Maternal care before birth? Cell Mol Immunol 2010;8:1-11.
3. LeBouteiller P, Tabiasco J. Killers become builders during pregnancy. Nat Med 2006;12:991-2.
4. Pröll J, Bensussan A, Goffin F, Foidart JM, Berrebi A, Le Bouteiller P. Tubal versus uterine placentation: Similar HLA-G expressing extravillous cytotrophoblast invasion but different maternal leukocyte recruitment. Tissue Antigens 2000;56:479-91.
5. Meisser A, Chardonnens D, Campana A, Bischof P. Effects of tumour necrosis factor-alpha, interleukin-1 alpha, macrophage

colony stimulating factor and transforming growth factor beta on trophoblastic matrix metalloproteinases. Mol Hum Reprod 1999;5:252-60.

6. Stewart C, Kaspar P, Brunet LJ, Bhatt H, Gadi I, Köntgen F, Abbondanzo S. Blastocyst implantation depends on maternal expression of leukemia inhibitory factor. Nature 1992;359:76-9.

7. Song JH, Houde A, Murphy BD. Cloning of leukemia inhibitory factor (LIF) and its expression in the uterus during embryonic diapause and implantation in the mink (Mustela vison). Mol Reprod Dev 1998;51:13-21.

8. Ace CI, Okulicz WC. Differential gene regulation by estrogen and progesterone in the primate endometrium. Mol Cell Endocrinol 1995;115:95-103.

9. Le Bouteiller P, Blaschitz A. The functionality of HLA-G is emerging. Immunol Rev 1999;167:233-44.

10. Fuzzi B, Rizzo R, Criscuoli L, Noci I, Melchiorri L, Scarselli B, et al. HLA-G expression in early embryos is a fundamental prerequisite for the obtainment of pregnancy. Eur J Immunol 2002;32:311-5.

11. Menezo Y, Elder K, Viville S. Soluble HLA-G release by the human embryo: An interesting artefact? Reprod Biomed Online 2006;13:763-4.

12. Sargent I, Swales A, Ledee N, Kozma N, Tabiasco J, LeBouteiller P. sHLA-G production by Human IVF embryos: Can it be measured reliably? J Reprod Immunol 2007;75:128-32.

13. Martal J, Chêne N, Huynh L, L'Haridon R, Reinaud P, Guillomot M, Charlier M, Charpigny G. IFN-tau: A novel subtype I IFN. Structural characteristics, nonubiquitous expression, structure-function relationships, a pregnancy hormonal embryonic signal and cross-species therapeutic potentialities. Biochimie 1998; 80:755-77.

14. Hansen PJ, Tekin S. Pregnancy-associated immunoregulatory molecules discovered in ruminants and their possible relevance to other species. Chem Immunol Allergy 2005;88:109-16.

15. Bany BM, Cross JC. Molecular complexity in establishing uterine receptivity and implantation. Cell Mol Life Sci 2005;62:1964-73.

16. Whaley AE, Meka CS, Harbison LA, Hunt JS, Imakawa K. Identification and cellular localization of unique interferon mRNA from human placenta. J Biol Chem 1994;269:10864-8.

17. Mohamed OA, Jonnaert M, Labelle-Dumais C, Kuroda K, Clarke HJ, Dufort D. Uterine Wnt/beta-catenin signaling is required for implantation. Proc Natl Acad Sci USA 2005;102:8579-84.

18. Lédée N, Frydman R, Osipova A, Taieb J, Gallot V, Lombardelli L, et al. Levels of follicular G-CSF and interleukin-15 appear as non-invasive biomarkers of subsequent successful birth in modified natural in vitro fertilization/intracytoplasmic sperm injection cycles. Fertil Steril 2011;95:94-8.

19. Lédée N, Munaut C, Sérazin V, Perrier d'Hauterive S, Lombardelli L, Logiodice F, et al. Performance evaluation of microbead and ELISA assays for follicular G-CSF: a non-invasive biomarker of oocyte developmental competence for embryo implantation. J Reprod Immunol 2010;86:126.

20. Lédée N, Petitbarat M, Rahmati M, Dubanchet S, Chaouat G, Sandra O, Perrier-d'Hauterive S, et al. New preconception immune biomarkers for clinical practice: interleukin-18, interleukin-15 and TWEAK on the endometrial side, G-CSF on the follicular side. J Reprod Immunol 2011;88:118-23.

21. Sanford TR, De M, Wood G. Expression of colony-stimulating factors and inflammatory cytokines in the uterus if CD1 mice during days 1 to days 3 of pregnancy. J Reprod Fert 1992;94: 213-20.

22. Mac Master MT, Newton RC, Sudhanski K, Dey, Andrews GK. Activation and distribution of inflammatory cells in the mouse uterus during the preimplantation period. J Immunol 1992;148: 1699-705.

23. Simon C, Frances A, Piquette GN, Danasouri IE, Zurawski G, Dang W, Polan ML. IL-1 receptor antagonist prevents successful implantation in mice. Endocrinology 1994;134:521.

24. Abbondanzo SJ, Cullinan EB, McIntyre K, Labow MA, Stewart CL. Reproduction in mice lacking a functional type 1 IL-1 receptor. Endocrinology 1996;137:3598-3601.

25. Simon C, Mercader A, Gimeno MJ, Pellicer A. The interleukin 1 system and human implantation. Am J Reprod Immunol 1997;37:64-72.

26. Delage G, Moreau J-F, Taupin J-L, Freitas S, Hambartsoumian E, Olivennes F, et al. In vitro endometrial secretion of human interleukin for DA cells/leukaemia inhibitory factor by explant cultures from fertile and infertile women. Hum Reprod 1995; 10:2483-8.

27. Laird SM, Tuckerman EM, Dalton CF, Dunphy BC, Lil TC, Zhang X. The production of leukemia inhibitory factor by human endometrium: presence in uterine flushings and production by cells in culture. Hum Reprod 1997;12:569-74.

28. Steck T, Giess R, Suetterlin MW, Bolland M, Wiest S, Poehls UG, Dietl J. Leukaemia inhibitory factor (LIF) gene mutations in women with unexplained infertility and recurrent failure of implantation after IVF and embryo transfer. Eur J Obstet Gynecol Reprod Biol 2004;112:69-73.

29. Kralickova M, Sima R, Vanecek T, Sima P, Rokyta Z, Ulcova-Gallova Z, et al. Leukemia inhibitory factor gene mutations in the population of infertile women are not restricted to nulligravid patients. Eur J Obstet Gynecol Reprod Biol 2006;127:231-5.

30. Delage G, Moreau J-F, Taupin J-L, Hambartsoumian E, Frydman R, Tartakowsky B, Chaouat G. Abnormal endometrial reactivity to colony-stimulating factor 1 and leukemia inhibitory factor dependent female infertility. Contracep Fertil Sex 1997;25:711-6.

31. Robb L, Li R, Hartley L, Nandurkar H, Koetgen F, Begley CG. Infertility in female mice lacking the receptor for interleukin-11 is due to a defective uterine response to implantation. Nat Med 1998;4:303-8.

32. Laird SM, Tuckerman EM, Li TC. Cytokine expression in the endometrium of women with implantation failure and recurrent miscarriage. Reprod Biomed Online 2006;13:13-23.

33. Dimitriadis E, Stoikos C, Stafford-Bell M, Clark I, Paiva P, Kovacs G, Salamonsen LA. Interleukin-11, IL-11 receptor alpha and leukemia inhibitory factor are dysregulated in endometrium of infertile women with endometriosis during the implantation window. J Reprod Immunol 2006;69:53-64.

34. Ledee-Bataille N, Dubanchet S, Kadoch J, Castelo-Branco A, Frydman R, Chaouat G. Controlled natural in vitro fertilization may be an alternative for patients with repeated unexplained implantation failure and a high uterine natural killer cell count. Fertil Steril 2004;82:234-6.

35. Bartocci A, Pollard JW, Stanley ER. Regulation of colony stimulating factor 1 during pregnancy. J Exp Med 1986;164:956-61.

36. Robertson SA, Roberts CT, Farr KL, Dunn AR, Seamark RF. Fertility impairment in granulocyte-macrophage colony-stimulating factor-deficient mice. Biol Reprod 1999;60:251-61.

37. Wegmann TG. Fetal protection against abortion: Is it immuno suppression or immuno stimulation? Ann Immunol Inst Pasteur 1984;135D:309-11.

38. Chaouat G, Menu E, Dy M, Minkowski M, Clark DA, Wegmann TG. Control of fetal survival in CBA × DBA/2 mice by lymphokine therapy. J Fertil Steril 1990;89:447-58.

39. Robertson SA, O'Leary S, Armstrong DT. Influence of semen on inflammatory modulators of embryo implantation. Reprod Suppl 2006;62:231-45.

40. Jasper MJ, Tremellen KP, Robertson SA. Primary unexplained infertility is associated with reduced expression of the T-regulatory cell transcription factor Foxp3 in endometrial tissue. Mol Hum Reprod 2006;12:301-8.

41. Moldenhauer LM, Diener KR, Thring DM, Brown MP, Hayball JD, Robertson SA. Cross-presentation of male seminal fluid antigens elicits T cell activation to initiate the female immune response to pregnancy. J Immunol 2009;182:8080-93.

42. Zenclussen AC, Blois S, StumpoR, Olmos S, AriasaK, Malan Borel I, et al. Murine abortion is associated with enhanced interleukin-6 levels at the feto-maternal interface. Cytokine 2003:24:150-60.

43. Jasper MJ, Tremellen KP, Robertson SA. Reduced expression of IL-6 and IL-1alpha mRNAs in secretory phase endometrium of women with recurrent miscarriage. J Reprod Immunol 2007;73:74-84.

44. Wegmann TG, Lin H, Guilbert L, Mossman TH. Bidirectional cytokines interactions in the materno fetal relationship: successful allopregnancy is a Th2 phenomenon. Immunol Today 1993;14:353-5.

45. Lin H, Mossmann TR, Guibert L, Tuntipopat S, Wegmann TG. Synthesis of T helper-2 cytokines at the maternal fetal interface. J Immunol 1993;151:4562-73.

46. Chaouat G, Assal Meliani A, Martal J, Raghupathy R, Elliot J, Mossmann T, Wegmann TG. Il-10 prevents inflammatory cytokine-mediated foetal death and is inducible by tau interferon. J Immunol 1995:152:2411-20.

47. Clark DA, Chaouat G, Arck PC, Mittruecker HW, Levy GA. Cytokine dependent abortion in CBA × DBA/2 mice is mediated by the procooagulant fgl/2 prothrombinase. J Immunol. Cutting edge 1998;160:550-5.

48. Gorczynski RM, Hadidi S, Yu G, Clark DA. The same immuno-regulatory molecules contribute to successful pregnancy and transplantation. Am J Reprod Immunol 2002;48:18-26.

49. Cadavid A, Peña B, García G, Botero J, Sánchez F, Ossa J, Beer A. Heparin plus aspirin as a single therapy for recurrent spontaneous abortion associated with both allo- and autoimmunity. Am. J Reprod Immunol 1999;41:271-8.

50. Szekeres-Bartho J, Polgar B, Kozma N, Miko E, Par G, Szereday L, Barakonyi A, Palkovics T, Papp O, Varga P. Progesterone-dependent immunomodulation. Chem Immunol Allergy 2005; 89:118-25.

51. Szekeres-Bartho J. Progesterone-mediated immunomodulation in pregnancy: its relevance to leukocyte immunotherapy of recurrent miscarriage. Immunotherapy 2009;1:873-82.

52. Hill JA. T helper 1 immunity to trophoblast: Evidence for a new immunological mechanism for recurrent abortion in women. Hum Reprod 1995;10:114-20.

53. Raghupathy R. Pregnancy: success and failure within the Th1/Th2/Th3 paradigm. Semin Immunol 2001;13:219-27.

54. Jenkins C, Roberts J, Wilson R, MacLean MA, Shilito J, Walker JJ. Evidence of a T(H) 1 type response associated with recurrent miscarriage. Fertil Steril 2000;73:1206-8.

55. Piccinni MP, Scaletti C, Vultaggio A, Maggi E, Romagnani S. Defective production of LIF, M-CSF and Th2-type cytokines by T cells at fetomaternal interface is associated with pregnancy loss. J Reprod Immunol 2001;52/1:3543.

56. Winger EE, Reed JL. Treatment with tumor necrosis factor inhibitors and intravenous immunoglobulin improves live birth rates in women with recurrent spontaneous abortion. Am J Reprod Immunol 2008;60:8-16.

57. Winger EE, Reed JL, Ashoush S, Ahuja S, El-Toukhy T, Taranissi M. Treatment with adalimumab (Humira) and intravenous immunoglobulin improves pregnancy rates in women undergoing IVF. Am J Reprod Immunol 2009;61:113-20.

58. Chaouat G. Comment: Primum non-Nocere. Am J Reprod Immunol 2008;60:17-8.

59. Winger EE, Reed JL, Ashoush S, El-Toukhy T, Ahuja S, Taranissi M. Degree of TNF-α/IL-10 cytokine elevation correlates with IVF success rates in women undergoing treatment with Adalimumab (Humira) and IVIG. Am J Reprod Immunol 2011;65:610-8.

60. Scarpellini F, Sbracia M. Use of granulocyte colony-stimulating factor for the treatment of unexplained recurrent miscarriage: a randomised controlled trial. Hum Reprod 2009;24:2703-8.

61. Ostojic S, Dubanchet S, Mjihdi A, Truyens C, Capron F, Chaouat G. Demonstration of the presence of IL-16, IL-17 and IL-18 at the murine fetomaternal interface during murine pregnancy. Am J Reprod Immunol 2003;49:101-13.

62. Guimond MJ, Luross JA, Wang B, Terhorst C, Danial S, Croy BA. Abscence of natural killer cells during murine pregnancy is asociated with Reproductive compromise in TgE26 mice. Biol Reprod 1997;56:169-79.

63. Guimond MJ, Wang B, Croy BA. Engraftment of bone marrow from severe combined immunodeficiency (SCID) mice reverses the reproductive deficit in Natural Killer cells deficient TgE26 mice. J Exp Med 1998;187:217-23.

64. Leonard S, Murrant C, Tayade C, van den Heuvel M, Watering R, Croy BA. Mechanisms regulating immune cell contributions to spiral artery modification—facts and hypotheses—a review. Placenta. 2006;27 Suppl A:S40-6.

65. Barber EM, Pollard JW. The uterine NK cell population requires IL-15 but these cells are not required for pregnancy nor the resolution of a Listeria monocytogenes infection. J Immunol 2003;171:37-46.

66. Miyazaki S, Tanebe K, Sakai M, Michimata T, Tsuda H, Fujimura M, Nakamura M, Kiso Y, Saito S. Interleukin 2 receptor gamma chain [gamma(c)] knockout mice show less regularity in estrous

cycle but achieve normal pregnancy without fetal compromise. Am J Reprod Immunol 2002;47:222-30.

67. Zhou Y, Genbacev O, Fisher SJ. The human placenta remodels the uterus by using a combination of molecules that govern vasculogenesis or leukocyte extravasation. Ann N Y Acad Sci 2003;995:73-83.

68. Girling JE, Rogers PA. Recent advances in endometrial angiogenesis research. Angiogenesis 2005;8:89-99.

69. Licht P, Fluhr H, Neuwinger J, Wallwiener D, Wildt L. Is human chorionic gonadotropin directly involved in the regulation of human implantation? Mol Cell Endocrinol 2007;269:85-92.

70. Sengupta J, Lalitkumar PG, Najwa AR, Charnock-Jones DS, Evans AL, Sharkey AM, et al. Reproduction 2007;133:1199-211.

71. Li XF, Charnock-Jones DS, Zhang E, Hiby S, Malik S, Day K, et al. Angiogenic growth factor messenger ribonucleic acids in uterine natural killer cells. J Clin Endocrinol Metab 2001;86:1823-34.

72. Wang C, Tanaka T, Nakamura H, Umesaki N, Hirai K, Ishiko O, Ogita S, Kaneda K. Granulated metrial gland cells in the murine uterus: Localization, kinetics, and the functional role in angiogenesis during pregnancy. Microsc Res Tech 2003;60:420-9.

73. Lash GE, Schiessl B, Kirkley M, Innes BA, Cooper A, Searle RF, Robson SC, Bulmer JN. Expression of angiogenic growth factors by uterine natural killer cells during early pregnancy. J Leukoc Biol 2006;80:572-80.

74. Xie X, He H, Colonna M, Seya T, Takai T, Croy BA. Pathways participating in activation of mouse uterine natural killer cells during pregnancy. Biology of Reproduction 2005;73:510-8.

75. Hirchenhain J, Huse I, Hess A, Bielfeld P, De Bruyne F, Krüssel JS. Differential expression of angiopoietins 1 and 2 and their receptor Tie-2 in human endometrium. Mol Hum Reprod 2003;9:663-9.

76. Hiby SE, Walker JJ, O'shaughnessy KM, Redman CW, Carrington M, Trowsdale J, Moffett A. Combinations of maternal KIR and fetal HLA-C genes influence the risk of preeclampsia and reproductive success. J Exp Med 2004;200:957-65.

77. Plaisier M, Dennert I, Rost E, Koolwijk P, van Hinsbergh VW, Helmerhorst FM. Decidual vascularization and the expression of angiogenic growth factors and proteases in first trimester spontaneous abortions. Hum Reprod 2009;24:185-97.

78. Moffett A, Hiby S. Influence of activating and inhibitory killer immunoglobulin-like receptors on predisposition to recurrent miscarriages. Hum Reprod 2009;24:2048-9.

79. Le Bouteiller P, Fons P, Herault JP, Bono F, Chabot S, Cartwright JE, Bensussan A. Soluble HLA-G and control of angiogenesis. J Reprod Immunol 2007;76:17-22.

80. Madeja Z, Yadi H, Apps R, Boulenouar S, Roper SJ, Gardner L, et al. Paternal MHC expression on mouse trophoblast affects uterine vascularization and fetal growth. Proc Natl Acad Sci USA. 2011;108:4012-17.

81. Ledee-Bataille N, Dubanchet S, Coulomb-L'hermine A, Durand-Gasselin I, Frydman R, Chaouat GA. New role for natural killer cells, interleukin (IL)-12, and IL-18 in repeated implantation failure after *in vitro* fertilization. Fertil Steril 2004;81:59-65.

82. Ledee-Bataille N, Bonnet-Chea K, Hosny G, Dubanchet S, Frydman R, Chaouat G. Role of the endometrial tripod interleukin-18, -15, and -12 in inadequate uterine receptivity in patients with a history of repeated *in vitro* fertilization-embryo transfer failure. Fertility and Sterility 2005;83:598-605.

83. Lédée N, Petitbarat M, Rahmati M, Dubanchet S, Chaouat G, Sandra O, et al. New pre-conception immune biomarkers for clinical practice: interleukin-18, interleukin-15 and TWEAK on the endometrial side, G-CSF on the follicular side. J Reprod Immunol 2011;88:118-23.

84. Petitbarat M, Rahmati M, Sérazin V, Dubanchet S, Morvan C, Wainer R, et al. TWEAK appears as a modulator of endometrial IL-18 related cytotoxic activity of uterine natural killers. PLoS One. 2011;6:e14497

85. Mas AE, Petitbarat M, Dubanchet S, Fay S, Ledée N, Chaouat G. Immune regulation at the interface during early steps of murine implantation: involvement of two new cytokines of the IL-12 family (IL-23 and IL-27) and of TWEAK. Am J Reprod Immunol 2008;59:323-38.

86. Tometten M, Blois S, Arck PC. Nerve growth factor in reproductive biology: Link between the immune, endocrine and nervous system? Chem Immunol Allergy 2005;89:135-48.

87. Clark DA, Blois S, Kandil J, Handjiski B, Manuel J, Arck PC. Reduced uterine indoleamine 2,3-dioxygenase versus increased Th1/Th2 cytokine ratios as a basis for occult and clinical pregnancy failure in mice and humans. Am J Reprod Immunol 2005;54:203-16.

88. Wang WJ, Hao CF, Yi-Lin, Yin GJ, Bao SH, Qiu LH, Lin QD. Increased prevalence of T helper 17 (Th17) cells in peripheral blood and decidua in unexplained recurrent spontaneous abortion patients. J Reprod Immunol 2010;84:164-70.

89. Chegini N, Ma C, Roberts M, Williams RS, Ripps BA. Differential expression of interleukins (IL) IL-13 and IL-15 throughout the menstrual cycle in endometrium of normal fertile women and women with recurrent spontaneous abortion. J Reprod Immunol 2002;56:93-110.

90. Niedbala W, Wei XQ, Cai B, Hueber AJ, Leung BP, Mc Innes IB, Liew FY. IL-35 is a novel cytokine with therapeutic effects against collagen-induced arthritis through the expansion of regulatory T cells and suppression of Th17 cells. Eur J Immunol 2007;37:3021-9.

91. Aluvihare VR, Kallikourdis M, Betz AG. Regulatory T cells mediate maternal tolerance to the fetus. Nature Immunol 2004; 5:266-71.

92. Kallikourdis M, Betz AG. Periodic accumulation of regulatory T cells in the uterus: Preparation for the implantation of a semi-allogeneic fetus? PLoS ONE 2007;18;2:e382.

93. Kallikourdis M, Andersen KG, Welch KA, Betz AG. Alloantigen-enhanced accumulation of CCR5+ 'effector' regulatory T cells in the gravid uterus. Proc Natl Acad Sci USA 2007;104:594.

94. Arruvito L, Sanz M, Banham AH, Fainboim L. Expansion of CD4+ CD25+ and FOXP3+ regulatory T cells during the follicular phase of the menstrual cycle: implications for human reproduction. J Immunol 2007;178:2572-8.

95. Das C, Basak S. Expression and regulation of integrin receptors in human trophoblast cells: role of estradiol and cytokines. Indian J Exp Biol 2003;41:748-55.

96. Girardi G, Yarilin D, Thurman JM, Holers VM, Salmon JE. Complement activation induces dysregulation of angiogenic factors and causes fetal rejection and growth restriction. J Exp Med 2006;203:2165-75.

97. Tartakovsky B, Ben-Yair E. Cytokines modulate preimplantation development and pregnancy. Dev Biol 1991;146:345-52.

98. Baines MG, Gendron RL. Natural and experimental animal models of reproductive failure. in. Immunology of pregnancy Chaouat G (ed). Boca Raton, CRC Press 1993:173-203.

99. Girardi G. Guilty as charged: All available evidence implicates complement's role in fetal demise. Am J Reprod Immunol 2008; 59:183-92.

100. Girardi G. Pravastatin prevents miscarriages in antiphospholipid antibody-treated mice. J Reprod Immunol 2009;82:126-31.

101. Girardi G. Role of tissue factor in pregnancy complications: Crosstalk between coagulation and inflammation. Thromb Res 2011;127 Suppl 3:S43-6.

102. Kumasawa K, Ikawa M, Kidoya H, Hasuwa H, Saito-Fujita T, Morioka Y, Takakura N, Kimura T, Okabe M. Pravastatin induces placental growth factor (PGF) and ameliorates pre-eclampsia in a mouse model. Proc Natl Acad Sci USA 2011;108:1451-5.

103. Clark DA, Manuel J, Lee L, Chaouat G, Gorczynski RM, Levy GA. Ecology of danger-dependent cytokine-boosted spontaneous abortion in the CBA × DBA/2 mouse model. I. Synergistic effect of LPS and (TNF-alpha + IFN-gamma) on pregnancy loss. Am J Reprod Immunol 2004;52:370-8.

104. Chaouat G, Petitbarat M, Bulla R, Dubanchet S, Valdivia K, Ledée N, et al. Early regulators in abortion and implications for a preeclampsia model. J Reprod Immunol 2009;82:131-40.

105. Oger P, Bulla R, Tedesco F, Portier A, Dubanchet S, Bailly M, et al. Higher interleukin-18 and mannose-binding lectin are present in uterine lumen of patients with unexplained infertility. Reprod Biomed Online 2009;19:591-8.

106. Altmäe S, Martínez-Conejero JA, Salumets A, Simón C, Horcajadas JA, Stavreus-Evers A. Endometrial gene expression analysis at the time of embryo implantation in women with unexplained infertility. Mol Hum Reprod 2010;16:178-87.

107. Zhang P, Zucchelli M, Bruce S, Hambiliki F, Stavreus-Evers A, Levkov L, Skottman H, Kerkelä E, Kere J, Hovatta O. Transcriptome profiling of human preimplantation development. PLoS One 2009;4:e7844.

108. Paidas MJ, Krikun G, Huang SJ, Jones R, Romano M, Annunziato J, Barnea ER. A genomic and proteomic investigation of the impact of preimplantation factor on human decidual cells. Am J Obstet Gynecol 2010;202:459.e1-8.

109. He K, Zhao H, Wang Q, Pan Y. A comparative genome analysis of gene expression reveals different regulatory mechanisms between mouse and human embryo preimplantation development. Reprod Biol Endocrinol 2010;8:41.

110. Chaouat G, Rodde N, Petitbarat M, Bulla R, Rahmati M, Dubanchet S, et al. An insight into normal and pathological pregnancies using large-scale microarrays: Lessons from microarrays. J Reprod Immunol 2011;89:163-72.

Endometrial Cancer and Wish of Pregnancy: Is Conservative Treatment Possible?

Priya Selvaraj, Kamala Selvaraj

OVERVIEW

Endometrial carcinoma is one of the most common malignancies of the female genital tract with an incidence of 2 percent to 14 percent in women less than 45 years of age. According to the last annual report released by International Federation of Gynecology and Obstetrics (FIGO), the five years survival rate is 90 percent for surgical stage I. It is more often seen in postmenopausal women, often presenting as bleeding. The dilemma arises in the young premenopausal woman who has not commenced her reproductive career. In this group, the tumor seems to be more hormone-dependent, which is why prolonged estrogen exposure has been implicated in its etiology. Interestingly, a higher incidence has been related to consumption of diets rich in saturated and unsaturated fatty acids, while intake of antioxidant-rich fruits and vegetables and naturally occurring phytoestrogens seemed to reduce the risk. Several screening procedures exist but those commonly performed are the Pap smear and endometrial biopsy. Of these, the Pap smear is not very reliable or specific to endometrial cancer as much as it helps in detecting cervical cancer. The most valuable test then becomes the endometrial biopsy followed by a confirmatory fractional curettage. The diagnostic value of these methods approaches 95 percent. All the other tests, namely ultrasound and magnetic resonance imaging (MRI) are adjuncts or of value in staging. The diagnosis of the 5 percent of women under the age of 40 years that do suffer from this form of cancer is early owing to better detection, differentiation as well as being receptor positive. Hence, as a fertility preserving option in these women, progestin therapy is the mainstay prior to any form of ovulation induction, ovarian hyperstimulation and oocyte retrieval procedures for ART. Other drugs, such as gonadotropin-releasing hormone (GnRH) agonists, progesterone-releasing intrauterine device and partial endometrial resection, have all been proved in literature to cause remission or cure in order to allow for pregnancy. Infertile women at risk were always the polycystic ovary syndrome (PCOS) group owing to chronic anovulation and persistence of an estrogen effect on the endometrium. Hence, a thorough surveillance of these candidates, as well as close monitoring helps to pick up early signs of the disease and also speeds up the fertility treatment process.

INTRODUCTION

The prevalence of gynecologic malignancies is generally higher in postmenopausal than in premenopausal age groups. However, the rising incidence among women in the reproductive age group poses a threat to their fertility potential, thereby causing a major concern. The evolving lifestyle changes and career options, which delay childbearing in women, are also contributory. Most often, the treatment of these malignancies is radical, resulting in surgical removal/clearance of the uterus and appendages. These days, when women desiring childbearing are afflicted, it only becomes imperative that fertility-preserving modalities of treatment become available or researched.

Being one of the most common malignancies of the female genital tract with an incidence of 2 percent to 14 percent in women lesser than 45 years,[1] endometrial carcinoma primarily affects postmenopausal women and its virulence increases with age. When it does affect younger premenopausal women, the tumor is hormone-dependent, whereby prolonged exposure to estrogen, either exogenous or endogenous, has been implicated.

Risk Factors

- Early menarche and late menopause.
- Nullipara
- *Polycystic ovary syndrome (PCOS):* Menstrual irregularity coupled with unopposed estrogen action on the endometrium.

- *Obesity:* Increased consumption of fatty foods can result in altered estrogen metabolism, and fatty deposits themselves increase the peripheral conversion of estrogen, increasing the risk for endometrial cancer.
- Estrogen only-hormone replacement therapy.
- Diabetes mellitus.
- Atypical endometrial hyperplasia.

Other Risk Factors

- *Age:* 95 percent of endometrial cancers occur above 40 years of age.
- Personal history of breast or ovarian cancer.
- *Tamoxifen therapy:* Although primarily antiestrogenic, it has estrogen-like effects on the endometrium leading to hyperplasia and subsequent cancer (1 in 500).
- Ethnicity
- *Hereditary nonpolyposis colorectal cancer:* Women can inherit a mutation from their parents and it may be worth testing for mutations if a woman has a particularly strong family history of endometrial or colon cancer.

Symptomatology

Endometrial cancer is almost always a primary cause when a postmenopausal woman has vaginal bleeding. As the disease progresses, it can produce a variety of problems.[2]
- Postmenopausal vaginal bleeding.
- Abnormal bleeding, including intermenstrual bleeding, or polymenorrhagia.
- Abnormal vaginal discharge, which may be foul smelling.
- Pelvic or back pain
- Pain on urination
- Dyspareunia
- Melena or hematuria.

Nutrition and Cancer Risk

While a diet high in animal fats has been implicated in endometrial cancer, a diet rich in fruits and vegetables may have a small preventive effect. It has also been suggested that diets high in naturally occurring phytoestrogens, as in soy products, may decrease the risk. However, further studies need to be performed before these nutritional recommendations can be made regarding prevention. Ecological studies have shown a positive correlation between per capita fat and animal protein consumption and the incidence of endometrial cancer. In an analysis of cancer incidence rates and mean nutrient intakes among five ethnic groups in Hawaii, endometrial cancer was positively related to consumption of saturated and unsaturated fat and animal protein.[3]

Obesity is an important determinant of EC, probably because of its effect on the hormonal milieu of both pre-and postmenopausal women. Randomized and observational studies of diet and sex hormones indicate that low fat diets may be associated weakly with decreased estrogen levels, and thus, a lowering of EC risk. In the large prospective American Cancer Society (ACS) study, mortality from endometrial cancer was also markedly affected by obesity. The risk increased with increasing obesity. The most obese women had more than four times the risk of dying from endometrial cancer than women of average weight. In postmenopausal women, obesity is positively related to the risk of both breast and endometrial cancer. Additionally, obesity is associated with increased estrogen production secondary to increased peripheral aromatization. In postmenopausal women, this effect is proportionately more significant because the ovaries no longer contribute to production of estrogen.[4]

Screening Procedures

At present, the following modalities described are the available screening procedures to detect early malignancy in the general population. A more intensive approach may be needed for those women who have a familial predisposition to genital tract cancers. In general, an annual pelvic examination with additional procedures, like Pap smear and a transvaginal pelvic ultrasound, is recommended for women as part of healthcare. Though this speaks largely for ovarian and cervical cancers, additional tests, such as a diagnostic curettage, may be offered for those with risk factors or symptomatology. Currently, the American Cancer Society recommends that women with Lynch Syndrome (it is also called Hereditary non-polyposis colorectal cancer syndrome - HNPCC) get annual endometrial biopsies starting at age 35 years. Endometrial biopsies can be done in an office setting, thereby making it a daycare procedure.[2]

The Pap smear is not very reliable as a screening procedure for endometrial cancer, although a retrospective study found a strong correlation between positive cervical cytology and high risk disease (i.e. high-grade tumor and deep myometrial invasion) as well as an increased risk of nodal involvement.[5] The degree of tumor differentiation has an important impact on the prognosis and on the selection of appropriate therapy.

Endometrial Biopsy

It is the primary test in evaluating a patient with abnormal uterine bleeding or suspected endometrial pathology. The diagnostic accuracy of endometrial biopsy is 95 percent when compared with subsequent findings of dilatation and curettage (D and C) or even hysterectomy.

Pap Smear

A pap test is not a very reliable diagnostic test, since only 30 to 50 percent of patients with endometrial cancer will have abnormal Pap test results.

Hysteroscopy

Hysteroscopy forms a valuable tool for the evaluation of the endometrial cavity prior to recruiting patients for treatment cycles. The accuracy of hysteroscopy is debatable, with some clinicians preferring an initial evaluation with dilatation and curettage owing to the risk of spread into the abdominal cavity, causing the staging to shift to stage III disease.[1] However in hyperplasias that are a prelude to cancer, this diagnostic method offers a sensitivity of 86.4 percent and a specificity of 99.2 percent, although the accuracy seems to be higher in diagnosing cancer than in excluding it.[1] In any case, the value of hysteroscopy still remains important in those patients with cervical stenosis or low patient tolerance to an outpatient aspiration biopsy. It can also be used as a follow-up tool for the evaluation of recurrent bleeding after a negative biopsy or if a specimen obtained by biopsy is inadequate to explain the pathology, in which case, the problematic area can be directly visualized and biopsied.

Dilatation and Curettage/Fractional

If the biopsy sample does not provide enough tissue or information despite persistence of symptoms then D and C must be done to rule out cancer, the advantage being that a larger area of endometrium is studied. Office endometrial sampling is probably sufficient for patients who will undergo hysterectomies. However, a D and C should be performed on all patients with endometrial carcinoma prior to the institution of conservative therapy. Better agreement with final grade and detection of occult malignancy can be achieved on tissue obtained at a D and C.[6]

Transvaginal Ultrasound (TVUS)

It is a useful adjunct to endometrial biopsy for evaluating abnormal uterine bleeding. It is of great help in those whose bleeding is caused by premenopausal anovulation, post-menopausal atrophy and in patients with significant amounts of endometrial tissue or polyps who are in need of further evaluation. The findings of an endometrial thickness greater than 5 mm, a polypoid endometrial mass, or a collection of fluid within the uterus definitely require further evaluation.

Magnetic Resonance Imaging

Non-contrast magnetic resonance imaging (MRI) is 88 to 92 percent accurate in staging endometrial carcinoma, and myometrial invasion is hardly ever found histologically when MRI shows the tumor to be limited to the endometrium.

The addition of contrast to MRI has proven to be essential to distinguish among the tumor, endometrium, and myometrium. MRI has been shown to be superior to transvaginal ultrasonography (TVUS) and computed tomography (CT) in assessing the depth of myometrial invasion in all patients who underwent TVUS, CT, and noncontrast MRI prior to surgery.[6] According to Chiva, et al.[1] prework of early well-differentiated disease, an MRI (contrast) to rule out myometrial invasion and suspicious pelvic or para-aortic nodes is imperative. Additionally, the presence of any co-existing ovarian tumors or pathology should be ruled out. In the presence of any doubt, serum ovarian tumor markers may also be included.

Staging

It is important to review the staging systems in order to have an idea of early and late stages of endometrial cancer, which will definitely influence the treatment options for those who wish to retain their potential for fertility. There are two main groups of women in whom the prognosis and treatment plan will differ according to the behavioral pattern of the tumor (Tables 70.1 to 70.3).

Prognostic Factors

For all practical purposes, most of the literature review concerning fertility sparing treatment options in endometrial cancer, has been directed only towards atypical hyperplasias and stage 1, grade 1 tumors. This group has a lower recurrence rate following medical therapy and also responds better in IVF treatment cycles (Table 70.4).

Table 70.1: Hormonal status	
Estrogen-dependent	*Estrogen-independent*
Young/perimenopausal women	Old, thin and postmenopausal women
Exposure to estrogen–exogenous/endogenous	No source of estrogen
Begin as hyperplasia	Atrophic endometrium
Better differentiated with good prognosis	Less differentiated with poor prognosis

Table 70.2: International Federation of Gynecology and Obstetrics (FIGO) definition for grading of endometrial carcinoma	
Histopathologic degrees of differentiation	
G 1	≤ 5% non-squamous or non-morular growth pattern
G 2	6-50% non-squamous or non-morular growth pattern
G 3	50% non-squamous or non-morular growth pattern

Table 70.3: 1988 FIGO surgical staging for endometrial carcinoma		
Stage I A	G 123	Tumor limited to endometrium
Stage I B	G 123	Invasion to less than one-half of the myometrium
Stage I C	G 123	Invasion to more than one-half of the myometrium
Stage II A	G 123	Endocervical glandular involvement only
Stage II B	G 123	Cervical stromal invasion
Stage III A	G 123	Tumor invades serosa and/or adnexa and/or positive peritoneal cytology
Stage III B	G 123	Vaginal metastasis
Stage III C	G 123	Metastasis to pelvic and/or para-aortic lymph nodes
Stage IV A	G 123	Tumor invasion of bladder and/or bowel mucosa
Stage IV B		Distant metastasis including intra-abdominal and/or inguinal lymph nodes

Table 70.4: Prognostic factors for endometrial carcinoma

Prognostic variables in endometrial carcinoma[1]

Age	Lymph node metastasis
Histological type	Intraperitoneal tumor
Histological grade	Tumor size
Myometrial invasion	Peritoneal cytology
Lymph-vascular space invasion	Hormone receptor status
Isthmus-cervix extension	DNA ploidy/proliferative index
Adnexal involvement	Oncogene amplification/expression

CLINICAL DISCUSSION

Fertility Options

Endometrial carcinoma, especially in young patients, has been found to be hormone-dependent and with a favorable prognosis. Studies done as early as 1960's, have clearly demonstrated the advantages of progesterone therapy in the regression of early stages of endometrial carcinoma.[7] Endometrial adenocarcinoma in the child bearing age has been found to be relatively uncommon, unless in the presence of predisposing risk factors like obesity, chronic anovulation due to PCOS or an estrogen producing tumor and infertility. Many patients with endometrial carcinoma are in their 50's and only 5 percent of them are under age 40. The main underlying pathophysiology is long-term unopposed estrogen exposure, especially in infertile women with PCOS, which leads to differing grades of endometrial hyperplasia, progressing to carcinoma. Anovulation,

manifesting as amenorrhea or oligomenorrhea, occurred in 21 percent of infertile women with ovulatory dysfunction causing subfertility in 15 to 20 percent of couples. Salha, et al.[8] reported that the risk of endometrial carcinoma was increased 4.8-fold in infertile women when compared to a rise of 10.3-fold in those with chronic anovulation. Hence, it is essential to evaluate the endometrial disease thoroughly during the infertility work-up in these patients.[8]

The standard treatment for endometrial carcinoma is total abdominal hysterectomy (TAH), however, in a young woman who wishes to bear a child, conservative treatment with progestins has been attempted, and successful pregnancies have also been reported. As mentioned earlier, the virulence of the disease in younger patients (age under the 40 years) is generally associated with a better prognosis because of early detection, better differentiation and being receptor positive. In such a setting, high-dose progestins followed by therapeutic as well as diagnostic curettage to rule out cancer may be the alternative treatment in those patients who wish to preserve fertility.[9]

Conservative Management

Selection Criteria

Grade 1 tumors, which are limited to the endometrium and not involving the cervix or myometrium, can be selected for conservative treatment. Moreover, the progesterone receptors in well-differentiated tumors are in a much higher concentration than the poorly differentiated ones (85–90% vs 55–60%, respectively). Hence, the response to medical therapy is an additional benefit. This pathological feature gives these patients a better survival rate than the other groups.[1]

Conservative management of endometrial carcinoma is mostly based on the presence of hormone receptors in the tumor and their sensitivity to manipulation with hormonal therapy. A large number of endometrial cancers express estrogen (E) and progesterone (P) receptors. The hyperestrogenic variety of cancers usually strongly expresses both these receptors, while the virulent hypoestrogenic variety do not express these. It has also been demonstrated that 80 percent of these cancers express receptors for GnRH analog (Table 70.5).[10]

Progestins

They have been in use as palliative therapy in advanced or recurrent endometrial adenocarcinoma with a 20 to 40 percent response rate. Quite a few studies have demonstrated its efficacy in conservative management of the same, with Megestrol acetate (40–160 mg/day) and Medroxyprogesterone acetate (200–600 mg/day) as the most commonly used agents. The response rates to progestin vary from 83 to 94 percent for atypical complex hyperplasia and from 57 to 75 percent for endometrial adenocarcinoma. The recurrence

Table 70.5: Conservative treatment of endometrial adenocarcinoma and atypical complex hyperplasia by progestins[10]

	N	Treatment	Duration	Regression	Recurrence	Pregnancy
Adenocarcinoma						
Kim 1997	7	Megestrol acetate (160 mg/day)	3 months	4/7 57%	2/4 50%	0/7
Kim's review 1997	14	Megestrol acetate or MPA	Up to 1 year	9/14 64%	1/9 11%	2/14 14%
Randall 1997	12	Megestrol acetate or MPA	3–18 months	9/12 75%	1/9 11%	3/12 25%
Kaku 2001	12	MPA 200 to 800 mg/day	2–14 months	9/12 75%	2/9 22%	2/12 16%
A typical complex hyperplasia						
Randall 1997	17	Megestrol acetate or MPA	3–18 months	16/17 94%	2/16 12,5%	2/17 12%
Kaku 2001	18	MPA 100 to 600 mg/day	1–23 months	15/18 83%	2/15 13%	5/18 28

rates were 13 percent for the former and 11 to 50 percent for the latter. High doses of progesterone may also change lipid metabolism leading to a greater risk of atherogenesis. Other known side effects, such as loss of libido, weight gain and mood changes, must also be taken into consideration.[10,11]

GnRH Agonists

Jedoul, et al.[10] and Grigoris, et al.[11] reported the use of GnRH agonist for a period of 6 months on 56 patients with endometrial hyperplasia. The regression of hyperplastic to normal endometrium was observed in 86.5 percent of patients with simple hyperplasia and 85.5 percent in patients with complex hyperplasia with persistence of the hyperplastic endometrium in 14.5 percent in the former and 7.1 percent in the latter groups. Most other studies have reported the use of agonist in the management of metastatic or recurrent disease. The most serious side effect was bone loss when the therapy was extended beyond 6 months.[10,11]

Progesterone Containing Intrauterine Device

The Levonorgestrel intrauterine system is indicated for those with early endometrial cancer who cannot tolerate systemic therapy. The efficacy of this intrauterine device (IUD) in treating well-differentiated early stage is unclear. Montz, et al.[13] reported its use in 12 women with stage IA1 endometrial cancer. They were observed for up to 36 months, with biopsies of endometrium negative in 7 of 11 at 6 months and in 6 of 8 at 12 months. No IUD-related complications occurred except for expulsion. Although this may seem to eliminate the presence of grade I cancer, the risk of residual invasive disease cannot be ruled out completely.[12,13] Minig, et al.[15] tested the efficacy of Levonorgestrel IUD plus gonadotropin-releasing hormone (GnRH) for conservative treatment in young women with atypical endometrial hyperplasia (AEH) or FIGO stage IA endometrioid endometrial cancer. The complete response rate was 95 percent in patients with AEH and 57.1 percent in those with endometrial cancer. In the case of cancer, the recurrence rate was 14.3 percent and the progression rate was 28.6 percent; these results are in accordance with rates in the literature.[15]

Gotlieb, et al.[14] reported their findings on the conservative management with progestins in 13 premenopausal women (mean age 31 years) with endometrial cancer and found a recurrence rate of 46 percent (6/13). However, the subsequent response to a second course of progestin therapy was favorable in 3 patients. Fertility treatment was also initiated as soon as the endometrial sampling was negative. There were totally 7 conceptions with 9 viable deliveries following conservative management.[14]

Jadoul, et al.[10] in his analysis of 70 articles and personal experience found that conservative management was beneficial in women with atypical endometrial hyperplasia or endometrial adenocarcinoma. Seven young women between 27 and 38 years of age with endometrial adenocarcinoma or complex atypical hyperplasia were treated by partial endometrial resection and GnRH agonist. Two of these patients showed persistent disease at the end of 3 months and were treated with a second course of GnRH agonist. Five patients were initiated for IVF of whom four conceived in the first attempt.[10]

Women with anovulatory cycles (PCOS) have been known to be at high risk for endometrial carcinoma and hence, highlight the need for early detection and fertility-sparing therapy. Increased body mass index (BMI), which is also a common feature of this syndrome, is also strongly related to the risk of cancer. This is because the adipose tissue is the primary site for conversion of adrenal androstenedione. Obesity has also been related to lower levels of sex hormone binding globulin leading to greater bio-availability of estrogen.[8] Given the high incidence of chronic anovulation and infertility in women with endometrial cancer, it is always better to enrol them in an assisted reproductive techniques (ART) program. The advantages of the long protocol are suppression of the endometrium by an agonist, multiple follicular recruitment, a higher yield of oocytes and more available embryos to work with. The advent of cryopreservation has also revolutionized the future of these patients, who could still have their biological child through surrogacy or in their own womb following successful therapy. Several live births have been reported following conservative management in these women primarily through IVF or ICSI.[16] Pinto et al.[17] reported successful pregnancies through IVF after controlled ovarian hyperstimulation (COH),[17] while Yarali, et al.[18] reported a live birth following ICSI.[18] Yet another interesting case, reported by Park, et al.[9] was one of a heterotopic pregnancy, achieved following IVF in a 36-year-old woman with stage I, grade I cancer suppressed by initial progestin therapy. A right salpingectomy was performed and she delivered uneventfully at 38 weeks.[9] Salha, et al.[8] reported the detection of endometrial carcinoma, manifested by bleeding at the time of embryo transfer, following which, the procedure was deferred and the embryos were cryopreserved.[8]

Revel et al.[19,20] have reported an interesting case where a 43 year old woman, clinically proven as PCOS and suffering from secondary infertility came for fertility treatment. During the evaluation, it was found that she had well- differentiated endometrial cancer and, considering the risk at her age, TAH with bilateral salpingo-oophorectomy (BSO) was performed. The authors subsequently isolated her ovaries in phosphate buffered saline postsurgery, and were able to harvest immature oocytes from the antral follicles that were previously imaged during the work-up. Subsequently, 17 oocytes retrieved were matured with conventional *in vitro* maturation (IVM) medium to yield MII oocytes, which were injected and cleavage stage embryos were cryopreserved for future use in a surrogacy program. The author also opined that oophorectomy in reproductive age patients, who still have a desire for fertility, can be performed for malignant disease or for the purpose of fertility preservation prior to ovariotoxic chemotherapy.[19,20]

One of the major difficulties encountered is in establishing the distinction between atypical hyperplasia and invasive carcinoma while interpreting the results of conservative management of well-differentiated endometrial cancer in young patients. Nevertheless, the real issue is whether there is a biologic difference between these two entities and if there are some histologically well-differentiated carcinomas that will behave in a more aggressive fashion. Molecular markers may contribute to make a more educated selection. Walter, et al.[14] are presently comparing molecular markers in the tumors of those patients who responded early and tumors did not recur as compared with those who responded late or in whom the tumors recurred (Fig. 70.1).[14] He has also put forth certain unresolved issues pertaining to the work-up, conservative medical therapy for fertility- sparing treatment, safety concerns of assisted reproduction and need for maintenance therapy.

Unresolved Issues

- Possible treatment of grade 2 tumors.
- Pretreatment evaluation—MRI, CA 125, hysteroscopy, laparoscopy.
- Optimal treatment regimen with progestins-dose, duration, local intrauterine administration.
- Safety of fertility treatments.
- Maintenance-oral contraceptives, intrauterine progestins.
- Need for hysterectomy after childbearing.
- Oophorectomy at the time of hysterectomy.

Our experience till date has been limited to mainly treating patients with complex and mild atypical hyperplasia with Medroxyprogesterone acetate (MPA) 20 mg/day for 12 days a month and for three consecutive cycles. In most cases, the repeat endometrial biopsy always showed a normal study. Only about 2 cases were actually diagnosed with adenomatous carcinoma that we referred for an oncology opinion and these cases were subsequently lost to follow-up. Currently, in October 2006, we harvested 40 oocytes from a 29-year-old infertile patient, who was diagnosed with complex hyperplasia with mild atypia and who had already been treated with progestins. Since there was no improvement in the endometrium, a surrogacy program with embryo cryopreservation was carried out.

It is always advisable to use extreme caution when advising conservative management with progestins, as one cannot eliminate any potential sign of spread of the tumor or possibly associated ovarian cancer. A careful clinical approach with good common medical sense is absolutely essential.

Recent Research

The last few years have seen increasing research in tumor markers or marker genes capable of predicting the clinical outcome and response to hormonal therapy. The concept is based on immunohistochemical analysis of molecules, such as phosphatase and tensin homologue (PTEN), phospho-Akt, p53, and estrogen and progesterone receptors. PTEN has been described as a tumor-suppressor gene, which is mutated in 30 to 55 percent of endometrial carcinomas. By upregulating PTEN proteins, positive discussion surrounds the possibility of an antitumor effect of progestins.

Garg, et al.[21] have proposed that loss of DNA mismatch repair (MMR) protein defects may be associated with high-grade tumors and unfavorable clinical results. These tumors show lowered estrogen/progesterone receptor expression and more aggressive behavior, explaining how 22 percent of patients with abnormal MMR died of disease compared with 4 percent in a group without the loss of these proteins.[21] The study of MMR can be applied for selecting suitable candidates for fertility preservation or conservative treatment as a part of screening tests.

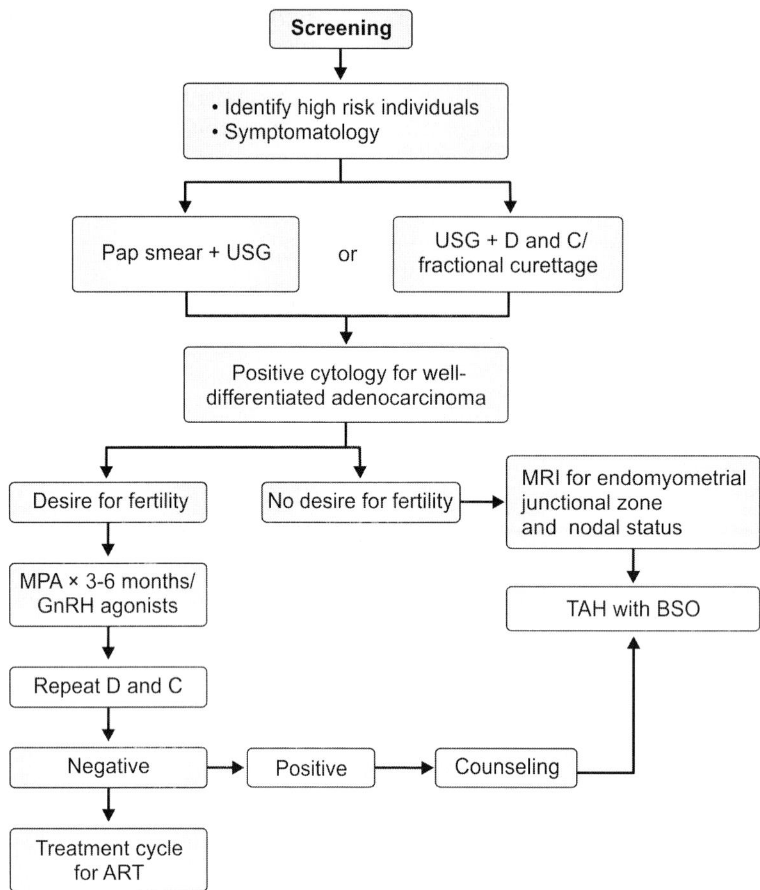

Fig. 70.1: Management steps for early endometrial carcinoma

CONCLUSION

Fertility-preserving treatment is an option in endometrial cancer patients, if carefully selected, and assisted reproductive techniques would be helpful. Based on the review of literature and the use of progestins, it seems safe to practise conservative management in those with well-differentiated endometrial carcinomas without the threat of worsening prognosis. In most studies, it has been seen that ART procedures are a better option than conventional ovulation induction protocols or natural methods. One should have a careful clinical approach and also counsel the patient adequately regarding follow-up evaluations and possible future surgical approach.

REFERENCES

1. Chiva LM, Alonso S. Fertility-preserving management of endometrial carcinoma. Eur J Obs Gyn 2011;6:47-51.
2. The American cancer society all about endometrial cancer. Detailed Guide. www.cancer.org.
3. Goodman MT, Hankin JH, Wilkens LR, Lyu LC, McDuffie K, Liu LQ, Kolonel LN. Diet, body size, physical activity and the risk of endometrial cancer. Cancer research 1997;57:5077-85.
4. Richard J, Hershcopf H, Leon Bradlow. Obesity, diet, endogenous estrogens, and the risk of hormone-sensitive cancer. Am J Clin Nutr 1987;45:283-9.
5. DuBeshter B, Deuel C, Gillis S, Glantz C, Angel C, Guzick D. Endometrial cancer: The potential role of cervical cytology in current surgical staging. Am J Obstet Gynecol 2003;101: 445-50.
6. Leitao MM Jr, Chi DS. Fertility-sparing options for patients with gynecologic malignancies. Oncologist 2005;10:613-22.
7. Muechler EK, Bonfiglio T, Choate J, Huang KE. Pregnancy induced with menotropins in a woman with polycystic ovaries, endometrial hyperplasia, and adenocarcinoma. Fertil Steril 1986;46:973-5.
8. Salha O, Martin-Hirsch P, Lane G, Sharma V. Endometrial carcinoma in a young patient with polycystic ovarian syndrome: first suspected at time of embryo transfer. Hum Reprod 1997; 12:959-62.
9. Park JC, Cho CH, Rhee JH. A successful live birth through *in vitro* fertilization program after conservative treatment of FIGO Grade I endometrial cancer. J Korean Med Sci 2006;21:567-71.

10. Jadoul P, Donnez J. Conservative treatment may be beneficial for young women with atypical endometrial hyperplasia or endometrial adenocarcinoma. Fertil Steril 2003;80:1315-24.
11. Grimbizis G, Tsalikis T, Tzioufa V, Kasapis M, Mantalenakis S. Regression of endometrial hyperplasia after treatment with the gonadotropin-releasing hormone analogue triptorelin: a prospective study. Hum Reprod 1999;14:479-84.
12. Liou WS, Yap OWS, Chan JK, Westphal LM. Innovations in fertility preservation for patients with gynecologic cancers. Fertil Steril 2005;84:1561-73.
13. Montz FJ, Bristow RE, Bovicelli A, Tomacruz R, Kurman RJ. Intrauterine progesterone treatment of early endometrial cancer. Am J Obstet Gynecol 2002;186:651-7.
14. Gotlieb WH, Beiner ME, Shalmon B, Korach Y, Segal Y, Zmira N, Koupolovic J, Ben-Baruch G. Outcome of fertility-sparing treatment with progestins in young patients with endometrial cancer. Obstet Gynecol 2003;102:718-25.
15. Minig L, Franchi D, Boveri S, et al. Progestin intrauterine device and GnRH analogue for uterus-sparing treatment of endometrial precancers and well-differentiated early endometrial carcinoma in young women. Ann Oncol 2011;22:643-9.
16. Shibahara H, Shigeta M, Toji H, Wakimoto E, Adachi S, Ogasawara T, Takemura T, Koyama K. Successful pregnancy in an infertile patient with conservatively treated endometrial adenocarcinoma after transfer of embryos obtained by intra cytoplasmic sperm injection. Hum Reprod 1999;14:1908-11.
17. Pinto AB, Gopal M, Herzog TJ, Pfeifer JD, Williams DB. Successful *in vitro* fertilization pregnancy after conservative management of endometrial cancer. Fertil Steril 2001;76:826-9.
18. Yarali H, Bozdag G, Aksu T, Ayhan A. A successful pregnancy after intracytoplasmic sperm injection and embryo transfer in a patient with endometrial cancer who was treated conservatively. Fertil Steril 2004;81:214-6.
19. Revel A, Safran A, Benshushan A, Shushan A, Laufer N, Simon A. *In vitro* maturation and fertilization of oocytes from an intact ovary of a surgically treated patient with endometrial carcinoma: Case report. Hum Reprod 2004;19:1608-11.
20. Revel A, Schenker JG. Ovarian tissue banking for cancer patients: Is ovarian cortex cryopreservation currently justified? Hum Reprod 2004;19:1-6.
21. Garg K, Shih K, Barakat R, Iasonos A, Soslow RA. Endometrial carcinomas in women aged 40 years and younger: tumors associated with loss of DNA mismatch repair proteins comprise a distinct clinicopathologic subset. Am J Surg Pathol 2009;33:1869-77.

Current Concepts in the Treatment of Male Infertility

Managing Azoospermia

Rajeev Kumar

OVERVIEW

Azoospermia is diagnosed in about one in six of all men undergoing evaluation for infertility. Advances in diagnostic and therapeutic techniques have significantly improved the fertility potential of these men and a careful, tailored evaluation can help choose men suitable for surgical intervention and those who need to proceed directly with assisted reproduction.

The primary goal of evaluation is to separate patients with abnormalities of sperm production or non-obstructive azoospermia from those with normal sperm production but abnormalities in sperm delivery. Non-obstructive azoospermia is rarely amenable to surgical or medical therapy. Most of these patients will require assisted reproduction with *in vitro* fertilization (IVF). Patients with non-obstructive azoospermia have varying degree of sperm production and sperms can often be retrieved from the testis for IVF.

Delivery abnormalities are primarily due to an anatomic obstruction in sperm passage. The site of obstruction could be the epididymis, vas deferens or the ejaculatory ducts. These patients are candidates for surgical correction to either relieve or bypass the obstruction. Success following such surgery depends on the site of obstruction, its etiology, duration of obstruction and technical skill of the surgeon. Ejaculatory dysfunction is another, uncommon cause of azoospermia.

Patients who fail surgical or medical therapy and those who are primarily not suitable for such therapy are candidates for assisted reproduction with sperm retrieval either from the epididymis in patients with distal obstruction or the testis in men with non-obstructive azoospermia.

INTRODUCTION

Azoospermia is the total absence of sperm in the semen. It is present in about 15 percent of all semen samples analyzed from men undergoing evaluation for infertility. Azoospermia results from either impairment in sperm production or an abnormality in delivery them through the semen (Fig. 71.1). Abnormalities of sperm production are known as non-obstructive azoospermia (NOA) while abnormalities of delivery are known as obstructive azoospermia (anatomical block to the passage of normally produced, mature sperms) or faulty expulsion of semen through the urethra. Differentiating NOA from delivery abnormalities is crucial to the evaluation and management of azoospermia since, while the former has minimal therapeutic options, the latter can often be surgically cured.

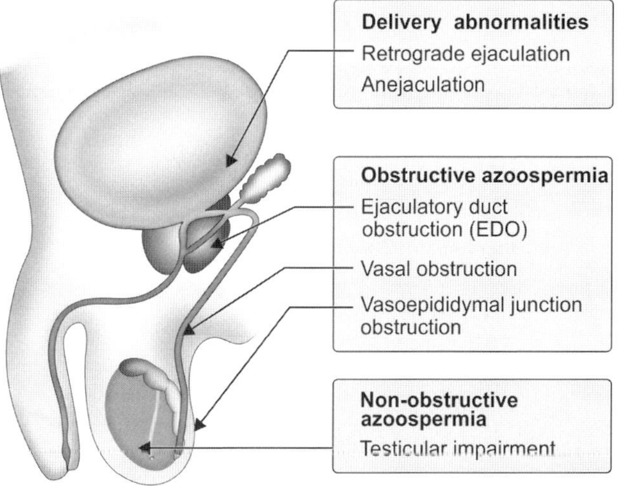

Fig. 71.1: Azoospermia causes

Etiologic Causes

Non-obstructive Azoospermia

Normal spermatogenesis is controlled by the reproductive axis that consists of the hypothalamus, pituitary and the testis. Pulsatile secretion of gonadotropin-releasing hormone (GnRH), luteinizing hormone (LH) and follicle stimulating hormone (FSH) stimulate and maintain both spermatogenesis and testosterone production in the testis. The testis measures about 15 to 25 mL in volume and about 80 percent of this volume is made up of seminiferous tubules within which spermatogenesis occurs. Each testis contains about 600 to 1200 tubules arranged in a loop with both ends opening in the rete testis. The rete testes open into the ductuli efferentes, which in turn coalesce into one epididymal tubule. The epithelium of the seminiferous tubules normally produces greater than 20 million sperms per day.[1] Briefly, spermatogenesis consists of two phases, the initial phase, whereby the germinal stem cells (spermatogonia) divide to produce haploid spermatids and the second phase of spermiogenesis wherein the spermatids turn into mature spermatozoa. This entire cycle requires about 64 days. It is important to remember this duration because ejaculated sperm reflect insults that may have been sustained upto three months earlier and any medical therapy may also not manifest effects till at least a new cycle of spermatogenesis has been completed.

Impaired spermatogenesis may result from either an imbalance in the hormonal control or due a primary abnormality within the testis (Table 71.1). Primary hormonal abnormalities occur in less than 3 percent of azoospermic men. Genetic abnormalities are seen in a similarly small group of men and among the chromosomal abnormalities, Klinefelter's syndrome is the most common etiology. However, this in itself is responsible for less than 1 percent of all cases of male infertility. The other large group of genetic abnormalities is microdeletions of the Y chromosome.[2] Varicoceles have also been described as a cause of azoospermia, however, this diagnosis should be considered in extremely rare circumstances and correction of varicoceles in the hope of reversing azoospermia is, most often, futile.[3]

Patients with non-obstructive azoospermia due to any cause may have certain common phenotypic and laboratory findings. These include small-sized testis, poor development of secondary sexual characteristics and a raised serum FSH level. Testicular size is small because of atrophy of the seminiferous tubules that form the major part of the testis. A concurrent decrease in the production of testosterone may result in poorly developed secondary sexual characters. FSH rises due to a lack of feedback inhibition from the Sertoli cells within the testis.

Delivery Abnormalities

After production within the seminiferous tubules, sperm undergo maturation over a period of 2 to 12 days while they transit through the epididymis. Epididymal transit is associated with increasing sperm motility and may be associated with increasing fertilization potential.[4] Sperm may be retained within the cauda epididymis for a variable period of time depending on the sexual activity. The tail of the epididymis opens into the vas deferens that is about 30 to 35 cm long and terminates into a common opening with the seminal vesicles. Seminal vesicle fluid and sperm then pass through the ejaculatory ducts into the posterior urethra during emission. Emission is followed by ejaculation that is caused by rhythmic contraction of the bulbo-cavernosus muscles of the bulbar urethra that force the deposited ejaculate antegrade through the urethral meatus. This antegrade expulsion is accompanied by closure of the bladder neck to prevent retrograde flow of the ejaculate into the bladder. Anatomic obstruction of any of these passages results in obstructive azoospermia while problems in ejaculation of the sperm from the posterior urethra is called ejaculatory dysfunction (Table 71.2).

Obstructive Azoospermia

Obstruction to sperm passage may occur at the level of the epididymis, the vas deferens or the ejaculatory ducts (Fig. 71.1). Obstruction is diagnosed in about a third of all cases of azoospermia. The etiology of obstruction is extremely variable in differing populations with vasectomy being the commonest cause among the Western populations, where this is the preferred method of sterilization. On the other hand, in countries, such as India, where vasectomy is used as a method of contraception by only about 2 percent of the couples, the etiology of obstruction remains undiagnosed in the majority of cases.

Table 71.1: Non-obstructive azoospermia

1. Endocrine abnormalities
    a. Hypogonadotropic hypogonadism
        i. Pituitary tumors
        ii. Congenital abnormalities
2. Testicular impairment
    a. Genetic causes
        i. Chromosomal abnormalities (Klinefelter's syndrome, etc.)
        ii. Y chromosome microdeletions
    b. Gonadotoxins
    c. Radiation, chemotherapy
    d. Infective (*orchitis*)
    e. Cryptorchidism
    f. Idiopathic

Table 71.2: Delivery abnormalities

1. Obstructive azoospermia
   a. Vasal obstruction
      i. Congenital
         1. Congenital bilateral absence of vas deferens (CBAVD)
         2. Unilateral absence of the vas (the other vas is often atretic/dysfunctional)
         3. Ectopic vas
      ii. Acquired
         1. Vasectomy
         2. Post surgery (hernia/hydrocele/retroperitoneal)
         3. Trauma
         4. Infective
         5. Idiopathic
   b. Ejaculatory duct obstruction
      i. Traumatic (transurethral surgery)
      ii. Inflammatory
   c. Epididymal dysfunction
2. Ejaculatory dysfunction
   a. Retrograde ejaculation
   b. Anejaculation

- *Vasal obstruction*: Vasal obstruction is probably the most common cause of obstructive azoospermia. The paired nature of the testis and the vas deferens means that the obstruction may to occur in either both the vasa deferentia or in the vas of the solitary functional testis.
- *Congenital bilateral absence of the vas deferens (CBAVD)*: Bilateral absence of vas deferens is a congenital developmental anomaly, usually associated with defects in the cystic fibrosis transmembrane regulator (CFTR) gene. Defects in CFTR gene can be transmitted to the offspring, who may manifest the disorder with full blown cystic fibrosis if the female partner is also a carrier of the CFTR mutation. Absence of vas deferens is associated with the absence of seminal vesicles that have a common embryologic origin with the vas. Seminal vesicle secretions form the bulk of the semen volume and also make the semen alkaline and rich in fructose. Lack of seminal vesicle secretion results in the semen being low-volume and acidic. Even an anatomically normal seminal vesicle in such patients is hypofunctional and the volume of semen remains low.[5] Patients with a unilateral absent vas deferens may also present with findings similar to CBAVD since the opposite vas deferens is usually atretic. These patients also have a higher incidence of associated renal anomalies and an ultrasound examination of the abdomen is routinely indicated.
- *Vasectomy*: Surgical vasectomy for contraception is one of the most popular methods of contraception among

Western nations. It is also the commonest cause of azoospermia in these populations.

- *Surgical trauma*: Surgical trauma continues to be one of the common causes of obstructive azoospermia in underdeveloped nations. This is often the result of an improperly performed bilateral hernia or hydrocele surgery, often in the prepubertal age group. The site of injury in hernial surgeries is the inguinal canal. Extensive retroperitoneal surgeries may also result in an injury to the vas deferens during its abdominal course.
- *Infective and idiopathic*: In the majority of a cases diagnosed with obstructive azoospermia in India, the cause may not be clearly determined.[6] Infections, such as *Chlamydia, Mycoplasma* or tuberculosis, may cause obstructive azoospermia due to an obstruction at various levels within the reproductive tract.[7] A definitive history of such infections cannot usually be elicited and the patients are treated as having an idiopathic obstruction. The presence of bilateral hydrocele or a history of bilateral hydrocele surgery may also be consistent with obstruction due to infection rather than through traumatic vasal transection since the inflammatory process itself may destroy the patency of the epididymal tubule.
- *Ejaculatory duct obstruction*: Obstruction at the level of the ejaculatory ducts may result from either surgical trauma or infection. Transurethral surgeries can result in an injury to the paired ejaculatory duct openings, resulting in fibrosis. Among the infective causes, tuberculosis is among the few infections that may be diagnosed through a history of tuberculosis of the genitourinary tract. Most other causes cannot be clearly elucidated during evaluation. Since the seminal vesicles and the vas deferens open together through the ejaculatory ducts, obstruction at this level results in a low-volume, acidic ejaculate lacking in fructose. However, contrary to CBAVD, the vas deferens is palpable in the scrotum.
- *Epididymal dysfunction*: Transit of the sperms through the epididymis is necessary for them to obtain functional maturity. Current knowledge about the mechanism of this transformation is limited as are tests for epididymal dysfunction.

Ejaculatory Dysfunction

Ejaculatory dysfunction may result in either retrograde propulsion of the ejaculate into the urinary bladder or a total lack of ejaculation. Retrograde ejaculation may occur in patients who have undergone previous surgeries on the bladder neck or in the retroperitoneum with damage to the sympathetic innervation. These include surgeries such as retroperitoneal lymph node dissection or sacral rectopexy. Anejaculation is a complex situation, often arising from lack of adequate genital stimulation, excessively inhibited sexual life or a neurologic abnormality. These may present as infertility with azoospermia rather than as anejaculation. The 'ejaculate' in such men actually consists of only urethral secretions or urine that the patient has forcibly evacuated during an attempted masturbation. In both these groups of patients, the volume of the ejaculate is low and acidic with a palpable vas deferens in the scrotum.

Evaluation

Evaluation of azoospermia can be broadly divided into two steps. The first step is to separate obstructive azoospermia and ejaculatory dysfunction from non-obstructive azoospermia. This in itself consists of primary decision-making based on the history, physical examination and the semen report (Table 71.3) followed by investigations based on the primary findings. The next step is to identify the specific etiology of azoospermia.

Step 1: Obstructive versus Non-obstructive Azoospermia

Primary decision-making: Before embarking on evaluating the cause for azoospermia and its management, it is imperative to ensure the validity of the report of azoospermia. This is because the presence of a few dead sperm in even one report rules out obstructive azoospermia. However, since non-obstructive azoospermia and severe oligozoospermia form a continuum with similar etiologies, patients who otherwise have reports of azoospermia may occasionally have a report of a few sperm present. It is also important to ensure that the finding of azoospermia is persistent and repeated in multiple samples since natural variability of semen parameters may present as azoospermia on rare occasions. This is particularly likely in men who have had a recent illness or stress that can

result in transient depression of spermatogenesis. The sample must have been collected into a wide mouth container with no spillage after an abstinence period of at least three days. Low abstinence periods or spillage may result in a falsely low-volume of the ejaculate that would confound the evaluation algorithm. Important primary decision-making findings in the semen analysis include the semen volume, pH and presence of fructose. Patients with a low seminal volume, acidic semen with absent fructose would be suspected to have either obstructive azoospermia or dysfunctional ejaculation. Rarely, hypogonadism may cause non-obstructive azoospermia with a low ejaculate volume.

The history may provide important pointers to the cause of azoospermia. A history of orchiopexy, orchidectomy, radiation therapy, chemotherapy or orchitis suggests testicular impairment. Previous vasectomy, hernia, hydrocele surgery or retroperitoneal surgery would indicate obstructive azoospermia. A history of genital tuberculosis or infections may also indicate obstruction. A family history of infertility could be present in patients with genetic abnormalities. Poor libido, decreased secondary sexual characters, headaches and visual impairment would suggest hormonal abnormalities.

The physical examination can be diagnostic of the cause of azoospermia in patients with bilaterally absent vas deferens. Poor secondary sexual characteristics suggest a low testosterone level that may occur in patients with hypogonadism. Bilaterally small testes are seen in patients with testicular failure. Undescended testes may also be picked up from examination for infertility. Normal-sized testis with fullness of the epididymis would indicate obstructive causes of azoospermia. Palpable nodularity of the vas deferens or the epididymis would indicate obstructive azoospermia, possibly secondary to infections or tumors.

Table 71.3: Azoospermia evaluation algorithm: Primary decision-making

1.	Semen analysis:		
	a.	Confirm azoospermia versus severe oligozoospermia, persistent	
	b.	Confirm complete collection and adequate abstinence	
	c.	Low volume ejaculate, acidic:	Consider obstructive
2.	History:		
	a.	Vasectomy, hernia or hydrocele surgery:	Consider obstructive
	b.	Cryptorchidism, orchiopexy:	Consider NOA
	c.	Low libido, poor sexual characteristics:	Consider NOA: hypogonadism
	d.	Radiation or chemotherapy:	Consider NOA
3.	Physical examination:		
	a.	Poor secondary sexual characteristics:	Consider NOA
	b.	Absent or atretic vas:	Consider obstructive: CBAVD
	c.	Small testes bilaterally:	Consider NOA
	d.	Distended epididymis, normal testis	Consider obstructive
	e.	Epididymal or vasal nodules	Consider obstructive; infective

Secondary Evaluation

Low volume ejaculate: The initial decision-making parameter of secondary evaluation is the semen characteristics. Low volume, acidic ejaculate with absent fructose is a distinct diagnostic category consisting of vas aplasia, ejaculatory duct obstruction or ejaculatory dysfunction (Flow chart 71.1). In such patients, it is important to determine their subjective assessment of ejaculatory volume. If they routinely ejaculate only a few drops and have never ejaculated more, this is consistent with an absent vas. The physical examination confirms non-palpable vas deferens in the scrotum. Additional investigations usually play no role in reaching the diagnosis.[8] However, in patients with a postinflammatory scrotum that is difficult to evaluate or a palpable atretic vas, a transrectal ultrasound may demonstrate the absence of the seminal vesicles. It is important to remember that even if the seminal vesicles are anatomically present, this is not inconsistent with the diagnosis of absent vas and therefore, this investigation needs careful interpretation in the light of semen analysis and physical examination findings.[5]

On the other hand, an earlier normal ejaculate volume (roughly teaspoonful) that has subsequently decreased may be due to a secondary ejaculatory duct obstruction (EDO). A history of genitourinary infections, transurethral surgery or prostatitis would be supportive of this diagnosis.[9] A clinical examination should be performed to confirm the presence

of both vas deferens. These patients require a transrectal ultrasound (TRUS) to look for dilatation of the ejaculatory ducts and seminal vesicles. Presence of such dilatation confirms the diagnosis of EDO.

Dilatation of the ejaculatory ducts and seminal vesicles may be absent in cases of EDO who have a diffusely fibrotic inflammation. The diagnosis of EDO in such cases is one of exclusion and it is important to rule out retrograde ejaculation as the cause of low volume ejaculate. A history of retroperitoneal or bladder-neck surgery would support the possibility of retrograde ejaculation. These patients require the examination of a postejaculatory urine specimen for sperm. The urine is alkalinized for two days using oral potassium citrate or soda-bicarbonate and the patient then attempts ejaculation through masturbation. Immediately after ejaculation, the patient passes urine into a sterile container and both the ejaculate and urine sample are assessed for presence of sperms. Absence of sperms in the ejaculate along with the presence of even a few sperms in the urine confirms retrograde ejaculation.

Normal volume ejaculate: Patients with a normal volume azoospermia are further categorized on the basis of their hormone profile and testicular histology (Flow chart 71.2).

Raised FSH, small testis: The presence of bilaterally small testes would indicate testicular failure. This can be confirmed without performing invasive investigations if the serum FSH is more than 2 to 3 times the upper limit of normal. Such patients require no further diagnostic investigation. Serum testosterone levels should also be evaluated if they have either a history of erectile dysfunction, poor libido or poor secondary sexual characteristics.

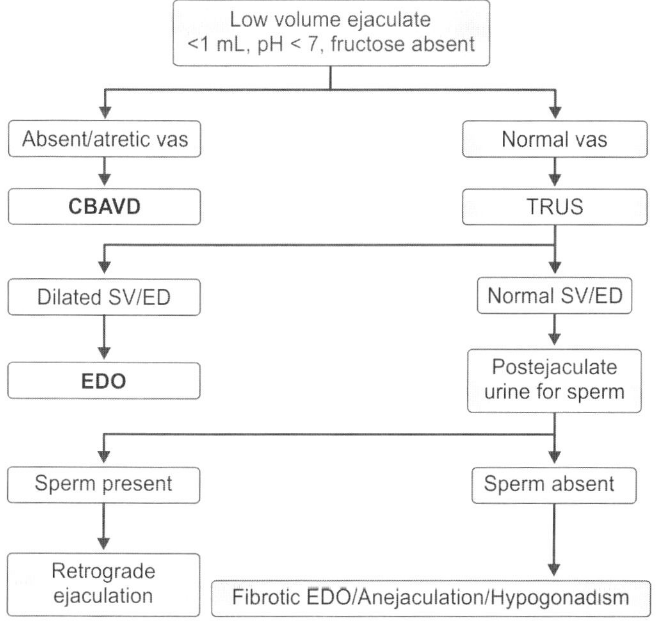

Flow chart 71.1: Low volume ejaculate—algorithm

Abbreviations: TRUS: transrectal ultrasound; SV: seminal vesicle; ED: ejaculatory ducts; EDO: ejaculatory duct obstruction; CBAVD: congenital bilateral absence of the vas deferens

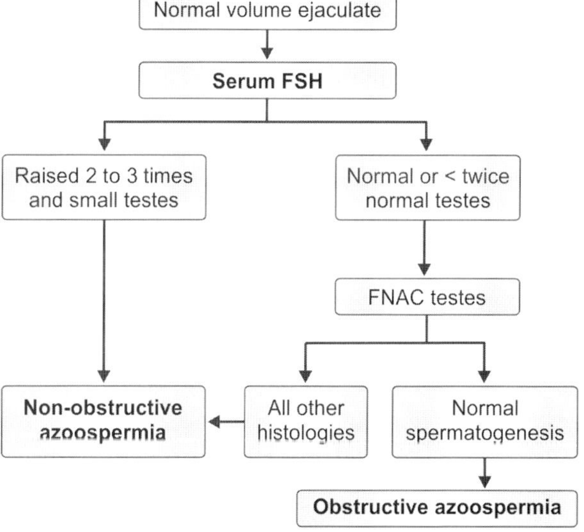

Flow chart 71.2: Normal volume azoospermia

Abbreviation: FNAC: fine needle aspiration cytology

Normal FSH or normal testis size: Testis size may be normal in patients with both obstructive and non-obstructive azoospermia. The majority of these patients have normal or borderline raised FSH. These patients require an evaluation of their testicular histology to differentiate obstructive from nonobstructive azoospermia. A serum FSH value twice above normal would indicate testicular failure. However, the presence of normal testicular size would necessitate confirmation of impaired spermatogenesis through testicular histology.

Testicular histology: Normal spermatogenesis on testicular histology along with azoospermia is the sine-qua-non of obstructive azoospermia. Fine needle aspiration cytology (FNAC) is a quick, out-patient procedure performed under local infiltrative anesthesia. The procedure is usually performed using a 22 to 23 gauge needle attached to a 10 mL syringe held in a specialized plunger controlling device. Through a single skin puncture, multiple passes are made through the substance of the testis without releasing the suction pressure. The aspirate is placed on a glass slide, air dried and stained with May-Grunwald-Giemsa stain. An adequate aspirate is confirmed if there are at least 2000 cells or 100 clusters of 20 cells each.[10] Based on the number of germ cells, Sertoli cells and spermatozoa, the aspirates are reported as normal spermatogenesis, hypospermatogenesis, maturation arrest or only Sertoli cells seen. Additional reports may include testicular fibrosis or atrophic testis.

FNAC provides an accurate assessment of spermatogenesis and numerous studies comparing its results with those of a standard open testicular biopsy confirm its efficacy and safety.[11-13] In rare cases, where adequate tissue is not obtained through the fine needle, or there is lack of expertise in evaluating these slides, a testicular biopsy may be considered. Shrivastava et al.[14] have recommended omitting the serum FSH estimation in men with azoospermia since the final diagnosis depends only on the testicular histology.[14] This recommendation is acceptable in most cases except those with bilaterally small testis where a significantly raised FSH would confirm testicular failure and the patients could avoid a diagnostic FNAC.

The presence of normal spermatogenesis is mandatory for the diagnosis of obstructive azoospermia. Patients with hypospermatogenesis or maturation arrest have various degrees of sperm maturation and may even show the presence of normal sperm in the aspirate. However, these are not due to obstructive azoospermia and would not benefit from surgical reconstruction. An FNAC report stating 'all stages of maturation seen' or 'mature sperm seen' does not indicate obstruction and a quantitative assessment with the statement of 'normal spermatogenesis' must be made to diagnose obstruction. All other reports would suggest non-obstructive azoospermia. Further, there are no clinical parameters that can definitively diagnose obstruction and evaluation of testicular histology must be performed before surgical exploration.[15]

Step 2 : Etiology of Azoospermia

Determining the etiology of azoospermia is important both, to tailor the therapy and prognosticate the likely outcome of interventions.

Obstructive Azoospermia

For obstructive azoospermia, the possibilities include ejaculatory duct obstruction, vasal obstruction and epididymal obstruction. EDO and delivery abnormalities have already been discussed under low-volume ejaculate. A history of vasectomy, hernia surgery or retroperitoneal surgery could be associated with vasal injury. Palpable nodularity of the epididymis or vas deferens indicates postinflammatory obstruction. FNAC from such nodules may lead to the diagnosis of the cause of infertility, particularly in granulomatous infections. Rarely, testicular tumors may also be diagnosed as the cause of such nodules. However, in the majority of patients, the site of obstruction is not identifiable. In such cases, it is presumed that obstruction exists at the vasoepididymal junction. The vasoepididymal junction is particularly susceptible to obstruction, both primarily in cases with idiopathic obstruction and secondarily, as a blow-out in patients with more distal vasal obstruction, and patients planned for a vasovasostomy may instead require a vaso-epididymal anastomosis due to the secondary obstruction.[16]

Vasography: Vasography involves the injection of iodinated contrast medium into the vas lumen to identify the site of obstruction. This investigation is rarely required in the evaluation of azoospermia. It does not aid in the diagnosis of the site of obstruction and may cause further obstruction due to the surgical trauma or inflammation from the contrast agents. In rare, complex reconstructions with suspected multiple site blocks, vasography may be performed on table during surgical reconstruction.

Non-obstructive Azoospermia

As with obstructive azoospermia, despite extensive investigations, the cause is often not determinable. Only two sets of investigations are generally recommended for further categorization.

Hormonal evaluation: A detailed hormonal investigation, including serum testosterone, LH and Prolactin is indicated in patients with a history of poor libido, poor secondary sexual characteristics or signs and symptoms of a pituitary

Table 71.4: Hormonal evaluation for non-obstructive azoospermia

	FSH	LH	Testosterone	Prolactin
Normal	N	N	N	N
Hypogonadotropic hypogonadism	Low	Low	Low	N
Hypergonadotropic hypogonadism	High	N-High	Low-N	N
Hyperprolactinemia	Low-N	Low-N	Low-N	High

adenoma. Diagnostic categories following hormonal estimation would include hypogonadotropic hypogonadism, hyperprolactinemia, hypergonadotropic hypogonadism or normal (Table 71.4).

Genetic testing: While the overall incidence of genetic abnormalities in infertile men is less than 3 percent, this may rise to 10 to 12 percent in men with azoospermia. Genetic abnormalities consist of large chromosomal abnormalities that can be detected through karyotyping or small microdeletions, particularly in the Y chromosome, that require more advanced polymerase chain reaction (PCR) tests for diagnosis. Genetic abnormalities cannot be treated presently. However, diagnosing them is imperative since they are transmissible to the offspring. Therefore, genetic testing with a karyotype and screening for Y chromosome microdeletions should be performed in all non-obstructive azoospermia patients planned for *in vitro* fertilizations (IVF).[17]

Therapy

The advent of *in vitro* fertilization (IVF) with intracytoplasmic sperm injection (ICSI) has created significant therapeutic options for men with azoospermia. At the same time, improvements in diagnostic methodologies and micro-surgical techniques have also improved the results of corrective surgeries for a subgroup of patients with obstructive azoospermia. Correction of reversible abnormalities should take precedence over bypassing them with assisted reproduction. This not only reduces the overall cost of treatment, but allows natural selection of the better sperm, does not require repetitive intervention and is psychologically more acceptable to the couple. It also removes 'the burden of treatment and risk from the female partner for a male problem'.[17]

Obstructive Azoospermia

CBAVD: Patients with CBAVD usually have a palpable caput of the epididymis while the remainder of the epididymis and vas are absent. Spermatogenesis in such patients is also normal. Since the vas deferens cannot be artificially created, these patients require assisted reproduction. Earlier therapy for such patients used to be the creation of an alloplastic spermatocele or sperm retrieval from a naturally formed spermatocele. The pregnancy rates using these techniques are extremely poor and they are no longer recommended. Current recommendations are the use of IVF with or without ICSI following retrieval of sperm from either the palpable caput epididymis or the testis. Since nearly all patients of CBAVD harbor an abnormality in the CFTR gene, genetic testing and counseling prior to assisted reproduction techniques (ART) is mandatory.

Vasoepididymal junction obstruction (VEJO): VEJO is one of the surgically correctable causes of azoospermia. Microsurgical techniques, using high magnification, allow a fine, two-layered mucosa to mucosa anastomosis between the non-obstructed epididymal tubule and the distal vas. The surgery is performed under local infiltrative or day-care general anesthesia. The testis is exposed through a longitudinal scrotal incision and the dilated, non-obstructed segment of the epididymis is identified. The vas deferens is isolated and divided distal to its convoluted portion. Patency of the distal vas is confirmed by injecting 10 to 20 mL of normal saline through the vas lumen. Free flow of the fluid confirms distal patency and a formal vasogram is not required. Anastomosis of the vas to the epididymal tubule can be achieved through a number of differing techniques. The modified two-stitch invagination technique, based on the original description of Marmar, is simple and easy to perform.[18,19] This technique uses two double-armed, 10 to 0 Nylon sutures to provide a four point fixation between the epididymal and vas mucosa. An outer layer of sturdier 8 to 0 or 9 to 0 Nylon sutures supports the mucosal anastomosis.

Early patency rates following this technique in patients with idiopathic obstruction may be up to 48 percent.[6] Much higher patency rates have been reported for surgeries performed for secondary blow-outs after a vasectomy.[6,20] Following a vasoepididymal anastomosis (VEA), sperm may appear in the ejaculate upto two years after the surgery.[20] The decision to declare the procedure a failure would thus need to be taken after a reasonable follow-up period. Unfortunately, there are few parameters that can be used to predict the outcome following surgery. The presence of motile sperm at the site of anastomosis and the technical satisfaction of the surgeon with the quality of the anastomosis may be the only independent predictors of success.[21] Following VEA for idiopathic obstruction, upto 40 percent couples may achieve a spontaneous pregnancy. However, such surgeries are heavily dependent on the skills of the surgeon and should only be performed by trained microsurgeons.[22]

Vasectomy reversal: Vasectomy reversal can be an extremely rewarding surgery with high patency and pregnancy rates.

Under an operating microscope, the ligated segment of the vas deferens is identified and the proximal and distal ends separated. Distal patency of the vas deferens in confirmed as in a VEA. The fluid from the proximal end of the vas is inspected for the presence of sperm before the anastomosis. A two or three-layered anastomosis is performed using 10 to 0 Nylon for the mucosal and 8 to 0/9 to 0 Nylon for the serosal layer.[23] An additional adventitial layer may be anastomosed to strengthen the repair. In occasional cases, absence of sperm and fluid at the proximal end of the vas may suggest a secondary blow-out at the vasoepididymal junction, necessitating an ipsilateral VEA. Up to 75 percent couples may achieve a spontaneous pregnancy following vasectomy reversal.[22] The interval since vasectomy plays a significant predictive role in the outcome of reversal surgery. An interval greater than 15 years may indicate poorer outcomes. However, even in these patients, the pregnancy rate may still be greater than that achievable after IVF.[24]

Vasectomy reversal can also be performed using a single-layered technique without the use of a surgical microscope. However, upto 48 percent patients who have a failed vasectomy reversal surgery have an unsuspected secondary vasoepididymal junction block as the cause of this failure.[25] It is therefore, preferable that only surgeons skilled in microsurgical VEA perform vasectomy reversals so that there would be no need for repeat surgeries and loss of time due to an inadequate primary surgery.

Vasal injuries: Vasal injuries following surgery may also be amenable to a surgical correction. The possibility depends on the level of obstruction, length of vasal defect and duration of obstruction. Techniques similar to those described for vasectomy reversal and VEA are employed, particularly for injuries within the inguinal canal. Injuries in the retroperitoneum are unlikely to be surgically correctable.

Ejaculatory duct obstruction (EDO): Management of EDO depends upon the cause of the obstruction and the findings on the TRUS examination. Patients with a discrete obstruction at the exit of the ejaculatory ducts would have a dilated ejaculatory duct and seminal vesicles on the TRUS. These patients are amenable to a transurethral resection of the ejaculatory ducts (TURED). This procedure involves the insertion of a transurethral resectoscope and identification of the obstructed ejaculatory ducts. The site of obstruction is resected and the dilated portion of the ducts is marsupialized into the posterior urethra. Identification of the ejaculatory ducts within the urethra can be difficult. One way to achieve this is through blind, tentative cuts in the region of the normally placed ducts. Alternatively, a dye, such as methylene blue, can be injected transrectally under ultrasound guidance into each of the seminal vesicles. This dye is then seen emanating from the ejaculatory ducts when digital rectal pressure is applied over the seminal vesicles during resection. Once the openings of the ducts have been identified, a portion of the prostatic tissue overlying it is removed using the resectoscope loop. Efflux of copious, thick fluid confirms the diagnosis and a successful procedure. Patients with a fibrotic type of EDO with no dilatation of the ejaculatory duct do not respond to this therapy and are more suited to assisted reproduction with sperm retrieval and IVF.

Ejaculatory dysfunction: Ejaculatory dysfunction responds poorly to medical therapy. Patients with retrograde ejaculation due to causes such as diabetes or neurologic abnormalities may be given a trial of sympathomimetic drugs (pseudoephedrine, imipramine) to be taken prior to ejaculation in an attempt to cause closure of the bladder neck and antegrade propulsion of the ejaculate. Regular therapy for about two weeks before the ovulatory period of the partner may enhance response rates. Men with surgical causes of retrograde ejaculation, such as bladder neck surgery, do not respond to medical therapy. Alternative management requires alkalinization of the urine followed by retrieval of postejaculatory sperm from urine and their preparation and use for assisted reproduction. Sperm recovery may be enhanced by deposition of sperm culture medium into the urinary bladder prior to ejaculation.

Anejaculation can occasionally be treated by the use of penile vibratory stimulators with visual sexual stimuli. This therapy is particularly useful in patients with situational anejaculation and spinal cord injuries above the T10 level. Electroejaculation under anesthesia is an alternative therapy for patients wishing to avoid surgical sperm retrieval prior to ART. Sperm retrieved through bladder collection, penile vibratory stimulation or electroejaculation are often low in number and of poor quality. While an initial attempt at intrauterine insemination (IUI) is justifiable, most would require IVF.

Non-obstructive Azoospermia

Varicoceles: Non-obstructive azoospermia is generally not amenable to surgical correction. There have been a number of reports of return of sperm to the ejaculate in azoospermic men with varicoceles.[26-28] The azoospermia in these cases is non-obstructive. However, these cases are an exception to the rule that varicoceles are rarely responsible for azoospermia. At the current moment, there are no predictive factors to determine which patients with azoospermia and varicoceles will respond to a varicocelectomy, and varicocele surgery for non-obstructive azoospermia cannot be considered a standard therapy.

Hypogonadotropic hypogonadism: Testosterone replacement is required for achieving virilization in hypogonadic teenaged males. However, this therapy is insufficient to induce spermatogenesis. Gonadotropin therapy, using human chorionic gonadotropin (hCG), 2000 IU, subcutaneously thrice a week, will initiate spermatogenesis in men with hypogonadotropic hypogonadism. The addition of FSH is required to complete and maintain spermatogenesis. Recombinant FSH (rFSH), 75IU, thrice a week, is added about 6 months after the initiation of hCG therapy. A number of these men will convert from azoospermia to oligozoospermia and may also achieve spontaneous pregnancy.

Hyperprolactinemia: Imaging of the pituitary is required before initiating therapy for hyperprolactinemia. The majority of these patients are likely to respond to oral Bromocriptine or Cabergoline therapy. Refractory patients, or those with pituitary tumors causing pressure symptoms, would require decompressive surgery.

Genetic abnormalities: Patients with genetic abnormalities are not amenable to corrective therapy and require ART. Counseling and genetic testing of the partner and fetus may be required since most of these defects are transmissible.

Chemotherapy and radiation: Both chemotherapy and radiotherapy have deleterious effects of varying magnitude on spermatogenesis. A number of patients have a return of their fertility after completion of therapy. This improvement in fertility is generally mirrored by a decline in the FSH levels that may have risen during the therapy. Return of fertility may occur 4 years or more after the end of therapy. Sperm banking is advisable in all such men prior to planned therapy. After completion of therapy, they should generally avoid natural conception until 2 to 4 years to prevent adverse effects of the therapy in the offspring.

Idiopathic non-obstructive azoospermia: Idiopathic non-obstructive azoospermia is not amenable to medical or surgical therapy. Treatment trials with gonadotropins, antiestrogens, testosterone and antioxidants have shown no benefit. On the contrary, androgen therapy may actually further suppress spermatogenesis and decrease the chances of successful sperm retrieval from the testis. All these patients require assisted reproduction.

Assisted Reproduction

The arguments favoring treatment of the primary abnormality rather than direct ART have been briefly presented above. However, most patients with non-obstructive azoospermia and a significant number of patients with delivery abnormalities will require assisted reproduction. Among the ART modalities, nearly all will require IVF since only rarely can enough sperm be made available for an IUI. Pregnancy rates following ICSI with surgically retrieved sperm from the testis are about 50 percent and delivery rates are about 25 to 30 percent.[23] Modalities of sperm retrieval are discussed later in this book.

CONCLUSION

Azoospermia management requires determination of its etiology and development of a comprehensive treatment plan based on the etiology. Obstructive azoospermia is amenable to surgical correction with good results. This requires the intervention of a surgeon skilled in microsurgical techniques. The American Urological Association and the American Society for Reproductive Medicine recommend surgical reconstruction over ART in all men with a history of vasectomy of less than 15 years duration.[23] They also recommend that VEA should be performed by expert microsurgeons. ART may be the preferred modality in patients with advanced age, associated female partner abnormality and in most men with non-obstructive azoospermia. These recommendations do not take into consideration the cost of each therapeutic modality which, at times, may lead to the choice of one modality over another.

REFERENCES

1. Amann RP, Howards SS. Daily spermatozoal production and epididymal spermatozoal reserves of the human male. J Urol 1980;124:211-5.
2. Ferlin A, Arredi B, Foresta C. Genetic causes of male infertility. Reprod Toxicol 2006;22:133-41.
3. Kumar R, Shah R. Varicocele and male infertility: current status. J Obstet Gynecol India 2005;55:505-16.
4. Moore HD, Hartman TD, Pryor JP. Development of the oocyte-penetrating capacity of spermatozoa in the human epididymis. Int J Androl. 1983;6:310-8.
5. Goldstein M, Schlossberg S. Men with congenital absence of the vas deferens often have seminal vesicles. J Urol 1988;140:85-6.
6. Kumar R, Gautam G, Gupta NP. Early patency rates following the two-stitch invagination technique of vasoepidiymal anastomosis for idiopathic obstruction. BJU Int. 2006;97:575-7.
7. Kumar R, Hemal AK. Bilateral epididymal masses with infertility. ANZ J Surg 2004;74:391.
8. Kumar R, Thulkar S, Kumar V, Jagannathan NR, Gupta NP. Contribution of investigations to the diagnosis of congenital vas aplasia. ANZ J Surg 2005;75:807-9.
9. Dohle GR. Inflammatory-associated obstructions of the male reproductive tract. Andrologia 2003;35:321-4.
10. Meng MV, Cha I, Ljung BM, Turek PJ. Testicular fine-needle aspiration in infertile men: correlation of cytologic pattern with biopsy histology. Am J Surg Pathol 2001;25:71-9.
11. Ali MA, Akhtar M, Woodhouse N, Burgess A, Faulkner C, Huq M. Role of testicular fine-needle aspiration biopsy in the evaluation of male infertility: cytologic and histologic correlation. Diagn Cytopathol 1991;7:128-31.

12. al-Jitawi SA, al-Ramahi SA, Hakooz BA. Diagnostic role of testicular fine needle aspiration biopsy in male infertility. Acta Cytol 1997;41:1705-8.

13. Aridogan IA, Bayazit Y, Yaman M, Ersoz C, Doran S. Comparison of fine-needle aspiration and open biopsy of testis in sperm retrieval and histopathologic diagnosis. Andrologia 2003;35:121-5.

14. Shrivastava A, Raghavendran M, Jain M, Gupta S, Chaudhary H. Fine-needle aspiration cytology of the testis: can it be a single diagnostic modality in azoospermia? Urol Int 2004;73:23-7.

15. Kumar R, Gautam G, Gupta NP, Aron M, Dada R, Kucheria K, Gupta SK, Mitra A. Role of testicular fine-needle aspiration cytology in infertile men with clinically obstructive azoospermia. Natl Med J India 2006;19:18-20.

16. Goldstein M. Vasovasotomy: surgical approach, decision-making and multilayer microdot technique. In: Goldstein M (Ed). Surgery of Male Infertility. WB Saunders Company, Philadelphia, 1995. pp. 46-60.

17. Sigman M, Jarrow JP. Male infertility. In: Walsh PC, Retil AB, Vaughan ED Jr, Wein AJ (Eds). Campbell's Urology, 8th edn. Saunders, Philadelphia 2002. pp. 1475-1531.

18. Kumar R, Mukherjee S, Gupta NP. Intussusception vasoepididymostomy with longitudinal suture placement for idiopathic obstructive azoospermia. J Urol 2010;183:1489-92.

19. Marmar JL. Modified vasoepididymostomy with simultaneous double needle placement, tubulotomy and tubular invagination. J Urol. 2000;16:483-6.

20. Matthews GJ, Schlegel PN, Goldstein M. Patency following microsurgical vasoepididymostomy and vasovasostomy: Temporal considerations. J Urol. 1995;154:2070-3.

21. Gautam G, Kumar R, Gupta NP. Factors predicting the patency of two-stitch invagination Vasoepididymal anastomosis for idiopathic obstruction. Indian J Urol 2005;21:112-5.

22. Male Infertility Best Practice Policy Committee of the American Urological Association; Practice Committee of the American Society for Reproductive Medicine. Report on management of obstructive azoospermia. Fertil Steril. 2004;82 (Suppl 1): S137-41.

23. Kumar R, Mukherjee S. 4 × 4 vasovasostomy: A simplified vasectomy reversal technique. Indian J Urol 2010;26:350-2.

24. Boorjian S, Lipkin M, Goldstein M. The impact of obstructive interval and sperm granuloma on outcome of vasectomy reversal J Urol 2004;171:304-6.

25. Chawla A, O'Brien J, Lisi M, Zini A, Jarvi K. Should all urologists performing vasectomy reversals be able to perform vasoepididymostomies if required? J Urol 2004;172:1048-50.

26. Pasqualotto FF, Lucon AM, Hallak J, et al. Induction of spermatogenesis in azoospermic men after varicocele repair. Hum Reprod 2003;18:108-12.

27. Schlegel PN, Kaufmann J. Role of varicocelectomy in men with nonobstructive azoospermia. Fertil Steril 2004;81:1585-8.

28. Cakan M, Altug U. Induction of spermatogenesis by inguinal varicocele repair in azoospermic men. Arch Androl 2004;50: 145-50.

The Effect of Smoking on Semen Quality in Infertile Men

Mete Isikoglu, Murat Seleker, Kemal Ozgur

OVERVIEW

Smoking is probably the most extensively practised potentially hazardous social habit across the world. Since there is more or less an association between cigarette smoking and fertility, advice to give up smoking will be prudent on the basis of current knowledge, especially before enrolling the couples in assisted reproductive technique (ART) programs.

INTRODUCTION

Smoking is one of the most extensively practised potentially hazardous social habit throughout the world that is more common among men compared to women. Owing to the fact that cigarette smoke contains known mutagens and carcinogens, there has been much concern that smoking may have unfavorable effects on male reproduction. Although an association between semen characteristics and smoking, tobacco chewing and other hazardous chemicals has been reported, results in the literature are inconclusive. There is a consistent association between cigarette smoking and fertility in women.[1-4] However, the data on cigarette smoking and measures of male fertility are less clear.

CLINICAL DISCUSSION

Several studies have revealed that in some parts of the world, average sperm counts have dropped by as much as 50 percent since the 1940s.[5,6] Occupational exposure, environmental exposure to hazardous substances, or both, have been blamed as etiologic factor(s) for this.[7]

Dikshit et al.[8] have reported no change in semen volume due to tobacco consumption.[8] However Holzki et al.[9] found significantly lower semen volumes in smokers compared to non-smokers of the same age.[9] Saaranen et al.[10] also reported lower semen volumes in smokers with no additional effects on sperm parameters.[10] We did not find any negative effect of smoking on semen volume in our laboratory data.

A majority of the studies has reported decreased sperm concentration due to smoking,[11-14] but contradictory results exist[8] in this regard. Osser et al.[15] have also found no statistically significant effect of cigarette smoking on sperm density. However, there was a difference between heavy smokers and non-smokers.[15] We, at our clinic, did not find any statistically significant difference between the three groups (non-smokers, light smokers and heavy smokers) in terms of sperm density. However, interestingly enough, our results show that heavy smoking seems to have an enhancing effect on the percentage of rapid progressive sperm motility in infertile men compared to light smoking. This finding concurs with that of Adelusi et al.[16] while not with other studies.[8,11,12,15,17] Although the study of Adelusi et al.[16] was confined to less than 100 patients, our study group included nearly 300 patients. There was no significant difference in our study between non-smokers and heavy smokers in terms of motility. Possible explanations for the enhancement of rapid progressive motility due to heavy smoking in comparison with light smoking are:

1. A definite number of cigarettes per day may constitute a threshold for the enhancement of rapid progressive motility in smokers.
2. Although none of the study patients had a history of urological operations, infections or maldescended testes, the effect may have been due to an undetermined characteristic of the heavy smoking group other than heavy smoking or the that mentioned in the medical history.

3. This may just be due to chance and related neither to heavy smoking nor to other factors. Additional studies with extended study populations are needed to clarify if this is a coincidental finding.

The effects of cigarette smoking on sperm morphology were also evaluated in several studies. While some studies did not find any correlation between smoking and sperm morphology.[15,17] However, others reported a lower percentage of normal sperm morphology,[13,14] especially increased headpiece abnormalities.[13] Our study is one of the few that correlated smoking and sperm morphology according to strict criteria. In our study, tail anomalies and percent of coiled tails were found to be higher in the heavy smokers than in nonsmokers (p < 0.05). All the other morphologic parameters were similar between the study subgroups. We did not find any effect of smoking on the other semen characteristics.

A literature review of the epidemiology indicates that cigarette smoking is associated with modest reductions in semen quality, including sperm concentration, motility and morphology. It also reveals that the associations between smoking and sperm concentration and motility are stronger among studies of 'healthy' men (e.g. volunteers and sperm donors) than among men from infertility clinic populations.[18] In our study, the tail seems to be the affected part of the spermatozoon. Since motility does not seem to be affected negatively by smoking in our study, it is difficult to claim a reduction in the chance of natural pregnancy in smokers based only on the tail anomalies.

Case Studies

Several inconsistent results in the published literature have revealed indecisive conclusions on the effect of smoking on sperm parameters. Experimental studies have indicated that in male rats exposed to smoking, serum levels of nicotine and cotinine were increased, which adversely affected spermatogenesis and sperm fertilizing potential.[19,20] Some studies found negative effects of smoking on sperm density,[11,12,21] motility[11,12,17] or morphology.[13] There are also studies that have claimed a relation between cigarette smoking and decreased semen volume.[9,10] Merino et al.[22] found smoking to have a negative effect on all the parameters of sperm quality,[22] while some authors did not find any effect of smoking on any of the sperm characteristics.[14,15] Zhang et al.[23] showed that semen volume, sperm density, viability and forward progression were much lower in smokers than in nonsmokers.[23] When smokers were divided into subgroups according to the amount and duration of smoking, it was found that there was a negative correlation between the amount[23,24] and duration[23] of smoking and the sperm density, viability and forward progressive motility.

Seminal zinc (Zn) levels were found to be lower in smokers.[23,24] Reduction in Zn secretion may decrease the chromatin Zn content and thereby, sperm chromatin stability; this may in turn contribute to reproductive failure.[25] In addition, smoking increases the production of free radicals that will impair the synthesis and/or augment the consumption of superoxide dismutase.[26]

We conducted a retrospective study to reveal the effect of smoking on semen volume, sperm concentration, motility and percentage of normal morphology according to strict criteria and percentage of specific sperm abnormalities in an infertile Turkish population. Medical records of 627 infertile couples, who presented to Antalya IVF in 2002, were reviewed. Semen parameters including volume, motility, concentration and morphology were documented. Thirty-seven patients, who were diagnosed with azoospermia, were not included in the study. Two hundred and ninety-four patients were excluded from the study because of insufficient data, especially about smoking. The remaining 296 patients were triaged according to smoking status as non-smokers, light smokers and heavy smokers. Non-smokers were men who never smoked (Group 1). Light smokers included men who currently smoked 1 to 19 cigarettes per day on an average (Group 2) and heavy smokers were men who currently smoked 20 or more cigarettes per day (Group 3). All smokers had smoked for at least a year. Smoking history of the patients was obtained by the attending physician at the time of the initial visit. None of these 296 infertile males had a history of prostatitis, orchitis, urological operations or cryptorchidism.

All but 5 of the semen specimens were provided at Antalya IVF, by masturbation after a sexual abstinence period of 3 to 7 days. Five patients (1 from the second group and 4 from the third group) provided semen at home and all the semen samples were examined within one hour. Semen analyses comprised semen volume, sperm concentration, motility and morphology. The motility of each spermatozoon was graded as +4, +3, and +2 according to whether it showed rapid progressive motility, slow or sluggish progressive motility or non-progressive motility. Sperm morphology was assessed after Diff-Quick staining. Anomalies were basically classified into 5 groups as head, acrosome, midpiece, tail and mixed anomalies. Kruger's strict criteria were used for the morphological assessment. Specimens with a sperm concentration below 2 million/mL were not evaluated in terms of morphology. All the semen analyses were performed by the same technician.

A total of 296 patients constituted the study population. Since semen specimens with a concentration below 2 million/mL were not evaluated morphologically, the total number decreased to 258 in morphologic assessment. Three patients from Group 2 and four patients from the Groups 1 and 3 each had a history of varicocelectomy.

Age of the patients, sexual abstinence period, semen volume, sperm concentration, liquefaction time and number of round cells/mL were all similar in the three groups (Table 72.1). The number of cigarettes smoked per day was different between all the three groups (p < 0.05). The ratio rapid progressive sperm motility was significantly greater in Group 3 compared to Group 2 (p < 0.05). Descriptive characteristics and part of the basic semen parameters are shown in Table 72.1.

Sperm morphological evaluation revealed better results in non-smokers than heavy smokers in terms of tail anomalies and percent of coiled tails (p < 0.05) (Table 72.2D).

All the other morphologic assesment parameters were similar in the three group of patients (Tables 72.2A to C and 72.2E).

RECENT ADVANCES AND CONCLUSION

Majority of the published studies support the view that smoking affects the semen quality of infertile men, particularly in heavy and long-term smokers. Our results regarding the effect of smoking on semen characteristics in infertile Turkish men corroborates reports of the detrimental effects of cigarette smoking on some of the sperm morphology characteristics, especially tail anomalies, in infertile males. Prospective studies with larger study populations are needed to come to a decision whether smoking really affects semen quality and fertilizing capacity.

Nevertheless, advice to give up smoking will be prudent in the light of current knowledge, especially before enrolling the couples in ART programs.

Table 72.1: Descriptive characteristics and basic semen parameters of the study population (mean ± SD)

	Non-smokers	Light smokers	Heavy smokers	p value
No. of patients	98	82	116	
Age	32.3 ± 5.3	32.4 ± 6.5	32.3 ± 5.3	0.986
Cigarettes/day	0	9.4 ± 4.7	23.5 ± 8.5	0.000*
Abstinence period (days)	4.0 ± 1.5	3.8 ± 1.1	3.9 ± 1.4	0.513
Volume (cc)	3.6 ± 1.6	3.9 ± 2.0	3.5 ± 2.1	0.475
Concentration (mill/mL)	54.5 ± 57.9	55.4 ± 60.4	68.3 ± 65.8	0.192
Total motility (%)	45.7 ± 20.6	44.6 ± 19.8	49.6 ± 19.3	0.168
+4 motility (%)	8.1 ± 8.1	6.8 ± 7.3	9.7 ± 7.5	0.029*
+3 motility (%)	18.3 ± 11.6	18.5 + 10.6	21.7 ± 12.1	0.056
+2 motility (%)	19.4 ± 9.4	19.3 ± 10	18.6 ± 8.4	0.794
Liquefaction time (min)	24.3 ± 3.7	24.7 ± 2.5	24.8 ± 2.5	0.493
Round cell/mL	2.2 ± 1.6	2.5 ± 2.8	2.7 ± 2.6	0.308

* Statistically significant (p < 0.05)

Table 72.2A: Head anomalies (% mean ± SD)

	Non-smokers	Light smokers	Heavy smokers	p value
No. of patients	83	69	106	
Pin	1.18 ± 1.49	1.28 ± 1.51	1.56 ± 1.80	0.257
Small	4.01 ± 3.25	3.99 ± 3.60	5.06 ± 5.63	0.175
Large	1.93 ± 2.15	2.58 ± 2.56	2.41 ± 2.46	0.208
Amorphous	9.47 ± 4.91	10.59 ± 5.13	9.15 ± 4.14	0.128
Tapered	3.37 ± 3.20	3.13 ± 2.94	3.65 ± 2.75	0.514
Elongated	5.93 ± 8.32	4.54 ± 4.23	4.91 ± 4.94	0.330
Round	2.93 ± 3.35	2.12 ± 2	3.09 ± 3.29	0.090
Pyriform	4.93 ± 4.44	5.28 ± 4	5.49 ± 4.59	0.682
Double	0.63 ± 1	0.90 ± 1.35	1.03 ± 1.65	0.141
Vacuolated	0.63 ± 1.21	0.77 ± 1.45	0.71 ± 0.99	0.763
Other	0.65 ± 1.51	0.51 ± 1.43	0.25 ± 0.82	0.088
Total	35.81 ± 10.50	35.68 ± 9.92	37.25 ± 11.19	0.539

Table 72.2B: Acrosome anomalies (% mean ± SD)

	Non-smokers	*Light smokers*	*Heavy smokers*	*p value*
No. of patients	*83*	*69*	*106*	
Small acrosome	2.54 ± 3.21	2.75 ± 3.24	2.62 ± 2.83	0.914
Large acrosome	0.37 ± 1.13	0.48 ± 1.27	0.25 ± 0.69	0.358
Vacuolated acrosome	3.36 ± 3.39	4.13 ± 4.12	3.29 ± 3.39	0.279
No acrosome	0.99 ± 2.10	0.70 ± 1.88	0.85 ± 1.79	0.646
Total	7.27 ± 6.16	8.07 ± 6.18	7.08 ± 5.70	0.547

Table 72.2C: Midpiece anomalies (% mean ± SD)

	Non-smokers	*Light smokers*	*Heavy smokers*	*p value*
No. of patients	*83*	*69*	*106*	
Cytoplasmic droplet	3.60 ± 3.21	3.49 ± 2.69	3.24 ± 2.73	0.668
Bent	3.39 ± 2.53	3.23 ± 2.49	3.48 ± 2.33	0.804
Thick	2.29 ± 2.05	2.43 ± 2.61	2.37 ± 2.05	0.921
Thin	0.29 ± 0.60	0.26 ± 0.50	0.46 ± 0.75	0.071
Amorphous	4.42 ± 3.66	4.68 ± 2.71	5 ± 2.73	0.430
Non-axial	2.76 ± 2.42	2.88 ± 2.85	2.78 ± 2.52	0.952
Total	16.75 ± 7.60	17.04 ± 7.61	17.38 ± 6.90	0.840

Table 72.2D: Tail anomalies (% mean ± SD)

	Non-smokers	*Light smokers*	*Heavy smokers*	*p value*
No. of patients	*83*	*69*	*106*	
No tail	2.40 ± 3.45	2.33 ± 2.88	2.26 ± 3.68	0.965
Coiled	8.42 ± 6.10	7.43 ± 5.42	5.90 ± 5.74	0.011*
Double	0.88 ± 1.24	0.90 ± 1	1.04 ± 1.41	0.642
Short	3.55 ± 3.17	3.78 ± 4.72	2.91 ± 3.41	0.265
Long	0.29 ± 0.69	0.38 ± 1.02	0.51 ± 1.82	0.524
Thick	0.57 ± 1	0.93 ± 1.46	0.88 ± 1.73	0.231
Dag defect	2.93 ± 4.30	2.99 ± 3.20	2.26 ± 2.84	0.290
Total	19.20 ± 9.76	18.74 ± 10.36	15.71 ± 9.38	0.029*

* Statistically significant (p < 0.05)

Table 72.2E: Mixed anomalies and total normal morphology (% mean ± SD)

	Non-smokers	*Light smokers*	*Heavy smokers*	*p value*
Mixed anomalies	15.57 ± 9.55	17.48 ± 8.87	17.78 ± 9.89	0.251
Total normal morphology	4.33 ± 3.76	3.17 ± 3.12	4.08 ± 3.66	0.116

(*Source:* Zhang JP, Meng OY, Wang O, Zhang LJ, Mao YL, Sun ZX. Effect of smoking on semen quality of infertile men in Shandong, China. Asian J Androl 2000;2:143-6).

REFERENCES

1. Olsen J, Rachootin P, Schiodt AV, Damsbo N. Tobacco use, alcohol consumption and infertility. Int J Epidemiol 1983; 12:179-84.

2. Hughes EG, Brennan BG. Does cigarette smoking impair natural or assisted fecundity? Fertil Steril 1996;66:679-89.

3. Augood C, Duckitt K, Templeton AA. Smoking and female infertility: a systematic review and meta-analysis. Hum Reprod 1998;13:1532-9.

4. Jensen TK, Henriksen TB, Hjollund NH, Scheike T, Kolstad H, Giwercman A, et al. Adult and prenatal exposures to tobacco smoke as risk indicators of fertility among 430 Danish couples. Am J Epidemiol 1998;148:992-7.

5. Carlsen E, Giwercman A, Keiding N, Skakkebaek NE. Evidence for decreasing quality of semen during the past 50 years. Br Med J 1992;305:609-13.

6. Auger J, Kunstmann JM, Czyglik F, Jouannet P. Decline in semen quality among fertile men in Paris during the past 20 years. N Engl J Med 1995;332:281-5.

7. Bigelow PL, Jarrell J, Young MR, Keefe TJ, Love EJ. Association of semen quality and occupational factors: comparison of case-control analysis and analysis of continuous variables. Fertil Steril 1998;69:11-8.

8. Dikshit RK, Buch JG, Mansuri SM. Effect of tobacco consumption on semen quality of a population of hypofertile males. Fertil Steril 1987;48:334-6.

9. Holzki G, Gall H, Hermann J. Cigarette smoking and sperm quality. Andrologia 1991;23:141-4.

10. Saaranen M, Suonio S, Kauhanen O, Saarikoski S. Cigarette smoking and semen quality in men of reproductive age. Andrologia 1987;19:670-6.

11. Handelsman DJ, Conway AJ, Boylan LM, Turtle JR. Testicular function in potential sperm donors: normal ranges and the effects of smoking and varicocele. Int J Androl 1984;7:369-82.

12. Vine MF, Tse CK, Hu P, Truong KY. Cigarette smoking and semen quality. Fertil Steril 1996;65:835-42.

13. Chia SE, Ong CN, Tsakok FM. Effects of cigarette smoking on human semen quality. Arch Androl 1994;33:163-8.

14. Osser S, Beckman-Ramirez A, Liedholm P. Semen quality of smoking and nonsmoking men in infertile couples in a Swedish population. Acta Obstet Gynecol Scand 1992;71:215-8.

15. Goverde HJ, Dekker HS, Janssen HJ, Bastiaans BA, Rolland R, Zielhuis GA. Semen quality and frequency of smoking and alcohol consumption: an explorative study. Int J Fertil Menopausal Stud 1995;40:135-8.

16. Adelusi B, al-Twaijiri MH, al-Meshari A, Kangave D, al-Nuaim LA, Younnus B. Correlation of smoking and coffee drinking with sperm progressive motility in infertile males. Afr J Med Med Sci 1998;27:47-50.

17. Rantala ML, Koskimies AI. Semen quality of infertile couples: comparison between smokers and nonsmokers. Andrologia 1987;19:42-6.

18. Vine MF. Smoking and male reproduction: a review. Int J Androl 1996;19:323-7.

19. Yamamoto Y, Isoyama E, Sofikitis N, Miyagawa I. Effects of smoking on testicular function and fertilizing potential in rats. Urol Res 1998;26:45-8.

20. Reddy A, Sood A, Rust PF, Busby JE, Varn E, Mathur RS, et al. The effect of nicotine on *in vitro* sperm motion characteristics. J Assist Reprod Genet 1995;12:217-23.

21. Chia SE, Xu B, Ong CN, Tsakok FM, Lee ST. Effect of cadmium and cigarette smoking on human semen quality. Int J Fertil Menopausal Stud 1994;39:292-8.

22. Merino G, Lira SC, Martinez-Chequer J. Effects of cigarette smoking on semen characteristics of a population in Mexico. C Arch Androl 1998;41:11-5.

23. Zhang JP, Meng OY, Wang O, Zhang LJ, Mao YL, Sun ZX. Effect of smoking on semen quality of infertile men in Shandong, China. Asian J Androl 2000;2:143-6.

24. Wang SL, Wang XR, Chia SE, Shen HM, Song L, Xing HX, et al. A study on occupational exposure to petrochemicals and smoking on seminal quality. J Androl 2001;22:73-8.

25. Oldereid NB, Thomassen Y, Purvis K. Seminal plasma lead, cadmium and zinc in relation to tobacco consumption. Int J Androl 1994;17:24-8.

26. Zhang JP, Zhang LJ, Meng QY, Sun ZX, Chen Y. The effects of smoking on the level of seminal plasma superoxide dismutase and its relationship to male infertility. J Labour Med 1999;16:93-4.

Is there an Ideal Sperm Retrieval Technique?

Rupin Shah, Hemant Bhanudas Nemade, Devendra Patil

OVERVIEW

In azoospermic men, sperm can be retrieved surgically from the epididymis or the testis and used for intracytoplasmic sperm injection (ICSI). A variety of techniques (open and percutaneous) are available. The ideal method will vary with the clinical situation. For each case, one should use that method, which can procure an adequate number of sperm in the least invasive manner, with the least damage to the testis. This review describes the various techniques with their advantages and disadvantages, and thus, helps identify the ideal sperm retrieval technique for a given situation. In most cases of obstructive azoospermia, percutaneous epididymal sperm aspiration (PESA) is the procedure of choice, followed by a needle aspiration biopsy (NAB) of the testis if the PESA does not succeed. In non-obstructive azoospermia, one starts with testicular NAB; if several NABs fail to procure sperm then an open method like the single seminiferous tubular (SST) biopsy technique or the testicular micro-dissection technique can be tried.

INTRODUCTION

With the advent of ICSI, it has become possible for an azoospermic man to father a child using sperm aspirated from the testis or epididymis.[1] Many methods of operative sperm retrieval have been described. The purpose of this review is to identify the best method of sperm retrieval in a given clinical situation.

Indications for Sperm Retrieval

Surgical retrieval of sperm is required in the following situations:

a. *Obstructive azoospermia:* Where reconstruction is not possible or has failed, or the couple prefers ICSI to reconstructive surgery.
b. *Non-obstructive azoospermia:* In these cases, there is a 30 percent chance that the testis will have focal areas of spermatogenesis;[2] these sperm are too few to emerge in the ejaculate but can be extracted through multiple testicular biopsies.
c. *Ejaculatory failure:* This may be due to psychological or physiological causes; if it does not respond to vibrator therapy or electroejaculation then sperm can be aspirated from the testis and used for ICSI.[3]

d. *Necrozoospermia:* Even when all the ejaculated sperm are dead, testicular sperm tend to be viable; hence, in necrozoospermia, testicular sperm (motile or immotile) are preferred to immotile ejaculated sperm.

In obstructive azoospermia, sperm can be retrieved from the epididymis or testis, while in non-obstructive azoospermia sperm can be retrieved only from the testis and not from the epididymis. Retrieval techniques may be percutaneous or may involve an open surgical procedure.

CLINICAL DISCUSSION

Requirements of an Ideal Technique

A procedure for sperm retrieval should ideally be:
- Non-invasive
- Simple
- Atraumatic
- Efficient
- Painless
- Repeatable.

In the following section, we will describe the pros and cons of commonly used techniques for sperm retrieval and identify which method comes closest to the ideal.

Sperm Retrieval Techniques

Epididymal Sperm Retrieval—Open Methods

Microsurgical epididymal sperm aspiration (MESA)

Method: The epididymis is exposed through a scrotal incision. Under magnification, using an operating microscope, the epididymal tunica is incised and a single distended loop of ductule on the epididymal head is dissected free. The ductule is incised and the effluxing fluid is aspirated using a micro-cannula. The fluid is checked for sperm. Once adequate sperm are retrieved, the ductular incision is closed using 10 to 0 nylon.[4,5] If there are no sperm, or only immotile sperm, then other ductules are exposed and incised.

Advantages: Since the procedure is performed under vision, it allows optimal sperm retrieval,[6] while minimizing damage to the ductule.[7]

Disadvantages: This is a complex, time-consuming procedure that needs an operating microscope. There is no advantage in suturing the ductular incision—the incised ductule may still fibrose after being sutured, and since many other adjacent ductules are available if the procedure has to be repeated, the ductular closure is a waste of time. Also, usually a large number of sperm are retrieved and cryopreserved; these are sufficient for multiple cycles and hence, a repeat MESA procedure is not required.

Open epididymal sperm aspiration (OESA)

Method: This is the non-microsurgical version of MESA. The epididymis is exposed through a scrotal incision. Through an avascular area in the caput, a distended ductule is punctured with an insulin syringe bearing a 26G needle. A small quantity of fluid is aspirated. As the needle is withdrawn, more spermatic fluid pours out of the puncture hole on the epididymal surface. This fluid is aspirated into several insulin syringes by placing the bevel of the needle on the fluid on the epididymal surface and applying gentle suction.[8,9]

Advantages: Like MESA, this technique allows direct aspiration of spermatic fluid under vision, with no contamination by blood, so that a large number of good quality sperm can be retrieved. Since the tubule is punctured through the intact tunica, it quickly seals itself and is not prone to fibrosis or occlusion. Thus, it is an easy and effective procedure that is much quicker and simpler than MESA.

Disadvantages: Its only disadvantage is that it is an open procedure. Compared to MESA, it has no disadvantages.

Epididymal Sperm Retrieval—Percutaneous Methods

Percutaneous epididymal sperm aspiration (PESA)

Method: The caput of the epididymis is stabilized between thumb and forefinger. An insulin syringe with a 26G needle is used (other authors have used 22G or 24G scalp vein needles). 0.1 mL of medium is aspirated into the syringe keeping 0.1 mL of air between the medium and the rubber stopper of the syringe's plunger. The needle is passed through the stretched skin into the epididymis. Suction is created by pulling the plunger of the syringe. The needle is slowly advanced through the epididymis and then withdrawn gradually while rotating the syringe so that the bevel of the needle points in different directions. One more pass is made in the same direction, The suction is released and the needle is pulled out of the epididymis while a little amount of suction remains.[10] The fluid is examined for sperm. If no sperm are seen, the procedure is repeated at another location on the head. Sometimes, several aspirations have to be performed before an adequate number of motile sperm are obtained.

Advantage: This method is quick, simple, efficient,[11] avoids an incision and is atraumatic enough to be repeated several times, if required.[12,13]

Disadvantage: PESA may fail if the epididymis is very atretic (as in some cases of vas aplasia) or extensively damaged by previous surgery or fibrosis (posthydrocelectomy).

Testicular Sperm Retrieval—Open Methods

Conventional open biopsy

Method: The testis is exposed through a scrotal incision. A small incision is made in the tunica, avoiding any visible vessels. Testicular tissue pops out. This is excised using a fine scissors. The tunical incision is closed using 6 to 0 prolene.

Advantage: This is a simple procedure that can be done without special training. A large piece of testicular tissue can be obtained.

Disadvantage: It is an open surgical procedure. The suture on the tunica can be painful, especially if a thick, reactive suture like 3 to 0 catgut is used. While incising and suturing the tunica it is possible to damage subtunical testicular vessels. Since the testicular arterioles are end-vessels, any damage will devascularize an area of the testis. Several studies have shown that when multiple testicular biopsies are taken by the conventional method it results in significant, measurable testicular damage.[14-16]

Testicular microdissection

Method: The entire testis is exposed through a scrotal incision. A long incision is made through the tunica allowing the testicular tissue to prolapse out. The tissue is dissected under an operating microscope and the seminiferous tubules are examined. Atrophic tubules are ignored.[17] 'Healthy-looking' tubules are biopsied and examined for sperm. If no sperm are found then promising tubules from other sites are biopsied. Once sperm are found, or the entire testicular tissue has been searched, the tunical incision is closed with a running prolene stitch.

Advantages: This method allows the entire testicular tissue to be searched for focal areas of spermatogenesis and high rates of sperm retrieval in men with non-obstructive azoospermia have been reported. Additionally, it has been claimed that this method is atraumatic since only a small amount of tissue is biopsied.[18]

Disadvantages: It is an open surgical procedure and is complex, time-consuming and needs an operating microscope and expertise. Though only a small amount of tissue is removed, the extensive dissection causes significant testicular fibrosis. The long incision on the tunica increases the possibility of damage to subtunical blood vessels, and also increases post-operative discomfort.

Single seminiferous tubule (SST) technique

Method: The testis is exposed through a scrotal incision. An avascular area of the testis is punctured with a 26G needle. The prong of an atraumatic microsurgical forceps is used to dilate the puncture hole just enough to allow a single seminiferous tubule to pop out. The tubule is grasped with the forceps and a length of tubule is pulled out of the testis. This is cut flush with the tunica and the tubule is examined for sperm. If sperm are found, more tubule is pulled out from the puncture hole. If no sperm are found, then another puncture is made a little distance away and another piece of tubule is pulled out and checked. The procedure is repeated all over the testicular surface till sperm are found or 8 to 16 tubular biopsies (depending on the size of the testis) have been taken and evaluated. There is no need to close the puncture openings.[19]

Advantages: This is a very atraumatic method of obtaining testicular tissue since the tunica is not cut or sutured and only a single tubule is pulled out. It allows for extensive sampling of the testicular tissue.[14,20] Since there are no sutures on the tunica, there is no pain postoperatively.

Disadvantages: It is an open surgical procedure. It samples only the surface of the testis; the deeper tissues are not biopsied. In very small fibrotic testes, no tubule may pop out of the puncture hole.

Testicular Sperm Retrieval—Percutaneous Methods

Fine needle aspiration cytology (FNAC)

Method: Classically, this involves the single passage of a 24G needle through the testicular parenchyma while applying strong suction. The aspirated fluid is checked for sperm.[21] However, other authors make multiple passages with the needle, almost macerating the tissue to get a sizeable aspirate.[22]

Advantage: It is a simple, easy method that does not involve open surgery.[23,24]

Disadvantage: It is not a very efficient method of sperm retrieval. Compared to a biopsy, FNAC retrieves fewer sperm, and, in cases of testicular failure, has a lower positive sperm retrieval rate.[25,26]

Needle aspiration biopsy (NAB)

Method: The scrotal skin is stretched firmly over the testis. An 18G scalp vein needle is inserted into the testis. Suction is created using a 10 mL syringe connected to the tubing. While maintaining the suction, the needle is passed in and out of the tissue a few times taking care to stay within the parenchyma. The direction of the needle is constant, the goal being to suck tubules into the needle, and not to macerate the testicular tissue. The tubing is clamped and the needle is slowly withdrawn out of the testis. A strand of testicular tissue will be seen between the scrotal skin and the needle.[9] This is grasped with an atraumatic microsurgical forceps and more tissue is pulled out of the testis till the tubule snaps. Additional tissue is recovered by flushing the tubing. The end result is a long strand of testicular tissue that is usually as large as an open biopsy. Pressure is applied for five minutes to achieve hemostasis and meanwhile, the tissue is checked for sperm. If no sperm are found, additional biopsies are taken from other locations.[27]

Advantage: This is quick, simple, involves no incision, is easy to learn and perform and delivers a piece of tissue that is as large as an open biopsy. It can be repeated at different locations, thus sampling the entire testis quite adequately. Testicular tissue is obtained from both, the surface and the interior of the testis.

Disadvantage: Since it is a blind procedure, there is some risk of puncturing a testicular blood vessel and causing an internal hematoma or a hematocele.

Cutting needle biopsy

Method: A standard biopsy needle, like the true-cut needle, can be used to cut a core of testicular tissue.[28]

Advantage: It is a relatively simple, percutaneous method of obtaining testicular tissue.

Disadvantage: Since it cuts through the tissue (unlike the NAB method which aspirates a long intact tubule) it causes a lot of internal damage and the amount of tissue obtained is much lesser than what the NAB method can procure.

Ideal Technique

In *Obstructive azoospermia:* PESA is the preferred method and has all the characteristics of an ideal procedure. If PESA fails due to epididymal fibrosis, then the NAB technique will always yield an adequate number of sperm.

In *Non-obstructive azoospermia:* The NAB procedure is able to obtain adequate tissue in the most cases and meets the requirements of an ideal technique. If no sperm are found after taking several NAB biopsies, then the SST open method is used. If that fails to find sperm, then the microdissection procedure can be tried. By following this step-wise approach, one can maximize the chances of sperm retrieval while minimizing the invasiveness of the procedure and damage caused.

In *Ejaculatory failure:* PESA will damage the epididymal ductule and often fails to retrieve sperm in a non-obstructed epididymis. Hence, the NAB procedure is the preferred method in this case. A single NAB biopsy will retrieve enough sperm. There is no need for an open procedure.

In *Necrozoospermia:* In this case, testicular sperm are needed and NAB is the ideal procedure.

CONCLUSION

While some of the procedures meet the 'ideal' criteria, they are not always applicable in every case. Thus, rather than seeking a single ideal technique, one should have an ideal plan for sperm retrieval; the plan will incorporate a sequence of procedures that would optimize the chances of sperm retrieval, starting with the simplest techniques first, and then utilizing more complex and invasive procedures if required.

REFERENCES

1. Tarlatzis B, Bili H. Clinical outcome of ICSI: Results of the ESHRE Task Force. In: Filicori M, Flamigni C (Eds). Treatment of infertility: The new frontiers. New Jersey: Communications Media for Education, 1998.
2. Silber SJ, Nagy Z, Devroey P, Tournaye H, Van Steirteghem AC. Distribution of spermatogenesis in the testicles of azoospermic men: The presence or absence of spermatids in the testes of men with germinal failure. Hum Reprod 1997;12:2422-88.
3. Shah R. Management of anejaculation. In: Pandian N (Ed.). Handbook of Andrology. Chennai: TR Publishers; 1999. pp.129-39.
4. Silber SJ, Nagy ZP, Liu J, Godoy H, Devroey P, Van Steirteghem AC. Conventional *in vitro* fertilization versus intracytoplasmic sperm injection for patients requiring microsurgical sperm aspiration. Hum Reprod 1994;9:1705-9.
5. Girardi SK, Schlegel P. Microsurgical epididymal sperm aspiration: Review of techniques, preoperative considerations and results. J Androl 1996;17:5-9.
6. Sheynkin YR, Ye Z, Menendez S, Liotta D, Veeck LL, Schlegel P. Controlled comparison of percutaneous and microsurgical sperm retrieval in men with obstructive azoospermia. Hum Reprod 1998;13:3086-9.
7. Nicopoullos JD, Gilling-Smith C, Almida PA, Norman-Taylor J, Grace I, Ramsay JW. Use of surgical sperm retrieval in azoospermic men; a meta-analysis. Fertil Steril 2004;82:691-701.
8. Lania C, Grasso M, Fortuna F, De Santis L, Fusi F. Open epididymal sperm aspiration (OESA): minimally invasive surgical technique for sperm retrieval. Arch Esp Urol 2006;59:313-6.
9. Shah RS. Surgical and Non-Surgical Methods of Sperm Retrieval. In: Hansotia M, Desai S, Parihar M (Eds). Advanced Infertility Management. New Delhi:Jaypee Brothers; 2002. pp.253-8.
10. Shrivastav P, Nadkarni P, Wensvoort S, Craft I. Percutaneous epididymal sperm aspiration for obstructive azoospermia. Hum Reprod 1994;9:2058-61.
11. Craft I, Tsirigotis M, Bennett V, Taranissi M, Khalifa Y, Hogewind G, Nicholson N. Percutaneous epididymal sperm aspiration and intracytoplasmic sperm injection in the management of infertility due to obstructive azoospermia. Fertil Steril 1995;63:1038-42.
12. Rosenlund B, Westlander G, Wood M, Lundin K, Reismer E, Hillensjo T. Sperm retrieval and fertilization in repeated percutaneous epididymal sperm aspiration. Hum Reprod 1998;13:2805-7.
13. Meniru GI, Gorgy A, Batha S, Clarke RJ, Podsiadly BT, Craft IL. Studies of percutaneous epididymal sperm aspiration (PESA) and intracytoplasmic sperm injection. Hum Reprod Update 1998;4:57-71.
14. Schlegel PN, Su LM. Physiological consequences of testicular sperm extraction. Hum Reprod 1997;12:1688-92.
15. Manning M, Junemann KP, Alken P. Decrease in testosterone blood concentrations after testicular sperm extraction for intracytoplasmic sperm injection in azoospermic men . Lancet 1998;352:37.
16. Schlegel PN. Testicular sperm extraction: microdissection improves sperm yield with minimal tissue excision. Hum Reprod 1999;14:131-5.
17. Dardashti K, Williams RH, Goldstein M. Microsurgical Testis Biopsy: a novel technique for retrieval of testicular tissue. J Urol 2000;163:1206-7.
18. Craft I, Tsirigotis M. Simplified recovery, preparation and cryopreservation of testicular sperm. Hum Reprod 1995;10:1623-6.
19. Shah RS. Operative sperm retrieval for ART. In: Goenka ML, Goenka D (Eds). Recent Advances in Infertility Management. Guwahati: Goenka; 2001. pp.179-83.
20. Ramasamy R, Yagan N, Schlegel PN. Structural and functional changes to the testis after conventional versus microdissection testicular sperm extraction. Urology 2005;65:1190-4.
21. Craft I, Tsirigotis M, Courtauld E, Farrer-Brown G. Testicular needle aspiration as an alternative to biopsy for the assessment of spermatogenesis. Hum Reprod 1997;12:1483-7.
22. Turek PJ, Givens CR, Schriock ED, Meng MV, Pedersen RA, Conaghan J. Testis sperm extraction and intracytoplasmic sperm injection guided by prior fine-needle aspiration mapping in patients with nonobstructive azoospermia. Fertil Steril 1999;71:552-7.

23. Tournaye H, Clasen K, Aytoz A, Nagy Z, Steirteghem A, Devroey P. Fine needle aspiration versus open biopsy for testicular sperm recovery: A controlled study in azoospermic men with normal spermatogenesis. Hum Reprod 1998;13:901-4.
24. Friedler S, Raziel A, Strassburger D, Soffer Y, Komarvosky D, Ron-El R. Testicular sperm retrieval by percutaneous fine needle aspiration compared with testicular sperm extraction by open biopsy in men with nonobstructive azoospermia. Hum Reprod 1997;12:1488-93.
25. Aridogan IA, Bayazit Y, Yaman M, Ersoz C, Doran S. Comparison of fine-needle aspiration and open biopsy of testis in sperm retrieval and histopathologic diagnosis. Andrologia 2003;35:121-5.
26. Tournaye H, Camus M, Goossens A, Goossens A, Liu J, Nagy P, et al. Recent concepts in the management of infertility because of nonobtructive azoospermia. Hum Reprod 1995;10:115-9.
27. Altay B, Hekimgil M, Cikili N, Turna B, Soydan S. Histopathological mapping of open testicular biopsies in patients with unobstructed azoospermia. Brit J Urol Int 2001; 87:834-7.
28. Morey AF, Deshon GE Jr, Rozanski TA, Dresner ML. Technique of biopsy gun testis needle biopsy. Urology 1993;42:325-6.

Why are We Still Ligating Varicoceles?

Kishore Nadkarni, Dharmesh Kapadia, Purnima Nadkarni

INTRODUCTION

Varicocele is the elongation, tortuosity and pathological dilatation of the veins of the pampiniform plexus, which is normally secondary to internal spermatic vein reflux. Varicocele is found in approximately 15 percent of the general population, 35 percent of men with primary infertility and 80 percent of men with secondary infertility. It is more common on the left side and frequently bilateral. Unilateral right-sided varicocele is rare. In adolescents, the incidence is approximately 15 percent.

Varicocele has for long been identified as one of the main causes of male infertility.[1] A study by the World Health Organization (WHO) on nearly ten thousand men showed that varicoceles are commonly accompanied by decreased testicular volume, impaired sperm quality and a decline in Leydig cell function.[2] There are conflicting reports on the association between varicocele and infertility.[3,4] Peng et al.[5] postulate the cofactor theory in which varicocele can cause subfertility in association with a cofactor like nicotine in which both the factors need treatment.[5] Varicocele usually results in oligoasthenoteratozoospermia (OAT), in which all three sperm parameters viz. count, motility and morphology are affected. Total azoospermia is rare in varicoceles and when present, may be associated with some testicular factor. Result after varicocele ligation in such cases is poor.[6]

History

Varicocele was first recognized as a clinical problem in the sixteenth century. Ambroise Pare (1500–1590), the most celebrated surgeon of the Renaissance, described this vascular abnormality as the result of melancholic blood. Barfield, a British surgeon, first proposed the relationship between infertility and varicocele in the late 19th century.

Shortly thereafter, other surgeons reported an association of varicocele with an arrest of sperm secretion and the subsequent restoration of fertility following repair. Through the early 1900s, reports by other surgeons continued to describe the association of varicocele with infertility. In the 1950s, the idea of surgically correcting varicoceles as a clinical approach to male infertility gained support among surgeons.

Pathophysiology

The exact mechanism by which varicocele causes impaired testicular function remains poorly understood. Theories include incompetent or absent valves in the internal spermatic vein, resulting in reflux,[7] high scrotal temperature, hypoxia due to venous stasis, dilution of intracellular substrate (e.g. testosterone), imbalances of the hypothalamic-pituitary-gonadal axis and reflux of renal and adrenal metabolites down the spermatic vein. Data exist to both, support and refute each of these possibilities. In addition, nitric oxide,[8] reactive oxygen species[9] and regulators of apoptosis[10] have all recently been implicated in the pathophysiology of varicoceles. It has been suggested that varicoceles impair thermoregulation by disrupting the countercurrent heat exchange mechanism in the pampiniform venous plexus (Fig. 74.1). Reversal of testicular blood flow abnormalities and a drop in testicular temperature have been reported following varicocele repair.[11] Varicoceles induced a characteristic stress pattern, which shows an increased number of tapered forms and immature cells and decreased motility and lower mean sperm count.

Diagnosis

The diagnosis of varicocele is made clinically by examination of the patient in a supine and standing position. A bunch of veins resembling a bag of worms is seen above the testis in the

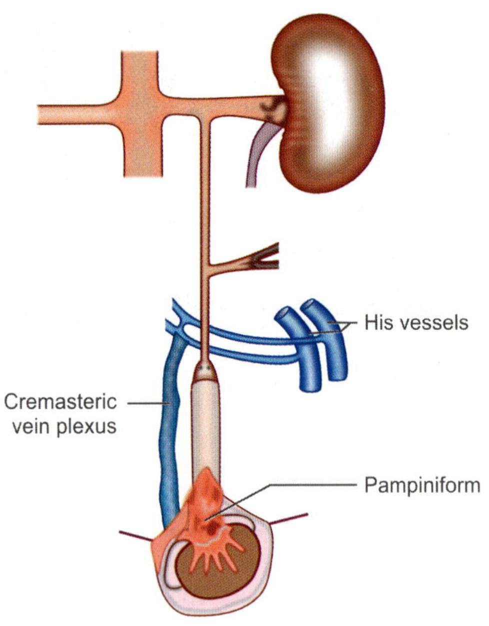

Fig. 74.1: Disruption of the countercurrent heat exchange mechanism in the pampiniform plexus

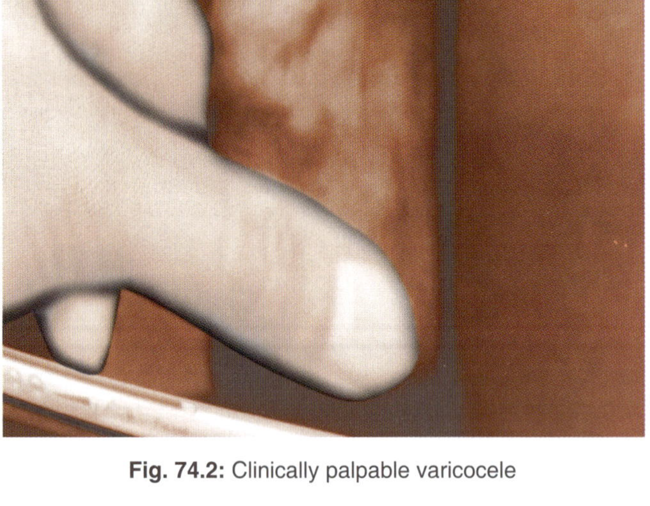

Fig. 74.2: Clinically palpable varicocele

cord, which gives a thrill on coughing and a palpable reflux on performing Valsalva maneuver. The varicoceles are clinically graded as grade 1, 2 and 3 as under.

Subclinical varicocele — (Not palpable)
       Doppler reflux on Valsalva and vein size greater than 2.8 mm.

Clinical Varicocele — (Palpable) (Fig. 74.2)

Grade 1: Small, palpable with Valsalva maneuver only.

Grade 2: Medium and palpable at rest without Valsalva but invisible.

Grade 3: Large, easily visible.

Reflux must be present in the venous system before any venous dilation is termed as varicocele. This reflux may be visible, palpable clinically or Doppler audible and can be demonstrated by color Doppler echography, retrograde venography or a radioisotope venous scintigraphy. There may be concomitant dilatation of a cremasteric system in advanced varicoceles.

High-resolution real time ultrasonography, using a 7 to 10 mHz probe, defines a varicocele as a hollow tubular structure that increases in size following Valsalva maneuver. This is the gold standard investigation to confirm the reflux.

Color-flow Doppler ultrasonography defines the anatomic and physiologic aspects of varicoceles by using real-time ultrasonography and pulsed Doppler in the same scan. The color of the signal identifies the blood flow and direction within the varicocele. The characteristic reverse flow of varicoceles is confirmed by prolonged flow augmentation within a colored flow area; the flow changes color (i.e. reverses) on real-time imaging (Figs 74.3A and B). Although the exact size definition is controversial, most surgeons consider a varicocele to be a vein 3 mm in diameter or larger while the patient is at rest. McClure et al.[12] define a varicocele as the presence of 3 or more veins, with one having a minimum resting diameter of 3 mm or an increase in venous diameter with the Valsalva maneuver.[12]

CLINICAL DISCUSSION

Why do We Need to Ligate a Varicocele in the Era of Assisted Reproduction?

In the era of sophisticated assisted reproductive techniques (ART), is the role of varicocelectomy in the treatment of male factor infertility outdated? Paul Devroey et al.[13] assert, 'Conventional treatment for male factor infertility has little value and has been revised and abandoned'. They further contend that intracytoplasmic sperm injection (ICSI) is an effective treatment even for cases of extreme cases of OAT, and should replace ineffective conventional therapies. In fact, Prof. Devroey proclaimed in 1995 that ICSI has rendered clinical andrology obsolete. Certainly, treatment at the gamete level is exciting but should not be unconditionally applied to all males seeking treatment for male factor infertility. A multifactor analysis, including outcomes, cost and morbidity,

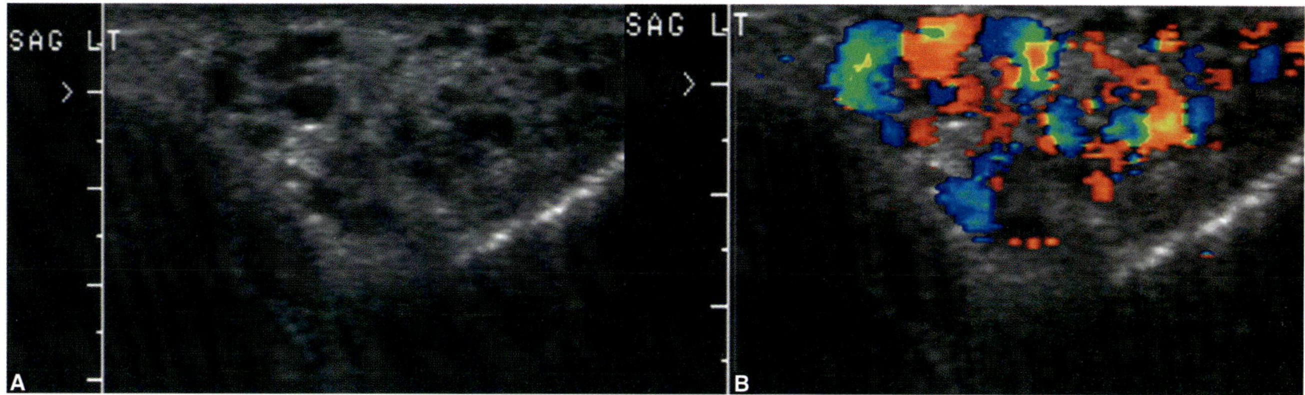

Figs 74.3A and B: Color-flow Doppler ultrasonography identification of a varicocele

all lend support to the fact that varicocele ligation still has a role in the treatment of the subfertile male.[14]

In male factor infertility, a count of at least 5 to 8 million postwash is needed to achieve pregnancy by natural methods, including intrauterine insemination (IUI). This is known as the total motile count (TMC). A TMC of less than 5 million usually necessitates advanced reproductive technologies like *in vitro* fertilization (IVF) or ICSI. If we are to avoid an inevitable ART outcome, all these borderline cases of male subfertiliy must be aggressively treated, so that these patients can achieve a pregnancy in a cost-effective way. Varicoceles, genital tract infections and nicotine are some of the very few factors, which are known to cause OAT. Most of the times, the cause of low sperm counts and declining sperm counts (spermatopause) are not known. Environmental cofactors adding to underlying genetic factors are believed to be the cause of this idiopathic condition. Thus, every attempt must be made to treat the known factors in order to avoid an inevitable ART outcome. Hence, varicoceles must be treated aggressively.

Indications for Surgical Treatment of Varicocele

Majority of men with varicoceles remain fertile and asymptomatic. Hence, treatment of all varicoceles is clearly unnecessary. Surgical correction is indicated in the following:
1. Clinically dectectable varicoceles with abnormal semen parameters (OAT) in infertile couples following appropriate evaluation of the female partner.
2. Varicoceles associated with azoospermia and severe oligozoospermia.
3. Palpable varicoceles in adolescent boys with ipsilateral testicular atrophy.
4. Varicoceles associated with debilitating testicular pain.

Surgical Procedures

- Surgical ligation
- Laparoscopic ligation
- Microsurgical ligation
- Percutaneous occlusion of the internal spermatic vein.

Surgical Ligation (Figs 74.4A and B)

1. *The scrotal approach:* The operation is obsolete today. The veins in the pampiniform plexus are individually ligated through an incision on the scrotum. However, because the veins are too many, too close and thin, the chances of hematoma formation and the chances of damage to the spermatic artery, with resulting testicular damage, is very high and hence, this approach has been abandoned.
2. *Inguinal approach (Ivanissavich 1960):[15]* In this approach, the veins of the pampiniform plexus are ligated within the inguinal canal. A 3 cm incision is taken at the level of the mid-inguinal point. The external oblique aponeurosis is cut. The cord is identified and elevated out of the way. The thin layer of fascia on the cord is cut and the veins carefully dissected out of the cord. They are then cut and ligated. Care is taken to protect the artery, which lies posteriorly. Some people prefer to cut and ligate a single vein at the internal ring or just behind it.
3. *Suprainguinal approach (High ligation) (Palomo, 1949):[16]* A transverse lower abdominal incision is made just above the anterior superior iliac spine. Layers cut include deep fascia and external oblique, internal oblique and transverses aponeurosis is split to expose the peritoneum. The peritoneum is retracted to expose the internal spermatic vein on its under surface. The vein, usually single, is identified, isolated, ligated and cut. In the modified Palomos operation, about 2 to 3 cm of the vein

The operations-schematic

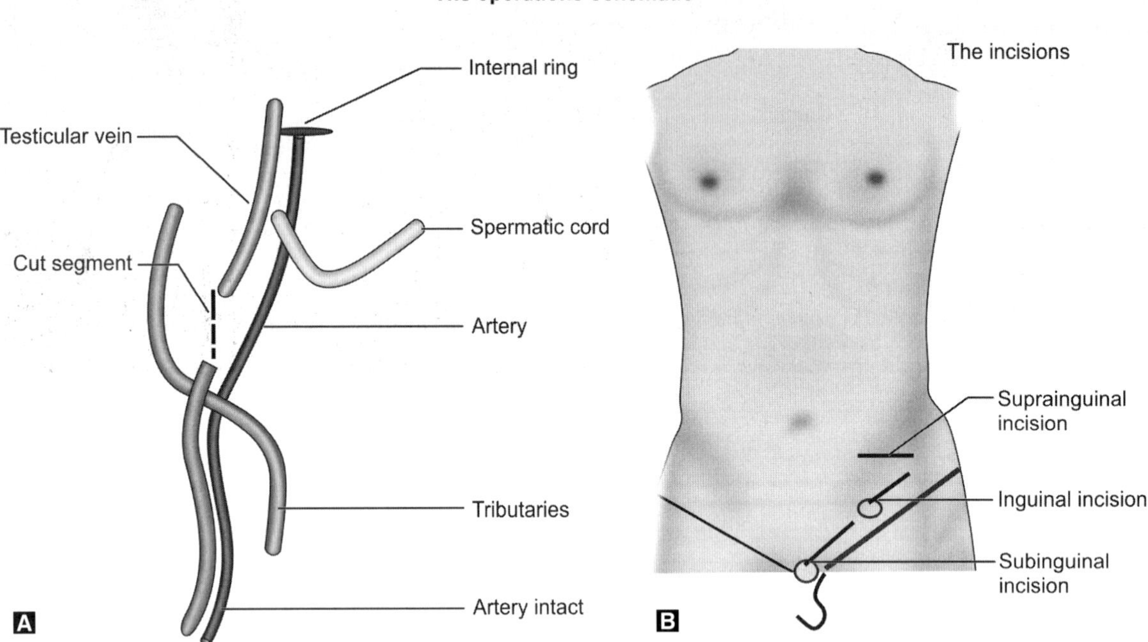

Figs 74.4A and B: Surgical ligation of the varicocele

is excised and the two ends approximated. This helps to hitch the sagging pampiniform plexus. This is the most popular method next to microsurgical varicocelectomy, which today, is the gold standard.

Advantages:
1. Less chances of damage to the spermatic artery, which is some distance away.
2. Vein is dilated, turgid (2–3 mm), single and can be easily isolated.
3. Even damage to the spermatic artery at this level causes little testicular dysfunction, because of extensive anastomosis between the spermatic and the cremasteric arterial systems.
4. There is a tributary, which anastomoses with the superficial circumflex iliac, the epigastric and the pudendal veins, and thus, with the caval system. Ligation below this tributary prevents return of the varicocele.

Disadvantage:
The disadvantage is that the varicocele involving the cremasteric venous system cannot be ligated or even inspected in this approach.

Laparoscopic Ligation

Laparoscopic ligation is gaining in popularity,[17,18] with more and more surgeons having a laparoscopic set-up and expertise. The vein is identified laparoscopically at the deep inguinal ring and obliterated by bipolar diathermy or clips.

Advantages include less morbidity, early discharge from the hospital and total safety.

Disadvantages are the requirement of a proper set-up and expertise, inability to deal with the cremasteric veins and chances of injury to vas.

Subinguinal Microsurgical Ligation

Microsurgical varicocele ligation involves ligation of each dilated vein in the spermatic cord and is carried out through a 2 cm incision just between the external ring and the base of the scrotum. A window is made and each individual vessel is ligated or coagulated. The artery is identified and protected.

Advantage is that accurate individual ligation is possible and recurrence is rare, and this operation is associated with a higher pregnancy rate.

Disadvantages are it requires microsurgical expertise, and a microscope, and lymphatics can be mistaken for veins, hence, the chances of hydrocele are more likely and it is possible that if the level changes, the same vein will be encountered twice or thrice.

Technique of Microsurgical Varicocelectomy

After standard preparation and draping of the patient, the position of the external inguinal ring is marked as 'X' on the skin. The incision extends about 2 cm from the mark following natural skin line. The size of the incision depends somewhat on the obesity of the patient and the size of the testicle being delivered.

The spermatic cord is exposed by hooking an index finger under the external inguinal ring while sliding a small Richardson retractor in the incision along the dorsum of the index finger and pulling in the opposite direction. The cord is encircled with a Babcock clamp. With gentle traction the cord is exposed, encircled with a Babcock clamp and delivered. The ilioinguinal and genital branches of the genitofemoral nerve are excluded and preserved. The Babcock clamp is replaced with a Penrose drain and the testis is delivered.

The gubernaculum is carefully inspected and any veins encountered are either electrocoagulated or clipped and divided depending on their size. All perforating external spermatic veins and gubernacular veins are also divided. The gubernacular veins have been demonstrated radiographically, to account for 10 percent of varicocele recurrences.

Delivery of the testicle enables the surgeon to identify and ligate these vessels, which are responsible for some varicocele recurrences.

Once all external spermatic perforators and gubernacular veins have been divided, the testicle is returned to the scrotum and the spermatic cord remains elevated over a large penrose drain for stabilization in preparation for microscopic examination.

The operating microscope is then brought into the operating field and the cord is examined under 8 to 15-power magnification. The internal and external fascias are opened longitudinally and the cord is examined. The magnification is increased to 15 power and 1 percent Papaverine is dripped over the cord. The testicular artery is identified by its pulsation and is dissected free from all surrounding tissues, tiny veins and lymphatics using a fine-tipped, non-locking microneedle holder and Perse tissue forceps. The pulsation is confirmed by observing a pulsating column of blood that appears just over the needle holder. The artery is identified and then encircled with a zero silk suture to preserve it. Any additional artery encountered is also identified and preserved in this manner. All remaining internal spermatic veins, with the exception of the vasal veins, are clipped with hemoclips or ligated and divided. Care is taken to preserve a majority of lymphatics, as these can contribute to hydrocele formation postoperatively when divided.

On completion of varicocelectomy, the cord should contain only the testicular artery or arteries, vas deferens and associated vessels, cremasteric muscle (with its veins ligated and artery preserved), and spermatic cord lymphatics.

The meticulous approach to varicocelectomy requires extensive training and the use of a high-quality operating microscope. Even loupe magnification is inadequate for the reliable identification of the tiny vascular channels and lymphatics of the spermatic cord. An experienced surgeon can perform this procedure in less than 30 minutes per side, and the procedure is always performed on an ambulatory basis.

Percutaneous Approach

The percutaneous approach to the internal spermatic vein is either through the jugular or right femoral vein via the inferior vena cava. Using a standard Seldinger needle, a catheter is introduced under radiological guidance. Small substances, such as steel coils, Dacron plugs, silicon miniballoons or fibrin plugs, may be injected to plug the spermatic vein. Sclerosants, such as sodium morohaute and sodium teradecyl sulfate or phenol, may also be used.

Complications of Varicocele Surgery

Complications of varicocele surgery include hematoma, testicular atrophy following damage to the spermatic artery, damage to vas deferens, hydrocele formation and of course, recurrence.

Hydrocele formation is the most common complication reported after non-microsurgical varicocelectomy, with an average incidence of about 7 percent.[19] Hydroceles form secondary to ligation of the testicular lymphatics. At least half of all postvaricocelectomy hydroceles grow to a size that produce sufficient discomfort to warrant surgical hydrocelectomy. The effect of hydrocele function on spermatogenesis and fertility is unknown. Theoretically, large hydroceles may impair testicular function by insulating the testes and preventing normal thermoregulation. Use of the operating microscope has essentially eliminated the development of hydroceles following varicocelectomy.[20]

Testicular artery ligation is also a common complication of non-microsurgical varicocelectomy, although its true incidence is unknown. Injury or ligation of the testicular artery may cause testicular atrophy, impaired spermatogenesis or both.[21] Optical magnification and/ or the use of a fine-tipped Doppler probe facilitates identification and preservation of the testicular artery.

The incidence of varicocele recurrence following surgical repair varies from 1 to 45 percent. The incidence of recurrence depends upon the type of procedure performed and the use of magnification. Venographic studies have shown that recurrent varicoceles are caused by periarterial, parallel inguinal, mid-retroperitoneal, gubernacular and transcrotal collateral veins.[19] The only approach equipped to deal with these vessels is the inguinal or subinguinal microscopic technique with delivery of the testis. A comparision of the various approaches to varicocelectomy is summarized in Table 74.1. Microscopic subinguinal technique comes nearest to being the preferred operation for varicocele.

Results and Cost-effectiveness

Increasing evidence suggests that varicocele ligation improves semen quality and pregnancy rates. However, the bulk of this data comes from retrospective, poorly controlled studies.

Table 74.1: A comparison of the various approaches to varicocelectomy

Technique	Artery preserved	Hydrocele (%)	Recurrence (%)	Potential for serious morbidity
Microscopic inguinal	Yes	0	1	No
Retro-peritoneal	No	7	15–25	No
Conventional inguinal	No	3–30	5–15	No
Laparoscopic	Yes	12	5–15	Yes
Balloon	Yes	0	7–25	Yes

Only two randomized, controlled prospective studies have been performed, which report increased semen quality and pregnancy rates, by Nieschlag and colleagues[22] and Medgar et al.[23] Overall, varicocelectomy results in significantly improved semen parameters in 60 to 80 percent of men and pregnancy rates of 20 to 60 percent.[24]

It is also important to remember that varicoceles cause a progressive decline in testicular function, both spermatogenesis and steroidogenesis with time. Thus, for couples desiring more than one child, the ability of varicocelectomy to prevent further deterioration may be even more important than the procedure's early beneficial effects.

Since 1992, with the emergence of ICSI as a treatment modality for severe male factor sterility and with its rising success rate and widespread availability, there is a tendency by some gynecologists to bypass both evaluation and treatment of the male, while proceeding straight to assisted reproduction. This is unfortunate because many cases of male infertility are caused by surgically correctable varicoceles.

Schlegel et al.[25] recently performed a comparision of ICSI and varicocelectomy for the treatment of varicocele-associated infertility using a cost per delivery analysis.[25] The total hospital costs, including delivery and any complications as well as costs attributable to multiple gestations were taken into account, along with published pregnancy and delivery rates for the two procedures. The overall cost per delivery for varicocelectomy averaged $26,300 compared to a striking $89,000 per delivery for ICSI in 1994. The European experience was similar. Comhaire et al.[26] had estimated that varicocelectomy is seven times more cost-effective than ICSI.[26] Although ICSI can clearly facilitate pregnancies in couples with varicocele-associated infertility, it is a very expensive alternative.

According to Dr Turek, in the final analysis, the answer to varicocelectomy versus ART may depend on the preoperative total motile count (p-TMC). If the p-TMC is below 10 million, varicocelectomy is more cost-effective and if the p-TMC is between 10 and 20 millions, then ART seems to be more cost-effective.

Controversial and Debatable Areas

1. *Should varicoceles with azoospermia and with severe oligoasthenozoospermia be operated?*
   Yes, the incidence of the above condition is reported to range from 4.8 to 13.8 percent and prospective controlled studies have demonstrated an improvement in semen quality and enhancement of spermatogenesis. Evidence-based medicine[27,28] suggests that varicocele repair must be considered in all men with azoospermia with palpable varicoceles, and due to considerable risk of relapsing into azoospermia after initial improvement in semen quality, sperm cryopreservation should be considered.

2. *Should subclinical varicoceles associated with subfertility be operated?*
   This is truly a controversial area and existing scientific evidence is compelling but not definitive in establishing the efficacy of varicocelectomy.[29]

3. *Is ICSI safer than varicocele repair?*
   The complication rate for varicocele repair is well-established. Much less obvious, however, are the complications associated with ICSI. Apart from procedural complications and fear of ovarian hyperstimulation syndrome (OHSS), there are several ICSI concerns. Some of these are outlined below.
   - Does ICSI bypass natural selection barriers?
   - Can ICSI introduce foreign material into the oocyte?
   - Does ICSI induce or perpetuate birth defects?
   - Is ICSI associated with a higher miscarriage rate?
   - Does ICSI induce or perpetuate chromosomal abnormalities in children?
   - Does ICSI affect childhood development?
   - Will ICSI babies be able to produce their own sperm?

   In view of the above concerns, varicocele surgery appears safer.

CONCLUSION

Aggressive varicocele surgery is indicated in varicocele-associated infertility. Inguinal and suprainguinal approaches to surgery are the most popular, easy and less costly. However, microsurgical varicocelectomy comes near to being an ideal operation.

In a developing country like India, every attempt must be made to improve sperm counts and achieve pregnancies the natural way and by IUI before submitting the patient to an inevitable ART outcome. Improvement in sperm counts occur 6 to 8 months after surgery and there is a significant relapse rate, hence, sperm cryopreservation should always be considered. Varicocele surgery is indeed a cost-effective option.

REFERENCES

1. Tulloch WS. Varicocele in subfertility: Results of treatment. Br Med J 1955;2:356-8.
2. World Health Organization: The influence of varicocele on parameters of fertility in a large group of men presenting to infertility clinics. Fertil Steril 1992;57:1289.
3. Nilsson S, Edvinson A, Nilsson B. Improvement of semen and pregnancy rate after ligation and division of internal spermatic vein; fact or fiction? Br J Urol 1979;51:591-6.
4. Nieschlag E, Hertle L, Fischedick A, Behre HM. Treatment of varicocele: counselling as effective as occlusion of the vena spermatica. Hum Reprod. 1995;10:347-53.
5. Peng BCH, Tomashevsky P, Nagler HM. The co factor effect: varicocele and infertility. Fertil Steril 1990;54:145-8.
6. Foresta C, Ruzza G, Rizzoti A, Lembo A, Valente ML, Mastrogiacomo I. Varicocele and infertility. Preoperative prognostic elements. J Androl 1984;5:135-47.
7. Braedel HU, Steffens J, Ziegler J, Polsky MS, Platt ML. A possible ontogenic etiology for idiopathic left varicocele. J Urol 1994;151:62.
8. Mitropoulos D, Deliconstantinos G, Zervas A, Villiotou V, Dimopoulos C, Stavrides J. Nitric Oxide synthase and xanthine oxidase activities in the spermatic vein of patients with varicocele. A potential role for nitric oxide and peroxinitrite in sperm dysfunction. J Urol 1996;156:1952.
9. Sharma RK, Agarwal A. Role of reactive oxygen species in male infertility. Urology 1996;48:835-50.
10. Baccetti B, Collodel G, Piomboni P. Apoptosis in human ejaculated cells (notulae seminologicae 9). Submicrosc Cytol Pathol 1996;28:587.
11. Wright EJ, Young GPH, Goldstein M. Reduction in testicular temperature after varicocelectomy in infertile men. Urology 1997;50:257-9.
12. McClure RD, Khoo D, Jarvi K, Hricak H. Subclinical varicocele: the effectiveness of varicelectomy. J Urol 1991;145:789-91.
13. Devroey P, Vandervorst M, Naggy P, Van Steiteghem A. Do we treat the male or his gamete? Hum Reprod 1998;13:175-85.
14. Cocuzza M, Cocuzza MA, Bragais FM, Agarwal A. The role of varicocele repair in the new era of assisted reproductive technology. Clinics (Sao Paulo). 2008;63:395-404.
15. Ivanissavich O. Left varicocele due to reflux. Experience with 4709 operative cases in 42 years. J Int Col Surg 1960;34:1287-90.
16. Palamo A. Radical care due to varicocele by a new technique: Preliminary report. J Urol 1949;61:604-7.
17. Winfield HN, Donovan JF. Laparoscopic varicocelectomy. Semin Urol 1992;10:152-60.
18. Tan SM, Ng FC, Ravintharan T, Lim PH, Chang HC. Laparoscopic varicocelectomy: Technique and results. British J Urol 1995; 75:523-8.
19. Szabo R, Kessler R. Hydrocele following internal spermatic vein ligation: A retrospective study and review of the literature. J Urol 1984;132:924.
20. Goldstein M, Gilbert BR, Dicker AP, et al. Microsurgical inguinal varicocelectomy with delivery of the testis: an artery and lymphatic sparing technique. J Urol 1992;148:1808.
21. Wosnitzer M, Roth JA. Optical magnification and Doppler ultrasound probe for varicocelectomy. Urology 1983;22:24.
22. Nieshlag E, Hertle L, Fischedick, Abshagen K, Behre HM. Update on treatment of varicocele: Counseling as effective as occlusion of the vena spermatica. Hum Reprod 1998;13:2147-50.
23. Madgar I, Weissenberg R, Lunenfeld B, Lunenfeld B, Karasik A, Goldwasser B. Controlled trial of high spermatic vein ligation for varicocele in infertile men. Fertil Steril 1995;63:120-4.
24. Pryor JL, Howards SS. Varicocele. Urol Clin North Am 1987;14:499-513.
25. Schlegel PN. Is assisted reproduction the optimal treatment for varicocele-associated male infertility? A cost-effectiveness analysis. Urology 1997;49:83-90.
26. Comhaire F. Economic strategies in modern male subfertility treatment. Hum Reprod 1995;10 (Suppl. 1):103.
27. Kadioglu A, Tefkeli A, Cayan S, Kendirali E, Erdemir F, Tellaloglu S. Microsurgical inguinal varicocele repair in azoospermic men. Urol 2001;57:328-33.
28. Kim ED, Leibman BB, Grinblat DM, Lipshultz LI. Varicocele repair improves semen parameters in azoospermic men with spermatogenic failure. J Urol 1999;162:737-40.
29. McClure R, Khoo D, Jarvi K, Hricak H. Sub clinical varicocele: effectiveness of varicocelectomy. J Urol 1991;145:789-91.

Is Cryopreserved Retrieved Sperm the Gold Standard for ART?

Luís Arturo Ruvalcaba Castellón, Martha Isolina García Amador, Jorge Eduardo Montoya Sarmiento, Humberto Aguirre Famanía, Henry Mateo Sanez, Marco Antonio Flores Miranda, Sandra Cubillos Gracía, Silvio Cuneo Pareto

OVERVIEW

Currently, we know that sperm cryopreservation is a good method to preserve male fertility. It is a widely used method across the world in assisted reproductive techniques (ART) for many reasons: to have a back-up sample, to avoid repetitive sperm surgical retrievals, to perform ART with donor sperm samples, for sperm banking and for research.

It is still controversial if the results in terms of the pregnancy rates using frozen sperm are similar to fresh sperm, and also if the cryodamage after thawing can affect the offspring. Better techniques for cryopreserving sperm with minimum possible damage and to identify DNA damage post-thaw still need to be developed.

It is also important to establish studies to detect DNA fragmentation prior to freezing the sperm samples, to avoid poor quality of the embryos resulting from oocytes being fertilized with such frozen sperm.

RATIONALE

There are many studies to evaluate the utility of the thawed spermatozoa. The studies show that the pre-thaw characteristics might be an important indicator of post-thaw quality.

One of the preferred parameters to cryopreserve a sperm sample is the finding of normal motility prior to capacitation, as frozen sperm have a lower potential of fertilizing an oocyte than fresh sperm (46% vs 65%). Also, the use of immotile spermatozoa is one of the foremost reasons for failure of fertilization.[1]

Something to consider is the fact that the cryopreservation procedure is not a procedure entirely without risk; the semen sample could be damaged during the thawing process because the DNA can be damaged in the process of forming intracellular ice crystals.[2]

Over 45 percent of the total sperm motility can be affected by the cryopreservation procedure. The use of pentoxifylline and 2-deoxyadenosine can improve the sperm mobility after sperm thawing.[3]

The pregnancy rates do not seem to be significantly affected by an intracytoplasmic sperm injection (ICSI) procedure when frozen-thawed or fresh sample is used (23.7% vs 35.2% respectively).[4] The success rates with the use of frozen sperm samples for insemination procedures are found to be lower than those with fresh sperm (5% vs 18% respectively).[5]

It is possible to use a frozen-thawed semen sample in ICSI procedures, but in patients with severe oligozoospermia, it is difficult to use the sample, because the probability of finding good quality spermatozoa is low. Sperm can be obtained either from an ejaculate or a surgically retrieved sample. When epididymal aspirations or a testicular biopsy are performed, the procedure involves risks such as hematoma formation, infections, fibrosis, etc. The possibility of a devascularization with consequent androgenic deficiency needs to be considered.

One of the most important concerns lies in the consequences of bringing a child with future genetic problems into the world. Considering all of these situations, we mostly use, if possible, sperm obtained from an ejaculate.

By analyzing different groups of sperm samples according to the severity of the oligozoospermia, we can evaluate the total sperm in the frozen samples with respect to the fertilization, implantation and pregnancy rates. A common finding is a difference in testicular size between patients with cryptozoospermia and control groups. Also, only in 62 percent of patients with cryptozoospermia, it is possible to freeze their ejaculate sample. The patients with cryptozoospermia needed 2.4 ejaculations more than an oligozoospermic patient to yield the minimum amount necessary to obtain a useful sample with the criteria for cryopreservation.[6]

Another important point to consider is type of surgical procedure used to obtain the sample. The use of microscopic testicular sperm extraction (TESE) has a higher miscarriage rate than the percutaneous epididymal sperm aspiration (PESA). ICSI done with sperm obtained from a PESA procedure has a 20 percent probability of ending in a miscarriage when compared to a 50 percent chance if the sample is obtained by TESE. For patients less than 30 years, these miscarriage rates were 10 percent vs 25 percent for PESA or TESA, respectively.[7]

INTRODUCTION

The first reported case of sperm freezing was by an Italian physician, named Lazaro Spallanzani, who used snow.[8] It was not until the end of 1930s and the beginning of 1940s, that investigators found that the sperm samples survived better when frozen to a temperature of –160°C. Thereafter, investigators in Veterinary Medicine developed techniques to freeze sperm samples using cryoprotective substances such as glycerol to confer protection to the sperm against damage during the cryopreservation procedure.

In 1953, the first newborn conceived with frozen-thawed sperm sample was reported[9] and in 1963 the technique of cryopreservation was published using nitrogen vapor with a temperature of –196°C. Since that time, the technologies have been improved day by day and we can now successfully use a thawed sample from a semen bank to perfom oocyte fertilization, thanks to the development of intracytoplasmatic sperm injection (ICSI).

CLINICAL DISCUSSION

The European Society of Human Reproduction and Embryology (ESHRE) drafted ethical and moral guidelines for the cryopreservation of gametes in 2004. In this paper, ESHRE emphasized basic and ethical principles: Adult persons are free to decide and plan their fertility to undergo procedures of family planning like vasectomy, cryopreservation of seminal sample, and also to seek treatment for pathologies in order to plan their life.

In the case of minors, ideally the consent must be given by the child, the parents and the tutors, providing clear information about the risk and benefits of each of the alternatives. An important point to evaluate is the risk of re-introducing carcinogenic cells in autologous transplantations, the transmission of viruses from a xenograft transplantation and the risk of too prolonged a culture of the genetic information *in vitro*.[10]

In addition to the evaluation of the ethical guidelines, preventive strategies also need to be developed to decrease the risks associated with the procedure. When we refer to a preventive guideline to avoid a risk, we look for methods to identify adverse events earlier on, and identify preventive steps. We thus try and include the identification and implementation of specific control strategies to decrease any hazards.

It is important to calculate the risks involved in each event, be it a financial, natural or a human resource problem.

Any risk in each event is calculated on a basic scale and classified depending on its relevance. It is possible to make a better evaluation of the risk by using the formula of the Australian/New Zealand model (Risk = consequence × probability).

In the case of sperm cryopreservation, to guarantee the quality of the procedure in the laboratory, we need to focus special attention on the next aspects: careful Physics, adequate nitrogen supply, a qualified staff, patient's serology studies, etc.

It is essential to maintain double tanks of liquid nitrogen to ensure basic security, thereby reducing the possibility of infections such as Hepatitis B. Additional measures include the use of PVC covers, ionoméric resins and blister glass. Liquid nitrogen is preferred to nitrogen vapor because the latter contains a risk of development of pathogens. In contrast, the major advantage of the liquid form is a constant contact with the tissue, maintaining a stable temperature of –160°C, and the elimination of bacterial or viral cross contamination.

The guidelines must be followed in detail to prevent possible accidents and to ensure patient security and efficient sample cryopreservation. One option is to offer the patients, the possibility of cryopreserving the sample in two different geographic locations in order to minimize the risk of loss due to accidents like fire or other natural disasters.[11]

Another important measure of security is to ask for a semen culture. This serves two purposes: to investigate the etiology of the infertility and to treat the infection and guarantee a sterile sample prior to use in the assisted reproduction technique (ART). For sperm cryopreservation, the security guidelines recommend a serology assay for human immunodeficiency virus (HIV), Hepatitis virus B and C, and *Treponema pallidum* (Syphilis). Levy et al.[12] suggested in 2004 the utilization of seminal culture as a new indication to ensure seminal control and then rule out a bacterial contamination before the sample is cryopreserved.[12] Something to consider is the fact that not all samples with a positive culture are infected, and sometimes, bacteriospermia can be a consequence of urethral colonization without pathogenic evidence.

It is important to note that liquid nitrogen does not prevent contamination by all fungi as the *Aspergillus* species can easily colonize the cryopreservation tanks. A good strategy is to wash the seminal sample with a gradient system in the case of bacterial colonization. *U. urealyticum, C. trachomatis* and *E. coli* are the most common bacteria found in semen. It is also possible to find samples with a mixed colonization of *Ureaplasma* and *Streptococcus anginosus*. An important fact

Table 75.1: Indications for sperm freezing	
Indication	*Example*
Donor sperm	Sperm bank, Donor inseminations
Preventive	Cancers, Chemotherapy before surgery
Patient's convenience	Before vasectomy
Oligoasthenoteratozoospermia	Before beginning ART treatment

is the presence of *E. coli* in the seminal sample of patients, who have been started on chemotherapy, therefore this group of patients must receive antibiotic therapy prior to starting chemotherapy, to guarantee the sterility of the sample before cryopreservation. In any case, it is possible to detect pathogens in 10 percent of all cases before cryopreserving the sample.[12]

Case Studies

Sperm cryopreservation still represents a valuable clinical aid in the management of infertility. Its current principle indications include are presented in Table 75.1.

Donor Sperm Insemination

The impact of age on donor insemination outcome in terms of live birth delivery does not seem to be significant as there are acceptable cumulative delivery rates after donor insemination even in older age subgroups. Many women in industrialized societies want to delay reproduction because they give priority to their careers or simply did not meet the right partner. This trend is also present in women seeking treatment.[13] Age is therefore, the most important limiting factor for the success of reproductive treatments. Unfortunately, in the literature, few reports deal with the effect of age on the outcome of donor insemination. A study of 6139 artificial insemination cycles with donor spermatozoa investigated only the cumulative pregnancy rates but not the cumulative delivery rates. They described cumulative pregnancy rates after 3, 6 and 12 months but not after each cycle as in this study. Overall, 928 deliveries were observed, i.e. a delivery rate of 14 percent per cycle and an expected cumulative delivery of 77 percent after 12 cycles. Subgroup analysis showed an expected cumulative delivery after 12 cycles of 87 percent for the group 20 to 29 years, 77 percent for the age group 30 to 34 years, 76 percent for the age group 35 to 37 years, 66 percent for the age group 38 to 39 years and 52 percent for the age group 40 to 45 years. Drop-out analysis in the latter subgroup showed that only one patient discontinued treatment because of medical reasons. In contrast to age, neither indication nor ovarian stimulation protocol had any significant effect on the delivery rate. Our study corroborates the impact of age on donor insemination outcome. Nevertheless, even in some older age subgroups, acceptable expected cumulative delivery rates were observed. Despite this, the main reason for discontinuing treatment, however, was the anticipated low success rate. Women, up until 42 years of age, could be encouraged to continue treatment.[14]

Freezing before Cancer Therapy to Maintain Reproductive Capacity

Semen cryopreservation is possible not only for most adults but also for adolescents and, regardless of disease type, may be a means of preserving fertility prior to gonadotoxic treatment that might impair the spermatogenesis process.[15,16] For instance, some studies show that in adolescents, cryopreservation was possible in 88.5 percent of the cases. Azoospermia was detected in 2.6 percent of the patients at the time of diagnosis. Malignant disease accounted for 84 percent of our male adolescents. In this type of disease, semen parameters were significantly altered only among patients with metastatic malignant bone tumors. After treatment, nine patients presented with azoospermia, five patients achieved pregnancy spontaneously, to achieved it after assisted reproductive techniques, using fresh ejaculated spermatozoa and one following sperm donation. Three failed with cryopreserved sperm.[15] Oncologists offer semen cryopreservation to about 25 percent of their adolescent patients.[17] They consider this procedure to be less effective in adolescents, especially for the youngest males and they generally underestimate the toxicity of cancer therapy to the male gonad. They also do not feel they have enough time to discuss and propose sperm banking because therapy cannot be delayed.[18] In agreement with other studies,[19-22] only a relatively small proportion of patients (2.2%) returned to use their cryopreserved samples for ART. Despite the low rate of straw utilization, most authors have concluded that sperm banking might be strongly encouraged for patients with malignant disease.[23]

With the view of preserving fertility, the technique of cryopreserving male germinal cells has been used. Such candidates are divided into two groups: prepubertal and postpubertal. In the case of the prepubertal group, it is possible to freeze testicular tissue and in the future, use it for autologous transplantation or for *in vitro* maturation.

Thus, sperm cryopreservation should be offered routinely to adolescents exposed to gonadotoxic treatment. Age must not be a discriminative parameter. It is generally difficult to predict which patients will remain azoospermic after treatment, except in the case of treatment for bone marrow transplantation. In general, authors recommended semen cryopreservation for adolescent males, whatever the disease type, before gonadotoxic treatment, which may impair spermatogenesis.[23]

Patient's Convenience

Sometimes, a patient decides to freeze sperm just to have a spare sample or before undergoing a vasectomy, or for personal reasons.

Safe Sperm in Patients with Different Degrees of Oligoasthenoteratozoospermia (OAT)

Cryopreservation of surgically retrieved spermatozoa from the epididymis and testis is a valuable component in effective treatment and management of male infertility, reducing the necessity of repeat surgeries. However, there are lower rates of survival and pregnancy reported. In the last review of several studies, 30 reports were identified, including 9 carriers for cryopreservation of small quantities/numbers of human spermatozoa (7 non-biological and 2 biological carriers). A wide variety of cryopreservation vehicles were reported. The recovery rate of spermatozoa cryopreserved in a known small number varied widely from 59 to 100 percent. Fertilization rates were in the range of 18 to 67 percent. Frozen-thawed spermatozoa, using this method, were subsequently used for intracytoplasmic sperm injection in only five studies, with few pregnancies reported so far. To date, there remains no consensus as to the ideal carrier for cryopreservation of small number of spermatozoa for clinical purposes. Cryopreservation of individual or small numbers of human spermatozoa may replace the need for repeated surgical sperm retrieval. A controlled multicenter trial with sufficient follow-up would provide valid evidence of the potential benefit of this approach.[24]

Methodology of Sperm Cryopreservation

Dr Sherman at the University of Arkansas was the first to utilize cryopreservation in early 1950s. He reported the first successful birth of a child following the use of a cryopreserved semen sample. His technique involved the addition of 10 percent (v/v) glycerol gradually for 2 to 3 min directly to the ejaculate. The glycerolated semen was then packaged into 0.8 mL vials or 0.5 mL straws and frozen in liquid nitrogen vapor. Subsequently, Dr Graham at the University of Minnesota in the early 1970s successfully cryopreserved semen with TEST yolk media, containing as an additive, 12 percent glycerol (freezing media; Irvine Scientific, Santa Ana, CA 92705). He gradually added an equal volume of freezing medium for 2 to 3 min directly to the ejaculate. Similar to the aforementioned procedure, the semen mixture was then packaged into 0.8 mL vials or 0.5 mL straws and frozen in liquid nitrogen vapor.

Cryopreservation, at present, can be implemented through many different methods (Table 75.2). Such variables as cryopreservative additives and media, semen packaging, freezing rate, storage and various thawing and sperm washing procedures are outlined below.

Table 75.2 Methods of sperm cryopreservation	
Indication	*Comments*
Programmed freezing method	More accurate
Manual freezing method	Less expensive
Vitrification	Less ice formation

Cryopreservation: Of the two available methods, the most relevant one must be chosen depending on the laboratory equipment.

Method 1: Programmed Freezing Method

If a controlled-rate freezer is available, place the vials or straws containing the semen inside and initiate the following pre-programmed freezing cycle:
- Starting temperature 20°C (or room temperature)
- Cooling rate of 1°C/minute to +5°C
- Cooling rate of 10°C/minute to –80°C
- Hold at –80°C for 10 min
- Plunge into liquid nitrogen (–196°C).

Method 2: Manual Freezing Method

If a controlled-rate freezer is not available, then:
- Cool slowly (–0.5°C); the glycerolated semen is ultimately lowered to 5°C.
  Note: Such cooling can be facilitated with the use of a 250 mL beaker containing 150 mL water. Then place entire beaker into refrigerator for 30 to 45 min.
- Package as 0.8 mL vials or 0.5 mL straws.
- Place vials or straws approximately 2.5 cm (1 inch) above the liquid nitrogen level (about –75°C) in a covered container.
- Hold at this position for 10 min.
- Plunge into liquid nitrogen.
- Store frozen semen samples in liquid nitrogen.
  Note: Do not store in liquid nitrogen vapor or any temperature higher than –140°C. At such higher temperatures, water molecular kinetic energy will cause recrystallization, inducing cellular injury. There are some variants like liquid vapor and drops pellet.

Method 3: Vitrification

The method of vitrification used has been described in detail by Isachenko, et al.[25] The same concentration of TEYG (test yolk buffer) as for slow freezing was used for vitrification in the presence of a cryoprotectant. Drops (20 ± 2 µL) of sperm samples were placed on copper loops of 5 mm diameter. These cryoloops were then plunged into liquid nitrogen and stored for at least 24 h. After the storage period, the samples were warmed by plunging the copper loops into a 15 mL tube containing 10 mL of medium with human serum albumin (HSA) at 37°C and mixing thoroughly. After warming, five loops per tube, the tubes were placed in a CO_2 incubator for 5 ± 10 min. The spermatozoa were then concentrated by centrifugation at 380 g for 10 min. The pellet was resuspended in 100 mL of medium.[25]

RECENT ADVANCES

Vitrification is a process of super quick freezing in a short time without ice crystal formation. This is possible by quickly submerging the sample in liquid nitrogen. Despite these technologies, there are some problems with the technique, one of them being during the thawing process, because it can form intracellular ice crystals similar to those resulting from a slow thawing process. New techniques, attempting to avoid this problem, have been utilized and one such maneuver is the creation of cryoprotective agents. A technique with ultra-quick freezing with a low volume of semen sample, using 'cryoloops', that are special devices for cryopreservation, reduce the freezing time to 5 minutes or less. With this procedure, it is possible to reduce sperm damage.[26]

Cryodamage

The nature of sperm cryodamage still remains to be elucidated. Several aspects of sperm freezing are important like the development of new technical approaches for cryopreservation, analysis of the stimulatory effect of cryoprotectant additives and selection and optimization of end-points for the analysis of cryodamage.

Human sperm DNA fragmentation is associated with an increase in oxidative stress during cryopreservation, rather than the activation of caspases and apoptosis.[27] The general composition of the cryoprotectant media available for semen/sperm cryopreservation in particular, has remained unchanged for many years. This is in stark contrast to the media available for embryo and oocyte cryopreservation, which is constantly the subject of new research. Apoptosis may play a role in cryoinjury to sperm DNA as the process of cryopreservation has been shown to increase the activation of particular aspartic acid-directed cysteine proteases, called caspases, in both human[28,29] and bull spermatozoa.[30] Caspases, particularly caspases 1, 3, 8 and 9, are known to play a key role in the cellular apoptotic cascade and eventual cell death.[31] Oxidative stress represents another potential mechanism by which DNA fragmentation can be induced in spermatozoa,[32] and as the process of cryopreservation does seem to increase the level of reactive oxygen species (ROS) generation in spermatozoa,[33,34] it is possible that oxidative stress is also responsible for cryo injury to sperm DNA.

The design of protocols for the cryopreservation of sperm from the various species should contain several elements: first, the consideration of spermatozoon as an integrated set of membrane-bound compartments, with an assay for the evaluation of the functionality of each; second, high concentrations of glycerol are likely to alter many aspects of the system in addition to the colligative properties of bulk solvent; third, each and every compartment may have its own relationship to both, temperature and potential interaction with the diluent, predisposition to osmotic swelling and resultant damage, and ATP requirements; and the fourth solution to these potential problems will require the successful development of a complex multifactorial equation.[35]

Cryopreservation of spermatozoa by equilibrium cooling usually consists of the following steps: (1) cells in suspension are placed in a solution of a cryoprotective agent (CPA); (2) the cells are cooled to temperatures near 0°C; (3) they are then cooled to subzero temperatures at a moderately low rate of about 5° to 10°C/min to an intermediate subzero temperature (about –75°C for spermatozoa) and then plunged into liquid nitrogen at –196°C for storage; (4) to restore their function, cryopreserved cells are warmed and thawed and the CPA removed. Any one or all of these steps may damage cells during the entire sequence of cryopreservation. Spermatozoa, in particular, are especially sensitive to these fluctuations of temperature and of osmolalities of solutions because of the delicate nature of the acrosome, the function of which is to disassemble during fusion of the spermatozoon with the oocyte. Nevertheless, it seems reasonable to assume that all cells of a given type ought to respond similarly to the same conditions of freezing and thawing. One might theorize that the same procedure should be reliable and reproducible for spermatozoa of all males of a given species. That clearly, is not the case.[36]

CONCLUSION

Currently, we know that cryopreservation is a good method to preserve the fertility to help solve many infertility problems, and to preserve fertility in other pathologies like cancer. Before these methods were developed, there was no possibility of preserving the fertility of these patients and now they have the possibilty to develop their future fatherhood.

It is still necessary to develop better technologies to cryopreserve sperm with the minimum possible damage and a method to identify if DNA damage has occurred. This is the reason to include new methods to detect DNA sperm fragmentation in routine sperm analysis to know the possibility of having poor embryo development due to poor sperm quality.

Also, it is interesting to develop gene therapy methods to treat sperm cells with previous damage or a damage provoked by the freeze-thaw process.

REFERENCES

1. Verheyen G, Vernaeve V, Van Landuyt L, et al. Should diagnostic testicular sperm retrieval followed by cryopreservation for later ICSI be the procedure of choice for all patients with nonobstructive azoospermia? Hum Reprod 2004;19:2822-30.

2. Witt MA. Sperm banking. In: Infertility in the Male, 3rd edn. Edited by Lipshultz LI and Howardds SS, St Louis: Moosby-Year Book, Inc., Chapt. 1997;32:501.

3. Tash-Anger J, Gilbert B, Goldstein M. Cryopreservation of sperm: Indications, methods and results. J Urol. 2003;170:1079-84.

4. Kuczynski W, Dhont M, Schlegel P N, Grochowski D, Wołczyñski S, Szamatowicz M. The outcome of intracytoplasmic injection of fresh and cryopreserved ejaculated spermatozoa: A prospective randomized study. Hum Reprod 2001;16:2109-13.

5. Richter MA. Haning RV, Shapiro SS. Artificial donor insemination: fresh versus frozen semen; the patient as her own control. Fertil Steril 1984;41:277.

6. Koscinski I, Wittemer C, Lefebvre-Khalil V, Marcelli F, Defossez A. Optimal management of extreme oligozoospermia by an appropriate cryopreservation programme. Hum Reprod 2007; 2679-84.

7. Buffat C, Patrat C, Merlet F, Guibert J, Epelboin S, Thiounn N, et al. ICSI outcomes in obstructive azoospermia: Influence of the origin of surgically retrieved spermatozoa and the cause of obstruction. Hum Reprod 2006;21:1018-24.

8. Mahony MC, Morshedi M, Scott RT, et al. Role of spermatozoa cryopreservation in assisted reproduction. In: Human Spermatozoa in Assisted Reproduction. Edited by AA Acosta, RJ Swanson, SB Ackerman, TAF kruger JA Van Zyl, R Menkveld. Baltimore: Williams & Wilkins Co, Chapt 10 p 100, 1990.

9. Bunge RG, Sherman JK. Fertilizing capacity of frozen human spermatozoa, Nature 1953;172:767.

10. The ESHRE task force on ethics and law. Taskforce 7: Ethical considerations for the cryopreservation of gametes and reproductive tissues for self use. Hum Reprod 2004;19:460-2.

11. Tomlinson M. Managing risk associated with cryopreservation. Hum Reprod 2005;20:1751-6.

12. Levy R, Grattard F, Maubon I, Ros A, Pozzetto B. Bacterial risk and sperm cryopreservation. Andrologia 2004;36:282-5.

13. De Brucker M, Haentjens P, Evenepoel J, Devroey P, Collins J, Tournaye H. Cumulative delivery rates in different age groups after artificial insemination with donor sperm. Hum Reprod 2009;24:1891-9.

14. Botchan A, Hauser R, Gamzu R, Yogev L, Paz G, Yavetz H. Results of 6139 artificial insemination cycles with donor spermatozoa. Hum Reprod 2001;16:2298-304.

15. Menon S, Rives N, Mousset-Siméon N, Sibert L, Vannier JP, Mazurier S, Massé L, et al. Fertility preservation in adolescent males: experience over 22 years at Rouen University Hospital. Hum Reprod 2009;24:37-44.

16. Crha I. Survival and infertility treatment in male cancer patients after sperm banking. Fertil Steril. 2009;91:2344-8.

17. Schover LR, Brey K, Lichtin A, Lipshultz LI, Jeha S. Oncologists' attitudes and practices regarding banking sperm before cancer treatment. J Clin Oncol 2002;20:1890-7.

18. Ogle SK, Hobbie WL, Carlson CA, Meadows AT, Reilly MM, Ginsberg JP. Sperm banking for adolescents with cancer. J Pediatr Oncol Nurs 2008;25:97-101.

19. Lass A, Akagbosu F, Brinsden P. Sperm banking and assisted reproduction treatment for couples following cancer treatment of the male partner. Hum Reprod 2001;7:370-7.

20. Agarwal A, Ranganathan P, Kattal N, Pasqualotto F, Hallak J, Khayal S, Mascha E. Fertility after cancer: a prospective review of assisted reproductive outcome with banked semen specimens. Fertil Steril 2004;81:342-8.

21. Chung K, Irani J, Knee G, Efymow B, Blasco L, Patrizio P. Sperm cryopreservation for male patients with cancer: An epidemiological analysis at the University of Pennsylvania. Eur J Obstet Gynecol Reprod Biol 2004;113(Suppl 1):7-11.

22. Pacey AA. Fertility issues in survivors from adolescent cancers. Cancer Treat Rev 2007;33:646-55.

23. Hallak J, Sharma RK, Thomas AJ Jr, Agarwal A. Why cancer patients request disposal of cryopreserved semen specimens posttherapy: a retrospective study. Fertil Steril 1998;69:889-93.

24. AbdelHafez F, Bedaiwy M, El-Nashar SA, Sabanegh E, Desai N. Techniques for cryopreservation of individual or small numbers of human spermatozoa: a systematic review. Hum Reprod Update 2009;15:153-64.

25. Isachenko E, Isachenko V, Katkov II, Rahimi G, Schöndorf T, Mallmann P, et al. DNA integrity and motility of human spermatozoa after standard slow freezing versus cryoprotectant-free vitrification. Hum Reprod 2004;19:932-9.

26. Schuster TG, Keller LM, Ohl DA, Smith GD. Ultra-rapid freezing of sever oligospermic samples using cryoloops. Fertil Steril 2002;76:S129.

27. Thomson LK, Fleming SD, Aitken RJ, De Iuliis GN, Zieschanj JA, Clark AM. Cryopreservation-induced human sperm DNA damage is predominantly mediated by oxidative stress rather than apoptosis. Hum Reprod 2009;24:2061-70.

28. Paasch U, Sharma RK, Gupta AK, Grunewald S, Mascha EJ, Thomas AJ Jr, Glander HJ, Agarwal A. Cryopreservation and thawing is associated with varying extent of activation of apoptotic machinery in subsets of ejaculated human spermatozoa. Biol Reprod 2004b;71:1828-37.

29. Wundrich K, Paasch U, Leicht M, Glander H-J. Activation of caspases in human spermatozoa during cryopreservation: an immunoblot study. Cell Tissue Bank 2006;7:81-90.

30. Martin G, Sabido O, Durand P, Levy R. Cryopreservation induces an apoptosis-like mechanism in bull sperm. Biol Reprod 2004;71:28-37.

31. Thornberry NA, Lazebnik Y. Caspases: Enemies within. Science 1998;281:1312-6.

32. Aitken RJ, De Iuliis GN, McLachlan RI. Biological and clinical significance of DNA damage in the male germ line. Int J Androl 2009;32:45-56.

33. Mazzilli F, Rossi T, Sabatini L, Pulcinelli FM, Rapone S, Dondero F, Gazzaniga PP. Human sperm cryopreservation and reactive oxygen species (ROS) production. Acta Eur Fertil 1995;26:145-8.

34. Wang AW, Zhang H, Ikemoto I, Anderson DJ, Loughlin KR. Reactive oxygen species generation by seminal cells during cryopreservation. Urology 1997;49:921-5.

35. Hammerstedt RH, Graham JK, Nolan JP. Cryopreservation of mammalian sperm: what we ask them to survive. J Androl 1990;11:73-88.

36. Stanley P Leibo, Helen M Picton, Roger G Gosden. Cryopreservation of human spermatozoa Gamete source, manipulation and disposition. Current practices and controversies in assisted reproduction Report of a meeting on 'Medical, Ethical and Social Aspects of Assisted reproduction' held at WHO headquarters in geneva, switzerland 17–21 september 2001 edited by Effy Vayena Patrick J. Rowe p. David Griffin world health organization Geneva 2002.

Ultrasonography in Infertility

3D Ultrasound and Infertility: Evaluating the Uterus of the Infertile Patient

L Gindes, Yaron Zalel

OVERVIEW

Three-dimensional (3D) sonography has, in the recent years, become a very useful diagnostic tool for the infertile patient. As the technology advanced, this new, non-invasive equipment, has replaced some surgical diagnostic procedures. Pelvic examination by two-dimensional (2D) ultrasound (US) allows insertion of the vaginal probe and rotation of the probe in inclination. The pictures demonstrate the sagittal and axial aspect of the uterus, but not the coronal aspect. With the three-dimensional modality, there are different and new angles of viewing the internal organs as a 3D structure, the coronal plane being the most valuable addition to the imaging of the uterus. By navigating a volume and post-processing, many options are opened to present the structure of interest. Rotating the volume and inverting it upside down cuts parts that hide the inspected organ (MagiCut), enabling an internal view of the volume by the 'Niche view', and measures the volume with 'Vocal II', spreading it like in computerized imaging (CT) with tomographic ultrasound imaging (TUI) software. There is an option for the amplification or attenuation of different echoes in the image setting, thus enabling better enabling of the inspected organ.

INTRODUCTION

Initial reports regarding the three-dimensional ultrasound (3DUS) began in the late 1980s and early 1990s.[1] The first 3D scanner that was commercially available (Voluson 350; Kretztechnik. Zipt, Austria) was presented at the International Radiology Congress, held in Paris in 1989. Image acquisition was accomplished by mechanical sweeping of the 2D transducer along the area of interest. The images were stored on a computer hard disk parallel to each other and equally spaced.[2] Today, ultrasound acquires and constructs volumetric images in real time—upto 40 volumes per second. Volume ultrasound not only improves the 3D/4D capabilities, it enhances the 2D imaging as well.

The advantage of 3DUS as compared to other 3D techniques [computerized tomography (CT), magnetic resonance imaging (MRI), and positron emission test (PET)] is that, it allows real time visualization of the structures and flexibility in viewing images from a different orientation. Although most anatomic structures and pathologies can be visualized by 2DUS, the interpretation and demonstration is much better with the 3DUS.

3DUS can overcome some limitations of 2DUS, like the patient's position, orientation and location of the pathology. 3DUS can increase the diagnostic confidence level and patient understanding and insight. The greatest strength of the 3DUS is the multiplanar image, which enables inspection of the structure from 3 directions at the same time. The 'C-plane' display demonstrates the anatomy parallel to the transducer surface, a view that cannot be obtained by 2DUS. Once the complete volume has been stored, the data can be accessed and re-examined even via telecommunication.

Limitations of the 3DUS do exist. The size of the volume is limited (typical volume size may be 1283 voxels), hence, a large organ or mass would be visualized by few different volumes, which is time-consuming and less accurate for translation. For a higher resolution, the ROI (Region of Interest) should be smaller and a longer time of acquisition should be taken. 3DUS has the same artifacts as 2DUS, however, some artifacts that are unique to the 3DUS include disruption or 'amputation' of organs, part of which are out of the sample volume.

CLINICAL DISCUSSION

Ultrasound Acquisition of Data

We have to choose few possessions before starting a volume acquisition:

- Getting a good B-mode image.
- The region of interest (ROI).
- The angle of the acquired volume.
- The quality of acquisition (this dictates time of acquisition).
- The primary plane of acquisition–longitudinal or transverse.
- 3D or 4D.

After considering all these parameters, it is time for taking the volume acquisition:

- The first step—Acquisition
- The second step—Optimization (minimum transparency for cystic structures, maximum for bony renderings, surface texturing for soft tissues.)
- The third step—Navigation
- The fourth step—Analyzation
- Storage and Recall.

3DUS in Gynecologic Pelvic Examination

The Uterus

The uterus is the first organ to be localized in the pelvic examination. In most women, the uterus is anteverted, but it can be retroverted, deviated and even rotated laterally, especially in the postoperation pelvis with adhesions. Transvaginal ultrasound is the best way to demonstrate the endometrium and myometrium due to the proximity of the probe to the vaginal fornices. Depending on the uterine size, the sweep of the ultrasound waves do not always allow acquisition of the whole organ. For the most part, the ultrasonographic demonstration of the uterus and its cervix has to be divided, with the uterine fundus and corpus on one scan and the isthmic part and the cervix on another one. In some cases of large fibroid uterus, the transabdominal transducer is superior or complementary, since the uterus is located in the abdomen and not in the pelvis. The endometrium is an echodense tissue. Endometrial pathologies are best visualized by 3DUS in the middle of the menstrual cycle, when it is at the end of the proliferative phase. By using the coronal plane, the triangular shape of the endometrium is visualized (Fig. 76.1).

The best imaging of the pelvis is by transvaginal ultrasound (TVS) transducer. Three-dimensional ultrasound (3DUS) overcomes the two dimensional ultrasound (2DUS) limitation of the minor tilting of the transducer in the vagina, and allows the coronal plane of the pelvic organs to be examined. The evaluation of the infertile patient can reveal congenital uterine malformations, and endometrial filling defects like

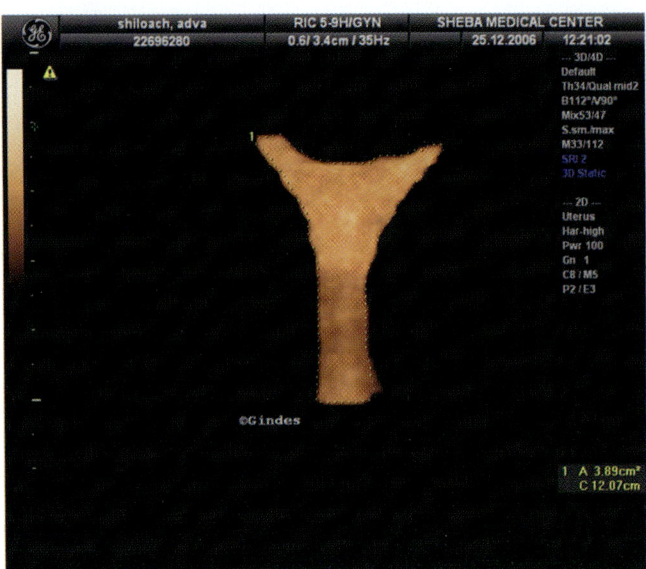

Fig. 76.1: Coronal plane of normal endometrium

polyps, submucus myomas, adenomyosis, adhesions, and left intrauterine defects (IUD).

Uterine pathology

Identification of uterine anomalies is important in the work-up of infertility patients to achieve the proper treatment. It is also important to be familiar with uterine anomalies before pregnancy to avoid unnecessary obstetrical complications, like cervical incompetence and preterm delivery. In the work-up of the infertile patient, the sonographer should examine carefully the corpus, the endometrium, and look for Müllerian abnormalities. The examination can be transvaginal, trans-perineal/translabial, transabdominal, or integrated.

Congenital Müllerian malformations

Most of the uterine malformations are asymptomatic, pending fertility is required. Uterine anomalies were identified in 0.17 percent of the fertile women and in 3.5 percent of infertile women in a meta-analysis of 47 studies from 14 countries.[3] The prevalence of uterine anomalies in the general population was 0.50 percent. Their distribution was: 7 percent arcuate, 34 percent septate, 39 percent bicornuate, 11 percent didelphic, 5 percent unicornuate, and 4 percent hypoplastic/aplastic/solid and other forms. In other publications, septate uterus accounted for upto 90 percent of all uterine anomalies.

During a routine check-up by 3DUS of 267 *in vitro* fertilization (IVF) patients, a uterine abnormality was suspected in 108 patients (40.4%),[4] which led to diagnostic hysteroscopy. The detection rate of submucus myoma, endometrial polyp, arcuate and septate uterus was 100 percent. The intrauterine synechiae detection rate was only 25 percent (one patient was diagnosed by 3DUS, and the other 3 were diagnosed by hysteroscopy). In other studies, the detection rate of minor uterine anomalies by 3DUS was

92 to 100 percent.[5,6] It is disputable weather these minor uterine abnormalities affect the implantation rate.

Congenital abnormalities of the Müllerian ducts are relatively common (incidence of 4–5%), and contribute to problems of infertility, recurrent pregnancy loss, and poor pregnancy outcome (encountered in approximately 25% of women with uterine anomalies).[7,8] Anomalies can result from arrested development, abnormal formation, or incomplete fusion of the Müllerian ducts.

Uterine anomalies can be organized into categories[9] (Table 76.1). Cases of hypoplasia of the Müllerian duct and diethylstilbestrol (DES)-related anomalies can be diagnosed with 3DUS. DES-related uterus have a normal external contour, but the endometrium is hypoplastic and T-shaped (Figs 76.2A and B). Mayer-Rokitansky-Kuster-Hauser syndrome

is lack of Müllerian development, a relatively common cause of primary amenorrhea (Figs 76.3A and B). These patients have an absence or hypoplasia of the internal vagina and usually, an absent or rudimentary uterus and Fallopian tubes.

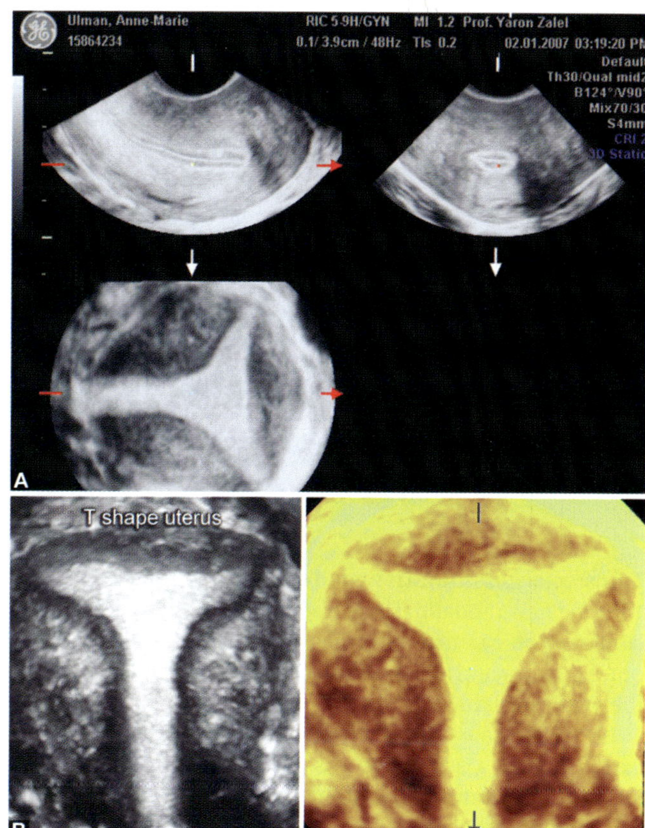

Figs 76.2A and B: T-shaped uterus, after DES exposure

Table 76.1: ASRM classification of Müllerian anomalies

	Classification	Anomaly
Class I	Agenesis/ hypoplasia	Vagina
		Cervix
		Fundus
		Tubes
		Combined
Class II	Unicornuate	Communicating horn
		Non-communicating horn
		No cavity
		No horn
Class III	Didelphys	
Class IV	Bicornuate	Complete partial
Class V	Septate	Complete partial
Class VI	Arcuate	
Class VII	DES-related	

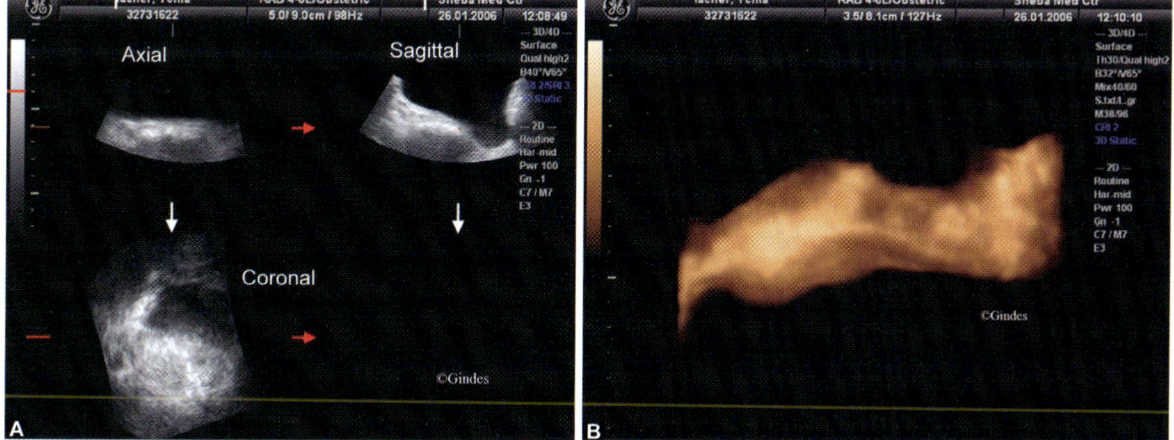

Figs 76.3A and B: Mayer-Rokitansky-Kuster-Hauser syndrome—lack of Müllerian development.
(A) Sectional plane of rudimentary uterus; (B) Render mode of rudimentary uterus

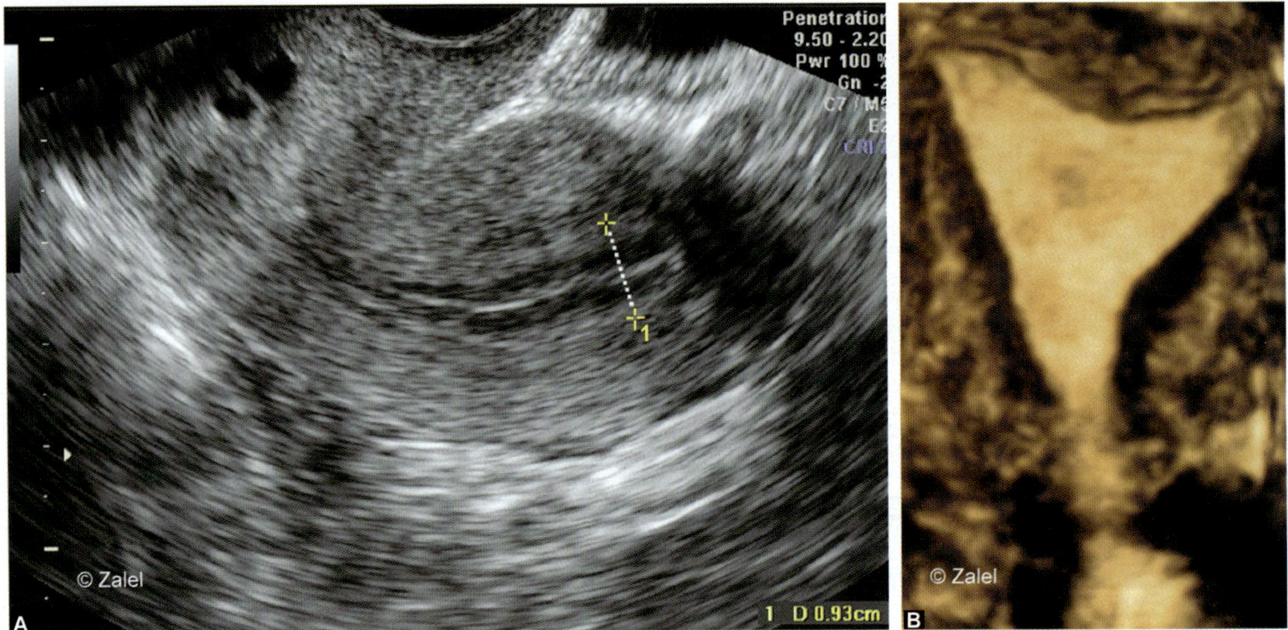

Figs 76.4A and B: Normal uterus; (A) Normal uterus 2DUS; (B) Normal uterus 3DUS

Transrectal ultrasound is a good option for the diagnosis,[10] but with the new modalities, the transperineal approach with 3D construction can make the diagnosis. It reveals an abnormal outer contour and an abnormal or absent endometrium. Both the ovaries usually are normal.

A bicornuate uterus correlates with obstetric complications, while a septate uterus correlates with reproductive failure, depending on the extent of the septum. It is important to differentiate between these anomalies, as hysteroscopic septectomy can be done in cases of receptivity failure, while bicornuate uterus is unoperable. In the era of 2DUS, hysteroscopy and laparoscopy were the examinations of choice to diagnose between these two conditions. With 3DUS, the correct diagnosis can made easily. By taking a volume of the entire the uterus, the volume is rotated to the position of the coronal plane. As described by Salim et al.[11] The endometrial shape and the outer contour of the uterus are seen at the same time. The normal uterus has a fundus that is straight convex and an external contour that is uniformly convex or with indentation of less than 10 mm (Figs 76.4A and B). Arcuate uteri have the same external contour but the fundal contour is concave with indentation with an obtuse angle (Fig. 76.5). Septate uteri have normal outer contour (convex), but a septum divides the cavity from the fundus toward the cervix, completely or partially (Figs 76.6A and B). A bicornuate uterus has fundal indentation in the external part that is more than 10 mm, with two well-formed uterine cornua (Figs 76.7A and B). Uterus didelphys results from lack of fusion of the two Müllerian ducts. There is duplication of

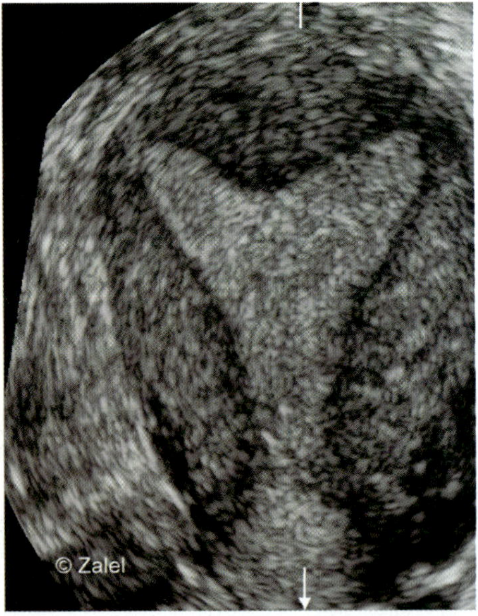

Fig. 76.5: Arcuate uterus

the corpus and cervix (Figs 76.8A to D). Occasionally, this pathology is associated with an obstructed hemivagina and ipsilateral renal agenesis. Unicornuate uterus is a single uterine cavity, and the external contour has a rudimentary horn (Figs 76.9A to C).

In an examination of 3850 infertile patients, 23.2 percent had uterine abnormalities,[12] detected by 3DUS. Uterine septum

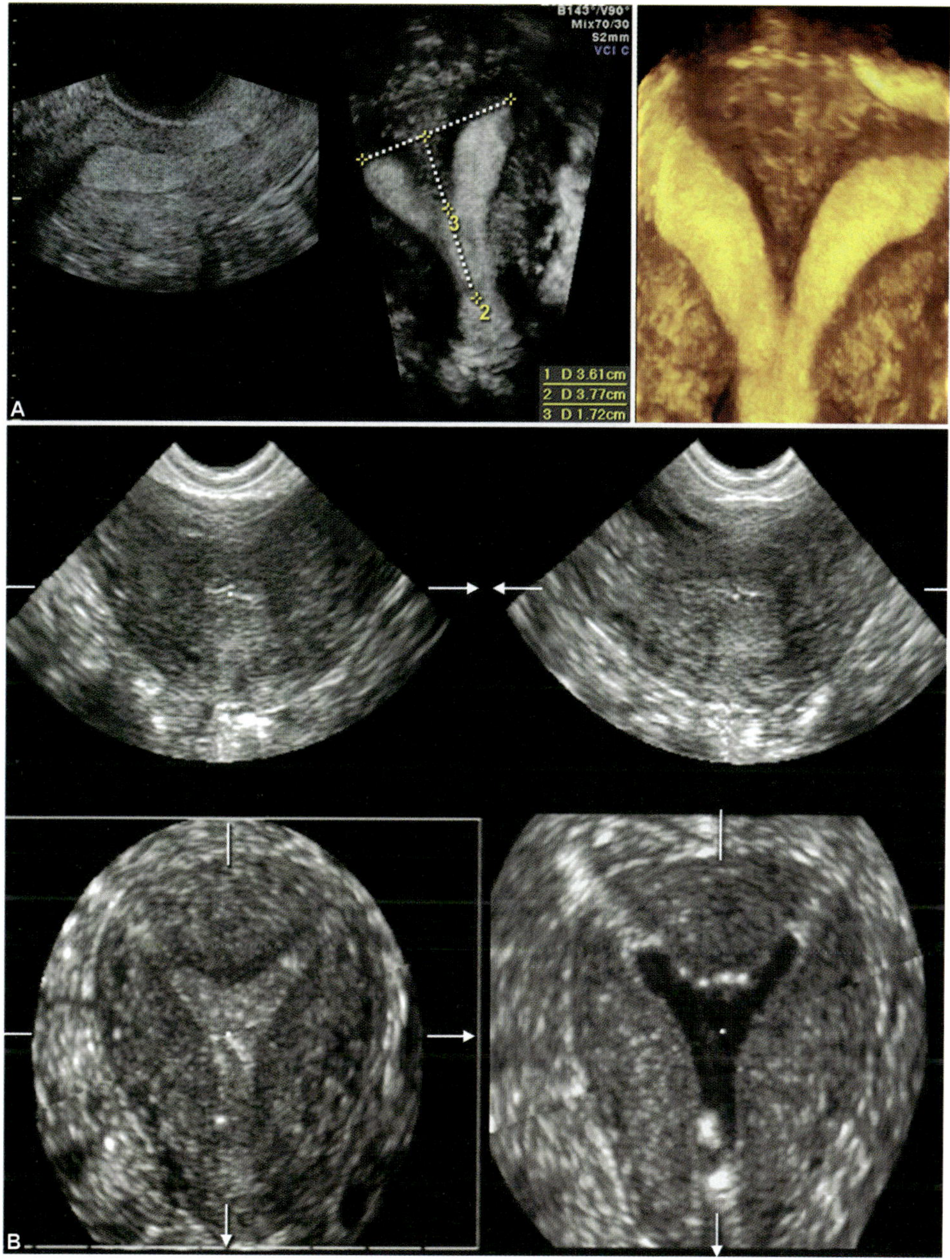

Figs 76.6A and B: Septate uterus. (A) VCI-C; (B) 3D sonohysterography (SHG)

was the most common uterine abnormality, accounting for 77.1 percent of the intracavitary lesions. The rate of spontaneous miscarriages dropped from 41.7 percent before to 11.9 percent after hysteroscopic resection of the septum.

A comparison between hysterosalpingography (HSG) and ultrasound in 61 patients with a history of recurrent miscarriage or infertility,[13] showed that 3DUS agreed with hysterosalpingography in all cases of arcuate uterus and major congenital anomalies. The advantage of the 3DUS over hysterosalpingography is its ability to visualize both, the uterine cavity and the myometrium, that facilitates the diagnosis of uterine anomalies and enables easy differentiation between septate and bicornuate uteri.

Further evaluation of patients with Müllerian duct anomalies should include abdominal US and radiologic studies. Approximately one-third of the patients have urinary tract abnormalities and 12 percent or more have skeletal anomalies.[14,15]

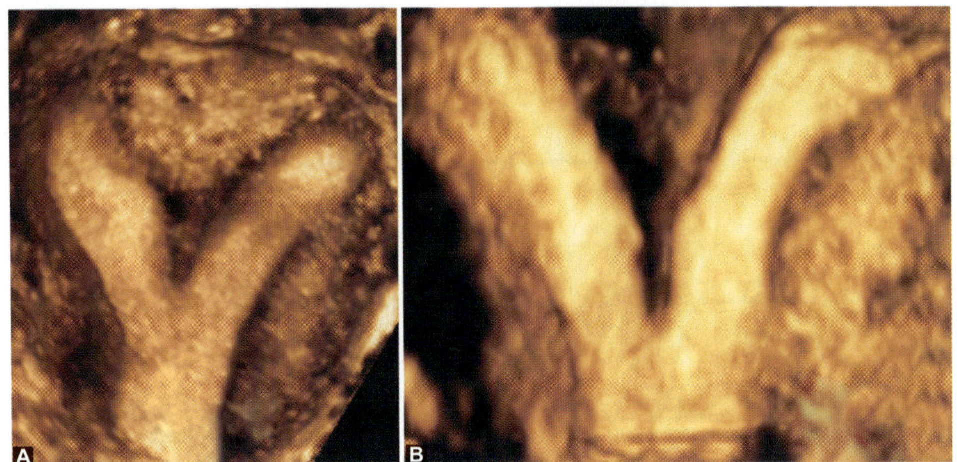

Figs 76.7A and B: Bicornuate uterus

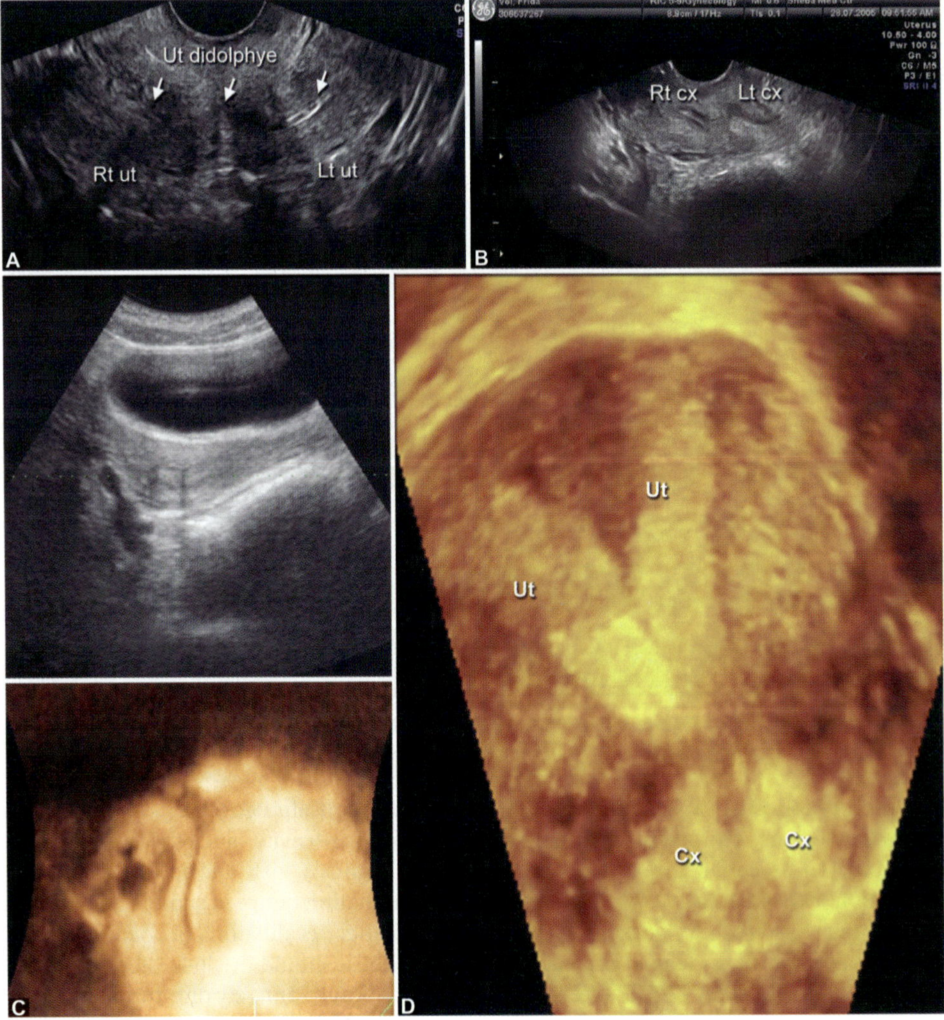

Figs 76.8A to D: Uterus didelphys. (A) Two uteri by 2DUS; (B) Two cervices by 2DUS; (C) 3DUS VCI-C; (D) 3DUS – render mode

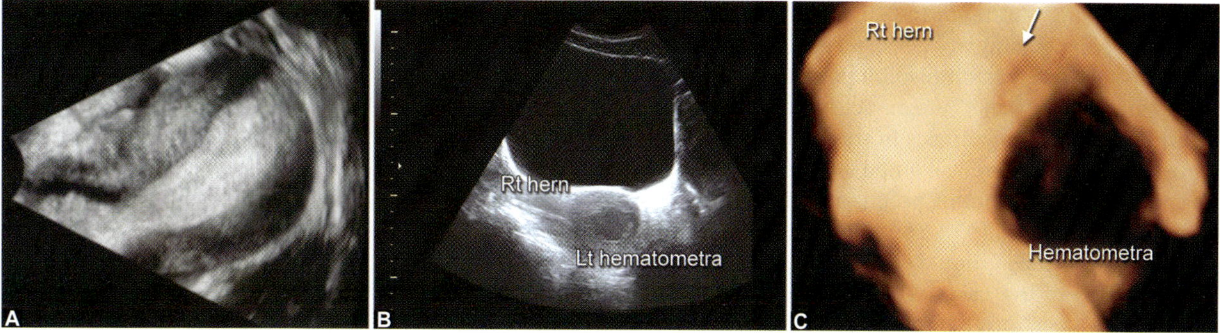

Figs 76.9A to C: Unicornuate uterus. (A) One horn VCI-C; (B) Complex uterine anomaly: Non-communicating horn 2D; (C) Complex uterine anomaly: Non-communicating horn 3D

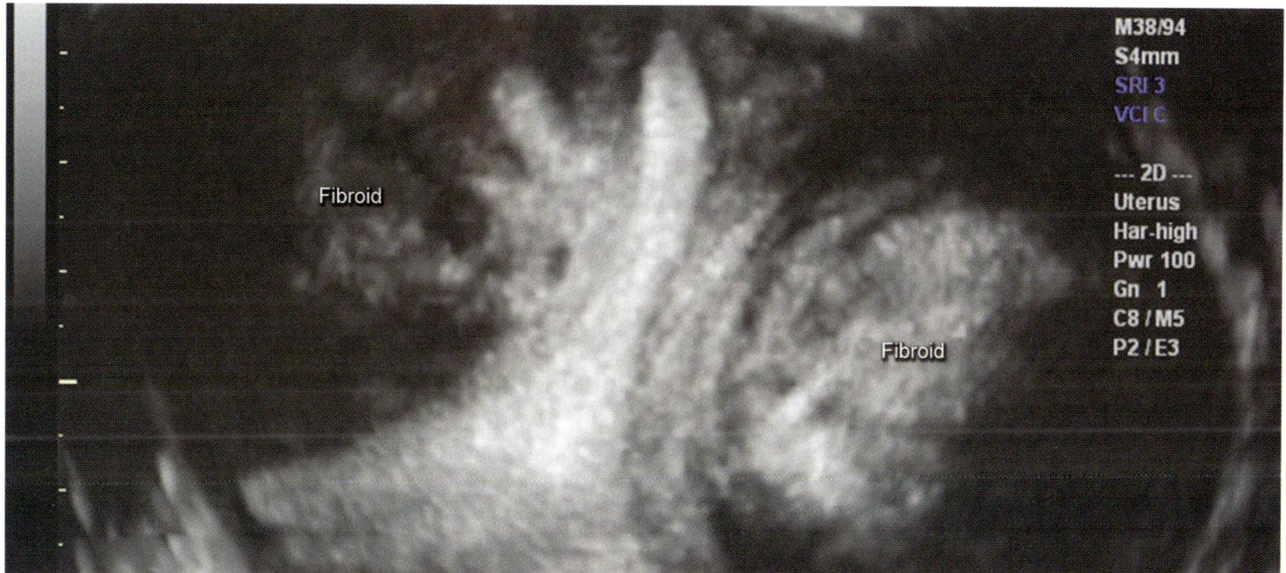

Fig. 76.10: Fibroid uterus

Endometrial filling defects

Endometrial filling defects may be due to intracavitary findings like polyps, submucous myomas, malignant tumors and intrauterine adhesions. A rare cause can also be a forgotten intrauterine device. The diagnosis of these defects is much easier when using 3DUS. By 3D examination, it is possible to localize the pathology, to measure the volume and the amount of pathology protruding to the uterine space.

Myometrium-uterine myomas: Leiomyoma is the most common gynecological tumor that affects 20 to 50 percent of women aged 30 years or more. Most of the myomas are asymptomatic, but submucous myomas can create infertility, most probably due to impaired receptivity. By 2DUS, the leiomyomas are echogenic and round with a clear border. The submucous myoma can change the endometrial contour.

2DUS can define the location of the myoma (submucous, etc.), the size of the myoma and can assist the surgeon/hysteroscopist pre and intraoperatively (Fig. 76.10). 3DUS adds information on the relationship of the fibroid to the endometrial cavity and the deformity of the uterine shape. 3DUS allows volume measurement of the myoma and follow-up of shrinkage after treatment [gonadotropin-releasing hormone (GnRH) analogs, surgery or high intensity focussed ultrasound (HIFUS)].

Endometrial polyps: It is not clear whether endometrial polyps affect fertility and whether polypectomy improves fertility (Figs 76.11A and B). In a prospective randomized study, 215 infertile women with ultrasonographically diagnosed endometrial polyps were divided randomly into two groups before undergoing intrauterine insemination (IUI).[16] Hysteroscopic polypectomy was performed in the study group. Diagnostic hysteroscopy and polyp biopsy was performed in the control group. A total of 93 pregnancies occurred after four IUI cycles, 64 and 29 pregnancies in the study group and in the control group respectively. Women in the study group had a better possibility of becoming pregnant after polypectomy, with a relative risk of 2.1 (95% confidence interval 1.5–2.9). Pregnancies in the study group were obtained before the first IUI in 65 percent of the cases. The authors suggested that hysteroscopic polypectomy before IUI is an effective measure.

In a study that compared conventional 2D and 3D scanning of the uterine cavity with or without saline contrast medium in the detection and evaluation of focal endometrial polyps, 23 patients out of 642 women were suspected with intrauterine anomalies at routine transvaginal sonography (TVS).[17] 2D transvaginal ultrasound diagnosed 23 polyps versus 16 confirmed at hysteroscopic and histological examinations, revealing a specificity of 69.5 percent; 2D TVS and hysterosalpingography (HSG) diagnosed 17 polyps, with a specificity of 94.1 percent; 3D TVS sonography diagnosed 18 polyps, with a specificity of 88.8 percent; 3D sonohysterography (SHG) diagnosed 16 polyps according to hysteroscopic and histological findings, with a specificity of 100 percent.[17]

In a prospective study that measured the accuracy of 3DUS in detecting intrauterine lesions in a group of 59 patients, who had hysteroscopy, the sensitivity of the 2D SHG and 3D SHG were 98 percent and 100 percent, with a positive predictive value of 95 percent and 92 percent, respectively.[18] The authors concluded that if 2D and 3D SHG are normal, invasive diagnostic procedures, such as hysteroscopy could be avoided. According to our experience, 3DUS can define the exact location and size of the polyps. The accuracy of this technique should be defined, and then it can replace diagnostic hysteroscopy.[18]

Do we still need HSG? There is no good answer, but most probably, the use of this technique will be reduced, mostly due to its inability to differentiate between a septate and bicornuate uterus, as it will be of value only in special cases of complicated uterine anomalies and for evaluating the patency of the Fallopian tubes.

Intrauterine Device

A rare cause of infertility is a missing or forgotten intrauterine device. Although 2DUS can detect the intrauterine device (IUD) that is in place, it can be difficult to find a missing IUD. Perhaps, the 3DUS has added value (Figs 76.12A and B). The appearance of the Mirena (Levonogestrel-releasing IUD) in 2DUS includes both proximal and distal ends of the vertical arm of the device, which extend into the internal cervical os and fundal region, respectively. Acoustic shadowing between both ends defines the location of the device.[19,20]

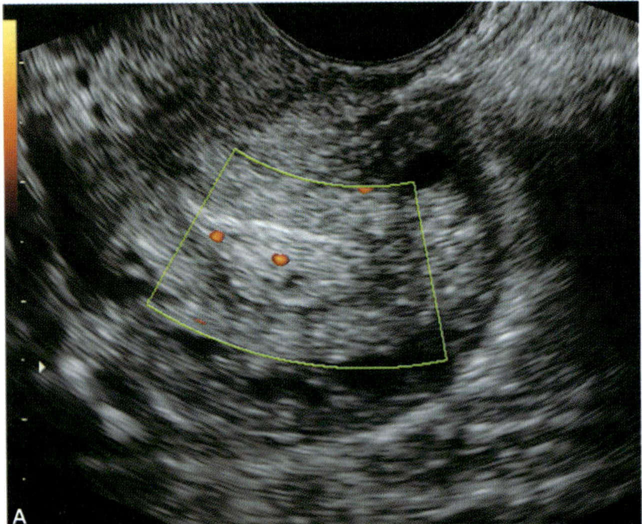

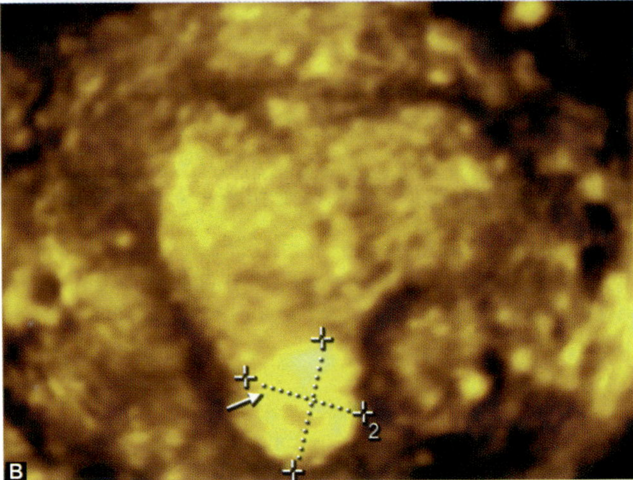

Figs 76.11A and B: Endometrial polyp. (A) 2DUS; (B) 3DUS

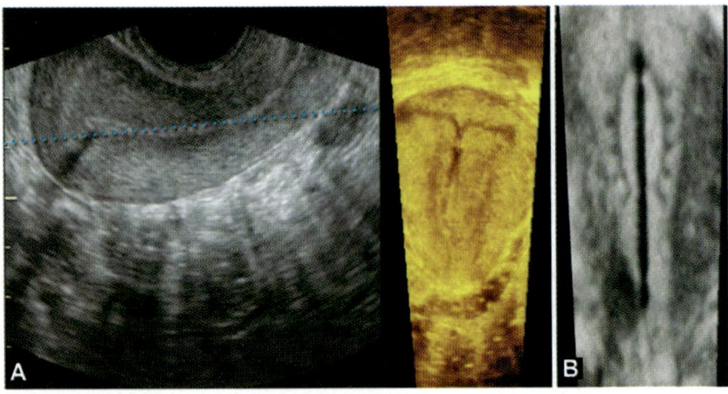

Figs 76.12A and B: Intrauterine device (IUD). (A) Mirena; (B) Copper IUD

Although we have demonstrated the 2D features of the Mirena, still, the Mirena is one of the major reasons for 'a missing IUD', and 3DUS can accurately demonstrate the Mirena.

Endometrial Receptivity

Endometrial receptivity can be evaluated by histological examination of an endometrial biopsy, endometrial proteins in uterine flushing, or more commonly, non-invasive ultrasound examination of the endometrium. Different ultrasound parameters have been used to assess endometrial receptivity during IVF treatment, including endometrial thickness, endometrial pattern, endometrial volume, Doppler of endometrial blood flow.

The 3D ultrasound with power Doppler provides a unique tool with which to examine the blood supply towards the whole endometrium and the subendometrial region. Raine-Fenning et al.[21] performed 3DUS throughout a spontaneous cycle of 27 normal women. Endometrial and subendometrial blood flow increased during the proliferative phase, peaking around 3 days prior to ovulation before decreasing to a nadir 5 days postovulation. Moreover, the subendometrial flow index (FI) was significantly lower in women 31 years of age and significantly higher in parous women. Smoking was associated with a significantly lower subendometrial

vascularization index (VI) and vascularization flow index (VFI).

Examination of the effect of women's type of infertility (i.e. primary or secondary), causes of infertility and serum estradiol (E2) concentration on endometrial and subendometrial blood flows, as measured by a three-dimensional power Doppler ultrasound, during IVF treatment, revealed no significant differences in endometrial and subendometrial blood flow among different causes of infertility.[22]

Neither endometrial volume nor endometrial thickness is suitable for predicting pregnancy in a statistically significant manner. However, the pregnancy rate in patients with an endometrial volume ≥ 2.5 mL was significantly higher than that in patients with an endometrial volume <2.5 mL (P=0.012).[23] Because pregnancies were also observed at a minimum endometrial thickness of 8 mm, no significant cut-off value could be determined for endometrial thickness. When a cut-off point for endometrial volume of <2.5 mL was used, poor specificity resulted (38.9%). In a prospective study, Raga, et al.[24] reported a significantly lower pregnancy rate among IVF patients with an endometrial volume <2.0 mL. No pregnancy was seen in patients with an endometrial volume <1.2 mL. 3DUS can define and measure uterine volume, mainly with the VOCAL technique (Fig. 76.13).

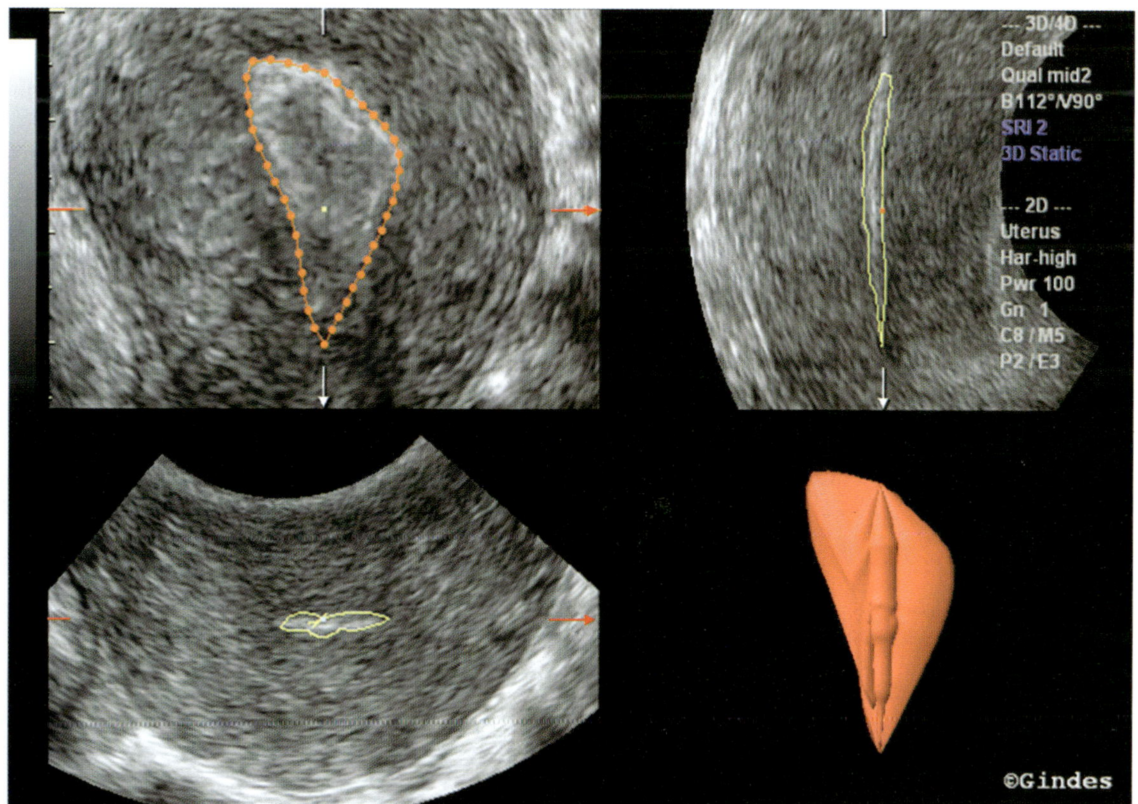

Fig. 76.13: Endometrial volume with VOCAL II

Adenomyosis

Uterine adenomyosis results from heterotopic endometrial glands and stroma in the myometrium, with adjacent myometrial hyperplasia. It is an important cause of infertility and cyclic pelvic pain in women. Focal adenomyosis has been diagnosed when a poorly defined area of abnormal echo-texture is present in the myometrium (increased or decreased echogenicity, including myometrial cysts). The ultrasonic characteristics of adenomyosis include ill-defined regions of mixed textural changes, asymmetric myometrial thickening, streaky shadowing posterior, and no calcifications. Sub-endometrial cysts, less than 3 mm in diameter, are commonly associated with adenomyosis. These cysts represent dilated endometrial glands that enlarge and shrink alternately during the menstrual cycle.

Transvaginal sonography in symptomatic patients, can be sensitive but not specific for the diagnosis of adenomyosis (Figs 76.14A and B). Because adenomyosis usually manifests as an area of abnormal echogenicity within the myometrium, abnormality will usually be wrongly ascribed to fibroid disease.[25]

Another study compares the accuracy of TVS and magnetic resonance imaging (MRI) in the diagnosis of adenomyosis. The authors prospectively studied 119 consecutive patients undergoing hysterectomy. The TVS scans and MRI images were interpreted independently in a double-blind fashion. At histopathologic examination, adenomyosis was found in 28 of the 119 patients (24%). Sensitivity and specificity was 89 percent for TVS and 89 percent for MRI imaging. There was no statistically significant difference between the sensitivities (P = 0.65) and specificities (P = 0.75) of TVS and MRI imaging. TVS was as accurate as MRI imaging in the diagnosis of uterine adenomyosis.[26] 3DUS cannot define diffuse adenomyosis better than 2DUS. However, as shown in Figures 76.15A and B, it can demonstrate the unique sub-type of adenomyosis, i.e. adenomyotic cysts, a well-defined area of adenomyosis within the myometrium.

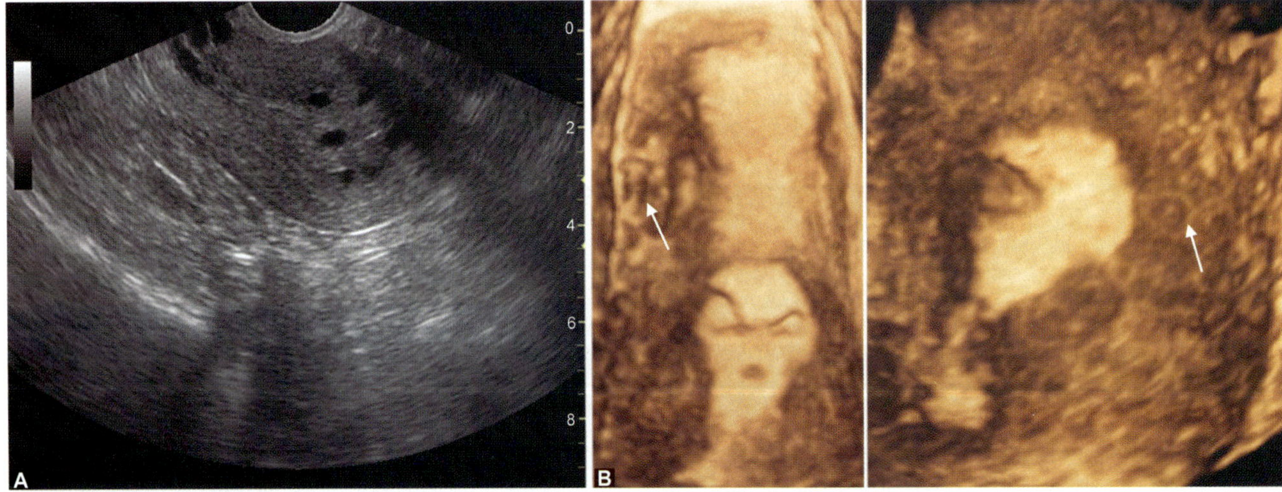

Figs 76.14A and B: Adenomyosis. (A) 2DUS; (B) 3DUS

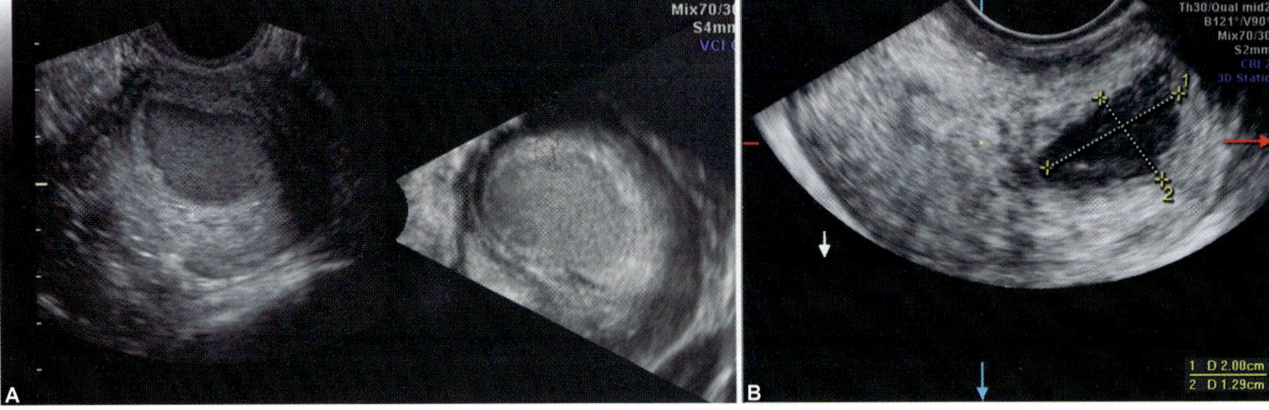

Figs 76.15A and B: Adenomyotic cyst. (A) 2DUS; (B) 3DUS

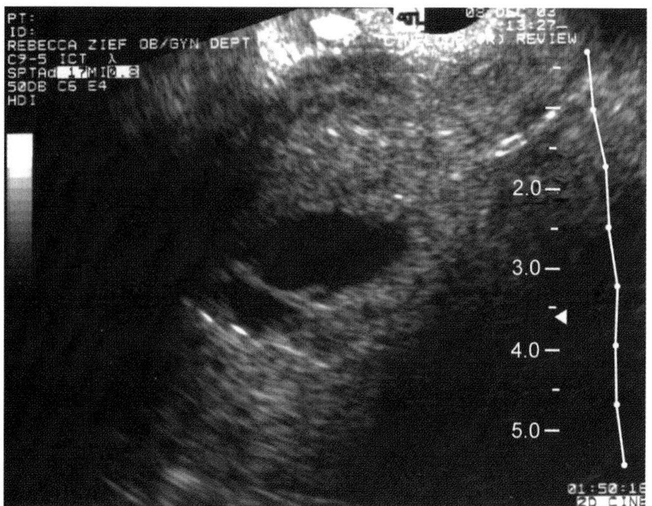

Fig. 76.16: Intrauterine adhesions

Intrauterine Adhesions

Adhesions are often not visualized at any imaging modality except if fluid is present on both sides (Fig. 76.16).

CONCLUSION

We are at the beginning of a new era of diagnostic procedures in Gynecology. Using the 3DUS modalities in any examination reveals more accurate information of the pelvic organ. The improvement in the 2DUS, and the ability to reconstruct of a volume of images by 3DUS is an upgradation in the knowledge and understanding of uterine pathology while evaluating the infertile patient. We already need less and less invasive studies for diagnosis and follow-up. It is doubtful whether the fertility rate will be increased, but the evaluation and treatment most probably, will be more suitable and satisfactory.

REFERENCES

1. Hamper UM, Trapanotto V, Sheth S, DeJong MR, Caskey CI. Three-dimensional US: preliminary clinical experience. Radiology 1994;191:397-401.
2. Maymon R, Herman A, Ariely S, Dreazen E, Buckovsky I, Weinraub Z. Three-dimensional vaginal sonography in obstetrics and gynecology. Hum Reprod Update 2000;6:475-84.
3. Nahum GG. Uterine anomalies. How common are they, and what is their distribution among subtypes? J Reprod Med 1998;43:877-87.
4. Radoncic E, Funduk-Kurjak B. Three-dimensional ultrasound for routine check-up in *in vitro* fertilization patients. Croat Med J 2000;41:262-5.
5. Raga F, Bonilla-Musoles F, Blanes J, Osborne NG. Congenital Mullerian anomalies: Diagnostic accuracy of three-dimensional ultrasound. Fertil Steril 1996;65:523-8.
6. Wu MH, Hsu CC, Huang KE. Detection of congenital mullerian duct anomalies using three-dimensional ultrasound. J Clin Ultrasound 1997;25:487-92.
7. Raga F, Bauset C, Remohi J, Bonilla-Musoles F, Simon C, Pellicer Reproductive impact of congenital Mullerian anomalies. Hum Reprod 1997;12:2277-81.
8. Pedro Acién. Reproductive performance of women with uterine malformations. Hum Reprod 1993;8:122-6.
9. The American Society of Reproductive Medicine. Classification of Müllerian Anomalies. Fertil Steril 1989;51:199-201.
10. Timor-Tritsch IE, Monteagudo A, Rebarber A, Goldstein SR, Tsymbal T. Transrectal scanning: an alternative when transvaginal scanning is not feasible. Ultrasound in Obstetrics and Gynecology 2003;21:473-9.
11. Salim R, Woelfer B, Backos M, Regan L, Jurkovic D. Reproducibility of three-dimensional ultrasound diagnosis of congenital uterine anomalies. Ultrasound Obstet Gynecol 2003;21:578-82.
12. Kupesic S, Kurjak A, Skenderovic S, Bjelos D. Screening for uterine abnormalities by three-dimensional ultrasound improves perinatal outcome. J Perinat Med 2002;30:9-17.
13. Jurkovic D, Geipel A, Gruboeck K, Jauniaux E, Natucci M, Campbell S. Three-dimensional ultrasound for the assessment of uterine anatomy and detection of congenital anomalies: a comparison with hysterosalpingography and two-dimensional sonography. Ultrasound in Obstetrics and Gynecology 1995;5:233-7.
14. Letterie GS, Wilson J, Miyazawa K, Magnetic resonance imaging of müllerian tract abnormalities. Fertil Steril 1988;50:365.
15. Fekele L, Dorta M, Brioschi D, Giudici MN, Candiani GB. Magnetic resonance imaging in Mayer-Rokitansky-Kuster-Hauser syndrome. Obstet Gynecol 1971;37:408.
16. Perez-Medina T, Bajo-Arenas J, Salazar F, Redondo T, Sanfrutos L, Alvarez P, Engels V. Endometrial polyps and their implication in the pregnancy rates of patients undergoing intrauterine insemination: A prospective, randomized study. Hum Reprod 2005;20:1632-5.
17. La Torre R, De Felice C, De Angelis C, Coacci F, Mastrone M, Cosmi EV. Transvaginal sonographic evaluation of endometrial polyps: A comparison with two-dimensional and three-dimensional contrast sonography. Clin Exp Obstet Gynecol 1999;26:171-3.
18. Sylvestre C, Child TJ, Tulandi T, Tan SL. A prospective study to evaluate the efficacy of two- and three-dimensional sonohysterography in women with intrauterine lesions. Fertil Steril 2003;79:1222-5.
19. Zalel Y, Kreizer D, Soriano D, Achiron R. Sonographic demonstration of a levonorgestrel-releasing IUD (Mirena). Harefuah 1999;137:30-1,86.
20. Zalel Y, Kreizer D, Achiron R. Sonographic images of a lost intrauterine device. Ultrasound Obstet Gynecol 1999;13:376-7.
21. Raine-Fenning NJ, Campbell BK, Kendall NR, Clewes JS and Johnson IR. Quantifying the changes in endometrial vascularity throughout the normal menstrual cycle with three-dimensional power Doppler angiography. Hum Reprod 2004;19:330-8.
22. Ernest Hung Yu Ng1, Carina Chi Wai Chan, Oi Shan Tang, William Shu Biu Yeung and Pak Chung Ho. Factors affecting

endometrial and subendometrial blood flow measured by three-dimensional power Doppler ultrasound during IVF treatment. Human Reproduction 2006;21:1062-9.

23. Yaman C, Ebner T, Sommergruber M, Pölz W, Tews G. Role of three-dimensional ultrasonographic measurement of endometrial volume as a predictor of pregnancy outcome in an IVF-ET program: A preliminary study. Fertility Steril 2000; 74:797-801.

24. Raga F, Bonilla-Musoles F, Casan EM, Klein O, Bonilla F. Assessment of endometrial volume by three-dimensional ultrasound prior to embryo transfer: Clues to endometial receptivity. Hum Reprod 1999;14:2851-4.

25. Reinhold C, Atri M, Mehio A, Zakarian R, Aldis AE, Bret PM. Diffuse uterine adenomyosis: Morphologic criteria and diagnostic accuracy of endovaginal sonography. Radiology 1995;197:609-14.

26. Reinhold C, McCarthy S, Bret PM, Mehio A, Atri M, Zakarian R, Glaude Y, Liang L, Seymour RJ. Diffuse adenomyosis: Comparison of endovaginal US and MR imaging with histopathologic correlation. Radiology 1996;199:151-8.

Color Doppler and Prediction of Success in ART

Anoop Kumar Gupta

OVERVIEW

With the changing lifestyle and ever changing epidemiology, the known diseases that caused infertility are now affected by a new set of problems. Rapid technological advances in their treatment have totally overshadowed the conventional methods that were practised for years.

Assisted reproductive techniques (ART) have become a much discussed science, not only amongst infertility specialists, but also amongst patients, their relatives, the press and the ethics group. With advances in techniques has come the added responsibility of producing reasonably good success rates, which have somehow flattened off since long. The rate-limiting factors affecting success are far from clear, or not effectively co-ordinated, making the prediction of success in ART a continuing enigma.

The promise of new imaging technologies for assessing ovarian and endometrial function to increase the predictive value over the last two decades has ushered a quiet revolution in research approaches to the study of ovarian structure and function and so also to endometrial receptivity that determines the ultimate success in ART. The most significant changes in our understanding of the ovary have resulted from the use of ultrasonography (USG), which has enabled sequential analyses. Computer-assisted image analysis and mathematical modeling of the dynamic changes within the ovary has permitted exciting new avenues of research with readily quantifiable endpoints. Spectral, color-flow and power Doppler imaging now facilitate physiologic interpretations of vascular dynamics over time. Similarly, magnetic resonance imaging (MRI) is emerging as a research tool in ovarian imaging. New technologies, such as three-dimensional ultrasonography (3D USG) and MRI, ultrasound-based biomicroscopy and synchrotron-based techniques, each have the potential to enhance our real-time picture of ovarian function to the near-cellular level. Collectively, information available in ultrasonography, MRI, computer-assisted image analysis and mathematical modeling heralds a new era in our understanding of the basic processes of female and male reproduction.

Although the above list sounds great, what is practically available with an infertility physician is a mere ultrasonography, or at the most, color Doppler and hence, the attempt to find reasonable clues using the above to predict the success in ART.

INTRODUCTION

What is Color Doppler Ultrasound?

Color Doppler ultrasound is an ultrasound technique that takes advantage of the changing frequencies of a moving object. In Medicine, it is used to assess blood flow in veins, arteries and the heart.

Contribution of Ovarian and Uterine Color Doppler to Medically-assisted ART

Along the menstrual cycle and during pregnancy, small blood vessels proliferate within the uterus and the ovulating ovary.

Angiogenic factors, such as vascular endothelial growth factor (VEGF), are involved in this phenomenon. In the ovulating ovary, neoangiogenesis spreads progressively inside the dominant follicle wall and plays a role in the maintenance of the corpus luteum under the influence of luteinizing hormone (LH) or human chorionic gonadotropin (hCG) during pregnancy. This neoangiogenesis is also important in the endometrium and, in particular, for embryo implantation. In ART, a measure of the blood flow is interesting, since it correlates with the number and quality of harvested oocytes. Follicle hypoxia may impair chromosomal organization and separation within the oocyte. Doppler ultrasound enables the estimation of endometrial receptivity, especially in *in vitro* fertilization (IVF) cycles. It is assumed that the chance for an ongoing pregnancy is almost zero if the endometrial thickness is < 8 mm and uterine artery pulsatility index (PI) is > 3. Doppler ultrasound is a useful imaging modality and even a mandatory complement to standard vaginal USG in ART. It can be viewed as an indicator of the endometrial and follicular 'well-being'.[1]

Ovarian Follicular Dynamics: From Basic Science to Clinical Practice

The management of low responders (LR) to ovarian stimulation in cycles of assisted reproduction (AR) is a difficult challenge. Aging of the ovary and poor response to ovarian stimulation are coincidental in many situations and poor response may also be a feature in young patients undergoing ART. In fact, poor response is a recognized cause of infertility today. There is evidence that the function of the granulosa cells, as well as the quality of oocytes and resulting embryos, are affected in an aged ovary. Similarly, in young LR, though the production of inhibin is affected, there is no evidence that the quality of oocyte and/or the resulting embryo is affected. We retrospectively analyzed our data and observed that the quality of oocytes and embryos was similar between young and old LR and normal responders (NR).

Studies using color Doppler vaginal ultrasound have shown that the PI and the resistance index (RI) were increased in LR as compared with NR, suggesting that there is some degree of vascular resistance to flow. Treatment of LR is also a difficult challenge and oocyte donation is a successful treatment option in LR, since cumulative birth rates are > 85 percent with four attempts of embryo transfer. The future may be promising for LR once new technologies are introduced into clinical practice. The use of recombinant gonadotropins and genetically engineered human gonadotropin derivatives may be of considerable help for LR. Similarly, non-gonadotropin hormones, such as cytokines or growth factors, may be shown to play a role in the stimulation of the ovary in the near future, and may therefore, open new frontiers for treatment of LR.[2]

CLINICAL DISCUSSION

Ultrasonography as a Predictor of Embryo Implantation after *In Vitro* Fertilization

Variables related to patients' clinical and treatment characteristics, ovarian response, oocyte retrieval, embryo transfer, ultrasonographic and Doppler endometrial measurements, and uterine blood flow have been proposed as potential predictors of implantation and hence, ART outcome.[2]

The only significant differences between groups were the type-A endometrium and the absence of a protodiastolic notch in the uterine arteries, both of which were more frequently found in the group that responded. However, a considerable overlap existed between conception and non-conception cycles regarding both the variables. Ultrasonographic parameters, as predictors of implantation in assisted reproduction, have a limited value in the clinical setting.[3]

Relationship Between Uterine Blood Flow and Endometrial and Subendometrial Blood Flows During Stimulated and Natural Cycles

Uterine pulsatility and resistance indices have been found to be negatively correlated with subendometrial vascularization, flow, and vascularization flow indices in both stimulated and natural cycles, whereas uterine resistance index was negatively correlated with endometrial vascularization and flow indices in natural cycles only. Subendometrial vascularization and vascularization flow indices were significantly lower in patients with a uterine resistance index ≥0.95 compared to those with a uterine resistance index <0.95. Hence, uterine blood flow is a poor reflector of subendometrial blood flow during stimulated and natural cycles and its measurement cannot reflect endometrial blood flow during stimulated cycles.[4]

The 3D vascular status of the follicle after hCG administration is qualitatively rather than quantitatively associated with its reproductive competence. A qualitative (FI) rather than quantitative (VI) relationship exists between vascular status and functional quality of the follicle after hCG administration.[5]

Endometrial and Subendometrial Perfusion are Impaired in Women with Unexplained Subfertility

Endometrial and subendometrial vascularity are significantly reduced in women with unexplained subfertility during the mid to late follicular phase irrespective of estradiol or progesterone concentrations and endometrial morphometry.[6]

The Role of Endometrial and Subendometrial Blood Flows, Measured by Three-Dimensional Power Doppler Ultrasound, in the Prediction of Pregnancy during IVF Treatment

A good blood supply towards the endometrium is usually considered to be an essential requirement for implantation.

Patients undergoing the first IVF cycle were recruited. A three-dimensional (3D) ultrasound examination with power Doppler was performed on the day of oocyte retrieval to determine endometrial thickness, endometrial pattern, pulsatility index (PI) and resistance index (RI) of the uterine vessels, endometrial volume, vascularization index (VI), flow index (FI) and vascularization flow index (VFI) of the endometrial and subendometrial regions.[7]

Endometrial and subendometrial blood flow, measured by 3D power Doppler ultrasound, were not good predictors of pregnancy if they were measured at one time-point during IVF treatment.[7]

The Role of Ultrasonography in the Evaluation of Endometrial Receptivity Following Assisted Reproductive Treatments: A Critical Review

The ultrasonographic prognostic indicators for implantation evaluated included periovulatory endometrial thickness and pattern and Doppler measurements of uterine artery blood flow. Sonographic parameters had a high negative predictive value and sensitivity, but a limited positive predictive value and low specificity. Several confounding factors may influence the interpretation of reports, and the statistical evaluation sometimes lacks calculation of the positive and negative predictive values of the parameters examined. Although ultrasonographic parameters of endometrial receptivity have a strong negative value in setting some minimum criteria, their value as prognostic indicators for implantation following embryo transfer has yet to be proved.[8]

Endometrial Evaluation in Superovulation Programs: Relationship with Successful Outcome

It is well-known that adequate endometrial receptivity is required for successful implantation in both natural and assisted reproductive cycles. In particular, a brief 'implantation window', during which the endometrium undergoes anatomical and molecular changes, necessary for embryo implantation, has been observed. The hormonal treatment applied to induce ovulation seems to be able to modify the normal development of the prenidatory endometrium, with a possible negative effect on the implantation rate. For this reason, several attempts have been made to identify specific markers of endometrial receptivity, useful for predicting implantation outcome in clinical practice. Even if different histological, immunohistochemical, and ultrasonographic parameters are studied, none unfortunately, has been unequivocally shown to be predictive of pregnancy outcome. Therefore, the evaluation of endometrial receptivity remains a challenge in clinical practice.[9]

Doppler Evaluation of the Uterine and Spiral Arteries from Different Sampling Sites and Phases of the Menstrual Cycle during Controlled Ovarian Hyperstimulation

There were no significant differences in PI and RI values of the uterine and spiral arteries at different sampling sites, phase of the menstrual cycle or age. The higher PI values tended to occur in the lateral uterine artery and posterior spiral artery, during the mid-menstrual phase and in the older age group. The PI and RI values of the mid-uterine and fundal spiral artery sampling sites are representative of the whole uterine artery and spiral artery, respectively.[10]

Transvaginal Color Flow Doppler in the Assessment of Ovarian and Uterine Blood Flow in Infertile Women

There are changes in the flow velocity patterns of the uterine and ovarian arteries during the normal ovulatory menstrual cycle. Because these changes in flow velocity begin before ovulation, it can be suspected that they may involve angiogenesis as well as hormonal factors. The changes noted in these studies are statistically significant, but may be too small to be used as a diagnostic tool in the study of infertility problems.[11]

Endometrial Receptivity in the Light of Modern Assisted Reproductive Techniques

Endometrial receptivity cannot, as yet, be directly assessed. Circumstantial evidence suggests that receptivity declines with age, is adversely affected by controlled ovarian hyperstimulation (COH), and is possibly affected by ovarian function. Future studies will have to focus on molecular cell biology and physiology of the endometrium.[12]

Endometrial Thickness, Morphology, Vascular Penetration and Velocimetry in Predicting Implantation in an *In Vitro* Fertilization Program

Women undergoing *in vitro* fertilization (IVF) treatment were studied on the day of human chorionic gonadotropin (hCG) administration by transvaginal ultrasonography with color and pulsed Doppler ultrasound. Endometrial thickness, endometrial morphology, presence or absence of subendometrial or intraendometrial color flow, intraendometrial vascular penetration and subendometrial blood flow velocimetry on the day of hCG administration were assessed and related to the pregnancy rates.[13]

It was observed that absent subendometrial and intraendometrial vascularization on the day of hCG administration appears to be a useful predictor of failure of implantation in IVF cycles, irrespective of the morphological appearance of the endometrium.[13]

REFERENCES

1. Yang JH, Wu MY, Chen CD, Jiang MC, Ho HN, Yang YS. Association of endometrial blood flow as determined by a modified colour Doppler technique with subsequent outcome of *in vitro* fertilization. Hum Reprod 1999;14:1606-10.

2. Pellicer A, Gaitán P, Neuspiller F, Ardiles G, Albert C, Remohí J, Simón C. Ovarian follicular dynamics: from basic science to clinical practice. J Reprod Immunol 1998;39:29-61.

3. Coulam CB, Bustillo M, Soenksen DM, Britten S. Ultrasonographic predictors of implantation after assisted reproduction. Fertil Steril 1994;62:1004-10.

4. Ng EH, Chan CC, Tang OS, Yeung WS, Ho PC. Relationship between uterine blood flow and endometrial and subendometrial blood flows during stimulated and natural cycles. Fertil Steril 2006;85:721-7.

5. Lozano DH, Frydman N, Levaillant JM, Fay S, Frydman R, Fanchin R. The 3D vascular status of the follicle after hCG administration is qualitatively rather than quantitatively associated with its reproductive competence. Hum Reprod 2007;22:1095-9.

6. Raine-Fenning NJ, Campbell BK, Kendall NR, Clewes JS, Johnson IR. Endometrial and subendometrial perfusion are impaired in women with unexplained subfertility. Hum Reprod 2004;19:2605-14.

7. Ng EH, Chan CC, Tang OS, Yeung WS, Ho PC. The role of endometrial and subendometrial blood flows measured by three-dimensional power Doppler ultrasound in the prediction of pregnancy during IVF treatment. Hum Reprod 2006;21: 164-70.

8. Friedler S, Schenker JG, Herman A, Lewin A. The role of ultrasonography in the evaluation of endometrial receptivity following assisted reproductive treatments: a critical review. Hum Reprod Update 1996;2:323-35.

9. Tropea A, Miceli F, Minici F, Orlando M, Lamanna G, Gangale M, et al. Endometrial evaluation in superovulation programs: relationship with successful outcome. Ann N Y Acad Sci 2004;1034:211-8.

10. Hsieh YY, Chang FC, Tsai HD. Doppler evaluation of the uterine and spiral arteries from different sampling sites and phases of the menstrual cycle during controlled ovarian hyperstimulation. Ultrasound Obstet Gynecol 2000;16:192-6.

11. Kurjak A, Kupesic-Urek S, Schulman H, Zalud I. Transvaginal color flow Doppler in the assessment of ovarian and uterine blood flow in infertile women. Fertil Steril 1991;56:870-3.

12. Yaron Y, Botchan A, Amit A, Peyser MR, David MP, Lessing JB. Endometrial receptivity in the light of modern assisted reproductive technologies. Fertil Steril 1994;62:225-32.

13. Zaidi J, Campbell S, Pittrof R, Tan SL. Endometrial thickness, morphology, vascular penetration and velocimetry in predicting implantation in an *in vitro* fertilization program. Ultrasound Obstet Gynecol 1995;6:191-8.

Uterine Contractility and Ultrasound

Jude Jose, Anil Gudi, Amit Shah

OVERVIEW

The possibility of assessing uterine contractility non-invasively in the non-pregnant uterus, using ultrasound scans, has improved the understanding of hormonal regulation and the influence of uterine contractility on human embryo implantation in both natural and ovarian stimulation cycles. Contractions of the non-pregnant uterus presumably partake in the *in vivo* fertilization and embryo implantation processes in humans. Interventions aimed at either stimulating or inhibiting uterine contractions could be instrumental in pregnancy rates following assisted reproductive techniques (ART).

INTRODUCTION

Embryo implantation is undoubtedly the greatest limiting factor in the success of *in vitro* fertilization (IVF) and embryo transfer (ET). Governed by complex mechanisms,[1] the interaction between the embryo and endometrium depends on the quality of each factor.[2] Uterine contractility is known to affect embryo implantation in animals[3] and uterine contractility during pregnancy has been extensively studied. However, there is limited data regarding the role of uterine contractions in the non-pregnant uterus in human reproduction.

The invasiveness of the available methods, like intra-uterine pressure measurements and electromyography, has limited use in clinical studies investigating natural and assisted reproduction. The use of ultrasound scans to visualize uterine contractions has opened a new era in the study of the possible relationship between uterine contractility and human reproduction.[4,5]

Studies using three-dimensional ultrasound[6] conclude that the contractions of the non-pregnant uterus are influenced by ovarian hormones and presumably partake in the *in vivo* fertilization and embryo implantation processes in human. There is a belief that interventions aimed at inhibiting these contractions could possibly improve pregnancy rates in assisted reproductive techniques (ART).

CLINICAL DISCUSSION

Physiology of Uterine Contractions in the Non-pregnant Uterus

Uterine contractility undergoes periodic variations with the different phases of the menstrual cycle, possibly under the influence of varying levels of estrogen and progesterone.

Follicular Phase

A progressive increase in the uterine frequency is observed in traditional and transvaginal ultrasound studies[7-13] during the follicular phase. This culminates in the preovulatory period when the frequency reaches a rate of 3 to 5 contractions/minute. Estradiol is the primary uterine stimulant and it is the rising levels of estradiol during late follicular phase that has been attributed to the preovulatory increase in uterine contractility. In support of this, the administration of estrogens to women lacking ovarian function as a result of surgical menopause[14] or primary amenorrhea induces a normal preovulatory pattern of uterine contractions.

Mid-luteal Phase

After ovulation, under the influence of progesterone secreted by the corpus luteum, the uterus goes into a state of relative quiescence, with small, slow and superimposed uterine contractions. The results from vaginal ultrasonography of uterine contractions, hysterosalpingoscintigraphy and documentation of embryo implantation sites in natural and artificial cycles show that this implantation window, created by uterine quiescence, facilitates the fundal implantation of the blastocyst.[15]

End Luteal Phase–early Follicular Phase

Low frequency uterine contractions of 2 to 3 per minute but with high mean amplitude of up to 60 mm Hg have been observed during this phase in studies using 3D ultrasound and intrauterine pressure (IUP) recording. The mean resting tone is also elevated at approximately 40 mm Hg. The highest value was found during the menstrual cycle. Interestingly, uterine contractility during early follicular phase is predominantly antegrade, propagating from the fundus to the cervix.[16] This pattern of uterine contractility is instrumental in the forward emptying of menstrual blood as well as in hemostasis.

Uterine Contractility and Conception

The effect of uterine contractility on conception in natural and IVF cycles was studied by Ijland et al.[7,17] In spontaneous conception cycles, there is a predominance of endometrial waves propagating from cervix to fundus in the periovulatory phase. Conception cycles also show an overall dampening of endometrial wave activity during consecutive cycle phases. The authors concluded that the dampening and fine-tuning of the activity patterns in the mid-cycle appear to be the prerequisites for successful implantation.

In IVF cycles, there is a definite correlation between the endometrial wave pattern and the occurrence of pregnancy. Most of the IVF cycles showed a switch from fundus to cervix to cervix to fundus waves, known as wave direction switch (WDS). A premature WDS has been associated with a reduced pregnancy rate (29%), while a late WDS favors a better pregnancy prognosis (88%).[18] The persistence of fundus to cervix waves until the day of human chorionic gonadotropin (hCG) administration appears to assist in good quality implantation.[17]

Ijland and co-researchers[17] found that endometrial activity was more pronounced in IVF cycles than in spontaneous cycles, thus confirming the role of estrogen predominance in enhancing uterine contractions. They also found no correlation between the frequency of endometrial waves and the occurrence of pregnancy in IVF cycles. Contrary to this, Fanchin et al.[19] using a transvaginal 3D-derived system, concluded that the clinical pregnancy rate and implantation rate correlated negatively with the frequency of endometrial waves on the day of embryo transfer. They also observed that the overall mean uterine contraction frequency during the early luteal phase of ovarian stimulation (4.3 contractions/minute on the day of embryo transfer) appeared to be higher than that measured during the corresponding phase of the menstrual cycle (2.5–3 contractions/minute). On the day of

hCG administration the overall uterine frequency remained at menstrual cycle level (4.6 uterine contractions/minute). However, the uterine contraction frequency remains almost unchanged on the day of embryo transfer, without the marked decrease seen in the natural menstrual cycle.[19]

Uterine Contractions and Sperm Transport

The passage of sperm from the vagina to the Fallopian tubes in a few minutes cannot be attributed to sperm motility alone.[20,21] It is likely that external factors, particularly uterine contractions assist sperm transport. The increased frequency of uterine contractions noted during the late follicular phase is consistent with this hypothesis. Additionally, the direction of uterine contractions is observed to be retrograde (from cervix to fundus) during this phase of menstrual cycle, which facilitates sperm transport.[17] Seminal fluid, which is rich in prostaglandins, is also likely to stimulate uterine contractility, thereby providing favorable conditions for sperm ascension. To elucidate this aspect, Kunz et al.[21] introduced technetium-labelled, sperm sized spheres into the cervix at different times of follicular phase. Using hysterosalpingoscintigraphic control, the authors observed a progressive increase in the movement of the spheres towards the Fallopian tubes from the early to the late follicular phase of the menstrual cycle.[21]

While the increasing uterine contractions during the periovulatory phase help sperm transport, uterine dyskinesia could hamper sperm ascension and reduce the probability of fertilization. In line with this, Brown et al.[22] studied the effect of administering Misoprostol (400 µg) vaginally at the time of intrauterine insemination (IUI). An overall improvement in pregnancy rates was observed and was attributed to the prostaglandin-induced uterine contractions. Another possible approach, which needs further evaluation, is the role of estradiol during the periovulatory phase, which can possibly increase uterine contractions and thereby, augment sperm ascension.[22]

Uterine Contractility on the Day of Blastocyst Transfer

Fanchin et al.[23] studied the frequency of uterine contractions on the day of blastocyst transfer in IVF cycles. In this study, 43 subfertile women undergoing IVF treatment with gonadotropin-releasing hormone (GnRH) agonist and follicle stimulating hormone (FSH) were evaluated using three-dimensional (3D) transvaginal ultrasound. Two minute-sagittal uterine scans were obtained with a 7.5 MHz transvaginal probe and uterine contraction frequency was assessed on the day of human chorionic gonadotropin (hCG) administration, the day of non-cavitating embryo transfer (hCG + 4 days) and the day of blastocyst transfer (hCG + 7 days). The results of this study demonstrated a small, yet significant, decrease in uterine contraction frequency from the day of hCG (4.4+/- 0.2 contractions/minute) to hCG +4 days (3.5 ± 0.2 contractions/minute), while a marked decrease

(P < 0.003) in uterine contractions occurred on hCG +7 days (1.5 ± 0.2 contractions/minute). The authors concluded that the near quiescent contractility status of the uterus on the day of blastocyst transfer favors embryo positioning in the endometrial cavity and therefore, assists in implantation.[23] This data supports the high implantation rates reported after blastocyst transfer.[24,25] Based on these results, it is reasonable to recommend blastocyst transfer instead of 2 to 8 cell embryos in women who demonstrate high uterine contraction frequencies (>4 contractions/minute) on the day of non-cavitating embryo transfer.

Role of Hormones in Uterine Contractility

Effect of Estrogen

Uterine contractility during the follicular phase is attributed to the role of estrogen. However, there is limited data supporting the clinical use of estrogen in augmenting sperm ascension during periovulatory phase.

Effect of Vaginal Progesterone

There is convincing evidence to prove that vaginal administration of progesterone provides direct access of the hormone to the uterus, leading to a high uterine tissue concentration of progesterone.[26-28] Fanchin et al.[29] looked into the effect of early use of vaginal progesterone in women undergoing IVF treatment. In this study, 84 women were recruited and on the day of oocyte retrieval; they were randomly assigned to either early (Group A, n=43) or conventional (Group B n=41) luteal support. Women in the two groups were matched for age, indications for IVF and ovarian reserve. Embryological and ovarian stimulation parameters were similar between the groups.

Women in group A were given vaginal progesterone gel soon after oocyte retrieval, while those in group B received the same treatment on the evening of embryo transfer. In both groups, vaginal progesterone treatment was continued either until confirmation of pregnancy or until pregnancy was ruled out by a negative serum hCG measurement.[29]

Three-dimensional ultrasound was used to study uterine contractility and serum estradiol and progesterone concentrations were measured on the day of hCG administration and prior to embryo transfer.

Serum estradiol levels fell from the day of hCG administration to embryo transfer in both the groups. Progesterone concentrations progressively increased following hCG administration in both the groups, but slightly higher concentrations were noted in women who started progesterone supplementation on the day of egg retrieval. Uterine contraction frequency was similar in Groups A and B (4.6 ± 0.3 and 4.5 ± 0.3 contractions/minute, respectively) on the day of hCG administration but declined significantly (P<0.001) at the time of embryo transfer in Group A (2.8 ± 0.2 contractions/minute). Uterine contraction frequency remained unchanged in Group B (4.1 ± 0.3 contractions/minute). The study also observed a trend for higher pregnancy and implantation rates in women who received early luteal support with progesterone.

Overall, the study concluded that early vaginal progesterone administration, starting two days before embryo transfer, significantly reduces the uterine contraction frequency at the time of embryo transfer and facilitates embryo positioning in the endometrial cavity, therefore assisting in implantation.[29]

Assessment of Uterine Contractility

The methodology used in the initial studies,[30-33] which looked into the contractility of the non-pregnant uterus can be classified into two categories:
1. Intrauterine pressure (IUP)
2. Electromyography (EMG).

Intrauterine Pressure

The intrauterine pressure (IUP) is recorded either by means of miniature pressure transducers introduced into the uterine cavity or by fluid filled cannulas connected to pressure recorders that remain outside the uterine cavity. Multiple tip catheters are available, which can record the IUP in the fundal, middle and lower uterine sections. This will also determine the direction of uterine contractility displacement by analyzing the time lags between the peak of uterine contractions recorded at different set points in the uterus.

Using the triple-ended catheters, Martinez-Gaudio, et al.[34] demonstrated retrograde displacement of IUP waves (from cervix to fundus) during the late follicular phase.

The advantage of IUP methods is that they provide information on the amplitude, duration and frequency of uterine contractions. The obvious disadvantage of these methods is their invasiveness. Furthermore, the devices used in this method can possibly influence the characteristics of uterine contractions, thus altering the reliability of the results.

Electromyography

Electromyography (EMG) involves the measurement of the electromechanical activity of the uterus.[35] In this method, with the help of multiple intrauterine electrodes, the changes in slow waves and rapid spikes, generated by the uterus, are studied. It provides information on uterine contractility because electrical activity, in particular, the action potential of the uterus, takes part in the triggering of uterine contractions. The disadvantages of EMG are, however, the same as the IUP method.

High-resolution Transvaginal Ultrasound

More recently, high-resolution transvaginal ultrasound has emerged as a reliable alternative to these methods. Ultrasound was first used to study uterine contractility by Birnholz[4] in 1984. It has been proven to be a reliable method for studying uterine contraction frequency and it benefits from being non-invasive. Ultrasound images are first recorded on tapes or digitized sequences and then analyzed in fast motion to identify and quantify the uterine contraction. Different researchers have used various approaches with regard to the video recording methodologies with no uniformity in the duration of recordings and playbacks, the latter sometimes varying by a five to ten (Table 78.1). A number of studies have focused on different characteristics (Table 78.2), and uterine contractions have not necessarily been uniformly classified in all studies (Table 78.3).

This, however, can raise the question of subjectivity, which can alter the reliability of the data. To overcome this, an original approach using a three-dimensional (3D) reconstruction software was developed by Fanchin et al.[36] Using the 3D technique, ultrasound images are initially digitized online at

Table 78.1: Ultrasound studies of movements in the non-pregnant human uterus

Author	Year	TAS	TVS	n	Observations	Type of cycle	Time in the cycle	Record time	Video	Replay X Normal speed
De Vries et al.	1990	+	+	35	35	Spontaneous	1st and 2nd half of cycle	120s	+	5X
Lyons et al.	1991	–	+	18	328	Spontaneous	Menstrual follicular, periovulatory, luteal	120s	+	5X
Leyendecker et al.	1996	–	+	66	a 15 b 27 c 39 d 19 e 18	Spontaneous Endometriosis	a. Menstruation b. Early follicular c. Mid follicular d. Late follicular e. Luteal	5 min	+	5X
Ijland et al.	1996	–	+	16	23 cycles	Spontaneous	Early, mid and late follicular; early, mid and late luteal	3–15 min	+	4X
Fanchin et al.	1998	–	+	209	209	IVF	Before ET	5 min	+	10X
Bulleti et al.	2000	–	+	30	180	Spontaneous	Early follicular, late follicular, periovulatory, early luteal, late luteal and menstrual period	2 min	+	10X

Abbreviations: TAS: transabdominal sonogram; TVS: transvaginal sonogram; IVF: *in vitro* fertilization; ET: embryo transfer
Source: Data from Bulleti, et al.[38] and Van Gestel, et al.[39]

Table 78.2: Description of uterine movements in the non-pregnant human uterus by ultrasound

Author	Year	Uterine movement description	Direction
Birnholz	1984	Endometrium stripping movements	ND
Oike et al.	1990	Endometrial movements	Towards fundus
De Vries et al.	1990	Inner 1/3 myometrium contractions	Antitrade/retrograde
Abromowicz and Archer	1990	Endometrial peristalsis	ND
Lyons et al.	1991	Subendometrial myometrial contractions	ND
Chalubinski et al.	1993	Myometrial contractions	Towards fundus and cervix
Fakuda and Fakuda	1994	Endometrial echo-free space	Horizontal, vertical
Salamanca and Beltran	1995	Subendometrial contractility	Antegrade, retrograde
Kunze et al. and Leyendecker et al.	1996	Uterine peristalsis	Fundo-cervical, cervico-fundal
Ijland et al.	1996	Endometrial waves	Cervix to fundus, fundus to cervix, opposing, random
Fanchin et al.	1998	Uterine contractions	Antegrade, retrograde, antagonistic, nonpropagated
Bulletti et al.	2000	Uterine contractions/endometrial waves	Cervix to fundus, fundus to cervix, opposing, random

Abbreviation: ND: no data. *Source:* Data from Bulleti, et al.[38] and Van Gestel, et al.[39]

Table 78.3. Aspects of movements in the non-pregnant human uterus studied by ultrasound						
Author	*Year*	*General*	*Direction*	*Frequency (movements/minute)*	*Amplitude, strength, symmetry*	*Effect of uterine contractions displacements*
Birnholz	1984	Most movements in first half of cycle				ND
Oike et al.	1990	No movements after ovulation	Towards fundus; late proliferative	Ovulation 3.9 Late proliferative 4.5	Increased amplitude to ovulation	ND
De Vries et al.	1990		Antegrade, menstruation Retrograde, all phases of cycle	Antegrade 2.3 Retrograde 3.3	First half of cycle symmetrical Second half of cycle asymmetrical	ND
Abramowicz et al.	1990	Gross movements score, average score (1.5), highest at mid-cycle			Increase in strength from early follicular to mid-cycle	ND
Lyons et al.	1991	>80% of contractions periovulatory	Direction towards fundus	Ovulation 2.5–3.5	Increase amplitude in follicular phase, decrease after ovulation	ND
Chalubinski et al.	1993		Towards cervix, menstruation Towards fundus, all phases	Cycle day 2, 1–3 Cycle day 7/8 <1 Ovulation, 10 Cycle day 20/22, 2–5	Ovulation Symmetrical mid-follicular and luteal, dysrhythmic	ND
Fakuda and Fakuda	1994	Late follicular most movements				ND
Salamanca and Beltran	1995	Endometriosis patients 87.5% retrograde contractions versus 4.8% in control group				ND
Kunz et al.	1996		Fundo-cervical contractions decrease in favor of cervico-fundal contractions in the follicular phase	Early follicular 1.2 Mid follicular 1.6 Late follicular 1.8	Increased intensity on follicular phase	ND
Leyendecker et al.	1996			Early follicular 1.2 Midfollicular >1.5 Late follicular 2.5		ND
Ijland et al.	1996	Spontaneous cycles	FC waves in follicular phase not after ovulation CF waves in periovulatory phase and luteal phase	FC-waves: Mid follicular, 2.99 ± 0.88; Late follicular, 3.90 ± 0.95 CF waves: Mid follicular 2.99 ± 0.86 Late follicular, 4.08 ± 1.24 Early luteal, 4.35 ± 1.48		ND
Fanchin et al.	1998	IVF cycles	Increased retrograde and decreased antagonistic contractions from low (a) to high (d) frequency group	Before ET a<3.0 (antagonistic) b3.1–4.0 c4.1–5.0 d>5.0 (retrograde)		ND

Contd...

Contd...

Author	Year	General	Direction	Frequency (movements/minute)	Amplitude, strength, symmetry	Effect of uterine contractions displacements
Ijland et al.	1999	IVF cycles	FC waves before hCG and not after hCG	FC waves: hCG –6,8.12 ± 4.5 hCG 7.15 ± 5.2 CF waves hCG –6,7.11 ± 4 hCG, 9.4 ± 5.7 ET, 10.1 ± 5.0		ND
Bulletti et al.	2000	Frequency of UCs comparable in ultrasound and intrauterine pressure recordings	Retrograde contractions most frequent at mid-cycle Opposing contractions dominant in luteal phase	Early and late luteal 1.8 ± 1.9 contractions/min	ND	ND
Bulletti et al.	2001	Frequency of UCs in patients with endometriosis	Increased retrograde UCs	Menstrual period	Increased retrograde bleeding	Decreased recurrence rate of endometriosis after endometrial ablation
Bulletti et al.	2002	Frequency of UCs in patients with endometriosis	Increased retrograde UCs. Increased retrograde bleeding with viable endometrial cells	Menstrual period	Increased retrograde UCs. Increased retrograde bleeding with viable endometrial cells	Extraction and culture of viable endometrial stromal and epithelial cells from the pelvic cul-de-sac

Abbreviations: FC: fundus to cervix; CF: cervix to fundus; IVF: *in vitro* fertilization; ET: embryo transfer; hCG: human chorionic gonadotropin; UC: uterine contraction. *Source:* Data from Van Gestel, et al.[38]

a rate of two images/second using a computer-assisted image analysis system. The uterine contraction frequency is then assessed on time mode graphs, which are generated using the 3D reconstruction software.

RESEARCH PROSPECTS

In an addition to hormonal treatment, a wide range of drugs with different properties has been tested to reduce the myometrial contractile activity prior to embryo transfer. These include cyclo-oxygenase inhibitors, beta-2-adrenoreceptor agonists, calcium channel blockers, phosphodiesterase inhibitors and oxytocin antagonists. Pierzynski et al.[37] observed a noticeable decrease in uterine contractility following the infusion of a potent oxytocin antagonist for one hour, before embryo transfer in an infertile woman. She had previous multiple IVF failures but became pregnant after receiving the uterorelaxing treatment. Nevertheless, further prospective randomized control trials are required to prove the efficacy of these drugs in IVF treatment cycles.[37]

CONCLUSION

Uterine contractility in a non-pregnant uterus is known to have a definite impact on spontaneous and assisted conception cycles. With wider availability of the 3D ultrasound-derived system, the clinical application of this knowledge will become more prevalent in the management of subfertility. In future, more research is needed to look into the role of uterine relaxants in enhancing the success rate of assisted conception treatment cycles.

REFERENCES

1. Tabibzadeh S, Babaknia A. The signals and molecular pathways involved in implantation, a symbiotic interaction between blastocyst and endometrium involving adhesion and tissue invasion. Hum. Reprod 1995;10:1579-602.
2. Paulson RJ, Sauer MV, Lobo RA. Factors affecting embryo implantation after human invitro fertilisation: a hypothesis. Am J Obstet Gynecol 1990;163:2020-3.

3. Rogers PA, Murphy CR, Squires KR, MacLennan AH. Effects of relaxin on the intrauterine distribution and antimesometrial positioning and orientation of rat blastocysts before implantation. J Reprod Fert 1983;68:431-5.

4. Birnholz JC. Ultrasonic visualisation of endometrial movements. Fertil Steril 1984;41:157-8.

5. Oike K, Obata S, Tagaki, et al. Observations of endometrial movement with transvaginal sonography. Journal of Ultrasound in medicine 1988;7:99.

6. Fanchin R, Ayoubi JM. Uterine dynamics:impact on the human reproductive process. Reprod Biomed Online 2009;18 (Suppl 2): 57-62.

7. Ijland Mm, Evers JL, Dunselman GA, van Katwijk C, Lo CR, Hoogland HJ, et al. Endometrial wavelike movements during the menstrual cycle. Fertil Steril 1996;65:746-9.

8. Lyons EA, Taylor PJ, Zheng XH, Ballard G, Levi CS, Kredentser JV, et al. Characterisation of subendometrial myometrial contractions throughout the menstrual cycle in normal fertile women. Fertil Steril 1991;55:771-4.

9. Abramowicz JS, Archer DF. Uterine endometrial peristalsis: A transvaginal ultrasound study. Fertil Steril 1990;54:451-4.

10. Hendricks CH. Inherent motility patterns and response characteristics of the nonpregnant human uterus. Am J Obstset Gynecol 1996;96:824-43.

11. Csapo AI, Pinto-Dantas CR. The cyclic activity of the non pregnant uterus. A new method for uterine pressure. Fertil Steril 1966;17:34-8.

12. Garett WJ. Some observations on the human myometrial cycle. J Physiol 1956;132:553-8.

13. Henry JS, Browne JSL. The contractions of the human uterus during the menstrual cycle. Am J Obstet Gynecol 1943;45:927.

14. Henry JS, Browne JS, Venning eH. Some observations on the relationships of estrogens and progesterone to the contractions of the nonpregnant and pregnant human uterus. Am J Obstet Gynecol 1950;60:471-82.

15. Kunz G, Beil D, Huppert P, Leyendecker G. Control and function of uterine peristalsis during the human luteal phase. Reprod Biomed Online 2006;13:528-40.

16. De Ziegler D, Bulleti C, Fanchin R, Epiney M, Brioschi PA, et al. Contractility of the nonpregnant uterus: The follicular phase. Ann NY Acad Sci 2001;943:172-84.

17. Ijland MM, Evers JLH, Dunselman GAJ, Volovics L, Hoogland HJ, et al. Relation between endometrial wavelike activity and fecundability in spontaneous cycles. Fertil Steril 1997;67:492-6.

18. Ijland MM, Hoogland HJ, Dunselman GAJ, Lo CR, Evers JL, et al. Endometrial wave direction switch and the outcome of *in vitro* fertilisation. Fertil Steril 1999;71:476-81.

19. Fanchin R, Righini C, Olivennes F, Taylor S, de Ziegler D, Frydman R, et al. Uterine contractions at the time of embryo transfer alter pregnancy rates after *in vitro* fertilizsation. Hum Reprod 1998;13:1968-74.

20. Hunter RH. Human fertilisation *in vivo*, with special reference to progression,storage and release of competent spermatozoa. Hum Reprod 1987;2:329-32.

21. Kunz G, Beil D, Deininger H, Wildt L, Leyendecker G, et al. The dynamics of rapid sperm transport through the female genital tract: evidence from vaginal sonography of uterine peristalsis and hysterosalpingoscintigraphy. Hum Reprod 1996;11:627-32.

22. Brown SE, Toner JP, Schnorr JA, Williams SC, Gibbons WE, de Ziegler D, Oehninger S, et al. Vaginal Misopristol enhances intrauterine insemination. Hum Reprod 2001;16:96-101.

23. Fanchin R, Ayoubi JM, Righini C, Olivennes F, Schönauer LM, Frydman R, et al. Uterine contractility decreases at the time of blastocyst transfers . Hum Reprod 2001a;16:1115-9.

24. Gardner DK, Vella P, Lane M, et al. Culture and transfer of human blastocysts increases implantation rates and reduces the need for multiple embryo transfers. Fertil Steril 1998;69:84-8.

25. Menezo Y, Veiga A, Benkhalifa M. Improved methods for blastocyst formation and culture. Hum Reprod 1998;13(Suppl. 4):256-65.

26. Cicinelli E, de Ziegler D, Bulletti C, Matteo MG, Schonauer LM, Galantino P, et al. Direct transport of progesterone from vagina to uterus. Obstet Gynecol 2000;95:403-6.

27. De Ziegler D, Bulletti C, De Monstier B, Jaaskelainen As. The first uterine pass effect. Ann N Y Acad Sci 1997;828:291-9.

28. Miles RA, Paulson RJ, Lobo RA, Press MF, Dahmoush L, Sauer MV, et al. Pharmacokinetics and endometrial tissue levels of progesterone after administration by intramuscular and vaginal routes: A comparative study. Fertil Steril 1994;62:485-90.

29. Fanchin R, Ayoubi JM, Olivennes F, Righini C, de Ziegler D, Frydman R, et al. Hormonal influence on the uterine contractility during ovarian stimulation. Hum Reprod 2000;15(Suppl.1):90-100.

30. Rucker MP. Contractions of a nonpregnant mutiparous human uterus. Am J Obstet Gynecol 1925;9:255.

31. Wilson L, Kurzok R. Studies on the motility of the human uterus *in vivo*. Endocrinology 1938;23:79.

32. Jacobson E, Lackner JE, Sinykin MB. Electrical and mechanical activity of the human nonpregnant uterus. Am J Obstet Gynecol 1939;38:1008.

33. Bickers W. Uterine contraction patterns: Effect of psychic stimuli on the myometrium. Fertil Steril 1956;7:268-75.

34. Martinez-Gaudio M, Yoshida T, Bengtsson LP. Propagated and nonpropagated myometrial contractions in menstrual cycles. Am J Obstet Gynecol 1973;115:107-11.

35. Shafik A. Electrohysterogram: Study of the electromechanical activity of the uterus in humans. Eur J Obstet Gynecol Reprod Biol. 1197;73:85-9.

36. Fanchin R, Righini c, de Ziegler D, Olivennes F, Ledée N, Frydman R, et al. Effect of vaginal progesterone administration on uterine contractility at the time of embryo transfer. Fertil Steril 2001b;75:1136-40.

37. Pierzynski P, Reinheimer TM, Kuczynski W. Oxytocin antagonists improve infertility treatment. Fertil Steril 2007; 88:e219-213e.222.

38. Bulleti C, deZiegler D, Polli V, Diotallevi L, Del Ferro E, Flamigni C, et al. Uterine contractility during the menstrual cycle. Hum Reprod 2000;15(Suppl):81-9.

39. Van Gestel I, Ijland MM, Hoogland HJ, Evers JL. Endometrial wavelike activity in the nonpregnant uterus. Hum Reprod Update 2003;9:131-8.

Batch IVF

Does Batch IVF Compromise the IVF Laboratory?

Jayant G Mehta

OVERVIEW

The success of any *in vitro* fertilization (IVF) program is primarily dependent on the clinical and the laboratory excellence. In India, the majority of the assisted reproductive techniques (ART) laboratories function once every six to eight weeks on a patient-batched basis requiring these clinics to switch off all the laboratory equipment at the end of each batch and only to turn them on just few days prior to the first egg collection of the following batch. This prevents routine documented monitoring of the functional capacity of the laboratory equipments. There are two purposes of a quality control program, the first and the most important one is the reproducibility of results. In any IVF laboratory, there are literally hundreds of variables that must be controlled. The second reason for establishing a quality control program is the issue of 'standard of care'. Implementation of a comprehensive quality control program which includes infection control and protective measures, use of correct and in date consumables, records and protocols, maintenance, calibration and equipment monitoring, positive pressured aircondition system and staffing requirements would provide the base for ensuring that the IVF laboratory is not compromised. Periodic retrospective analysis of the program can only make a good program better.

INTRODUCTION

The success of any *in vitro* fertilization (IVF) program is primarily dependent on the clinical and laboratory excellence. Louise Brown, born after many attempts with IVF and embryo transfer techniques in 1978,[1] highlights this excellence.[2-5]

In India, the majority of the assisted reproductive techniques (ART) laboratories function once every six to eight weeks on a patient-batched basis. This may be due to the lack of patients or non-availability of a trained in-house embryologist. It is also a normal practice in these clinics to switch off all the laboratory equipment at the end of each batch and only to turn them on just few days prior to the first egg collection of the following batch. This prevents routine documented monitoring of the functional capacity of the laboratory equipments. Although not an ideal scenario, pregnancy rates in excess of 50 percent have been reported by most of these clinics, indicative of no compromise to IVF laboratory (verbal communication). More than drugs used for treatments, equipment choice or even personnel, a good laboratory practice (Table 79.1), developed on the 'backbone' of a sensible and user-friendly quality control program, would

ensure no compromise to the IVF laboratory and ultimately determine the success of the IVF program.[6]

There are two purposes of a quality control program. The first and the most important one is the reproducibility of results. In any IVF laboratory, there are literally hundreds of variables that must be controlled. The second reason for establishing a quality control program is the issue of 'standard of care'. In the medical and legal sense, 'standard of care' is defined by what is appropriate procedure and practice in your locale and in your speciality. The European Society of Human Reproduction and Embryology (ESHRE), recognizing a need for standardization, has constituted guidelines for good laboratory practice in IVF laboratories, allowing the embryologist to implement a quality control system.[6] Although such guidelines are valuable, they are inevitably subjective and reflect the local practices of the country or region in which they were produced. In India, the Indian Council of Medical Research (ICMR), has debated and revised Indian ART guidelines. Until there is a legal working regulatory body in India, it is left to each laboratory to institute a strict quality control program, which will help maintain good pregnancy rates and not compromise the IVF laboratory.[6-12]

Table 79.1: Infection control in the ART laboratory - laboratory procedures

All blood and body fluids (i.e. semen) should be treated as potentially infectious and due care observed

1. Either laboratory coats or theater greens should be worn.
2. Eating, drinking, smoking and application of cosmetics should not be permitted.
3. Food should be stored in a separate refrigerator in a non-clinical area.
4. Gloves should be worn for direct contact with all clinical specimens (including blood, semen and serum) and for cleaning all spills.
5. Hands should be washed after manipulating the biological specimen.
6. Mouth pipetting should be avoided.
7. Aerosalization of fluids should be minimized (include use of caps in the centrifuge).
8. Needles and disposal sharps should be placed in an appropriate containers.
9. All blood/body fluid contaminated specimens and laboratory ware should be separately bagged.
10. Disposable plastic ware and glassware should be used for all laboratory procedures involving blood or semen.
11. Blood/body fluid spills should be cleaned immediately with 1:10 solution of bleach or phenolic disinfectant/detergent followed by a 70 percent methanol clean.
12. Personnel should be vaccinated against Hepatitis B and C.

Over the past two decades, there has been a significant increase in our knowledge in gamete physiology, requiring laboratory protocols to be updated. At the molecular level, this includes the role played by various intracellular components in generating a competent mature, fertilizable grade A embryo for transfer, leading to a successful pregnancy. Further, the role of culture media i.e. sequential and embryo transfer media, such as 'embryo glue', and the influence of extrinsic factors on the culturing system have also contributed to the final outcome.

Some difficulties, which once seemed insurmountable, are now common knowledge and points, which were once the focus of our attention, are now past history. Although, there is still a lot to learn, the foundation of our knowledge has improved considerably and is more established now. Technical aspects seem to be less important for IVF due to recent advances in technology and instrumentation. However, these skills are essential for ICSI as it is an invasive procedure.

This chapter addresses various components of a comprehensive quality control program which, if observed, would provide the base for ensuring that the IVF laboratory is not compromised in batched IVF.

CLINICAL DISCUSSION

Infection Control and Protective Measures

Infection control and protective measures in the ART (and Andrology) laboratories are essential for success as well as for mediolegal reasons.[6] All ART procedures involve handling biological material and pose potential hazards of transmitting diseases to personnel. Semen is a known carrier of infectious diseases.[13-15] Gloves should be worn all the time and care taken to prevent aerosol formation (bubble formation and potential spraying) during sperm preparation.[15] Care should also be taken to avoid contamination of laboratory personnel as well as equipment, which will come into contact with patients, who are carriers for Hepatitis B/C surface antigens[16] or are HIV positive. It is therefore, mandatory to culture the gametes and sperm of infected patients in a separate incubator and not with gametes or embryos of other non-infected patients.[16,17] In case of seropositivity for Syphilis, appropriate treatment has to be given before *in vitro* fertilization (IVF).

In addition, some IVF patients may have a history of pelvic inflammatory or tubal disease that may be associated with specific infectious components. IVF failure has been attributed to Chlamydial infection.[18] Cross-contamination with infectious material from one patient to another remains a strong possibility. This is more evident during cryopreservation of semen samples using straws, sealing them with powder and passing them into liquid nitrogen storage containers. Similarly, embryos of patients with positive HIV, Hepatitis B and Hepatities C, status need to be stored in separate liquid nitrogen storage tanks.[19] It is therefore necessary to screen all IVF patients and treat them appropriately if the pathogen can be isolated prior to treatment being offered (Tables 79.1 and 79.2).

Consumables

The laboratory should maintain written records of all the consumables used for the IVF program. The record should monitor the supplier, batch number, shipment date and

Table 79.2: Suggested infectious disease screens for patients undergoing IVF

1. All women scheduled for IVF-ET should have
   a. Serological testing for sexually transmitted diseases, i.e. Syphilis
   b. Cervical culture for *Neisseria gonorrhea*
   c. Rubella titers
2. Participants at high-risk for diseases
   a. Hepatitis B and C surface antigens
   b. Cervical culture for Herpes simplex virus
   c. Cervical or urethral culture for *Chlamydia*
   d. HTLV-III ELISA antibody titers
   e. HIV.

conditions of shipment when received. As chemicals and plasticware may vary from batch to batch, it is best to be able to go back and verify whether a change in a supplier, a new batch of chemicals or inappropriate storage and shipment may have contributed to a bad outcome.[20]

Similarly, records must be maintained for culture media. Culture media on receipt should be stored refrigerated at 2 to 8°C. It must be ensured that the cold-chain was not broken at any stage of shipment and a human sperm survival test must be carried out at 4h and 24h with oil and oil-free culture at 37°C in a 5 percent CO_2 atmosphere.[21] It is also important not to use expired media and never to mix media from two different sources or manufacturers for any given ART procedure. For a given batch, adequate media should be ordered. If any turbidity or color change (with Phenol) is observed in the media, contamination should be suspected and a sample should be sent for culture and sensitivity test before discarding it. All the media must be handled in an aseptic manner to prevent any contamination (Table 79.3).

Records and Protocols

A procedures manual is one of the most important components of the quality control program.[6] Explicit step-by-step instructions of every protocol in the laboratory from glassware washing to IVF should be developed. Specific instructions about reagent preparation and expiry dates, calibration procedures, equipment operation, the procedure itself and quality control measures should also be included. This will help in keeping track that every step of every protocol is followed correctly and any deviation from it will help with any troubleshooting. Table 79.4, summarizes the components of a written protocol, including the principle of the test requirements for specimen handling.

The following should be analyzed between different batches: (a) fertilization, (b) embryo quality, (c) pregnancy rates, (d) multiple pregnancy rates and (e) implantation rates.[22-24] The analyses results will help prevent bias due to patient variation for the purpose of quality control. Each

Table 79.3: Troubleshooting guide for the preparation and use of culture media in an ART program

Outcome	Probable reason	How to overcome
Failed fertilization and/or embryo development	Problem with media or problem with protein source in media	Check the following parameters • Quality of H_2O used to make media • pH of media • Osmolarity • Ability to support mouse embryo development • Check incubator gas concentrations • Check for infection in the incubator • Contamination of the media • Check if there was a break in cold-chain during transportation of commercially prepared media • Check the expiry date and turbidity of the media
Sperm do not survive	Problem with media and/or serum source	Check above parameters • Check the sperm preparation protocols • Check the glass/plastic-ware used and possible contribution of endotoxins • Check the temperature of heating block in which media was warmed
Sperm agglutinate	Presence of antisperm antibodies	Test serum source for the presence of antibodies, use different serum source if necessary
Formation of a white precipitate in media	Precipitation of $CaCO_3$	Add Ca^2 lactate and $NaHCO_3$ as dilute solutions while stirring
Bacterial growth in media	Improper use of laminar flow hood Dirty laminar flow hood Incubator contamination Cap placed on culture tubes too loosely Rupture of sterilizing filter Damage to the container during transit of commercially prepared media	• Use proper tissue culture technique in hood • Clean hood and check filters • Clean incubator • Make sure cap is screwed on but loose • Use a hand-operated vacuum pump, check rest of filters for damage • Check for leaked media on receipt • Check with the supplier if there was a problem in the shipment • Breakdown in cold-chain during transportation • Improper storage during transport

Table 79.4: Components of written protocols that should form the basis of good laboratory practice

1. Principles of the test, including a brief statement of purpose and reaction involved
2. Specimen handling and preparation procedure
   a. Method of obtaining the sample
   b. Criteria for an acceptable sample
   c. Handling conditions
   d. Identification and storage
3. Reagent preparation
   a. Specific methods
   b. Detailed listing of materials needed
   c. Documentation of batch and supplier
   d. Identification and labeling
   e. Expiry date and procedure for discarding.
4. Calibration procedure
   a. Standards used where appropriate
   b. Acceptable tolerance limits and procedures to be followed if the results fall outside these limits.
   c. Expiry dates for the standards used.
5. Procedure—A detailed description of the exact procedure (including safety or biological hazards)
6. Calculations—Presented in a stepwise fashion with a specific example
7. Quality control
   a. State reference material used
   b. State minimum frequency of performing standards and performing the procedure
   c. State corrective action and trouble shooting activities to be followed
   d. State number of replicates, etc. that are necessary
8. Reporting of results
   a. State expected and/or normal range
   b. State any information about methodology that may be important to the interpretation of results
   c. Establish a system for flagging 'absurd' values and or critical values
   d. Report the results in an acceptable format and file them in a method that permits easy access
9. Procedural notes
   a. List possible sources of donors
   b. Plan for alternate means of handling specimens should the procedure fail
10. References for the procedures.

laboratory should have their own benchmarks (Table 79.5), which would help understand deviations from the expected values between batches and allow the correction of any poor results within IVF and andrology laboratories. Clinics should therefore develop protocols for every single procedure that is performed in the laboratory. On number of occasions, failure in IVF is due to seemingly insignificant aspect(s) of laboratory operation(s). Since the IVF laboratory is non-functional between batches, it is important that a detailed start-up protocol be established. Procedures for sanitizing the water system, glassware washing and sterilization, handling and preparation of transfer catheters and aspiration needles should be included in this protocol.[20]

The IVF laboratory will not be compromised if various commonly encountered problems in ART procedures are avoided (Tables 79.6 to 79.8).

Maintenance Calibration and Equipments Monitoring

The maintenance manual is an essential part of the record keeping for troubleshooting and for accreditation purposes. Maintenance must be documented in writing at prescribed time intervals (Table 79.9). This exercise is mandatory for clinics offering batch IVF and would not have any records for the period between batches. In my opinion, the best maintenance protocols should provide a system of checks and balances to determine, when any portion of the equipment is malfunctioning. For example, consider the incubator, the two main functions of which are to maintain a constant gas environment and temperature. A daily written log (not possible for clinics offering batch IVF) of the temperature of the incubators should be kept. However, one should know that a digital read out is not necessarily accurate. Therefore, a thermometer inside the incubator is necessary to verify the digital read out. In addition, the incubator temperatures can be monitored on an ongoing basis by equipping incubators with thermo tubes connected by a radio modem to a computer.[12]

Similarly, the percentage of gas content of the incubator is also registered in a digital form, and it is as good as the calibration of your incubator. However, if your incubator was calibrated with CO_2 in the chamber, your digital readout is incorrect. For example, if your incubator has been set to run at 5 percent CO_2 but the incubator was zeroed with 2 percent carbondioxide in the chamber, then the actual gas content of the chamber will be 7 percent CO_2. The best way to verify the CO_2 content of an incubator is by performing multiple checks. Daily measurements, using either a CO_2 Drager tube values or CO_2 digital sensor recordings, will allow you to determine the percentage of CO_2 content of the incubator and compare them against the digital display. Any discrepancy between the two has to be adjusted. It should be noted that the values of CO_2 for a humidified incubator would be different from that of an incubator run dry. Zero the incubator reading depending on which mode of operation you prefer to use: dry or humidified. Care should also be taken to allow humidity to a saturation point within the incubator chamber prior to calibration. Normally, calibration is carried out 24 hours after setting up the incubator on completion of a disinfection cycle. In addition, to check whether the pH control of the media is adequate, it can be monitored by placing a tube of culture

Table 79.5: Bench marks that need verification once every 4 months	
Embryology procedures	*Acceptable levels*
Normal Fertilization IVF	> 65%
ICSI	> 80%
Polyspermic rate IVF	< 10%
ICSI	< 1%
ICSI degeneration rates	< 5%
Embryo cleavage rate	> 80%
4 cells after 40–48 hrs	> 60%
> 8 cells after 72 hours	> 60 %
> Blastocyst on day 5	> 60%
Cryopreservation survival rates	> 50%
Ongoing pregnancy IVF	> 40%
rates ICSI	> 60%
Implantation rates IVF	> 20%
ICSI	> 35%
FET	> 25%
Assisted hatching	> 50%
Sperm concentration	+/– 5% of the mean
Sperm morphology	+/– 2% of the mean
Sperm motility	+/– 5% of the mean

Abbreviations: IVF: *in vitro* fertilization; ICSI: intracytoplasmic sperm injection; FET: frozen embryo transfer

Table 79.6: Troubleshooting guide for the preparation of semen sample for human IVF		
Outcome	*Probable reasons*	*How to overcome*
Sperm count very low	Oligozoospermia, inappropriate abstinence time	• Wash sperm by centrifugation and re-suspension or reduce overlay volume for swim-up wash • Inseminate multiple eggs in a single culture dish • Inseminate eggs at a higher sperm concentration
Ejaculate displaying high viscosity	Abnormal semen characteristics	• Use a Pasteur pipette to break up the sample
Ejaculate displaying slow liquefaction times	Abnormal semen characteristics	• Use a Pasteur pipette to break up the sample • Leave the sample in the incubator at 37°C for 30 minutes
Husband unable to provide a semen specimen	Stress-related factor(s)	• Ensure that semen sample is provided before oocyte retrieval • Tell the husband to relax and assure him that you can wait for the specimen • Try to freeze a back up for the next cycle
All sperm dead in the ejaculate	Some factor(s) involved in the method of semen collection	• Use frozen sperm back up if it is available • If unavailable, determine potential collection problem and request another sample after two hours

media (containing phenol red indicator) in the incubator and checking change in the color of the media each morning. Whatever the method used for calibration, its limitations must be recognized as fluctuations have disastrous consequences for the embryos.

A minimum number of two incubators are recommended and the gas cylinders should be placed outside or in a separate room and connected to an automatic switch-over system. Critical items of equipment, including incubators and frozen embryo storage facilities, should be appropriately equipped with alarms and monitored. In countries experiencing frequent power failures, it is necessary to have all the laboratory equipment connected to an automatic emergency generator back-up. It is necessary to ensure that all the laboratory equipment is functional and calibrated before the first egg collection. It is recommended that the disinfection

Table 79.7: Troubleshooting human oocyte fertilization

Outcome	Probable reasons	How to overcome
Failed fertilization—no motile sperm, no cumulus dispersal	Bad media, male factor	• Check media pH, osmolarity, sperm survival or fertilizing potential by penetration assay
No PN	Bad sperm or egg	• Re-inseminate with husband or perhaps donor sperm or ICSI with husband's sperm
Motile sperm cumulus dispersal	Post or immature eggs, male factor	• Re-inseminate • ICSI • Screen couple for *Chlamydia*
Agglutinated sperm cumulus dispersal	Antisperm antibody	• Collect sperm in culture media to minimize antibody contact • ICSI
Polyspermic fertilization-3 or more PN	High inseminating motile sperm concentrations, immature or aged oocyte	• Culture but do not transfer • Reconstitute PN number by removal of excess PN by micromanipulation
Fragmentation or 1 PN + premature and often irregular cleavage	Proper culture conditions not observed, or activation due to injecting pipette	• Culture but do not transfer • Try to remove fragments using micromanipluation techniques
Cracked zona	Excessive stress during aspiration, postmature oocytes	• Check negative pressure used during aspiration should be approx 100 mm Hg • Check follicular recruitment and timing of hCG injection • ICSI

Abbreviations: PN: pronuclei; ICSI: intracytoplasmic sperm injection

Table 79.8: Troubleshooting early embryonic development, observation at 40 hrs postinsemination/injection

Outcome	Probable reason	How to overcome
2–4 cell	Successful fertilization and early cleavage	Prepare for ET
16 cell or greater, unequal blastomeres	Activation without sperm penetration	Discard; re-evaluate follicular recruitment schedule if frequent and persistent
2 PN – failed cleavage: cleavage arrest	Heat or temperature shock, abnormal oogenesis, unknown causes	• Optional for ET • Observe meiotic spindle damage • Polar body preimplantation genetic diagnosis (PGD) • Check incubator temperature and concentration of gases • Check the pH of media and osmolarity
3 or more PN with cleavage	Polyspermic penetration	• Correct PN number by micromanipulation • Culture *in vitro* and cryopreserve for subsequent ET if normal blastocyst results

Abbreviations: PN: Pronuclei; ET: Embryo transfer

cycle and calibration of the incubator is done 72 hours prior to the egg collection.

Staffing Requirements

The successful functioning of the IVF laboratory depends totally on the knowledge of the laboratory staff. Since batch IVF clinics do not have resident laboratory staff, it is paramount that the staff providing laboratory services be experienced in both Embryology/Tissue culture and Andrology. In a discipline in which burnout comes early, it is very important to provide adequate support to the personnel and free up the embryologist from the day-to-day routine aspects of performing IVF. While media preparation (if not using commercially available) and testing, insemination of eggs, observing the fertilization and cleavage of embryos should be under the strict control of the senior embryologist, the day-to-day support activity, such as glassware washing, pipette sterilization and all the other monumental aspects

Table 79.9: Periodic check of laboratory quality control items

Laboratory quality control items checked on a monthly basis
Centrifuge timer clock (5 minutes ± 15 secs)
Hot plate cleaned
Air flow cabinet cleaned
Heating block calibrated
Door seal on all incubators checked and approved

Laboratory procedures conducted weekly in an IVF Laboratory

Heating block disinfected
Interior of all incubators cleaned
Circulating fan of incubators checked
Over-temperature safety thermostat on incubators checked

Laboratory procedures conducted at the end of the day in an IVF laboratory

Still H_2O system off
H_2O bath off
Oven off
Freezing machine off
Bench cleaned
Microscopes covered
Liquid N_2 levels approved

of supporting an IVF program, can best be assigned to appropriate support personnel. Personnel attuned to quality control and documentation of laboratory activities should be preferred. In selecting personnel, it is important to evaluate transferable experience or skills. Attributes should include microbiology, tissue culture, quality control and laboratory documentation experience, and manual dexterity. Individual responsibilities of each member of staff and line of responsibilities have to be indicated in a written procedure. This one single aspect of a trained embryologist will influence the final outcome in batch IVF program.

Air Conditioning System

It is assumed that most ART laboratories will have an adequate clean air supply considering the level of both organic and non-organic pollution in the air. The nature of clean air needs to be discussed since it plays a significant role in the percentage of pregnancies achieved, and especially, for those units where batch IVF is offered.[25] In my Unit, we have specifically designed our air handling system to remove both particulate matter and volatile organic gases. Our air handling system is a dedicated air conditioning unit exclusively for the IVF laboratory, which effectively removes 99 percent of 0.25μm and larger particles. A series of high efficiency gas phase filters have been installed to remove gas contaminants. Two inches pleated pre-HEPA filters as well as postcarbon filters effectively remove both large dust particles and any volatile organic gaseous contaminants from outside as well as recirculated internal air. Our system allows us for

10 air changes per hour and provides positive pressure in the laboratory relative to the external surroundings. The air is not mixed with other supplies and is not recirculated. Air in our laboratory is monitored every four months to determine the efficiency of our carbon and HEPA filters. Carbon filters are changed every 10 months while HEPA filters are only changed every 18 months. Timely changes of the filters have coincided with an increase in pregnancy rates in our Unit. It is therefore, important that, as part of your troubleshooting, the efficiency of the filters be checked at prescribed intervals.[25]

Although a central air conditioning unit with positive pressure is preferred, many units may only have split air conditioning with no positive pressure capabilities. In order to ensure filtered ambient air, such laboratories should install devices, which allow an ambient air filtration. Bacteriological samples of air and surfaces taken, using Gelose Count Tact (Biomerieux, Lyon, France), will ensure that the required conditions of asepsis were duly maintained.

CONCLUSION

An optimum embryo culture environment is important for the success of an IVF-ET program. Gametes and early embryos are sensitive to small changes in temperature, pH and physical properties of culture media. Any batch IVF, therefore, has a potential of compromising the IVF laboratory unless strict attention to the general components of a quality control program (Table 79.10) with written documentation, is observed. This will ensure that the laboratory operations

Table 79.10: Components of a quality control program

1. Written procedures and policies manual
   a. Detailed description of all procedures
   b. Sample handling protocols
2. Documentation and reporting of results
   a. Acceptable limit for results
   b. Documentation of corrective action
   c. Record keeping
3. Equipment maintenance
   a. Daily equipment monitoring
   b. Monthly/yearly preventive maintenance
   c. Establishment of acceptable operation standards
   d. Documentation of corrective action taken
   e. Instrument calibration
4. Safety procedures (including appropriate storage of materials)
5. Infection control measures
6. Staffing requirements
   a. Credentials of staff
   b. In service and continuing education
   c. Evaluation and performance appraisal
   d. Orientation procedures
7. Documentation of suppliers and sources of chemicals and supplies

Table 79.11: Components of a quality control program for *in vitro* fertilization

1. Equipment monitoring
   a. Daily monitoring of incubator function including temperature and gas content
   b. Daily monitoring of maintenance and operations of other laboratory equipment
   c. Emergency generator back-up to all equipment
   d. Regular recalibration scheduling including use of internal standards (i.e. thermometers)
2. Disposable supplies
   a. Documentation of supplier and batch/laboratory number
   b. Testing of all disposables, which come in contact with culture media for ability to sustain mouse embryo development
   c. Rinsing of disposable supplies (e.g. transfer catheters, etc.) with culture media before use
3. Non-disposable supplies
   a. Segregation for IVF use only
   b. Washing with ultrapure water (no tap water) heat sterilization (170°C for 2 hours) where possible, avoiding autoclaving where gas sterilization is used, allowing equipment to degas for 48 hours before use, rinsing vigorously with culture media
   c. All non-disposable supplies should be replaced at predetermined intervals.
4. Culture media preparation and testing
   a. Batch, storage and expiration requirements on all culture media should be documented in writing.
   b. ACS grade chemicals should be purchased for media modifications.
   c. Water used for preparations should be from an unopened bottle or freshly obtained from the point of delivery.
   d. All culture media and serum should be tested in the mouse embryo culture bioassay.
   e. Media should be discarded seven days after the completion of testing.
   f. All plastic ware should be tested to determine its ability to support mouse embryo development.
5. Written protocols should be prepared for every step of the procedure.
6. Written records should be kept of
   a. Induction protocol including ultrasound and estradiol monitoring
   b. Number of follicles aspirated
   c. Number of oocytes obtained and their stage of maturation
   d. Detailed analysis of semen parameters
   e. Number of oocytes fertilized
   f. Number of fertilized oocytes cleaved
   g. Number of embryos transferred and fate of extra embryos

Table 79.12: Summaries of quality control criteria

1. Perform all procedures using known reference material. The individual performing the tests must record the date and sign the results.
2. Assay controls are often enough to ensure the reliability of test results.
3. Compare results of quality control studies with previously established values. Identify and document any discrepancies.
4. Evaluate the components of the procedures for which discrepancies are identified.
5. Document the appropriate corrective action after identifying the cause for the discrepancy.
6. Repeat the quality control procedures and document acceptability of the repeated results before repeating procedures on patient material.
7. Document the use of preventive maintenance schedules and equipment service records.
8. Perform internal and external testing and control programs.
9. Perform systematic retrospective review of services to include.
   a. Technical and professional services
   b. Delivery systems
   c. Appropriateness of services
   d. Adherence to established protocols by all practitioners as appropriate.

spell' when these occur; a rational approach to correcting problems is a return to the basics (Table 79.11).

Table 79.12 highlights the general principles of quality control through which the troubleshooting of problems in the IVF laboratory can be achieved. Comparisons of retrieved results against previous laboratory records, as well as literature values, will allow the identification of failures in the system. A human embryo that develops slowly compared to the established growth schemes would suggest possible problems. Documentation of corrective action prevents repetition of problems, allows one to trace where problems occurred and prevents a 'shotgun' approach, where many variables are changed at once.

After correcting a problem, the quality control procedures must be repeated to see how they affect a specific outcome, i.e. did recalibration of the incubator result in improved embryo development? Documentation of preventive maintenance can avoid problems that arise as the system is used over time. Internal and external controls of all procedures must be established. Finally, periodic retrospective analysis of the program can only make a good program better. Adherence to a stringent quality control program ensures continued success and helps pinpoint problems to troubleshoot. Laboratory personnel have to be adequately trained in Embryology/Tissue culture and Andrology as they contribute significantly to the final result. Batch IVF will not compromise the IVF laboratory as long as a strict quality control is followed.

continue within specific tolerance limits. As stated earlier, the goal of a quality control program is to ensure reproducibility of results. The biggest fear of a fledgling program is lack of success and the fear of the established program is a long 'dry

REFERENCES

1. Steptoe PC, Edwards RG. Birth after reimplantation of a human embryo. Lancet 1978;2:366.
2. Steptoe PC, Edwards RG. Reimplantation of a human embryo with subsequent tubal pregnancy. Lancet 1976;1:880.
3. Edwards RG. Test tube babies. Nature 1981;293:253-6.
4. Asch RH, Ellsworth LR, Balmaceda JP, Wong PC. Pregnancy after translaproscopic gamete intrafallopian transfer. Lancet 1980;2:1034.
5. Jones HR, Jr Jones GS, Andrews MC, Acosta A, Bundren C, Garcia J, et al. The program of *in vitro* fertilization at Norfolk. Ferti Steril 1982;38:14-21.
6. Gianaroli L, Plachot M, Kooij RV, Al-Hasani S, Dawson K, DeVos A, et al. ESHRE guidelines for good practice in IVF laboratories. Hum Reprod 2000;15:2241-6.
7. Wikland M, Sjoblom C. The application of quality systems in ART programs. Molecular and Cellular Endocrinology 2000; 166:3-7.
8. Wiemer K, Anderson A, Weikert L. Quality control in IVF laboratory. In Textbook of Assisted Reproductive Techniques: Laboratory and Clinical Perspectives. Martin Dunitz, London, 2001. pp.27-33.
9. Alper MM, Brinsden PR Fischer R, Wikland M. Is your IVF programme good? Hum Reprod 2002;17:8-10.
10. Kastrop P. Quality management in the ART laboratory. Reprod Biomed Online 2003;7:691-4.
11. Land J, Evers J. Risks and complications in assisted reproduction techniques: report of an ESHRE consensus meeting. Hum Reprod 2003;18:455-7.
12. Frydman N, Fanchin R, Le Du A, Bourrier MC, Tachdjian G, Frydman R. Improvement of IVF results and optimisation of quality control by using intermittent activity. Reprod Biomed Online 2004;9:521-8.
13. Mascola L, Guinan ME. Screening to reduce transmission of sexually transmitted diseases in semen used for artificial insemination: N Engl J Med 1986;314:1354-9.
14. Baccetti B, Benedetto A, Burrini, AG, Collodel G, Ceccarini EC, Crisà N. HIV-particles in spermatozoa of patients with AIDS and their transfer into oocyte. J Cell Biol 1994;127:903-14.
15. World Health Organization. WHO laboratory manual for the examination of human semen and sperm-cervical mucus interaction. Cambridge University Press. Cambridge 1999.
16. Axelrod P and Talbot GH. Infection control considerations for *in vitro* fertilization and embryo transfer programs. Infect Control 1986;7:373-8.
17. Barriera P, Lopes P, Boiffard JP, L'Hermite A, Lerat MF. An unusual cause of failure of *in vitro* fertilization report of a case. J In Vitro Fert Embryo Transf 1985;2:170-1.
18. Ronland GF, Forsey T, Moss TR, Steptoe PC, Hewitt J, Darougar S. Failure of *in vitro* fertilization and embryo replacement following infection with *Chlamydia trachomatis*. J In Vitro Fert Embryo Transf 1985;2:151-5.
19. Tedder RS, Zuckerman MA, Goldstone AH, Hawkins AE, Fielding A, Briggs EM. Hepatitis B transmission from contaminated cryopreservation tank. Lancet 1995;346:137-9.
20. Schiewe M, Schmidt P, Bush M, Wildt D. Toxicity potential of absorbed/retained ethylene oxide residues in culture dishes on embryos development *in vitro*. J Anim Sci 1985;60:1610-9.
21. Franco J, Mauri A, Petersen C, Baruffi RL, Campos MS, Oliveira JB. Efficacy of the sperm survival test for the prediction of oocytes fertilization in culture. Hum Reprod 1993;8:916-8.
22. Cummins JM, Breass TM, Harrison KL, Shaw JM, Wilson LM, Hennessey JF. A formula for scorring human embryo growth rates in *in vitro* fertilization: its value in predicting pregnancy and in comparison with visual estimates of embryo quality. J In Vitro Fert Embryo Transf 1986;3:284-95.
23. Van Royen E, Mangelschots K, DeNeubourg DI, Valkenburg M, Van de Meerssche M, Ryckaert G, et al. Characterization of top quality embryo, a step towards single embryo transfer. Hum Reprod 1999;14:2345-9.
24. Mayer J, Jones E, Dowling-Lacey D, Muasher SJ, Gibbons WE, Oehninger SC. Total quality improvement in the IVF laboratory: choosing indicators of quality. Reprod BioMed Online 2003;7:192-6.
25. Cohen J, Gilligan A, Esposito W, Schimmel T, Dale B. Ambient air and its potential effects on conception *in vitro*. Hum Reprod 1997;12:1742-9.

Marketing and Advertising in IVF

Web Marketing for IVF Clinics

Aniruddha Malpani

OVERVIEW

Every *in vitro* fertilization (IVF) clinic needs its own website. This is good for both, the clinic and for infertile couples as it helps to promote transparency. Information therapy represents the heart of good Medicine and a website is a very cost-effective investment in helping IVF clinics to promote their practice and keep their patients happy.

Why You Need a Website?

In vitro fertilization (IVF) is a very competitive business and getting patients can be extremely hard work. IVF costs a lot of money and because so much is at stake, patients are very careful about which IVF clinic they will select. Also, competition is not restricted to the clinics in one's own town anymore. Infertile couples can be very motivated and because they are willing to travel half-way across the globe to complete their families, all IVF clinics are potential competition.

Moreover, infertile couples are thirsty for information. They will spend a lot of time doing research and choosing the best clinic, to maximize their chances of getting pregnant. Thanks to the Web, it has become much easier for patients to compare clinics and to shop around, and an increasing number of infertile couples spend a lot of time on the net routinely.

Since infertile couples spend so much time online, and because other IVF clinics have a strong Web presence, this means that you simply cannot afford not to have your own website anymore.

In the past, getting on the internet meant learning how to surf the Web, and having your own email address was considered to be a status symbol. However, today, this is no longer enough—you need to have your own website. This rapid pace of change is symbolic of how quickly things are changing in today's world. In fact, it is my contention that IVF clinics can no longer afford not to have their own website. Just like you need a telephone line to practise Medicine, a website has become an integral part of IVF practice, and doctors who are not proactive are likely to get left behind.

How Your Website Helps You?

You are a busy doctor, so why should you take the time and trouble of setting up your own website ?

Every good doctor knows that keeping his/her patients happy and providing excellent patient care is key to success. A website enables you provide many value-added services for your patients. It can provide basic details such as:
- The timings of your clinics
- Directions as to how to get to your clinic
- Information on the specialized services you offer
- Why you are better than other IVF clinics
- Answers to patient's commonly asked questions (FAQs)
- Post procedure instructions.

This means you can use your website to serve your patients round the clock without requiring them to call or visit, making your website a valuable support/contact center.

Your website allows you to answer your patient's queries by email. Patients are thirsty for information about their illness, and many will use the internet to find information. Please do not underestimate your patient's intelligence. Many will spend hours hunting for information, in order to help them to get better. Even if they do not have a personal computer (PC), they can go to the cyber café. And even illiterate patients do have relatives who can do an internet search for them. However, most patients would much rather get information from their own doctor, and if you provide this information on your website, your patients know they can trust it. Your website will also save you a lot of time. Most doctors have now started seeing patients coming with internet print outs of pages and pages of unreliable and irrelevant information. If you put up your own website, you can guide your patients to reliable sources of information, thus saving your patients the frustration of wading through pages of garbage and misinformation. By providing this information, you establish yourself as a credible expert. You can 'refer' patients to your website at the end of the consultation, so they can educate themselves. Patients appreciate this and word of mouth will help you get more patients.

Your website can help you to attract new patients. Indian medical care is very cost-effective, and a website is very valuable for informing non-resident Indians (NRIs) of your medical expertise. Soon, it will become routine for patients in India to do 'research' about their doctors, as it is in USA, and your website can help patients to find you. At our website at http://www.DrMalpani.com, we answer over 20 queries a day, as a result of which, we get direct patient referrals from all over the world. Remember that internet positive patients may be slightly different from your average patient. They are well-informed, used to getting second opinions, and can be quite demanding. Most are affluent, and know exactly what they want.

However, website benefits are not restricted to practice promotion only. For example, we sell ovulation test kits and self insemination kits on our website, allowing infertile couples in India to buy fertility tools they cannot get otherwise. This is an additional revenue stream for us. Our website at www.TheBestMedicalCare.com allows us to publicize our book, 'How to Get the Best Medical Care—A Guide for the Intelligent Patient'. We now get orders from all over the world for this book – and get paid in US dollars too for this.

Our first website, www.healthlibrary.com is a purely educational site, and by putting up over 20 full-textbooks on Ayurveda and Yoga online in our reading room, we are helping to promote Indian healing systems internationally. Patients all over the world are very interested in alternative medicine, and websites can allow Indian doctors to treat patients from all over the globe.

Putting up a website has become very easy, and many companies provide free web hosting. However, it's well worth spending about ₹ 20,000 to get your own domain name and a commercial web host. This lets your patients know that you are professional and serious about the services you offer. This is an excellent return on investment, which one should not scrimp on.

Promoting Your Website—An Ongoing Effort

You need to have realistic expectations of what your website can do for you. Just because you publish a website does not mean patients will start pouring in. Just having a website is not enough. It is important to remember that there are over a million websites out there. You need to promote your website actively and this is a challenging task. It is important not to underestimate the difficulty and necessary to budget for this. It is very cost-effective to do so, so one should think of it as an investment, rather than as an expense.

Online promotion usually means registering the site with all the relevant search engines, so people can 'find' you. Offline promotion is even more important, and you need to tell everybody about it. The website address (URL) must be printed on your business cards and your stationery and displayed in your waiting room. Patients should be encouraged to use your website and evidently, most will be happy to follow their doctor's orders. And if your website has content which is useful to them, and which is updated on a regular basis so it is fresh and new, many will happily visit it regularly and even refer many of their friends to your site as well.

You can also design a monthly magazine, to keep patients coming back to your site. Your staff should constantly be on the lookout for interesting pieces for the next month's issue. This creates a direct link to your website, but does require a commitment to keep the content fresh. You can employ a webmaster to do this for you, to ensure you do a good job.

The web changes all the time, and your website also needs to evolve. Social media and Web 2.0 is the current flavor of the time and if you have your own website, it is very easy to use these clever new tools to reach out to infertile couples.

As electronic medical records (EMRs) and personal health records (PHRs) become increasingly popular, it is now possible to integrate these in your website by providing patients with their own patient portal to your site, so they can get updated information about their laboratory results and medical treatment.

Are there any downsides? The major one for doctors in the US is that of legal liabilities. Protecting patient privacy and confidentiality is a major concern, and while this is still not an issue in India as yet, it is likely to become important as the world shrinks even further. Using simple common sense electronic security measures (just like banks do for online transactions) can prevent problems.

It is true that putting up a website and updating it can be time consuming and you might want to consider outsourcing it. Your website is an image of your clinic hence, it is important that you make sure you do a professional job. Typing errors, poor grammar and deadlinks all create a poor impression. Also, it is important that queries and emails are promptly answered. It is a good idea to check out competing websites, so you can see what they are doing. This can also provide you with an incentive to upgrade your own services. Your website can help to keep you on your toes both, professionally, because you need to update your medical knowledge to provide fresh content for your website and to answer queries received by email from patients in all parts of the world, which means this is a great method of continuing medical education (CME); and technologically, because you will need to keep abreast with computer and internet technology. A website is valuable even for doctors in rural areas, who are often cut off from the rest of the world. This is a valuable way of 'keeping in touch' and contributing to the medical knowledge base.

The Indian government has started encouraging doctors and hospitals to export their services, and medical services can be a major area of foreign exchange revenue for the future. By encouraging doctors and clinics to put up their own websites, the Indian Health Ministry can help the Indian medical industry to export their specialized medical services and knowledge without contributing to brain drain. This can be a valuable source of foreign exchange for the country, and our hospitals can be actively promoted as medical centers of excellence. Indian doctors have the expertise—we just need the infrastructure and the promotion.

Some doctors are worried that having their own website may be misconstrued as a form of advertising. However, the internet is a very valuable means of educating patients, and doctors need to be in the forefront for providing reliable information to their patients. After all, if we do not take up the responsibility of educating patients, then who will?

CONCLUSION

The future of medical care is e-healthcare, with the promise of online medical records, online pharmacies, telemedicine, patient education and an ever-expanding list of exciting opportunities. The opportunity to help our patients navigate the wealth of information on the Worldwide Web and better educate themselves is now in our hands. We owe it to ourselves and our patients to meet the challenge that lies before us all, for if we fail to do so, the friendly competitor down the road will and will take away all our patients.

Role of Mass Media in Marketing Your IVF Center

Jayant G Mehta

OVERVIEW

Mass media refers collectively to tools for the transfer of information, concepts, and ideas to both general and specific audiences. It is an important tool in advancing public awareness of your clinic's goals; it may be health-related issues or may involve treatment offered by your *in vitro* fertilization (IVF) center. Currently, societies worldwide depend on mass media to deliver health-related information. Mass media is capable of facilitating short, intermediate, and long-term effects on audiences. Further, mass media also performs three key functions: educating, shaping public relations, and advocating for a particular policy or point of view. Types of media that can be employed include television, radio, internet, newspaper, magazines and other print media such as pamphlets, brochures and posters.

Billboards and signs, placards inside and outside of commercial transportation modes, flying billboards (e.g. signs in tow of airplanes), blimps, and skywriting constitute outdoor media and are very effective. Whatever the mass media used for marketing your IVF clinic, it is important to understand the basic principles involved in composing an effective message. Decades of studies on the consequences of mass media exposure demonstrate that effects are varied and reciprocal—the media impacts audiences and audiences also impact media by the intensity and frequency of their usage.

The three effects or functions of media namely (1) the knowledge gap, (2) agenda setting, and (3) cultivation of shared public perceptions have been identified to be crucial in marketing the clinic. Although mass media is important for disseminating your clinic's messages and encouraging an adoption of successful outcome, they currently fall short of their potential. The realization of this potential in the future depends, in part, on increasing the media advocacy skills of public health authorities, improving understanding of competing anti-health media messages and organizing channels for an optimal media mix.

INTRODUCTION

In advancing public awareness of your clinic's goals, including health-related issues or treatment aspects, mass media, through the transfer of information, concepts, and ideas to both general and specific audiences, serves as a significant tool. Although communicating about health through mass media is complex, it challenges professionals in diverse disciplines to understand the basic principles involved in marketing. Winett and Wallack[1] wrote, 'using the mass media to improve public health can be like navigating a vast network of roads without any street signs—if you are not sure where you are going and why, chances are you will not reach your destination.' On the other hand Krep and Thornton[2] believe that mass media extends 'people's ability to communicate, to speak to others far away, to hear messages, and to see images that would be unavailable without media'. At the same time, mass media can also be counterproductive if the channels used to market your clinic are not audience-appropriate, or if the message being delivered is too emotional, fear arousing or controversial. Undesirable side effects usually can be avoided through proper formative research, knowledge of the audience, experience in linking media channels to audiences and message testing. This chapter addresses types and functions of mass media, its advantages and shortcomings understanding the importance of media effects and how to implement them in marketing your IVF clinic.

CLINICAL DISCUSSION

Types and Functions of Mass Media

Currently, societies worldwide depend on mass media to deliver health-related information. Marketing an IVF program is no different; essentially, it is delivery of specialized health-related information. It follows that employment of mass media to disseminate health news (or matters related to your clinic) has, in effect, reduced the size of the world. The value of health news is related to what gets reported and how it gets reported.

Mass media is capable of facilitating short-term, intermediate-term, and long-term effects on audiences. Short-term objectives include exposing audiences to your clinic's information and concepts, creating awareness and knowledge of the treatments offered and the results achieved, altering outdated or incorrect knowledge and enhancing audience recall of particular treatments only being offered through your clinic. Intermediate-term objectives include all of the above, as well as documenting changes in attitudes, behaviors, and perceptions of the potential patients. Finally, long-term objectives should incorporate all of the above-mentioned tasks, in addition to focused restructuring of perceived patient norms, and maintenance of behavior changes. Evidence of achieving these three tiers of objectives will help in evaluating the effectiveness of mass media in marketing your IVF clinic.

Further, mass media also performs three key functions: educating, shaping public relations, and advocating for a particular policy or point of view. As education tools, media not only imparts knowledge, but can be part of larger efforts (e.g. cervical cancer) to promote social health-related issues. As a public relations tools, media assists organizations in achieving credibility and respect among opinion leaders, stakeholders, and other gatekeepers in the field of Assisted Reproductive Medicine. As an advocacy tool, mass media assists clinicians in setting a policy agenda, shaping debates about controversial issues and gaining support for particular viewpoints. All these exposures help identify the clinician with the clinic and the clinic with assisted reproductive policies.

Types of Media that can be Employed in Marketing your IVF Clinic

Television

Television is a powerful medium for appealing to mass audiences—it reaches people regardless of age, sex, income or educational level. In addition, television offers sight and sound, and it makes dramatic and life-like representations of people and products. Focused television coverage of public health has been largely limited to crises. However, for audiences of the late 1950s, the 1960s, and the 1970s, television presented or reinforced certain health messages through product marketing. Some of these messages were related to toothpaste, hand soaps, multiple vitamins, fortified breakfast cereals and other items. A more focused coverage of health matters occurred in the 1990s as a result of two events: (1) an expansion of 'health segments' on news broadcasts,

which included the hiring of 'health' reporters, and (2) the expansion and wider distribution of cable television (CATV) and satellite systems. As a result, television has become a very powerful global medium, surpassing all expectations of marketing norms, and just like any other product, the IVF clinic should be considered as a product to be marketed.

However, television coverage of health issues has revealed some of the medium's weaknesses as an educator. Health segments incorporated into news broadcasts are typically one to three minutes in length—the consumer receives only a brief report or 'sound bite', while the broadcaster remains constrained by the fact that viewers expect the medium to be both visual and entertaining. Fortunately, with the advent and maturation of CATV, more selected audience targeting has become possible. The Health Network on the cable is dedicated entirely to health matters, while other cable networks (e.g. Discovery Channel) devote significant amounts of broadcast time to health. Although this narrow casting allows the medium to reach particular market segments, the proliferation of cable channels decreases the volume of viewers for a given channel at any point in time.

The main consumer effect of messages occurs through repetition and brand familiarity. Most health messages do not have the exposure level that brands of toothpaste, soap or antiperspirant receive, for public health groups rarely can sustain the cost of television, thereby limiting the penetration of their message. For all its potential strengths, TV suffers many shortcomings. The cost of placing your clinic's messages on TV is high, not only because of the expense of purchasing airtime, but because of production time by 'Production Service Association' (PSA) member's creation. Televised messages are fleeting, aired in most instances for only 15 to 30 seconds, and for 13 to 17 minutes of every hour, viewers are bombarded with messages, creating a clutter that makes retention difficult.[3] This medium may not be an effective way of marketing your IVF program.

Radio

Radio also reaches mass and diverse audiences. The specialization of radio stations by listener age, taste and even gender permits more selectivity in reaching audience segments. Since placement and production costs are lesser for radio than for TV, the radio is able to convey your clinic's messages in greater detail. Thus, the radio is sometimes considered to be more efficient. Radio requires somewhat greater audience involvement than television, creating the need for more mental imagery or 'image transfer'.[3]

Radio message campaigns have been effective in developing countries, especially when combined with posters and other mass media. However, care has to be taken to ensure that the large number of radio stations do not fragment the audience for the delivery of your clinic's message.

Internet

The advent of the Worldwide Web and the massive increase in Internet users offers IVF clinics enormous opportunities and challenges to interact with potential patients. The Internet places users in a firmer autonomous control of which messages are accessed and when they are accessed. It is therefore, possible to put virtually anything online and disseminate it to any location having Internet access, but the user has little control over quality and accuracy. Internet search engines can direct users to tens of thousands of websites after the user's introduction of one or more keywords. The most important challenge for any IVF clinic is to make it easier for potential patients to discriminate information of other Internet-based IVF clinics and to encourage them to use your clinic's websites more often. Efforts are therefore needed to stop short of censorship, thus balancing accuracy, quality and protection of free speech.

Unlike the television or radio, which are available in nearly all households, Internet access requires some technical skill, as well as the resources to purchase hardware and Internet subscription services. As with its predecessor technologies, the Internet suffers from a certain 'legacy of fear' about its impact on children, youth and others.[4] Unlike some other mass media, the Internet is presently not universally available across socioeconomic strata due to cost and other barriers. It is possible that this lack of universality has already contributed to the existing information gaps between society's 'haves' and 'have-nots.' The Internet's utility for conveying the clinic's information can be best illustrated by creating a very interactive user-friendly web page(s), that should have factual information about the infrastructure of the clinic, educational and specialization details of the main clinician(s), embryologist(s) and nursing staff. There should be appropriate links to more detailed information on a given subject. The clinic's research interests and publications posted on the web would endorse the academic stature of the clinic. Details about any conferences and training workshops conducted by the clinic raises the awareness within the IVF fraternity. One most important area, not to be ignored, is a patient feedback—question answer section. It allows individual patients to submit questions anonymously and receive a response, and also serves as a service monitor for the clinic. Display of visual images from different areas of your clinic can be helpful to portray the state-of-the-art facility with pleasant ambience.

Although, the internet offers all of the audio and visual strengths of other electronic media, plus interactivity and frequent updates, speculating about its future is not easy. The challenge is to increase its availability and augment the skills of Internet users.

Newspapers

It is estimated that more than 70 percent of households and more than 90 percent of high-income household read the newspaper daily.[3] Newspapers permit a level of detail in reporting not feasible with broadcast media. Whereas one can miss a television broadcast about your IVF program, and thus, lose its entire message, one can read the same (and more detailed) message in a newspaper at one's choice of time and venue. Although newspapers permit consumer flexibility concerning what is read, and when, they do have a brief shelf life. In many households, newspapers seldom survive more than one or two days.

Newspapers are available in daily and weekly formats in local and regional languages as local, regional and national publications. There are also numerous special audience newspapers (e.g. various ethnic groups, women and feminist-related, gay and lesbian, geography-specific, and neighbourhood). Consequently, messages about your clinic contained in newspapers can reach many people and diverse groups. However, newspapers often fall short of their dissemination potential. While educating people about your clinical activities, programs, results and special events, it is important that deliberate efforts are made directly to educate other media and politicians.[4]

Few stories call for individual or community policy or action, and even fewer present a local angle.[4] It is therefore, essential to choose the correct newspaper for marketing your IVF program.

Magazines

Magazines have been divided into three varieties: consumer (e.g. Reader's Digest, Newsweek, People), farm (e.g. Farm Journal, National Hog Farmer, Beef), and business (professional, industrial, trade, and general business publications).[3] Magazines have several strengths, including audience selectivity, reproduction quality, prestige, and reader loyalty. Furthermore, magazines have a relatively long shelf life—they may be saved for weeks or months, and are frequently re-read and passed on to others. Magazine reading also tends to occur at a less hurried pace than newspaper reading. Messages about your clinic in relation to treatment modalities or a general article on women's health issues therefore, can receive repeated exposure. Like the newspaper, it is important to choose the correct magazine with a large circulation that is published in the language most commonly understood to market your clinic. It is always important to know the target audience as the response to any marketing will depend on the perception of the audience.

Other Print Media

Pamphlets, brochures and posters constitute other print media used to disseminate simple but accurate messages about your clinic. These devices can be circulated among your local neighbourhood or made available at most public health agencies, offices of private practitioners, health care institutions, and voluntary health organizations. Though widely used, their actual utility is infrequently evaluated (e.g. units distributed versus changes in awareness, cost analysis). Until the 1990s, few of these print media were developed with the assistance of target audiences, few contained varied messages, were culturally tailored, or employed readability and face validity techniques. The extent to which persons read, re-read, and keep these devices or circulate them to other readers is difficult to evaluate. Thus, their permanence is unknown. The person responsible for marketing your IVF clinic needs to have some mechanism in place to monitor the response to such devices on an ongoing basis. These devices allow you to control what information and in which format it is disseminated. It costs much less compared to other media discussed here and should be considered as the first choice and an ongoing marketing channel.

Outdoor Media

Outdoor media include billboards and signs, placards inside and outside of commercial transportation modes, flying billboards (e.g. signs in tow of airplanes), blimps, and skywriting. Commercial advertisers, such as Goodyear, Fuji, Budweiser, Pizza Hut and Blockbuster, all make extensive use of their logo-bearing blimps around sports stadiums. In the United States, none of these outdoor modes are used extensively to convey health messages, although billboards and transit placards are the most likely forms to contain health information. For people who regularly pass by billboards or use public transportation, these media provide repeated exposure to your clinic's messages.

In their 1994 Chicago-based study, Hackbarth, et al.[5] revealed how billboards promoting tobacco and alcohol were concentrated in poor neighbourhoods. Similar themes were seen in other urban centers (Baltimore, Detroit, St. Louis, New Orleans, Washington DC, San Francisco) where alcohol and tobacco billboards were much more concentrated in African-American neighbourhoods than in White neighbourhoods. The tobacco industry now pursues the same strategy in developing countries. Billboard advertisement can be expensive; however, selective location for the target audience will bring positive response to your messages. The messages should be very simple but precise and factual. There should be a proper balance of color and they should be appealing even to the non-targeted audience. Too much information can be counter-productive.

Composing Effective Messages for Specific Channels

Whatever mass media is used for marketing your IVF clinic, it is important to understand the basic principles involved in composing an effective message.

1. It is important to focus on patients needs by stepping into their shoes. For example, when targeting a woman's magazine, a story that is of interest to their readers must be thought of, especially if they were your potential patients. When targeting a late afternoon radio show a story that is of interest to the people driving home from work, listening to the radio, must be targeted. If you were reading the publication or listening to the radio show, what would jump out and appeal to you? If you can answer that question, you have got the subject for your effective message.

2. The headline of the message needs to be bold and interesting, and above all, it needs to stand out from all the other messages on the same page or the same edition, or for that matter, on the billboards. Your best option is to write it in the style of the headlines of the publication you are targeting. For example, if you were selling a new supplement to help indigestion, which of these messages do you think would get the best response: 'New Supplement Helps Ease Indigestion' or 'Why Some Foods Explode in Your Stomach?'. The reason that newspapers use bold, attention-grabbing headlines is that they work. You can deploy the same strategy to grab the attention of the audience you are trying to reach.

3. Messages must be formatted correctly. Here are my Golden Rules for formatting messages: (a) Make sure the headline is big and bold, (b) aim to fit the message(s) on one page, (c) use short paragraphs, and (d) use language that will appeal to the type of media that you are going to employ and the audience for which it has been targeted. You may want to write different messages for different media, for example, use different wording for targeting a tabloid than you would for a technical business publication.

4. One most important area is to be recognized as an opinion leader overnight. Most people think that the only way to get good message(s) across is to come up with a story. But there is another way. This involves positioning yourself as an expert in your specialized area. Whatever your profession, there is an area that you are an expert in. As an IVF specialist, contact the media during the next National Fertility Week and respond to any IVF-related controversial news; for example, creation of a human clone or Women's Day being celebrated to bring awareness of certain health issues, related to women's health. Tell the media about your interest in the subject and organize an interview to discuss it further. At the time of interview, ensure that the media has a chance to see your clinic

and enough photographs are taken to demonstrate the ambience of your clinic, availability of the state-of-the-art equipment in your assisted reproductive techniques (ART) laboratory and the facilities in your operating theater(s). These photographs would normally be filed by the media for future news casting, which would give your clinic and yourself frequent exposures.

5. By hosting scientific conferences, not only you are exposing your clinic to your fraternity but also demonstrating your international standing in the field of Reproductive Medicine. In India, patients love international exposure, especially being treated by a renowned clinician who has collaboration with clinics abroad.

6. Finally, because of the inherent properties of various mass media, message designers of your clinic should also consider a series of questions, relative to the choice of channels:
   a. Which channels are most appropriate for the health problem/issue and message?
   b. Which channels are most likely to be credible to and accessible by the target audience?
   c. Which channels fit the program purpose (e.g. inform, influence attitudes, change behavior)?
   d. Which and how many channels are feasible, considering your time and budget?

Understanding How to Interact with Media

Media Effects

Decades of studies on the consequences of mass media exposure demonstrate that effects are varied and reciprocal— the media impacts audiences and audiences also impact media by the intensity and frequency of their usage. The results of mass media for promoting social change, especially in developing countries, have become important for public health. Three effects or functions of media, namely: (1) the knowledge gap, (2) agenda setting, and (3) cultivation of shared public perceptions have been identified to be crucial in marketing your clinic.[6]

The Knowledge Gap

Health knowledge, or for that matter, your clinic's message is differentially distributed in the population, resulting in knowledge gaps. Unfortunately, mass media is insufficient for distributing information in an egalitarian fashion— changes in social structure and institutions are also necessary for this to occur. Thus, the impact of mass media on audience knowledge gaps is influenced by such factors as the extent to which the content is appealing, the degree to which information channels are accessible and desirable, and the amount of social conflict and diversity there is in a community. Hence, the clinic's message(s) through media campaigns are more effective when structural factors that impede the distribution of knowledge are addressed.

Agenda Setting

The selective nature of what members of the media choose for public consumption influences how people think about your clinic's message(s), and what they think about them. A related theme is the extent to which the media sets the public's perception of health risks and how they interact with your clinic's message. According to Davis,[7] when risks are highlighted in the media, particularly in great detail, the extent of agenda setting is likely to be based on the degree to which a public sense of outrage and threat is provoked. Where mass media can be especially valuable is in the framing of issues. 'Framing' means taking a leadership role in the organization of public discourse about an issue. Media, of course, is influenced by pressures to offer balance in coverage, and these pressures may come from persons and groups with particular political action and advocacy positions. It has been reported that 'groups, institutions, and advocates compete to identify problems, to move them onto the public agenda, and to define the issues symbolically'.[6] Thus, persons who desire to access mass media's agenda-setting potential must be aware of the competition. It is therefore, necessary to be aware of your competitor's strength and weaknesses.

Cultivation of Perceptions

Cultivation is the extent to which media exposure shapes audience perceptions over time. Television is a common experience, especially in the United States, and it serves as a 'homogenizing agent'.[8] However, the effect is often based on several conditions, particularly socioeconomic factors.

The Relationship of Mass Media to Other Forms of Communication

The interaction between media messages and interpersonal communication can be divided into a two-step flow hypothesis. Media effects are moderated principally by interpersonal encounters. Community opinion leaders scan the media for information, and then communicate that information to others in interpersonal contexts. It is in this second step, interpersonal interaction, which opinion leaders wield enormous power, influencing others not only by what they choose to reveal but also the slant that they use in conveying the message. Similarly, message(s) communicated by a clinic can take advantage of this process and as an opinion leader, you can wield enormous influence on the outcome.

The two-step model can further be expanded to include multistep models, most notably, information diffusion models. Media influence is undeniably linked to complex interpersonal dynamics. A shared influence likely results when people are exposed to the clinic's messages and then converge together in contexts that influence what they say to one another (and even how they say it), as well as what they selectively think.

Gerbner[9] described three-component framework essential for interaction with mass media. The first component is Semiotics, the study of signs, symbols, and codes. Language comprises one such set of symbols and codes that can be further embellished by sights, sounds and other visual and aural cues. The second aspect of the framework relates to behaviors and interactions associated with exposure to your clinic's messages. Psychologists, marketing agents, and others attempt to predict behavior based on specially designed messages. The third element examines how communication is organized around social systems and the extent to which history and human experience influence society's institutions.

Designers of your clinic's messages need to consider such models and frameworks in creating an effective marketing strategy. Modern views of health behavior change acknowledge eclectic approaches and consider multiple aspects of human experience from the individual level to the community level. Individual channels of communication (e.g. face-to-face encounters) offer personal support and may invoke trust, but are labor intensive, have limited reach and may require ancillary materials. Although mass media channels transmit information rapidly and to general or specific audiences, they can set agendas, but questions have been raised concerning their impartiality and integrity. Community channels (e.g. coalitions, community action groups, and the like) have less 'reach' than mass media but they reinforce, expand and localize media messages and offer institutional and social support. Knowledge of the complementary strengths of various channels helps to optimize the penetration and effectiveness of your clinic's messages.

CONCLUSION

Mass media is a very effective tool for marketing your IVF center by educating, shaping public relations and advocating for a particular policy or your clinic's point of view. Mass media is capable of facilitating short-term, intermediate-term and long-term effects on audiences. Although, mass media includes, television, radio, internet, newspaper, magazines, other print media and billboards, to name few, internet has been proven to be the most effective global vehicle for marketing your IVF center. Successful marketing of your IVF clinic will also depend on the budget and the time allocated for proper mix of channels to disseminate your clinic's information. Messages need to be short, informative, varied and appealing to the targeted audience. Understanding the effects of mass media and monitoring its influence on the targeted audience should be an integral part of marketing. Finally, the knowledge gap, agenda setting and cultivation of shared public perceptions needs to be explored for the successful outcome of your marketing strategy.

Although mass media is important for disseminating your clinic's messages and encouraging the adoption of a successful outcome, it currently falls short of potential. The realization of this potential in the future depends, in part, on increasing the media advocacy skills of public health authorities, improving understanding of competing anti-health media messages, and organizing channels for an optimal media mix.

REFERENCES

1. Winett LB, Wallack L. Advancing public health goal through the mass media. Journal of Health Communication 1996;1:173-96.
2. Kreps GL, Thornton BC. Health communication theory and practice. 1992; Prospect Heights, IL: Waveland Press.
3. Belch GE, Belch MA. Introduction to advertising and promotion. 1995; 3rd edition. Chicago: Irwin.
4. McDermott RJ. Health education research: evolution or revolution (or maybe both)? Journal of Health Education 2000;33:264-71.
5. Hackbarth DP, Silvestri B, Cosper W. Tobacco and alcohol billboards in 50 Chicago neighborhoods: market segmentation to sell dangerous products to the poor. Journal of Public Health Policy 1994;16:213-30.
6. Finnegan JR Jar, Viswanath K. Communication theory and health behaviour change: the media studies framework. Health Behaviour and Health Education (2nd edn). In: Glanz K, Lewis FM, Rimer BK (Eds). San Francisco: Jossey-Bass Publishers, 1997.
7. Davis JJ. Riskier than we think? The relationship between risk statement completeness and perceptions of direct to consumer advertised prescription drugs. Journal of Health Communication 2000;5:349-70.
8. Littlejohn SW. Theories of Human Communication. 1989; Belmont, CA: Wadsworth Publishing Company.
9. Gerbner G. Field Definitions: Communication Theory. In 1984–85 U.S. Directory of Graduate Programs. 1983; 9th edition. Princeton, NJ: Educational Testing Service.

Cross-border Reproductive Care: A Worldwide Phenomenon

Daniel S Seidman, Guy Israel Seidman

OVERVIEW

Cross-border Reproductive Care indicates, according to the European Society for Human Reproduction and Embryology (ESHRE) Task Force on Ethics and Law, the movements by patients looking for infertility treatment from one country or jurisdiction, where treatment is unavailable for them, to another country or jurisdiction where they can obtain the treatment they need. It was suggested that the terms 'reproductive' or 'procreative tourism' should be avoided because of their negative connotations, and that, the neutral term 'cross-border reproductive care' should be used instead. Multiple authors have recently pointed out in the medical literature that cross-border reproductive care represents an urgent and challenging issue to tackle from medical, legal, psychological and ethical perspectives.

The main reasons patients seeking cross-border reproductive care include the pursuit of high quality care, absence of local availability, differences in laws and regulations, cost, social support concerns and ethnic needs. The most important motivators behind the recent rapid expansion in the demand for cross-border reproductive care include: 1. Easy dissemination of information on reproductive procedures in foreign countries enabled by new information technology; 2. International travel currently more comfortable and affordable; 3. Patients from foreign countries now actively seeked by IVF clinics in certain countries through advertisements in airline magazines or international satellite TV channels; 4. Convenient all-inclusive packages, now offered by fertility centers, that not only include the reproductive procedures, but also flight tickets, escorted transport, hotels, interpreters and local recreational tours; 5. A very cost-effective and efficient way provided by the internet for patients to compare the foreign clinic's services and unique merits in terms of cost, expertise in reproductive technologies and local policies; 6. More patients seeking treatment forbidden by law in the couple's own country or inaccessible to the couple because of their demographic or social characteristics. As this relatively new phenomena seems unstoppable, growing concerns remain with regard to the lack of international regulations and quality assurance.

INTRODUCTION

Fertility tourism is a relatively new phenomenon that occurs when aspiring parents travel from their home country, in which advanced reproductive techniques (ART) are expensive and legally awkward, to nations where the procedures are cheaper and legally more obtainable. The first well-publicized case of fertility tourism was that of an American couple, the Rios, seeking *in vitro* fertilization (IVF) treatment in Australia in the early 1980s[1] and the term 'procreative tourism' was coined by Knoppers and LeBris in 1991.[2]

The extent of '*in vitro* fertilization tourism' is unknown since smuggling an embryo back home in ones womb is difficult for a customs official to detect. In this way, IVF tourism differs, for example, from international child adoption which is easier to monitor and is subject to both national and international law standards. Most of the available data on reproductive tourism is therefore, based not on methodical assessments, but on anecdotal reporting by specific clinics. For instance, it has been estimated that over 1000 Japanese couples travel every year to California alone to seek reproductive care. This is mainly a direct consequence of the restrictions imposed on egg donation and surrogacy in Japan.

IVF clinics in the USA have also reported an impressive rise in non-U.S. donor-egg recipients. For example, the Center for Fertility and Reproductive Endocrinology at Virginia Mason Medical Center in Seattle recently reported that while five years ago, 16 percent of the donor-egg recipients, who came to their center, were Canadian, today it is 33 percent. The Somerville, Massachusetts-based 'Tiny Treasures' egg donation agency reported that, currently, couples from

Table 82.1: The main reasons behind the recent rapid expansion in reproductive tourism
1. New information technology allows easy dissemination of information on reproductive procedures in foreign countries.
2. International travel is currently more comfortable and affordable.
3. IVF clinics in certain countries are now actively seeking patients from foreign countries through advertisements in airline magazines or international satellite TV channels.
4. Fertility centers now offer convenient all-inclusive packages that include not only the reproductive procedures, but also flight tickets, escorted transport, hotels, interpreters and local recreational tours.
5. The internet allows a very cost-effective and efficient way for patients to compare the foreign clinic's services and unique merits in terms of cost, expertise in reproductive techniques and local policies.

abroad, typically Australia and the UK, account for about 10 of the 100 couples that they assist each year. Three years ago, just one or two of their clients were not from the USA. Dr Zev Rosenwaks has also been recorded stating that the number of Europeans has significantly increased over the past five years at the Center for Reproductive Medicine and Infertility of the Weill Medical College of Cornell University in New York.

CLINICAL DISCUSSION

The Increase in Reproductive Tourism

The recent increase in the extent of international travel for reproductive technique services has been attributed to several factors (Table 82.1). First, following the current revolution in information technology, patients can readily obtain data and compare figures regarding the cost and the availability of different infertility services in countries around the world. Second, patients are now more used to international travel, which has become, in some ways, more comfortable and affordable in recent years. Third, IVF clinics in many countries are more aware of their relative advantages in terms of price and type of services rendered compared to other countries, and are actively seeking to attract patients from foreign countries. Currently, these centers often offer comprehensive packages to facilitate access by foreign patients. Such packages often include not only the reproductive procedures, but also flight tickets, local escorted transport, hotels, interpreters and local recreational tours. Fourth, the improved use of the internet offers IVF clinics, through their multi-language websites, a very cost-effective and efficient way to disseminate information regarding the clinic's services and unique merits in terms of cost, expertise in reproductive techniques and local policies. Moreover, it is currently not rare to find business advertisements posted by fertility clinics in airline magazines or international satellite television channels, aimed at luring clients worldwide.

Reasons for International Travel for IVF Treatment

It is fair to note that people have always traveled in search of medical treatments that were unavailable, unaffordable or

Table 82.2: The main reasons patients choose to travel for advanced reproductive techniques to foreign countries
1. Pursuit of high quality care
2. Absence of local availability
3. Difference in laws and regulations
4. Cost
5. Social support concerns
6. Ethnic needs

illegal to carry out in their own countries. There are at least six major reasons leading people to travel to foreign countries in pursuit of reproductive care (Table 82.2):

Quality of Care

Although IVF has to a large extent, become a rather standardized procedure, with readily available 'over-the-counter' equipment and disposables, large differences remain in the results achieved. The variability in established success rates is found, not only when comparing small-sized IVF units in developing countries to large, well-established centers, but also among major world famous centers. Gleicher, et al.[3] recently showed that large differences are found in the results obtained by various countries. The ART outcomes were compared between Europe and the US for the year 2001. US patients experienced significantly higher clinical pregnancy rates (P < 0.001) and delivery rates per started cycle (P < 0.001) than European patients. The better pregnancy and live birth outcomes in the US could not be explained by the transfer of larger embryo numbers alone.[3]

Local Availability

Many countries, especially Africa and South America, simply do not have advanced IVF programs in place. Other centers may lack modern equipment or have limited knowledge and experience in current reproductive techniques. In certain countries, long waiting times exist for IVF cycles covered by health insurance. This is often an additional major hurdle for couples interested in reproductive care.

Law and Regulations

IVF tourism is merely another example of the familiar phenomenon of 'medical treatment shopping', where people travel in search of medical care unavailable in their own country for, among other things, legal reasons. A familiar example is travel for the purpose of obtaining an abortion. Seeking a legally banned medical treatment in a foreign country raises complex questions of law and public policy of which, we will mention four. For the purpose of our discussion, we will assume that the medical procedure is banned in country A, from which the IVF tourists travel, but allowed in country B, where they seek treatment.

This is not merely a theoretical example. Take, for example, the case of Italy. In 2004, Italy introduced a controversial law, which permits access to ART within very limited confines of stable heterosexual couples of a fertile age, who may use only their own, and not donor, gametes. The legislative vacuum that existed until 2004 meant, in essence, that all scientific techniques were legal. Italy, now, has the most restrictive access to reproductive techniques in Europe, and between 2004 and 2006, the restrictions imposed in Italy increased fertility tourism by three-fold.[4]

We would like to make several more observations on the legal ramifications of fertility tourism:

First: Addressing the efficacy of the legal ban as a practical matter, we believe it is not realistic for the authorities of country A to monitor IVF procedures undertaken in other countries without extreme infringement on the human and civil rights of IVF tourists. Moreover, adding new travel limitations seems unlikely; bear in mind that travel within North America and Europe is almost unrestricted, and that, the resources available for monitoring the ever-expanding international tourism are focused on criminal and terror-related trafficking. It is noteworthy that such measures were taken in Europe in the context of abortions in the early 1990s, yet, were condemned by the European Parliament in 1991.[5]

Second: There is a question of both domestic and international public policies; how strongly does nation A view its ban on IVF procedures as a matter of national law, and is it willing to strain international relations by banning travel to certain countries for the purpose of receiving such treatment? To our knowledge, only few examples are known where countries have sought to constrain IVF tourism by arresting physicians and patients believed to be involved in such practice, and trying to prevent the transfer of fresh and frozen embryos between countries. It is worth noting, historically, that Ireland's law once went so far as to make it illegal for an Irish woman to travel to another country where

abortion is legal and obtain one there. It is also worth noting that Ireland still only permits a legal abortion in exceptional cases, and many women still travel abroad to obtain one.[6] State B could, however, chooses to respect state A's law and offer controversial medical procedures only to its citizens.

Third: The legal question of extra-territorial criminal liability, i.e. whether a country can bring charges against its citizens when they return for alleged criminal actions carried out outside its territory, is highly problematic and controversial. In brief, nations are highly selective in deciding which of their citizens they will charge and for what crimes. Sanctioning soldiers for misconduct abroad or criminal charges against sexual-predators acting outside the state, where they reside, are such extreme instances. It seems unlikely that women seeking advanced fertility treatments will face similar charges.

Indeed, given the diversity of regulation worldwide, it is doubtful whether any single jurisdiction can, in fact, continue to enforce its own rules.[7] That said, however, it is known that several physicians involved in the practice of egg donation in Eastern Europe have been warned not to travel to certain countries as they might be arrested for 'organ trafficking'. As Prof. Pennings observed, 'Only a worldwide consensus would eliminate the problem of regulating assisted conception and that is, to put it mildly, highly unlikely'.[5]

Fourth: There are several further social aspects to the situation where country A bans a medical practice within its borders yet, allows its citizens to carry out such procedures elsewhere. One is that forcing women to travel in order to obtain medical treatment will likely, raise the cost of the treatment and make it unavailable for women who cannot travel. In Italy, there is concern that for women who cannot afford fertility tourism, procreative 'adultery' may become an option. A black market for gametes and possibly, even babies may be developed and illegal surrogacy arrangements contracted.[4] This is one of the most frequently expressed worries of critiques concerning the availability of abortion services in the United States, as is clearly true with IVF tourism.[8] By allowing citizens to travel to other countries, country A increases the demand for healthcare in other countries, perhaps without bearing the added costs; if country B does not charge country A or its citizens for the use of its resources, it is subsidizing country A. This may be acceptable on a small basis and for humanitarian reasons, not as a systemic solution.

Fifth: What is nation B to think of Nation A, which allows its citizens to leave its borders to practice 'unlawful' practices within the borders of nation B? If this was a matter of sexual practices or drug abuse, nation B would likely be offended; in the case of IVF treatment, it is likely that nation B would simply view itself as a leader in cutting-edge technology and of more advanced social norms than other nations, where such treatments are unavailable.

Indeed, this is how scholars explain the phenomenon of European fertility tourism, suggesting that it 'owes its existence to the interplay between member states' individual (some would say idiosyncratic) policies on 'responsible' procreation and the globalist policy of free movement of persons within Europe, thought to be essential to the continued integration and internationalization of European nations.'

Many restrictions on various reproductive procedures are currently in place in various countries (Table 82.3). In some countries like Canada, Italy or Germany, egg donation is strictly prohibited, several countries, including Israel, allow egg donation only from IVF patients ('egg sharing'), a few countries like Sweden prohibit donor anonymity in the interest of the future child, while other countries prohibit revealing the identity of the donor and do not allow egg donation from family members or young friends.

An even more controversial procedure is sex selection by prenatal genetic diagnosis (PGD). The practice is banned by many countries, while other countries, for instance Australia and Israel, allow sex selection of embryos only to avoid an inherited disease. Consequently, Canadian couples seeking a girl and Chinese couples desiring a boy are now commonly seen visiting clinics in the USA, where sex selection by PGD is widely and openly marketed. This has led the bioethicist Arthur Caplan, from the University of Pennsylvania Center for Bioethics, to dub the USA as 'the Wild West of reproductive technology.'

Cost

Advanced reproductive care is clearly an expensive medical treatment, often making it beyond the reach of many couples in need. This state of affairs is not only found in poor and less developed countries, but also in the wealthiest of nations, where the cost of such treatment can quickly accumulate to over US$ 50,000. Furthermore, while some countries, like Israel, offer comprehensive national health insurance that fully covers an almost unlimited number of IVF cycles, most countries offer, at best, only a limited number of IVF cycles at the public expense.

Not surprisingly, patients with a desperate need for these expensive treatments, often opt to international comparisons, seeking more affordable reproductive care. On June 30, 2004, Caroline Ryan of the BBC News described this new trend under the headline 'EU faces reproductive tourism threat'. She went on to report how the European Union (EU) enlargement could encourage 'fertility tourists' to travel to Eastern Europe for cheap IVF. She stated that IVF treatment in countries, such as Hungary and Slovenia, costs around 2,400 Euros (£1,608), compared to between £2,000 and £4,000 in the UK. Ryan interviewed Western European doctors, who admitted that IVF success rates are as good in Eastern Europe as elsewhere, but warned that these clinics are often unregulated.

Many clinics in countries, like Russia and Slovenia, currently employ the internet to attract fertility tourists with promises of cut-rate *in vitro* fertilization treatments, high success rates, liberal reproductive policies and little administrative oversight. From my own experience, it seems that there is a wide discrepancy in Eastern Europe between small poorly equipped IVF units and larger clinics with the most up-to-date setting and very satisfactory results. Additionally, claims of success seem to be clearly exaggerated by some Eastern European clinics, as their reported success rates of 70 to 100 percent have not yet been achieved even by the world's most reputed centers.

Silvia Spring of Newsweek Magazine reported on April 12, 2006, that cheaper prices, high-quality health care and the availability of donor eggs and surrogates are drawing an increasing number of couples to Thailand, Eastern Europe, Russia, China and India. She specifically noted that in the English-speaking world, India has a big advantage because of the availability of English-speaking doctors.

Apparently, infertile couples are drawn to India, largely because of the lower cost of treatments and lighter regulations.

Table 82.3: Examples of types of reproductive procedures prohibited or unaffordable in certain countries, thereby attracting medical tourism to countries offering them		
Country of origin	*Country of destination*	*Reproductive procedure*
Israel	Ukraine, Cyprus	Egg donation
Sweden	Denmark	Anonymous sperm donation
USA	India	Ethnic Indian egg donors
Australia, China	USA	Sex selection
Germany	Belgium	PGD
Italy	Spain	IVF for non-married women
Moslem countries	Europe	Sperm donation
Uganda	South Africa	IVF and ICSI
Britain	India	Surrogacy
Japan	USA	Egg donation

One of the biggest attractions offered by Indian ART clinics is maternal surrogacy. The number of surrogate births in India has more than doubled in the past three years, fertility clinics report. I am personally aware of several Israeli patients, who recently decided to undergo surrogacy in India, either due to financial considerations or due to the less rigid regulations allowing, for instance, homosexual couples to have a child by combining egg donation and surrogacy. The British Human Fertilisation and Embryo Authority (HFEA) has outlawed payments to surrogates, but they can be (and usually are) reimbursed for expenses upto $18,000 at private clinics in Britain, which perform 70 percent of all the IVF treatment. On the other hand, the Indian Council of Medical Research (ICMR) allows Indian surrogates to claim monetary compensation, as well as expenses, but these usually do not amount to more than $5,400. Indian clinics offer the same treatment for around $7,200, including plane tickets and a hotel stay in the bargain. Another example of the more lax rules in India is the observation that whereas British clinics allow doctors to implant only two embryos into the uterus in a treatment cycle, the limitations set by the ICMR Guidelines, Code of Practice, Ethical Considerations and Legal Issues (Section 3.2.7: Use of gametes and embryos) on the transfer of no more than three embryos in a woman in any one cycle, regardless of the procedure/s used, is far from regulated, resulting in clinics far exceeding the limit. Indian ART centers are also willing to treat women who have been deemed too old or overweight by the British National Health Service (NHS) for IVF treatment. Consequently, Indian clinics are performing a growing number of IVF treatments for foreigners frustrated with disappointing results and soaring costs at home. The Newsweek Magazine article points out that by some counts, the reproductive tourism industry brings more than $450 million a year into India.

This soaring practice in India has drawn concern in Britain and other foreign countries. First, transferring multiple embryos has lost favor in Europe and is considered a dangerous practice, significantly associated with a high chance for risky multiple gestations. Second, besides the health risks faced directly by surrogate mothers, the practice is also a legal minefield. Because the Indian Council of Medical Research has not issued any guidelines to deal with foreign clients using Indian surrogates, couples who take part in this procedure must adopt their child under the Indian law, and because India does not fall under the Hague Convention on International Adoption, an adoption in India is not recognized under the British law.

Social

Many people trust the reputation of their home country and are interested in traveling to where they will have family support. In the age of global immigration, many couples prefer, when in need of costly and complex ART care, to go back to their countries of origin to undergo the required fertility treatment.

Ethnic Needs

It is a common expectation that patients, when in need for sperm or egg donation, would elect to travel back to their country of ethnic origin, where gametes of ethnically similar genetic make-up can easily be obtained.

Is IVF Tourism a Good or a Bad Phenomenon?

Reproductive tourism has recently drawn growing attention and noteworthy criticism (Table 82.4). Media exposure has set the beacon on what was deemed exploitation of poor egg donors by clinics selling oocytes to rich Western clients. Specifically, the Daily Mail and British television apparently exposed a plot, where a Romanian fertility clinic in Bucharest was selling oocytes to elderly (i.e. women in their early sixties) women from more affluent countries, mainly Britain, USA and Israel. It seems that the relatively aggressive and open way that the specific clinic was advertising on the Web in order to lure American and British clients may have been too enthusiastic, leading to scrutiny by the media. Yet, without investigating the specific claims, they seem to be overstated. Such claims appeared in the Daily Mail on the 17th of July 2006, in an article by Fran Abrams titled 'The misery of the baby trade.' The journalist condemns the travel of citizens of developed countries to less developed countries in order to seek IVF care as going by the innocent-sounding name of 'fertility tourism.' The article described women who paid up to £11,000 for treatment abroad in order to side-step a British law, which bans payment for egg donations. The journalist proclaimed that their donors were paid between £150 and £300 for their trouble, and presented a grim outlook of the egg donation trade:

'This lucrative trade thrives on the desires of vulnerable women in Britain and in other Western countries, desperate to fulfill their dreams of a family. But it thrives, too, on the vulnerability of other desperate women in poor countries who sell their eggs. Those who come in search of a child are not told about the terrible risks imposed on egg donors, and even more scandalously, in some cases, neither are the donors themselves. Too often, those women are left damaged by the procedures they undergo, and a growing number have been robbed, as a result, of the chance to have families of their own. The doctors at the Romanian clinic, which had links with a leading London fertility center, and where Alina was paid £150 for her eggs, left her ovaries so damaged and scarred that she is now infertile.'

Further criticism has been presented by opponents of reproductive tourism, claiming that the practice does not simply represent travel by people seeking a better bargain but rather, amounts to medical tourism for designer babies and therefore, should alarm lawmakers.[9]

Table 82.4: The pros and cons of medical tourism in IVF practice

The Pros

- Allows patients access to more affordable treatment.
- Provides patients a mean to fulfill their autonomy by obtaining services, such as sex selection, prohibited in their country of residence.
- Provides poor patients an honorable means of earning money by selling their eggs or renting their uteri as surrogate mothers.
- Offers poor patients a way to pay for their expensive fertility treatment through 'egg sharing' programs funded by wealthy foreign patients.
- Creates an influx of revenue that might bolster the health care industry in developing countries, providing an opportunity for them to repatriate health care professionals.
- Encourages competition, in terms of excellence and price, among the world's reproductive centers.

The Cons

- Exploits poor women by unknowingly exposing them to the risks of egg donation and surrogacy.
- Provides a mean for patients to obtain ethically disputable and prohibited reproductive services in poorly regulated countries.
- Many foreign reproductive centers poorly regulated.
- Some foreign centers, willing to undertake practices considered dangerous like transferring a high number of embryos despite the risk of multiple gestations, considered dangerous.
- Legal obstacles when surrogates are used in countries that do not fall under the Hague convention on International adoption.

Sex selection of embryos remains the most controversial issue. American doctors, who freely offer such services for about $20,000, claim they are merely serving the marketplace and helping nature, not playing God. Dr. Jeffrey Steinberg, who provides sex selection at the Fertility Institutes of Los Angeles and Las Vegas, says that people will be less alarmed as sex selection becomes more routine. His website promises 'near 100 percent (99.99%) effective gender selection methods to help balance families.' Dr. Steinberg claims his international push has been highly successful with his web page on sex selection, generating 140,000 hits a month from China, and the only country outpacing China's interest is Canada. In an interview, he said that in one recent week, his clinics performed the procedure on eight women from abroad and consulted with 12 new foreign patients from China, Germany, Canada, the Czech Republic, Guam, Mexico and New Zealand.

The concern regarding medical tourism for ART services has led some groups to call for regulation of the practice and its marketing. Sujatha Jesudason of the Center for Genetics and Society, a non-profit information and public-affairs organization in Oakland, California has been quoted claiming that: 'Right now, the market is driving practices rather than social and ethical concerns, people who have money to pay for it are getting the children of their choice.' However, she does not view reproductive tourism as a problem, since she seems to believe that 'it contributes to a peaceful coexistence of different ethical and religious views in Europe.'

Guido Pennings, a Professor of Ethics and Bioethics at the University of Ghent, Belgium, has also stated at the European Society for Human Reproduction and Embryology (ESHRE) Conference, Copenhagen, 2005, that 'contrary to some existing views, it may increase justice by giving people, who cannot pay for the treatment at home, the ability to look for cheaper treatment elsewhere'. Furthermore, he claimed that "We should not condemn 'reproductive tourism' in Europe but regard it as a 'safety valve' that can help to avoid moral conflict." In his view '...laws should not be harmonized in order to seek to prevent such tourism'. Rather than harmonizing laws on reproductive medicine across Europe, we should accept the existing diversity.[10]

Another concern that has recently been raised is whether the growing number of visits by citizens from high income countries adversely affects residents of developing countries. However, a current analysis by a World Bank economist[11] suggested that the risk was minimal and that, the influx of revenue associated with this practice might bolster the health care industry in developing countries, providing an opportunity for them to repatriate health care professionals, who currently account for a substantial fraction of the physician and registered-nurse workforces in the USA.[11]

CONCLUSION

Medical tourism in IVF serves couples in many ways. It allows patients to seek centers with better results and often, at more affordable prices. Occasionally, international travel merely presents the wish of immigrants to return to their country of origin in order to receive care within a more supportive family environment and ethnic background. The most controversial aspect of reproductive tourism is when it takes place in order to seek services that are locally banned for religious or ethical reasons (Table 82.3). Since the demand for the ability to become a parent is extremely strong, it is very doubtful that new laws and regulation are likely to succeed in limiting international travel for reproductive services. This is especially true among those barred from treatment in their own country, including single women, homosexual men and women, and older women. Even more contentious reproductive services, including sex selection, surrogacy and egg donation, are likely to follow the laws of demand even if unacceptable to many.[10] It seems that the international community of reproductive care providers should work together, demanding better regulation and transparency of IVF units providing such procedures, including supplying patients with information regarding the actual compensation provided to the surrogate mothers and egg donors,[12] as well as long-term follow-up, allowing centers working in less developed countries to offer reliable outcome results.[13]

Whittaker and Speier,[14] from Australia, have criticized reproductive tourism, claiming it was a reflection of the 'commodification of reproductive bodies'. Storrow[15] has recently claimed that cross-border reproductive travel fails to promote moral and political pluralism in democratic states. He noted three primary reasons: first, the opportunity for patients to go abroad for treatment tempers organized resistance to the law and allows government to pass stricter regulations than it otherwise might. Second, cross-border reproductive care has been shown to have deleterious extraterritorial effects that undermine the articulated rationales behind restrictive reproductive laws. Third, laws that generate demand for cross-border reproductive care often fail to satisfy the standard of proportionality that restrictions on human reproduction must meet.[15]

As long as some people are determined to obtain certain reproductive services, such as donated eggs or surrogate wombs, and others are willing to sell them, the trade will be impossible to stop.[16] Hence, it makes better sense to regulate the business than to drive it underground or to limit it to countries, like the USA, where few limitations exist but reproductive procedures are affordable only to a selected group of very well-off people.

REFERENCES

1. Storrow RF. Quests for conception: fertility tourists, globalization and feminist legal theory. Hastings Law J 2005;57:295-330.
2. Knoppers BM, LeBris S. Recent advances in medically assisted conception: legal, ethical and social issues. Am J Law and Med 1991;17:329-61.
3. Gleicher N, Weghofer A, Barad D. A formal comparison of the practice of assisted reproductive technologies between Europe and the USA. Hum Reprod 2006;21:1945-50.
4. Fenton RA. Catholic doctrine versus women's rights: the new Italian law on assisted reproduction? Med Law Rev 2006;14:73-107.
5. Pennings G. Reproductive tourism as moral pluralism in motion. Med Ethics 2002;28:337-41.
6. Campbell M, Sahin-Hodoglugil NN, Potts M. Barriers to fertility regulation: a review of the literature. Stud Fam Plann 2006;37:87-97.
7. Brazier M. Regulating the reproduction business? Med Law Rev 1999;7:166-93.
8. Davis DS. The role of religion in health law and policy symposium: the Puzzle of IVF. Houston J Health Law Policy 2006;6:275-97.
9. Blyth E, Farrand A. Reproductive tourism – a price worth paying for reproductive autonomy? Critical Social Policy 2005:25:91-114.
10. Pennings G. Legal harmonization and reproductive tourism in Europe. Hum Reprod 2004;19:2689-94.
11. Mattoo A, Rathindran R. How health insurance inhibits trade in health care. Health Aff (Millwood) 2006;25:358-68.
12. Heng BC. Ethical issues in transitional 'mail order' oocyte donation. Int J Ob Gyn 2006;95:302-4.
13. Heng BC. Should fertility specialists refer local patients abroad for shared or commercialized oocyte donation? Fertil Steril 2007;87:6-7.
14. Whittaker A, Speier A. 'Cycling overseas': care, commodification, and stratification in cross-border reproductive travel. Med Anthropol 2010;29:363-83.
15. Storrow RF. The pluralism problem in cross-border reproductive care. Hum Reprod 2010;25:2939-43.
16. Spar LD. The baby business: how money, science and politics drive the commerce of conception. Harvard Business School Press, Boston, 2006.

ART Regulation

Is there a Worldwide Need for ART Regulatory Guidelines?

Jyothi Pillai, Kamini A Rao

Laws and policies may facilitate or inhibit women's access to reproductive health care.
"You will find no justification in any of the language of the Constitution for delay in the reforms which the mass of the American people now demand."

–Franklin D Roosevelt

INFERTILITY AND HEALTH CARE SYSTEMS

Health care systems now represent one of the largest sectors in the world economy. Health, as defined in the constitution of the World Health Organization (WHO), is not merely the absence of disease or infirmity but a state of complete physical, mental or social well-being. Patients do perceive the suffering from infertility as very real, and as compromising their health. There are countries, which develop laws with a particular goal in reproductive health care. The General Assembly of the International Federation of Obstetrics and Gynecology (FIGO) on 5th September 2000 adopted a resolution on women's rights relating to reproductive and sexual health. The resolution affirmed that improvements in women's health need more than better science and health care; they require state action to correct injustice to women.[1]

Health care providers, health policy makers and lawyers address reproductive health from different perspectives. It can be said that four factors or four Ps contribute to the determination of health in general and reproductive health in particular: providence, people, politicians and providers of health services.[2]

Health professionals have to abide by the laws in their countries. However, they have two obligations. They have to understand the limits of the law, which may not be as restrictive as sometimes perceived. Also, where the laws appear to be dysfunctional in practice, health professionals have an obligation to work with the legal profession, women's group and other progressive forces in the society.[2]

In the current scenario, there are many countries practising medically assisted reproduction, some of them having:

- Set laws
- Established rules and regulations
- National guidelines
- States having set none of the above.

While in the United States, IVF programs operate under voluntary guidelines, programs in many other countries are subject to regulations that monitor many aspects of *in vitro* fertilization (IVF) practice. In such settings, regulations may dictate:[3]

- The number of oocytes that can be fertilized.
- The number of embryos that can be transferred.
- The use of cryopreservation.
- The use of third party reproduction.
- The ability to perform tests or interventions on the embryo.

In 2004, the Government of Italy made it a crime to freeze human embryos or to perform preimplantation diagnosis (PGD).

Ethical Issues

Ethical issues raised by medically assisted reproduction have been considered so profound that several countries, particularly those where the more advanced reproductive technologies are applied, have created national commissions to address them and propose legal, regulatory and other responses. The major issues raising ethical concerns include:[3,4]

- Bypassing the natural method of conception
- Creating life in the laboratory
- Fertilizing more embryos than will be needed
- Discarding excess embryos
- Unnatural environment for embryos
- Using untested technology
- Not affordable for many
- Misallocation of medical resources.

Legal Status of Embryo

Another concern is the status of an embryo as a person/commodity. Heated debates are still on regarding:
- Creating embryos, freezing them, and keeping them 'in limbo'.
- Exposing embryos to unnatural substances.
- Destroying embryos in research.
- Potential to create embryos for medical purposes.
- Potential to select embryos by PGD or to modify embryos.

There has been concern that financial rewards for IVF doctors dissuade them from recommending other methods to couples.

In what is called 'reproductive tourism' in India, couples, many of them of Asian origin, find arranging for surrogate mothers in India far cheaper than the thousands of pounds they spend on fertility treatment in Britain. Campaigners in Britain have reportedly questioned the ethics of such businesses. The report claimed that the Indian Council for Medical Research (ICMR) did not have any guidelines to deal with foreign clients using Indian surrogates, but added that a study was being prepared to assess the issue. It added that any child born to an Indian woman through such a process would not automatically get a British passport.

By medically assisted reproduction (MAR), it is now possible for a child to have upto five parents: a genetic father, a rearing father, a genetic mother, a gestating mother and a rearing mother. There are concerns about the nature of medical practice, since the demarcation between experimental and established procedures is not always clear. The quality assurance of services in many countries leaves something to be desired.

Israel is the only country from the Asian region that provides IVF to single mothers. In Europe, this policy is found in Belarus, Italy and Netherlands. The status of genetic parents when surrogates are involved is another area of controversy. Laws differ on the status of children born by gamete and embryo donation. Laws relating to lesbian reproductive rights should be also well-defined.

Presence of National Guidelines

Statutory regulation will give entrepreneurs the legal and economic security they need to corporatize procreation. Also, with the backbone of definite guidelines, better customer care is ensured, curbing commercialization. All the assisted reproductive technique (ART) centers should be registered and regulated by a national body.

Absence of Guidelines

In the states having no set regulations and laws there can be:
- Far-reaching assumptions about the nature of children.
- That they are property, that their genetic heritage is unimportant, and that they have no inherent right to a natural mother and father.
- Privileges to the desire of an adult for a child above a child's need for a family.

Strict guidelines should be established on the medical and social criteria of the eligibility to donate, requirements of anonymity to recipients or allowance of designated donors and subsequent identification of donors to their biological children. Donations should be altruistic rather than for profit. The number of times that an individual donation can be used should be limited. The donation records should be preserved.

CONCLUSION

Regulation and supervision of the function of ART clinics becomes easier in the presence of established guidelines or laws. Additionally, regulations help the ART clinics in providing safe and ethical services to the needy infertile couples.

REFERENCES

1. FIGO resolution on Womens Rights related to reproductive and sexual health, 2000.
2. Cook RJ, Dickens BM, Fathalla MF. Reproductive Health and Human Rights: Integrating Medicine, Ethics, and Law.
3. Caplan A. The future of human reproduction: Ethics, choice, and regulation. BMJ 1999;318:948A.
4. European Journal of Contraception and Reproductive Health Care: Millenium edition 1999. pp. 212-6.

Ethical Issues in Gamete Donation and Surrogacy

RS Sharma

INTRODUCTION

The birth of the world's first baby conceived by assisted reproductive techniques (ART) occurred on 25th July 1978, in UK. The world's second baby conceived by ART was born 67 days later on 3rd October 1978 in Kolkata, West Bengal, India. India's first scientifically documented IVF-ET (*In vitro* fertilization and embryo transfer) baby was born on August 6, 1986 in Mumbai through the support of the Indian Council of Medical Research (ICMR). Since then, over one and a half million babies have been born around the world though ART.

It is well evident that any new technology that affects mankind raises several technical and moral dilemmas and poses many ethical, technical and even moral challenges. ART also raises these challenges from time to time all over the world, and including India. In India, where infertility is a social stigma and infertile patients look up to ART as the last resort to parenthood, many infertile couples are prepared to go to any extent to achieve their life's ambition. Unfortunately, ART has not reached a stage where all forms of infertility can be treated and clinically offer a 100 percent success. Even the ART service provider is often faced with technical challenges of trying to select the right treatment for a particular type of infertility problem, knowing fully well that none of the available techniques offer 100 percent success.

The ART practitioner is also faced with the moral responsibility of trying to convince the infertile couple of this fact and letting them know the chances of success and failure of the particular treatment that is being offered. The increasing demand for ART has resulted in mushrooming of infertility clinics in India. Though ART has enhanced the possibility of pregnancy, at the same time it also raises certain problems. ART requires enormous technical expertise and infrastructure, which in turn, taxes the infertile couple's endurance physically, emotionally and monetarily. There are possible misuses of this highly sophisticated technology and hence, ART raises ethical, safety and at the same time, even moral issues. The absence of guidelines and the lack of control by the government leads to more critical problems. The ICMR has developed National Guidelines for Accreditation, Supervision and Regulation of ART clinics in India, which have been accepted by the government of India. All issues related to ART have been described in the document and ethical issues related to gamete donation and surrogacy are summarized in this chapter.[1]

CLINICAL DISCUSSION

The following are general ethical issues in gamete donation and surrogacy.[1]

- *Confidentiality:* Any information about clients and donors must be kept confidential. No information about the treatment of couples, provided under a treatment agreement, may be disclosed to anyone other than the accreditation authority or persons covered by the license, except with the consent of the person(s) to whom the information relates, or in a medical emergency concerning the patient, or a court order. It is the above person's right to decide what information will be passed on and to whom, except in the case of a court order.
- *Information to patient:* All relevant information must be given to the patient before a treatment is given. Thus, before starting treatment, information should be given to the patient on the limitations and results of the proposed treatment, possible side effects, the techniques involved, comparison with other available treatments, the availability of counseling, the cost of the treatment, the rights of the child born through ART, and the need for the clinic to keep a register of the outcome of a treatment.
- *Consent:* No treatment should be given without the written consent of the couple to all the possible stages of that treatment, including the possible freezing of

supernumerary embryos. A standard consent form, recommended by the accreditation authority, should be used by all ART clinics. Specific consent must be obtained from couples who have their gametes or embryos frozen, with regard to what should be done with them if he/she dies, or becomes incapable of varying or revoking his or her consent.

- *Counseling:* People seeking licensed treatment must be given a suitable opportunity to receive proper counseling about the various implications of the treatment. No one is obliged to accept counseling but it is generally recognized as being beneficial, and couples should be encouraged to go through it. The provision of facilities for counseling in an ART clinic (of Levels 1B, 2 or 3) is, therefore, mandatory. Couples should be referred for support or therapeutic counseling as appropriate.
- *Use of gametes and embryos:* No more than three oocytes or embryos may be placed in a woman in any one cycle, regardless of the procedure(s) used, excepting under exceptional circumstances (such as elderly women, poor implantation, adenomyosis, or poor embryo quality), which should be recorded. No woman should be treated with gametes or with embryos derived from the gametes of more than one man or woman during any one treatment cycle.
- *Storage and handling of gametes and embryos:* The 'highest possible standards' in the storage and handling of gametes and embryos with respect to their security, and with regard to their recording and identification, should be followed.

In addition to the above, there are other issues, specially pertaining to gamete donation and surrogacy, and are described below.[1]

Gametes donations

Donation of gametes is a process by which a person voluntarily offers his or her gametes for the process of procreation.

Artificial Insemination with Donor Semen

The indications for artificial insemination with donor semen (AID) are when there is (a) non-obstructive azoospermia; (b) the husband has a hereditary genetic defect; or (c) when the couples have Rh incompatibility.

The main advantage of AID is that it enables a couple to achieve pregnancy even though the husband is not the biological father. However, the possible transmission of diseases from the donor to the future child and the risk of consanguinity, constitute some drawbacks that must be brought to the notice of the patients. It is necessary to get the informed consent of both the partners after they are counseled about the possible psychological conflict they may face later in their life, with the knowledge that one of them is not the biological parent of their child.[1]

Artificial insemination with donor semen involves the placing of a donor's semen into the uterine cavity of the female. AID is an ethically acceptable procedure, provided there is a medical indication and psychological confirmation for its use. Also, the normal conditions of anonymity and screening of the donor must be met and only frozen sperm samples that have passed appropriate quarantining for infectious diseases, such as HIV, Hepatitis B and C, and Syphilis, should be used.[1]

Common indications

- Husband has non-obstructive azoospermia.
- Husband has a hereditary genetic defect.
- The couple has Rh incompatibility.
- The woman is iso-immunized and has lost previous pregnancies and intrauterine transfusion is not possible.
- Husband has severe oligozoospermia and the couple does not wish to undergo any of the sophisticated ART procedures, such as intracytoplasmic sperm injection (ICSI).

Requirements for a sperm donor

- The individual must be free of HIV and Hepatitis B and C infections, hypertension, diabetes, sexually transmitted diseases, and identifiable and common genetic disorders such as thalassemia.
- The age of the donor must not be below 21 or above 45 years.
- An analysis must be carried out on the semen of the individual, preferably using a semen analyzer, and the semen must be found to be normal according to WHO method manual for semen analysis,[2] if intended to be used for ART.
- The blood group and the Rh status of the individual must be determined and placed on record.
- Other relevant information in respect of the donor, such as height, weight, age, educational qualifications, profession, color of the skin and the eyes, record of major diseases, including any psychiatric disorder, and the family background with respect to the history of any familial disorder, must be recorded in an appropriate proforma.[1]

Oocyte Donation or Embryo Donation

Oocyte donation means an ART procedure performed with third-party oocytes. Oocyte donation would necessitate using the husband's semen for fertilization and transferring the resultant embryos to the infertile female partner.

Embryo donation means the transfer of an embryo, resulting from gametes that did not originate from the recipient and/or her partner.[1]

Embryo donation would obviate the necessity of using the husband's semen. The choice of oocytes and embryos for oocyte or embryo donation, respectively would depend entirely on the circumstances prevalent at the time the infertile couple comes for treatment and the access of the infertility clinic to frozen oocytes or embryos.

Indications for oocyte or embryo donation:

- Gonadal dysgenesis.
- Premature ovarian failure.
- Iatrogenic (due to ovarian surgery or radiation, or chemical castration) ovarian failure.
- Women who have resistant ovary syndrome, or who are poor responders to ovulation induction.
- Women who are carriers of recessive autosomal disorders.
- Women who have attained menopause.[1]

Donors should be healthy (as determined by medical and psychological examination, screening for STDs, and absence of HIV antibodies) women in the age group of 18 to 35 years. Oocytes may be obtained for donation, mostly by surgical intervention from women participating in an IVF program, or those undergoing elective sterilization or surgery.

The recipient should be a healthy woman (determined by medical and psychological examination) having normal genitalia (as determined by physical examination) and uterine cavity (as determined by hysterosalpingography). In case of oocyte donation, the semen characteristics of the husband must be determined to see if they are in conformity with those associated with normal fertility. The blood group of the donor should be noted; the donor should also be tested for antibodies to Rubella, HIV, Hepatitis, Cytomegalovirus (CMV), gonorrhea, syphilis, *Chlamydia, Mycoplasma* and *Trichomonas*.[1]

Ovum/embryo donation can be carried out in menopausal women with no surviving child and desiring to have a child. The endometrium of menopausal women has the ability to respond to sex hormones and provide a receptive environment for the implantation of an embryo.

Various protocols are now available to prepare the endometrium of the recipient for oocyte donation (OD) or embryo donation (ED) with estrogens and progestogens until the placenta takes over the function of maintaining the gestation.[1]

Other Issues in Gamete Donation

- The donor must be informed that the offspring will not know his identity but a child born through ART has a right to seek information about his genetic parents/surrogate mother on reaching 18 years, except individual personal identity.
- A third party donor and surrogate mother must relinquish in writing all parental right concerning the offspring and vice versa.
- Use of sperm/oocytes donated by a relative or a known friend of either the wife or the husband shall not be permitted.[1]

- Consent must be a true informed consent, witnessed by a person who is in no way associated with the clinic.
- It will be the responsibility of the ART clinic to obtain sperm from appropriate semen banks; neither the clinic nor the couple shall have the right to know the donor's identity and address, but both the clinic and the couple, however, shall have the right to have the fullest possible information from the semen bank on the donor, such as height, weight, skin color, educational qualification, profession, family background, freedom from any known diseases or carrier status (such as Hepatitis B or HIV infection), ethnic origin, and the DNA fingerprint (if possible), from the semen bank before accepting the donor semen. It will be the responsibility of the semen bank and the clinic to ensure that the couple does not come to know the identity of the donor. The ART clinic will be authorized to appropriately charge the couple for the semen provided and the tests done on the donor semen.
- The ART clinic must not be a party to any commercial element in donor programs or in gestational surrogacy.[1]

Surrogacy

Surrogacy is an arrangement in which a woman agrees to carry a pregnancy that is genetically not related to her and her husband with the intention to carry it to term and hand over the child to the genetic parents for whom she is acting as a surrogate.[1]

Surrogacy, by ART, should normally be considered only for infertile patients for whom it would be physically or medically impossible/undesirable to carry a baby to term. A surrogate mother, carrying a child biologically unrelated to her, must register as a patient in her own name. While registering, she must mention that she is a surrogate mother and provide all the necessary information about the genetic parents such as names, address, etc. She must not use/register in the name of the person for whom she is carrying the child as this would pose legal issues, particularly in the untoward event of maternal death (in whose name will the hospital certify this death).[1]

The birth certificate shall be in the name of the genetic parents. The clinic however, must also provide a certificate to the genetic parent giving the name and address of the surrogate mother. All the expenses of surrogate mother during the period of pregnancy and postnatal care relating to pregnancy should be borne by the couple seeking surrogacy. The surrogate mother would also be entitled to a monetary compensation from the couple for agreeing to act as a surrogate. The exact value of this compensation should be decided by discussion between the couple and the proposed surrogate mother. An oocyte donor cannot act as a surrogate mother for the couple to whom the oocyte is being donated. A surrogate mother, as well as a third party donor, must relinquish in writing all parental rights concerning the offspring and vice versa.

In addition to the above, the following are the general considerations, which should also be considered under surrogacy.[1]

General Considerations in Surrogacy

- A child born through surrogacy must be adopted by the genetic (biological) parents, unless they can establish through genetic (DNA) fingerprinting (of which the records will be maintained in the clinic) that the child is theirs.
- Surrogacy, by assisted conception, should normally be considered only for patients for whom it would be physically or medically impossible/undesirable to carry a baby to term.
- Payments to surrogate mothers should cover all genuine expenses associated with the pregnancy. Documentary evidence of the financial arrangement for surrogacy must be available. The ART center should not be involved in this monetary aspect.
- Advertisements regarding surrogacy should not be made by the ART clinic. The responsibility of finding a surrogate mother, through advertisement or otherwise, should rest with the couple, or a semen bank (see 3.9.1.1; 3.9.2 of ICMR ART guidelines).[1]
- A surrogate mother should not be over 45 years of age. Before accepting a woman as a possible surrogate for a particular couple's child, the ART clinic must ensure (and put on record) that the woman satisfies all the testable criteria to go through a successful full-term pregnancy.
- A relative, a known person, as well as a person unknown to the couple may act as a surrogate mother for the couple. In the case of a relative acting as a surrogate, the relative should belong to the same generation as the woman desiring the surrogate.
- A prospective surrogate mother must be tested for HIV and shown to be seronegative for this virus just before embryo transfer. She must also provide a written certificate that (a) she has not had a drug intravenously administered into her through a shared syringe, (b) she has not undergone blood transfusion; and (c) she and her husband (to the best of her/his knowledge) has had no extramarital relationship in the last six months. (This is to ensure that the person would not come up with symptoms of HIV infection during the period of surrogacy.) The prospective surrogate mother must also declare that she will not use drugs intravenously, and not undergo blood transfusion, excepting of blood obtained through a certified blood bank.
- No woman may act as a surrogate more than thrice in her lifetime.[1]

Possible Misuse of ART—Sale of Embryos and Stem Cells

There is a growing interest in embryonic stem cells because of their potential use for developing spare organs or replacing defective tissues, such as parts of the brain destroyed due to Alzheimer's disease, or pancreatic cells in diabetic patients. The range of their potential use is limited only by one's imagination. ART clinics are the only source of embryonic stem cells. Spare embryos are either frozen or returned to the infertile couple for replacement during a later cycle, donated to another infertile couple, or discarded after five years, using a suitable protocol (Section 3.11 of ART Guidelines).[1]

USA has banned all federal support for embryonic stem cell research, unless the laboratories could demonstrate that they had developed embryonic stem lines before August 10, 2001. However, private funding is allowed, which encourages scientists in the USA to procure stem cells from abroad. Germany has banned all research on embryos produced in that country but permits the use of embryos brought from abroad. The stand taken by the foreign governments on embryo research opens up the possibility of embryos from developing countries that do not have appropriate national guidelines in this area, being commercially exploited and sold to foreign countries.[1]

Therefore, sale or transfer of human embryos or any part thereof, or of gametes in any form and in any way, that is, directly or indirectly, to any party outside the country must be prohibited. Within the country, such embryos or gametes could be made available to bonafide researchers only as a gift, with both parties (the donor and the donee) having no commercial transaction, interest or intent.[1]

Rights of a Child Born Through Various ART Techniques

- A child born through ART shall be presumed to be the legitimate child of the couple, having been born in wedlock and with the consent of both the spouses. Therefore, the child shall have a legal right to parental support, inheritance, and all other privileges of a child born to a couple through sexual intercourse.
- Children born through the use of donor gametes, and their 'adopted' parents, shall have a right to available medical or genetic information about the genetic parents that may be relevant to the child's health.[1]
- Children born through the use of donor gametes shall not have any right whatsoever to know the identity (such as name, address, parentage, etc.) of their genetic parent(s). A child thus born will, however, be provided all other relevant information (mentioned under requirements for a sperm donor) about the donor as and when desired by the child, when the child becomes an adult. While the couple will not be obliged to provide the above 'other'

information to the child on their own, no deliberate attempt will be made by the couple or others concerned to hide this information from the child as and when asked for by the child.

- In the case of a divorce during the gestation period, if the offspring is of a donor program, be it sperm or ova, the law of the land, as pertaining to a normal conception, would apply.[1]

FUTURE CHALLENGES

In addition to the technical and ethical issues, there are a few issues remaining to be resolved, especially in those cases where a third party has been involved in the way of (a) gamete donation, (b) embryo donation and (c) surrogacy.

Under such types of situations, the question remains to be answered whether parenting in these families is different from parenting in families with natural reproduction. To answer such questions it is necessary that surveillance should include (a) the quality of parenting, (b) family functioning and (c) child psychological development.

REFERENCES

1. Sharma RS, Bhargava PM, Chandhiok N, Saxena NC (Eds). National Guidelines for Accreditation, Supervision and Regulation of ART Clinics in India. ICMR, New Delhi, 2005.
2. World Health Organization (WHO) Laboratory Manual for the Examination of Human Semen and sperm-certhical mucus Interaction. Cambridge University, Press, Cambridge, 1999.

Accreditation and Supervision of ART Clinics: Worldwide Trends

Kulvinder Kochhar Kaur, Gautam N Allahbadia

OVERVIEW

Since the first *in vitro* fertilization (IVF) birth, assisted reproductive techniques (ART) mushroomed all over the world and the need for legislation and accreditation was recognized after experiments were carried out by scientists despite legislation. The most important issues requiring legislation revolve around the number of embryos transferred, donation of gametes or embryos, the cryopreservation of gametes, embryos, gonadal tissue and preimplantation genetic screening (PGS) of embryos.

Importantly, two significant scenarios have emerged with supervision, inspection and accreditation in developing countries, mainly to ensure ethical practices in the ART procedure, and proper labeling systems for gametes and embryos similar to that in technologically advanced developed countries to avoid mixing of gametes. Accreditation is required to keep a check on the ethics of advanced reproductive procedures and the future effect on mankind of stem cell research, cloning and preimplantation genetc diagnosis (PGD).

Although most of Europe has acquired a 100 percent reporting system, there are still 5 to 6 countries with poor reporting, e.g. Estonia, Romania, Kazakhstan, Moldova and Bosnia, and laws, like those in Italy, do not help to improve but rather, decrease the pregnancy rates and increase cross-border reproductive tourism.

INTRODUCTION

Initial History of IVF

In the USA, IVF research began as early as the 1930's, when Pincus and Enzmann at Harvard were involved in attempts at IVF in the rabbit. In the 1940's, John Rock attempted human IVF with 138 human oocytes without success. In 1965, Bob Edwards was with Georgeanna and Howard Jones at Johns Hopkins, where attempts were made to fertilize oocytes *in vitro.*

Following the birth of Louise Brown in 1978, live births after IVF occurred in Australia in 1980, in the USA in 1981, and in Sweden and France in 1982. Following the first IVF birth in Australia, the Government of Victoria established a review of IVF Research and Practice, which lead to the proclamation of the Infertility (Medical Procedures) Act 1984, the first legislation to regulate IVF and its associated human embryo research. Despite such restriction, IVF doctors and scientists from Victoria, especially those under the leadership

of Carlwood, Alan Trounson and Ian Johnston, continued to initiate new treatments for infertility and new methods for delivering this treatment. Clinical IVF began in earnest in the USA in 1980 with the first birth in 1981, achieved by the use of human menopausal gonadotropin (hMG)—a first succeeded use with IVF. In France, two groups Frydman and Testart (Clamart) and Cohen, Mandelbaum and Plachot (Sevres) focussed their research in particular directions In 1981, the Clamart group developed a plasma assay for the initial rise in LH. The Sevres group developed a transport technique. Plachot produced a long series of cytogenetic analysis of oocytes and human embryos. Mandelbaum described the microstructures of the human oocyte. The start of IVF in France benefitted with the help of animal researchers from the Institute National de la Recherche Agronomique. The first babies were born in Clamart in February 1982 and in Sevres in June 1982.[1] Important contributions to the development of IVF from the Nordic countries include techniques of ovarian stimulation, sonographic techniques of monitoring and vaginal oocyte retrieval and also, unique possibilities for monitoring IVF safety. Since then, IVF spread globally with a lot of advances in the field from 1978 till date, namely, oocyte donation, intracytoplasmic sperm injection (ICSI), preimplantation genetic diagnosis (PGD), embryo cryopreservation, semen cryopreservation, stem cell research, cloning, etc.

Assisted reproduction raises complex ethical, legal and social dilemmas.[2] Controversial issues in Reproductive Medicine concern the restriction of assisted reproduction techniques (ART), based on age or sexual orientation, the impact of multiple births on health and health resources, the donation of gametes or embryos, the cryopreservation of gametes, embryos, or gonadal tissue and the preimplantation genetic screening (PSG) of embryos.[3] Criticism of assisted reproduction arises in the context of a broad spectrum of cultural, religious and social attitudes in societies towards technical intervention.[4]

Although the necessity for some form of regulation in Reproductive Medicine is obvious, there has been ongoing debate in society regarding the best approach to regulate assisted reproduction.[5] Many countries have opted for national legislation on assisted reproduction.[6] The recent legislative interventions of the Italian government to regulate Reproductive Medicine, restricting and banning several common procedures to assist human reproduction, are well-known.[7,8] Although restrictive reproductive laws can impose strict limitations on the practice of assisted reproduction, it is argued that legislation is inappropriate to deal adequately with the continuing rapid technological advances in Reproductive Medicine.[6]

The development of clinical practice guidelines may be a more effective approach to regulate assisted reproduction. On the one hand, subfertility guidelines can assist healthcare professionals interested in clinical practice guidelines and increasingly support the development of guidelines for Reproductive Medicine.

Given the potential detrimental consequences of low quality guidelines for Reproductive Medicine, such guidelines should meet basic quality criteria (The AGREE Collaboration, 2003).[9] However, the development of high quality guidelines requires specific expertise and considerable resources.[10] International collaboration offers opportunities for sharing some elements of the expensive and time-consuming process of guideline development activities in Reproductive Medicine.

CLINICAL DISCUSSION

Accreditation

Accreditation is an external professional audit by which an independent accreditation body gives formal recognition that the medical laboratory is competent to provide high quality services that are compliant with rigorous professional standards. *In vitro* medical laboratories have pioneered quality control and quality assurance in health care. The International Organization for Standardization (ISO) IS189 Standard is the first developed, especially for accreditation of medical laboratories, and emphasizes the laboratory client interface. Certification of health care services, according to ISO 9001 standards in Hungarian[11] hospitals, is not sufficient to prove professional competence of medical laboratories. The primary aim of accreditation is the improvement of the quality of diagnostic services by voluntary participation, professional peer review, continuous training and education and compliance with professional standards, and its introduction in Hungary, helps to improve, quality, efficiency and effectiveness of laboratory services during the course of Hungary's accession to the European union. The Japan Accreditation Board for Conformity Assessment (AB) and the Japanese Committee for Clinical Standards (CCLS) are jointly developing the program of accreditation of medical laboratories (ISO15189).[12] Requirements consist of two parts; one is management requirements and the other is technical requirements. The former includes the requirements of all parts of ISO9001, Moreover, it includes the requirements of conformity assessment body, for example, impartiality and independence from any other party. The latter includes the requirements of laboratory competence (e.g. personnel, facility, instrument and examination methods). Moreover, it requires that laboratories shall participate in proficiency testing(s) and laboratories examination results shall have traceability of measurements and implement uncertainty of measurement.

Accreditation in India and the Subcontinent

In our article on accreditation in India and the other subcontinent countries, the authors highlighted how pathetic the situation of supervision is, let alone accreditation in India.[13] Having been born in a country where population explosion was the biggest worry, the government had initially little time or money to spend in this direction. However, despite a high population, any infertile human being has a right to have a baby. But seeing the malpractices that started in the name of IVF and ART, the government was forced to pay attention to this field and few guidelines were released by the Government of India, which address the following issues.[14,15]

   i. Ensure the ethical practice of ART.

  ii. Maintain a national registry of all ART clinics

 iii. Accredit and license ART clinics.

 iv. Supervise the performance of ART clinics regularly.

  v. Regulate the functioning of ART clinics and take punitive action against erring clinics.

 vi. Make ART affordable to the economically weak.

 vii. Draw up guidelines for the use of spare embryos.

viii. Support training and research in ART.

Although these guidelines are on paper, one is waiting for the day when they will be implemented. Few clinics, like ours, have got our clinics accredited on our own by ISO 9002 to maintain and upgrade our standards and keep transparency, and we are the ones who still have to compete with quacks/ every other medico, who considers him/herself an infertility specialist, for getting patients for infertility treatment, although having the ISO 9002 helps us in getting non-resident Indian (NRI) patients under the banner of reproductive tourism on our website and with Indians spread all over the globe. Although this does not represent a big chunk of our IVF fraternity, we have some IVF centers run by bright brains. However, because of the above-mentioned facts, mistrust is always there in any research coming from India, so much so, that the first IVF baby apparently came from Calcutta, India, but because of rampant jealousy and corruption, it was not highlighted.

Recently, Anand[16] highlighted that India, with its diverse ethnic and social background and with various religious practices spread over a wide canvas, in which almost all of major religions are represented, Hindus are the majority. Such population diversity makes it difficult to identify a common Indian viewpoint on the moral and philosophical aspects of assisted reproduction.

In USA

For several years now, the College of American Pathologists (CAP) and the American Society of Reproductive Medicine (ASRM) have collaborated to accredit ART laboratories, to comply the Clinical Laboratory Improvement Act of 1988 (CLIA), affiliated with standards as rigid or even more rigid than laboratories inspected by the Clinical Laboratory Agency (CLA), affiliated with the Health Care Finance Administration (HCFA), although only CLIA can certify a clinical laboratory.[17] Only the states of Washington, Oregon, and New York are CLIA exempt, in which case, a CLIA-authorized state agency performs these functions.[17] The ASRM strongly advocated CAP accreditation since the early 1990's, although a recent survey of ART laboratory practices indicates that only approximately one-third of respondent laboratories are accredited by CAP.[18] Smith[19] reported a decrease in take home baby rates in accredited laboratories as compared to non-accredited ones. From a list of 91 CAP accredited laboratories, the national statistics for live births per cycle for women of age <35, 35 to 39, and >39 years from all 300 reporting national laboratories are 28.7 percent, 21.3 percent and 8.7 percent respectively.

Toner[20] subsequently reported much better results as compared to Europe, 20 years after the birth of Louise Brown. Adamson[21] further described the regulation of ART in USA, saying that, it was felt that ART was not well-regulated in USA as it did not have statutory national bodies like, Reproductive Technology Accreditation

Commitetee (RTAC) Australia, or the Human Fertilisation and Embryology Authority (HFEA) in England. Further, he described the Regulations under the headings Mandatory General Medical Regulations affecting ART, Mandatory Clinical ART Specific Regulations, Mandatory Non-specific Regulation of Clinical ART, Mandatory Laboratory Regulations, ART Research Regulations, Mandatory Regulation of Somatic Cell Nuclear Transfer, Mandatory Regulation of Genetics Testing and Treatment, and Mandatory Regulation of ART Human Subject Research. For details read Adamson.[21]

Professional Accomplishments that have Enhanced Oversight of ART

The numerous initiatives of CAP/ASRM laboratory accreditation have been taken by professional societies associated with ART in the USA. The ASRM was founded in 1944 and has been actively involved in research, education, and setting standards for practice in Reproductive Medicine, including ART. Founded in 1987, the Society for Assisted Reproductive Techniques (SART), is an affiliate society of the ASRM; it published in 1989 clinic-specific success rates on a voluntary basis, and has continued annual publications since then. Both SART and ASRM worked with the congressman, Wyden to support the FCSRCA, which was passed in 1992. With the College of American Pathologists, SART and ASRM have developed the CAP/ASRM Reproductive Laboratory Accreditation Program (RLAP). The RLAP includes strict standards, collaboratively developed by professionals in the field in 1992, and on site laboratory inspections by CAP/ASRM/RLAP inspectors. Over 200 SART clinics have now been accredited on a voluntary basis by this national accrediting body. As a result of changes in SART by laws, in December 1998, accreditation became mandatory for all SART programs; programs must apply for accreditation to CAP/ASRM, JCAHO, or the state of New York. Those IVF clinics that do not become accredited or do not apply for accreditation lose their membership in SART. At this time, essentially, all SART clinics have completed accreditation or are in the process of completing accreditation.

Professional Society Guidelines and Practice

The ASRM and SART have collaboratively developed professional society guidelines and practice standards, shown in Table 85.1. The American College of Obstetricians and Gynaecologists (ACOG) has also developed technical bulletins and practice opinions on ART procedures (Table 85.2).

Professional Society Ethical Guidelines

Recognizing the social context in which ART must be practiced ASRM, SART and ACOG have not confined their

Table 85.1: ASRM and SART guidelines and practice standards

- Minimum standards for IVF (1984)
- Minimum standards for GIFT (1988)
- Revised minimum standards for IVF, GIFT, and related procedures (1990)
- Guidelines for Human Embryology and Andrology laboratories (1992)
- Guidelines for practice, including gamete donation (1993)
- Statement on intracytoplasmic sperm injection (1994)
- Guidelines for the provision of infertility services (1996)
- Elements to be considered in obtaining informed consent for ART (1997)
- Induction of ovarian follicle development and ovulation with exogenous gonadotropins (1998)
- Guidelines for number of embryos transferred (1998)
- Guidelines for gamete and embryo donation (1988)
- Revised minimum standards for *in vitro* fertilization, gamete intrafallopian transfer, and related procedures (1998)
- Position statement on nurses performing limited ultrasound in a gynecology/infertility setting (1997)
- Intravenous immunoglobulin (IVIG) and recurrent spontaneous pregnancy loss (1998)
- Guidelines on number of embryos to transfer (1999)
- Antiphospholipid antibodies do not affect IVF success (1999)
- Who is to report ART cycles (1999)
- Optimal evaluation of the infertile female (2000)
- The role of assisted hatching in IVF: a review of the literature (2000)
- Repetitive oocyte donation (2000)
- Does intracytoplasmic sperm injection (ICSI) carry inherent genetic risks? (2000)
- Blastocyst production and transfer in clinical assisted reproduction (2001)
- Salpingectomy for hydrosalpinx prior to IVF (2001)
- Preimplantation genetic diagnosis (2001)

(Adopted from Adamson. Regulation of ART in the US. Fertil Steril 2002.)

Table 85.2: ACOG technical bulletins and practice opinions

- Technical bulletin on infertility (1989)
- Technical bulletin on new reproductive technologies (1990)
- Technical bulletin male infertility (1990)
- Practice opinion on ZIFT (1993)
- Technical bulletin male infertility (1994)
- Practice opinion on use of frozen sperm (1994)

(Adopted from Adamson. Regulation of ART in the US. Fertil Steril 2002.)

Table 85.3: Professional society and ethical guidelines

- ASRM and SART: ethical considerations of the assisted reproductive techniques (1986, 1988, 1990, 1994, 1997)
- 1994 report with complete statements on over 29 topics
- 1997 report with statements on :

  disposition of abandoned embryos

  oocyte donation to postmenopausal women

  embryo splitting for infertility treatment

  the use of fetal oocytes in assisted reproduction

  posthumous reproduction
- ASRM and SART: ethical issues with respect to specific ART practices including IVF, GIFT, ZIFT gamete donation, surrogacy, cryopreservation of embryos, and research
- ASRM and SART: guidelines addressing quality assurance and formation of public policy
- Definition of 'experimental' (1993)
- Definition of 'infertility' (1993)
- ACOG committee on ethics and opinions on IVF (1986), surrogacy (1990) and research on preimplantation embryos (1993)
- The National Advisory Board on Ethics in Reproduction (NABER) [Originally organized through the cooperative efforts of ACOG and ASRM in 1991, then became independently incorporated and funded and had broad representation before disbanding in 1998 because of lack of funding: Informed consent and the use of gametes and embryos for research 1997]
- ASRM and SART: Shared-risk or refund programs in assisted reproduction (1998)
- Guidelines for advertising by ART programs (1998, 1999)
- Sex selection and preimplantation genetic diagnosis (1999)
- Financial incentives in recruitment of oocyte donors (2000)
- Human somatic cell nuclear transfer-cloning (2000)
- Preconception gender selection for non-medical reasons (2001)

(Adopted from Adamson. Regulation of ART in the US. Fertil Steril 2002.)

concerns regarding ART just to the clinical and laboratory practice of Medicine. Considerable time, effort and expertise have been devoted to developing ethical guideline initiatives that have created standards for self-regulation. Because most practitioners follow these guidelines, they have been important in directing the ethical practice of ART (Table 85.3).

In Canada

Gunby and Daya[22] presented the latest data available from Canada and for 2003. The Canadian ART Register achieved 100 percent (24/24) voluntary participation from Canadian ART Centers. Success rates were higher (clinical pregnancy rates 41.6 percent and live birth rates was 31.4%) and multiple birth rates lower (36.5%).

Monitoring Reproductive Health in Europe

The main impact of the World Health Organization's (WHO) health for the 2000 program was probably related to its focus upon using health indicators as health policy goals rather than productivity or cost alone. The vision was that healthcare planning would be prepared with expertise in Public Health, Clinical Medicine as well as Economics and Management. Health professionals should outline the paths to achieve these goals, and the managers should estimate how much it would cost and let the politicians make the final decisions. The hope was that the decision process would be related to health parameters and that, the progress would be transparent for the taxpayers, so that achievements could be monitored. The philosophy of this approach is still worth pursuing, but the first condition for such a planning process is to identify relevant health indicators that can be monitored over time. If we have no such indicators, we do not know whether we are on the right track; we may not even know where we are. In many European countries, there are few reproductive health indicators that are measured routinely. We have reports on age at first childbirth, fertility and maternal mortality. However, not many other indicators of reasonable validity exist for Europe, even among European Union (EU) member states. This prevents comparisons over time or between countries. EU now has the finance, and they gave 'Reprostat'[23] an ad hoc committee of clinicians and public health experts, the task to suggest a set of indicators in reproductive health (Final Technical Report, 2003; supplementary data file1), that can also be obtained by sending an e-mail to the co-ordinator of the task force, Dr Miguel da Silva(mos@fm.ul.pt). We encourage views from all with an interest in reproductive health. However, the question is: what kind of indicators do we need in reproductive health and not for reproductive healthcare that we deliver in our clinics? Only a few of these indicators, such as Reprostat 11 can be used as proxy measures for reproductive healthcare: the proportion of deliveries associated with ART. Monitoring reproductive health care in the opinion of Nelen et al.[24] by quality indicators is also important, because it gives insight into the overall quality of delivered subfertility care, it gives the opportunity to compare the delivered care with the recommended care in evidence-based guidelines, and determination of sub-standard reproductive healthcare can easily guide improvement of this care. Therefore, to improve reproductive healthcare,

a comprehensive set of clinical practice guidelines, valid quality indicators and effective strategies to implement the guidelines are needed. Clinical practice guidelines provide clinicians easily accessible information regarding optimal reproductive health care. They are a tool to bridge the gap between evidence from the literature and the daily practice. However, clearly, the availability of evidence-based guidelines by itself, does not result in the delivery of optimal patient care.[25,26] Implementation of the key recommendation of these guidelines requires more than just their publication and dissemination. Well-developed and evaluated strategies are necessary to facilitate this implementation. Quality indicators, defined as measurable elements of practice performance, for which there is evidence or consensus that they can be used to assess the quality of care,[27] are crucial in this field; they measure the application of guidelines in daily practice and provide ammunition for feedback and development of implementation strategies (Fig. 85.1).[24]

Role of ESHRE

In 2005, some new clinical guidelines were published by the European Society of Human Reproduction and Embryology and (ESHRE) about, e.g. endometriosis, preimplantation genetic diagnosis (PGD) and recurrent miscarriage.[28] Although these evidence-based guidelines were well-developed, unfortunately, they were not accompanied by a set of quality indicators. Recently, Haagen et al.[29] finding a surprisingly small number of IUI guidelines in Europe, recommended a central body with expertise to update guideline development methodology and sufficient resources could be established.

In Europe, for central selection and international exchange of evidence, in support guideline recommendations. Europe has a European IVF Monitoring Program (EIM) and the latest paper in the fifth annual ESHRE publication on

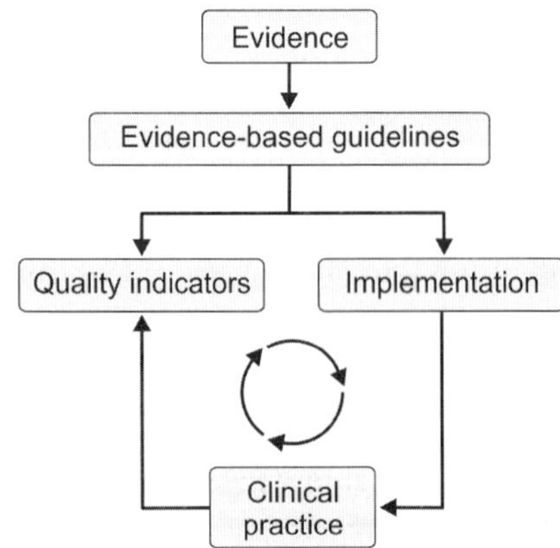

Fig. 85.1: Schematic representation of the different steps from clinical evidence to the implementation in clinical practice *(Adopted from Nelon, et al. Human Reproduction 2006.)*

European data on ART. The four previous reports published in Human Reproduction (ESHRE 2001 a,b, 2002, 2004) covered treatment cycles during 1997, 1998, 1999 and 2000.[30] Data have been collected from 23 European countries and cover IVF, ICSI, frozen embryos replacements (FERs), egg donations (EDs) and PGD, initiated during 2001. Data on intrauterine insemination (IUI) with husband semen (IUI-H) or donor sperm (IUI-D) were also included for 15 countries. The number of clinics reporting IUI data may differ from the number of clinics presenting data on the *in vitro* techniques. Data from each participating country are sent to ESHRE once a year. A draft report is made and then scrutinized by all the consortium members. A fourth consortium meeting was held in Berlin in July 2004, with representatives from participating countries, where the present and future reporting systems were discussed. Here, it was noticed that Germany reported a marked increase in the coverage in their register. Austria and Czech Republic would not be able to provide data for 2001. The consortium stressed that efforts should be made to include the Balkan countries and have better coverage in East Europe. Subsequently, the numbers have increased to 33 countries[31] and 36 countries from 2007 [11th European IVF Monitoring report (EIM) to 2008 (12th EIM report),[32] with the entry of new countries like Bosnia in 2007 to Estonia, Moldova, Kazakhistan and Romania in 2008.

But in Europe in, 2004, the Italian government enacted a law regarding medically assisted reproduction (MAR). Although the law recognizes as legal certain ART techniques, several other procedures are implicitly or explicitly banned, such as oocyte or sperm donation, using embryos for scientific research purposes and reproductive cloning.[6] Critics of the 2004 legislation have pointed out that oocyte and sperm donation are legal in many European countries. In fact France, Great Britain, Spain, Greece and Belgium allow oocyte and sperm donation. Consequently, Italian couples are able to seek treatments that are not allowed in Italy by traveling to other EU Countries, circumventing the prohibition by resorting to so called 'reproductive tourism'.[33] European couples living in countries with more restrictive regulations have sought MAR treatments in more liberal countries.[34-36] It is very likely that the very restrictive Italian law will increasingly force couples to seek treatment for infertility in foreign countries. Although reproductive tourism may be seen as an opportunity to enjoy moral pluralism,[33] it raises domestic issues of inequality of access to healthcare, which is covered by public health insurance and thus, accessible to all citizens. Besides the moral issue, reproductive tourism also raises constitutional issues. The constitutional rights to health care and to equal protection (Italian constitution, 1947, ART3 and 29) are jeopardized if access to some medical treatments for infertility depends upon the economic means of infertile couples and their ability to secure those treatments in a foreign country. In a 5-year study by Levi-Setti, et al.[37] that analyzed 10,706 cycles after the imposition of a restrictive law, the delivery rate per started cycle fell from 20 to 16 percent.[37]

Finally, surrogate motherhood is prohibited. Consequently, all surrogate mother contracts, which require the mother to consent to third party adoption of the child following birth and to facilitate the transfer of child custody, are null under the Italian civil code (1942, ART 1325), because the law views them as being against public policy. For details of Italian law, refer to Boggio.[6]

In UK

Public reaction to breakthroughs in fertility treatment and embryo research tends to be extremely mixed, revealing an often ambivalent attitude to science itself. After 12 years of intense public debate about the ethics of IVF and human embryo research, parliament passed the HFEA Act. The aims of the HFEA are to regulate licensed clinics in a rigorous but sensitive way; to protect patients who may be vulnerable to exploitation, whether intended or inadvertent, of the possibility to enable this in a responsible way, and to reassure the public of the possibility between the practitioner's right to clinical freedom and scientific progress against protection, future offspring and the limits of public acceptability, or the right of access to treatment against the need to maintain acceptability, respectability and safety. In the last 8 years, several issues have arisen that challenge society's view of what is normal or acceptable in human reproduction, and this will undoubtedly continue to happen in the future. These issues have been difficult for society to accommodate, and have presented serious challenges to conventional ideas. However, the HFEA has been able to assure both the public and legislators that clinics are acting reasonably and that there are adequate controls in place.[37] Through the Code of Practice it produces and the licensing system it operates, the HFEA both, protects and supports good clinical decision-making within the ART community.[38] Deech[39] describes the details of regulation of therapeutic cloning in UK.

In Sweden

A quality control (QC) system is needed in ART units to assure reproducibility of all methods and competence in all duties performed by the personnel.

Systems for Quality Control (QC)

Systems for QC have been employed within the production industry since the Second World War. QC systems, originally created for the industry, have later, also been employed in other activities, such as management of organizations and services like healthcare, including in different type of laboratories.

Over the years, different national and international standards for QC systems have been developed. Examination of such standards that have been used for health care are the ISO 9000 series[40] and the EN 45000 series.[41] National and International bodies have been established to further develop standards to be more general so they can be applied to different activities and try to harmonize standards between different countries. These bodies can also act as a third party for auditing QC systems. In Europe, there is an organization called European Co-operation for Accreditation (EA), which approves accreditation bodies for each of the member countries. In Sweden, the authority for accreditation, according to certain QC standards, is called SWEDAC (Swedish Board for Accreditation and Conformity Assessment), which is a member of EU. In Sweden, SWEDAC is a governmental authority responsible for accreditation to standards such as ISO or EN,[42] QC in the Swedish healthcare and specifically in ART.

In Sweden there has been an Act since 1989 (Swedish National Board of Health and Welfare 1989) controlling what is allowed within the field of ART. Furthermore, there are clinical and laboratory guidelines for ART in the Nordic countries (NFOG1997). These guidelines are minimal standards for an ART clinic and laboratory, which have been put together by an expert group within the Nordisk Forening for Obstetrik och Gynekolog (NFOG). However, so far, in the Nordic countries, there is no group or body for auditing ART clinics.[42]

In Australia

As ART expanded globally, several countries introduced prescribed requirements for the treatment and monitoring of outcomes, as well as licensing or accreditation requirement. While it is common for ART laboratories to be required to have an effective quality control system, the remainder of the clinic is often under less stringent regulation. Furthermore, when treatment conditions are prescribed, the standards tend to be conservative and clinics may choose to establish their own standards. Total quality management systems are now being used by an increasing number of ART clinics. In Australia and New Zealand, it is now a requirement to have a quality management system in order to be accredited and to help meet customer demands for improved delivery of ART services in these two countries.[43] In 2003, the Australian government passed a legislation that regulates the method of production and use of human embryos. This includes prohibited practices such as cloning, flushing of embryos from the uterus, etc. Research, utilizing excess embryos, now requires a licence and there are many conditions that that need to be met for a licence application to be successful. Central to the Australian legislation is that, the purpose of creating a human embryo is to establish a pregnancy. Only when the couple no longer requires their excess embryos to establish a pregnancy, or when an embryo is deemed incapable of establishing a pregnancy, can it be used for another purpose. Nevertheless, within Australia, different states have varying levels of legislature (ranging from none to highly regulated), which in the relatively new federal legislative environment, primarily deals with who can access ART treatment and for what reason. For example, in the state of New South Wales, a relatively unregulated state, social sexing of embryos 'for family balancing', is not restricted (as there is no state legislation restricting access), yet, in the other states, such as Victoria, such activity is prohibited. In Victoria, the range of ART services is far more limited. The Victorian clinics uniformly restricted access of single and lesbian women to ART services and did not offer social sex selection procedures.[44] It was also found that reproductive tourism was prevalent in South Wales and restrictions were circumnavigated by patients with assistance from clinics.[45] Intriguingly, this occurs against the background of a large proportion of the costs of treatment met by the federally funded medical benefit scheme. Finally, the Fertility Society of Australia administers the national accrediting body, which oversees the practice of ART treatment in both Australia and New Zealand. This involves regular site inspections and auditing of procedures to follow 'Best Practice' principles. Three embryos is the maximum number recommended for transfer by the Australian National Accrediting Authority. Such a number is reserved for difficult cases, such as repeated IVF failure. Unfortunately, it is also available for a woman receiving treatment if she is greater than 38 years old who has already had 3 children.

Egg Sharing (Pros and Cons)

Assisted reproduction carries with it known and putative medical and surgical risks. Exposing healthy women to these risks in order to harvest eggs for donation when a safer alternative exists, is morally and ethically unacceptable. Egg sharing minimizes this risk and provides a source of eggs for donation. Anonymity protects all parties involved and should not be removed.[46] However, consent for egg donation is a must. The fear that the ethics and practice of egg sharing will be undermined by the growing success of oocyte cryopreservation is not based on published evidence. Separate contracts and directed counseling of donors and recipients, as required by law in the UK, provide protection against pitfalls with egg sharing. The cost and wasting of time with egg donation might even fall should oocyte cryopreservation become a practicable procedure.[47] Egg sharing does not compromise the chance of achieving a pregnancy or live birth for the egg sharer or the recipient as compared to standard IVF/ICSI patients. The egg sharers were not at a higher potential risk of ovarian hyperstimulation syndrome (OHSS), and there was no imbalance of egg allocation.[48]

CONCLUSION

In a nutshell, supervision, inspection, and accreditation are required in two different scenarios in the world. One is in the developing countries, where it is required mainly to ensure ethical practice of the ART procedure (IUI/IVF/ICSI) itself and to ensure that there is proper labeling of gametes and no mixing of gametes, with proper labeling systems. The second one is in the developed countries that have technologically advanced so much that accreditation is required to keep a check on the ethics of the advanced procedures, like preimplantation diagnosis,[49] stem cell research,[50] cloning[39] and the like, and their future consequences on mankind. Harsher rules, like those in Italy, need to be relaxed as, in any case, they are available in the neighbouring countries but just at a higher cost.

REFERENCES

1. Cohen J, Trounson A, Dawson K, Jones H, Hazekamp J, Nygren KG, Hamberger L. The early days of IVF outside the UK. Hum Reprod Update 2005;11:439-59.
2. Sozos J, Fasoulioutis, Joseph G. Schenker Social aspects in assisted reproduction. Human Reproduction Update 1999;1:26-39.
3. Kaariainen H, Evers-Kiebooms G, Coviello D. Medically assisted reproduction and ethical challenges. Toxicol Appl Pharmacol 2005;207:684-8.
4. Fasouliotis SJ, Schenker JG. Ethics and assisted reproduction. Eur J Obstet Gynecol Reprod Biol 2000;90:171-80.
5. Fasouliotis SJ, Schenker JG. Social aspects in assisted reproduction. Eur J Hum Reprod Update 1999;5:26-39.
6. Boggio A. Italy enacts new law on medically assisted reproduction. Hum Reprod 2005;20:1153-7.
7. Turone F. Italy to pass new law on assisted reproduction. BMJ 2004;328:9.
8. Ragni G, Allegra A, Anserini P, Causio F, Ferraretti AP, Greco E, Palermo R, Somigliana E. The 2004 Italian legislation regulating assisted reproduction technology: a multicenter survey on the results of IVF cycles. Hum Reprod 2005;20:2224-8.
9. The AGREE Collaboration Development and validation of an international appraisal instrument for assessing the quality of clinical practice guidelines: the AGREE project. Qual Saf Health Care 2003;12:18-23.
10. Grol R, Wensing M, Eccles M. Improving Patient Care. The Implementation of Change in Clinical Practice. Elsevier Butterworth Heinemann, Oxford, UK. 2005.
11. Hovrath, Ar, Endroczi E, Miko T. Quality improvement of medical diagnostic laboratories. Orv Hetil. 2003;144:1389-95.
12. Aoyagi T. ISO 15189 medical laboratory accreditation. Rinsho Byori 2004;52:860-5.
13. Allahbadia GN, Kaur K. Accreditation, supervision, and regulation of ART clinics in India—a distant dream. A Journal of Asst Reprod Genet 2003;20:276-80.
14. Anand Kumar TC. Proposed legislation for assisted reproductive technology clinics in India. Reprod Biomed Online 2002; 5:351-2.
15. Anand Kumar TC. The Indian Council of Medical Research issues a statement on assisted. reproductive techniques. Reprod Biomed Online 2001;2:88.
16. Anand Kumar TC. Ethical aspects of assisted reproduction: An Indian viewpoint Reprod Biomed Online 2007;Suppl 1;140-2.
17. Clinical Laboratory Improvement Amendments of 1988, Public Law, 100-578.
18. Practice Committee for the American Society for Reproductive Medicine. Revised minimum standards for *in vitro* fertilization, gamete intrafallopian transfer, and related procedure. Fertil Steril 1998;70 (2suppl):1s-5s.
19. Smith AL. College of American Pathologistss and American Society for Reproductive Medicine Accreditation of Assisted Reproduction Technology (ART) laboratories is associated with a dectrease in take home baby rates of reporting ART laboratories. Fertil Steril 2000;73:173-4.
20. Toner JP. Progress we can be proud of: U.S. trends in assisted reproduction over the first 20 years. Fertil Steril 2002;78:943-50.
21. Adamson D. Regulation of Assisted reproductive technologies in the United States. Fertil Steril 2002;78:932-42.
22. Gunby J, Daya S. IVF Directors Group of the Canadian Fertility and Andrology Society. Assisted reproductive technologies (ART) in Canada: 2003 results from the Canadian ART Register. Fertil Steril 2007;88:550-9.
23. Jahn A, Bloemenkamp KWM, Hannaford P, Olsen J, da Silva MO, Temmerman M. Monitoring reproductive health in Europe–What are the best indicators of reproductive health? Hum Reprod 2006;21:2199-200.
24. Nelen WLDM, Hermens RPMG, Mourad SM, Haagen EC, Grol RPTM, JAM Kremer. Monitoring reproductive health in Europe: What are the best indicators of reproductive health? A need for evidence-based quality indicators of reproductive health care. Hum Reprod Advance access published 2006;15:1-3.
25. Grimshaw JM, Russell IT. Effect of clinical guidelines on medical practice: a systematic review of rigorous evaluations. Lancet 1993;42:1317-22.
26. Bero LA, Grilli R, Grimshaw JM, Harvey E, Oxman AD, Thomson MA. Closing the gap between research and practice: an overview of systematic reviews of interventions to promote the implementation of research findings. The Cochrane Effective Practice and Organization of Care Reveiw Group. BMJ 1998;317:465-8.
27. Donabedian A. The quality of care. How can it be assessed? JAMA 1988;60:1743-8.
28. Jauniaux E, Farquharson RG, Christiansen OB, Exalto N. Evidence-based guidelines for the investigation and medical treatment of recurrent miscarriage. Hum Reprod 2006;21: 2216-22.
29. Haagen EC, Hermens RPMG, Nelen WLDM, Braat DDM, Grol RPTM, Kremer JAM. Subfertility guidelines in Europe: the quantity and quality of intrauterine insemination guidelines. Hum Reprod 2006;2103-9.
30. Anderson AN, Gianaroli L, Felberbaum R, de Mouson J, Nygren KG. Assisted reproductive technology in Europe, 2001. Results generated from European registers by ESHRE. Hum Reprod 2005;20:1158-76.
31. de Mouzon J, Goossens V, Bhattacharya S, Castilla JA, Ferraretti AP, Korsak V, et al. European IVF-Monitoring (EIM);

Consortium for the European Society on Human Reproduction and Embryology (ESHRE). Assisted reproductive technology in Europe, 2007: results generated from European registers by ESHRE. Hum Reprod 2012;27:954-66.

32. Ferraretti AP, Goossens V, de Mouzon J, Bhattacharya S, Castilla JA, Korsak V, et al. European IVF-monitoring (EIM); Consortium for European Society of Human Reproduction and Embryology (ESHRE). Assisted reproductive technology in Europe, 2008: results generated from European registers by ESHRE. Hum Reprod 2012;27:2571-84.

33. Pennings G. Legal harmonization and reproductive tourism in Europe. Hum Reprod 2004;19:2689-94.

34. Pennings G. The loss of sperm donor candidates due to the abolition of the anonymity rule: analysis of an argument. J Assist Reprod Genet 2001;18:617-22.

35. Baetens P, Devroey P, Camus M, Van Steirteghem A, Ponjaert Kristoffersen. I counseling couples and donors for oocyte donoation: the decision to use either known or anonymous oocytes. Hum Reprod 2000;15:476-84.

36. Vandervorst M, Staeseen C, Sermon K, et al. Th Brussel's experience of more than 5 years of clinical preimplantation genetic diagnosis. Hum Reprod Update 2004;6:364-73.

37. Levi Setti PE, Albani E, Matteo M, Morenghi E, Zannoni E, Baggiani AM, et al. Five years (2004–2009) of a restrictive law-regulating ART in Italy significantly reduced delivery rate: analysis of 10,706 cycles. Hum Reprod. 2012 Nov 21. [Epub ahead of print].

38. Deech R. Regulating reprod: the art of decision-making in ART: Reprod Biomed Online 2001;3:94-7.

39. Deech R. Regulation of therapeutic cloning in the UK. Reprod Biomed Online 2000;5:7-11.

40. Haeckel R, Kindler M. Effect of current and forthcoming European legislation and standardization on the setting of quality specifications by laboratories. Scand J Clin Lab Invest 1999;59:569-73.

41. Libeer JC. Total quality management for clinical laboratories: a need or a new fashion? Acta Clin Belg 1997;52:226-32.

42. Wikland M, Sjoblom C. The application of quality systems in ART programs. Molecular and Cellular Endocrinology 2000; 166:3-7.

43. Warnes GM, Norman RJ. Quality management systems in ART: are they really needed? An Australian clinic's experience. Best Pract Res Clin Obstet Gynaecol 2007;21:41-55.

44. Jeremy G, Thompson. A mixed bag: a perspective on the regulation of IVF in Australia Human Fertility 2005;8:69-70.

45. Petersen K, Baker HW, Pitts M, Thorpe R. Assisted reproductive techniques: professional and legal restrictions in Australian clinics. J Law Med 2005;12:373-85.

46. Ahuja KK, Simons EG. Advanced oocyte cryopreservation will not undermine the practice of ethical egg sharing. Reprod Biomed Online 2006;12:282-3.

47. Ahuja KK, Simons EG, Nair S, Rimington MR, Armar NA. Minimizing risk in anonymous egg donation. Reprod Biomed Online 2003;7:504-5.

48. Thum MY, Gafar A, Wren M, Faris R, Ogunyemi B, Korea L, Scott L, Abdalla HI. Does egg sharing compromise the chance of donors or recipients achieving a live birth? Hum Reprod 2003;18:2363-7.

49. De Wert G. Preimplantation genetic diagnosis: the ethics of intermediate cases. Hum Reprod 2005;20:3261-6.

50. Wert GD, Mumerry C. Human embryonic stem cells: research, ethics and policy. Hum Reprod 2003;18:672-87.

The Uterus in Third Party Reproduction: Medicolegal Status and Ethical Concerns

Nikhil D Datar

INTRODUCTION

The word 'mother' is defined as a person who conceives, gives birth to, or raises and nurtures a child. The word mother and its legal meaning was never a question of law. So far, all the roles of the mother from the conception to giving birth were expected to be carried out by the same woman. Interestingly, surrogacy was not unknown to the society. A female would conceive a child, deliver and hand it over to someone to raise. The situation, whereby a male and a female with their own genetic material conceive a child, which is nurtured and raised in someone else's womb, and handed over back to the genetic parents was a scientific fiction few years back. With the advent of assisted reproductive techniques (ART), it is possible that the genetic material comes from a different set of individuals and the biological mother may be different. This has posed various legal and ethical issues in before the medical and legal community and society at large. This article, as the name suggests, shall deal with the legal, ethical and practical situations, where the genetic and biological mothers are different. In the process of ART, there can be potentially three parties namely; the party that gives genetic material, that is sperm or oocytes, the party that nourishes the fetus *in utero*, and the party that wants the child to be born, namely the commissioning parents.

CLINICAL DISCUSSION

What is Surrogacy?

Surrogacy is an arrangement whereby a woman agrees to become pregnant for the purpose of gestating and giving birth to a child for others to raise. The word surrogate, from Latin 'surrogare', means 'elect as a substitute'.[1] She may or may not be the child's genetic mother. In the past, the female would conceive by sexual intercourse with a man, or she would be impregnated by the artificial insemination and later, hand over the child to the couple. In such cases, the genetic and biological mother would be the same. This arrangement is called as 'traditional surrogacy'. Whereas, when the genetic material comes from the parents and the surrogate only lends her uterus to raise the child, it is called 'gestational surrogacy'.

In the Indian context, it is interesting to note the guidelines of Indian Council of Medical Research (ICMR).[2] The section 3.5.4 states that:

'An oocyte donor cannot act as a surrogate mother for the couple to whom the oocyte being donated'.

Thus, in India, traditional surrogacy arrangements are not allowed.

Is Surrogacy Recognized in India?

There is no legislation that specifically states that surrogacy is legal. It also does not expressively prohibit surrogacy. It must be submitted that there is no special law governing surrogacy in India to date. The ICMR has set forth its guidelines on the subject. These guidelines lay down the minimum standards and procedures in relation to assisted reproductive techniques (ART) and surrogacy. Based on the ICMR guidelines, the draft bill, called 'ART draft bill' has been prepared by the Ministry of Health. The ICMR guidelines also give a model draft for surrogacy contracts. Thus, it can be said that India recognizes 'surrogacy.'

The guidelines state that all ART techniques should be employed only when pregnancy is undesirable or impossible by other routes. It may be argued that surrogacy is not a matter of right and should be employed only when medical need exists. However, it must be submitted that there has not been any case contested in the apex court challenging the validity of the surrogacy contract so far. The contract, that complies with all the legal formalities, need not be legitimate and legal.

Section 23 of the Indian Contract Act provides that the contract may be termed as 'void' if the object or the consideration of the contract is opposing the public policy. In the surrogacy contract, the surrogate is obliged to hand over the child to commissioning parents. This may be for consideration or otherwise. It may be argued that the surrogacy contract may commodify motherhood; womb renting may become a business and poor women may become womb renting machines. Some feel that surrogacy is worse than prostitution as one rents the body for nine months at a stretch. Thus, it may be argued that the surrogacy contract is against public policy.

However, the concept of public policy is never a static one. It is dynamic and ever-changing. A contract, which has the tendency to injure public interests or public welfare, would depend upon the times and climes. The social mileu in which the contract is sought to be enforced will decide the factum, the nature and the injury.[3]

To procreate is a natural urge. To pass on the genetic material to the next generation is the natural phenomenon. Over and above in a country like India, where childlessness is a taboo and a common cause for marital disharmony, the steps taken towards achieving motherhood cannot be termed as 'illegal or unlawful'. The author submits that a great deal of judicial activism is needed in this aspect.

Is Commercial Surrogacy Unethical?

The ICMR guideline, in section 3.10.3, expressively provides for financial consideration to the surrogate. According to the section 3.10.6, a relative, a known person, as well as unknown person may act as a surrogate. A known person or relative may or may not expect monetary compensation and may choose to be a surrogate out of love and affection. However, when an unknown woman decides to be a surrogate, it is quite likely for her to expect monetary.

Money seems to be a crucial factor for many surrogates.[4] In the United States, surrogate arrangements are enforceable by law. However, if commercial surrogacy were to become an alternative to adoption, it would be so only for the wealthy. Poorer people, who might be just as deserving, or even more so, could never afford the fees demanded. What we may see in the future is a class of breeder women, probably poor women, who rent their wombs to wealthy people.

Elizabeth Kane, the first commercial surrogate in the United States, now active in the National Coalition against Surrogacy, writes 'A woman (surrogate mother) feels like a flesh covered test tube during the entire experience. As the fetus grows, the woman is depersonalized; she becomes fragmented from the whole person, merely a vehicle for breeding babies!'[5]

One therefore, treats a woman's womb as a commodity to house the fetus. Women are used as human incubators. The relation between the surrogate and the child is commercial rather than emotional.

As stated above, since money is a crucial factor that prompts women to be surrogates, it inevitably leads to their financial exploitation. Is it morally right for a woman to offer herself for a fee, procreate and then sell the child? In some cases, money may not change hands. In altruistic surrogacy one woman, say a relative or known person, carries the pregnancy for another just out of love and affection and not for financial gains. But in any case, the surrogate is contracting her body and herself.

In a civilized society, sexual interactions between couples are perceived as something very private and permissible within acceptable ethos. It is only when pregnancy and childbirth come into focus that the society becomes vocal. Medical ethicists are divided on the propriety of commercial surrogacy. Some liken commercial surrogacy to 'baby selling'. 'Baby selling' is when one sells a born child to another person. The surrogacy agreement is made even before conception has occurred.

Does the Surrogacy Contract Infringe upon the Right to Life and Liberty?

The right to life and liberty is a fundamental right enshrined in Article 21 of the Indian Constitution. The right to privacy is also a fundamental right derived from the Article 21.

In surrogacy agreements, the surrogate is contractually obliged to act as per the norms of the agreement. These agreements may impose personal restrictions, such as not to drink alcohol, not to smoke and even sometimes, not to consume certain medications, etc. The question here is whether these terms of contract, though mutually accepted, amount to infringement upon personal liberty.

Since it is not her own child, the surrogate may not adhere to these restrictions that strictly. Hence, if in case there is a suit for non-performance, what should be the remedy? The remedy should be limited so as to preserve the right of the privacy and procreative autonomy.[6]

Right to Abort

The woman has right to abort, that flows from Article 21. The Medical Termination of Pregnancy Act is in place to guard the right of woman to abort, provided that certain conditions are fulfilled.

In surrogacy arrangements, who has the right to exercise the right to abort? Does the right vest in the surrogate or the genetic mother? In the Johnson versus Calvert case, it was held that the right is extended only to the intending parents and not to the surrogate mother, as she was not exercising her right to procreate.[7]

But what if the surrogate wants to abort the fetus? In the Planned Parenthood versus Danfurth case, it was decided that since the state cannot prohibit abortion, it cannot delegate this responsibility to another person.[8] The existing MTP Act has no answer to these questions. The rules framed under the MTP Act imply that the husband of the woman cannot veto the decision of the woman to abort the child, provided that the requirements of the law are fulfilled. Thus, an unrelated genetic couple cannot have the right to prohibit the surrogate from abortion. In such an event, the commissioning parents can sue the surrogate for non-performance of the contract and for damages at the most.

Does the Child have the Right to Find his/her Genetic Parents?

The gametes in a surrogacy arrangement may not necessarily come from the commissioning couple. In such a situation, does the child have the right to know his genetic parents?

The medical and genetic information may be of great importance to the child. This may depict the inheritance and probability of certain diseases. Most importantly, there is a potential risk that the child born out of donated gametes may unknowingly marry another person who is a genetic sibling. Thus, it is of paramount importance to know such information.

On the other hand, the donor has a right to privacy and he/she is assured of maintaining strict secrecy about the gamete donation. Genetic information has been recognized to be entitled to the highest expectation of privacy.[9] The interest of the offspring to have knowledge of the genetic and gestational roots is in total conflict with the freedom and privacy of the donor and surrogate. Thus, the right 'to know' may invade someone's right to privacy![10] It may be stated that if the right to know is further pressed too far, it may inhibit the gamete donation and surrogacy both.

So the question; does the child have right to know his genetic parents?

The Human Fertilisation and Embryology Act (HFEA), 1990 in the United Kingdom, in Section 31 (3), embodies the right to the person above age 18 and born by ART, to check all the records maintained by the authority (if the applicant has received counseling). The Indian judiciary has held that the right to health will override the right of privacy of another.[11] In India, the ICMR guidelines have clarified the position. The children born by ART have the right to know the medical and genetic information that may be relevant to a child's health. In this connection, the Sections 3.12.3, 3.4.8 and Section 3.16.1 of the ICMR guidelines can be collectively read to deduce as under:

- The gamete donors shall have no parental rights or duties in relation to the child.

- The child born shall not have the right to know the identity, such as name, address, parentage, etc. of the donor.
- The child has a right to seek relevant information, including a DNA fingerprint, but not the details about identity.

Custody of the Child

The most famous suit on the subject matter was the 'Baby M' case between the surrogate mother, Mary Beth Whitehead, and the people with whom she originally arranged to give her baby, William and Elizabeth Stern. In this case, heard by the courts in 1987, the Sterns hired Mary Beth Whitehead to be a surrogate mother. After Ms Whitehead bore the child, she changed her mind about giving the baby to the Sterns, asked for the child back and ran away with the baby to Florida.

A lower court awarded custody of the child to the Sterns and made Mrs Stern an adoptive mother. The New Jersey Supreme Court overturned the adoption in May of 1988 but left custody of the child with the Sterns. Whitehead was allowed visitation rights.

The surrogate mother is the de facto mother of the child. The presumption under section 112 of Indian Evidence Act states that the natural mother shall have the custodial rights. This presumption needs to be shifted. As per the ICMR guidelines the birth certificate is expected to be issued in the name of the genetic parents hence, it can be said that the above presumption is rebutted.

Section 13 (1) of the Hindu Minority and Guardianship Act and Section 17 (1) of the Guardians and Wards Act imply that the while declaring guardianship, the best interest of the child be taken into consideration .Since the intending parents would have more love and affection, the custody would pass on to the intending parents. However, the question is what if the commissioning parents refuse to take the custody. As per section 25 of the Guardians and Wards Act, if the ward is removed from the custody of the guardian, the court may in the best interest, order the custody to the natural mother.

A unique situation may arise, whereby the commissioning couple may split due to the death of the spouse or otherwise. The question is whether the commissioning father can contest for the custody against the surrogate? The father does have a right of custody arising out of the contract. Hon'ble Supreme Court in Veena Kapoor versus Verinder Kapoor has stated 'In matters concerning the custody of minor children, the paramount consideration is the welfare of the minor and not the legal rights of this or that party'.[12] Most of the courts have decided in favor of the mother while deciding the custody.

Unresolved Issues

The author will like to flag, following unresolved issues in this article. ART and surrogacy can pose many tricky problems that have an impact on various laws and their interpretations. It is interesting to note that if the commissioning couple wants to insure the surrogate in the event of the surrogate's death, etc. no insurance company today is ready to insure the life.

It will be important to know as to what would be the rights and liabilities of the husband of the surrogate?

If by using frozen gametes, one wants to procure the child after the death of the partner, what would be the position of the law? What would be its effect on the inheritance laws of the land?

Complicating Issues Further

The author submits that ART and surrogacy pose various ethical and legal dilemmas.

The surrogate undergoes a phenomenon of carrying the pregnancy till term, and delivering the baby, and not of nurturing the baby. Does the baby have a right to be breast-fed?[13] The matter also has close connection to the child's well-being! But on the other hand, would allowing breast feeding develop an emotional bond with the surrogate, which may complicate the situation further?

Would the surrogate have the right to choose the mode of delivery or the same shall vest in the genetic parents?

India has a 'two child norm' for population control. However, a woman can become a surrogate for three times in life. In surrogacy, the medical situation becomes more complicated due to multifetal pregnancy, fetal reductions, etc. India has been fighting issues such as maternal mortality, gender discrimination and the like.

CONCLUSION

The various assisted reproductive techniques have opened up a pandora's box of conflicting rights and liabilities. The parties involved, namely donor, commissioning parents and surrogate and lastly, the child have their unique positions, sometimes conflicting with each other. It is important that all these issues be addressed thoughtfully.

It is said that 'Law is blessed with conservatism and science with dynamism'.

The existing laws are quiet insufficient to address these issues. The judges will have to show an ingeniousness and judicial activism while making decisions and interpreting the status in the events of legal conflicts. The parties would expect speedy remedy in matters of legal issues related to surrogacy, mainly so, when matters related to specific performance of surrogacy contracts are being tried. The pace of judicial machinery may turn out to be too slow in dealing with such matters.

In India, ART and surrogacy is being practised routinely. In spite of that, the parliament has not yet passed the law in this regard. This means that the patients and practitioners remain at the mercy of this uncertainty all the time and can be easily abused by the administrative machinery.

The time has come to define the word 'mother' again. Is she the one who imparts genetic material to the offspring? Or, is she the one who nourishes and gives birth to the offspring? Or, is she the one who nourishes and imparts love and affection to the child later? What actually defines the 'mother' is an ethical, legal, moral and even emotional question.

REFERENCES

1. Soanes, Catherine. Compact Oxford Dictionary Thesaurus & Wordpower guide. s.l.: Oxford University Press, 2005.
2. [Online] [Cited: December 25, 2012.] http://icmr.nic.in/art/art_clinics.htm.
3. http://www.indiacourts.in/RATTAN-CHAND-HIRA-CHAND-Vs.-ASKAR-NAWAZ-JUNG-%28DEAD%29-BY-L.RS.-AND-ORS._940ac556-5f78-4e02-9d2e-6795dd094a0d. [Online] [Cited: December 2012, 26.].
4. Mason JK, Smith McCall. The management of infertility and childlessness. Law and medical ethics. s.l.: Rutterworth, 1994.
5. Allis T. The moral implications of motherhood by hire. Issues Med Ethics 1997;5:21-2.
6. Jerome, Nishant Parikh. Vishnu. Surrogacy arrangements: A conundrum of conflivting rights and liabilities. Health care Policy, Ethics, Law Vol 6. 2000.
7. http://faculty.law.miami.edu/zfenton/documents/Johnsonv.Calvert.pdf. [Online] [Cited: December 26, 2012].
8. http://www.law.cornell.edu/supct/html/historics/USSC_CR_0428_0052_ZS.html. [Online].
9. http://www.ncbi.nlm.nih.gov/pubmed/11648435. [Online] [Cited: December 27, 2012].
10. Basu S. Genetic privacy: resolving the conflict between the donor and the child. Curr Sci 2004;86:1363-5.
11. http://www.indiacourts.in/Mr.-%22X%22-Vs.-Hospital-%22Z%22_b8bf0129-7245-4e9f-9a22-47bf02b7edda. [Online] [Cited: December 27, 2012].
12. Kapoor Veena, Kapoor V. Varinder. http://www.indiankanoon.org/doc/373752/. [Online] [Cited: December 27, 2012].
13. Qadeer I. The ART of marketing babies. Indian J Med Ethics. 2010;7:209-15.

The Future of ART

Anti-Müllerian Hormone: Insights into a Novel Biomarker of the Ovarian Follicular Status

Michael Grynberg, Estelle Feyereisen, C Ferretti, René Frydman, Renato Fanchin

OVERVIEW

In contrast to most hormonal biomarkers of the follicular status, anti-Müllerian hormone (AMH) is exclusively produced by the granulosa cells of a wide range of follicles (primary to the early antral stages), presumably follicle stimulating hormone (FSH)-independently and with little susceptibility to disorders of antral follicle growth during the luteal-follicular transition. This paper summarizes the authors' clinical research on the role of AMH as a marker of ovarian functioning. It shows that the relationship between antral follicle counts (AFCs) and serum AMH concentrations is stronger than that observed with FSH, inhibin B and estradiol on day 3, and that, intercycle reproducibility of AMH measurements is better than the latter parameters. In addition, peripheral AMH concentrations decline during ovarian stimulation, thus confirming that maturing follicles lose progressively their ability to produce AMH. Indeed, follicular fluid (FF) AMH concentrations in small antral follicles are thrice as high as AMH in preovulatory follicles. Further, human chorionic gonadotropin (hCG)-driven luteinization additionally curtails follicular AMH production. Finally, AMH production, measured in FF from individual follicles, is increased in women having normal follicular counts and responsiveness to ovarian stimulation. Together, these data reinforce the soundness of AMH measurements as a quantitative and possibly, qualitative marker of granulosa cell activity and health.

INTRODUCTION

Anti-Müllerian hormone (AMH) is a glycoprotein that belongs to the transforming growth factor β superfamily.[1] AMH, produced by the Sertoli cells of the fetal testis, induces the regression of the Müllerian ducts, the anlagen of the female reproductive tract.[2] However, after birth, this sex-dimorphic expression pattern is lost and AMH is also expressed in granulosa cells of growing follicles in the ovary.[3] Yet, the precise physiological role of AMH in adult women remains poorly understood. Studies in rodents have suggested that AMH might be involved in both the inhibition of primordial to primary follicle growth[4] and the follicular responsiveness to FSH.[5] Moreover, previous experiments conducted in animals have suggested that AMH, probably via its specific type II receptors expressed in granulosa and theca cells, may reduce both, aromatase activity and the number of luteinizing hormone (LH) receptors in FSH-stimulated granulosa cells,[6] and inhibit testosterone production by theca cells.[7] Ovarian AMH production is probably modulated by the degree of gonadic development. Indeed, AMH expression only begins in the perinatal period,[8] remains low throughout reproductive life and becomes undetectable after menopause.[9] Moreover, the stage of follicular growth is likely to influence AMH expression which starts in the columnar granulosa cells of primary follicles immediately after differentiation from the flattened pregranulosa cells of primordial follicles. Expression is highest in granulosa cells of preantral and small antral follicles, and gradually diminishes in the subsequent stages of follicle development. AMH is no longer expressed during the FSH-dependent final stages of follicle growth.[4,10] Data from ovarian physiology indicate that AMH exhibits at least three biological characteristics that are not shared by the conventional hormonal predictors of follicular status and that are clinically worthy : expression in the granulosa cells of a wide variety of follicles (from large primary to early antral stages), the loss of capacity to express AMH in follicles that grow beyond the early antral follicle[10] and a production, probably FSH-independent.[11] Therefore, peripheral AMH measurements may provide information on the activity of a larger span of follicles under little or no influence of the hormonal-follicular dynamics at the luteal-follicular transition, which is likely to spare AMH from noticeable intra- and inter-cycle variations. Taken together, these characteristics single AMH out as a promising biomarker of ovarian follicular status. Indeed, controversies have been raised with regard to the predictability of the classical hormone triad represented by FSH,[12] inhibin B[13] and estradiol concentrations,[14] measured on day 3 of the menstrual cycle. The rationale for these hormone measurements is essentially based on the ability of early antral follicles to produce inhibin B and estradiol in response to FSH and on the modulating action of both the hormones on FSH secretion during the luteal-follicular transition in the menstrual cycle. By definition, these hormonal tests disregard the status of other follicles that are barely or not sensitive to FSH and/or have not yet reached the antral stage, but which contribute to the functioning of subsequent menstrual cycles and to women's fertility potential.[15] In addition, they are reportedly biased by confounding variables linked to the status of follicular growth and to size discrepancies of early antral follicles during the early follicular phase. It is conceivable that these limitations of traditional hormonal tests explain, at least in part, the noticeable variability of their results from one cycle to another.[16-18] Recent studies have suggested that AMH would be a more sensitive predictive parameter of ovarian status than the usual markers. Some investigators[19] have demonstrated that serum AMH concentrations on cycle day 3 decrease progressively along with age and become undetectable after menopause. This suggests that peripheral AMH concentrations are a valuable parameter to monitor the relative follicular exhaustion due to ovarian aging. Consistently, clinical data have indicated that peripheral AMH concentrations, during the early follicular phase of the menstrual cycle, is a useful reflector of the number of oocytes retrieved in subsequent ovarian stimulation cycles.[20] In line with this, reports have shown that day 3 serum AMH concentrations were positively related to the pregnancy rate in *in vitro* fertilization (IVF) and embryo transfer (ET) cycles.[11,21]

CLINICAL DISCUSSION

Serum AMH Concentration is a Marker of the Ovarian Follicular Status

The first investigation compared the relationship between serum AMH levels and other markers of ovarian function (serum concentrations of inhibin B, estradiol, FSH and LH) with early antral follicle count on day 3.[22] A total of 75 normo-ovulatory infertile women was studied prospectively. On cycle day 3, serum levels of AMH, inhibin B, estradiol (E2), FSH and LH levels were measured, and the number of early antral follicles (2–10 mm in diameter) estimated at ultrasound scanning to compare the strengths of hormonal-follicular correlations. The aim of the ultrasound examination was to evaluate the number and sizes of early antral follicles and to

calculate the mean ovarian volume. In an attempt to optimize the reliability of ovarian follicular assessment,[23] the ultrasound scanner used was equipped with a tissue harmonic imaging system that allowed improved image resolution and adequate recognition of follicular borders.[23] Serum AMH concentrations were determined using 'first generation' ultrasensitive enzyme-linked immunosorbent assay (ELISA) (Beckman-Coulter, Villepinte, France) as described previously.[24] The results showed that median (range) serum levels of AMH, inhibin B, E2, FSH and LH were 1.39 ng/mL (0.24–6.40), 90 (16–182) pg/mL, 31 (15–111) pg/mL, 7.0 (2.9-19.3) mIU/mL and 4.7 (1.2-11.7) mIU/mL, respectively, and the follicular count was 12 (1–35). Median day 3 serum concentrations of AMH were slightly and negatively related to age ($r = -0.22$, $P < 0.04$), but this did not apply to serum concentrations of inhibin B, estradiol, FSH or LH ($r = 0.06$, $r = 0.09$, $r = -0.13$ and $r = -0.02$ respectively). Unlike serum concentrations of estradiol and LH ($r = -0.08$ and $r = 0.05$), those of AMH, inhibin B and FSH were significantly related to the number of early antral follicles on cycle day 3. Serum AMH levels were more strongly correlated ($P < 0.001$) with follicular count ($r = 0.74$, $P < 0.0001$) than were serum levels of inhibin B ($r = 0.29$, $P < 0.001$), or FSH ($r = -0.29$, $P < 0.001$). In agreement with this, serum AMH concentrations showed a stronger relationship ($P < 0.001$) with ovarian volume ($r = 0.43$, $P < 0.0001$) than did those of inhibin B ($r = 0.11$, not significant), estradiol ($r = 0.13$, not significant), FSH ($r = -0.27$, $P < 0.02$) and LH ($r = 0.02$, not significant). This study confirmed that serum AMH levels were more robustly correlated with the number of early antral follicles than inhibin B, E_2, FSH and LH on cycle day 3. This suggests that AMH may reflect ovarian follicular status better than the usual hormone markers. These results also indicate that early antral follicles (2–12 mm) are probably a major source of AMH in adult women. These results not only corroborate, but also expand clinical data reported by other investigators.[11,20,25,26] Yet, the contribution of smaller follicles is supposed to also influence serum AMH concentrations. If this hypothesis is true, AMH production by FSH-independent follicles could reduce the intercycle variability of peripheral AMH measurements.

Serum AMH: A Reproductive Intercycle Measurement

Fanchin, et al.[27] compared the intercycle reproducibility of serum AMH measurements with that of other conventional markers of follicular status such as serum inhibin B, estradiol, FSH and early antral follicle counts on cycle day 3.[27] The study included 47 normo-ovulatory, infertile women, who underwent measurements of serum AMH, inhibin B, estradiol and FSH, and early antral follicle counts by transvaginal ultrasound on cycle day 3 during three consecutive menstrual cycles. Reproducibility of measurements was estimated using intraclass correlation coefficient (ICC) calculation. The study also evaluated for each parameter the number of repeated measurements needed to reach satisfactory reliability (ICC ≥ 0.80). Serum AMH showed significantly higher reproducibility (ICC, 0.89; 95% confidence interval, 0.83–0.94) than inhibin B (0.76; 0.66–0.86; P < 0.03), estradiol (0.22; 0.03–0.41; P < 0.0001), FSH levels (0.55; 0.39–0.71; P < 0.01), and early antral follicle counts (0.73; 0.62–0.84; P < 0.001), and reached satisfactory reliability with a single measurement. These findings indicated that the intercycle variability of AMH concentrations was lower compared with that of the other markers of ovarian follicular status on cycle day 3.[27] This phenomenon may be, at least in part, explained by the putative differences in the AMH regulation as compared with that of inhibin B, estradiol and FSH during the luteal-follicular transition in the menstrual cycle. These differences may be attributable to the reduced susceptibility of some AMH-producing follicles to cyclic changes, and stresses the cost-effectiveness of AMH measurements in the prediction of the fertility potential.

Dynamics of Serum AMH Concentrations During the Menstrual Cycle and the Final Follicle Maturation and Luteinization

Dynamics of Serum AMH Levels during the Menstrual Cycle

Non-significant variations of AMH throughout the menstrual cycle have been reported by several groups.[28-31] On the other hand, others have reported significant cyclical fluctuations in AMH levels with a rapid decrease in the early luteal phase.[32,33] However, excursions from mean levels of +3 percent to –19 percent have been calculated.[32,33] These variations are similar to the reported intercycle variability for AMH.[28,31] Hence, in the clinical setting, the inter- and intracycle variability in serum AMH levels may be considered to be low enough to permit random timing of AMH measurement during the menstrual cycle.

In women, AMH levels seem to be unmodified under conditions in which endogenous gonadotropin release is substantially diminished, such as during pregnancy,[34] GnRH agonist treatment[35] and short-term oral contraceptive administration,[31,36,37] indicating that non-cyclic FSH-independent ovarian activity persists even when pituitary FSH secretion is suppressed.

Consequences of Final Follicle Maturation on Serum AMH Concentrations

To investigate possible changes in serum AMH levels during the final maturation process from early antral stage to the ovulatory follicle, and their possible relationship with follicular development and other ovarian hormones, Fanchin, et al.[38] studied prospectively 93 women undergoing controlled

ovarian hyperstimulation (COH) with GnRH agonist and FSH.[38] Indeed, COH constituted an attractive model, since it is characterized by the thorough transformation of small antral follicles into maturing follicles as a result of exogenous FSH. Indeed, this process is not reproduced during the menstrual cycle, in which the early antral follicle cohort remains nearly intact throughout the follicular phase and only a single follicle reaches maturation. Also, given that large antral follicles may express AMH only weakly,[10] the multiplicity of maturing follicles could be instrumental in exacerbating overall serum AMH concentrations and improving their detection. In this study, serum levels of AMH, inhibin B, estradiol (E2), progesterone, testosterone and delta 4-androstenedione were measured when pituitary suppression was achieved (baseline), on days 6 and 8 of FSH treatment, and on the day of human chorionic gonadotropin (hCG). The number of small (<12 mm) and large (≥12 mm) antral follicles were estimated using ultrasound. Serum AMH levels declined progressively (baseline, 1.21 ± 0.11 ng/mL; day 6, 0.91 ± 0.09 ng/mL; day 8, 0.77 ± 0.08 ng/mL; and day of hCG, 0.53 ± 0.06 ng/mL), in parallel with a decrease in the number of small antral follicles (16.6 ± 0.6, 10.8 ± 0.6 and 4.0 ± 0.4 follicles <12 mm in diameter on baseline, day 8 and day of hCG, respectively). In the same time, the other hormone levels increased during FSH treatment. Throughout COH, serum AMH levels correlated positively with the number of small but not large antral follicles (r = 0.73, P < 0.0001; r = 0.65, P < 0.0001 and r = 0.73, P < 0.0001 on baseline, day 8 and day of hCG, respectively), and with inhibin B serum levels, respectively. No correlation between AMH and the other hormones was observed. Nevertheless, AMH concentrations were positively related to the total number of oocytes retrieved, in particular, at baseline (r = 0.43, P < 0.0001). Afterwards, the strength of such a relationship declined progressively (r = 0.42, P < 0.0002 on day 6; r = 0.27, P < 0.03 on day 8, and r = 0.22, not significant on day of hCG). These findings indicate that serum AMH levels decline gradually during multiple follicular maturation, probably reflecting the dramatic reduction in the number of small antral follicles due to COH, and confirming the scarce AMH expression by larger follicles. Thus, this study provides support to the hypothesis that the differentiation of granulosa cells during follicular growth is likely to alter their ability to express AMH.[10]

Consequences of Follicle Luteinization and Corpus Luteum Formation on Serum AMH Concentrations

Beyond the preovulatory stage, the possible effects of granulosa cell luteinization and corpus luteum formation on AMH production by the granulosa cells in women remained to be documented. To investigate the dynamics of serum AMH levels during the luteal phase of COH and its possible association with follicle development, thirty-four women undergoing COH with GnRH agonist and FSH were prospectively studied.[39] On the day of hCG (dhCG), serum AMH, estradiol (E2), progesterone and hCG levels were measured, and ovarian follicles were sorted into three size classes: small (3–11 mm in diameter), intermediate (12–15 mm in diameter), and large (16–22 mm in diameter). Hormonal measurements were repeated 4 days (hCG + 4) and 7 days (hCG + 7) after hCG. From dhCG to hCG + 4, a decline in serum AMH levels was observed (– 64 ± 3%; P < 0.0001), which paralleled that of E2 levels. From hCG + 4 to hCG + 7, an increase in AMH levels occurred (82 ± 28%; P < 0.02), whose magnitude was correlated with the number of small follicles (r = 0.68; P < 0.0001) but not with other follicle size classes nor with the remaining hormone levels. Incidentally, as expected, serum estradiol concentrations were positively related to the total number of follicles (r = 0.44, P < 0.009) on the day of hCG administration, but the strength of such a relationship tended to decrease as the follicle size increased (small follicles, r = 0.35, P < 0.04; intermediate follicles, r = 0.32, P < 0.05; large follicles, r = 0.21, not significant). The authors concluded that after hCG, AMH levels initially decline, presumably as an effect of the putative adaptations that granulosa cells undergo during the follicle luteinization process, and then increase during the mid-luteal phase. Although the mechanisms implicated in the mid-luteal AMH increase are unclear, its positive association with small follicle count, but not with luteal progesterone and E2 levels, supports the hypothesis that AMH levels might reflect luteal follicle development.[39]

Serum AMH: A Qualitative Marker of the Ovarian Follicular Status

In an effort to challenge the results of the preceding study, it was decided to investigate the possible changes that occur in intrafollicle AMH concentrations along with the follicular maturation process. In addition, it still remained unclear whether increased peripheral AMH concentrations reflect exclusively the number of early antral follicles or were also due to increased per-follicle AMH secretion. To investigate the possible influence of follicular maturation and luteinization on AMH secretion and the relationship between per-follicle AMH levels, ovarian follicular status and responsiveness to COH,[38] *in vitro* fertilization/embryo transfer (IVF-ET) candidates undergoing COH using a long GnRH agonist protocol, were propectively studied.[40] On the day of oocyte retrieval, serum samples and follicular fluids from two small (8–12 mm in diameter) and two large (16–20 mm in diameter) follicles were collected for AMH, E2, and progesterone (P4) measurements. To avoid possible bias due to follicular fluid volume variability, hormone concentrations in the follicular fluid were adjusted to its protein content,[41] and were expressed as ng/g of protein for AMH and as µg/g of protein for estradiol and progesterone. Small follicles secreted AMH levels (111.0 ng/g of protein, range: 21.7–656.2 ng/g of protein)

that were approximately three times as high as large follicles (40.6 ng/g of protein, range:14.4–108.0 ng/g of protein; P < 0.0001). Follicular fluid AMH and P4 levels were negatively correlated to each other both, in small and large follicles. Per-follicle AMH levels in both small and large follicular classes were positively correlated with the antral follicle count on cycle day 3 before COH (r = 0.37, P < 0.03; and r = 0.63, P < 0.0001 respectively), with growing follicles on the day of hCG administration (≥ 12 mm, r = 0.32, P < 0.05; and r = 0.45, P < 0.005, respectively) and oocytes retrieved (r = 0.31, P < 0.05; and r = 0.56. P < 0.0003, respectively), but were negatively related to the total recombinant FSH dose required for ovarian stimulation (r = –0.30, P < 0.05; and r = –0.48, P < 0.003 respectively). Thus, both final follicular maturation and luteinization interfere with granulosa cell AMH production in individual follicles. The observed relationship between AMH content in individual follicles and the surrounding follicular status, as represented by the number of early antral follicles on day 3 and their responsiveness to ovarian stimulation, is remarkable. It indicates that peripheral AMH concentrations are not exclusively dependent on the number of follicles but also modulated by the ability of individual follicles to produce AMH. Hence, elevated peripheral AMH concentrations indicate not only that the number of antral follicles is increased, but also that, each follicle probably produces more AMH individually. This contributes to the understanding of the reported association between peripheral AMH concentrations and the ovarian fertility potential, and leads to speculation that serum AMH measurements could reflect not only quantitative but also qualitative ovarian responsiveness to ovarian stimulation.[41]

CONCLUSION

All these data, generated up to the time of writing this manuscript in 2007, lead to the following assumptions:

- The relationship between antral follicle counts and serum AMH concentrations is more reliable than that observed with FSH, inhibin B and estradiol on cycle day 3.
- Serum AMH measurements on cycle day 3 are more reproducible from one cycle to another than the remaining parameters.
- Peripheral AMH concentrations decline during ovarian stimulation confirming that maturing follicles progressively lose their ability to produce AMH. This observation is corroborated by follicular fluid measurements that showed a higher AMH content in small versus preovulatory antral follicles.
- hCG-driven luteinization additionally curtails AMH production by granulosa cells.
- Per-follicle measurements indicate that AMH production is increased in follicles from women exhibiting a normal follicle count and responsiveness to ovarian

stimulation. These data reinforce the clinical soundness of AMH measurements, not only as quantitative but maybe, a qualitative marker of granulosa cell activity and health. From a practical standpoint, predictability of AMH overcomes that of the usual markers.[21,22,42] Yet, uncertainties persist with respect to the control of granulosa cell AMH production and its physiological role during the final maturation. The understanding of these key issues will be helpful to refine future clinical applications of AMH measurements in evaluating the fertility potential of women and monitoring infertility treatments. In addition, the results showing that AMH concentrations, measured after pituitary suppression by GnRH agonists, remain predictive of ovarian stimulation outcome, and may encourage further investigation on the value of AMH measurements during ovarian stimulation in the evaluation of ovarian responsiveness to exogenous gonadotropins, follicular quality and perhaps, also embryo implantation outcome, although this latter event involves extraovarian mechanisms.[43]

- Further studies, possibly looking at the fate of oocytes and embryos derived from individual follicles containing high or low AMH concentrations, are also required to verify the hypothesis that serum AMH measurements might provide not only quantitative but also qualitative information about the ovarian follicular status.

REFERENCES

1. Cate RL, Mattaliano RJ, Hession C, Tizard R, Farber NM, Cheung A, et al. Isolation of the bovine and human genes for Müllerian inhibiting substance and expression of the human gene in animal cells. Cell 986;45:685-98.
2. Lee MM, Donahoe PK. Müllerian inhibiting substance: A gonadal hormone with multiple functions. Endocrine Reviews 1993;14:152-64.
3. Vigier B, Picard JY, Tran D, Legeai L, Josso N. Production of anti-Müllerian hormone: Another homology between Sertoli and granulosa cells. Endocrinology 1984;114:1315-22.
4. Durlinger AL, Gruijters MJ, Kramer P, Karels B, Ingraham HA, Nachtigal MW, et al. Anti-Müllerian hormone inhibits initiation of primordial follicle growth in the mouse ovary. Endocrinology 2002;143:1076-84.
5. Durlinger AL, Gruijters MJ, Kramer P, Karels B, Kumar TR, Matzuk MM, et al. Anti-Müllerian hormone attenuates the effects of FSH on follicle development in the mouse ovary. Endocrinology 2001;142:4891-9.
6. di Clemente, N, Ghaffari S, Pepinsky RB, Karels B, Kumar TR, Matzuk MM, et al. A quantitative and interspecific test for biological activity of anti-Müllerian hormone: the fetal ovary aromatase assay. Development 1992;114:721-7.
7. Teixeira J, Maheswaran S, Donahoe PK. Müllerian inhibiting substance: An instructive developmental hormone with diagnostic and possible therapeutic applications. Endocrine Reviews 2001;22:657-74.
8. Rajpert-De Meyts E, Jørgensen N, Graem N, Müller J, Cate RL, Skakkebaek NE. Expression of anti-Müllerian hormone during normal and pathological gonadal development: association with differentiation of Sertoli and granulosa cells. J Clin Endocrinol Metab 1999;84;3836-44.
9. Hudson PL, Dougas I, Donahoe PK, Cate RL, Epstein J, Pepinsky RB, MacLaughlin DT. An immunoassay to detect human Müllerian-inhibiting substance in males and females during normal development. J Clin Endocrinol Metab 1990;70:16-22.
10. Baarends WM, Uilenbroek JT, Kramer P, Hoogerbrugge JW, van Leeuwen EC, Themmen AP, Grootegoed JA. Anti-Müllerian hormone and anti-Müllerian hormone type II receptor messenger ribonucleic acid expression in rat ovaries during postnatal development, the estrous cycle, and gonadotropin-induced follicle growth. Endocrinology 1995;136:4951-62.
11. Eldar-Geva T, Ben-Chetrit A, Spitz IM, Rabinowitz R, Markowitz E, Mimoni T, et al. Dynamic assays of inhibin B, anti-Müllerian hormone and estradiol following FSH stimulation and ovarian ultrasonography as predictors of IVF outcome. Hum Reprod 2005;20:3178-83.
12. te Velde ER, Scheffer GJ, Dorland M, Broekmans FJ, Fauser BC. Developmental and endocrine aspects of normal ovarian aging. Mol Cell Endocrinol 1998;145:67-73.
13. Hall JE, Welt CK, Cramer DW. Inhibin A and inhibin B reflect ovarian function in assisted reproduction but are less useful at predicting outcome. Hum Reprod 1999;14:409-15.
14. Vazquez ME, Verez JR, Stem JJ, Gutiérrez Najar A, Asch RH. Elevated basal estradiol concentrations have no negative prognosis in young women undergoing ART cycles. Gynecol Endocrinol 1998;12:155-9.
15. Gougeon A. Regulation of ovarian follicular development in primates: facts and hypotheses. Endocrine Reviews 1996;17:121-55.
16. Scott RT Jr, Hofmann GE, Oehninger S, Muasher SJ. Intercycle variability of day 3 follicle-stimulating hormone concentrations and its effect on stimulation quality in *in vitro* fertilization. Fertil Steril 1990;54:297-302.
17. Hansen KR, Morris JL, Thyer AC, Soules MR. Reproductive aging and variability in the ovarian antral follicle count: application in the clinical setting. Fertil Steril 2003;80:577-83.
18. Kwee J, Schats R, McDonnell J, Lambalk CB, Schoemaker J. Intercycle variability of ovarian reserve tests: results of a prospective randomized study. Hum Reprod 2004;19:590-5.
19. van Rooij IA, Tonkelaar I, Broekmans FJ, Looman CW, Scheffer GJ, de Jong FH, et al. Anti-Müllerian hormone is a promising predictor for the occurrence of the menopausal transition. Menopause 2004;11:601-6.
20. Seifer DB, MacLaughlin DT, Christian BP, Feng B, Shelden RM, et al. Early follicular serum Müllerian-inhibiting substance concentrations are associated with ovarian response during assisted reproductive technology cycles. Fertil Steril 2002;77: 468-71.
21. Hazout A, Bouchard P, Seifer DB, Aussage P, Junca AM, Cohen-Bacrie P. Serum anti-Müllerian hormone/Müllerian-inhibiting substance appears to be a more discriminatory marker of assisted reproductive technology outcome than follicle-stimu-

lating hormone, inhibin B, or estradiol. Fertil Steril 2004;82: 1323-9.

22. Fanchin R, Schonauer LM, Righini C, Guibourdenche J, Frydman R, Taieb J. Serum anti-Müllerian hormone is more strongly related to ovarian follicular status than serum inhibin B, estradiol, FSH and LH on day 3. Hum Reprod 2003a;18:323-7.

23. Thomas JD, Rubin DN. Tissue harmonic imaging: why does it work? J Am Soc Echocardiogr 1998;11:803-8.

24. Long WQ, Ranchin V, Pautie P, Belville C, Denizot P, Cailla H. Detection of minimal concentrations of serum anti-Müllerian hormone during follow-up of patients with ovarian granulosa cell tumor by means of a highly sensitive enzyme-linked immunosorbent assay. J Clin Endocrinol Metab 2000;85:540-4.

25. Grynberg M, Genro V, Gallot V, El-Ali A, Frydman R, Fanchin R. Early follicle development during the luteal-follicular transition affects the predictability of serum follicle-stimulating hormone but not anti-Müllerian hormone levels on cycle day 3. Fertil Steril 2010;94:1827-31.

26. Grynberg M, Feyereisen E, Scheffer JB, Koutroubis P, Frydman R, Fanchin R. Early follicle development alters the relationship between antral follicle counts and inhibin B and follicle-stimulating hormone levels on cycle day 3. Fertil Steril 2010;93:894-9.

27. Fanchin R, Taieb J, Lozano DH, Ducot B, Frydman R, Bouyer J. High reproducibility of serum anti-Müllerian hormone measurements suggests a multi-staged follicular secretion and strengthens its role in the assessment of ovarian follicular status. Hum Reprod 2005a;20:923-7.

28. La Marca A, Stabile G, Artenisio AC, Volpe A. Serum anti-Müllerian hormone throughout the human menstrual cycle. Hum Reprod 2006a;21:3103-7.

29. Hehenkamp WJ, Looman CW, Themmen AP, de Jong FH, Te Velde ER, Broekmans FJ. Anti-Müllerian hormone levels in the spontaneous menstrual cycle do not show substantial fluctuation. J Clin Endocrinol Metab 2006;91:4057-63.

30. Tsepelidis S, Devreker F, Demeestere I, Flahaut A, Gervy CH, Englert Y. Stable serum levels of anti-Müllerian hormone during the menstrual cycle: A prospective study in normo-ovulatory women. Hum Reprod 2007;22:1837-40.

31. Streuli I, Fraisse T, Pillet C, Ibecheole V, Bischof P, de Ziegler D. Serum anti-Müllerian hormone levels remain stable throughout the menstrual cycle and after oral or vaginal administration of synthetic sex steroids. Fertil Steril 2008;90:395-400.

32. Wunder DM, Bersinger NA, Yared M, Kretschmer R, Birkhäuser MH. Statistically significant changes of anti-Müllerian hormone and inhibin levels during the physiologic menstrual cycle in reproductive age women. Fertil Steril 2008;89:927-33.

33. Streuli I, Fraisse T, Chapron C, Bijaoui G, Bischof P, de Ziegler D. Clinical uses of anti-Müllerian hormone assays: Pitfalls and promises. Fertil Steril 2009;91:226-30.

34. La Marca A, Giulini S, Orvieto R, De Leo V, Volpe A. Anti-Müllerian hormone concentrations in maternal serum during pregnancy. Hum Reprod 2005b;20:1569-72.

35. Mohamed KA, Davies WA, Lashen H. Anti-Müllerian hormone and pituitary gland activity after prolonged down-regulation with goserelin acetate. Fertil Steril 2006;86:1515-7.

36. Arbo E, Vetori DV, Jimenez MF, Freitas FM, Lemos N, Cunha-Filho JS. Serum anti-Müllerian hormone levels and follicular cohort characteristics after pituitary suppression in the late luteal phase with oral contraceptive pills. Hum Reprod 2007;22: 3192-6.

37. Somunkiran A, Yavuz T, Yucel O, Ozdemir I. Anti-Müllerian hormone levels during hormonal contraception in women with polycystic ovary syndrome. Eur J Obstet Gynecol Reprod Biol 2007;134:196-201.

38. Fanchin R, Schonauer LM, Righini C, Frydman N, Frydman R, Taieb J. Serum anti-Müllerian hormone dynamics during controlled ovarian hyperstimulation. Hum Reprod 2003b;18:328-32.

39. Fanchin R, Mendez Lozano DH, Louafi N, Achour-Frydman N, Frydman R, Taieb J. Dynamics of serum anti-Müllerian hormone concentrations during the luteal phase of controlled ovarian hyperstimulation. Hum Reprod 2005b;20:747-51.

40. Fanchin R, Louafi N, Mendez Lozano DH, Frydman N, Frydman R, Taieb J. Per-follicle measurements indicate that anti-Müllerian hormone secretion is modulated by the extent of follicular development and luteinization and may reflect qualitatively the ovarian follicular status. Fertil Steril 2005c;84:167-73.

41. Franchimont P, Hazee-Hagelstein MT, Hazout A, Frydman R, Schatz B, Demerlé F. Correlation between follicular fluid content and the results of *in vitro* fertilization and embryo transfer. I. Sex steroids. Fertil Steril 1989;52:1006-11.

42. van Rooij IA, Broekmans FJ, Scheffer GJ, Looman CW, Habbema JD, de Jong FH. Serum anti-Müllerian hormone concentrations best reflect the reproductive decline with age in normal women with proven fertility: a longitudinal study. Fertil Steril 2005;83:979-87.

43. Urman B, Yakin K, Balaban B. Recurrent implantation failure in assisted reproduction: how to counsel and manage. A. General considerations and treatment options that may benefit the couple. Reprod Biomed Online 2005;11:371-81.

In Vitro Maturation of Oocyte: Will it Ever Replace the Traditional IVF Program?

Sulochana Gunasheela

INTRODUCTION

When Robert Edwards and Patrick Steptoe produced their first ever baby by *in vitro* fertilization (IVF), they had already mastered the art of taking out immature ova from ovaries, removed either totally or by slices. These were all small antral follicles, which were matured *in vitro* and later fertilized. The eggs cleaved to 4 cells, then to the 8 cell stage and in course of time, developed into blastocysts. After the announcement of the birth of Louise Brown following transfer of a single cleaving embryo after the aspiration of a single egg from an ovary, several other workers, including Trounson of Monash University, put forth the possibility of increasing pregnancy rates by collecting multiple eggs from stimulated ovaries and transferring multiple embryos with the hope of successful implantation of at least one of them. This was the beginning of controlled ovarian hyperstimulation (COH) in an assisted reproductive techniques (ART) program. As COH became popular, several centers, anxious to produce high rates of pregnancies, went overboard. Multiple embryos were introduced into the uterine cavity at a single event of embryo transfer (ET). Ovaries were stimulated with gonadotropic hormones with such great enthusiasm that they frequently saw high order multiple pregnancy and also witnessed the horror of ovarian hyperstimulation syndrome (OHSS) with a severe degree of morbidity and sometimes, even mortality. Cancellation of cycles rose to 22 to 25 percent, either because of the fear of hyperstimulation or because of a premature luteinizing hormone (LH) surge, caused by increasing levels of estrogen produced by multiple follicular production.

To circumvent the latter event gonadotropin-releasing hormone (GnRH) analogs were introduced to downregulate the activity of pituitary gonadotrops so that the ovaries came under the control of the exogenous supply of gonadotropic hormones. Cancellation rates certainly fell, since there was little scope for endogenous pituitary interference. Human chorionic gonadotropin (hCG) could be given at a flexible time so as to organize the ovum pick-up at a comfortable time for all. But unfortunately, the danger of the onset of OHSS did not reduce with the use of GnRH analogs; it probably even increased when the clinicians, having overcome the fear of premature LH surge, started using gonadotropic hormones even more confidently resulting in a higher incidence of OHSS.

OHSS not only threatened the life of the patient, but it also reduced the implantation rate and increased the abortion rate.[1] These problems have brought forth new enthusiasm for the collection of human oocytes from unstimulated ovaries, pushing the ART program back to the *in vitro* maturation (IVM) of human oocytes, first demonstrated by Edwards in 1965.[2] The greatest advantage of collecting such oocytes is that one can totally circumvent the complications of OHSS.

There are many advantages in establishing the program of immature oocytes, which is patient-friendly as there is no pretreatment program. It encourages sympathetic friends and relatives to offer their own oocytes for donation. There is no need for monitoring follicular growth, thus making labor less intensive. There is of course, total freedom from the complications of OHSS.

The disadvantages of *in vitro* maturation are that:
- Ovum pick-up from unstimulated ovaries is much more difficult than in stimulated ovaries.
- Identification of oocytes in the laboratory is more time-consuming because the oocyte corona cumulus complex (OCCC) is very much smaller in the immature oocyte than in the mature one, making it difficult to identify them even under microscope.
- There is a percentage of loss of oocytes during maturation, which takes anywhere between 24 and 48 hrs. This adds an extra step to the laboratory program of oocyte culture.
- As of today, the pregnancy rate of IVM is much lesser than that of IVF.

Oocyte maturation amounts to continuation of the first meiotic division and progression to metaphase II accompanied by cytoplasmic reaction within the oocytes, which is essential for fertilization and support of early development. Nuclear maturation results in a haploid chromosomal complement from the previous diploid status. When meiosis resumes the germinal vesicle (GV—the visible nucleus) breaks down and the chromatin mass changes into a meiotic spindle at metaphase I. The separation is complete at metaphase II, which is recognized by the presence of the first polar body besides the disappearance of the nucleus.

The oocyte is arrested at the metaphase II stage until the penetration of sperm occurs, resulting in extrusion of the second polar body. The formation of oocyte with two pronuclei oocyte completes the picture of oocyte fertilization. *In vitro* maturation of oocytes denotes the act of culturing and maturating oocytes that have been harvested in an immature state.

Polycystic ovary syndrome (PCOS) is one of the most common reproductive disorders, seen among women of child-bearing age. Women with PCOS frequently present with anovulatory infertility and a varied type of response to exogenous gonadotropin treatment. While some women are resistant to gonadotropin treatment, most PCOS women over respond to gonadotropin stimulation, resulting in the production of a large number of follicles, which secrete high estrogen levels, resulting in significant risk of OHSS.[3]

About 15 percent of ART cases are canceled due to inappropriate response to exogenous gonadotropins. This group of patients may also benefit from IVM. IVM is also applicable for young women undergoing anticancer therapy, which frequently destroys gonadal functions. Such women may opt for cryopreservation of oocytes and ovarian tissue. Immature oocytes may be isolated, frozen, thawed and matured later when required.

Pregnancies have been reported using immature oocytes that were retrieved during a conventional ovarian stimulation with follicle stimulating hormone (FSH) and human chorionic gonadotropin (hCG) administration.[4] However, these are really oocytes, which had failed to develop along with the mature cohort, resulting in erratic development, probably with advanced oocyte cytoplasmic maturation and delayed nuclear maturation. There have been reports[5,6] on PCO patients who were administered a single injection of hCG without previous FSH administration between days 10 to 12 of the cycle. The hCG injection was followed by ovum pick-up 36 hrs later. These were maturated within next 24 to 36 hrs and intracytoplasmic sperm injection (ICSI) conducted soon after. This resulted in clinical pregnancy rates of approximately 39 percent.[6] In another extreme, immature oocytes, collected without giving even hCG injection, have been maturated and clinical pregnancies obtained.[7] However, these pregnancies

resulted in a live birth rate of 5 percent. Chian, et al.[6] showed that the maturation rate of immature oocytes retrieved from women with PCOS improved by hCG priming.

The first report of pregnancy following IVM of immature oocyte and IVF was made in 1994.[8] In 1995, a pregnancy was reported from a group of PCOS patients treated with IVM combined with ICSI and assisted hatching.[9] However, only 60 percent of immature oocytes from PCO patients matured in vitro and the pregnancy rates were approximately 22 percent.[10] Chian, et al.[6] showed that injection of hCG 36 hrs before immature oocyte retrieval in unstimulated PCO patients gave a maturation rate of 84.3 percent, a fertilization rate of 90.7 percent and a cleavage rate of 94.9 percent, resulting in 5 clinical pregnancies out of 13 cycles (38.5%). At the same time, oocytes recovered without previous hCG priming showed a maturation rate of 69.1 percent, fertilization rate of 83.9 percent, cleavage rate or 95.7 percent and a clinical pregnancy in 3 out of 11 cycles with a pregnancy rate of 27.3 percent. Oocytes primed with hCG matured in 24 hrs, whereas most oocytes obtained without hCG priming took anywhere between 36 and 48 hrs in culture.

Thus, IVM of immature oocytes can be done from oocytes picked up from unstimulated ovaries or partially stimulated ovaries primed with hCG.

Collection of immature oocytes: Immature oocytes may be obtained from patients undergoing operations for variety of indications like tuboplasty, cesarean section, hysterectomy or tubal sterilization. Further, oocytes have been collected from surgically removed ovaries. Oocytes are aspirated by puncturing visible follicles with a 21-gauge needle attached to a syringe filled with culture medium. This can be done from a whole ovary or from ovaries, which can be sliced.[11] Cha et al.[11] collected 270 immature oocytes, aspirated from 23 women aged between 22 and 50 years. An average of 11 oocytes were removed during each operation. Table 88.1 shows the age-wise distribution of the number of oocytes collected from ovaries removed. It may be noted that the number of oocytes collected remained the same between the age of 20 and 40 years with a sudden deterioration from 41 years onwards.[11]

Table 88.1: Age-wise distribution of the number of oocytes collected from ovaries removed				
S. No.	*Age*	*No. of ovaries removed*	*Total no. of oocytes*	*Per ovary*
1.	26–30 years	02	36	18 (± 0)
2.	31–35 years	03	47	15.7 (± 7)
3.	36–40 years	07	99	14.1 (± 10.0)
4.	41–45 years	09	78	8.7 (± 5.3)
5.	46–50 years	02	10	5.0 (± 0)

(Adopted from Cha et al.[11])

Ovaries were washed with 37°C saline to remove adhering blood clots. Oocytes were aspirated by puncturing follicles between 2 and 5 mm in diameter with a 21-gauge needle attached to a syringe filled with culture medium. Follicular fluid was obtained from women attending the IVF program. The fluid was double filtered and stored at –20°C.[11]

Maturating media consisted of modified Ham's F10 with 20 percent fetal cord serum (FCS) or 50 percent mature follicular fluid, obtained from follicles of a traditional IVF program. Oocytes were cultured for 32 to 48 hrs and later transferred into culture medium containing modified Ham's F10 (Gibco) with 10 percent of FCS and then inseminated. The fertilized eggs were then cultured in modified Ham's F10 for 24 to 48 hrs.[11]

The results in Table 88.1 show that the number of oocytes collected from 23 ovaries ranged from 0 to 32 with a mean of 11 oocytes per ovary. There was no significant difference between the rate of healthy oocytes and degenerative oocytes regardless of age. However, the number of collected oocytes significantly declined as the age of the donor increased. There was no difference in number or quality of oocytes, whether they were removed in the follicular phase or the luteal phase. The maturation rate and fertilization rate of oocytes, cultured in modified Ham's F10, which contained follicular fluid, was higher than that with FCS.[11]

Cha's work[11] showed that *in vitro* maturation of follicular oocytes might be readily accomplished in an environment that simulates the preovulatory stage. Therefore, to enhance the maturation of immature oocytes, gonadotropins, steroid hormones, serum and follicular fluid have all been added to culture media by various workers. Follicular fluid collected after the leutinizing hormone (LH) surge has adequate level of gonadotropins and steroid hormones for maturation and this was thought to be the reason why modified Ham's F10 with added follicular fluid did better than the same media with addition of FCS. Cha et al.[11] produced a triplet pregnancy in a recipient woman after transferring embryos produced from IVM oocytes, aspirated from surgically removed ovarian tissue.[11]

Although there is a case for the use of immature oocytes in ART, clinicians are still unwilling to adopt this method for the fear that it may reduce their pregnancy rates. One also has to be careful to watch the outcome of IVM babies before changing over to a new method. This has to be again weighed against the danger of impending OHSS in several types of patients, particularly the PCO patients and some of the extreme forms of hypo-gonadotropic women.

What are the Strategies Available to Prevent OHSS Today?

- Cancellation of cycle when there is a threat of impending OHSS, either on ultrasound or in terms of soaring levels of estradiol or both. This is most unacceptable to both the patients and the infertility practitioners.

  The grievance of the patient is understandable when her cost of medication is not even reimbursable.
- 'Careful' stimulation protocol?
    - By using the technique of step-up and step-down protocol (estradiol level going up and down can cause break-through bleeding).
    - Coasting during stimulation frequently results in a sudden drop in estradiol level and is sometimes accompanied by total disappearance of all follicles amounting to cycle cancellation only.
    - Sometimes ovum pick-up (OPU) after coasting has produced a variety of oocytes, including atretic, degenerate, postmature, immature and non-fertilizable (personal experience).
- The next alternative is to conclude stimulation, aspirate all oocytes, fertilize and cryopreserve all embryos, thus postponing embryo transfer (ET) to a subsequent cold cycle. There is no guarantee that this will stop OHSS even if one continues to give the agonist after OPU. In most centers, pregnancy rates after frozen embryo transfer (FET) are by no means comparable to the percentage of pregnancies obtained from fresh embryo transfer. The much touted antagonist has not prevented OHSS completely.

Hence, these are the patients who may be taken up for *in vitro* maturation of immature oocytes. Ovum pick-up can be made easy by partially stimulating the follicles for a period of 4 to 5 days until the average follicle reaches a diameter of 1.1 to 1.2 cm. hCG may be given at this stage and oocytes aspirated 36 hrs later. The follicle would have grown up to 1.4 to 1.5 cm at the time of OPU and the oocytes still remain immature. The idea of giving hCG is to loosen the oocyte corona cumulus complex (OCCC) from the follicular wall and remove the oocyte maturation inhibiting (OMI) factor.

The success of IVM in ART depends upon the ability to retrieve large number of oocytes because there is a percentage of loss of oocytes during maturation itself although there is still a high percentage of fertilization and cleavage. Table 88.2 shows the percentage of miscarriages, varying between 25 and 39 percent. This is surely not acceptable; but one must consider that most of the work on IVM has been done on PCOS patients, who have a low implantation rate and a higher miscarriage rate, even in traditional IVF.[12 14] This rate, added to cancellation rate for the fear of OHSS, reduces the take-home baby rate (THBR) per patient recruited in traditional IVF.

If one develops the technology of collecting oocytes from the whole ovary, removed by laparoscopy, one can also anticipate that there will be many more women willing for donation. If immature oocytes are retrieved from unstimulated ovaries, the patient must be given a hormone replacement therapy (HRT), similar to what is done for FET or oocyte/embryo donation programs.

Table 88.2: Clinical outcome of IVM cycles in PCO and PCOS patients: worldwide statistics

Author (Year)	Cycles (n)	Priming	Mean oocytes retrieved	Maturation (%)	Fertilization (%)	Cleavage (%)	Mean embryos transferred	Preg/ET (%)	Live births (n)	Abortion (%)
Cha et al. (2000)[15]	94	None	13.6	62.2	68	88	4.9	27.1	20	20
Cha et al. (2005)[16]	203	None	15.5	NA	NA	NA	5.0	21.9	24	37
Chian et al. (2000)[6]	13	hCG vs	7.8	84.3	90.7	94.9	2.8	38.5	03	40
	11	None	7.4	69.1	83.9	95.7	25	27.3	03	0
Child et al. (2002)[17]	107	hCG	10.3	76	78	74	3.2	21.5	17	26.1
Lin et al. (2003)[18]	35	FSH + hCG	21.9	76.5	75.8	89.4	3.8	31.4	21	13
	33	vs hCG	23.1	71.9	69.5	88.1	3.8	36.4	–	–
Gunasheela IVF Center 2006	77	FSH + hCG	9.94	63.83	57.66	89	2.64	19.4	06	53.8

Abbreviation: NA: Not applicable

At this stage, one must make a note of caution that IVM cannot be taken up as an optimal procedure in poor responders, like women with borderline ovarian failure, severe degree of endometriosis and chronic pelvic inflammatory diseases with a frozen pelvis. Such patients are better off with full stimulation and collection of mature eggs and there is no danger of these women ever reaching the stage of OHSS.

In vitro maturation can also be done on women who are being stimulated for the purpose of intrauterine insemination (IUI). The option of conversion to ART may be offered to them when they produce too many follicles. It is more difficult to reduce the risk of high order multiple pregnancy in IUI than in assisted reproduction.

If one goes to the world literature, the pregnancy rates have been improving steadily, with some authors reporting a 25 percent delivery rate.[6,15] Table 88.3 shows the experience of ART with IVM at Gunasheela IVF (GIVF) Center, Bangalore, Karnataka, India.

Table 88.2 show the clinical outcome of IVM cycles in PCO and PCOS patients.

Tables 88.4 and 88.5 show comparative studies of ART with IVM—worldwide statistics.

As of the date of writing this article, there are approximately 400 babies born out of IVM technology in the world.[22] Information is available on approximately 300 of these children, which includes both published and unpublished data.[23] The information is scattered and incomplete. Suikkari et al.[24] studied children born between the years 2000 and 2004 out of immature oocyte retrieval and IVM with ART. The results were as follows:

- Live birth rate after IVM was 15 percent.
- A total of 42 women delivered 45 infants; 39 singletons and 3 sets of twins; 2 infants were born after an FET cycle.

Table 88.3: GIVF Study of ART with IVM (Study period: June 2002 to September 2006)

1.	Total patients (n)	77
2.	Total oocytes (n)	766
3.	Oocytes per patient (n)	9.94
4.	MII oocytes in 24 hours	489 (63.83%)
5.	Oocytes fertilized	282 (57.66%)
6.	Fertilized oocytes cleaved	251 (89%)
7.	Total ETs done (n)	67
8.	Embryos transferred (n)	177
9.	Embryos per transfer (n)	2.64
10.	Pregnancies per ET	13/67 (19.4%)
11.	Deliveries per ET	6 (8%)
12.	Biochemical pregnancies (n)	03
13.	Clinical abortions (n)	03
14.	Ectopic pregnancies (n)	01

Abbreviation: ET: embryo transfer

- The mean gestational age of delivery was 40 weeks with a range of 35 to 42. The mean birth weight of singletons was 3532 g (range 2575–4250 g).
- After examining the children, 10 children showed minor developmental delay (MDD) in 1 to 3 developmental fields (DF) at the end of 12 months.
- One child, who demonstrated considerable delay and nystagmus, was found to have glioma of the optic nerve.
- Psychological assessment was done at 2 yrs of age. The MDI of the children examined was 104 ± 9.0.

Table 88.4: Comparative study of IVM characteristics worldwide IVM statistics

Author (Year)	Mean oocytes (n)	Maturation rate	Fertilization rate	Cleavage rate
Cha et al. (1999)[11]	15.2	63%	77% (ICSI)	89%
Trounson et al. (1994)[8]	13.1	81%	34% (IVF)	56%
Barnes et al. (1996)[19]	–	67%	32% (IVF)	62%
Russell et al. (1997)[20]	–	40.62%	75–76% (ICSI)	64–92%
Suikkari et al. (2000)[21]	11.2–11.5	64–78%	57–72% (ICSI)	72.77%
GIVF (UP) (Jun 2002–Sep 2006)	9.94	63.83%	57–66% (ICSI)	89%

Abbreviation: UP: Unpublished

Table 88.5: Comparative study of worldwide IVM statistics

Author (Year)	Cycles (n)	Embryos transferred	Pregnancies	Abortions	Ongoing deliveries
Cha et al. (2000)	85	3.9 ± 2.2	25/85 (29.4%)	6 (26%)	17 (20%)
Chian et al. (1994)	24	2.6 ± 1.0	8/24 (33%)	2 (25%)	6 (25%)
Tim Child et al. (2001)	121	–	32/119 (26.8%)	13 (39%)	19 (16%)
GIVF (UP) 2002 – 2006	77	2.64	13/67 (19.4%)	6 + 1(Ect. Preg) (53.8%)	6 (8%)

Abbreviation: UP: Unpublished

Table 88.6: Obstetrics, perinatal and developmental outcome of IVM babies

Study (Year) Time Period	Babies born	Gestational age at delivery	Mean birth weight	Congenital defects	Period of follow-up
Cha et al. (2000)[15] 1995–1998	20	> 37 wks	3 kgs	No defects	Triple test at 18 wks
Cha et al. (2005)[16] 1995–2001	28	37 wks (Sing) 34.6 wks (Twins)	3.2 kgs 2.4 kgs	1 Hydrops 1 Omphalocele 1 Cleft palate	Omphalocele showed mosaicism by amniocentesis
Mikkelsen et al. (2005)[23] 1999–2004	47	40 wks (Sing) 33 wks (Twins)		1 Cleft soft palate 1 Still birth at 42.3 wks	Inherited from father 21 babies followed up. All normal
Bucket 2004 1998–2003	48	3.5 wks (Sing) 2.44 wks (Twins)		1 Hip dislocation I VSD	All healthy till now
Suikkari et al. (2005)[24] 2000–2004	45	39 (Sing) 3 (Twins)			1 baby developed glioma
Le Du et al. (2005)[25] 2002–2003	05	Single			Follow-up 1 yr normal
GIVF (UP)	06	Single		All normal	Short-term follow-up

Abbreviation: UP: Unpublished

- It was concluded that the perinatal outcome of the children was good. The preliminary data acquired on neurological and neuropsychological follow-up of IVM children was reassuring. It was found to be within the normal range in all but one child upto 2 yrs of age.

The obstetric, perinatal and developmental outcome of IVM children reported by several authors can be seen in Table 88.6.

CONCLUSION

As the state of ART presents itself today, IVM is a safer option than IVF in patients who are extremely sensitive to gonadotropins. IVM certainly holds a great promise as another type of ART if the technology is whole-heartedly developed. It has tremendous advantages, which include socioeconomic factors, cost effectiveness and exclusion of gonadotropins and gonadotropin-releasing hormone analogs. The procedure is not only patient-friendly, but also donor-friendly. The small amount of additional difficulty in oocyte aspiration for the clinicians and its identification for laboratory technicians can be overcome by experience. It is a small price to pay for total avoidance of complications caused by induction of ovulation.

REFERENCES

1. Papanikolaou EG, Tournaye H, Verpoest W, Camus M, Vernaeve V, Van Steirteghem A, Devroey P. Early and late ovarian hyperstimulation syndrome: early pregnancy outcome and profile. Hum Reprod 2005;20:636-41.
2. Edwards R.G. Maturation *in vitro* of human ovarian oocytes. Lancet 1965;2:926-9.
3. Bergh PA, Navot D. Ovarian hyperstimulation syndrome: A review of pathophysiology. J Assist Reprod Genet 1992;9:429-38.
4. Veeck LL, Wortham JW, Witmyer J. Maturation and fertilization of morphologically immature oocytes in a programme of *in vitro* fertilization. Fertil Steril 1983;39:594-602.
5. Chian RC, Buckett WM, Too LL, Tan SL. Pregnancies resulting from *in vitro* matured oocytes retrieved from patients with polycystic ovary syndrome after priming with human chorionic gonadotropin. Fertil Steril 1999;72:639-42.
6. Chian RC, Buckett WM, Tulandi T, Tan SL. Prospective randomized study of human chorionic gonadotropin priming before immature oocyte retrieval from unstimulated women with polycystic ovarian syndrome. Hum Reprod 2000;15:165-70.
7. Cha KY, Koo JJ, Ko JJ. Pregnancy after *in vitro* fertilization of human follicular oocytes collected from non-stimulated cycles, their culture *in vitro* and their transfer in a donor oocyte programme. Fertil Steril 1991;55:109-13.
8. Trounson A, Wood C, Kausche A. *In vitro* maturation, fertilization and developmental competency of oocytes recovered from untreated polycystic ovarian patients. Fertil Steril 1994;62:353-62.
9. Barnes FL, Crombie A, Gardner DK, Kausche A, Lacham-Kaplan O, Suikkari AM, et al. Blastocyst development and birth after *in vitro* maturation of human primary oocytes, intracytoplasmic sperm injection and assisted hatching. Hum Reprod 1995;10:3243-7.
10. Cha KY, Chian RC. Maturation *in vitro* of immature human oocytes for clinical use. Hum Reprod Update 1998;4:103-20.
11. Cha KY. *In vitro* fertilization using immature follicular oocytes harvested from ovarian tissue. Progress in Infertility (4th edn) In: Behrman SJ, Grant W Patton Jr, Gary Holtz (Eds). 1999. pp. 99-112.
12. Carlos Simon, Fidel Cano, Diana Valbuena, Remohí J, Pellicer A. Clinical evidence for a detrimental effect on uterine receptivity of high serum oestradiol concentrations in high and normal responder patients. Hum Reprod 1995;10:2432-7.
13. Paulson RJ, Sauer MV, Lobo RA. Embryo implantation after human IVF: Importance of endometrial receptivity. Fertil Steril 1990;53:870-4.
14. Forman R, Fries N, Testar J, Belaisch-Allart J, Hazout A, Frydman R. Evidence for an adverse effect of elevated estradiol concentrations on embryo implantation. Fertil Steril 1998;49:118-22.
15. Cha KY, Han SY, Chung HM, Choi DH, Lim JM, Lee WS, et al. Pregnancies and deliveries after *in vitro* maturation culture followed by *in vitro* fertilization and embryo transfer without stimulation in women with polycystic ovary syndrome. Fertil Steril. 2000;73:978-83.
16. Cha KY, Chung HM, Lee DR, Kwon H, Chung MK, Park LS, et al. Obstetric outcome of patients with polycystic ovary syndrome treated by *in vitro* maturation and *in vitro* fertilization–embryo transfer. Fertil Steril 2005;83:1461-5.
17. Child TJ, Simon J Philips, Ahmad Kamal Abdul-Jalil, et al. A comparision of *in vitro* maturation and *in vitro* fertilization for women with polycystic ovaries. Obstet Gynecol 2002;100:665-70.
18. Lin YH, Hwang JL, Huang LW, Seow KM, Chung J, Hsieh BC, et al. Combination of FSH priming and HCG priming for *in vitro* maturation of human oocytes. Hum Reprod 2003;18:1632-6.
19. Barnes F, Kauche A, Tiglias J, Wood C, Wilton L, Trounson A. Production of embryos from *in vitro* matured primary human oocytes. Fertil Steril 1996;65:1151-6.
20. Russell JB, Knezerich KM, Fabian KF, Dickson JA. Unstimulated immature oocyte retrieval: Early versus mid-follicular endometrial priming. Fertil Steril 1997;67:616-20.
21. Suikkari A, Tulppala M, Turri T, Hovatta O, Barnes F. Luteal phase start of low dose FSH priming of follicles results in an efficient recovery, maturation and fertilization of immature human oocytes. Hum Reprod 2000;15:747-51.
22. Marcus W. Jurema, Daniela Nugueira. *In vitro* maturation of human oocytes for assisted reproduction. Fertil Steril 2006;86:1277-91.
23. Mikkelsen AL. Strategies in human *in vitro* maturation and their clinical outcome. Reprod Biomed Online 2005;10:593-9.
24. Suikkari AM, Salokorpi T, Pihlaja M, et al. Healthy children born after *in vitro* maturation of oocytes. Hum Reprod 2005;20: i105.
25. Le Du A, Kadoch IJ, Bourcigaux N, Bourrier MC, Chevalier N, Fanchin R, et al. *In vitro* maturation for the treatment of infertility associated with polycystic ovarian syndrome: The French experience. Hum Reprod 2005;20:420-4.

Stem Cell Therapeutic Potential: Miles to go Before We Sleep

Jayant G Mehta

OVERVIEW

Treatment of monocellular deficiency diseases by pluripotent stem cell replacement therapies, either directly at the site of damage or in a manner such that the cells home to the appropriate sites, has been reported. For example, transplantation of fetal tissue containing dopaminergic neurons has been shown to, at least partially, ameliorate symptoms in Parkinson's sufferers. Further, a wide range of additional potential targets has been identified, including stroke, spinal cord injuries, multiple sclerosis, motor neuron disease, macular degeneration, liver and muscle regeneration, diabetes and restoration of immune function. The basic requirement for cell therapy is a supply of safe, highly pure, defined cell populations in adequate numbers for transplantation. However, a major limitation in the advance of such therapies has been problems associated with purification of sufficient numbers of the appropriate cell types from donors. Whether human stem cells are of embryonic, fetal or adult origin, the donor source must be carefully screened. Pedigree evaluation and/or genetic testing will help establish whether the human stem cells in question are suitable for use in the context of a particular clinical situation. The integrity, uniformity and reliability of establishing and maintaining human stem cells in culture, intended for clinical use, can be ensured by following rigorous controlled, standardized practices and procedures. Like every new area of Biomedical Science, stem cell research is under considerable pressure from patient groups to develop human therapies as rapidly as possible. In the area of laboratory and preclinical testing, a great deal of work still needs to be done to develop appropriate assays for cell differentiation, migration and functional integration. Both same-species and inter-species testing has to be carried out to determine the relevance of species-specific signaling and host environment and to select the most appropriate animal models for human disease. Unless proper clinical trials are conducted, treatment with stem cells should not be offered to patients.

INTRODUCTION

The potential therapeutic applications of stem cells and the ethical issues surrounding the generation of human embryonic stem (ES) cell lines from human embryos have been a focus of recent media attention and political scrutiny. Proponents of this technology claim that human ES[1] cells may revolutionize the fields of Transplantation and Regenerative Medicine, promising cures for many of the major diseases facing society today, including diabetes, cardiovascular disease,[2] neurodegenerative disease,[3,4] and cancer. However, the embryo destruction, associated with derivation of ES cells from human embryos raises a number of ethical concerns and other stem cell sources, such as adult stem cells,[5] are being considered as useful alternatives. This chapter discusses the potential applications of stem cells and safety issues that need to be addressed in order to develop products suitable for clinical application.

Cell Therapy and Regenerative Medicine

Many serious human diseases are caused by cell loss, damage or dysfunction. A possibility therefore exists that transplantation or replacement of the deficient cell population would restore normal function. Clinical studies involving the transplantation of blood-restoring, or hematopoietic, stem cells have been underway for a number of years.[6] Reconstituting the blood and immune systems through stem cell transplantation is an established practice for treating hematological malignancies such as leukemia and lymphoma. Transplantation of hematopoietic stem cells, resident in the bone marrow or isolated from cord blood or circulating peripheral blood, is used to counter the destruction of certain bone marrow cells caused by high-intensity chemotherapeutic regimens used to battle various solid tumors. Moreover, clinical trials are being conducted to assess the safety and efficacy of using hematopoietic stem cell transplantation to treat various autoimmune conditions, including multiple sclerosis, lupus and rheumatoid arthritis.[6]

It is only recently that proof of concept for the treatment of monocellular deficiency diseases by pluripotent stem cell replacement therapies; either directly at the site of damage or in a manner such that the cells home to the appropriate sites, has been reported.[1] For example, transplantation of fetal tissue containing dopaminergic neurons has been shown to, at least partially, ameliorate symptoms in Parkinson's sufferers.[4] Transplantation of pancreatic Islet cells from cadavers has been shown to restore insulin levels in diabetes patients. Further, a wide range of additional potential targets has been identified, including stroke, spinal cord injuries, multiple sclerosis, motor neuron disease, macular degeneration, liver and muscle regeneration and restoration of immune function.[1] While these reports confirm the therapeutic potential of stem cells, no single report of proper clinical trials, addressing the safety issues using human stem cells in clinical setting exists.[7] For human stem cells to advance to the stage of clinical investigation, a virtual safety net composed of a core set of safeguards is required.

The basic requirement for cell therapy is a supply of safe, highly pure, defined cell populations in adequate numbers for transplantation. However, a major limitation in the advance of such therapies has been problems associated with purification of sufficient numbers of the appropriate cell types from donors. Each step in the human stem cell development must therefore, be carefully scrutinized to include the derivation, expansion, manipulation, and characterization of human stem cell lines, as well as preclinical efficacy and toxicity testing in appropriate animal models. Being able to trace back from the cell population prepared for transplantation to the source of the founder human stem cells also allows each safety checkpoint to be connected, one to the other.

CLINICAL DISCUSSION

Screening of Donor Sources

Whether human stem cells are of embryonic, fetal or adult origin, the donor source must be carefully screened. Although the risk of infectious disease transmission from the donor to recipient is common to all types of tissue and organ transplants, with increasing donor age, this risk reaches new dimensions. Potentially transmissible diseases from donors of any age include infections, congenital disorders and acquired illnesses like autoimmune diseases or malignancies of hematological or non-hematological origin.[8] Routine testing should be done to guard against the inadvertent transmission of infectious diseases. Additionally, pedigree assessment and molecular genetic testing appear to be warranted. This is arguably the case when human stem cells,

intended for transplantation, are derived from an allogeneic donor, that is, someone other than the recipient, and especially if the cells are obtained from a master cell bank that has been established using human embryonic stem or human embryonic germ cells.

The purpose of pedigree evaluation and/or genetic testing is to establish whether the human stem cells in question are suitable for use in the context of a particular clinical situation. For example, embryos derived from a donor with a family history of diabetes may not be the best suited for the derivation of Islet cells intended to repair damaged pancreas. Similarly, the use of molecular genetic analysis could detect a mutation in the gene for alpha-synuclein. This gene is known to be responsible for the rare occurrence of early onset of Parkinson's disease. Detecting such a genetic abnormality in neuronal progenitor cells, derived from an established embryonic germ cell line, could block the use of those cells as a treatment for a number of neurodegenerative conditions, including Parkinson's disease.[4]

Although the number of genes, known to be directly responsible for causing disease or anomalous physiologic function is relatively small, analysis using advanced molecular techniques could detect a mutation in a given gene responsible for a particular disease. Clearly, it will eventually not be possible, or even necessary, to screen every source of human stem cells for the entire panoply of disease-associated genes. The screening of targeted genes will be conducted within the context of the relevant clinical population.

Setting Standards for Cultured Human Stem Cell Lines

The integrity, uniformity and reliability of establishing and maintaining human stem cells in culture, intended for clinical use, can be ensured by following rigorous controlled, standardized practices and procedures.[9]

Human stem cells from virtually every source other than blood-derived hematopoietic stem cells are maintained in tissue culture for some defined period of time. This is necessary to obtain a sufficient number of cells for use in clinical studies involving transplantation. Culturing human stem cells requires the use of formulated liquid media supplemented with growth factors and other chemical substances that promote cellular replication and govern the differentiation of the cultured human stem cells. Since human stem cells are a dynamic biological entity, failure to standardize procedures for maintaining and expanding cells in culture could result in unintended alterations in the intrinsic properties of the cells. The characteristics of human stem cells, maintained in the culture, is highly dependent on the initial seeding density ART the cells, the frequency with which the culture medium is replenished, and the density cells are permitted to achieve before subdividing. Further, altering the concentrations of supplemental growth factors and chemical substances, even switching from one supplier to another, may lead to changes in cell growth rate, expression of defined cell markers, and differentiation potential. It is therefore likely that the behavior and effectiveness of the cells transplanted could be influenced by the use of non-standardized culture practices.

One common addition to liquid culture media is serum derived from cows. Although serum produced from cows, reared in countries, certified to be free of bovine serum albumin (BSA) is used, there is always a fear of the serum being contaminated. Since BSA results in the relentless destruction of brain tissue and is invariably fatal, it would be both irresponsible and devastating if neural stem cells contaminated with the BSA infectious agent were transferred in a patient's nervous system to investigate cellular-replacement therapies for neurological disorders. Serum-free, chemically defined liquid media that obviates risks associated with the use of bovine serum has recently been used.[9]

Culturing without a Feeder Layer of Animal Cells Improve Safety

To maintain human embryonic stem cells and embryonic germ cells in a proliferating, undifferentiated condition, it has been a common practice to layer these cells directly onto a bed of irradiated mouse feeder cells. Transplanting into humans, stem cell preparations, derived from founder cells that have been in direct, intimate contact with non-human animal cells, constitutes xenotransplantation—the use of organs, tissues and cells derived from animals to treat human disease. The principal concern of xenotransplantation is the unintended transfer of animal viruses into humans.[10]

Researchers in the UK, Korea, Singapore[10] and Australia have recently grown human stem cell lines on various extra cellular matrices, such as Fibronectin and Metrigel, for support of the cells.[9] It has been reported that human embryonic stem cells, seeded on a commercially available basement membrane matrix, in media conditioned by feeder cells, retain their proliferative potential and capacity to form all three embryonic germ layers (mesoderm, endoderm, and ectoderm). This suggests that human embryonic stem cells, maintained in the absence of direct culture on a mouse feeder cell layer, are comparable to human embryonic stem cells co-cultured with mouse feeder cells.

Importance of Detailed Characterization of Human Stem Cell Populations

Identifying the cells that make up the human stem cell population intended for clinical study requires identifying cells exhibiting the desired phenotype within the preparation, as well as those that do not. This poses considerable challenges because human embryonic stem and embryonic germ cells have the capacity to give rise to all differentiated cell types, while adult human stem cells, though generally more restricted in their plasticity, are capable of generating all cell types that make up the tissue from which they were derived.

Among the many biological properties, human stem cells have potential to differentiate along multiple lineages and give rise to a variety of cell types. Detailed characterization of stem cell preparations will require a panel of orthogonal assessments.[11] Some of the parameters that will prove useful in establishing identity include: (1) cell morphology (visual microscopic inspection of cells to assess their appearance), (2) expression of unique cell-surface antigens (as is the case for CD34+ hematopoietic stem cells), (3) characterization of biochemical markers such as tissue-specific enzymatic activity (e.g. enzymes that produce neurotransmitters for nerve cells), and (4) expression of genes that are unique to a particular cell type. Further, analysis of the nuclear chromosomal karyotype may be used to assess the genetic stability of established human embryonic stem and embryonic germ cell lines maintained in culture for extended periods of time. Continued development and standardization of DNA-microarray analysis (simultaneous screening for many genes) and proteomics[12] (protein profiling) technologies has significantly enhanced stem cell characterization.

In order to evaluate the extent to which the purity of a human stem cell preparation predicts efficacy after transplantation, it is necessary to explore quantitative identification of cell types within a heterogeneous population of differentiating human stem cells. The interaction of various phenotypic cell types within a preparation of progenitor cells, obtained after the controlled differentiation of cultured human embryonic stem cells, needs to be actively investigated. Alterations that occur outside what is expected due to normal biologic variation could reflect the introduction of genetic mutations as a consequence of culture conditions used to promote expansion and to induce differentiation of the progenitor cell population.

Before clinical studies involving human stem cell transplantation can be done, it is essential to demonstrate that human stem cell preparations possess relevant biological activity. The bioassay provides a quantitative measure of the potency of a cell preparation and ensures that cells destined for transplantation are not inert. Assays may be based on a biologic activity such as insulin release from pancreatic islet-like cells, glycogen storage by cells intended for regeneration of liver tissue, or synchronous contraction in the case of stem cell-derived cardiomyocytes to be used for repairing damaged heart muscle. When cells that have not acquired fully differentiated functionality are to be transplanted, it may be appropriate to use surrogate markers that predict the acquisition of the intended biologic activity upon further differentiation. For example, counting tyrosine hydroxylase-expressing neural progenitor cells in a mixed population of cells intended to provide dopaminergic neurons for treating Parkinson's disease, could predict the acquisition of relevant biologic activity after transplantation.

Assessment of Human Stem Cell Safety in Animal Models of Human Diseases

A critical element of the safety net is the transplantation of human stem cells into animals to demonstrate that the therapy does what it is supposed to do ('proof of concept')[13] and to assess toxicity. Admittedly, animal models of human disease are imperfect because most human maladies do not spontaneously occur in animals. Chemical, surgical and immunologic methods are used to damage neurons, induce diabetes, simulate heart attacks, stroke and hypertension or compromise organ function. In situations when focal genetic lesions are known to cause disease, the creation of transgenic mouse colonies in which the culpable gene is either eliminated or over-expressed results in disease models that are capable of faithfully reproducing human disease-specific pathologies.

Human stem cells must be transplanted into animal models of human disease. Transplantation of neural stem cells should demonstrate measurable evidence of efficacy in models of neurodegenerative disease, such as Parkinson's disease, Huntington's disease, amyotrophic lateral sclerosis (ALS), Alzheimer's disease, as well as spinal cord injury and stroke. Improved liver function after transplantation of hepatocyte precursors should also be observed in an animal model of hepatic failure. Normalization of blood insulin concentrations and amelioration of diabetic disease symptoms should result from the transplantation of pancreatic islet progenitors in a mouse model of diabetes. It is likely that in all cases, immunosuppression will be required due to immunologic incompatibility between humans and the animal model species (usually mouse or rat).

In addition to efficacy, evidence for anatomic and functional integration of transplanted human stem cells should be assessed. Human stem cells, destined for transplantation, may be tagged with a marker, such as green fluorescent protein, that allows transplanted cells to be readily identified upon histological examination. A similar approach should be used to evaluate the migration of transplanted human stem cells from the site of injection into adjacent and more distant tissues. The migration of transplanted human stem cells to a non-target site and subsequent differentiation into a tissue type that is inappropriate for that anatomic location could be problematic.

Questions about the use of embryonic compared with adult stem cells with respect to robustness and durability should be addressed in animal-transplantation models.

Similarly, the issue of whether less-differentiated cells will be more effective than more differentiated cells following transplantation should be investigated. Continued advancements in non-invasive imaging technologies, such as magnetic resonance imaging (MRI) and positron emission tomography (PET scanning), will allow these events to be observed in real time with reasonable resolution and without having to use large numbers of animals.

From the perspective of toxicology, the proliferative potential of undifferentiated human embryonic stem and embryonic germ cells evokes the greatest level of concern. A characteristic of human embryonic stem cells is their capacity to generate teratomas when transplanted into immunologically incompetent strains of mice. Undifferentiated embryonic stem cells are not considered suitable for transplantation due to the risk of unregulated growth. The question that remains is, at what point during differentiation does this risk become insignificant, if ever? Identifying the stage at which the risk for tumor formation is minimized will depend on whether the process of stem cell differentiation occurs only in a forward direction or is reversible. Before clinical trials can be initiated in humans, the issue of unregulated growth potential and its relationship to stem cell differentiation has to be evaluated. It is essential that careful toxicology studies, that are of the appropriate duration and that involve transplantation of undifferentiated or partially differentiated embryonic stem cells, as well as adult stem cells into immunocompromised animals, are performed.

CONCLUSION

Like every new area of Biomedical Science, stem cell research is under considerable pressure from patient groups to develop human therapies as rapidly as possible. In the area of laboratory and preclinical testing, a great deal of work still needs to be done to develop appropriate assays for cell differentiation, migration, and functional integration. Both same-species and inter-species testing has to be carried out to determine the relevance of species-specific signaling and host environment and to select the most appropriate animal models for human disease. Follow-up times in animal experiments will have to take into account the problem of potential tumor formation. The question of how much animal testing should be executed before human trials may ethically proceed will be difficult to resolve, given that cell-based therapy is a relatively new paradigm and appropriate assays and outcomes have yet to be defined. The Food and Drug Administration (FDA) has published a document on 'Regulation of stem cell-based-therapies,'[14,15] which outlines the specific criteria necessary for safety and toxicity testing in the first Phase I clinical trials. Unless these guidelines are strictly adhered to, the pace of the transition from the laboratory to clinical research will be very slow. Although, claims of successful clinical treatments have been reported, none of them have taken into account the safety issue discussed here. Unless proper clinical trials are conducted, treatment with stem cells should not be offered to patients.

REFERENCES

1. Scadden DT. The stem cell niche as an entity of action. Nature 2006;441:1075-9.
2. Srivatara D, Ivey KN. Potential of stem cell-based therapies for heart diseases. Nature 2006;441:1097-9.
3. Muotri AR, Gage FH. Generation of neuronal variability and complexing. Nature 2006;441:1087-3.
4. Lindvall O, Kokaia Z. Stem cells for the treatment of neurological disorders. Nature 2006;441:1094-6.
5. Randon TA. Stem cells, ageing and quest for immortality. Nature 2006;441:1080-6.
6. Bordignon C. Stem cells therapies for blood diseases. Nature 2006;441:1100-2.
7. Dawson L, Bateman-House AS, Agnew DM, Bok H, Brock DW, Chakravarti A, et al. Safety issues in cell-based intervention trials. Fertil Steril 2003;80:1077-84.
8. Niederwieser D, Gentilini C, Hegenbart U, Lange T, Moosmann P, Pönisch W, et al. Transmission of donor illness by stem cell transplantation: Should screening be different in older donors? Bone Marrow Transplant 2004;34:657-65.
9. Brivanlou AH, Gage FH, Jaenisch R, Jessell T, Melton D, Rossant J. Setting standards for human stem cells. Science 2003;300:913-6.
10. Wang W, Sun X. Human embryonic stem cell lines are contaminated what should we do? Hum Reprod 2005;20:2987-9.
11. Richards M, Fong CY. Chan WK, Wong PC, Bongso A. Human feeders support prolonged undifferentiated growth of human inner cell masses and embryonic stem cells. Nat Biotechnol 2002;20:933-6.
12. Trounson A. The production and directed differentiation of human embryonic stem cells. Endocr Rev. 2006;27:208-19.
13. Vodicka P, Skalnikova H, Kovarova H. The characterization of Stem Cell proteomes. Curr Opin Mol Ther 2006;8:232-9.
14. Committee on Guidelines for Human Embryonic Stem Cell research. Guideline for Human Embryonic Stem Cell Research. 2005; National Academic Press Washington Publication. www.nap.edu.
15. Halme DG, Kessler DA. FDA regulation of Stem-cell-based therapies. N Engl J Med 2006;355:16.1730-5.

Page numbers followed by *f* refer to figure and *t* refer to table, respectively.